THE BIPOLAR BOOK

THE BIPOLAR BOOK

HISTORY, NEUROBIOLOGY, AND TREATMENT

EDITED BY

Ayşegül Yildiz, MD

Pedro Ruiz, MD

Charles B. Nemeroff, MD, PhD

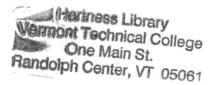
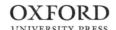
OXFORD
UNIVERSITY PRESS

OXFORD
UNIVERSITY PRESS

Oxford University Press is a department of the University of
Oxford. It furthers the University's objective of excellence in research,
scholarship, and education by publishing worldwide.

Oxford   New York
Auckland   Cape Town   Dar es Salaam   Hong Kong   Karachi
Kuala Lumpur   Madrid   Melbourne   Mexico City   Nairobi
New Delhi   Shanghai   Taipei   Toronto

With offices in
Argentina   Austria   Brazil   Chile   Czech Republic   France   Greece
Guatemala   Hungary   Italy   Japan   Poland   Portugal   Singapore
South Korea   Switzerland   Thailand   Turkey   Ukraine   Vietnam

Oxford is a registered trademark of Oxford University Press
in the UK and certain other countries.

Published in the United States of America by
Oxford University Press
198 Madison Avenue, New York, NY 10016

© Oxford University Press 2015

First issued as an Oxford University Press paperback, 2016

Library of Congress Cataloging-in-Publication Data
The bipolar book : history, neurobiology, and treatment / edited by Ayşegül Yildiz, Pedro Ruiz, and Charles B. Nemeroff.
p. ; cm.
Includes bibliographical references.
ISBN 978–0–19–930053–2 (hardcover : alk. paper); 978–0–19–062001–1 (paperback : alk. paper)
I. Yildiz, Ayşegül, editor.   II. Ruiz, Pedro, 1936– , editor.   III. Nemeroff, Charles B., editor.
[DNLM: 1. Bipolar Disorder. WM 207]
RC516
616.895—dc23
2014028538

To our patients, to the giants in the field whose shoulders we have stood on, and to our students and junior colleagues. All of these individuals have taught us and in some fashion helped make this book possible.

A.Y. and P.R. and C.B.N.

To my mother Zekiye Yıldız and sister Sultan Tınastepe for their unconditional love and support and to my mentors Perry F. Renshaw, Kamil Uğurbil, and especially Gary S. Sachs for their guidance and encouragement in my quest of science and research.

A.Y.

To my wife Angela and my four grand kids who have always being a source of inspiration for me.

P.R.

To my wife Gayle and our children Sarah Frances, Ross, Amanda and Michael for their ongoing support and love.

C.B.N.

CONTENTS

SECTION III
CURRENT TREATMENTS

PREFACE

Charles B. Nemeroff, Ayşegül Yildiz, Pedro Ruiz

Bipolar disorder, one of the major and most severe psychiatric disorders, remains a key focus of clinical practice and research. This volume is a testimony to the remarkable progress we have made in understanding this group of disorders, as well as highlighting the substantial gaps in our knowledge. For the psychiatric disorder with the greatest genetic contribution to disease vulnerability, we are only now beginning to identify its molecular and genetic underpinnings as, for example, exemplified by the recent genome-wide association study findings of novel single nucleotide polymorphisms (Muhleisen et al., 2014; Nurnberger et al., 2014). The precise neurobiological mechanisms by which these and other genetic variations lower the threshold for bipolar disorder remain obscure. In addition to the profound genetic influence on disease vulnerability is the recent finding that similar to major depression and posttraumatic stress disorder, early adverse life experiences, such as child abuse and neglect, increase both the risk for development of bipolar disorder and worsens its course—including an earlier age of onset and more severe course (Gilman et al., 2014; Nemeroff & Binder, 2014). In many ways, bipolar disorder is indeed the quintessential gene × environment driven complex medical disorder. There are a myriad of unresolved issues related to management of bipolar disorder, including its increased risks of dying not only by suicide, which is roughly 20 times more common in this population, but also from prevalent medical disorders with a consequent shortening in life expectancy of 10 to 13.6 years relative to the general population of same age (Laursen, 2011; Leboyer et al., 2012) and how to recognize the warning signs of an imminent episode or suicide attempt, to the remarkably high rate of nonadherence to recommended treatment. In terms of treatment, a myriad of issues emerge. These include the implementation of evidence-based treatments into community practice, a major problem worldwide, as well as much needed new data on long-term management. The remarkable underutilization of lithium, the gold standard of treatment, is a case in point. The good news is that we are actually quite good at managing acute mania with a combination of mood stabilizers and antipsychotics; the bad news is that the treatment of bipolar depression remains a significant challenge in spite of novel approved treatments including lamotrigine, lurasidone, and quetiapine. The role of antidepressants in the management of bipolar depression remains controversial. Unfortunately, many patients do not achieve remission and some only for brief periods. The precise role of psychotherapy and, most important, what form of psychotherapy remains a much heated topic of debate. We would also be remiss if we did not address the controversy associated with diagnosis of bipolar disorder with some suggesting that the diagnosis is used too freely—that is, overdiagnosis as the fundamental problem of including individuals who are no more than hyperthymic—and others who claim that the disorder is terribly underdiagnosed, especially in patients diagnosed with unipolar major depression. In our view, both schools of thought are undoubtedly correct.

We are grateful to the authors, all world authorities in bipolar disorder, who agreed to contribute to this book. Its purpose simply is to provide a relatively comprehensive update on bipolar disorder that will fill the gaps that remain since publication of the last edition of the "bible"— the Goodwin and Jamison textbook, *Manic-Depressive Illness: Bipolar Disorders and Recurrent Depression* (second edition, 2007).

REFERENCES

Gilman, S. E., Ni, M. Y., Dunn, E. C., Breslau, J., McLaughlin, K. A., Smoller, J. W., & Perlis, R. H. (2014). Contributions of the social environment to first-onset and recurrent mania. *Molecular Psychiatry*. Advance online publication, doi:10.1038/mp.2014.36

Laursen, T. M. (2011). Life expectancy among persons with schizophrenia or bipolar affective disorder. *Schizophrenia Research, 131*(1–3), 101–104.

Leboyer, M., Soreca, I., Scott, J., Frye, M., Henry, C., Tamouza, R., & Kupfer, D. J. (2012). Can bipolar disorder be viewed as a multi-system inflammatory disease? *Journal of Affective Disorders, 141*(1), 1–10.

Muhleisen, T. W., Leber, M., Schulze, T. G., Strohmaier, J., Degenhardt, F.,. . . Cichon S. (2014). Genome-wide association study reveals two new risk loci for bipolar disorder. *Nature Communications, 5,* 3339. doi:10.1038/ncomms4339.

Nemeroff, C. B., & Binder, E. (2014). The preeminent role of childhood abuse and neglect in vulnerability to major psychiatric disorders: Towards elucidating the underlying neurobiological mechanisms. *Journal of the American Academy of Child & Adolescent Psychiatry, 53,* 395–397.

Nurnberger, J. I., Koller, D. L., Jung, J., Edenberg, H. J., Foroud, T., Guella, I., . . . Kelsoe, J. R. (2014). Identification of pathways for bipolar disorder: A Meta-analysis. *JAMA Psychiatry, 71,* 657–664.

CONTRIBUTORS

Erika Abrial, PhD
Department of Psychiatry and Behavioral Sciences
University of Miami Miller School of Medicine
Miami, Florida, USA

Gabriella M. Ahle, BA
Department of Psychiatry
Icahn School of Medicine at Mount Sinai
New York, New York, USA

Alessandra Alciati, MD
Department of Clinical Neurosciences,
Albese con Cassano
Como, Italy

Guillermo Perez Algorta, PhD
Department of Psychiatry
The Ohio State University
Columbus, Ohio, USA

Ana Cristina Andreazza, MD
Centre for Addiction and Mental, Ontario, Canada
Departments of Pharmacology and Psychiatry,
University of Toronto
Toronto, Canada

Jean-Michel Azorin, MD
Department of Psychiatry,
Ste Marguerite Hospital
Marseille Cedex, France

Christopher R. Bailey MD
Department of Internal Medicine,
Johns Hopkins University School of Medicine
Baltimore, Maryland, USA

Ross J. Baldessarini, MD
International Consortium for Bipolar Disorder Research,
McLean Hospital, Belmont, Massachusetts USA;
Department of Psychiatry, Harvard Medical School,
Boston, Massachusetts USA

Richard Balon, MD
Departments of Psychiatry and Behavioral Neurosciences
and Anesthesiology
Wayne State University School of Medicine
Detroit, Michigan, USA

Michael Bauer, MD, PhD
Department of Psychiatry and Psychotherapy
University Hospital Carl Gustav Carus
Technische Universität Dresden
Dresden, Germany

Raoul Belzeaux, MD
Department of Psychiatry
Ste Marguerite Hospital
Marseille Cedex, France

Eleonore Beurel, PhD
Department of Psychiatry and Behavioral Sciences
University of Miami Miller School of Medicine
Miami, Florida, USA

Mimi C. Briggs, BA
Department of Psychiatry
Icahn School of Medicine at Mount Sinai
New York, New York, USA

Joseph R. Calabrese, MD
Department of Psychiatry
Case Western Reserve University School of Medicine/
University Hospitals Case Medical Center
Cleveland, Ohio, USA

Danielle S. Cha, HBSc
Mood Disorders Psychopharmacology Unit,
University Health Network, Toronto, Ontario;
Institute of Medical Science, University of Toronto,
Toronto, Ontario, Canada

Kiki Chang, MD
Department of Psychiatry and Behavioral Sciences
Stanford University Medical Center
Stanford, California, USA

Elizabeth A. Crocco, MD
Department of Psychiatry and Behavioral Sciences
University of Miami, Miller School of Medicine
Miami, Florida, USA

Rosie E. Curiel, PsyD
Department of Psychiatry and Behavioral Sciences
University of Miami, Miller School of Medicine
Miami, Florida, USA

Melissa P. DelBello, MD, MS
Department of Psychiatry and Behavioral Neuroscience
University of Cincinnati College of Medicine
Cincinnati, Ohio, USA

Colin A. Depp, PhD
Department of Psychiatry
University of California, San Diego
San Diego, California, USA

Timothy Dinan, MD
Department of Psychiatry
University College Cork
Cork, Ireland

James C. Eliassen, PhD
Center for Imaging Research
University of Cincinnati College of Medicine
Cincinnati, Ohio, USA

David E. Fleck, PhD
Department of Psychiatry & Behavioral Neuroscience
University of Cincinnati College of Medicine
Cincinnati, Ohio, USA

Konstantinos N. Fountoulakis, MD
Department of Psychiatry, School of Medicine
Aristotle University of Thessaloniki
Thessaloniki, Greece

Keming Gao, MD, PhD
Department of Psychiatry
Case Western Reserve University School of Medicine/
University Hospitals Case Medical Center
Cleveland, Ohio, USA

Allison Greene, BA
John Hopkins University School of Medicine
Baltimore, Maryland, USA

Heinz Grunze, MD, PhD
Department of Psychiatry
Paracelsus Medical University & Christian Doppler
Klinik
Salzburg, Austria

Andrew Freeman, PhD
Department of Psychology
University of Nevada, Las Vegas
Las Vegas, Nevada, USA

Gabriel Rodrigo Fries, PhD
Department of Psychiatry and Behavioral Sciences
University of Texas Health Science Center at Houston
Houston, Texas, USA

Sabrina Maria Gippert, PhD
Department of Psychiatry and Psychotherapy
University Hospital
Bonn, Germany

Alexandrea L. Harmell, MS
Department of Psychiatry
University of California, San Diego
Department of Psychology
San Diego State University, San Diego
San Diego, California

Philip D. Harvey, PhD
Department of Psychiatry and Behavioral Sciences
University of Miami Miller School of Medicine
Miami, Florida, USA

Robert M.A. Hirschfeld, MD
Department of Psychiatry
Weill Cornell Medical College,
New York, New York, USA

Frank K. Hu, PhD
Department of Psychiatry and Behavioral Sciences
The University of Texas Health Science Center at
Houston
Houston, Texas, USA

Julie Hyman, MD
Department of Psychiatry & Behavioral Health
The Ohio State University College of Medicine
Columbus, Ohio, USA

Richard S. Jope, PhD
Department of Psychiatry and Behavioral Sciences
University of Miami Miller School of Medicine
Miami, Florida, USA

Flávio Kapczinski, MD, PhD
Bipolar Disorder Program
Hospital de Clínicas de Porto Alegre
Universidade Federal do Rio Grande do Sul, Brazil
INCT for Translational Medicine, Brazil

Sarah Kayser, MD, MSc
Department of Psychiatry and Psychotherapy
University Hospital
Bonn, Germany

Paul E. Keck, Jr., MD
Department of Psychiatry & Behavioral Neuroscience
Lindner Center of HOPE
Mason, Ohio, USA

Charles H. Kellner, MD
Department of Psychiatry
Icahn School of Medicine at Mount Sinai
New York, New York, USA

Levente Kriston, PhD
Department of Medical Psychology
University Medical Center
Hamburg-Eppendorf, Hamburg, Germany

Paul A. Kudlow, MD, BSc
Department of Psychiatry
University of Toronto
Toronto, Ontario, Canada

Eric Laber, PhD
Department of Statistics
North Carolina State University
Raleigh, North Carolina, USA

Lauren S. Liebman, BA
Department of Psychiatry
Icahn School of Medicine at Mount Sinai
New York, New York, USA

Alexandre Loch, MD, PhD
Mood Disorders Program, LIM-27, Institute and
Department of Psychiatry
University of Sao Paulo
Sao Paulo, Brazil

Rodrigo Machado-Vieira, MD, PhD
Mood Disorders Program, LIM-27, Institute and
Department of Psychiatry
University of Sao Paulo, Brazil;
Center for Interdisciplinary Research on Applied
Neurosciences (NAPNA)
University of Sao Paulo, Brazil

Carlo Maggini, MD
International Consortium for Bipolar Disorder Research,
McLean Hospital, Belmont, MA USA;
Department of Neuroscience, Faculty of Medicine,
University of Parma, Italy

Nina R. McCune, BA
Department of Psychiatry and Behavioral Neuroscience
University of Cincinnati College of Medicine
Cincinnati, Ohio, USA

Susan L. McElroy, MD
Department of Psychiatry & Behavioral Neuroscience
Lindner Center of HOPE
Mason, Ohio, USA

Roger S. McIntyre MD, FRCPC
Mood Disorders Psychopharmacology Unit, University
Health Network, Toronto, Ontario
Institute of Medical Science, University of Toronto,
Ontario;
Department of Psychiatry and Pharmacology, University
of Toronto
Toronto, Ontario, Canada

Kathleen R. Merikangas, PhD
Genetic Epidemiology Research Branch
Intramural Research Program
National Institute of Mental Health
Bethesda, Maryland, USA

Valeria Mondelli, MD
Institute of Psychiatry, King's College London
Department of Psychological Medicine
London, United Kingdom

Keitha Moseley-Dendy, MA
Department of Psychiatry
The University of Texas Medical Branch
Galveston, Texas, USA

Charles B. Nemeroff, MD, PhD
Department of Psychiatry and Behavioral Sciences
University of Miami Miller School of Medicine
Miami, Florida, USA

Alexander Neumeister, MD, PhD
Molecular Imaging Program for Mood and Anxiety
Disorders
Departments of Psychiatry and Radiology,
New York University School of Medicine
New York, New York, USA

D. Jeffrey Newport, MD, MS, MDiv.
Department of Psychiatry & Behavioral Health and
Obstetrics & Gynecology
The Ohio State University College of Medicine
Columbus, Ohio, USA

Dost Öngür, MD, PhD
Department of Psychitary
McLean Hospital
Harvard Medical School
Boston, Massachusetts, USA

Diana Paksarian, MPH, PhD
Genetic Epidemiology Research Branch
Intramural Research Program
National Institute of Mental Health
Bethesda, Maryland, USA

Carmine M. Pariante, PhD
Institute of Psychiatry, King's College London
Department of Psychological Medicine
London, United Kingdom

Marta Pardo, PhD
Department of Psychiatry and Behavioral Sciences
University of Miami Miller School of Medicine
Miami, Florida, USA

Luis R. Patino, MD, MSc
Department of Psychiatry and Behavioral Neuroscience
University of Cincinnati College of Medicine
Cincinnati, Ohio, USA

Roy H. Perlis, MD MSc
Center for Experimental Drugs and Diagnostics
Massachusetts General Hospital
Boston, Massachusetts

Jesus Pérez, MD, PhD
International Consortium for Bipolar Disorder Research,
McLean Hospital, Belmont, MA USA;
Department of Psychiatry,
University of Cambridge, Cambridge, UK;
CAMEO Early Intervention Services,
Cambridgeshire & Peterborough NHS Foundation Trust,
Cambridge, UK

Giampaolo Perna, MD, PhD
Department of Clinical Neurosciences, Villa San
Benedetto Menni
Albese con Cassano, Como, Italy;
Department of Psychiatry and Neuropsychology, Faculty
of Health, Medicine and Life Sciences
University of Maastricht, Maastricht, Netherlands;
Department of Psychiatry and Behavioral Sciences
Leonard Miller School of Medicine, University of Miami,
Miami, Florida, USA

Giulio Perugi, MD
Department of Clinical e Experimental Medicine, Unit of
Psychiatry,
University of Pisa, Pisa, Italy;
Institute of Behavioral Science "G. De Lisio"
Pisa, Italy

Dina Popovic, MD, PhD
Bipolar Disorders Program, Institute of Neuroscience
Hospital Clínic Barcelona, University of Barcelona,
Barcelona, Catalonia, Spain;
Department of Psychiatry, Sheba Medical Center,
University of Tel Aviv, Tel Aviv, Israel.

Robert M. Post, MD
Bipolar Collaborative Network
Bethesda, Maryland, USA

Michelle Primeau, MD
Department of Psychiatry and Behavioral Sciences
Stanford University;
Division of Sleep Medicine
Stanford University;
Sierra Pacific MIRECC, VA Health Care System
Palo Alto, California

Gislaine Tezza Rezin, PhD
Centre for Addiction and Mental, Ontario, Canada
Departments of Pharmacology and Psychiatry,
University of Toronto
Toronto, Ontario, Canada

Pedro Ruiz, MD
Menninger Department of Psychiatry and Behavioral
Sciences,
Baylor College of Medicine,
Houston, Texas, USA

Samir Sabbag, MD
Department of Psychiatry and Behavioral Sciences
University of Miami, Miller School of Medicine
Miami, Florida, USA

Ihsan Salloum, MD
Professor of Psychiatry and Behavioral Sciences
University of Miami Miller School of Medicine
Miami, Florida, USA

Paola Salvatore, MD
International Consortium for Bipolar Disorder Research,
McLean Hospital
Belmont, MA USA;
Department of Neuroscience,
University of Parma, Parma, Italy

Marsal Sanches, MD, PhD
Department of Psychiatry and Behavioral Sciences
The University of Texas Health Science Center at
Houston
Houston, Texas, USA

Marguerite Reid Schneider, BA
University of Cincinnati College of Medicine,
Cincinnati, Ohio, USA;
Neuroscience Graduate Program, University of Cincinnati
Cincinnati, Ohio, USA

Noreen A. Reilly-Harrington, PhD
Department of Psychiatry
Massachusetts General Hospital
Harvard Medical School
Boston, Massachusetts, USA

Jan Scott, PhD
Institute of Neuroscience, Newcastle University;
Centre for Affective Disorders, Institute of Psychiatry
London, United Kingdom

Emanuel Severus, MD
Department of Psychiatry and Psychotherapy
University Hospital Carl Gustav Carus
Dresden, Germany

Jair C. Soares, MD, PhD
Department of Psychiatry and Behavioral Sciences
The University of Texas Health Science Center at
Houston
Houston, Texas, USA

Trisha Suppes, MD, PhD
Department of Psychiatry
Stanford University School of Medicine
Palo Alto, California, USA

Louisa G. Sylvia, PhD
Department of Psychiatry
Massachusetts General Hospital
Harvard Medical School
Boston, Massachusetts, USA

Stephanie Roberts, PhD
Private Practice
Boston, Massachusetts, USA

Steven P. Roose, MD
Department of Psychiatry
Columbia University College of Physicians and Surgeons
New York State Psychiatric Institute
New York, New York, USA

Alice Russell, BSc
Institute of Psychiatry, King's College London
Department of Psychological Medicine
London, United Kingdom

Bret R. Rutherford, MD
Columbia University College of Physicians and Surgeons
New York State Psychiatric Institute
New York, New York, USA

Janusz K. Rybakowski, MD, PhD
Department of Adult Psychiatry
Poznan University of Medical Sciences
Poznan, Poland

Giacomo Salvadore, MD
Neuroscience Experimental Medicine
Janssen Research & Development, LLC
Titusville, New Jersey, USA

Gabriele Sani, MD
NeSMOS Department (Neurosciences, Mental Health, and Sensory Organs)
School of Medicine and Psychology, Sapienza University;
UOC Psychiatry, Sant'Andrea Hospital, Centro Lucio Bini
IRCCS Santa Lucia Foundation
Department of Clinical and Behavioural Neurology,
Neuropsychiatry Laboratory
Rome, Italy

Thomas Eduard Schlaepfer, MD, PhD
Department of Psychiatry and Psychotherapy, University Hospital
Bonn, Germany;
Departments of Psychiatry and Mental Health,
The Johns Hopkins University
Baltimore, Maryland, USA

Erica Snook, MD
Psychiatry Resident
Department of Psychiatry, The University of Texas
Medical Branch
Galveston, Texas, USA

Stephen M. Strakowski, MD
Department of Psychiatry & Behavioral Neuroscience
University of Cincinnati College of Medicine
Cincinnati, Ohio, USA.;
Center for Imaging Research,
University of Cincinnati College of Medicine
Cincinnati, Ohio, USA

Christina Switala, MSc
Department of Psychiatry and Psychotherapy
University Hospital
Bonn, Germany

Joshua Z. Tal, PhD
Department of Psychiatry and Behavioral Sciences
Stanford University
Stanford, California, USA

Jane M. Tandler, BA
New York State Psychiatric Institute
New York, New York, USA

Leonardo Tondo, MD, MSc
International Consortium for Bipolar and Psychotic
Disorders Research
McLean Hospital
Belmont, MA, USA;
Lucio Bini Mood Disorder Centers,
Cagliari and Rome, Italy;
Department of Psychiatry,
Harvard Medical School
Boston, Massachusetts, USA

Tatiana Torti, PhD
Department of Clinical Neurosciences
Albese con Cassano
Como, Italy

Katharina Trede, MD
International Consortium for Bipolar Disorder Research,
McLean Hospital
Belmont, MA, USA;
Department of Psychiatry, Tufts University School of Medicine,
Maine Medical Center
Portland, Maine, USA

Juan Undurraga MD, PhD
Department of Psychiatry,
Facultad de Medicina Clinica Alemana,
Universidad del Desarrollo, Santiago, Chile;
Early Intervention Program,
Instituto Psiquiátrico 'Dr Horwitz Barak', Santiago, Chile

Anna Van Meter, PhD
Ferkauf Graduate School
Yeshiva University
Bronx, New York, USA

Gustavo H. Vázquez, MD, PhD
International Consortium for Bipolar and Psychotic
Disorders Research,
McLean Hospital
Belmont, MA, USA;
Department of Neuroscience,
Palermo University
Buenos Aires, Argentina

Eduard Vieta, MD, PhD
Bipolar Disorders Program, Institute of Neuroscience
University of Barcelona, IDIBAPS, CIBERSAM
Barcelona, Catalonia, Spain

Jelena Vrublevska, MD
Department of Psychiatry and Narcology
Riga Stradins University
Riga, Latvia
Sarah Wooderson, PhD
Centre for Affective Disorders, Institute of Psychiatry
King's College London
London, United Kingdom

Janet Wozniak, MD
Department of Psychiatry
Harvard Medical School
Boston, MA, USA;
Massachusetts General Hospital
Boston, Massachusetts, USA

Fan Wu, PhD
Department of Statistics
North Carolina State University
Raleigh, North Carolina, USA

Renrong Wu, MD, PhD
Institute of Mental Health
the Second Xiangya Hospital of Central South University
Hunan, P. R. China

Ayşegül Yildiz, MD
International Consortium for Bipolar Disorder Research,
McLean Hospital, Belmont, MA USA;
Department of Psychiatry,
Dokuz Eylül University
Izmir, Turkey

Allan H. Young M.D., Ph.D.
Centre for Affective Disorders, Institute of Psychiatry
King's College London
London, United Kingdom

Eric A. Youngstrom, PhD
Department of Psychology
University of North Carolina at Chapel Hill
Chapel Hill, North Carolina, USA

Marcus V. Zanetti, MD, PhD
Mood Disorders Program, LIM-27
Institute and Department of Psychiatry
Center for Interdisciplinary Research on Applied
Neurosciences (NAPNA)
University of Sao Paulo
Sao Paulo, Brazil

THE BIPOLAR BOOK

THE HUMAN BOOK

SECTION I

CLINICAL PRESENTATION

1.

HISTORY OF BIPOLAR MANIC-DEPRESSIVE DISORDER

Ross J. Baldessarini, Jesús Pérez, Paola Salvatore, Katharina Trede,

and Carlo Maggini

Even though the classification of mental illness is a problem that has been occupying the best minds for unthinkable times, it has not been solved in a satisfactory manner. FLEMMING, *1844, p. 97*

INTRODUCTION

Bipolar manic-depressive disorder is arguably both the youngest and possibly also one of the oldest forms of major mental illness. Tradition has detected seeds of the concept in ancient Greco-Roman writings of physician-scholars on syndromes designated as *mania* and *melancholia*. Ancient texts include evidence that some observers perceived close relationships between these conditions and as arising in the same person at different times (Aretæus, 1861; Roccatagliata, 1986). These basic concepts were further elaborated by medieval Islamic scholars and later in Europe. However, the meaning of these terms in ancient and medieval times and their relationship to modern *major depression* and *mania* are uncertain: states of physical debility, as well as of emotional and behavioral excitation, are not specific and can be associated with a variety of neuromedical, metabolic, and toxic conditions, as well as arising spontaneously. Primary and secondary forms of depression and mania are unlikely to have been precisely and accurately differentiated in the distant past and continue to require careful diagnostic consideration even in modern times (Healy, 2008; Shorter, 2012).

A great deal of attention has been given to the acrimonious debate in Paris in the 1850s between Jean-Pierre Falret ("circular insanity") and Jules Baillarger ("insanity of double-form") about their claims of priority in describing cases involving mania and melancholia in the same person over time, though many such descriptions long preceded theirs. Even more attention has been given to the highly influential, though debated, division of idiopathic psychotic disorders into broad "manic-depressive" and "dementia præcox" groups by Emil Kraepelin in the 1890s. The Kraepelinian hypothesis continues to dominate modern psychiatric nosology with the tacit contrast of major disorders mainly of mood and behavior with an episodic or recurring pattern and relatively favorable long-term course and outcome versus those of a more chronic nature that involve profound dysfunctions of cognition, reasoning, perception, and motivation. The concept of *bipolar disorder* arose remarkably recently, since the mid-20th century, reaching acceptance in standard international diagnostic systems only in 1980.

Currently the concept of bipolar disorder remains an evolving and changing one, with efforts to extend its reach into the complex and challenging territory of pediatric disorders, as well as into conditions marked mainly by recurrent major depression with varying elements of excitation or agitation and even into conditions traditionally considered to represent personality disorders or temperaments (Trede et al., 2005). Such broad concepts had been considered previously, including in the "cyclothymia" of Kahlbaum and Hecker (Baethge, Salvatore, & Baldessarini, 2003a, 2003b). Tension arises between efforts to broaden the concept of bipolar disorder for nosological and potential clinical purposes versus inclinations to constrain it to relatively clearly defined conditions (phenotypes) appropriate for medical research.

This chapter briefly summarizes noteworthy highlights in the historical evolution of the bipolar disorder concept from ancient to current times. This history is complicated by the relative lack of documentation of concepts pertaining to mania and melancholia during the first millennium CE and by uncertainties arising from imperfect differentiation of primary mental illnesses from relatively nonspecific emotional and behavioral manifestations of neuromedical conditions. Moreover, it is always risky to approach history in search of earlier observations that seem to anticipate currently favored concepts.

ANCIENT CONTRIBUTIONS

Ancient physician-scholars of the Hippocratic school in ancient Greece used the terms *melancholia* and *mania* in the 5th century BCE, and the concepts may have been familiar even earlier (Marneros & Angst, 2000). However, ancient and later understanding of those terms probably differ considerably, as distinctions among illnesses presenting with depressed or excited mood and behavior were no doubt limited (Healy, 2008; Roccatagliata, 1986; Shorter, 2012). Nevertheless, even for ancient writers, mania and melancholia were abnormal behavioral states to be differentiated from febrile illnesses and forms of "phrenitis" that may have included delirium arising from toxic or metabolic conditions (Jackson, 1986; Marneros & Angst, 2000; Roccatagliata, 1986). Moreover, Hippocratic writers described behavioral conditions that might now be recognized as hypomania and mixed manic-depressive states (Marneros & Angst, 2000).

Most ancient writers on mania and melancholia or other mental disorders identified with an early clinical tradition in medicine that attempted to understand illnesses from a biological perspective, considered the brain as the seat of the problem, and eschewed spiritual explanations, such as demonic possession, that has continued to modern times (Marneros & Angst, 2001; Roccatagliata, 1986). A humoral "imbalance" theory was widely accepted, which was based on the essential humors of blood, yellow and black bile, and phlegm that probably dates to Middle Eastern cultures prior to classical Greek times. The humoral concept of human physiology as applied to mental illnesses may not be much less speculative than some modern theories in biological psychiatry involving ill-defined and unproved "chemical imbalances" (Baldessarini, 2013). The humoral theory was strongly popularized by the influential Greco-Roman physician Galen (Aelius Galenus of Pergamon, c. 129–208 CE), who is also credited with ascribing behavior, emotion, and thought to functions of the brain (Brain, 1986). The humoral theory, with variations and modifications, was largely retained until the 19th century. The balance of the four basic humors was believed to influence personality traits or temperament types (*sanguine* [pleasure-seeking, sociable], *melancholic* [analytical, thoughtful], *choleric* [ambitious, assertive], and *phlegmatic* [restrained, quiet]). Traditionally, melancholia was associated with an excess or maldistribution of black bile and mania with the influence of yellow or black bile (Arikha, 2007).

A particularly striking early description of mania and melancholia was given by the Greco-Syrian scholar *Posidonius* (c. 135–51 BCE). He proposed that mania was due to actions of "yellow bile on frontal portions of the brain, which alters the imagination and as a consequence, reason" (Roccatagliata, 1986). Posidonius wrote of those afflicted with mania or melancholia, suggesting that they may represent a single disorder:

> The patient laugh, sings, dances…he bites himself…sometimes is wicked and kills…sometimes he is anxious and seized by terror or hate…sometimes he is abulic…[it is] an intermittent disease…repeated…once a year or more often…melancholia occurs in autumn whereas mania in summer…mania occurs in young people and melancholia in adults…the melancholic is sad, afraid; he isolates himself and cries; he thinks…about death…he exaggerates his evils and his faults…and his illness; he thinks himself a terrible sinner…he feels desperate.
>
> ROCCATAGLIATA, *1986, p. 143.*

Aretæus of Cappadocia (c. 150 CE) was a physician believed to have been born in what is now central Turkey and trained in a Hellenistic medical tradition. He may have worked in Alexandria and probably died in Rome. He was a man of modest background and means and was not widely cited in his own era, owing largely to writing in the Ionian Greek dialect (Aretæus, 1861; Cordell, 1909; Jackson, 1986; Roccatagliata, 1986). Aretæus is widely credited with being among the first medical writers to describe what appear to be episodes or illness phases representing melancholia and mania in the same person at different times (Goldney, 2012; Healy, 2008; Jackson, 1986; Marneros & Angst, 2000; Pichot, 2006; Shorter, 2012). That Aretæus' conceptions of these conditions were not entirely nonspecific is indicated by his care in distinguishing them from febrile disorders, including "phrenitis," which also involved depressed or excited behaviors and psychotic thought, as well as distinguishing the melancholia of young adults from the dementias of the elderly and mania from delirious intoxication with alcohol or plant toxins. In addition, he distinguished what might be considered "endogenous" or autonomous melancholia as a disorder involving sadness and depression as well as depression and grief associated with stressful life events, such as the loss of a loved one (Aretæus, 1861, pp. 298–300).

However, it is less clear whether he or other ancient writers considered melancholia and mania to be different disorders or dissimilar presentations of a single disorder (Roccatagliata, 1986). Of note, Aretæus discussed melancholia and mania in separate sections of his writings

(Aretæus, 1861, pp. 298–300, 301–304). Mania for him seems sometimes to represent an extreme or late form of severe melancholia, but sometimes he found mania-like elements in milder phases of melancholia, and often found depressive elements in patients with mania. Aretæus (1861) provided somewhat ambiguous descriptions of characteristics of melancholic and manic patients:

> without fever... melancholia is the commencement and a part of mania.... [Melancholia] affects the head... [in which] abnormal irritability of temper change[s] to laughter and joy... [They] become mad rather from the increase of the disease... They are prone to change... readily... to become simple, extravagant, munificent... from the changeableness of the disease... The modes of mania are infinite in species, but one alone in genus. For it is altogether a chronic derangement of the mind, without fever... mania intermits, and with care ceases altogether... Those prone to [mania] are naturally passionate, irritable, of active habits, an easy disposition, joyous, puerile; likewise those whose disposition inclines to the opposite condition [to melancholia]... are sluggish, sorrowful, slow to learn but patient in labor... those likewise are more prone to melancholia who have formerly been in a mad [manic] condition.

His writings (Aretæus, 1861) also suggest that Aretæus associated particular personality traits with risks for mania or melancholia and associated specific seasons of the year (especially spring) with risk for recurrences. He also described loss of sleep, with tiredness in the morning, as well as decreased appetite in melancholia, and increases in mania along with increases of sexuality, behavioral disinhibition or aggression, and abuse of alcohol. He also found the risk for melancholia to be greater among women than men and that mania was most likely to begin in adolescence or early adulthood. There are even suggestions by Aretæus of episodes or illness phases that may resemble what have been considered "mixed" manic-depressive states over the past century, and he recognized severe versus moderate forms of mania (possible antecedents of modern-day hypomania) as well as periods of "demi-mania" in melancholia (possible antecedents of bipolar spectrum disorders; Merikangas, et al. 2007; Roccatagliata, 1986, p. 231; Salvatore et al., 2002). He described hallucinations as well as psychotic suspiciousness and easy frustration or anger in mania, contrasted to fearfulness, grief, fear of ill health, and a desire to die in melancholia (Aretæus, 1861, pp 199–301).

However, as already noted, there are definite risks of reading unwarranted modern interpretations into such ancient observations.

In the 6th century CE, *Alexander of Tralles* (c. 525–605 CE), brother of the architect of the reconstructed Hagia Sophia in Constantinople, wrote that melancholia and mania could occur in cycles (Kudlien, 1970). He sometimes observed admixtures of features of either condition and recognized an increased risk of suicide associated with what he may well have conceived as a single disorder. However, he and other early writers seem to have conceived of mania as a more intense or severe manifestation of an essentially melancholic disorder, rather than as a polar phase found early in the course of illness (Goldney, 2012; Roccatagliata, 1986).

Following the seminal observations of clinical conditions termed *melancholia* and *mania* by ancient Greco-Roman and Middle Eastern physician-scholars, reports pertaining to these conditions are hard to find until later in the first millennium CE, and mainly in the writings of Persian and Arabic physicians.

9TH TO 11TH CENTURIES: THE ISLAMIC WORLD

Contributions of several medieval Persian and Arabic physician-scholars to the understanding of mental illness are especially noteworthy. They had a lasting impact among their contemporaries and for centuries thereafter. These scholars not only assimilated ancient medical information of Egypt, Greece, and Rome but also adapted it to their needs and concepts and added their own empirical findings. The first known psychiatric hospitals (*maristans*) were founded by Persian and Arabic physicians in the 9th and 10th centuries and spread widely into North Africa and Moorish southern Spain (*Al-Andalus*) in the 14th century. Most were established by sultans, supported by donations and patient fees, and typically supervised by physicians; some were components of early academic medical centers (Pérez, Baldessarini, & Undurraga, 2012). Several medieval Islamic clinicians can be considered the first psychologists or psychiatrists, as detailed clinical information on various mental or behavioral disorders is found in their medical treatises. These include texts by *Ishaq Ibn Imran* (c. 848–906 CE), *Razes* (Muhammad ibn Zakariya al-Razi; c. 865–925 CE), *Avicenna* (Abu Ali al-Husayn ibn Abd Allah ibn Sina; 980–1037 CE), *Esmail Jorjani* (Sayyid Zayn al-Din Isma'il al-Husayni al-Jurjani; 1041–1136), and others (Omrani, Holtzman, Akiskal, & Ghaemi, 2012; Vakili & Gorji, 2006).

Medieval physicians in this Islamic tradition distinguished four major mental disorders: *melancholia, mania, ghotrah* (persecutory psychosis, paranoia), and *ishgh* (a combination of anxiety and depression). Mania was a state of raving madness with exalted mood, excitability, sleep disturbance, and sometimes violence. A particular type of mania, *daol-kahl*, involved aggression and unrestrained excitement, followed later by becoming calm and cooperative though not necessarily melancholic. In that era, melancholia and mania seem to have been viewed as different but related entities sometimes encountered in the same person at different times. For example, both Ishaq Ibn Imran (c. 908 CE) and Avicenna (1025) saw mania and melancholia as closely related or suggested that these states lay on a continuum and could pass from one to the other (Omrani et al., 2012; Vakili & Gorji, 2006). Nevertheless, it was unclear whether the disorders represented phases of a single illness or separate diseases.

12TH TO 16TH CENTURIES

The first half of the second millennium CE provides scattered comments in writings by scholarly European Christian physicians on possible associations of mania and melancholia, with influence by earlier writings of such predecessors as Galen and Avicenna. English physician and theologist, *John of Gaddesden* (c. 1280–1361) appears to have considered mania and melancholia as different forms of the same disorder (Gaddesden, 1314). A century later, *Johannes Manardus* (Giovanni Manardo) of Ferrara (1462–1536), an influential Italian physician who taught Swiss physician *Paracelsus* (1493–1541), observed the following in approximately 1500: "Melancholia manifestly differs from what is properly called mania; there is no doubt, however, that at some time or other, authorities agree that it replaces melancholia" (Whitwell, 1936, p. 205).

In the mid-16th century, *Felix Platter* (Platerus; 1536–1614) dean of the medical school of Basel, postulated a continuum between mania and melancholia, arising from a "perturbation" of what he called "the spirit of the brain" that could produce melancholia or mania depending on how it was influenced by other materials (Platter, 1549). Similarly, Dutch physician *Jason Pratensis* (1486–1558) discussed melancholia and mania in what may be the first textbook of neurology, *De Cerebri Morbis* of 1549 (Pestronk, 1988). Pratensis viewed mania as a mental corruption without fever that "carried a man outside his own mind and wretchedly beyond the use of all reason" (Pestronk, 1988). This statement may suggest a broad view of "mania"

as the approximate equivalent of "madness" or "psychosis." Nevertheless, Pratensis stated that mania and melancholia could not easily be distinguished because they proceeded from the same causes, despite their dramatic clinical dissimilarity. He further indicated that most physicians of his era considered mania and melancholia as one disorder.

Another remarkable contribution from this period is by Chinese encyclopedist and dramatist *Gao Lian* (Kao Lien; 16th century) who described clinical conditions marked by mania and melancholia as a specific form of mental illness (Maciocia, 2009).

17TH TO 18TH CENTURIES

In the 1600s and 1700s, influential European medical theorists included "iatromechanical" physicians who developed physical or mechanical theories for medical conditions. They proposed that bodily parts are connected by small canals conveying blood and other fluids considered central to humoral theories of illness. The postulated connectivity implied common causal mechanisms and continuity between different disorders, probably including melancholia and mania. Representatives of this movement include *Friedrich Hoffmann* of Germany (1660–1742), *Archibald Pitcairn* (1652–1713) of Scotland, and Dutch botanical expert *Hermann Boerhaave* (1668–1738). Pitcairn (1718) and Hoffman (1695) emphasized effects of humors on the brain as a basis of mental disorders, as well as of personality types. For example, a common view was that melancholia resulted from sluggishness of the circulation of blood in the brain (King, 1971).

Of considerable importance, Hoffman (1695) and Boerhaave (1735) considered melancholia and mania as alternating mental states or stages of the same disorder, with melancholia maintaining a primary role and mania sometimes viewed as a more severe, acute form of illness. Hoffman observed, "Mania can easily pass over into melancholy, and conversely, melancholy into mania" (p. 72). Later, he added, "Though usually reckoned different disorders, [they] appear to be rather different stages of one: mania being properly an exacerbation of melancholia, and leaving the patient melancholic in the calmer interval" (p. 298). In the same era, Boerhaave stated:

If melancholy increases so far, that from the great motion of liquid of the brain, the patient be thrown into a wild fury, it is called madness [mania] which differs only in degree from the sorrowful kind of melancholy, is its offspring, produced from the same causes. (pp. 323–324)

English physicians *Thomas Willis* (1621–1675), *Thomas Sydenham* (1624–1689), and *Richard Mead* (1673–1754), as well as the Italians *Giovanni Morgagni* (1682–1771) and, later, *Vincenzo Chiarugi* (1759–1820), also commented on the common recurrent, alternating course of patients with melancholia and mania, indicating that the concept was widely held even before the 18th century (Angst & Marneros, 2001; Haustgen, 1995).

Also, of interest, even earlier than theories postulated by iatromechanical theorists, *Théophile Bonet* (1620–1689), a French physician who moved from France to Geneva to escape the Counter-Reformation, reified a link between mania and melancholia by use of the term *maniaco-melancholicus* (Bonet, 1686). Similar concepts appeared a century later in the work of *Richard Mead* (1673–1754) of London and of *Anne-Charles Lorry* (1684–1766) of Montpellier, France, who used the term *mania-melancholica* (Lorry, 1765).

Both of these compound terms may have referred to mixed states rather than manic-depressive illness (Marneros & Angst, 2000). Nevertheless, by the early 1700s, ideas concerning close relationships between melancholia and mania evidently were widely accepted. Furthermore, the notion of a single mental illness was increasingly consolidated, usually with melancholia still considered as the main explanation for the overall condition.

Andres Piquer-Arrufat (1711–1772) was a prominent figure in Spanish medicine in the mid-18th century (Pérez, Baldessarini, Cruz, Salvatore, & Vieta, 2011). His writings acknowledge influence by the work of earlier writers, including Boerhaave, Hoffmann, Sydenham, and Willis. He became principal physician to the court of King Ferdinand VI in 1751 to 1759, with a simultaneous royal appointment as vice president of the Academy of Medicine in Madrid. Ferdinand VI (1713–1759) was of the Spanish Bourbon linage descended from the French Bourbons. Ferdinand was described as shy, cautious, and somewhat indolent as a boy. He developed a severe mental illness similar to that of his father (King Phillip V), with episodes of excitement and rages, typically alternating with periods of profound self-doubt, fearful preoccupations about his health, and melancholic depression. Shortly after Ferdinand's death, Piquer authored a monograph on the king's illness in 1759 that was not published until the early 1800s, with additional clinical observations on mania and melancholia reported in his textbook of 1764

(Piquer-Arrufat, 1764). Based on prolonged clinical observations of the royal family, the 1759 manuscript contains particularly detailed discussion of a severe psychiatric illness to which he applied a novel diagnostic term a century and a half before Kraepelin's "manic-depressive insanity": "The King suffered a melancholic-manic illness… affectio melancholico-maniaca…Melancholia and mania, although treated in many medical books separately, are the same disease" (Piquer-Arrufat, 1759, p. 8).

Piquer specifically acknowledged the proposals by Willis (1672) and probably also knew of the work of other English scholars, including *Robert James* (1705–1776) and *Richard Mead* (1673–1754), all of whom commented on alternation between melancholia and mania in the same patients over time (James, 1745; Mead, 1751; Willis 1672). These citations and Piquer's own writing suggest that the concept of alternation of clinical states in a single manic-depressive disorder of unknown cause was an accepted view in Europe by the 18th century. Nevertheless, this concept of alternating states appears variably to retain the view that mania represented an extreme expression of an essentially melancholic disorder (Pérez et al., 2011). Piquer's position differed from that of other predecessors or contemporaries: "Melancholia and mania are terms denoting a single disease accompanied by several disorders of mood. When the sick mind is moved by fear and sadness, we name this melancholia, and when it is by rage and audacity, mania" (Piquer-Arrufat, 1764, pp. 14–15).

Moreover, Piquer recorded several other characteristics of his *melancholic-manic* illness that resemble important elements of modern bipolar disorder. These include mixed manic-depressive, or rapidly alternating states of affective and behavioral instability, as well as seasonal mood changes and perhaps rapid cycling with several recurrences within one year—all of which are clearly described in his writings (Piquer-Arrufat, 1759, 1764). Importantly, and at variance with lingering Galenic humoral theories, even as modified by the iatromechanics, Piquer also introduced the concept of mental or brain "damage" as a consistent and fundamental etiological factor accounting for altered mood and behavior, particularly in later stages of melancholic-mania disorder (Pérez et al., 2011).

19TH-CENTURY FRANCE

Philippe Pinel (1745–1826) is well known for changing the inhumane conditions under which the severely mentally ill were treated, starting at the Bicêtre (for men) and later the

Salpêtrière (for women) hospitals in Paris for which he was responsible and in which he was influenced by his asylum manager *Jean-Baptiste Pussin* (1745–1811). Pinel worked to establish psychiatry as a specialty and led to expansion of humane mental hospitals in the early 1800s, similar to developments in many European countries and North America. The improved institutional environments probably facilitated his strongly encouraged practice of acquiring detailed knowledge of each patient's symptoms and clinical course and emphasis on the individual patient, perhaps more than his concern about diagnostic categories (Pinel, 1909). He also had a strong influence on the work of *Jean-Étienne Dominique Esquirol* (1772–1840) and a series of their students. One, *Louis-Victor Marcé* (1828–1865), produced a comprehensive treatise on perinatal psychiatry in 1859 that remained unsurpassed until the late 20th century (Trede, Baldessarini, Viguera, & Bottéro, 2009). The introduction to his general textbook (Marcé, 1862) notes difficulties in studying mental illness prior to Pinel's reforms:

> Patients were in prison, in asylums or unworthy sheds. Alienists [psychiatrists] were not able to conduct cohesive studies as the patients were dispersed. The humanitarian reform by Pinel allowed for real studies of mental ailments as the mentally ill were hospitalized in specialized mental hospitals.

Creating a place where many mentally ill could be treated and studied was pivotal for future developments of the concept of bipolar and other major psychiatric disorders. For Pinel mental disorders included manic, melancholic, demented, and idiotic clinical presentations that were not considered as separate entities but instead to be part of a single disease process, "mental alienation." Pinel's (1806) conceptualization of mania was virtually interchangeable with insanity and probably even delirium, although he recognized a periodic or episodic pattern to its longitudinal course: "The term mania indicates…a general delirium (délire général) with more or less agitation or a state of rage…Intermittent or periodical insanity is the most common form of [maniacal disorders] (pp. 4, 5, 145).

Pinel (1806) also recognized a close association of mania and melancholia but did not formulate the concept of their occurring in a single disorder:

> But some…[melancholic patients] who were endowed with greater mobility of character, from constantly seeing the extravagances of their more furious associates, became themselves decided maniacs. Others, after the lapse of some years and

for no evident cause, have undergone a thorough revolution of character…[with] a continuous ebb and flow of affections with happy or sad ideations, with threatening gestures or an air of benevolence. The facial traits therefore alternate…between fugacious passion, despair, terror, hate, desire for vengeance and appear like lightening and disappear without leaving any trace [p. 145].

Esquirol was a favored student of Pinel's and became a prominent clinician and teacher of psychiatry. In his textbook, Esquirol (1838) relied heavily on clinical observations and tabulations of illness types but without theoretical concepts (Lefebvre, 1988). He adhered to most of Pinel's classification but replaced Pinel's "partial delirium" with *lypémanias* and *monomanias*. Lypémanias were sad delusions or depressions; monomanias were delusions with a single theme, related to modern paranoid delusional disorders (Postel, 2004). Esquirol (1819) taught that mania and melancholia can occur separately over time in the same person but, like Pinel, did not incorporate them conceptually into a single entity: "Sometimes melancholia passes into mania; indeed it is the ease with which this transformation occurs that has led all the authors confuse melancholia with mania."

Jean-Pierre Falret (1794–1870) and *Jules Baillarger* (1809–1890) have been highly celebrated for their formulation of a single disorder marked by episodes of mania and melancholia (Pichot, 2006). In 1851 Falret reported in a very brief publication based on a series of lectures given at the Salpêtrière Hospital in 1850 that included his concept of *circular insanity*, marked by recurrences of episodes of mania and melancholia (Falret 1951a) and later elaborated on the concept, including periods of stability or wellness between recurrences of mania or melancholia (Falret, 1851a,b). These reports are often accepted as the birth of the modern concept of bipolar disorder (Marneros & Angst, 2000; Pichot, 2006; Sedler, 1983). Falret's circular insanity was characterized by cycles of depression and mania, separated by more or less stable intervals of variable duration, and the free interval was an integral part of the psychopathology.

In 1854, during a meeting of the Parisian Academy of Medicine, Baillarger (1854a) introduced his similar concept of *insanity of double form* (*folie à double forme*), further elaborated in a later report (Baillarger, 1954b). The illness was characterized by a sudden or progressive succession of depression and excitation, with or without illness-free intervals. At a subsequent Academy meeting in 1854, Falret claimed priority for essentially the same concept and emphasized an apparent hereditary contribution to its risk. Baillarger accused Falret of plagiarism. Falret subsequently showed great restraint in the controversy whereas Baillarger repeated his accusations until his death in 1890, sometimes using his position as editor of the influential *Annales Medico-Psychologiques* to support his position (Goldney, 2012; Pichot, 2006).

The concept was readily accepted and given a variety of similar names by French contemporaries, including *folie à formes alternes* (insanity of alternative forms), proposed by *Jean-Baptiste Delaye* (1789–1879), as well as *das circuläre irresein* (circular insanity) of *Richard von Krafft-Ebing* (1840–1902) in Germany (Goldney, 2012; Ritti, 1892) and *periodic insanity* by *Henry M. Hurd* (1843–1927), the first director of the Johns Hopkins Hospital in Baltimore (Hurd, 1882). Some contemporaries emphasized differences between Falret's *folie circulaire* and Baillarger's *folie à double forme*, although most observers and the authors themselves appeared to believe that the concepts were very similar, as is also indicated by the prolonged debate over priority (Goldney 2012). Marcé (1962), for example, diplomatically included a chapter titled "De la Folie à Double Forme ou Folie Circulaire" in his textbook to acknowledge both Falret and Baillarger.

In his own textbook, Falret (1864) significantly limited his *folie circulaire* to episodes of mania and melancholia "that have to alternate for a long time, in always the same order with a relatively short interval of normalcy" (pp. 456–461). This conceptualization evidently excluded irregularities in the types and timing of mood swings as well as cases in which features of mania and melancholia overlapped in mixed states. In addition, Falret (1862) separated himself from his teachers Pinel and Esquirol by proposing a different classification of mental illnesses:

> To enter this path of a new classification, to base the distinctions of mental illness on a group of subordinate features and on their course, evolution… means following one of the principles that can best bring us to a regular classification, an enlightened prognosis and a rational treatment. As long as we content ourselves with studying insanity in general, or even mania and melancholia…we will not find much usefulness in what we find…for science or for practice [p. 473].

Louis-Victor Marcé (1828–1865) was a student of Esquirol's. He lived a brief but intense life as a prolific scholar and writer who produced two important books, including his monograph on perinatal mental disorders of women in 1858 and a practical clinical textbook of general psychiatry in 1862, as well as approximately 25 scientific papers that included seminal work on anorexia nervosa (Trede et al. 2009). Marcé may have suffered from bipolar illness himself and is now believed to have committed suicide at age 36 following a bout of depression during the summer of 1865 (Luauté & Lempérière, 2012). Following his death, there was a striking silence about him and his considerable contributions.

Marcé (1862, p. 339) gave considerable attention to *folie circulaire* or *folie à double forme*. He also credited Willis for describing the alternations and successions between mania and melancholia nearly two centuries earlier (Goldney, 2012; Pordage, 1681; Willis, 1672). In addition, Marcé quoted German neuropsychiatrist *Wilhelm Griesinger* (1817–1868) of Berlin on the alternation of mania and melancholia in some cases (Griesinger, 1845). However, he did not discuss Griesinger's concept of unitary psychosis (*einheitpsychose*), which was not in keeping with emerging tendencies to seek evidence of separate and discrete syndromes or disorders.

This movement toward identifying discrete disorders became increasingly dominant in French and German psychiatry in midcentury, encouraged no doubt by the contributions of *Antoine Laurent Bayle* (1799–1858) to identifying general paresis of the insane as a discrete brain disease (Bayle, 1826). Marcé credited Falret and Baillarger with the concept of mania and melancholia as manifestations of a single disease process and with coining unique names for it but was also aware that similar ideas had been expressed far earlier. He also was more willing to accept a somewhat broader conceptualization of the manic-depressive entity with less restrictive clinical manifestations. For Marcé, episodes of mania and melancholia as well as periods of relative euthymia could be irregular in intensity and duration and could include forms that we might now recognize as cyclothymic disorder or recurrent melancholia alternating with mania of limited intensity (as in modern bipolar II syndrome), in evident anticipation of proposals by Kahlbaum on cyclothymia and later descriptions of a broad range of manic-depressive types by Kraepelin. Marcé (1862) noted that:

> What is infinitely more common is to see excitation and depression without going into manic or melancholic episodes. They simply constitute differences in levels of intellectual activities to the point where the illness can go unrecognized and can be seen for long periods of time as simple bizarreness of character…One could be tempted to suppose but should

not believe that there is always a perfect correlation between the intensity of the agitation and the intensity of depression. I have seen a melancholic episode with profound stupor followed by a period of excitation, characterized only by intellectual overactivity. In a similar way that a manic or excitation episode can be mild and yet correspond to a profound period of stupor, a very short manic episode can be followed by a very long melancholic episode

MARCÉ, *1862, pp. 343–345.*

In his monumental monograph on major mental illnesses of women during pregnancy and the postpartum, Marcé (1858) warned that sharp delineation of specific neuropsychiatric disorders was difficult, including the challenge that *mixed states* or prodromal phases could mislead the clinical observer:

> While attempting to provide sharp distinctions among the different forms of mental alienation that occur postpartum, I should point out some minor cautions. In particular, we find in the puerperal state a small number of [psychiatric] mixed states that are impossible to classify or to clearly define. We also find among postpartum insanities, curious morbid transformations that are found in other disorders [pp. 343–345].

His sensitivity to such subtle diagnostic details indicates that Marcé was aware of intimate and complex connections among mania and melancholia and of the challenge of differentiating other forms of relatively acute or episodic psychoses (Trede et al., 2009).

19TH-CENTURY GERMANY

German academic psychiatry of the 19th century was influenced by contemporary French psychiatry and routinely cited its literature. Prominent trends included a continuation of the evolution away from nosologically noncommittal approaches to insanity as a more or less unitary concept or one not readily organized into discrete disorders, as well as descriptions of numerous, largely idiosyncratically defined conditions and some combining of disorders with prominent similarities based on signs and symptoms, longitudinal course, and outcome. The unitary view was represented by Pinel, although it was challenged by the landmark description of general paresis of the insane by Bayle (1926) and such functional or idiopathic conditions as circular

insanity (Falret, 1851a,b). German psychiatry was influenced by the unitary-psychosis views of *Joseph Guislain* (1797–1860) of Belgium (who also accepted the idea of mixed manic-depressive states) (Guislain, 1833; Marneros & Angst, 2000) and the even stronger unitary views of *Ernst Albrecht von Zeller* (1804–1877) of Württemberg, who translated Guislain's textbook into German (Beer, 1996). Von Zeller did perceive various stages of insanity, typically starting with melancholia, later mania, yet later paranoia, and finally dementia.

The tradition of unitary psychosis also was vigorously espoused by *Johann Christian August Heinroth* (1773–1843), native of Leipzig educated initially in theology and later in medicine in Leipzig and Vienna. He was the first to hold a university chair of psychiatry in Germany but became a controversial figure, losing his job of 20 years at the University of Leipzig for not fulfilling his duties (Schmideler & Steinberg, 2004). He is known particularly for recommending a holistic approach to evaluating psychiatric patients, partly based on Protestant theology (Steinberg, 2013). Heinroth was deeply spiritual and believed that a wrongly conducted life or sin would lead to mental illness, noting for example that mania was likely to give way to melancholia as a result of remorse for violence done when manic (Jackson, 1986). In his textbook of psychiatry Heinroth (1818) considered melancholia and mania as separate clinical conditions and not as alternating stages of a single disorder. Nevertheless, he devoted an entire chapter of his book to "mixed mood disturbances" (*Gemischte Gemüthsstörungen*), including "melancholia with silliness" (*Melancholie mit Narrheit*), and "quiet rage" (*stille Wut*), and recognized rapid cycling (Heinroth, 1808, pp. 355–378). Mixed states may date to reports by physicians of classical Greece and were noted by 18th-century writers including *François Boissier de Sauvages* (1706–1777) of Montpellier and *William Cullen* (1710–1790) of Scotland (Marneros & Angst, 2000).

The concept of mixing of dissimilar symptomatic states was continued by *Carl Friedrich Flemming* (1799–1880), educated in medicine in Berlin, who worked in psychiatric institutions in both north Germany and Carinthia, Austria, and died at Wiesbaden. His contributions include the concept of "changeable dysthymia" (*dysthymia mutabilis*), which could shift from a depressive phase (*dysthymia atra*) or a hypomanic phase (*dysthymia candida*) or even include elements of both types simultaneously, such as in elated melancholia (*melancholia hilaris*; Flemming, 1844). He was concerned about how to classify common clinical conditions in which mania, melancholia, and delusional states (*Wahnsinn*) could predominate at different times (varying from hours to months) and indeed considered such poorly delineated, variable, or mixed states to be the most prevalent forms of mental illness and a major diagnostic challenge (Flemming, 1844).

Wilhelm Griesinger (1817–1868) followed von Zeller (1804–1877), with whom he worked briefly in Württemberg, in adopting the concept of "unitary psychosis" (*Einheitpsychose*), or the proposition that virtually all forms of major mental illnesses represented or originated in a single disease process. Griesinger separated depression or melancholia from exaltation or mania and considered them as different manifestations of a single disease process, noting that transitions between these states are quite common, even as had been described by Falret (Griesinger, 1861, p. 238). However, this view seems to be more a manifestation of his concept of there being particular manifestations of a single psychosis rather than considering a discrete manic-depressive syndrome. Nevertheless, he cited the work of Falret and accepted the concept of circular insanity (Marneros & Angst, 2000). He went further, in reporting that many cases of melancholia and mania develop into states of "mental weakness" (*psychische Schwächezustände*), suggesting that prognosis and outcome often were unfavorable (Griesinger, 1861, p. 214). Another vigorous supporter of the unitary-psychosis hypothesis was *Heinrich Neumann* (1814–1888), who trained in general medicine before switching to psychiatry and becoming the director of an asylum in Breslau in Silesia, where he was a teacher of *Carl Wernicke* (1848–1905) at the university. His unitary-psychosis views were quite flexible and were readily modified to include a range of clinical conditions, as well as to support early interventions (Engström, 2003).

Karl-Ludwig Kahlbaum (1828–1899) worked in a psychiatric hospital in Görlitz in eastern Germany most of his professional career, rather than in a university position. Nevertheless, he was a major contributor to 19th-century academic psychiatry. He espoused a clinical, descriptive, longitudinal approach to psychiatric nosology and psychopathology, which strongly influenced Kraepelin and many others (Baethge et al., 2003a,b). Kahlbaum introduced the term *catatonia* (or "tension insanity;" *die Katatonie oder das Spannungsirresein*; Kahlbaum, 1874). He also observed that similar clinical presentations do not necessarily share the same etiology, course, or outcome and emphasized efforts to differentiate organic versus functional disorders (Bräuning, 1999; Klosterkötter, 1999). Consistent with earlier French proposals of Falret and Baillarger, whose work he cited, for Kahlbaum cyclic insanity (*cyklisches Irresein*) was characterized by a primary disturbance of mood and represented a single disorder (Baethge et al., 2003a,b; Kahlbaum, 1882).

He also introduced the concept of *cyclothymia* as relatively benign form of circular insanity, accepted Flemming's concept of dysthymia, and considered cyclothymia as the alternation of the two. His colleague and brother-in-law, *Ewald Hecker* (1843–1909) of Görlitz elaborated and promoted this syndrome as well as Kahlbaum's catatonia (Baethge et al., 2003a,b; Kraam, 2004).

The conflict between "splitting" clinical illnesses into numerous subgroups versus "lumping" them into broad categories was central to the work of *Emil Kraepelin* (1856–1926) in Heidelberg and Munich. This struggle is well documented in his influential textbook through its nine editions between 1883 and 1926 (Trede et al., 2005). Writing the book evidently was stimulated initially by Kraepelin's need to raise money to enable his marriage. The first edition (the *Compendium*) relied heavily on contributions of various 19th-century German and French authors. Nevertheless, it began his lifelong process of consolidating different clinical presentations into larger groups, ideally based on causes to the limited extent that they could be identified, but usually based on course and outcome as well as symptomatic presentations. Even in the first edition of his textbook (1883), he noted that mania and circular or periodic insanity "are simply manifestations of a single pathological process...certain basic traits are found consistently, even though there are many external differences." He saw excitement or activation and inhibition, rather than mood, as unifying themes of these disorders, and he supported the idea of an underlying pathological predisposition that could lead to a range of clinical manifestations (Trede et al., 2005).

In the second edition of his textbook, Kraepelin (1889) introduced the concept of delusional disorders (*Wahnsinn*), in an effort to manage confusing and ambiguous cases with prominent affective and psychotic symptoms. In the fourth edition (Kraepelin, 1893), he began to consider mixed states in describing "manic stupor" as unusual stuporous states within the excited phase of circular conditions. This concept was greatly expanded in response to the thesis of his junior colleague *Wilhelm C. J. K. Weygandt* (1870–1939), who described simultaneous or rapidly alternating combinations of manic and melancholic features, as indicated by inclusion of portions of Weygandt's dissertation in the sixth edition of Kraepelin's (1899) textbook, with an emphasis on the protean nature of circular insanity, with fluctuations and complex admixtures of abnormalities of psychomotor activity, thought, and mood (Salvatore et al., 2002; Trede et al., 2005). The affiliations among mania, melancholia, periodic and circular insanity, and mixed states were initially accepted in Kraepelin's (1896) unifying concept of "the periodic constitutional disorders" in his fifth edition, leading to introduction of his new *manic-depressive insanity* concept in the sixth (Kraepelin, 1899), with its distinction from more chronic psychotic conditions termed *dementia præcox*.

In the sixth textbook edition, Kraepelin (1899) supported the categorization of major psychiatric disorders into his two broad syndrome groups by asserting that "we have no right to trace these endless varieties of clinical pictures back to fundamentally different basic mechanisms." The seventh edition (Kraepelin, 1903–1904) and multivolume eighth edition (Kraepelin, 1909–1915) of his textbook represent the final version of Kraepelin's *manic-depressive insanity*. Edition 8 includes involutional melancholia (previously held separate), as well as basic states and temperaments, into a broad concept of manic-depressive illness. Kraepelin's justification for this gathering of seemingly heterogeneous conditions was supported by his tendency to view them as united not simply by polarities of mood but by the shifting between states of heightened versus inhibited functioning in arousal, cognition, speech, and behavior, as well as mood, and by their tendency to follow an episodic course with a relatively favorable prognosis (Trede et al., 2005).

Modern psychiatry appears to view Kraepelin as a strict empiricist and a founder of phenomenological psychiatry, whose work led to the currently fashionable coding of diagnostic criteria as a basis for psychiatric nosology. However, in the eighth edition of his textbook, Kraepelin (1909–1915) noted the limitations of his dual system based on manic-depressive insanity and dementia præcox: "It is indisputable today that, despite honest efforts, we are still unable to categorize quite a vast number of cases within the frame of one of the known forms in the system." Severe limitations of his scheme, including the high prevalence of mixed, hybrid, or atypical cases were further acknowledged in his later writings (e.g., Kraepelin, 1920; Trede et al., 2005): "The mixed and transitional states make delineations impossible… these are the cases that push us to widen our knowledge." He acknowledged having made a sharp distinction between manic-depressive illness and dementia præcox mainly to simplify instruction of students and young physicians (Kraepelin, 1920).

20TH CENTURY

Even by Kraepelin's own descriptions, he indicated that manic-depressive patients with both mania and depression differed from those with recurrent depression, including by having a younger onset-age, briefer episodes, and a higher recurrence rate, but declined to separate them into discrete subgroups, at least until more was known (Trede et al., 2005). Manic-depressive illness had evolved into a theory concerning coherence of various clinical features and the tendency of common elements to alternate or mix unpredictably. Moreover, Kraepelin recognized chronic forms of manic-depressive illness and associated "fundamental states" or temperaments (Trede et al., 2005). In the very breadth and complexity of illnesses subsumed by the manic-depressive concept lay risk for tension between retaining its wholeness versus splitting into subgroups and differentiating other disorders characterized by an episodic course and lack of profound loss of reasoning and functioning. There also was a risk of ascribing a doctrinaire and rigid implication of Kraepelin's scheme that seems at variance with his own flexibility and tentativeness, as well as with his apparently greater interest in the fundamental dynamic instability of his manic-depressive illness rather than a concrete emphasis on polar states of mood, thought, and behavior (Marneros & Angst, 2000; Marneros & Akiskal, 2007). In short, the concept was ripe for classic tensions between "lumpers" and "splitters" (Vázquez, Tondo, & Baldessarini, this volume).

Early disagreement with a unified concept of manic-depressive illness arose in Scandinavia, where recurrent depression was a separate disorder, dating from the work of *Carl Georg Lange* (1834–1900), a contemporary of Kraepelin's (Lange, 1896; Marneros & Angst, 2000). An early major conceptual challenge to Kraepelin's perspective of a broad, unitary manic-depressive illness came from *Carl Wernicke* (1848–1905) (Wernicke, 1881). He proposed new entities with polarities, including hyperkinetic and akinetic forms of "motility psychosis." This move away from, or addition to, a unified manic-depressive concept went further, following the untimely sudden death of Wernicke, when *Karl Kleist* (1879–1960) and, later, his associate *Edda Neele* (1910–2005) proposed that manic-depression included both monopolar (*einpolige*; recurrent depressive) and bipolar entities (*zweipolige Erkrankungen*; bipolar manic-depressive disorder; Kleist, 1928; Neele, 1949). Kleist was skeptical that mania and melancholia, though often affiliated, were expressions of a single disorder. He also considered the concept of "the group of schizophrenias" proposed by *Paul Eugen Bleuler* (1857–1939) (Bleuler, 2011) excessively broad and insisted that many psychotic conditions fit poorly within the manic-depressive or the schizophrenia concepts. He proposed other recurrent disorders, including psychoses that alternate between agitated confusion and stupor, separate from both manic-depressive illness and schizophrenia (Kleist, 1928). His ideas were elaborated by *Karl Leonhard* (1904–1988) into several types of periodic or cyclical psychoses (Leonhard, 1979). The proposals of the Wernicke–Kleist–Leonhard school were not widely accepted, probably in part owing to their complexity and subtlety.

The trend toward "splitting" the nonchronic psychoses into various subtypes continued in the 20th century, despite occasional warnings of the difficulties in firmly establishing separate and distinct psychiatric disorders on a sound scientific basis (Bolton, 1908; Goldney, 2012). Notably, the monopolar/bipolar distinction in major mood disorders was supported by Leonhard in noting that a family history of psychotic illnesses (as well as depression) was differentially associated with bipolar mood disorders. Similar findings and conclusions were also supported by Swiss investigator *Jules Angst* (1926–; Angst, 1966), Italo-Swedish *Carlo Perris* (1928–2000; Perris 1966), and American *George Winokur* (1925–1996; Winokur, Clayton, & Reich, 1969). Many subsequent studies added differences in onset age (younger in bipolar disorder than in major depression), sex risk-ratio (nearly 1:1 in bipolar disorder, women more than men in unipolar depression), duration of episodes, and of cycles between recurrences (both shorter in bipolar disorder; Goodwin & Jamison, 2007). Other concepts introduced by Kleist and Leonhard include complex subtypes of depressive or episodic psychotic disorders. Again, their complexity and subtlety probably contributed to their limited impact, though they underscore the existence of many clinical conditions that do not fit neatly into Kraepelin's dualistic scheme, even though both his manic-depressive and dementia praecox groups were broad (Marneros & Angst, 2000). Nevertheless, the work of Leonhard, Angst, Perris, and Winokur led to broad acceptance of the concept of bipolar disorder by the late 1960s. By 1980, *bipolar disorder* (with mania) was accepted officially in the Diagnostic and Statistical Manual of the American Psychiatric Association in 1980 (third edtion; American Psychiatric Association, 1980) and bipolar II disorder into its fourth edition along with cyclothymic disorder (American Psychiatric Association, 1994); bipolar I and II disorders also are included in the *International Classification of Diseases* (tenth edition; World Health Organization, 1999).

Another factor that may well have contributed to the acceptance of bipolar disorder as a discrete clinical entity was the introduction of lithium carbonate as a relatively specific treatment for the disorder in 1949, of the antimanic-antipsychotic drugs in 1952, and of the antidepressants later in the 1950s (Baldessarini, 2013;

Cade, 1949; Schou, 2001). Prior to the introduction of these modern agents, treatment of mania, psychosis, and depression (sedatives, stimulants, electroconvulsive treatment, psychotherapy) had been largely nonspecific and of questionable efficacy. Novel and effective treatments and diagnoses can be mutually reinforcing (Baldessarini, 2013; Stoll. Baldessarini, Tohen, et al., 1993).

CURRENT STATE OF BIPOLAR DISORDER

Currently bipolar manic-depressive illness (bipolar disorder) is firmly established. It is one of the most longitudinally stable diagnostic entities among all major mental illnesses based on standard international diagnostic criteria (Salvatore et al., 2009). Studies of the disorder are encouraged by dedicated international associations (International Society for Bipolar Disorder, 1999; European Network of Bipolar Research Expert Centres, 2009, and others), as well as international scientific journals devoted exclusively to the topic (*Bipolar Disorders*, 1999) and others, most recently the *International Journal of Bipolar Disorders* (2013).

Along with wide international acceptance of the bipolar disorder concept, there have been many efforts to extend its range or to define subtypes. For example, a distinction has been made between cases with depression (D) predominantly preceding (DMI course-pattern) or following mania (MDI pattern, both with intervening euthymic intervals [I]), with evidence of inferior treatment responses with the DMI pattern (Koukopoulos, Reginaldi, Tondo, Visioli, & Baldessarini, 2013). In addition, the polarity of initial major episodes is highly predictive of future illness, notably in distinguishing patients predominantly experiencing manic, hypomanic, or psychotic episodes from those more likely to have depressions, mixed manic-depressive states, or episodes of anxiety disorders (Baldessarini, 2012; Baldessarini, Salvatore, et al. 2010; Baldessarini, Tondo & Visioli, 2014; Colom, Vieta, Daban, Pacchiarotti, & Sánchez-Moreno, 2006).

An important trend has been toward including a broader range of disorders within the concept of bipolar disorders. Indeed, the popularity of the bipolar concept has recently shown indications of becoming something of a clinical fad, possibly encouraged by hopes for a relatively optimistic prognosis and effective treatments (Healy, 2008). An unresolved aspect of the concept are cyclothymic conditions involving minor or moderate cycles or phases of increased and decreased mood, thinking, and activity that have been considered part of the cyclic or manic-depressive "spectrum" since the work of Kahlbaum and Hecker and of

Kraepelin reviewed earlier. A basic uncertainty is whether such phenomena represent a cyclothymic *disorder* or a personality type (Van Meter, Youngstrom, & Findling, 2012).

Since the concept of bipolar disorder without episodes of mania (bipolar II disorder) emerged in the 1970s (Fieve, Kumbaraci, & Dunner, 1976), there have been efforts to define a group of disorders characterized by recurrent episodes of major depression, with varying elements of hypomanic features, to define a "bipolar spectrum" of disorders (Marneros & Angst, 2000; Merkangas et al., 2007). This idea was anticipated in the work of Kahlbaum and Kraepelin and continued in the broad inclusion of subtly mixed states proposed by *Ernst Kretschmer* (1888–1964), Bleuler, and others (Marneros & Angst, 2000). Current extensions of the concept are exploring conditions traditionally considered to represent personality disorders, including borderline disorder (Gunderson & Elliott, 1985). It remains to be seen how broadening may add to effective formulation of long-term prognoses or guide more specific treatments. Some research findings support the hypothesis that depressed patients with elements of hypomania below requirements for a formal diagnosis of bipolar disorder may not respond well to antidepressant treatment (Akiskal & Pinto, 1999; Angst, 2007; Vázquez, Tondo, Undurraga, & Baldessarini, 2013).

Additional unresolved questions include the significance of cases initially presenting with depression, sometimes recurrent, before hypomania or mania are diagnosed. Is this pattern simply representative of a common early manifestation of the natural history of bipolar disorder, or is there an actual change in the illness, either arising spontaneously or, more speculatively, as a result of treatment with ubiquitous antidepressants and stimulants, perhaps particularly in juveniles? A related question is of the significance of hypomania or mania associated with treatment with mood-elevating drugs (antidepressants, corticosteroids, stimulants; Krauthammer & Klerman, 1978): Are these simple psychotoxic reactions to foreign chemicals or an indication of the presence of undiagnosed bipolar disorder with a potential for later spontaneous manic episodes?

There also are controversial efforts to extend bipolar disorder into juvenile populations, including in prepubertal children, despite many descriptive differences between juvenile versus typical, episodic, adult forms of the disorder (Papolos & Papolos, 2000). Emerging research suggests that variable proportions, sometimes only a minority, of young children given the diagnosis later prove to have a typical, adult bipolar disorder (e.g., Geller, Tillman, Bolhofner, & Zimerman, 2008; Wozniak et al., 2011). Nevertheless, there is great interest in defining the earliest indications of bipolar disorder and in distinguishing its early presentation from other adult mental illnesses, in part to support long-term clinical planning (Salvatore et al., 2014). More controversial, however, are considerations of early intervention in juveniles presumed to be at risk for bipolar disorder, possibly even before secure clinical expression of the disorder (Noto et al., 2013).

A related challenge is that the history of the past century underscores the limits to even broad and inclusive diagnostic categories, such as manic-depressive illness and schizophrenia, which leave many clinical conditions poorly accounted for, little studied, and inadequately treated. Late in his career Kraepelin noted that many, if not most, patients he had evaluated did not fit neatly into his dualistic scheme (Trede et al. 2005). Such illnesses include various acute psychotic disorders of relatively favorable prognosis, as well as the ill-defined category of "schizoaffective" disorders—all of which remain unreliable diagnostically and prognostically, as well as inadequately studied therapeutically (Goodwin & Jamison, 2007; Malhi, Green, Fagiolini, Peselow, & Kumari, 2008; Salvatore et al., 2009). Perhaps even more challenging is how to organize and make sense of the wide range of conditions left after typical bipolar disorders are removed from the broad manic-depressive group. There have been repeated suggestions that, in addition to unipolar recurrent major depressive disorders, there may be a syndrome of recurrent mania, possibly separable from bipolar disorder (Mehta, 2014).

As the limits of the bipolar disorder concept expand, there is a risk that compromises will arise in its clinical application to diagnosis, prognosis, and treatment. It seems highly unlikely that all cases currently labeled as "bipolar disorder" follow similar courses to a predictable outcome or achieve optimal treatment responses with standardized treatments. Indeed, a major challenge in contemporary therapeutics for the mood disorders is to define optimal treatments for the growing range of types and ages of bipolar disorder patients as well as for the very broad range of unipolar forms of depression. Particularly needed is clarification of how to treat bipolar depression, the major unresolved component of the disorder and a crucial contributor to disability and mortality (Baldessarini, Salvatore, et al., 2010; Baldessarini, Vieta, Calabrese, Tohen, & Bowden, 2010; Vázquez et al., 2013).

This historical overview (also see Table 1.1) should remind us that the nosological basis for clinical conditions considered to represent particular psychiatric disorders or diseases contrasts with most disorders of general medicine in lacking a tissue pathology or even a plausible pathophysiology. Instead, psychiatric diagnosis rests

Table 1.1. HIGHLIGHTS IN THE HISTORICAL EVOLUTION OF THE BIPOLAR DISORDER CONCEPT

CONTRIBUTOR	TIME AND PLACE	CONTRIBUTION
Hippocratic tradition	Greece, 5th cent. BCE	Descriptions of "mania" and "melancholia"
Posidonius (c. 135–51 BCE)	Syria, 2nd cent. BCE	Mania and melancholia may be a single disease
Aretaeus of Cappadocia (2nd century CE)	Alexandria and Rome, 2nd cent. CE	Mania and melancholia can occur in the same person over time (c. 150 CE)
Galen (c. 129–298)	Greece, 2nd cent. CE	Humoral theory of personality types and mental and other illnesses
Alexander of Tralles (c. 525–605)	Greece, 6th cent. CE	Mania and melancholia occur in cycles and features can mix; high suicide risk
Islamic scholars: Ishag ibn Imran (848–906), Razes (865–925), Avicenna (980–1037), Ismail Jorjani (1041–1136)	Middle-East and North Africa, 9th–11th cents. CE	Mania and melancholia closely related and perhaps on a continuum
John of Gaddesden (c. 1280–1361)	England, 14th cent.	Mania and melancholia as different forms of the same disorder; melancholia primary
Johannes Manardus (1462–1536)	Italy, 15th cent.	Mania "replaces" melancholia; melancholia primary
Felix Platter (1536–1614)	Switzerland, 1549	Mania and melancholia as brain disorders
Jason Pratensis (1486–1558)	Holland, 1549	Mania and melancholia hard to separate, arising from the same causes; melancholia primary
Gao-Lian (1500s)	China, 16th cent.	Mania and melancholia are manifestations of a single illness
Thomas Willis (1621–1675)	England, 17th cent.	Mania and melancholia alternate in a recurrent course
Théophile Bonet (1620–1689)	Switzerland, 17th cent.	Coined term *maniaco-melancholicus* for a single disorder
Iatromechanists: Friedrich Hoffmann (1660–1742), Archibald Pitcairn (1652–1713), Herman Boerhaave (1668–1738)	Germany, Scotland, Holland, 17th cent.	Mania and melancholia arise from specific personality types and represent effects of humors on the brain
English physicians: Thomas Sydenham (1624–1689), Richard Mead (1673–1754), Robert James (1703–1776)	England, 17th–18th cents.	Mania and melancholia follow a recurrent course; melancholia primary
Italian physicians: Giovanni Morgagni (1682–1771), Vincenzo Chiarugi (1759–1820)	Italy, 18th cent.	Mania and melancholia follow a recurrent course
Andrés Piquer-Arrufat (1711–1772)	Spain, 18th cent.	Coined term *affectio melancholico-maniaca* for a single, brain-based disorder; melancholia not primary
Phillipe Pinel (1745–1826)	France, early 19th cent.	Defined mania broadly; skeptical of separate forms of insanity but mania and melancholia closely related
Jean-Étienne Esquirol (1772–1840)	France, early 19th cent.	Coined term *lypemania* for depression
Johann Heinroth (1773–1843)	Germany, early 19th cent.	Described mixtures of melancholia + psychosis (including with mania): gemische Gemüthsstörungen (1819)
Laurent Bayle (1799–1858)	France, early 19th cent.	General paralysis of the insane as a distinct psychotic disorder
CarlFlemming (1799–1880)	Germany, mid-19th cent.	Described changeable dysthymia: dysthymia metabilis (1844)
Jean-Pierre Falret (1794–1870)	France, mid-19th cent.	Described circular insanity (1851)
Jules Baillarger (1809–1890)	France, mid-19th cent.	Described insanity of double form (1854)

(continued)

Table 1.1. CONTINUED

CONTRIBUTOR	TIME AND PLACE	CONTRIBUTION
Louis-Victor Marcé (1828–1865)	France, mid-19th century	Integrated "circular insanity of double form"
Wilhelm Griesinger (1817–1868)	Germany, mid-19th cent.	Skeptical about distinguishing specific psychotic disorders (*einheitpsychose*)
Karl Kahlbaum (1828–1899), Ewald Hecker (1843–1909)	Germany, mid-19th cent.	Described cyclothymia (moderate mania-melancholia)
L. Kirn (1800s)	Germany, late 19th cent.	Described periodic psychoses (including mania-melancholia) (1878)
E. E. Mendel (1800s)	Germany, late 19th cent.	Coined term *hypomania* (Mendel, 1881)
Wilhelm Weygandt (1870–1939)	Germany, late 19th cent.	Described mixed mania-depressive syndromes (die Mischzustände des manisch-depressiven Irreseins)
Emil Kraepelin (1856–1926)	Germany, late 19th cent.	Described a broad manic-depressive insanity group of disorders
Carl G. Lange (1834–1900)	Denmark, late 19th cent.	Described recurrent depression
Carl Wernicke (1848–1905)	Germany, early-20th cent.	Described novel "bipolar" syndromes, including motility psychoses
Karl Kleist (1879–1960), Edda Neele (1910–2005)	Germany, early 20th cent.	Distinguished monopolar (*einpolige*) and bipolar (*zweipolige*) manic-depressive disorders (from 1911 to 1930s)
Karl Leonhard (1904–1988)	Germany, mid-20th cent.	Periodic and cyclic psychoses (including cycloid); family studies to support separation of monopolar and bipolar types of manic-depressive disorders
John F Cade (1912–1980), Mogens Schou (1918–2005)	Australia (1949), Denmark (1950s–1960s)	Introduction of lithium carbonate as a selectively effective treatment for bipolar disorder
Jules Angst (living), Carlo Perris (1928–2000), George Winokur (1925–1996)	Switzerland, Italy-Sweden, United States	Provided further support for bipolar disorder (1966–1969)
Ronald Fieve (living), David Dunner (living)	United States, 1970s	Bipolar II disorder (depression with hypomania)
American Psychiatric Association	United States, *DSM–III* and *DSM–IV*	Inclusion of bipolar disorder (1980) and bipolar II disorder (1994)
Frederick K. Goodwin (living), Kay R. Jamison (living)	United States, 2000 and 2007	*Manic-Depressive Illness*, Oxford University Press
International Society for Bipolar Disorders	United States, 1999	Society founded

NOTE: DSM–III = Diagnostic and Statistical Manual of Mental Disorders (3rd ed.; American Psychiatric Association, 1980); DSM–IV = *Diagnostic and Statistical Manual of Mental Disorders* (4th ed.; American Psychiatric Association, 1994).

almost entirely on observation and description of symptoms, including detailed psychopathology, clinical course, treatment response, and long-term outcome, supported by such additional descriptors as onset age and family history. Manifestations of mania, in particular, can arise from various causes, including neuromedical disorders and intoxications. Expectations of modern medical science, including studies of genetic risk factors and neuroimaging or physiological measures, though important to pursue, have not yet served to place psychiatric diagnosis on a secure footing (Baldessarini, 2000a, 2013). Advances in biological research in themselves may prove to be inadequate as a basis of formulating clinical diagnoses and will still require matching to descriptive clinical syndromes, if only for clinical and administrative purposes (Berrios, 1999; Goldney, 2012; Healy, 2008). For psychiatric research, a fundamental problem is that most findings of the past century involve clinical entities of indubitable heterogeneity, rendering most findings insecure for improving understanding of particular psychiatric disorders. This challenge might be termed the *phenotype problem* for endeavoring to study clinical entities or phenomena with reasonable biological coherence. (See Table 1.1.)

CONCLUSION

A theme running through this brief summary of the history of bipolar disorder is that mania and melancholia are clinical entities recognized since the dawn of medical scholarship, at least as separate clinical conditions that probably have been far broader than current use of the terms may seem to imply. In addition, their close association in many of the same persons has been known for two millennia, but the significance of this relationship remained uncertain for centuries. Current nosological concepts have arisen largely in reaction to Kraepelin's bold declaration that a very wide range of clinical disorders could be gathered together into a "manic-depressive" group. There is much support for the existence of some forms of bipolar disorder that contrast to an extraordinarily diverse group of more or less unipolar depressive disorders (e.g., "major depressive disorder") that remains to be better defined and organized into clinically and scientifically meaningful subgroups.

Recent trends have been toward further broadening of the concept and inclusion of illnesses that until recently have been considered forms of depressive or even personality disorders and including conditions in juveniles that bear an uncertain relationship to typical adult bipolar disorder. To some extent this tendency is encouraged by efforts to define disorders of favorable prognosis for which there may be selectively effective treatments. However, diagnostic broadening risks loss of specificity. In turn, nonspecificity and heterogeneity complicate clinical diagnosis, prognosis, and treatment. Moreover, broad, heterogeneous diagnostic entities are an unsatisfactory basis for biomedical research.

ACKNOWLEDGMENTS

This chapter was supported in part by a grant from the Bruce J. Anderson Foundation and by the McLean Private Donors Psychiatric Research Fund (to RJB).

Disclosures: No author or any immediate family member has financial relationships with commercial organizations that might represent potential conflicts of interest with the material presented.

REFERENCES

Angst, J. (1966). *Zur Ätiologie und nosologie endogener depressiver psychosen: Eine genetische, soziologische und clinische studie* [On the etiology and nosology of depressive psychoses: A genetic, sociological and clinical study]. Berlin: Springer.

American Psychiatric Association. (1980). *Diagnostic and statistical manual of mental disorders* (3rd ed.). Washington, DC: Author.

American Psychiatric Association. (1994). *Diagnostic and statistical manual of mental disorders* (4th ed.). Washington, DC: Author.

American Psychiatric Association. (2000). *Diagnostic and statistical manual of mental disorders* (4th ed., text rev.). Washington, DC: Author.

Aretæus the Cappadocian. (1861). *The extant works of Aretaeus, the Cappadocian* (F. Adams, Trans. and Ed.). London: Sydenham Society.

Arikha, N. (2007). *Passions and tempers: A history of the humours.* New York: HarperCollins.

Baethge, C., Salvatore, P., & Baldessarini, R. J. (2003a). Cyclothymia, a circular mood disorder. *History of Psychiatry, 14*(55 Pt. 3), 377–390.

Baethge, C., Salvatore, P., & Baldessarini, R. J. (2003b). "On cyclic insanity" (1882) by Karl Ludwig Kahlbaum, MD: A translation and commentary. *Harvard Review of Psychiatry, 11*, 78–90.

Baillarger, J. G. F. (1854a). De la folie à double forme. *Annales Médico-psychologiques, 12*, 367–391.

Baillarger, J. G. F. (1854b). Notes on a type of insanity with episodes characterized by two regular periods, one of depression and one of excitation. *Annales Médico-psychologiques, 6*, 369–389.

Baldessarini, R. J. (2000a). American biological psychiatry and psychopharmacology 1944–1994. In R. W. Menninger & J. C. Nemiah (Eds.), *American psychiatry after World War II (1944–1994)* (pp. 371–412). Washington, DC: American Psychiatric Press.

Baldessarini, R. J. (2000b). Plea for integrity of the bipolar disorder concept. *Bipolar Disorder, 2*, 3–7.

Baldessarini, R. J. (2013). *Chemotherapy in psychiatry* (3rd ed.). New York: Springer.

Baldessarini, R. J., Salvatore, P., Khalsa, H. M., Gebre-Medhin, P., Imaz, H., González-Pinto. A.,…Tohen, M. (2010). Morbidity in 303 first-episode bipolar I disorder patients. *Bipolar Disorder, 12*, 264–270.

Baldessarini, R. J., Tondo, L., & Visioli, C. (2014). First-episode types in bipolar disorder: predictive associations with later illness. *Acta Psychiatrica Scandinavica 129*, 383–392.

Baldessarini, R. J., Undurraga, J., Vázquez, G. H., Tondo, L., Salvatore, P., Ha, K.,…Vieta, E. (2012). Predominant recurrence polarity among 928 adult international bipolar-I disorder patients. *Acta Psychiatrica Scandinavica, 125*, 293–302.

Baldessarini, R. J., Vieta, E., Calabrese, J. R., Tohen, M., & Bowden, C. (2010). Bipolar depression: Overview and commentary. *Harvard Review of Psychiatry, 18*, 143–157.

Bayle, A. L. J. (1826). *Traité des maladies du cerveau et de ses membranes* [Treatise on diseases of the brain and its membranes]. Paris: Gabon.

Beer, M. D. (1996). The endogenous psychoses: a conceptual history. *History of Psychiatry, 7*, 1–29.

Berrios, G. E. (1999). Classifications in psychiatry: A conceptual history. *Australian & New Zealand Journal of Psychiatry, 33*, 145–160.

Bleuler, E. (1950). *Dementia praecox or the group of schizophrenias* (J. Zinkin, Trans.). New York: International Universities Press, 1950. (Original work published 1911)

Boerhaave, H. (1735). *Aphorisms: Concerning the knowledge and cure of diseases.* London: W. and J. Innys.

Bolton, J. S. (1908). Maniacal-depressive insanity. *Brain, 31,* 301–318.

Bonet, T. (1686). *Medicina septentrionalis collatitia* [Compendium of medical practice in northern Europe]. Geneva: Sumptivus Leonardi Chouet & Socij.

Brain, P. (1986). *Galen.* Cambridge, UK: Cambridge University Press.

Bräuning, P. (1999). Images in psychiatry: Karl Ludwig Kahlbaum, MD, 1828–1899. *American Journal of Psychiatry, 156,* 989–989.

Cade, J. F. (1949). Lithium salts in the treatment of psychotic excitement. *Medical Journal of Australia, 2,* 349–352.

Colom, F., Vieta, E., Daban, C., Pacchiarotti, I., & Sánchez-Moreno, J. (2006). Clinical and therapeutic implications of predominant polarity in bipolar disorder. *Journal of Affective Disorders, 93*(1–3), 13–17.

Cordell, E. F. (1909). Aretaeus of Cappadocia. *Bulletin of the Johns Hopkins Hospital, 20,* 371–377.

Engström, E. J. (2003). *Clinical psychiatry in Imperial Germany.* Ithaca, NY: Cornell University Press.

Esquirol, J. E. D. (1819). Mélancholie. In L. J. Renauldin (Ed.), *Dictionnaire des sciences médicales* [Dictionary of Medical Sciences] (Vol. 39, pp. 147–183). Paris: Panckoucke.

Esquirol, J. E. D. (1838). *Traité des maladies mentales considérées sous le rapport médical, hygiénique et médico-légal.* [Treatise on mental illnesses in relation to medical, hygienic, and medicolegal considerations]. Paris: J Baillière.

Falret, J. P. (1851a). De la folie circulaire ou forme de maladie characterisée par l'alternative régulière de la manie et de la mélancholie. *Bulletin de l'Académie Nationale de Médecine, 19,* 382–400.

Falret, J. P. (1851b). De la folie circulaire ou forme de maladie mentale caracterisée par l'altérnative régulière de la manie et de la mélancholie. *Gazette des Hôpitaux de Toulouse, 24,* 18–19.

Falret, J. P. (1854). Mémoire sur la folie circulaire, forme de maladie mentale caractérisé par la reproduction successive et régulière de l'état maniaque, de l'état mélancholique, et d'un interval lucide plus ou moins prolongé. *Bulletin de l'Académie Nationale de Médecine, 19,* 382–415.

Falret, J. P. (1864). *Des maladies mentales et des asiles et d'aliénés* [Mental illnesses in the asylums of the insane]. Paris: J-B. Baillière et Fils.

Fieve, R. R., Kumbaraci, T., & Dunner, D. L. (1976). Lithium prophylaxis of depression in bipolar I, bipolar II, and unipolar patients. *American Journal of Psychiatry, 133,* 925–929.

Flemming, C. F. (1844). Über csassifikation der Seelenstörungen. *Allgem Zeitschr Psychiatrie, 1,* 97–130.

Gaddesden, J. (1492). *Rosa Anglica practica medicinae a capite ad pedes* [The English rose of medical practice, from head to foot]. Pavia, Italy: Franciscus Girardengus und Johannes Antonius Birreta.

Geller, B., Tillman, R., Bolhofner, K., & Zimerman, B. (2008). Child bipolar I disorder: Prospective continuity with adult bipolar I disorder. *Archives of General Psychiatry, 65,* 1125–1133.

Guislain, J. (1833). *Traité sur les phrenopathies* [Treatise on brain diseases]. Brussels: Hebbelynck.

Goldney, R. D. (2012). From mania and melancholia to the bipolar disorders spectrum: Brief history of controversy. *Australian & New Zealand Journal of Psychiatry, 6,* 306–312.

Goodwin, F. K., & Jamison, K. R. (2007). *Manic-depressive illness* (2nd ed.). New York: Oxford University Press.

Griesinger, W. (1845). *Die pathologie und therapie der psychischen krankheiten für ärzte und studierende* [Pathology and therapy of psychological diseases for physicians and students]. Stuttgart: Krabbe.

Gunderson, J. G., & Elliott, G. R. (1985). The interface between borderline personality disorder and affective disorder. *American Journal of Psychiatry, 142,* 277–288.

Haustgen, T. H. (1995). Les troubles bipolares dans l'histoire de la psychiatrie (Kraepelin excepté). In M. L. Bourgeois & H. Verdoux (Eds.), *Les troubles bipolares de l'humeur* [The bipolar mood disorders] (pp. 7–17). Paris: Masson.

Healy, D. (2008). *Mania: Short history of bipolar disorder.* Baltimore: Johns Hopkins University Press.

Heinroth, J. C. A. (1818). *Lehrbuch der störungen des seelenlebens* [Textbook on disorders of the psychic life]. Leipzig: FCW Vogel Verlag.

Hoffmann, F. (1783). *A system in the practice of medicine,* Vol. 2 (1695). London: J Murray Press.

Hurd, H. M. (1882). Treatment of periodic insanity. *American Journal of Insanity, 39,* 174.

Jackson, S. W. (1986). *Melancholia and depression: From Hippocratic to modern times.* New Haven, CT: Yale University Press.

James, R. (1745). *Medical dictionary.* London: T. Osborne.

Kahlbaum, K-L. (1874). *Die katatonie oder das spannungsirresein* [Catatonia or tension psychosis]. Berlin: Hirschwell.

Kahlbaum, K-L. (1882). Über cyclishes Irresein. *Die Irrenfreund, 24,* 145–157.

King, L. S. (1971). *Friederich Hoffmann's Fundamenta Medicinae (1695).* London: McDonald Press.

Kirn, L. (1878). *Die periodischen psychosen* [The periodic psychoses]. Stuttgart: Enke.

Kleist, K. (1928). Über zycloide, paranoide und epileptoide psychosen and über die frage der degenerationspsychosen. *Schweizer Archiv für Neurologie, Neurochirurgie und Psychiatrie, 23,* 3–37.

Klosterkötter, J. (1999). Psychiatric classification: Basic idea and development of an ongoing process (In German). *Fortschritte Der Neurologie Psychiatrie, 67,* 558–573.

Koukopoulos, A., Reginaldi, D., Tondo, L., Visioli, C., & Baldessarini, R. J. (2013). Course sequences in bipolar disorder: Depressions preceding or following manias or hypomanias. *Journal of Affective Disorders, 151,* 105–110.

Kraam, A. (2004). On the origin of the clinical standpoint in psychiatry: Dr. Ewald Hecker in Görlitz. *History of Psychiatry, 15*(59, Pt. 3), 345–360.

Kraepelin, E. (1920). Die erscheinungsformen des Irreseins. *Zeitschrift Gesampt für Neurologie und Psychiatrie, 62,* 1–29.

Krauthammer, C., & Klerman, G. L. (1978). Secondary mania: Manic syndromes associated with antecedent physical illness or drug. *Archives of General Psychiatry, 35,* 1333–1339.

Kudlien, F. (1970). Alexander of Tralles. In *Dictionary of Scientific Biography* (Vol. 1, p. 121). New York: Scribner's.

Lange, C. G. (1896). *Periodiske depressioner* [Periodic depressions]. Hamburg: Voss.

Leonhard, K. (1979). *Classification of endogenous psychoses and their differential etiology* (1st English ed.). New York: Irvington.

Lefebvre, P. (1988, April 16). *Le traité des maladies mentales d'Esquirol: Cent cinquante ans après* [Treatise on mental illness by Esquirol: 150 years later]. Paper presented at the Proceedings of the French Society of the History of Medicine.

Lorry, A-C. (2009). *De melancholia et morbis melancholicis* [On melancholia and melancholic illness] (Facsimile ed.). Whitefish, MT: Kessinger Press. (Original work published 1765)

Luauté, J. P., & Lempérière, T. (2012). *La vie et l'oeuvre pionnière de Louis-Victor Marcé* [The life and pioneering work of Louis-Victor Marcé]. Société, Histoire et Medicine Série. Paris: Editions Glyphe.

Maciocia, G. (2009). *The psyche in Chinese medicine.* New York: Elsevier.

Malhi, G. S., Green, M., Fagiolini, A., Peselow, E. D., & Kumari, V. (2008). Schizoaffective disorder: Diagnostic issues and future recommendations. *Bipolar Disorders, 10,* 215–230.

Manardus, J. (1542). *Epistolae medicinales* [Medical letters]. Venice.

Marcé, L. V. (1858). *Traité de la folie des femmes enceintes, des nouvelles accouchés et des nourrices, et des considerations medico-légales qui se rattachent à ce sujet* [Treatise on madness of pregnant women, with childbirth and nursing, and medicolegal considerations related to this subject]. Paris: J-B. Baillière et Fils.

Marcé, L. V. (1862). *Traité pratique des maladies mentales* [Practical treatise on mental illnesses]. Paris: J-B. Baillère et Fils.

Marneros, A., & Akiskal, H. S. (2007). *The overlap of schizophrenic and affective spectra.* New York: Cambridge University Press.

Marneros, A., & Angst, J. (2000). Bipolar disorders: Roots and evolution. In A. Marneros & J. Angst (Eds.), *Bipolar disorders: 100 years after manic-depressive insanity* (pp. 1–36). New York: Kluwer.

Mead, R. (1751). *Medical precepts and cautions*. London: Brindley.

Mehta, S. (2014). Unipolar mania: recent updates and review of the literature. *Psychiatry Journal 2014*: 261943 (6 pp).

Mendel, E. (1881). *Die manie* [The manias]. Vienna: Urban.

Merikangas, K. R., Akiskal, H. S., Angst, J., Greenberg, P. E., Hirschfeld, R. M., Petukhova, M., & Kessler, R. C. (2007). Lifetime and 12-month prevalence of bipolar spectrum disorder in the National Comorbidity Survey replication. *Archives of General Psychiatry, 64*, 543–652.

Neele, E. (1949). *Die Phasischen psychosen nach ihrem erscheinungs- und erbbild* [The phasic psychoses, according to presentation and family history]. Leipzig: Barth.

Noto, M. N., de Souza-Noto, C., de Jesus, D. R., Zugman, A., Mansur, R. B., Berberian, A. A.,…Brietzke, E. (2013). Recognition of bipolar disorder type I before the first manic episode: Challenges and developments. *Expert Review of Neurotherapeutics, 13*, 795–807.

Omrani, A., Holtzman, N. S., Akiskal, H. S., & Ghaemi, S. N. (2012). Ibn Imran's 10th century *Treatise on Melancholy*. *Journal of Affective Disorders, 141*, 116–119.

Pacchiarotti, I., Bond, D. J., Baldessarini, R. J.,…Vieta, E. (2013). International Society for Bipolar Disorders (ISBD) task force report on antidepressant use in bipolar disorders. *American Journal of Psychiatry 170*, 1249–1262.

Papolos, D., & Papolos, J. (2000). *The bipolar child*. New York: Random House.

Pérez, J., Baldessarini, R. J., Cruz, N., Salvatore, P., & Vieta, E. (2011). Andrés Piquer-Arrufat (1711–1772): Contributions of an eighteenth-century Spanish physician to the concept of manic-depressive illness. *Harvard Review of Psychiatry, 19*, 68–77.

Pérez, J., Baldessarini, R. J., & Undurraga, J. (2012). Origins of psychiatric hospitalization in medieval Spain. *Psychiatric Quarterly, 83*, 419–430.

Perris, C. (1966). Study of bipolar (manic-depressive) and unipolar recurrent depressive psychoses. *Acta Psychiatrica Scandinavica, 194*(Suppl.): 1–89.

Pestronk, A. (1988). The first neurology book: *De Cerebri Morbis* (1549) by Jason Pratensis. *Archives of Neurology, 45*, 341–344.

Pichot, P. (2006). Tracing the origins of bipolar disorder: from Falret to DSM-IV and ID-10. *Journal of Affective Disorders, 96*, 145–148.

Pinel, P. (1806). *Treatise on insanity in which are contained the principles of a new and more practical nosology of maniacal disorders* (D. Davis, Trans.). London: Todd, Cadell & Davis.

Pinel, P. (1909). *Traité medico-philosophique sur l'aliénation mentale* [Medical-philosophical treatise on mental alienation] (2nd ed.). Paris: Antoine Brossonz.

Piquer-Arrufat, A. (1759). *Discurso sobre la enfermedad del Rey Nuestro Señor Fernando VI (que dios guarde)* [Treatise on the illness of Our Lord King Fernando VI, whom God protect]. Unpublished manuscript, Biblioteca Nacional de España, Madrid.

Piquer-Arrufat, A. (1764). *Praxis medica ad usum scholae valentinae* [Practice of medicine for the Valentine Schools]. Madrid: Ediciones Joachim Ibarra.

Pitcairn, A. (1718). *Philosophical and mathematical elements of physik*. London: A. Bell.

Platter, F. (1664). *Histories and observations*. London: Culpeper and Cole. (Original work published 1549)

Pordage, S. (1681). *Opera Omnia: The extant medical works of that famous and renowned physician, Dr. Thomas Willis*. London: Dring, Harper, Leigh & Martin.

Postel, J. (2004). *Nouvelle histoire de la psychiatry* [New history of psychiatry]. Paris: Dunod.

Ritti, A. (1892). Circular insanity. In D. H. Tuke (Ed.), *Dictionary of psychological medicine* (Vol. 1, pp. 214–229). London: J. & A. Churchill.

Roccatagliata, G. (1986). *History of ancient psychiatry*. New York: Greenwood.

Salvatore, P., Baldessarini, R. J., Centorrino, F., Egli, S., Albert, M., Gerhard, A., & Maggini, C. (2002). Weygandt's *The Manic-Depressive Mixed States*: A translation and commentary on its significance in the evolution of the concept of bipolar manic-depressive disorder. *Harvard Review of Psychiatry, 10*, 255–275.

Salvatore, P., Baldessarini, R. J., Khalsa, H.-M. K., Vázquez, G. H., Pérez, J., Maggini, C., & Tohen, M. (2014). Antecedents of manic versus other first psychotic episodes in 263 bipolar I disorder patients. *Acta Psychiatrica Scandinavica, 129*, 275–285.

Salvatore, P., Baldessarini, R. J., Tohen, M., Khalsa, H.-M., Pérez, J. P., Zarate, C. A. Jr.,…Maggini, C. (2009). McLean-Harvard International First-Episode Project: Two-year stability of DSM-IV diagnoses in 500 first-episode psychotic disorder patients. *Journal of Clinical Psychiatry, 70*, 458–466.

Schmideler, S., & Steinberg, H. (2004). Psychiatrist Johann Christian August Heinroth's (1773–1843) practical work at St. George's prison, orphanage and madhouse in Leipzig. *Würzbrg Medizinhist Mitt, 23*, 346–375.

Schou, M. (2001). Lithium treatment at 52. *Journal of Affective Disorders, 67*(1–3), 21–32.

Sedler, M. J., & Dessain, E. C. (Trans.). (1983). Falret's discovery: The origin of the concept of bipolar affective illness. *American Journal of Psychiatry, 140*, 1127–1133.

Shorter, E. (2012). Bipolar disorder in historical perspective. In P. Parker (Ed.), *Bipolar II disorder: Modeling, measuring and managing* (2nd ed., pp. 1–9). New York: Cambridge University Press.

Steinberg, H. (2013). Johann Christian August Heinroth: Psychosomatic medicine eighty years before Freud. *Psychiatria Danubina, 25*, 11–16.

Stoll, A. L., Tohen, M., Baldessarini, R. J., Goodwin, D. C., Stein, S., Katz, S.,…McGlashan, T. (1993). Shifts in diagnostic frequencies of schizophrenia and major affective disorders at six North American psychiatric hospitals, 1972–1988. *American Journal of Psychiatry, 150*, 1668–1673.

Trede, K., Baldessarini, R., Viguera, A., & Bottéro, A. (2009). *Treatise on insanity in pregnant, postpartum, and lactating women* by Louis-Victor Marcé (1958): Commentary. *Harvard Review of Psychiatry, 17*, 157–165.

Trede, K., Salvatore, P., Baethge, C., Gerhard, A., Maggini, C., & Baldessarini, R.J. (2005). Manic-depressive illness: Evolution in Kraepelin's textbook, 1883–1926. *Harvard Review of Psychiatry, 13*, 155–178.

Vakili, N., & Gorji, A. (2006). Psychiatry and psychology in medieval Persia. *Journal of Clinical Psychiatry, 67*, 1862–1869.

Van Meter, A. R., Youngstrom, E. A., & Findling, R. L. (2012). Cyclothymic disorder: A critical review. *Clinical Psychological Review, 32*, 229–243.

Vázquez, G. H., Tondo, L., Undurraga, J., & Baldessarini, R. J. (2013). Overview of antidepressant treatment of bipolar depression. *International Journal of Neuropsychopharmacology, 16*, 1673–1685.

Wernicke, C. (1881). *Lehrbuch der gehirnkrankheiten für ärzte und studirende* [Textbook of brain diseases for physicians and students]. Kassel: Fischer Verlag.

Willis, T. (1672). *De anima brutorum* [On animal spirits]. Oxford: R. Davis.

Winokur, G., Clayton, P. J., & Reich, T. (1969). *Manic-depressive illness*. St. Louis: Mosby.

World Health Organization (WHO) (1999). International Classification of Diseases, tenth edition (ICD-10), Geneva: WHO.

Wozniak, J., Petty, C. R., Schreck, M., Moses, A., Faraone, S. V., & Biederman, J. (2011). High level of persistence of pediatric bipolar-I disorder from childhood into adolescent years: Four-year prospective longitudinal follow-up study. *Journal of Psychiatric Research, 45*, 1273–1282.

2.

UPDATE ON EPIDEMIOLOGY, RISK FACTORS, AND CORRELATES OF BIPOLAR SPECTRUM DISORDER

Kathleen R. Merikangas and Diana Paksarian

INTRODUCTION

In recent years there has been a proliferation of epidemiologic research, both in the United States and abroad, that has strengthened the evidence base on the magnitude, correlates, and consequences of bipolar disorder. This work has highlighted the dramatic personal and societal impact of bipolar disorders. In the World Health Organization World Mental Health (WHM) surveys, bipolar disorder was the second ranking cause of disability, measured by days spent out of role per year, among a range of physical and mental health conditions (Alonso et al., 2011). In 2004 it was the fourth leading cause of disability adjusted life years worldwide among young people ages 10 to 24, ranking above violence, alcohol use, HIV/AIDS, self-inflicted injury, tuberculosis, and lower respiratory infection (Gore et al., 2011). The aims of this chapter are (a) to summarize the frequency of occurrence of bipolar disorder from population-based studies of adults and youth, (b) to describe the patterns of comorbidity of bipolar disorder in the general population, and (c) to summarize the risk factors and correlates of bipolar disorder, as well as current knowledge regarding its genetic underpinnings.

DESCRIPTIVE EPIDEMIOLOGY

PREVALENCE

Comprehensive summaries of the prevalence of bipolar disorder have been provided in several recent publications (Bauer & Pfennig, 2005; Goodwin & Jamison, 2007; Waraich, Goldner, Somers, & Hsu, 2004). The lifetime prevalence of bipolar I disorder (BPI) is generally estimated at about 1.0% (Merikangas & Tohen, 2011). A summary of prevalence rates according to definition of bipolar disorder provided by recent community-based studies of adults is presented in Table 2.1. Total estimates range from 0.0% in Nigeria (Gureje, Lasebikan, Kola, & Makanjuola, 2006) to 3.3% in the United States (Grant et al., 2005). Twelve-month prevalence is generally estimated to be only slightly lower than lifetime prevalence, ranging from 0% to 2.0%. Recent studies have begun to include estimates for bipolar II (BPII) and bipolar spectrum (BPS) disorders as well as BPI (Bauer & Pfennig, 2005; Merikangas, Jin, et al., 2011). As would be expected, prevalence tends to increase with successively more inclusive disorder definitions (Waraich et al., 2004). For example, in the WMH surveys, the cross-national lifetime prevalence of BPS disorders was 2.4%; of which 0.6% met criteria for BPI, 0.4% for BPII, and 1.4% for subthreshold bipolar disorder (Merikangas, Jin, et al., 2011). In many (but not all) studies assessing BPII, its prevalence is lower than that of BPI (Merikangas, Jin, et al., 2011; Wittchen, Nelson, & Lachner, 1998); this may indicate that the majority of people who experience hypomanic episodes also experience manic episodes, or it may be explained by the major depressive episode requirement for diagnosis of BPII.

An increasing number of studies have begun to estimate the occurrence of bipolar disorder in youth. The results of the existing cross-sectional and prospective community-based studies of youth are shown in Table 2.2. Lifetime prevalence rates of bipolar disorder in youth range from 0.2% in the Great Smoky Mountains Study (Costello et al., 1996) to 2.9% for BPI or BPII in the National Comorbidity Survey—Adolescent supplement (NCS-A; Merikangas et al., 2010). Young adults ages 19 to 24 in the Canadian Community Health Survey (CCHS; Kozloff et al., 2010) had a lifetime prevalence of 3.8%. A few studies have also estimated 12-month prevalence rates of bipolar disorder, ranging from 1.3% (Wittchen et al., 1998) to 2.5% (Benjet, Borges, Medina-Mora, Zambrano, &

Table 2.1. PREVALENCE OF *DSM-IV* BIPOLAR DISORDERS IN COMMUNITY SAMPLES OF ADULTS

LOCATION	STUDY	AGE	N	METHOD	DIAGNOSIS	PREVALENCE (%)
Australia	Zutshi et al. (2011)	≥15	2004: 3,015 2008: 3,014	MDQ	BPS	2004 LT: 2.5 2008 LT: 3.3
China	Lee et al. (2007)	18–70	5,201	WMH-CIDI/*DSM-IV*	BPI/BPII	LT: 0.1
	Phillips et al. (2009)	≥18	63,004 screened	SCID/*DSM-IV-TR* 2nd stage	BPI BPII	1m: .099 1m: .026
Germany	Jacobi et al. (2004)	18–65	4,181	M-CIDI/*DSM-IV*	BPD	LT: 1.0 (0.8 m, 1.2 f); 12m: 0.8 (0.6 m, 1.1 f)
Iraq	Alhasnawi et al. (2009)	≥18	4,332	WMH-CIDI/*DSM-IV*	BPS	LT: 0.2; 12m: 0.2
Israel	Levinson et al. (2007)	≥21	4,859	WMH-CIDI/*DSM-IV*	BPI/BPII	LT: 0.7; 12m: 0.1
Italy	Carta et al. (2012)	≥18	3,398	MDQ ≥7	BPS	LT: 3.0 (3.4 m, 2.7 f)
Japan	Kawakami et al. (2005)	≥20	1,664	WMH-CIDI/*DSM-IV*	BPI/BPII	12m: 0.1
Lebanon	Karam et al. (2008)	≥18	2,857	CIDI 3.0/*DSM-IV*	BPD	LT: 2.4 (2.6 m, 2.3 f)
Mexico	Medina-Mora et al. (2007)	18–65	5,826	WMH-CIDI/*DSM-IV*	BPI/BPII	LT: 1.9
New Zealand	Wells et al. (2006)	16–64	12,992	CIDI 3.0/*DSM-IV*	BPS	12m: 2.2 (2.1 m, 2.3 f)
Nigeria	Gureje et al. (2006)	≥18	4,984	WMH-CIDI/*DSM-IV*	BPI/BPII	LT: 0.0; 12m: 0.0
Singapore	Subramaniam et al. (2013)	≥18	6,616	WMH-CIDI/*DSM-IV*	BPI BPII BPI/BPII	LT: 1.1; 12m: 0.5 LT: 0.06; 12m: 0.04 LT: 1.2 (1.2 m, 1.3 f); 12m: 0.6 (0.5 m, 0.7 f)
Switzerland	Angst et al. (2005)	40	591	SPIKE/*DSM-IV*	BPI BPII	CP: 0.6 (0.0 m, 1.0 f) CP: 0.9 (0.0 m, 1.8 f)
United States	Grant et al. (2005)	≥18	43,093	NESARC/*DSM-IV*	BPI	LT: 3.3 (3.2 m, 3.4 f); 12m: 2.0 (1.8 m, 2.2 f)
	Ford et al. (2007)	≥55	6,082	WMH-CIDI/*DSM-IV*	BPI/BPII	LT: 0.8; 12m: 0.4
	Hoertel et al. (2013)	≥18	43,093	AUDADIS/*DSM-IV*	BPI BPII Sub-BP	LT: 2.19; 12m: 0.87 LT: 1.12; 12m: 0.32 LT: 2.53; 12m: 1.84
	Kessler (2012c)	18–64	9,282	CIDI/*DSM-IV*	BPI BPII BPI/BPII	LT: 1.1 (0.9 m, 1.3 f); 12m: 0.7 LT: 1.4 (1.2 m, 1.6 f); 12m: 1.0 LT: 2.5 (2.1 m, 2.9 f); 12m: 1.7
	Merikangas et al. (2007)	≥18	9,282	CIDI/*DSM-IV*	BPI BPII Sub-BP	LT: 1.0 (0.8 m, 1.1 f); 12m: 0.6 LT: 1.1 (0.9 m, 1.3 f); 12m: 0.8 LT: 2.4 (2.6 m, 2.1 f)
11 Countries	Merikangas et al. (2011)	≥18[a]	61,392	WMH-CIDI/*DSM-IV*	BPI BPII Sub-BP BPS	LT: 0.6; 12m: 0.4 LT: 0.4; 12m: 0.3 LT: 1.4; 12m: 0.8 LT: 2.4; 12m: 1.5

NOTE: DSM-IV = *Diagnostic and Statistical Manual of Mental Disorders* (fourth ed.), *DSM-IV-TR* = *Diagnostic and Statistical Manual of Mental Disorders* (fourth ed., text rev.); LT = lifetime; 12m = 12-month; 1m = 1-month; BPS = bipolar spectrum disorder; BPI = bipolar I disorder; BPII = bipolar II disorder; BPD = subthreshold bipolar disorder; Sub-BP = subthreshold bipolar disorder; MDQ = Mood Disorder Questionnaire. WMH = World Mental Health. M = Munich. CIDI = Composite International Diagnostic Interview. NESARC = National Epidemiologic Survey on Alcohol and Related Conditions. AUDADIS = Alcohol Use Disorder and Associated Disabilities Interview Schedule. SPIKE = Structured Psychopathological Interview and Rating of Social Consequences of Psychic Disturbances for Epidemiology. SCID = Structured Clinical Interview for DSM-IV Disorders.

[a] In 9 countries; ≥16 in one country and ≥20 in one country.

Aguilar-Gaxiola, 2009). Prevalence rates of mania range from 0.4% (12-month; Roberts, Roberts, & Xing, 2007) to 2.0% (12-month; Cannon et al., 2002), and rates of hypomania range from 0.1% (lifetime; Costello et al., 1996) to 0.9% (6-month; Verhulst, van der Ende, Ferdinand, & Kasius, 1997). The results of longitudinal studies converge in estimating the prevalence of bipolar disorder at between 1.4% and 2.1%, which approximates cross-sectional prevalence rates in adult samples. This was confirmed by a recent meta-analysis of epidemiologic studies of bipolar disorder in children and adolescents, which reported a mean prevalence of 1.8% (Van Meter, Moreira, & Youngstrom, 2011).

INCIDENCE AND AGE OF ONSET

A number of recent studies have assessed the incidence of bipolar disorder in the general population (Chou, Mackenzie, Liang, & Sareen, 2011; de Graaf, ten Have, Tuithof, & van Dorsselaer, 2013; Grant et al., 2009). In the National Epidemiologic Survey on Alcohol and Related Conditions (NESARC), one-year incidence rates of BPI and BPII were 0.53% and 0.21%, respectively (Grant et al., 2009). The three-year incidence rate of bipolar disorder among adults age 18 to 64 in the Netherlands was 0.41% (de Graaf et al., 2013). Among adults age 60 and older

Table 2.2. PREVALENCE OF BIPOLAR DISORDERS IN COMMUNITY SAMPLES OF CHILDREN AND ADOLESCENTS

AUTHORS	STUDY NAME	SAMPLE SIZE	AGE	PREVALENCE
Cross-sectional				
Verhulst et al. (1997)	Dutch Adolescent Study	760	13–18	6m Mania: 1.9 6m Hypomania: 0.9
Costello et al. (1996)	Smoky Mountains Study	1,015	9, 11, 13	3m Mania: 0 3m Hypomania: 0.1
Roberts et al. (2007)	Teen Health 2000	4,175	11–17	12m Mania: 0.4 12m Hypomania: 0.8
Benjet et al. (2009)	Mexican Adolescent Mental Health Survey	3,005	12–17	12m BPI/BPII: 2.5
Kozloff et al. (2010)	Canadian Community Health Survey	5,673	15–18 19–24	LT BPI[a]: 2.1 LT BPI[a]: 3.8
Merikangas et al. (2010) Kessler et al. (2012b) Merikangas et al. (2012)	National Comorbidity Survey—Adolescent Supplement	10,123	13–18	LT Mania: 1.7 12m Mania: 1.3 LT BPI/BPII: 2.9 12m BPI/BPII: 2.1 30d BPI/BPII: 0.7
Longitudinal				
Wittchen et al. (1998)	Early Developmental Study of Psychopathology	3,021	14–24	BPI: LT: 1.4, 12m: 1.3 BPII: LT: 0.4, 12m: 0.4
Cannon et al. (2002)	Dunedin Longitudinal Study	980	26	12m Mania: 2.0
Johnson et al. (2000)	Children in the Community Study	717	T1: 9–18 T2: 11–20 T3: 17–26	T1 or T2 BPI: 2.0; Sub-BP: 1.4 BPI: 1.4; Sub-BP: 2.0
Lewinsohn et al. (2000)	Oregon Adolescent Depression Project	1,709 1,507 865	T1: 14–18 T2: 15–19 T3: 24	LT BPD: 0.9; LT Sub-BP: 4.4 LT BPD: 1.0; LT Sub-BP: 4.3 LT BPD: 2.1; LT Sub-BP: 5.3

NOTE: LT = lifetime; BPI = bipolar I disorder; BPII = bipolar II disorder; BPD = bipolar disorders; Sub-BP = subthreshold bipolar disorder.

[a] This study used a slightly looser duration requirement but the authors note that their diagnosis most closely resembles BPI.

in the United States, the three-year incidence of BPI was 0.54% and the incidence of BPII was 0.34% (Chou et al., 2011). Prospective studies of child and adolescent samples from population surveys also provide valuable information regarding the incidence of bipolar disorder. Lewinsohn, Seeley, Buckley, and Klein. (2002) found that the peak incidence of bipolar disorder is at age 14 in both males and females and decreases gradually thereafter. By age 21, the rate of bipolar disorder rose to 2% in the prospective cohort studies of youth who were followed for several years (Cannon et al., 2002; Lewinsohn, Klein, & Seeley, 2000). Indeed, emerging evidence indicates that the first onset of BPI generally begins in adolescence or early adulthood, with a mean age of onset of 18 years (Merikangas et al., 2007). This contrasts with the previously dominant belief, largely based on clinical studies, that onset begins in the third decade of life.

DIAGNOSTIC BOUNDARIES

As indicated here, there has been growing interest in testing the thresholds and boundaries of bipolar disorder in community samples. Among those with 12-month subthreshold bipolar disorder in the WMH surveys, 79.2% reported a clinically severe or moderate manic or hypomanic episode in the past year, with 79.3% reporting moderate to severe role impairment (Merikangas, Jin, et al., 2011). Using data from the NESARC, Hoertel, Le Strat, Angst, and Dubertret (2013) found that the lifetime prevalence of major depressive episode plus subthreshold manic symptoms was 2.53%, while the 12-month prevalence was 1.84. Participants in this group differed significantly from those with "pure" major depressive disorder (MDD) on the lifetime presence of a number of psychiatric comorbidities but differed from those diagnosed with BPII on only one. They also had a younger age at onset, had a greater number of episodes, met a greater number of *Diagnostic and Statistical Manual of Mental Disorders* (*DSM*) criteria, and were more likely to use alcohol to relieve their symptoms. They also had higher rates of any lifetime treatment seeking, 12-month treatment seeking, and lifetime use of medication compared to those with "pure" MDD (Hoertel et al., 2013). Likewise, expansion of the definition of hypomania in the NCS-R study yielded a lifetime prevalence rate of 4.5%. (Kessler et al., 2006; Merikangas et al., 2007). The severity of symptoms of depression and mania associated with subthreshold bipolar disorder suggested that the latter category did tap clinically significant manifestations of disorder that were comparable to people seeking treatment for these conditions in outpatient settings (Kessler et al., 2006). Similarly, among adolescents with a broad definition of 12-month bipolar disorder (including BPI and BPII as well as subthreshold bipolar disorder), less than half (43.1%) were rated as having mild severity as defined by the Children's Global Assessment Scale (CGAS). 30.5% of cases were rated as having serious severity (CGAS scores ≤50) while 26.5% had moderate severity (CGAS scores 51–60; Kessler, Avenevoli, Costello, Green, et al., 2012a).

SERVICE UTILIZATION

The majority of studies reviewed earlier in this chapter indicate that about 60% of those with BPI in US community samples receive mental health treatment. Across all countries in the WMH surveys, 68.7% of those with BPI reported any lifetime treatment, and 51.6% reported any lifetime specialty mental health treatment. Treatment rates were highest in high income countries. In low and middle income countries, 37.9% of those with BPI received any mental health treatment and only 22.3% received specialty mental health treatment (Merikangas, Jin, et al., 2011). There are also recent estimates of service utilization among youth. In a representative sample of US adolescents, only 22.2% of adolescents with BPI or BPII (26.5% of girls and 17.9% of boys) reported lifetime disorder-specific mental health service use (Merikangas, He, et al., 2011). Eighteen percent of those with 12-month bipolar disorder reported receiving any medication (14.2% received antidepressants), and 33.8% reported receiving any type of specialty mental health treatment (Merikangas, He, Rapoport, Vitiello, & Olfson, 2013). In the CCHS, 45.8% of 15- to 18-year-olds and 60.3% of 19- to 24-year-olds with bipolar disorder reported using mental health services (Kozloff et al., 2010). The relatively low rates of service utilization in some countries is alarming, as it suggests that a large proportion of individuals are not receiving adequate care. It also highlights the extent to which research conducted in treatment settings may fail to properly represent those with bipolar disorder in the general population.

PATTERNS OF COMORBIDITY

MENTAL DISORDERS

Recent epidemiologic surveys have highlighted the striking magnitude of comorbidity between bipolar disorder and other Axis I *Diagnostic and Statistical Manual of Mental Disorders* (fourth ed. [*DSM-IV*]; American Psychiatric Association, 1994) disorders. As shown in

Table 2.3, more than 90% of those with lifetime BPI or BPII disorder in the NCS-R also meet criteria for another lifetime disorder, and 70% of those with bipolar spectrum disorders have a history of three or more disorders (Merikangas et al., 2007). Comorbid anxiety disorders are very common; more than 80% of those with bipolar disorder also have a lifetime history of *DSM-IV* anxiety disorders, particularly panic attacks (61.9%) and social phobia (37.8%; Merikangas et al., 2007). Likewise, among those 18 years and older in the NESARC, 60% of individuals with bipolar disorder had at least one comorbid anxiety disorder, and 40% had two or more (Sala et al., 2012). This is also true cross-nationally. In the WMH surveys, the rates of any lifetime mental disorder

comorbidity were 88.2% for BPI, 83.1% for BPII, 69.1% for subthreshold bipolar disorder, and 76.5% for BPS (Merikangas, Jin, et al., 2011). The majority of those with BPI and BPII had three or more comorbid mental disorders; 76.5% of those with BPI and 74.6% of those with BPII had a comorbid anxiety disorder, the most common of which was panic attacks (57.9% of those with BPI and 63.8% of those with BPII; Merikangas, Jin, et al., 2011).

Bipolar disorder is also highly comorbid with substance use disorders. A recent review of alcohol misuse and bipolar disorder found that of eight epidemiologic studies, seven from Europe and North American reported that alcohol use disorders were significantly elevated among study participants with bipolar disorder; one

Table 2.3. COMORBIDITY OF BIPOLAR DISORDER IN THE NCS-R

COMORBIDITY CATEGORY	DISORDER	BIPOLAR DISORDER			
		%[a]	SE	OR[*b]	95% CI
Anxiety	Agoraphobia without panic	5.7	1.3	5.3	3.0–9.3
	Panic disorder	20.1	2.0	5.8	4.4–7.7
	Panic attacks	61.9	2.0	4.3	3.5–5.2
	Posttraumatic stress disorder	24.2	2.6	4.7	3.3–6.8
	Generalized anxiety disorder	29.6	2.5	6.1	4.6–8.1
	Specific phobia	35.5	2.8	4.0	3.1–5.2
	Social phobia	37.8	3.1	4.6	3.5–5.9
	Obsessive-compulsive disorder	13.6	3.1	10.2	4.6–22.9
	Separation anxiety disorder	35.4	2.0	5.4	4.6–6.5
	Any anxiety disorder	74.9	2.8	6.5	4.7–9.0
Substance use	Alcohol abuse	39.1	2.6	4.3	3.3–5.5
	Alcohol dependence	23.2	1.9	5.7	4.3–7.6
	Drug abuse	28.8	2.7	4.5	3.3–5.9
	Drug dependence	14.0	1.8	5.2	3.7–7.2
	Any substance	42.3	2.7	4.2	3.3–5.5
Any disorder	Any disorder	92.3	2.2	13.1	6.7–25.5
	Exactly one disorder	12.7	2.0	4.8	2.2–10.4
	Exactly two disorders	9.4	1.7	5.6	2.5–12.5
	Three or more disorders	70.1	2.5	26.4	13.7–50.8

NOTE: NCS-R = National Comorbidity Survey-Replication; SE = standard error; OR = odds ratio; CI = confidence interval.

[a] Mean (SE) prevalence of the comorbid disorder in respondents with bipolar disorder. [b] Based on logistic regression models with one *Diagnostic and Statistical Manual of Mental Disorders* (fourth ed.)/Composite International Diagnostic Interview disorder at a time as a predictor of lifetime bipolar disorder, controlling for age at interview (five-year intervals), sex, and race/ethnicity.

[*] Significant at the $\alpha = .05$ level, two-sided test.

study conducted in Asia found no such association (Di Florio, Craddock, & van den Bree, 2014). Likewise, in the NCS-R, 42.3% of those with bipolar disorder had any lifetime substance use disorder, the most common of which was alcohol abuse (Table 2.3). Among 19- to 24-year-olds with bipolar disorder in the CCHS, 46.0% had a 12-month substance use disorder (Kozloff et al., 2010). The onset of bipolar disorder generally precedes that of the substance use disorder. For example, using data from a 20-year prospective cohort study, Merikangas et al. (2008) demonstrated the dramatic increase in risk of alcohol dependence associated with symptoms of mania and bipolar disorder in early adulthood. In an analysis of the 10-year follow-up data from the National Comorbidity Survey, Swendson et al. (2010) found that baseline bipolar disorder was associated with the onset of nicotine, alcohol, and substance dependence; with the conversion to nicotine dependence among daily users; with the first onset of substance abuse among substance users; and with the onset of substance dependence among substance users.

These patterns of comorbidity also hold for youth with bipolar disorder. Among adolescents in the CCHS, 41.8% of 15- to 18-year-olds with bipolar disorder also met lifetime criteria for an anxiety disorder, 32.1% had a 12-month substance use disorder, and 54.6% reported lifetime suicidality (Kozloff et al., 2010). However, follow-up studies of children have shown that bipolar disorder is associated with multiple other disorders including attention deficit hyperactivity disorder (ADHD), anxiety disorders and/or oppositional defiant disorder, and conduct disorder (Lewinsohn et al., 2002; Youngstrom et al., 2005). An eight-year follow up study of a population sample of youth from New York state revealed that childhood anxiety disorders and depression, and to a lower extent disruptive behavior disorders, were significantly associated with the development of bipolar disorder in early adulthood (Johnson, Cohen, & Brook, 2000).

PHYSICAL DISORDERS

Epidemiologic studies indicate an elevated rate of physical comorbidities among individuals with bipolar disorder. In an analysis of NCS-R data that considered a range of mental and physical comorbidities, Gadermann, Alonso, Vilagut, Zaslavsky, and Kessler (2012) found that 94.6% of participants with 12-month bipolar disorder had at least one other physical or mental condition, and, among

those with comorbidity, the mean number of other disorders was 4.6. In the CCHS, those with a lifetime manic episode were more likely to report physician diagnoses of asthma, gastric ulcer, hypertension, chronic bronchitis, and migraine (McIntyre et al., 2006). Other studies have also found associations between migraine and bipolar symptoms/disorder (Saunders, Merikangas, Low, Von Korff, & Kessler, 2008). In a nationally representative cross-sectional survey in Singapore, 52.1% of those with BPI reported any physical comorbidity, the most common of which was chronic pain (28.3%; Subramaniam, Abdin, Vaingankar, & Chong, 2013).

The increasing use of health registries with national coverage for research purposes provides a valuable source of information about physical comorbidity. Although such studies rely on treated rates of disorder, this may present less of a problem in situations where medical services are provided without charge and for more severe forms of mental disorder. Using data from the Danish population and health registries, Laursen, Munk-Olsen, and Gasse (2011) presented risk ratios for a range of chronic physical conditions over 12 years of follow-up. Individuals with bipolar disorder had an elevated risk of 11 of the conditions presented, including diabetes, liver disease, congestive heart failure, chronic pulmonary disease, cerebrovascular disease, renal disease, and dementia.

CORRELATES AND RISK FACTORS

DEMOGRAPHIC CORRELATES

US population-based studies have traditionally found equal rates of bipolar disorder in males and females (Grant et al., 2009; Merikangas et al., 2007). In cross-national estimates from the WMH surveys, however, the lifetime prevalence of BPI and subthreshold bipolar disorder were higher in males, while the lifetime prevalence of BPII was higher in females (Merikangas, Jin, et al., 2011). This may reflect cultural differences in sex-specific expression of bipolar disorder. There is also emerging evidence of differences in expression between males and females in the United States. In the NCS-A, the prevalence of mania/hypomania with MDD and the prevalence of MDD alone were both higher among females than males, while the prevalence of mania alone was greater among males (Merikangas et al., 2012). However, among youth ages 15 to 24 in the CCHS, which used an inclusive definition of bipolar disorder comprising BPI, BPII, and BP–not otherwise specified, lifetime prevalence did not differ between males and females (Kozloff et al., 2010). This is consistent with the lack of sex differences reported for BPI and BPII in the NCS-A (Kessler, Avenevoli, Costello, Georgiades, et al., 2012b). Thus there could be sex-specific patterns of the emergence of bipolar disorder in adolescence and young adulthood that are visible only when the components of bipolar disorder are examined individually.

Although many early studies of treated samples suggest that bipolar disorder was more common in upper socioeconomic classes, the most recent US epidemiologic studies have typically failed to detect an association or found higher rates among those with lower income and education (Grant et al., 2005, 2009; Merikangas et al., 2007). Likewise, rates of bipolar disorders tend to be greater among those who are separated or divorced compared to those who are never married (e.g., Subramaniam et al., 2013). One potential explanation for these discrepancies is the distinction between socioeconomic status (SES) in the family of origin and individual SES at the time of illness onset. For example, using data from Danish population registries, Tsuchiya et al. (2004) differentiated between indicators of SES in the individual and in the individual's parents, both measured in the year prior to onset. Adjusting for sex and family history, those with bipolar disorder were more likely to be single and more likely to be lower on SES indicators such as employment and income. Their parents, however, were more likely to have higher levels of education and greater paternal wealth (Tsuchiya, Agerbo, Byrne, & Mortensen, 2004). Such findings should be interpreted with caution, however, as they are based on treated rates of disorder and may not capture the entire range of severity present in the population.

Studies have not generally found consistent racial or ethnic differences in rates of bipolar disorder. For example, no differences were found between racial groups in the United States in prevalence of bipolar disorder in the NCS-R (Merikangas et al., 2007). However, it may be difficult to distinguish racial and ethnic differences in many studies because of the need to include sufficiently large multiethnic samples. In the NESARC, which had a large sample size and thus enabled inclusion of several distinct ethnic subgroups, the lifetime prevalence of BPI was greater among Native Americans and lower among Hispanics and Asians and Pacific Islanders compared to Whites (Grant et al., 2005). In an analysis of mothers in the National Survey of American Life, Boyd (2011) reported significant associations between racial/ethnic group and both lifetime and 12-month bipolar disorder. African American mothers had higher lifetime and 12-month rates of bipolar disorder than White mothers and higher 12-month rates than Caribbean Black mothers (Boyd, Joe, Michalopoulos, Davis, & Jackson, 2011). Ethnic differences have also been reported in studies from New Zealand (Baxter, Kokaua, Wells, McGee, & Browne, 2006) and Singapore (Subramaniam et al., 2013).

ENVIRONMENTAL RISK FACTORS

Until recently there has been a relative dearth of consistent information regarding nongenetic etiologic risk factors for bipolar disorder (Tsuchiya, Byrne, & Mortensen, 2003). Despite apparent overlap in genetic underpinnings of bipolar disorder and schizophrenia (discussed later), there has traditionally been little evidence for overlap in environmental risk factors for the two disorders. Although exceptions exist, established risk factors for schizophrenia such as season of birth, urbanicity, parental age, migration status, and obstetric complications have generally not been implicated in the etiology of bipolar disorder (Demjaha, MacCabe, & Murray, 2012). Recently there has been renewed interest in the potential role of stressors in the etiology of bipolar disorder. Bipolar disorder may be more common among those who experienced childhood stressors such as the loss of a parent (Mortensen, Pedersen, Melbye, Mors, & Ewald, 2003). Furthermore, in the New Zealand Mental Health Survey, those who reported childhood physical abuse and those who reported childhood sexual abuse were more likely to meet criteria for both 12-month and lifetime bipolar disorder, and those who reported violence in the family during childhood were more likely to have 12-month bipolar disorder with frequent mood episodes and lifetime bipolar disorder (Wells, McGee, Scott, & Browne, 2010). A range of similar associations was reported based on data from the NCS-R (Nierenberg et al., 2010). For example, those with 12-month bipolar disorder were more likely to report childhood neglect, physical abuse, and sexual abuse, while those with other lifetime bipolar disorder were more likely to report sexual abuse; those with both 12-month and lifetime bipolar disorder were also more likely to report parental violence and criminal behavior (Nierenberg et al., 2010). In a recent analysis of NESARC data, Gilman et al. (2014) reported that childhood abuse, sexual maltreatment, and economic adversity predicted both incident and recurrent mania. In addition, there was evidence that childhood abuse potentiated the effect of recent stressors on mania onset.

There are two issues regarding research on childhood adversity that warrant note. First, many forms of childhood adversity appear to be nonspecific risk factors for adult mental disorder. Using NESARC data, Sugaya et al. (2012) found that childhood physical abuse increased risk for bipolar disorder after adjusting for socioeconomic characteristics and other psychiatric comorbidities, but it also increased risk of drug abuse, nicotine dependence, posttraumatic stress disorder, ADHD, generalized anxiety disorder, panic, MDD, and suicide attempt. This lack of specificity suggests the involvement of more general mechanisms underlying any potential causal effects of adversity.

A second issue relevant to this area of research is that assessment of childhood adversities often relies on retrospective recall, which introduces the potential for bias. To address this weakness, prospective studies, or studies using prospectively and independently collected exposure measurements, are needed. For example, Scott, Smith, and Ellis (2010) linked information from 16- to 27-year-old respondents in the New Zealand Mental Health Survey to the national electronic database of the New Zealand Child, Youth and Family agency. Using this measure of childhood maltreatment, they report associations with a number of 12-month and lifetime psychiatric disorders including major depression, social phobia, drug and alcohol use disorders, and posttraumatic stress disorder; they did not find associations with bipolar disorder, panic disorder, or generalized anxiety disorder. Population registry data provide another opportunity for studying the mental health effects of childhood exposures using prospectively and independently ascertained exposure information. Population registry from Denmark indicates that the loss of a parent due to death, particularly before age 12 and from unnatural causes, increases risk for bipolar disorder in adulthood (Laursen, Munk-Olsen, Nordentoft, & Bo Mortensen, 2007). Additional, prospectively designed studies are needed to help identify nongenetic risk factors for bipolar disorder in order to ultimately inform strategies for intervention.

FAMILY HISTORY AND GENETIC RISK FACTORS

Family and twin studies

A family history of bipolar disorder is one of the strongest and most consistent risk factors for the development of bipolar disorder. Controlled family studies indicated that first-degree relatives of probands with bipolar disorder have substantially increased risk of bipolar disorder compared to relatives of controls. Two recent family studies of the mood disorder spectrum confirmed that the familial loading for BPI is much higher than that of BPII or MDD (Merikangas, Cui, et al., 2013; C. L. Vandeleur, Merikangas, Strippoli, Castelao, & Preisig, 2014). Estimates of the familial aggregation of bipolar disorder have also recently been derived from population-based treatment registries. There was a 7-fold increased risk and a 6.5-fold increased risk of bipolar disorder among first-degree relatives of probands with bipolar disorder in the Swedish (Lichtenstein et al., 2009) and Dutch (Aukes et al., 2012) registries, respectively. In a recent meta-analysis of the familial loading of mood disorders, Wilde et al. (2014) reported close to an eight-fold increase in odds of bipolar disorder among first-degree relatives of one proband with the disorder. Likewise, a meta-analysis of bipolar disorder in children found that the odds of BPI were almost 7-fold in first-degree relatives of probands with pediatric bipolar disorder compared to control probands (Wozniak, Faraone, Martelon, McKillop, & Biederman, 2012).

Recent twin studies using modern definitions of bipolar disorder have reported concordance rates in monozygotic twins that are about 8 times those of dizygotic twins and have yielded high heritability estimates (Smoller & Gardner-Schuster, 2007). For example, a study of twins from the Maudsley Twin Registry reported a heritability estimate of 85% when employing a narrow definition of concordance and 89% when employing a broad definition (McGuffin et al., 2003). Such high heritability estimates indicate that a substantial proportion of phenotypic variation in bipolar disorder is attributable to genes.

Molecular genetic studies

Despite high heritability estimates for bipolar disorder, the search for specific causal variants has proven difficult. Recently, the results of several large-scale case-control studies of bipolar disorder in samples from the United Kingdom, United States, and Germany have emerged (Baum et al., 2008; Burton et al., 2007; Sklar et al., 2008). Although few loci exceeded genome-wide significance levels in these individual studies, meta-analyses of three initial studies yielded identified two genetic loci that exceeded genome-wide significance: ANK3 on chromosome 10 and CACNA1C on chromosome 12 (Ferreira et al., 2008). None of these studies confirmed the results of earlier candidate gene and linkage studies of bipolar disorder, and the effect sizes of these genes were quite small (odds ratio < 1.4). These studies also increased recognition of the need for larger samples because of the small effects of the loci on bipolar disorder and the need for built-in replication samples to reduce the false positive rates that have plagued earlier candidate gene and smaller studies of genes involved in bipolar disorder. Copy number variants that have been strongly implicated for schizophrenia have also been reported in bipolar disorder (Malhotra & Sebat, 2012), but these findings have not been replicated (Bergen et al., 2012).

The largest genome-wide association study of bipolar disorder was a multi-investigator collaborative study titled the Psychiatric Genome Wide Association of Bipolar Disorder Consortium (Sklar et al., 2011), which included 7,418 cases and 9,250 controls in Stage 1 and 11,974 cases and 51,792 controls in Stage 2. Analyses of this study yielded only two genome-wide significant loci: rs4765,913 near the CACNA1C locus identified in earlier studies with an odds ratio of 1.14, and rs12,576,775 near a gene ODZ4 on chromosome 11 with an odds ratio of 0.88. There are several possible explanations for the small number of findings. One explanation that is currently receiving a great deal of attention is the substantial heritability in the phenotypic presentation of bipolar disorder. This may be especially relevant to genome-wide association studies, which usually rely on a simple "case versus control" outcome definition, leaving the potential for substantial heterogeneity within the case group (Craddock & Sklar, 2013). One potential solution to this problem is the use of endophenotypes to define cases rather than disorder categories (Gottesman & Gould, 2003).

CROSS-DISORDER STUDIES

Evidence from both family and molecular genetic studies indicate some degree of genetic overlap between bipolar disorder and other purportedly distinct disorders such as MDD and schizophrenia. For example, offspring of probands with bipolar disorder have increased rates of major depression, although these are not usually as high as the increases in rates of bipolar disorder (Vandeleur et al., 2012; Wilde et al., 2014). Similarly, a recent meta-analysis found increased rates of depression, anxiety, disruptive disorders, substance use, and ADHD among offspring of parents with bipolar disorder (Rasic, Hajek, Alda, & Uher, 2014). Other evidence has come from families assembled using population registry data. For example, using data from the Swedish treatment registry, Lichtenstein et al. (2009) reported a significant genetic correlation between the two disorders of 0.60. However, two recent family studies failed to find evidence of cross-transmission between bipolar disorder and major depression and also demonstrated specificity of the core components of bipolar disorder, psychosis,

mania, and major depression (Merikangas, Cui, et al., 2013; Vandeleur et al., 2014). Likewise, Goldstein, Buka, Seidman, and Tsuang (2010) found substantial specificity of familial transmission of affective psychosis and schizophrenia in the New England Family Study.

Molecular genetic evidence for disorder overlap is based on single nucleotide polymorphism–based heritability. The Cross-Disorder Group of the Psychiatric Genetics Consortium recently reported high single nucleotide polymorphism coheritability between bipolar disorder and schizophrenia (0.68) and moderate coheritability between bipolar disorder and major depressive disorder (0.47; Lee et al., 2013). Although this suggests that there may be common genes underlying these two conditions, caution is advised in interpreting these results because of issues such as diagnostic misclassification and heterogeneity, the low attributable risk of common variants underlying bipolar disorder, and the assumptions underlying the analyses used. The whole of the evidence thus far suggests that a combination of specific and nonspecific factors underlie the development of mental disorders within families. Future efforts to distinguish between common and unique pathways to psychiatric disorders will be critical to our understanding of the major psychiatric disorders.

SUMMARY

In recent years there has been a substantial growth in research on both the descriptive and analytic epidemiology of bipolar disorder, as well as its genetic underpinnings. An increase in population-based studies in international settings, as well as large, cross-national collaborations, have provided insight into the magnitude of occurrence of bipolar disorder and its substantial impact. The average cross-national lifetime prevalence of bipolar disorder is estimated at 2% to 3% in adults and 2% in youth. The burden of bipolar disorder is especially pronounced among young people, consistent with recent evidence that first onset begins during adolescence and early adulthood. Despite its substantial impact, only about 50% of adults and 20% of adolescents receive specialty mental health care treatment.

There is growing recognition that bipolar disorder has a spectrum of expression, and prevalence estimates for this spectrum are often appreciably greater than for BPI. Delineating the diagnostic boundaries of bipolar disorder remains an important area for future research. This is especially evident when one considers the substantial magnitude of comorbidity of bipolar disorder with other mental and substance use disorders, evidence for familial overlap between bipolar disorder and other mental disorders such as depression and anxiety, and evidence from molecular genetic studies suggesting the presence of common genes underlying bipolar disorder and schizophrenia. Elucidation of the boundaries of bipolar disorder will also aid in the search for both genetic and nongenetic risk factors for bipolar disorder, areas of research that have been greatly expanded in recent years but in which further progress is needed. Greater advances in our understanding of the epidemiology of bipolar disorder will have important implications for prevention and treatment.

Disclosure Statement: The authors have no conflicts of interest to disclose. This work was supported by the Intramural Research Program of the National Institute of Mental Health. The views and opinions expressed in this article are those of the authors and should not be construed to represent the views of any of the sponsoring organizations, agencies, or the US government.

REFERENCES

Alhasnawi, S., Sadik, S., Rasheed, M., Baban, A., Al-Alak, M. M., Othman, A. Y., ... Kessler, R. C. (2009). The prevalence and correlates of DSM-IV disorders in the Iraq Mental Health Survey (IMHS). *World Psychiatry*, 8(2), 97–109.

Alonso, J., Petukhova, M., Vilagut, G., Chatterji, S., Heeringa, S., Ustun, T. B., ... Kessler, R. C. (2011). Days out of role due to common physical and mental conditions: results from the WHO World Mental Health surveys. *Molecular Psychiatry*, 16(12), 1234–1246. doi:10.1038/Mp.2010.101

American Psychiatric Association. (1994). *Diagnostic and statistical manual of mental disorders* (4th ed.). Washington, DC: Author.

Angst, J., Gamma, A., Neuenschwander, M., Ajdacic-Gross, V., Eich, D., Rossler, W., & Merikangas, K. R. (2005). Prevalence of mental disorders in the Zurich Cohort Study: a twenty year prospective study. *Epidemiologia E Psichiatria Sociale*, 14(2), 68–76.

Aukes, M. F., Laan, W., Termorshuizen, F., Buizer-Voskamp, J. E., Hennekam, E. A., Smeets, H. M., ... Kahn, R. S. (2012). Familial clustering of schizophrenia, bipolar disorder, and major depressive disorder. *Genetics in Medicine*, 14(3), 338–341.

Bauer, M., & Pfennig, A. (2005). Epidemiology of bipolar disorders. *Epilepsia*, 46, 8–13.

Baum, A. E., Hamshere, M., Green, E., Cichon, S., Rietschel, M., Noethen, M. M., ... McMahon, F. J. (2008). Meta-analysis of two genome-wide association studies of bipolar disorder reveals important points of agreement. *Molecular Psychiatry*, 13(5), 466–467.

Baxter, J., Kokaua, J., Wells, J. E., McGee, M. A., & Browne, M. A. O. (2006). Ethnic comparisons of the 12 month prevalence of mental disorders and treatment contact in Te Rau Hinengaro: The New Zealand Mental Health Survey. *Australian and New Zealand Journal of Psychiatry*, 40(10), 905–913.

Benjet, C., Borges, G., Medina-Mora, M. E., Zambrano, J., & Aguilar-Gaxiola, S. (2009). Youth mental health in a populous city of the developing world: Results from the Mexican Adolescent Mental Health Survey. *Journal of Child Psychology and Psychiatry*, 50(4), 386–395.

Bergen, S. E., O'Dushlaine, C. T., Ripke, S., Lee, P. H., Ruderfer, D. M., Akterin, S., ... Sullivan, P. F. (2012). Genome-wide association study in a Swedish population yields support for greater CNV and MHC involvement in schizophrenia compared with bipolar disorder. *Molecular Psychiatry*, 17(9), 880–886.

Boyd, R. C., Joe, S., Michalopoulos, L., Davis, E., & Jackson, J. S. (2011). Prevalence of mood disorders and service use among US mothers by race and ethnicity: Results from the National Survey of American Life. *Journal of Clinical Psychiatry*, 72(11), 1538–1545. doi:10.4088/Jcp.10m06468

Burton, P. R., Clayton, D. G., Cardon, L. R., Craddock, N., Deloukas, P., Duncanson, A., ... Collaborat, B. C. S. (2007). Genome-wide association study of 14,000 cases of seven common diseases and 3,000 shared controls. *Nature*, 447(7145), 661–678. doi:10.1038/Nature05911

Cannon, M., Caspi, A., Moffitt, T. E., Harrington, H., Taylor, A., Murray, R. M., & Poulton, R. (2002). Evidence for early-childhood, pan-developmental impairment specific to schizophreniform disorder: Results from a longitudinal birth cohort. *Archives of General Psychiatry*, 59(5), 449–456.

Carta, M. G., Aguglia, E., Balestrieri, M., Calabrese, J. R., Caraci, F., Dell'Osso, L., ... Hardoy, M. C. (2012). The lifetime prevalence of bipolar disorders and the use of antidepressant drugs in bipolar depression in Italy. *Journal of Affective Disorders*, 136(3), 775–780. doi:10.1016/j.jad.2011.09.041

Chou, K. L., Mackenzie, C. S., Liang, K., & Sareen, J. (2011). Three-year incidence and predictors of first-onset of DSM-IV mood, anxiety, and substance use disorders in older adults: results from Wave 2 of the National Epidemiologic Survey on Alcohol and Related Conditions. *Journal of Clinical Psychiatry*, 72(2), 144–155. doi:10.4088/Jcp.09m05618gry

Costello, E. J., Angold, A., Burns, B. J., Stangl, D. K., Tweed, D. L., Erkanli, A., & Worthman, C. M. (1996). The Great Smoky Mountains Study of youth—Goals, design, methods, and the prevalence of DSM-III-R disorders. *Archives of General Psychiatry*, 53(12), 1129–1136.

Craddock, N., & Sklar, P. (2013). Genetics of bipolar disorder. *Lancet*, 381(9878), 1654–1662. doi:10.1016/S0140-6736(13)60855-7

de Graaf, R., ten Have, M., Tuithof, M., & van Dorsselaer, S. (2013). First-incidence of DSM-IV mood, anxiety and substance use disorders and its determinants: Results from the Netherlands Mental Health Survey and Incidence Study-2. *Journal of Affective Disorders*, 149(1–3), 100–107. doi:10.1016/j.jad.2013.01.009

Demjaha, A., MacCabe, J. H., & Murray, R. M. (2012). How genes and environmental factors determine the different neurodevelopmental trajectories of schizophrenia and bipolar disorder. *Schizophrenia Bulletin*, 38(2), 209–214. doi:10.1093/schbul/sbr100

Di Florio, A., Craddock, N., & van den Bree, M. (2014). Alcohol misuse in bipolar disorder: A systematic review and meta-analysis of comorbidity rates. *European Psychiatry*, 29(3), 117–124. doi:10.1016/j.eurpsy.2013.07.004

Ferreira, M. A., O'Donovan, M. C., Meng, Y. A., Jones, I. R., Ruderfer, D. M., Jones, L., ... Wellcome Trust Case Control, C. (2008). Collaborative genome-wide association analysis supports a role for ANK3 and CACNA1C in bipolar disorder. *Nature Genetics*, 40(9), 1056–1058. doi:10.1038/ng.209

Ford, B. C., Bullard, K. M., Taylor, R. J., Toler, A. K., Neighbors, H. W., & Jackson, J. S. (2007). Lifetime and 12-month prevalence of Diagnostic and Statistical Manual of Mental Disorders, Fourth Edition disorders among older African Americans: Findings from the national survey of American life. *American Journal of Geriatric Psychiatry*, 15(8), 652–659.

Gadermann, A. M., Alonso, J., Vilagut, G., Zaslavsky, A. M., & Kessler, R. C. (2012). Comorbidity and disease burden in the National Comorbidity Survey Replication (NCS-R). *Depression and Anxiety*, 29(9), 797–806. doi:10.1002/Da.21924

Gilman, S. E., Ni, M. Y., Dunn, E. C., Breslau, J., McLaughlin, K. A., Smoller, J. W., & Perlis, R. H. (2014). Contributions of the social environment to first-onset and recurrent mania. *Molecular Psychiatry.* Advance online publication. doi:10.1038/mp.2014.36

Goldstein, J. M., Buka, S. L., Seidman, L. J., & Tsuang, M. T. (2010). Specificity of familial transmission of schizophrenia psychosis spectrum and affective psychoses in the New England Family Study's high-risk design. *Archives of General Psychiatry, 67*(5), 458–467.

Goodwin, F., & Jamison, K. (2007). *Manic-depressive illness* (2nd ed.). Oxford: Oxford University Press.

Gore, F. M., Bloem, P. J., Patton, G. C., Ferguson, J., Joseph, V., Coffey, C.,...Mathers, C. D. (2011). Global burden of disease in young people aged 10–24 years: A systematic analysis. *Lancet, 377*(9783), 2093–2102. doi:10.1016/S0140-6736(11)60512-6

Gottesman, I. I., & Gould, T. D. (2003). The endophenotype concept in psychiatry: Etymology and strategic intentions. *American Journal of Psychiatry, 160*(4), 636–645.

Grant, B. F., Goldstein, R. B., Chou, S. P., Huang, B., Stinson, F. S., Dawson, D. A.,...Compton, W. M. (2009). Sociodemographic and psychopathologic predictors of first incidence of *DSM-IV* substance use, mood and anxiety disorders: Results from the Wave 2 National Epidemiologic Survey on Alcohol and Related Conditions. *Mol Psychiatry, 14*(11), 1051–1066. doi:10.1038/mp.2008.41

Grant, B. F., Stinson, F. S., Hasin, D. S., Dawson, D. A., Chou, P., Ruan, W. J., & Huang, B. (2005). Prevalence, correlates, and comorbidity of bipolar I disorder and axis I and II disorders: Results from the National Epidemiologic Survey on Alcohol and Related Conditions. *Journal of Clinical Psychiatry, 66*(10), 1205–1215.

Gureje, O., Lasebikan, V. O., Kola, L., & Makanjuola, V. A. (2006). Lifetime and 12-month prevalence of mental disorders in the Nigerian Survey of Mental Health and Well-Being. *British Journal of Psychiatry, 188*, 465–471.

Hoertel, N., Le Strat, Y., Angst, J., & Dubertret, C. (2013). Subthreshold bipolar disorder in a U.S. national representative sample: Prevalence, correlates and perspectives for psychiatric nosography. *Journal of Affective Disorders, 146*(3), 338–347. doi:10.1016/j.jad.2012.09.016

Jacobi, F., Wittchen, H. U., Holting, C., Hofler, M., Pfister, H., Muller, N., & Lieb, R. (2004). Prevalence, co-morbidity and correlates of mental disorders in the general population: results from the German Health Interview and Examination Survey (GHS). *Psychol Med, 34*(4), 597–611.

Johnson, J. G., Cohen, P., & Brook, J. S. (2000). Associations between bipolar disorder and other psychiatric disorders during adolescence and early adulthood: A community-based longitudinal investigation. *American Journal of Psychiatry, 157*(10), 1679–1681.

Karam, E. G., Mneimneh, Z. N., Dimassi, H., Fayyad, J. A., Karam, A. N., Nasser, S. C.,...Kessler, R. C. (2008). Lifetime prevalence of mental disorders in Lebanon: First onset, treatment, and exposure to war. *PLos Medicine, 5*(4), 579–586. doi:10.1371/journal.pmed.0050061

Kawakami, N., Takeshima, T., Ono, Y., Uda, H., Hata, Y., Nakane, Y.,...Kikkawa, T. (2005). Twelve-month prevalence, severity, and treatment of common mental disorders in communities in Japan: preliminary finding from the World Mental Health Japan Survey 2002–2003. *Psychiatry and Clinical Neurosciences, 59*(4), 441–452.

Kessler, R. C., Akiskal, H. S., Angst, J., Guyer, M., Hirschfeld, R. M. A., Merikangas, K. R., & Stang, P. E. (2006). Validity of the assessment of bipolar spectrum disorders in the WHOCIDI 3.0. *Journal of Affective Disorders, 96*(3), 259–269. doi:10.1016/j.jad.2006.08.018

Kessler, R. C., Avenevoli, S., Costello, J., Green, J. G., Gruber, M. J., McLaughlin, K. A.,...Merikangas, K. R. (2012a). Severity of 12-month *DSM-IV* disorders in the National Comorbidity Survey Replication Adolescent Supplement. *Archives of General Psychiatry, 69*(4), 381–389.

Kessler, R. C., Avenevoli, S., Costello, E. J., Georgiades, K., Green, J. G., Gruber, M. J.,...Merikangas, K. R. (2012b). Prevalence, persistence, and sociodemographic correlates of *DSM-IV* disorders in the National Comorbidity Survey Replication Adolescent Supplement. *Archives of General Psychiatry, 69*(4), 372–380. doi:0.1001/archgenpsychiatry.2011.160

Kessler, R. C., Petukhova, M., Sampson, N. A., Zaslavsky, A. M., & Wittchen, H. U. (2012c). Twelve-month and lifetime prevalence and lifetime morbid risk of anxiety and mood disorders in the United States. *International journal of methods in psychiatric research, 21*(3), 169–184.

Kozloff, N., Cheung, A. H., Schaffer, A., Cairney, J., Dewa, C. S., Veldhuizen, S.,...Levitt, A. J. (2010). Bipolar disorder among adolescents and young adults: Results from an epidemiological sample. *Journal of Affective Disorders, 125*(1–3), 350–354. doi:10.1016/j.jad.2010.02.120

Laursen, T. M., Munk-Olsen, T., & Gasse, C. (2011). Chronic somatic comorbidity and excess mortality due to natural causes in persons with schizophrenia or bipolar affective disorder. *PLoS One, 6*(9): e24597.

Laursen, T. M., Munk-Olsen, T., Nordentoft, M., & Bo Mortensen, P. (2007). A comparison of selected risk factors for unipolar depressive disorder, bipolar affective disorder, schizoaffective disorder, and schizophrenia from a Danish population-based cohort. *Journal of Clinical Psychiatry, 68*(11), 1673–1681.

Lee, S., Tsang, A., Zhang, M. Y., Huang, Y. Q., He, Y. L., Liu, Z. R.,...Kessler, R. C. (2007). Lifetime prevalence and inter-cohort variation in DSM-IV disorders in metropolitan China. *Psychol Med, 37*(1), 61–71. doi:10.1017/s0033291706008993

Lee, S. H., Ripke, S., Neale, B. M., Faraone, S. V., Purcell, S. M., Perlis, R. H.,...Genetic, I. I. B. D. (2013). Genetic relationship between five psychiatric disorders estimated from genome-wide SNPs. *Nature Genetics, 45*(9), 984–994. doi:10.1038/Ng.2711

Levinson, D., Zilber, N., Lerner, Y., Grinshpoon, A., & Levav, I. (2007). Prevalence of mood and anxiety disorders in the community: results from the Israel National Health Survey. *Isr J Psychiatry Relat Sci, 44*(2), 94–103.

Lewinsohn, P. M., Klein, D. N., & Seeley, J. R. (2000). Bipolar disorder during adolescence and young adulthood in a community sample. *Bipolar Disorders, 2*(3), 281–293.

Lewinsohn, P. M., Seeley, J. R., Buckley, M. E., & Klein, D. N. (2002). Bipolar disorder in adolescence and young adulthood. *Child & Adolescent Psychiatry Clinics of North America, 11*(3), 461–475.

Lichtenstein, P., Yip, B. H., Bjork, C., Pawitan, Y., Cannon, T. D., Sullivan, P. F., & Hultman, C. M. (2009). Common genetic determinants of schizophrenia and bipolar disorder in Swedish families: A population-based study. *Lancet, 373*(9659), 234–239.

Malhotra, D., & Sebat, J. (2012). CNVs: Harbingers of a rare variant revolution in psychiatric genetics. *Cell, 148*(6), 1223–1241.

McGuffin, P., Rijsdijk, F., Andrew, M., Sham, P., Katz, R., & Cardno, A. (2003). The heritability of bipolar affective disorder and the genetic relationship to unipolar depression. *Archives of General Psychiatry, 60*(5), 497–502.

McIntyre, R. S., Konarski, J. Z., Soczynska, J. K., Wilkins, K., Panjwani, G., Bouffard, B.,...Kennedy, S. H. (2006). Medical comorbidity in bipolar disorder: Implications for functional outcomes and health service utilization. *Psychiatric Services, 57*(8), 1140–1144.

Medina-Mora, M. E., Borges, G., Benjet, C., Lara, C., & Berglund, P. (2007). Psychiatric disorders in Mexico: lifetime prevalence in a nationally representative sample. *The British Journal of Psychiatry, 190*(6), 521–528.

Merikangas, K. R., Akiskal, H. S., Angst, J., Greenberg, P. E., Hirschfeld, R. M., Petukhova, M., & Kessler, R. C. (2007). Lifetime and 12-month prevalence of bipolar spectrum disorder in the National Comorbidity Survey replication. *Archives of General Psychiatry, 64*(5), 543–552. doi:10.1001/archpsyc.64.5.543

Merikangas, K. R., Cui, L., Heaton, L., Nakamura, E., Roca, C., Ding, J.,...Angst, J. (2013). Independence of familial transmission of mania and depression: Results of the NIMH family study of affective spectrum disorders. *Molecular Psychiatry*, 19(2), 214–219.

Merikangas, K. R., Cui, L. H., Kattan, G., Carlson, G. A., Youngstrom, E. A., & Angst, J. (2012). Mania with and without depression in a community sample of US adolescents. *Archives of General Psychiatry*, 69(9), 943–951. doi:10.1001/archgenpsychiatry.2012.38

Merikangas, K. R., He, J. P., Burstein, M., Swanson, S. A., Avenevoli, S., Cui, L.,...Swendsen, J. (2010). Lifetime prevalence of mental disorders in U.S. adolescents: Results from the National Comorbidity Survey Replication–Adolescent Supplement (NCS-A). *Journal of the American Academy of Child & Adolescent Psychiatry*, 49(10), 980–989.

Merikangas, K. R., He, J. P., Burstein, M., Swendsen, J., Avenevoli, S., Case, B.,...Olfson, M. (2011). Service utilization for lifetime mental disorders in U.S. adolescents: Results of the National Comorbidity Survey Adolescent Supplement (NCS-A). *Journal of the American Academy of Child & Adolescent Psychiatry*, 50(1), 32–45.

Merikangas, K. R., He, J. P., Rapoport, J., Vitiello, B., & Olfson, M. (2013). Medication use in US youth with mental disorders. *JAMA Pediatrics*, 167(2), 141–148.

Merikangas, K. R., Herrell, R., Swendsen, J., Rossler, W., Ajdacic-Gross, V., & Augst, J. (2008). Specificity of bipolar spectrum conditions in the comorbidity of mood and substance use disorders. *Archives of General Psychiatry*, 65(1), 47–52.

Merikangas, K. R., Jin, R., He, J. P., Kessler, R. C., Lee, S., Sampson, N. A.,...Zarkov, Z. (2011). Prevalence and correlates of bipolar spectrum disorder in the world mental health survey initiative. *Archives of General Psychiatry*, 68(3), 241–251. doi:10.1001/archgenpsychiatry.2011.12

Merikangas, K. R., & Tohen, M. (2011). Epidemiology of bipolar disorder in adults and children. In M. T. Tsuang, M. Tohen, & P. Jones (Eds.), *Textbook of psychiatric epidemiology* (3rd ed., pp. 329–342). West Sussex, UK: Wiley.

Mortensen, P. B., Pedersen, C. B., Melbye, M., Mors, O., & Ewald, H. (2003). Individual and familial risk factors for bipolar affective disorders in Denmark. *Archives of General Psychiatry*, 60(12), 1209–1215. doi:10.1001/archpsyc.60.12.1209

Nierenberg, A. A., Akiskal, H. S., Angst, J., Hirschfeld, R. M., Merikangas, K. R., Petukhova, M., & Kessler, R. C. (2010). Bipolar disorder with frequent mood episodes in the National Comorbidity Survey Replication (NCS-R). *Molecular Psychiatry*, 15(11), 1075–1087. doi:10.1038/Mp.2009.61

Phillips, M. R., Zhang, J., Shi, Q., Song, Z., Ding, Z., Pang, S.,...Wang, Z. (2009). Prevalence, treatment, and associated disability of mental disorders in four provinces in China during 2001–05: an epidemiological survey. *Lancet*, 373(9680), 2041–2053. doi:10.1016/S0140-6736(09)60660-7

Rasic, D., Hajek, T., Alda, M., & Uher, R. (2014). Risk of mental illness in offspring of parents with schizophrenia, bipolar disorder, and major depressive disorder: A meta-analysis of family high-risk studies. *Schizophrenia Bulletin*, 40(1), 28–38. doi:10.1093/schbul/sbt114

Roberts, R. E., Roberts, C. R., & Xing, Y. (2007). Rates of *DSM-IV* psychiatric disorders among adolescents in a large metropolitan area. *Journal of Psychiatric Research*, 41(11), 959–967. doi:10.1016/j.jpsychires.2006.09.006

Sala, R., Goldstein, B. I., Morcillo, C., Liu, S. M., Castellanos, M., & Blanco, C. (2012). Course of comorbid anxiety disorders among adults with bipolar disorder in the U.S. population. *Journal of Psychiatric Research*, 46(7), 865–872. doi:10.1016/j.jpsychires.2012.03.024

Saunders, K., Merikangas, K., Low, N. C. P., Von Korff, M., & Kessler, R. C. (2008). Impact of comorbidity on headache-related disability. *Neurology*, 70(7), 538–547.

Scott, K. M., Smith, D. R., & Ellis, P. M. (2010). Prospectively ascertained child maltreatment and its association with *DSM-IV* mental disorders in young adults. *Archives of General Psychiatry*, 67(7), 712–719.

Sklar, P., Ripke, S., Scott, L. J., Andreassen, O. A., Cichon, S., Craddock, N.,...D, P. G. C. B. (2011). Large-scale genome-wide association analysis of bipolar disorder identifies a new susceptibility locus near ODZ4. *Nature Genetics*, 43(10), 977–U162. doi:10.1038/Ng.943

Sklar, P., Smoller, J. W., Fan, J., Ferreira, M. A., Perlis, R. H., Chambert, K.,...Purcell, S. M. (2008). Whole-genome association study of bipolar disorder. *Molecular Psychiatry*, 13(6), 558–569.

Smoller, J. W., & Gardner-Schuster, E. (2007). Genetics of bipolar disorder. *Current Psychiatry Report*, 9(6), 504–511.

Subramaniam, M., Abdin, E., Vaingankar, J. A., & Chong, S. A. (2013). Prevalence, correlates, comorbidity and severity of bipolar disorder: Results from the Singapore Mental Health Study. *Journal of Affective Disorders*, 146(2), 189–196. doi:10.1016/j.jad.2012.09.002

Sugaya, L., Hasin, D. S., Olfson, M., Lin, K. H., Grant, B. F., & Blanco, C. (2012). Child physical abuse and adult mental health: A national study. *Journal of Traumatic Stress*, 25(4), 384–392. doi:10.1002/Jts.21719

Swendsen, J., Conway, K. P., Degenhardt, L., Glantz, M., Jin, R., Merikangas, K. R.,...Kessler, R. C. (2010). Mental disorders as risk factors for substance use, abuse and dependence: Results from the 10-year follow-up of the National Comorbidity Survey. *Addiction*, 105(6), 1117–1128.

Tsuchiya, K. J., Agerbo, E., Byrne, M., & Mortensen, P. B. (2004). Higher socio-economic status of parents may increase risk for bipolar disorder in the offspring. *Psychological Medicine*, 34(5), 787–793.

Tsuchiya, K. J., Byrne, M., & Mortensen, P. B. (2003). Risk factors in relation to an emergence of bipolar disorder: a systematic review. *Bipolar Disorder*, 5(4), 231–242.

Van Meter, A. R., Moreira, A. L. R., & Youngstrom, E. A. (2011). Meta-analysis of epidemiologic studies of pediatric bipolar disorder. *Journal of Clinical Psychiatry*, 72(9), 1250–1256. doi:10.4088/Jcp.10m06290

Vandeleur, C., Rothen, S., Gholam-Rezaee, M., Castelao, E., Vidal, S., Favre, S.,...Preisig, M. (2012). Mental disorders in offspring of parents with bipolar and major depressive disorders. *Bipolar Disorders*, 14(6), 641–653.

Vandeleur, C. L., Merikangas, K. R., Strippoli, M. P., Castelao, E., & Preisig, M. (2014). Specificity of psychosis, mania and major depression in a contemporary family study. *Molecular Psychiatry*, 19, 209–213.

Verhulst, F. C., van der Ende, J., Ferdinand, R. F., & Kasius, M. C. (1997). The prevalence of *DSM-III-R* diagnoses in a national sample of Dutch adolescents. *Archives of General Psychiatry*, 54(4), 329–336.

Waraich, P., Goldner, E. M., Somers, J. M., & Hsu, L. (2004). Prevalence and incidence studies of mood disorders: A systematic review of the literature. *Canadian Journal of Psychiatry/Revue Canadienne de Psychiatrie*, 49(2), 124–138.

Wells, J. E., Browne, M. A. O., Scott, K. M., McGee, M. A., Baxter, J., & Kokaua, J. (2006). Prevalence, interference with life and severity of 12 month DSM-IV disorders in Te Rau Hinengaro: The New Zealand Mental Health Survey. *Australian and New Zealand Journal of Psychiatry*, 40(10), 845–854. doi:10.1080/j.1440-1614.2006.01903.x

Wells, J. E., McGee, M. A., Scott, K. M., & Browne, M. A. O. (2010). Bipolar disorder with frequent mood episodes in the New Zealand Mental Health Survey. *Journal of Affective Disorders*, 126(1–2), 65–74. doi:10.1016/j.jad.2010.02.136

Wilde, A., Chan, H. N., Rahman, B., Meiser, B., Mitchell, P. B., Schofield, P. R., & Green, M. J. (2014). A meta-analysis of the risk of major affective disorder in relatives of individuals affected by major depressive disorder or bipolar disorder. *Journal of Affective Disorders*, 158, 37–47. doi:10.1016/j.jad.2014.01.014

Wittchen, H. U., Nelson, C. B., & Lachner, G. (1998). Prevalence of mental disorders and psychosocial impairments in adolescents and young adults. *Psychological Medicine*, 28(1), 109–126.

Wozniak, J., Faraone, S. V., Martelon, M., McKillop, H. N., & Biederman, J. (2012). Further evidence for robust familiality of pediatric bipolar I disorder: Results from a very large controlled family study of pediatric bipolar I disorder and a meta-analysis. *Journal of Clinical Psychiatry*, 73(10), 1328–1334. doi:10.4088/Jcp.12m07770

Youngstrom, E., Meyers, O., Demeter, C., Youngstrom, J., Morello, L., Piiparinen, R., . . . Findling, R. (2005). Comparing diagnostic checklists for pediatric bipolar disorder in academic and community mental health settings. *Bipolar Disorders*, 7(6), 507–517.

Zutshi, A., Eckert, K. A., Hawthorne, G., Taylor, A. W., & Goldney, R. D. (2011). Changes in the prevalence of bipolar disorders between 1998 and 2008 in an Australian population. *Bipolar Disorders*, 13(2), 182–188. doi:10.1111/j.1399-5618.2011.00907.x

3.

PRESENTATION, CLINICAL COURSE, AND DIAGNOSTIC ASSESSMENT OF BIPOLAR DISORDER

Erica Snook, Keitha Moseley-Dendy, and Robert M. A. Hirschfeld

HISTORY OF THE DIAGNOSIS OF BIPOLAR DISORDER

The concepts of depression and mania date back over 2,000 years when Hippocrates attributed melancholia and mania to an excess of black bile and yellow bile, respectively. However, modern notions of bipolar disorder began with Emil Kraepelin's (1896) proposal that endogenous (i.e., due to altered physiologic function) psychoses be divided into two distinct categories—"manic-depressive insanity" and "dementia precox." He described manic-depressive insanity as having an episodic course with a better prognosis in contrast to the deteriorating course of dementia precox. This view of manic-depressive illness was widely accepted and is adhered to among today's clinicians.

In 1957 Leonhard coined the terms "bipolar" referring to patients who had both manic and depressive episodes and "monopolars," who had only depressive episodes. Jules Angst (1966) and Winokur, Clayton, and Reich (1969) independently proposed this distinction as well and included case studies and family history data. This separation of recurrent unipolar depression from bipolar illness was not universally accepted. One proponent of including recurrent unipolar and bipolar patients into the simple category of manic depressive illness was Fredrick Goodwin (Goodwin & Jamison, 2007). However a variety of clinical and genetic studies have not supported this position.

The third edition of the *Diagnostic and Statistical Manual of Mental Disorders* (*DSM-III*; American Psychiatric Association, 1980) was consistent with the separation of bipolar and unipolar disorder, and bipolar disorder was separated from major depressive depression in the "Mood Disorders" chapter. In the *DSM-III*, the only criterion distinguishing bipolar disorder was a history of mania. Around this time, Dunner, Gershon, and Goodwin

(1976) suggested the classification of bipolar patients into the categories bipolar I and bipolar II. Bipolar I required an episode of mania, whereas bipolar II required a history of hypomanic (symptoms interfered with normal functioning but were not severe enough to require hospitalization) and depressive episodes but no manic episodes.

The diagnosis of bipolar disorder has continued to evolve over the years. In the fifth edition of the *Diagnostic and Statistical Manual of Mental Disorders* (*DSM-5*; American Psychiatric Association, 2013), bipolar disorder has its own chapter, completely separate from the depressive disorders.

PRESENTATIONS OF BIPOLAR DISORDER

MANIA AND HYPOMANIA

General

In mania and hypomania, all aspects of being are accelerated and sharpened. Thought processes move swiftly. The rapid pace that may initially be invigorating can quickly lead to frustration. Activity parallels the increased mental activity, and manic patients seem to be fueled by an infinite reservoir of energy, bouncing quickly from one activity to another without need for rest.

Mood

Mood disturbance is a core feature of mania and hypomania and is usually elevated or irritable. Mood may also be described as angry, grandiose, expansive, or euphoric. As an episode progresses, irritability may become more predominant. Mood may change abruptly from euphoria to rage due to low frustration tolerance.

Behavior/psychomotor activity

Overactivity became a core criterion in the *DSM-5* for mania and hypomania because it occurs even more frequently in mania than in elevated mood. Specifically, overactivity in mania refers to increased time spent walking, increased goal-directed behavior, and socially disinhibited interactions (Perry et al., 2010). Several studies demonstrated the presence of overactivity to be the most highly correlated symptom with the diagnosis of mania or hypomania (Akiskal et al., 2001, Angst et al., 2003, Benazzi, 2007).

Social behaviors are strongly affected by mania. While manic patients are often eager to interact with others, they may not realize if they are behaving inappropriately or making others uncomfortable. Examples of impaired social behaviors in mania include inattention to social cues, inappropriate familiarity with strangers, overconfidence in abilities or opinions, and inability to allow others to speak in the conversation.

Sleep

Manic and hypomanic patients sleep less and have a decreased need for sleep. They may only sleep two to three hours per night yet feel alert and energetic in the morning. This differs from insomnia, whereby patients have difficulty sleeping and feel tired and sluggish the next day.

Speech

Speech may be pressured and increased in volume and rate. Patients feel compelled to share their thoughts and may be difficult to redirect or interrupt, often at the expense of irritating others around them.

Perceptual disturbances and thought content

By definition, psychotic features may only be present in mania, not hypomania. Two-thirds of patients with bipolar I have a lifetime history of at least one psychotic symptom (Goodwin & Jamison, 2007). Delusions are the most common psychotic symptom. Patients may become so preoccupied with religious, political, financial, or romantic thoughts that they become delusional. Examples include delusions of special or supernatural abilities or powers, carrying a divine message from God, wealth, or aristocratic ancestry. Hallucinations are usually fleeting and part of a delusion, such as a command hallucination from God.

Hallucinations are the symptom that disappear the fastest during recovery, followed by delusions (Goodwin & Jamison, 2007).

Disturbances of thought

Thinking is accelerated, distractible, and tangential. Patients may report feeling as if their thoughts are racing though their mind more quickly than they can be expressed. They often describe very rapid thoughts as a flight of ideas. In severe mania, as thoughts flow more quickly, associations may become loosened.

Alertness and orientation are not affected unless mania is severe. In the manic or depressed state, bipolar patients were found to demonstrate significant impairments in verbal memory and executive functioning (Mur, Portella, Martinez-Aran, Pifarre, & Vieta, 2008). Examples of impaired executive functioning include problems with keeping track of time, doing more than one thing at once, making plans, waiting to speak until called on in groups, knowing when to ask for help, and evaluating and reflecting on ideas.

Impulse control

In general, manic patients are very impulsive. Examples of impulsive behaviors frequent in mania include shopping sprees, hypersexual behavior, poor business investments, gambling, drug use, legal problems, and violent or assaultive behavior.

Insight and judgment

Both manic and hypomanic patients usually lack insight into their condition and often do not believe they need treatment. Impairments in judgment are also a feature of mania; examples are included in the previous section.

DEPRESSION

General

Although mania and hypomania are the signature and most recognizable characteristics of bipolar disorder, depression is its most frequent clinical presentation. This was dramatically demonstrated in a long-term follow-up study of 146 patients with bipolar disorder. Over 13 years, they spent about 40% of the time depressed. In contrast, they were manic or hypomanic less than 9% of the time and asymptomatic about half of the time (Judd et al., 2002).

Table 3.1. INDICATORS OF BIPOLAR DISORDER
IN DEPRESSED PATIENTS

1. Family history of bipolar disorder
2. Earlier onset of illness (early 20s)
3. Numerous past episodes
4. History of psychiatric hospitalization
5. History of suicide attempt
6. History of treatment-resistant depression
7. Seasonality
8. Mixed states
9. Mood reactivity
10. Switching on antidepressants

Cross-sectionally, bipolar depression is often indistinguishable from unipolar depression. Therefore a careful clinical history is crucial, including the age when symptoms were first noted, frequency of depressions, history of manic symptoms, and family history of bipolar disorder.

While there are no pathognomonic characteristics of bipolar depression compared to unipolar depression, certain characteristics tend to be more common to each type of depression. In general, in bipolar I depression, "atypical" depressive features such as hypersomnia, hyperphagia, and psychomotor retardation are more common than in unipolar depression (Mitchell, Goodwin, Johnson, & Hirschfeld, 2008). Psychotic features and mood lability are also more frequently found in bipolar depression (Mitchell et al., 2008).

Mood

The core mood disturbance is sadness, but it may also be experienced as apathy or "flatness," anxiety, or irritability. In general, there is no difference in the severity of bipolar versus unipolar depression (Mitchell et al., 2001). There is also no difference in the severity of the depressed phase of bipolar I and bipolar II disorder (Goodwin & Jamison, 2007).

Behavior/psychomotor activity

Patients with bipolar disorder when depressed are more likely to experience neurovegetative symptoms, particularly hypersomnia, increased appetite, and weight gain. Conversely, patients with unipolar depression are more likely to experience insomnia, either as trouble falling asleep or early morning awakenings (Mitchell et al., 2008).

Although psychomotor changes are rare in both unipolar and bipolar depression, bipolar I patients are significantly more likely to have this symptom, especially psychomotor retardation (Parker, Roy, Wilhelm, Mitchell, &

Hadzi-Pavlovic, 2000). Examples of psychomotor retardation include difficulty getting out of bed in the morning, feeling even the smallest task is too difficult or requires too much energy, feeling weak or sluggish, trouble concentrating, or having trouble making decisions. Leaden paralysis is a very severe form of psychomotor retardation where the limbs feel impossibly heavy and even minor tasks of daily activities seem impossible.

Patients with bipolar II disorder may be less likely to demonstrate psychomotor retardation (Benazzi, 2002). In a study of 379 bipolar II depressed and 271 unipolar depressed outpatients, psychomotor agitation occurred more frequently in the bipolar II group (Benazzi, 2002). Examples of psychomotor agitation include restlessness, pacing, hand-wringing, rapid speech, or racing thoughts.

Speech

Consistent with increased psychomotor slowing, patients may have increased latencies of response, slowed rate of speech, decreased speech volume, or poverty of speech, or they may answer questions with one-word answers (Mitchell et al., 2008, Sadock, Sadock, & Ruiz, 2009).

Disturbances of perception

Psychotic symptoms occur less often in depressive episodes than in manic episodes (Goodwin & Jamison, 2007, Sadock et al., 2009) but are more frequent in bipolar depression compared to unipolar depression (Mitchell et al., 2008). The primary psychotic symptom encountered in bipolar depressed patients is mood-congruent delusions of guilt, sinfulness, poverty, illness, or prosecution (Sadock & Sadock, 2007). Delusional depressions, especially in younger people, marked by severe psychomotor retardation or even stupor, raise suspicion for the diagnosis of bipolar disorder (Sadock et al., 2009).

Disturbances of thought

Thinking may be slowed, easily confused, distractible, and focused on ruminating. The core cognitive changes in depression or the "cognitive triad" as described by Aaron Beck are negative thoughts about the self, surroundings, and future. Automatic thoughts, also called cognitive distortions, occur due to these negative beliefs and cause the patient to negatively misinterpret external events (Sadock & Sadock, 2007).

Insight and judgment

Insight remains intact, but pessimism and negativity are heightened. Depressed patients may overemphasize their negative views and may believe improvement is impossible (Sadock & Sadock, 2007).

Other characteristics

Anhedonia, or the inability to experience pleasure, is also an important characteristic of bipolar depression. One woman's personal recollection of an episode of bipolar depression painfully reflects this sentiment: "I was unbearably miserable and seemingly incapable of any kind of joy or enthusiasm...Everything that once was sparkling was now flat" (Jamison, 1995, p. 110). Seasonality, with worsening of depression in the fall and winter and increased propensity for mania in the spring and summer, is typical of bipolar disorder and other cyclic depressions.

MIXED EPISODES/FEATURES

During a manic or depressed episode, patients often experience symptoms from the opposite pole. For example, patients who are primarily depressed may complain of symptoms related to mania, such as racing thoughts, decreased need for sleep, or impulsivity. Similarly, patients who are primarily manic or hypomanic may complain of depressive symptoms such as sadness, anhedonia, and decreased energy. Whether the predominant polarity of the mood episode is manic or depressive, a mixed episode is associated with a higher risk of suicide (Swann et al., 2013). The coupling of hopelessness with impulsivity and increased activation substantially increases (Swann et al., 2013).

A person's temperament, or innate personality, may create a predisposition for mixed states (Perugi et al., 1997). A patient with a depressive temperament but suffering from acute mania may present with symptoms of both depression and mania, which could be categorized as mania with mixed features. The same theory can apply to those with hyperthymic temperaments and depressive episodes presenting as depression with mixed features. In a controlled study of 118 patients with mania and 143 patients with mixed states, hyperthymic temperament was most strongly associated with mania (56.8% of manic patients had hyperthymic temperaments). Both depressive and hyperthymic temperaments were associated with an increased prevalence of mixed episodes (Perugi et al., 1997). A hyperthymic temperament was found in 28% of patients with mixed episodes, and a depressive temperament was found in 31.5%. This study concluded that a person's temperament, when opposite to the polarity of his or her mood episode, may contribute to the affective instability that characterizes mixed states.

Manic or hypomanic with mixed features

In the past, mania with three or more depressive symptoms was called dysphoric mania. The episodes included many of the manic symptoms such as racing thoughts, pressured speech, irritability, and impulsivity but in the absence of euphoria and grandiosity. A patient with mania or hypomania with mixed features may present with irritability and the increased speed of thought and speech typical of mania but also complain of depressed mood, increased guilt, anhedonia, and poor energy. Instead of feeling triumphant and invincible, a patient with mania or hypomania with mixed features may feel very edgy and uncomfortable.

Depressed with mixed features

Distinguishing depressed episodes with mixed features from episodes of major depression with agitation or irritability is a difficult task, but certain symptoms can help differentiate the two. Increased goal-directed activity (instead of purely increased activity of any kind or restlessness), decreased need for sleep (not insomnia), and impulsivity point toward the diagnosis of a depressed episode with mixed features (Ketter, 2010).

According to the International Society for Bipolar Disorders Task Force, anxiety symptoms are very common in both "pure" depression and episodes of depression with mixed features (Swann et al., 2013). There is no change in the frequency of psychotic symptoms in depressed episodes with mixed features as opposed to pure depression, but if they do occur, the content of the psychotic symptoms varies. In patients with bipolar I, mood-incongruent psychotic symptoms occur more often in a mixed episode than they do in a purely depressed episode (Swann et al., 2013).

DIAGNOSTIC AND STATISTICAL MANUAL FOR MENTAL DISORDERS, FIFTH EDITION

The preceding section describes key components of the clinical presentation of manic, hypomanic, and depressive episodes and mixed state. This section describes how the symptoms are organized into discreet diagnoses according to the *DSM-5* (American Psychiatric Association, 2013).

In the *DSM-5* for the first time, bipolar and related disorders have been separated from depressive disorders and given their own chapter. The rationale for this change was differences in symptomatology, family history, and genetics. Bipolar disorders are longitudinally defined disorders of mood that include episodes of highs characterized by euphoric, elevated, expansive, or irritable mood and increased energy and activity and depressive episodes characterized by depressed mood and/or loss of interest in pleasure and associated symptoms. Included diagnoses are bipolar I disorder, bipolar II disorder, cyclothymic disorder, substance/medication-induced bipolar and related disorder, bipolar and related disorder due to another medical problem, other specified bipolar and related disorder, and unspecified bipolar and related disorder.

BIPOLAR I DISORDER

To receive a diagnosis of bipolar I disorder, the person must have experienced a manic episode. Patients may also experience hypomanic or major depressive episodes, but they are not necessary for the diagnosis.

A manic episode is defined as "a distinct period of abnormally and persistently elevated, expansive, or irritable mood and abnormally and persistently increased goal-directed activity or energy, lasting at least one week and present most of the day, nearly every day (or any duration if hospitalization is necessary)" (Sadock & Sadock, 2007). The inclusion of increased goal-directed activity or energy as a core criterion for manic episode is new to *DSM-5* and represents a step forward. Thus it is necessary for a manic episode to have not only a mood disturbance but also a substantial change in behavior.

In addition to the core mood and activity criteria, an individual must exhibit at least three of other associated symptoms, including increased self-esteem or grandiosity, decreased need for sleep, being more talkative than usual or feeling pressure to keep talking, flight of ideas or subjective experience where thoughts are racing, distractibility, increase in goal-directed activity or psychomotor agitation, and/or excessive involvement in activities that have a high potential for painful consequences (e.g., unstrained buying sprees, sexual misbehavior, or foolish, risky business investments).

The mood disturbance must be sufficiently severe to cause marked impairment in social or occupational functioning or to necessitate hospitalization. It must also not be attributable to the physiological effects of a substance or a medical condition.

BIPOLAR II DISORDER

To receive a diagnosis of bipolar II disorder, the individual must have experienced at least one hypomanic episode and at least one major depressive episode. The individual may not have ever experienced a manic episode. Furthermore, the occurrence of the hypomanic episodes and expressive episodes may not be better explained by schizoaffective disorder, schizophrenia, schizophreniform, delusional disorder, or other specified or unspecified schizophrenia spectrum and other psychotic disorder.

A hypomanic episode is similar to a manic episode. It requires a distinct period of abnormally and persistently elevated, expansive, or irritable mood and abnormally persistently increased activity or energy, lasting at least four consecutive days and present most of the day nearly every day. It also requires at least three (four if the mood is only irritable) associated symptoms described previously in the definition of a manic episode. The episode must be associated with an unequivocal change in functioning that is uncharacteristic of the individual when not symptomatic. This change in mood and functioning must be observable by others.

However, the episode must not be severe enough to cause marked impairment in social or occupational functioning or to necessitate hospitalization. It must not include psychotic features. Furthermore, the episode may not be attributable to the physiological effects of a substance (e.g., of drug abuse, medication, or other treatment). An important clarification is that a hypomanic episode occurring during antidepressive treatment may be considered diagnostic for bipolar II if it persists at a fully syndromal level beyond the physiological effects of the treatment.

A major depressive episode requires at least five symptoms occurring within the same two-week period and represents a change in previous functioning. At least one of the symptoms must be either a depressed mood or loss of interest or pleasure. Other symptoms include depressed mood most of the day, nearly every day, markedly diminished interest or pleasure in almost all activity, significant weight loss when not dieting or weight gain or decreased and increase in appetite nearly every day, insomnia or hypersomnia nearly every day, psychomotor agitation or retardation nearly every day, fatigue or loss of energy nearly every day, feelings of worthlessness or excessive or inappropriate guilt nearly every day, diminished ability to think or concentrate or indecisiveness nearly every day, and recurrent thoughts of death, recurrent suicidal ideation without a specific plan, or a suicide attempt or a specific plan for committing suicide.

These symptoms must cause clinically significant distress and impairment in the social, occupational, or other important areas of functioning. The episode must not be attributable to the physiological effects of a substance or other medical condition.

An important change in *DSM-5* is that bereavement is not an exclusion for a major depressive episode. Thus if an individual meets criteria for a major depressive episode even if recently bereaved, then the diagnosis of a major depressive episode will be made.

CYCLOTHYMIC DISORDER

Cyclothymic disorder describes an individual who has experienced at least two years of both hypomanic and depressive periods without ever completely fulfilling the criteria for an episode of mania, hypomania, or major depression. To receive a diagnosis of cyclothymic disorder the individual must have had for at least two years numerous periods of hypomanic symptoms that do not meet full criteria for hypomanic episode and numerous periods of depressive symptoms that do not meet full criteria for major depressive disorder. The individual must have been experiencing hypomanic and depressive episodes at least half the time during the two years and had no period without symptoms lasting more than two months. The individual must not have experienced major depressive, manic, or hypomanic episode ever in his or her life. The symptoms may not be better explained by schizoaffective disorder, schizophrenia, schizophreniform disorder, delusional disorder, or other specified or unspecified schizophrenia spectrum or other psychotic disorder. Furthermore, the symptoms may not be attributable to the physiological effects of a substance or another medical condition. The symptoms must cause clinically significant distress or impairment in social, occupational, or important areas of functioning.

SUBSTANCE/MEDICATION-INDUCED BIPOLAR AND RELATED DISORDER

A diagnosis of substance/medication-induced bipolar and related disorder may be made when various substances or medical conditions lead to manic-like episodes. Specifically this occurs when there is a "prominent and persistent disturbance in mood that predominates in the clinical picture and is characterized by elevated, expansive, or irritable mood, with or without depressed mood, or markedly diminished interest or pleasure in all, or almost all activities" (From DSM 5 diagnostic criteria for substance/medication induced bipolar and related disorder, p. 142). This disturbance in mood must have occurred or developed during or soon after substance intoxication or withdrawal or after exposure to a medication. The involved substance or medication must be capable of producing these symptoms. The disturbance may not occur exclusively during the course of delirium and must cause clinical significant stress or impairment in social, occupational, or other important areas of functioning.

BIPOLAR AND RELATED DISORDER DUE TO ANOTHER MEDICAL CONDITION

This classification is similar to the substance/medication-induced bipolar and related disorder. To be diagnosed as having a bipolar and related disorder due to another medical condition requires a "prominent and persistent period of abnormally elevated, expansive, or irritable mood and abnormally increased activity or energy that predominates in the clinical picture" (From DSM 5 diagnostic criteria for bipolar and related disorder due to another medical condition, p. 145). This disturbance must be a direct pathophysiological consequence of another medical condition. Furthermore, the disturbance may not be better explained by another mental disorder, and it may not occur exclusively during the course of a delirium. As with other disorders, the disturbance must cause clinically significant distress or impairment in social, occupational, or other important areas of functioning or necessitate hospitalization.

OTHER SPECIFIED AND UNSPECIFIED BIPOLAR AND RELATED DISORDERS

These two categories include presentations characteristic of a bipolar or related disorder but do not meet the criteria of any of the previously described bipolar and related disorders. The reason for specifying why this condition is a bipolar or related disorder may or may not be included by the clinician.

Examples of other specified bipolar and related disorders are episodes of hypomania that are less than four days in duration or have fewer than three or four symptoms. Another example would be a history of hypomanic episodes without a history of major depressive disorders.

SPECIFIERS

DSM-5 includes a number of specifiers for bipolar and related disorders: anxious distress, mixed features, melancholic features, atypical features, psychotic features, catatonia, peripartum onset, and seasonal pattern.

As in the fourth edition (text revision) of the *Diagnostic and Statistical Manual of Mental Disorders* (*DSM-IV-TR*; American Psychiatric Association, 2000), rapid cycling is defined as the occurrence of at least four mood episodes in the previous twelve months.

The melancholic specifier is characterized by a loss of pleasure in nearly all activities, inability to respond to pleasurable stimuli, unchanging emotional expression, excessive or inappropriate guilt, early morning awakening, marked psychomotor retardation or agitation, and significant anorexia or weight loss. The atypical specifier is characterized by a brightened mood in response to positive events, increased sensitivity to rejection resulting in depressive overreaction to any perceived criticism or rejection, feelings of leaden paralysis or anergy, weight gain or increased appetite, and hypersomnia. In atypical depression, symptoms tend to worsen as the day progresses. The psychotic specifier is indicated in patients with delusions, often of having committed unpardonable sins or crimes, of harboring incurable or shameful disorders, or of being persecuted. Patients suffering from delusions may also have auditory or visual hallucinations such as hearing accusatory or condemning voices. If voices are heard in the absence of delusions, careful consideration should be given to whether the voices represent true hallucinations. The content of the delusions and or hallucinations may be consistent (mood-congruent psychotic features) or inconsistent (mood-incongruent psychotic features) with typical depressive themes. The catatonic specifier refers to a subgroup characterized by severe psychomotor retardation or excessive purposeless activity, withdrawal, and in some patients grimacing and mimicry of speech (echolalia) or movement (echopraxia). The seasonal pattern specifier applies to the recurrence of at least one type of episode (manic, hypomanic, or depressive) at a particular time of year (e.g., spring, winter).

The specifier with the most significant change from prior editions is mixed features. In *DSM-IV-TR* (American Psychiatric Association, 2000), a mixed episode required that criteria for a manic episode and a major depressive episode were met in full at the same time. However, many patients experience features of the both poles prominently during an episode but do not meet full criteria for the other pole episodes.

However, many patients experience prominent features of both poles during a single episode but do not meet criteria for both types of episodes. Therefore, the episode could not be labeled as mixed even though it was certainly not purely one type of episode. In the DSM 5, the mixed specifier replaces the mixed episode. For a manic or hypomanic episode with mixed specifier, full criteria are met for the manic or hypomanic episode. In addition, the individual must experience at least three of the following depressive symptoms occurring during the majority of days of the manic or hypomanic episode: prominent dysphoria or depressed mood, diminished interest or pleasure in all or almost all activities, psychomotor retardation nearly every day, feeling fatigue or loss of energy, feelings of worthlessness or excessive or inappropriate guilt, or recurrent thoughts of death, recurrent suicidal ideation without a specific plan, or a suicide attempt or specific plan for committing suicide.

A depressive episode with mixed features requires meeting full criteria for a major depressive episode and at least three manic or hypomanic symptoms present during the majority of days of the episode. These include elevated, expansive mood, inflated self-esteem or grandiosity, being more talkative than usual or feeling pressure to keep talking, flight of ideas or subjective experience, racing thoughts, increase in energy or goal-directed activity, increased or excessive involvement in activities that have a high potential for painful consequences, and decreased need for sleep. These mixed symptoms must not be attributable to the physiological effects of a substance.

Another addition is the anxious distress specifier. The anxious distress specifier is indicated when two or more of the following symptoms are present for the majority of days during the current or the most recent episode of mania, hypomania, or depression: feeling keyed up or tense, feeling unusually restless, difficulty concentrating because of worry, fear that something awful may happen, or feeling one may lose control of oneself. Based on the number of symptoms reported, the severity may be mild (two symptoms), moderate (three), moderate-severe (four or five), or severe (four or five with motor agitation). According to the *DSM-5*, high levels of anxiety are associated with increased risk of suicide, lengthier duration of illness, and greater risk of nonresponse to treatment.

ASSESSMENT

RATING SCALES

In the outpatient setting, patients with bipolar disorder are often indistinguishable from those with unipolar depression. Unipolar depression is much more prevalent (16.2%)

than bipolar spectrum disorders (4.4%), and, without appropriate evaluation, the patient with bipolar disorder may be misdiagnosed (Merikangas et al., 2007). Recognition of bipolar disorder in patients with depression may be improved by using screening instruments.

Screening instruments

Self-reported rating scales are helpful for efficient screening of patients presenting with depressive symptoms. A positive screen triggers the need for a comprehensive psychiatric evaluation. In the following list, tools described in 1 through 3 are screening instruments for bipolar disorder, and that described in number 4 is a screen for depression of any etiology.

1. The Mood Disorder Questionnaire (MDQ) is the most widely used screening instrument for bipolar disorder (Hirschfeld et al., 2000). It has been translated into 19 languages and cited in over 600 publications. It is a validated self-rated questionnaire that consists of 13 questions about manic and hypomanic symptoms the patient may have experienced in the past. It takes approximately 5 minutes to complete. In depressed samples, it has a sensitivity of 0.73 and specificity of 0.90.

2. The Hypomania/Mania Symptom Checklist (HCL-32; Angst et al., 2005) is another assessment used to screen for bipolar disorder. There are two introductory questions regarding the subject's current emotional state and usual mood and levels of energy and activity. Thirty-two questions follow, mostly regarding symptoms of mania and hypomania. It takes approximately 10 minutes to complete. In depressed samples it has a sensitivity of 0.80 and specificity of 0.51.

3. The Bipolar Spectrum Diagnostic Scale (BSDS) was created (Ghaemi et al., 2005) to better screen for bipolar II and bipolar not otherwise specified, but it also detects bipolar I with similar accuracy. For all bipolar spectrum disorders (bipolar I, II, and not otherwise specified), it has a sensitivity of 0.76 and specificity of 0.85. The BSDS is written in story format, with 19 sentences that describe symptoms of bipolar spectrum disorders. Following each sentence is a space for a checkmark. After reading the entire passage, test-takers are asked how much the passage describes them: *very well, fairly well, to some degree but not most,* or *not at all.* They are then asked to go back to the story and put a check after each sentence that definitely describes them. This test takes about 10 to 15 minutes to complete.

4. The Patient Health Questionnaire (PHQ-9) is used in the screening, diagnosis, and monitoring of depression occurring at the present time. It does not indicate whether the depression is part of bipolar disorder or major depression. The PHQ-9 differs from the MDQ and HCL-32 in that it focuses only on the depressive symptoms and only on the symptoms occurring at the present time, not on a lifelong basis. It has nine questions, each describing a symptom of depression. Each question is graded from zero to 3 depending on symptom frequency. The PHQ-9 takes less than 3 minutes to complete, and an abbreviated version, the PHQ-2, takes less than 1 minute to complete. The PHQ-9 has a sensitivity of 0.88 and specificity of 0.88 for major depression.

Symptom rating scales: Clinician administered

Clinician-administered symptom rating scales are useful for monitoring patient mood status over time and response to treatment. There are two clinician-administered rating scales for depression employed in both clinical and research settings: the Hamilton Depression Rating Scale (Ham-D)

Table 3.2. SENSITIVITY AND SPECIFICITY OF SCREENING ASSESSMENTS

	SENSITIVITY	SPECIFICITY
MDQ	0.73	0.90
HCL-32	0.80	0.51
BSDS	0.76	0.85

NOTE: MDQ = Mood Disorder Questionnaire; HCL-32 = Hypomania/Mania Symptom Checklist; BSDS = Bipolar Spectrum Diagnostic Scale

Table 3.3. PROBABILITY OF RELAPSE IN BIPOLAR DISORDER

	PROBABILITY OF RELAPSE		
EPISODE	BY 6 MONTHS (%)	BY 1 YEAR (%)	BY 5 YEARS (%)
Manic	20	48	81
Depressive	33	60	88
Mixed/ Cycling	36	57	91

NOTE: Reprinted with permission from Lippincott Williams & Wilkins. Keller et al. (1993).

and the Montgomery–Åsberg Depression Rating Scale (MADRS). The HAM-D is the most widely used assessment for clinician rated depression worldwide (Hamilton, 1960). It requires a clinically experienced rater to determine numerical ratings of 21 depressive symptoms and takes less than 20 minutes to complete. The MADRS is more sensitive to changes in the depressed clinical state and has been used in trials to assess efficacy of antidepressant medications (Montgomery & Åsberg, 1979). It is composed of 10 items, each of which may be rated from zero to 6 and takes less than 15 minutes to complete.

The Young Mania Rating Scale (YMRS) and the Bech Rafaelsen Mania Rating Scale (MAS) are the two most widely used clinician-rating scales for assessing severity of manic symptoms. The YMRS is a 15- to 30-minute interview that consists of 11 items to be rated from zero to 4. Four of the 11 items are given double weight and are rated from zero to 8. These four were considered to be core symptoms of mania and are irritability, speech, bizarre thought content, and disruptive or aggressive behavior. They are given double weight to account for lack of patient cooperation in the severely ill population. The YRMS takes 15 to 30 minutes to complete (Miller, Johnson, & Eisner, 2009).

The MAS is a clinical interview designed to cover the classic symptoms of mania. There are 11 items total: elevated mood, irritable or hostile mood, increased self-esteem, increased verbal activity, speech noise level, increased motor activity, increased social contacts, increased sexual activity, flight of thoughts, distractibility, increased self-esteem, and sleep disturbances. Each item is rated from zero to 44, and cut-off scores have been determined for hypomania, moderate mania, and severe mania (Bech, 2002). The MAS takes 10 to 20 minutes to complete.

CLINICAL COURSE

This section addresses what happens to people with bipolar disorder and their symptoms over time. Bipolar disorder is a recurrent and often lifelong illness. Its course varies considerably from person to person but for most is dominated by depressive symptoms (Judd et al., 2002). The initial presentation is around the age of 22 and is usually depressive (and therefore bipolar disorder should always be screened for when a patient presents with depression; Goodwin & Jamison, 2007). Even with the current treatments for bipolar disorder, its natural course remains highly recurrent. Patients with bipolar disorder also experience psychosocial functioning impairment that can progressively worsen over time.

Several long-term studies are responsible for what we know about the course of bipolar disorder today. Most of the information in this section focuses on these pioneering studies. The Zurich study followed 220 patients prospectively for up to 28 years (Angst, 1966). The Iowa 500 study was a 30- to 40-year follow-up of 685 patients with schizophrenic and affective disorders compared with nonpsychiatric patients (Tsuang, Woolson, & Fleming, 1979). The Cologne study followed 355 patients with affective, schizoaffective, and schizophrenic disorder for approximately 25 years (Marneros, Deister, & Rohde, 1990). The National Institute of Mental Health Collaborative Study of the Psychobiology of Depression (CDS study) is a prospective study following 955 patients (232 bipolar disorder patients) who were recruited from 1978 to 1981 (Katz & Klerman, 1979).

PRECIPITANTS OF EPISODES

Stress is a frequent precipitant of bipolar episodes (Goodwin & Jamison, 2007). Stress is more likely associated in early rather than late episodes and can cause increased sleeplessness, alcohol use, and drug use. Work-related events are also important precipitants of manic/hypomanic episodes. The relationship between stress and bipolar episodes is complicated because bipolar patients often create their own stressful events.

Pregnancy and the postpartum period are often very difficult for women with bipolar disorder: 30% to 50% of bipolar disorder women are depressed during the pregnancy or postpartum period, and mood instability is frequent during pregnancy (Akdeniz et al., 2003; Viguera & Cohen, 1998; Viguera, Cohen, Baldessarini, & Nonacs, 2002).

Another precipitant of mood episodes is substance use. This effect may be from the drug itself or from the sleep impairment it causes. The role of antidepressants in precipitating mania is controversial. The evidence suggests that older antidepressants, particularly the tricyclics, are much more likely to precipitate mania than the newer antidepressants (e.g., SSRIs; Pacchiarotti et al., 2013). Light and seasonality are also factors as mood fluctuates with the seasons. It is common for bipolar patients to experience depression in the winter and manic episodes in spring/summer.

DURATION OF EPISODE

A manic episode usually develops quickly in a matter of days. Some patients experience a period of hypomanic symptoms before the onset of mania called a "hypomanic alert" (Keitner et al., 1996; Winokur, 1976). Seventy-seven percent of patients experience sleep disturbance as a precursor to a manic onset.

Manic episodes typically last 6 to 12 weeks while mixed episodes typically last 17 weeks (Angst & Preisig, 1995; Coryell, Endicott, & Keller, 1990; Eaton et al., 1997; Keller, Lavorim, Coryell, Endicott, & Mueller, 1993). Hypomanic episodes may last several weeks to months (American Psychiatric Association, 2000).

A bipolar depressive episode may develop slowly over a period of weeks (Angst & Preisig, 1995; Winokur, 1976) and last around 11 to 15 weeks (Coryell et al., 1990; Keller et al., 1993).

CHRONICITY

Chronicity is defined as fully meeting criteria for an episode for a period greater than 2 years. A relatively high number of bipolar patients experience chronicity—16% according to the Zurich study (Angst & Sellaro, 2000). The CDS study found a similar percentage with 20% of patients experiencing chronicity during an entire 15-year follow-up (Coryell et al., 1998).

PATTERN

Kraepelin believed that interepisode periods became shorter over time, leading to more frequent episodes. Recent longitudinal studies do not support this assertion (Goodwin & Jamison, 2007). The current consensus is that cycle length does not change predictably with time, although it may shorten gradually in the initial stages of illness in some patients with more severe or atypical presentations.

There are three patterns of episodes of bipolar disorder: mania followed by depression and then an interval of wellness (MDI), depression followed by mania and then an interval of wellness (DMI), and continuous cycling (MDMD). MDI was thought to have the best outcome (Koukopoulos et al., 1980), although newer studies are somewhat inconsistent with this (Kessing, 1999). In a 15-year follow-up study the CDS (the longest study assessing polarity) did find DMI had worse outcome than MDI (Turvey et al., 1999). From these findings, we can cautiously conclude that patients who first exhibit depression then mania generally have a poorer long-term outcome.

RELAPSE/RECURRENCE

Relapse occurs rapidly and frequently in patients with bipolar disorder. Nearly half of patients with a manic episode

Table 3.4. AVERAGE NUMBER OF RECURRENT EPISODES IN BIPOLAR DISORDER

STUDY	NUMBER OF PATIENTS	LENGTH OF FOLLOW-UP	AVERAGE NUMBER OF EPISODES
Zurich	220	>25 years	9
Cologne	355	>25 years	5
CDS	165	10	5.5

NOTE: CDS = Collaborative Study of the Psychobiology of Depression. Adapted from Angst et al. (2000); Marneros et al. (1990); Solomon et al. (2010).

will relapse by one year, and nearly 60% of patients with depressive or mixed episodes will relapse by one year (Keller et al., 1993). Nearly 90% of all patients will have relapsed at least once by five years (see Table 3.3). By 10 years, 66% of bipolar I patients will have had at least one manic episode, and 34% of bipolar II patients will have had at least one hypomanic episode (Coryell et al., 1995). The likelihood of recurrence in the ensuing six months for bipolar I disorder has been shown to range from 36% when the preceding episode has ended 4 to 12 months previous, to 18% if one to two years has passed, to 10% if at least three years has past. Eventually, though, the likelihood of recurrence is high even for those who had at one point been in remission for at least three years. At seven years, 82% had experienced a new episode of mania or major depression.

Table 3.5. DEFINITIONS OF TREATMENT OUTCOMES IN BIPOLAR DISORDER

TREATMENT OUTCOME	DEFINITION
Response	50% reduction in symptoms from baseline as measured by a standardized scale (e.g. 50% decrease in MADRS)
Remission	Absence of minimal symptoms for at least one week
Recovery/Sustained Remission	At least 8–12 consecutive weeks of remission
Relapse/Recurrence	Return to full syndrome criteria following a remission of any duration
Roughening	Return of symptoms at subsyndromal level, perhaps representing a prodrome of an impending episode

NOTE: MADRS = Montgomery–Åsberger Depression Rating Scale. Adapted from Hirschfeld et al. (2007).

The Zurich study found that 82% of patients experienced a recurrence after recovery during the study period (up to 28 years). The average number of episodes was nine during that same follow-up period (Angst et al., 2000). The Cologne study followed patients for 25 years and found an average of five episodes (Marneros et al., 1990; see Table 3.4).

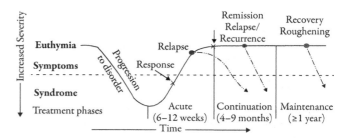

Figure 3.1 Clinical Course of Bipolar Disorder
Adapted from Frank et al. Arc Gen Psychiatry 1991; 48:851–855 and Hirschfeld et al. Psychopharmacology Bulletin 2007; 40:7–14.

LONG-TERM COURSE: SYMTOMATOLOGY OVER TIME

Bipolar is a highly episodic illness in which patients have been found to have several episodes in their lifetime (Goodwin and Jamison, 2007). Ninety-three percent of bipolar I patients and 98% of bipolar II patients will have another mood episode within 10 years of the initial episode (Judd et al., 2003). Bipolar disorder can also be chronic, and patients may be symptomatic most of their lives even when not experiencing an episode. In a 13-year prospective follow-up study, bipolar patients were found to have symptoms approximately half of the time (47% bipolar I and 56% for bipolar II disorder; Judd et al., 2002, 2003). Of that time spent ill, symptoms were depressive 67%, manic 20%, and mixed 13% of the time. Subsyndromal symptoms were more common than episodes (23% vs. 9% weeks during follow-up).

Over 30% of patients were found to have persisting symptoms in the Cologne study (Marneros et al., 1990). As previously mentioned, the CDS study found that bipolar disorder patients experience symptoms approximately half of the time (Judd et al., 2002, 2003). Only 12% of that 50% was an actual episode; the rest of the time patients experienced subsyndromal symptoms. For patients followed for 15 years, 20% experienced manic or depressive symptoms for the entire 15-year follow-up (Coryell et al., 1998). According to the CDS study, 1 in 10 bipolar patients remain chronically ill (Judd et al., 2002).

MORTALITY

Mortality risk is twice as high for bipolar patients in both natural and unnatural causes of death. The three most frequent natural causes of death for bipolar patients are cardiovascular disease, suicide, and cancer. The risk of suicide for bipolar patients is 30 times greater than the general population (American Psychiatric Association, 2002). An estimated 7% to 20% of bipolar patients have attempted suicide (Angst et al., 1999).

PSYCHOSOCIAL FUNCTIONING

Psychosocial functioning is substantially impaired with bipolar disorder (Hirschfeld, 2013). Over 60% of bipolar patients do not achieve full social and occupational recovery and do not return to their premorbid level after an episode (Martínez-Arán et al., 2004). Contributing to this functional impairment are neurocognitive deficits, as bipolar patients, whether in a manic state or a depressed state, have significantly impaired neuropsychological functioning compared to the general population (Martínez-Arán et al., 2004). Findings suggest significant cognitive dysfunction in verbal memory and in formal executive functioning (e.g., planning, problem-solving, verbal reasoning, and monitoring of actions). These cognitive deficits persisted even two years into remission with executive functioning and processing speed remaining impaired over time in patients who were well treated and euthymic (Mur et al., 2008; Tabarés-Seisdedos et al., 2008).

Table 3.5 lists the common definitions used to describe the course of bipolar disorder and Figure 3.1 illustrates their use.

Disclosure statement: Dr Snook and Mrs Moseley-Dendy have no conflicts of interests. For the 12-month period March 1, 2013 to February 28, 2014, Dr. Hirschfeld has received royalties from Jones and Bartlett and honorarium from CMEology, Equinox, CME Outfitters, and Merck Manual Editorial Board.

REFERENCES

Akdeniz, F., Vahip, S., Pirildar, S., Vahip, I., Doganer, I., & Bulut, I., (2003). Risk factors associated with childbearing-related episodes in women with bipolar disorder. *Psychopathology*, 36, 234–238.

Akiskal, H. S., Hantouche, E. G., Bourgeois, M. L., Azorin, J. M., Sechter, D., Allilaire, J. F., ... Lancrenon, S. (2001). Toward a refined phenomenology of mania: combining clinician-assessment and self-report in the French EPIMAN study. *Journal of Affective Disorders*, *67*, 89–96.

American Psychiatric Association. (1980). *Diagnostic and statistical manual of mental disorders*. (3rd ed.). Washington, DC: Author.

American Psychiatric Association. (2000). *Diagnostic and statistical manual of mental disorders*. (4th ed., text rev.). Washington, DC: Author.

American Psychiatric Association. (2002). Practice guideline for the treatment of patients with bipolar disorder (revision). *American Journal of Psychiatry*, *159*, 1–50.

American Psychiatric Association. (2013). *Diagnostic and statistical manual of mental disorders*. (5th ed.). Washington, DC: Author. http://dx.doi.org/10.1176/appi.books.9780890425596.910646

Angst, J. (1966). *Zur aetiologie und nosologie endogener depressiver psychosen: eine genetische*. Sociologische und Klinische Studie. Berlin: Springer.

Angst, J., Adolfsson, R., Benazzi, F., Gamma, A., Hantouche, E., Meyer, T. D., … Scott, J. (2005). The HCL-32: Towards a self-assessment tool for hypomanic symptoms in outpatients. *Journal of Affective Disorders*, *88*(2), 217–233. doi:10.1013/j.jad.2005.05.011

Angst, J., Angst, F., & Stassen, H. H. (1999). Suicide risk in patients with major depressive disorder. *Journal of Clinical Psychiatry*, *60*(Suppl. 2), 57–116.

Angst, J., Gamma, A., Benazzi, F., Ajdacic, V., Eich, D., & Rössler, W. (2003). Toward a re-definition of subthreshold bipolarity: Epidemiology and proposed criteria for bipolar-II, minor bipolar disorders and hypomania. *Journal of Affective Disorders*, *73*, 133–146.

Angst, J., & Preisig, M. (1995). Course of a clinical cohort of unipolar, bipolar and schizoaffective patients: Results of a prospective study from 1959 to 1985. *Schweizer Archiv fur Neurologie und Psychiatrie*, *146*, 5–16.

Angst, J., & Sellaro, R. (2000). Historical perspectives and natural history of bipolar disorder. *Biological Psychiatry*, *48*, 445–457.

Bech, P. (2002). The Bech-Rafaelsen Mania Scale in clinical trials of therapies for bipolar disorder: A 20-year review of its use as an outcome measure. *CNS Drugs*, *16*(1), 47–63.

Benazzi, F. (2002). Psychomotor changes in melancholic and atypical depression: Unipolar and bipolar II subtypes. *Psychiatry Research*, *112*(3), 211–220. doi:10.1016/S0165-1781(02)0024.x

Benazzi, F. (2007). Is overactivity the core feature of hypomania in bipolar II disorder? *Psychopathology*, *40*, 54–60. doi:10.1159/000096513

Coryell, W., Endicott, J., & Keller, M. (1990). Outcome of patients with chronic affective disorder: A five-year follow-up. *American Journal of Psychiatry*, *147*, 1627–1633.

Coryell, W., Endicott, J., Maser, J. D., Keller, M. B., Leon, A. C., & Akiskal, H. S. (1995). Long-term stability of polarity distinctions in the affective disorders. *American Journal of Psychiatry*, *152*, 385–390.

Coryell, W., Turvey, C., Endicott, J., Leon, A.C., Mueller, T., Solomon, D., & Keller, M. (1998). Bipolar I affective disorder: predictors of outcome after 15 years. *Journal of Affective Disorders*, *50*, 109–116.

Dunner, D. L., Gershon, B. M., & Goodwin, F. K. (1976). Heritable factors in the severity of affective illness. *Biological Psychiatry*, *11*, 31–42.

Eaton, W. W., Anthony, J. C., Gallo, J., Cai, G., Tien, A., Romanoski, A., … Chen, L. S. (1997). Natural history of Diagnostic Interview Schedule/DSM-IV major depression: The Baltimore Epidemiologic Catchment Area follow-up. *Archives of General Psychiatry*, *54*, 993–999.

Ghaemi, N. S., Miller, C. J., Douglas, A. B., Klugman, J., Rosenquist, K., & Pies, R. (2005). Sensitivity and specificity of a new bipolar spectrum diagnostic scale. *Journal of Affective Disorders*, *84*(2–3), 273–277. doi:10/1016/S0165-0327(03)00196-4

Goodwin, F. K., & Jamison, K. R. (2007). *Manic-depressive illness: Bipolar disorders and recurrent depression*. New York: Oxford University Press.

Hamilton, M. (1960). A rating scale for depression. *Journal of Neurology, Neurosurgery and Psychiatry*, *23*, 56–62.

Hirschfeld, R. M. (2013). The unrecognized side of bipolar disorder. *American Journal of Psychiatry*, *70*, 815–817.

Hirschfeld, R. M., Calabrese, J. R., Frye, M. A., Lavori, P. W., Sachs, G., Thase, M. E., & Wagner, K. D. (2007). Defining the clinical course of bipolar disorder: response, remission, relapse, recurrence, and roughening. *Psychopharmacological Bulletin*, *40*, 7–14.

Hirschfeld, R. M., Williams, J. B., Spitzer, R. L., Calabrese, J. R., Flynn, L., Keck, P. E., … Zajecka, J. (2000). Development and validation of a screening instrument for bipolar spectrum disorder: The Mood Disorder Questionnaire. *American Journal of Psychiatry*, *157*, 1873–1875.

Jamison, K. (1995). *An unquiet mind: A memoir of moods and madness*. New York: Random House.

Judd, L. L., Akiskal, H. S., Schettler, P. J., Endicott, J., Maser, J., Solomon, D. A., … Keller, M. B. (2002). The long-term natural history of the weekly symptomatic status of bipolar I disorder. *Archives of General Psychiatry*, *59*(6), 530–537. doi:10.1001/archpsyc.59.6.530.

Judd, L. L., Schettler, P. J., Akiskal, H. S., Maser, J., Coryell, W., Solomon, D., … Keller, M. (2003). Long-term symptomatic status of bipolar I vs. bipolar II disorders. *The International Journal of Neuropsychopharmacology*, *6*, 127–137.

Katz, M., & Klerman, G. L. (1979). Introduction: Overview of the clinical studies program. *American Journal of Psychiatry*, *136*, 47–51.

Keitner, G. I., Solomon, D. A., Ryan, C. E., Miller, I. W., Mallinger, A., Kupfer, D. J., & Frank, E. (1996). Prodromal and residual symptoms in bipolar I disorder. *Comprehensive Psychiatry*, *44*, 263–269.

Keller, M. B., Lavorim P. W., Coryell, W., Endicott, J., & Mueller, T. I. (1993). Bipolar I: A five-year prospective follow-up. *Journal of Nervous Mental Disorders*, *181*, 238–245.

Kessing, L. V. (1999). The effect of the first manic episode in affective disorder: A case register study of hospitalized episodes. *Journal of Affective Disorders*, *53*, 233–239.

Ketter, T. (2010). Handbook of diagnosis and treatment of bipolar disorders. Arlington, VA: American Psychiatric Publishing.

Koukopoulos, A., Reginaldi, D., Laddomada, P., Floris, G., Serra, G., & Tondo, L. (1980). Course of the manic-depressive cycle and changes caused by treatments. *Pharmakopsychiatrie, Neuro-Psychopharmakologie*, *13*, 156–167.

Kraepelin, E. (1896). *Psychiatrie* (5th ed.). Leipzig: Barth.

Leonhard, K. (1957). *Aufteilung der endogenen psychosen und ihre differenzierte aetiologie*. Berlin: Akademie-Verlag.

Marneros, A., Deister, A., & Rohde, A. (1990). Psychopathological and social status of patients with affective, schizophrenia and schizoaffective disorders after long-term course. *Acta Psychiatrica Scandinavica*, *82*, 352–358.

Martínez-Arán, A., Vieta, E., Reinares, M., Colom, F., Torrent, C., Sánchez-Moreno, J., … Salamero, M. (2004). Cognitive function across manic or hypomanic, depressed, and euthymic states in bipolar disorder. *American Journal of Psychiatry*, *161*, 262–270.

Merikangas, K. R., Akiskal, H. S., Angst, J., Greenber, P. E., Hirschfeld, R. M., Petukhova, M., & Kessler, R. C. (2007). Lifetime and 12 month prevalence of bipolar spectrum disorder in the National Comorbidity Survey Replication. *Archives of General Psychiatry*, *64*(5), 543–552. doi.10.1001/archpsych.64.5.543

Miller, C. S., Johnson, S. L., & Eisner, L. (2009). Assessment tools for adult bipolar disorder. *Clinical Psychology*, *16*(2), 188–201. doi:10.1111/j.1468-2850.2009.01158.x

Mitchell, P. B., Goodwin, G. M., Johnson, G. F., & Hirschfeld, R. M. A. (2008). Diagnostic guidelines for bipolar depression: A probabilistic approach. *Bipolar Disorders*, *10*(1), 144–152. doi:10.1111/j.1399-5618.2007.00559.x

Mitchell, P. B., Wilhelm, K., Parker, G., Austin, M. P., Rutgers, P., & Malhi, G. S. (2001). The clinical features of bipolar depression: A comparison with matched major depressive disorder patients. *Journal of Clinical Psychiatry, 62*, 212–216.

Montgomery, S. A., & Åsberg, M., 1979. A new depression scale designed to be sensitive to change. *British Journal of Psychiatry, 134*, 382–389.

Mur, M., Portella, M., Martinez-Aran, A., Pifarre, J., & Vieta, E. (2008). Long-term stability of cognitive impairment in bipolar disorder: A 2-year follow up study of lithium treated euthymic bipolar patients. *Journal of Clinical Psychiatry, 69*, 712–719.

Pacchiarotti, I., Bond, D. J., Baldessarini, R. J., Nolan, W. A., Grunze, H., Licht, R. M., ... Vieta, E. (2013). The International Society for Bipolar Disorders (ISBD) Task-Force report on antidepressant use in bipolar disorders. *American Journal of Psychiatry, 170*(11), 1249–1262.

Parker, G., Roy, K., Wilhelm, K., Mitchell, P., & Hadzi-Pavlovic, D. (2000). The nature of bipolar depression: Implications for the definition of melancholia. *Journal of Affective Disorders, 59*(3), 217–224. doi:10.1016/S0165-0327(99)00144-5.x

Perry, W., Minassian, A., Henry, B., Kincaid, M., Young, J. W., & Geyer, M. A. (2010). Quantifying over-activity in bipolar and schizophrenia patients in a human open field paradigm. *Psychiatry Research, 178*(1), 84–91. doi:10.1016/j/psychres 2010/04/032

Perugi, G., Akiksal, H., Micheli, C., Musetti, L., Paiano, A., Quilici, C., ... Cassano, G. (1997). Clinical subtypes of bipolar mixed states: Valicating a broader European definition in 143 cases. *Journal of Affective Disorders, 43*(3), 169–180 doi:10.1016/S0165-0327(97)01446-8

Sadock, B. Sadock, V., & Ruiz, P. (2009). *Kaplan and Sadock's comprehensive textbook of psychiatry* (9th ed.). Philadelphia, PA. Lippincott Williams & Wilkins.

Sadock, B., & Sadock, V. (2007). *Kaplan and Sadock's synopsis of psychiatry* (10th ed.). Philadelphia, PA. Lippincott Williams & Wilkins, p. 528.

Solomon, D. A., Leon, A. C., Coryell, W. H., Endicott, J., Li, C., Fiedorowicz, J. G., ... Keller, M. B. (2010). Longitudinal course of bipolar I disorder: Duration of mood episodes. *Archives of General Psychiatry, 67*, 339–347.

Swann, A. C., Lafer, B., Perugi, G., Frye, M., Bauer, M., & Bahk, W. M. (2013). Bipolar mixed states: An International Society for Bipolar Disorders Task Force Report of symptom structure, course of illness, and diagnosis. *American Journal of Psychiatry, 170*(1), 31–42. doi:10.1176/appi.ajp.2012.12030301.

Tabarés-Seisdedos, R., Balanzá-Martínez, V., Sánchez-Moreno, J., Martinez-Aran, A., Salazar-Fraile, J., Selva-Vera, G., ... Vieta, E. (2008). Neurocognitive and clinical predictors of functional outcome in patients with schizophrenia and bipolar I disorder at one-year follow-up. *Journal of Affective Disorders, 109*, 286–299.

Turvey, C. L., Coryell, W. H., Solomon, D. A., Leon, A. C., Endicott, J., Keller, M. B., & Akiskal, H. (1999). Long-term prognosis of bipolar I disorder. *Acta Psychiatrica Scandinavica, 99*, 110–119.

Tsuang, M. T., Woolson, R. F., & Fleming, J. A. (1979). Long-term outcome of major psychoses: I. Schizophrenia and affective disorders compared with psychiatrically symptom-free surgical conditions. *Archives of General Psychiatry, 36*, 1295–1301.

Viguera, A. C., & Cohen, L. S. (1998). The course and management of bipolar disorder during pregnancy. *Psychopharmacological Bulletin, 34*, 339–346.

Viguera, A. C., Cohen, L. S., Baldessarini, R. J., & Nonacs, R. (2002). Managing bipolar disorder during pregnancy: Weighing the risks and benefits. *Canadian Journal of Psychiatry, 47*, 426–436.

Winokur, G. (1976). Duration of illness prior to hospitalization (onset) in the affective disorders. *Neuropsychobiology, 2*, 87–93.

Winokur, G., Clayton, P., & Reich, T. (1969). *Manic depressive illness.* St. Louis, MO: C. V. Mosby.

4.

DIFFERENTIAL DIAGNOSIS AND BIPOLAR SPECTRUM DISORDERS

Jean-Michel Azorin and Raoul Belzeaux

INTRODUCTION

The view that bipolar disorder is a chronic disease with alternating episodes of mania and depression with free intervals has been gradually overtaken by an understanding of its heterogeneity and the need to identify phenotypic markers associated with subtypes (Azorin et al., 2013).

The most common classifications of the disorder have therefore shifted the emphasis in diagnosis away from polarity and toward other diagnostic validators (Katzow, Hsu, & Ghaemi, 2003). This has contributed to make the diagnosis process of bipolar disorder much more difficult than it was. At the same time, this process, including differential diagnosis, has become a controversial issue, as demonstrated by an expanding literature on this topic (Zimmerman, Ruggero, Chelminski, & Young, 2008). In this chapter we review the recent evolution in the classification of bipolar disorders together with the diagnostic issues the evolving classification may have raised.

BIPOLAR SPECTRUM DISORDERS

ORIGIN OF THE CONCEPT

A spectrum or continuum concept was already present in Kraepelin's (1921) descriptions of manic-depressive insanity, when he wrote that the latter included "certain slight and slightest colouring of mood, some of them periodic, some of them continuously morbid, which on the one hand are to be regarded as the rudiment of more severe disorders, on the other hand pass without sharp boundary into the domain of personal predisposition." Such a concept may allow the recognition of subsyndromal aspects of the illness and their potential merging into personality and temperament, as well as legitimate continuity between bipolar and unipolar forms (Goodwin & Jamison, 2007). During the previous century, Klerman (1981) was one of the first at the root of a revival of the concept. He differentiated six subtypes: mania (+/– depression), hypomania (+/–depression), hypomania + depressive symptoms, mania or hypomania secondary to substance abuse or somatic disease, depression with a family history of bipolar disorder, and unipolar mania (without depression). In a similar vein, Angst (1998) hypothesized a continuity between hypomania (m), cyclothymia (md), mania (M), mania + mild depression (Md), mania + major depression (MD), and major depression + hypomania (Dm).

Our research has also shown that hypomania could be briefer than usually admitted and that hyperactivity could have the same value as mood elevation for the diagnosis of (hypo)mania (Angst et al., 2003b). The spectrum concept was supported by the finding that "softer" definitions of the disorders were linked with as severe consequences as those found for "harder" criteria (Angst et al., 2003b). Disorders were included in the bipolar spectrum on the basis of a certain number of validators, among which the most common were family history, course, age at onset, response to antidepressants, and presence of comorbidity (Angst et al., 2003b). As noticed by some authors (Katzow et al., 2003), the bipolar spectrum concept shifts the emphasis in diagnosis of bipolar disorder away from polarity (presence of spontaneous manic episodes) and toward other diagnostic validators. However, difficulties with conceptual issues and diagnostic skills may emerge where no absolute consensus exists as to which specific symptoms or how many symptoms need to be present to diagnose a bipolar spectrum condition. In this regard, most clinicians may agree with the statement from Katzow et al. (2003) that "common sense…suggests that the more such signs are present, the most likely the diagnosis of a bipolar spectrum condition."

EPIDEMIOLOGICAL DATA

The lifetime prevalence of bipolar I disorder in community samples may vary from 0.4% to 1.6%, whereas that of bipolar II is about 0.5%. For cyclothymic disorders, studies have reported a lifetime prevalence of from 0.4% to 1%, which may range from 3% to 5% in mood disorders clinics. On a follow-up period of five years, 5% to 15% of bipolar II patients could present a manic episode, with a risk to develop bipolar I or II disorder of from 15% to 50% for cyclothymic disorder (American Psychiatric Association, 1994). The Epidemiologic Catchment Area study reported that mania and hypomania occur in 1.2% of the population over a lifetime, which is roughly one-fourth of the prevalence of major depression (Regier et al., 1995). However, a reanalysis of the Epidemiologic Catchment Area data to include all patients in the bipolar spectrum reported a lifetime prevalence rate of 6.4% (Judd et al., 2003).

Other studies conducted in Europe have found lifetime prevalence rates of from 0.3% to 3% for bipolar II disorder, 0.5% to 2.8% for cyclothymic disorder, and 2.2% to 5.7% for hypomania. For the whole bipolar spectrum, prevalence rates could vary from 2.6% to 7.8% (Angst et al., 2003b). However, if one uses less conservative criteria to define each disorder, these rates could reach 24% (Angst et al., 2003b). In clinical populations, the prevalence of bipolar disorders was reported to vary from 10% to 15% of psychiatric consultations, which is about half of the consultations needing care in the domain of affective disorders (Rouillon, 2005). Furthermore, the overall prevalence of bipolar disorders does not seem to vary according to gender, although a certain number of studies have shown a greater number of depressive episodes in women, whereas men display more (hypo)manic episodes (Nivoli et al., 2011).

CURRENT ISSUES

One of the most popular models for bipolar spectrum currently is that from Akiskal and Pinto (2000; Akiskal, 2007). Ten types are identified in this model, ranging from Type ½ to Type VI, if one considers schizophrenia representing Type 0.

Bipolar ½ refers to schizomanic or schizobipolar disorder and is considered a variety in which manic excitement occurs in association with mood-incongruent features beyond what could be permissible in bipolar I disorder. Bipolar I refers to full-blown mania. Bipolar I ½ means depression and protracted hypomania, depicting patients whose hypomanic periods cause trouble to them and significant others without reaching the destructive potential characteristic of the extreme excitement of full-blown

manic psychosis. Bipolar II disorder may be characterized by moderately to severely impairing major depressions, interspersed with hypomanic periods of at least four days duration without marked impairment.

Bipolar II ½ subtype refers to patients whose hypomanic episodes are shorter than four days and who fulfill the criteria for cyclothymic disorder. Compared to bipolar II, patients from this subtype were found to score higher on the so-called dark side of hypomania characterized by more traveling, imprudent driving, excessive shopping and spending, foolish behavior in business, irritability, attention easily distractible, increased sex drive and interest in sex, increased consumption of coffee and cigarettes, as well as increased consumption of alcohol (Akiskal, Hantouche, & Allilaire, 2003).

Bipolar III represents clinically depressed patients who experience hypomania solely during antidepressant treatment or other somatic treatment. Different from bipolar II patients, who may also develop hypomania during antidepressant treatment, bipolar III patients have more depressive than cyclothymic temperaments. Bipolar III ½ refers to patients whose periods of excitement are so closely linked with substance or alcohol use/abuse that it is not always easy to decide whether these periods would have occurred in the absence of such use/abuse. Bipolar IV depicts patients with depression occurring late in life and superimposed on a lifelong hyperthymic temperament. They often present with protracted depressive mixed states or "agitated depression." Bipolar V are patients presenting with major depressive episodes but who may share more subtle features of bipolarity. Finally, Type VI represents affectively disinhibited and mood labile states in the setting of early course of dementia.

Another popular model is that proposed by Ghaemi, Ko, and Goodwin (2002). This model establishes specific diagnostic criteria for bipolar spectrum disorders. Four criteria must be fulfilled: A, B, C, and D. Criterion A refers to the presence of at least one major depressive episode and criterion B to the absence of any spontaneous episode of mania or hypomania. Criterion C requires the presence of one of the following items, plus at least two items from criterion D, or two among the following items plus one item from criterion D: (a) family history of bipolar disorder in first-degree relatives, (b) mania or hypomania induced by antidepressant treatment. Criterion D states that if none among items from criterion C is present, six among the following nine items are required: (a) hyperthymic temperament, (b) recurrent major depressive episodes (> 3), (c) brief major depressive episodes (avg < 3 months), (d) atypical features (*Diagnostic and Statistical Manual of Mental Disorders*, fourth edition [*DSM-IV*] criteria; American

Psychiatric Association, 1994), (e) major depressive episodes with psychotic features, (f) early onset of first major depressive episode (< 25 years), (g) postpartum depression, (h) wearing off of antidepressant efficacy, (i) lack of response after at least three well-conducted antidepressant treatments.

This model is based on the idea that there may be some subtle features indicative of bipolarity in the absence of any spontaneous manic or hypomanic episode. In addition to those listed in the aforementioned criteria, one could mention substance abuse, seasonal pattern of depressive episodes, or the presence of hypomanic symptoms during a depressive episode (Kaye, 2005). Mood lability on antidepressants, as well as a history of suicide attempts, may also be predictive of bipolarity (Angst et al., 2011). The criteria proposed by Ghaemi et al. (2002) have received support from empirical studies (Smith, Harrison, Muir, & Blackwood, 2005). The same may hold true for the identifying features of bipolarity in presence of a major depressive episode (Angst et al., 2011; Kaye, 2005). Interestingly, the criteria from Ghaemi et al. can be considered as the development of Akiskal and Pinto's model (2000); both models highlight that in the vast majority of cases, clinicians have to reorganize bipolar disorder despite the absence of spontaneous manic and/or hypomanic episodes.

In keeping with previous research, Angst et al. (2003a) have also elaborated diagnostic criteria for bipolarity specifier. Bipolarity specifier criteria attribute a diagnosis of bipolar disorder in patients who experienced an episode of elevated mood, an episode of irritable mood, or an episode of increased activity with at least three of the symptoms listed under criterion B of the *DSM-IV-* associated with at least one of the three following consequences: (a) unequivocal and observed change in functioning uncharacteristic of the person's usual behavior, (b) marked impairment in social or occupational functioning observable by others, and (c) requiring hospitalization or outpatient treatment. No minimum duration of symptoms is required and no exclusion criteria are applied. Bipolar specifier criteria include all cases meeting *DSM-IV* criteria for bipolar I and bipolar II disorders, as well as additional cases excluded by *DSM-IV* exclusionary criteria (e.g., symptoms occurring during antidepressant treatment). In a recent multicenter, multinational, transcultural study conducted among 5,635 major depressive patients, 903 patients (16%) were found to fulfil *DSM-IV* criteria for bipolar disorder, whereas 2,647 (47%) met the bipolarity specifier criteria. Thus these criteria allowed the identification of an additional 31% of patients with major depressive episodes who scored positive on the bipolarity criteria. Their validity was established

by showing that using both definitions, significant associations (odds ratio > 2; $p < .001$) with bipolarity were observed with some well-recognized identifying features of bipolarity. The bipolarity specifier additionally identified significant associations for manic/hypomanic states while taking antidepressants, comorbid substance use disorder, and borderline personality disorder (Angst et al., 2011).

In a more recent analysis of this data set, patterns of concurrent comorbidities were found to differ between major depressive patients (*DSM–IV*) and those meeting bipolarity specifier criteria. In addition, specifier definition provided better discrimination between major depressive disorder and bipolar I, as well as bipolar II. Interestingly, eating and substance use disorders where clearly associated with bipolar I and bipolar II defined according to bipolarity specifier only, as well as attention deficit hyperactivity disorder (ADHD) and borderline personality disorder (Angst et al., 2013).

THE PROBLEM OF MISDIAGNOSIS

EPIDEMIOLOGICAL FINDINGS

A number of studies conducted in many countries worldwide have reported delays in correct diagnosis for bipolar disorder, as well as frequent misdiagnoses with other disorders. Two surveys were conducted a decade apart among members of the National Depressive and Manic-Depressive Association (DMDA) in the United States. The 1992 National DMDA constituent survey reported that long delays between the onset of symptoms, the seeking of treatment, and the receipt of an accurate diagnosis were common (Lish, Dime-Menan, Whybrow, Price, Hirschfeld, 1994). The survey was repeated in 2000 and displayed findings that were very similar to those reported nearly a decade earlier (Hirschfeld, Lewis, & Vornik, 2003). Nearly half of respondents who had been misdiagnosed at least once reported a lapse of several months up to five years between seeking their first treatment and diagnosis.

Over one-third of those who were initially misdiagnosed in both 1992 and 2000 did not receive a correct diagnosis for 10 or more years after seeking treatment. In 2000, 69% of respondents reported having been misdiagnosed; those who were misdiagnosed received a mean of 3.5 other diagnoses and consulted four physicians before receiving an accurate diagnosis. Before being diagnosed as having bipolar disorder, respondents were most likely to see either a psychiatrist (62%) or a physician for guidance and treatment. Nevertheless, a psychologist and counsellor or social worker were visited at the next highest levels of frequency, followed by clergy. In 2000, the most common incorrect diagnosis was unipolar depression (60%). Other frequently mentioned misdiagnoses included anxiety disorder (26%), schizophrenia (18%), borderline personality or antisocial personality disorder (17%), alcohol or substance abuse and/or dependence (14%), and schizoaffective disorder (11%).

A roughly comparable study was conducted in 2001 by GAMIAN-Europe, a pan-European federation of national patient organizations from 30 European countries (Morselli et al., 2003). The findings indicated that, on average, a bipolar patient was expected to wait for 5.7 years for a correct diagnosis from the first onset of symptoms, whereas a non-bipolar patient had a significantly lower delay (4.5 years). The respondents stated that the diagnosis was made in the vast majority of the cases by a psychiatrist and in a smaller percentage by the family doctor or a neurologist.

Two other studies dealing with the epidemiology of mania were conducted in France among patients hospitalized for a manic episode. The first of these studies recruited 104 manic patients (Akiskal et al., 1998). A delay (≥ 5 years) before correct diagnosis was found for 29% of patients with pure mania but for 40% of patients with probable dysphoric mania and 57% of those with definite dysphoric mania. The second study included 1,090 hospitalized manic patients (Hantouche, Akiskal, Azorin, Châtenet-Duchêne, & Lancrenon, 2006). It also found significantly longer delays before correct diagnosis of mixed mania compared to pure mania. The records of prior misdiagnoses revealed a global rate of patients with at least one prior diagnosis, which was significantly higher in mixed patients. These clustered basically into anxiety disorders and/or personality disorders in the mixed group. Interestingly, the 2000 National DMDA survey showed that, despite such high rates of misdiagnoses, more than 70% of respondents experienced at least one manic symptom prior to diagnosis, and more than three-quarters of respondents experienced various depressive symptoms (Hirschfeld et al., 2003).

CONSEQUENCES OF MISDIAGNOSIS

The consequences of misdiagnosis can be serious and even occasionally fatal. Misdiagnosis may lead to inappropriate treatment, which is particularly true when bipolar depression is not recognized and treated with antidepressants without the concomitant use of mood stabilizers (Kaye, 2005; Perlis, 2005). In this case patients may develop mood switches, which worsen the course of the disease and

sometimes contribute to the apparition of rapid cycling as well as mixed states (Perlis, 2005). Both conditions have been reported to be associated with diminished response to medication (Kaye, 2005). Cases were also reported in which, despite an initial response to antidepressants, a loss of response some months later may lead to dose increase (Perlis, 2005). Overall, in the absence of effective treatment patients may experience more episodes or more refractory episodes that may impair patients' functioning (Kaye, 2005; Perlis, 2005).

Delay in the start of mood stabilizers was found to be associated with increased health-care cost, including increased suicide attempts and higher rates of hospital use (Singh & Rajput, 2006). Estimates of completed suicide in persons with bipolar disorder are between 10% and 15%, with most suicides occurring during the depressive phase (Kaye, 2005; Singh & Rajput, 2006).

In a study assessing the impact of number of years undiagnosed on current morbidity in patients with bipolar disorder, the number of years undiagnosed was found to be associated with higher depression and lower quality of life within the physical and psychological domains (Gazalle et al., 2005). Economically, misdiagnosis of bipolar disorders was also shown to result in lost work days and productivity; as the onset of bipolar disorder is common in adolescence, misdiagnosis at that time may have a negative impact on the development of interpersonal skills, education, and earning potential (Singh & Rajput, 2006). Some authors (Zimmerman et al., 2008) have stressed that if there was a risk for bipolar disorder to be under- and misdiagnosed, the risk also exists to be overdiagnosed. This was based on the results of a study showing that fewer than half the patients who reported that they had been previously diagnosed with bipolar disorder received a diagnosis of bipolar disorder based on structured interview (Zimmerman et al., 2008). Consequences of overdiagnosis can be also profound. The main problems may be related to unnecessary side effects of mood stabilizers and atypical antipsychotics (Katzow et al., 2003; Perlis, 2005, Zimmerman et al., 2008). These drugs, which are used to treat bipolar disorder, may have potentially significant health complications affecting renal, endocrine, hepatic, immunologic, or metabolic function. Therefore overdiagnosing bipolar disorder can unnecessarily expose patients to serious drug-adverse effects (Zimmerman et al., 2008).

Overdiagnosis may also delay the use of more appropriate treatments. Borderline personality disorder, for example, was shown to be at increased risk of being misdiagnosed with bipolar disorder (Ruggero, Zimmerman, Chelminski, & Young, 2010). In this case, misdiagnosis with bipolar disorder could delay the indication of many new psychotherapeutic treatments shown to be effective to treat borderline personality disorder but not suitable to bipolar disorder (Ruggero et al., 2010).

CONTRIBUTORS TO MISDIAGNOSIS

Many factors are likely to contribute to misdiagnosis of bipolar disorder. They may be related to the patient, to the doctor, and/or to the illness (Perlis, 2005).

Patients were frequently found to underreport important symptoms, particularly during acute episodes. For example in the study conducted by Hirschfeld et al. (2003), it appeared that, during mania, only erratic sleeping was reported by more than half of the respondents, whereas less than one-third mentioned erratic eating, reckless behavior, excessive spending, and increased sexual interest. The same study showed that, as with manic symptoms but to a lesser extent, symptoms of depression were also underreported to physicians. This failure to report relevant symptoms has been related to lack of insight and/or fear of stigma (Perlis, 2005). In the Hirschfield et al. study, patients who were more likely to have unreported symptoms were those who experienced symptoms for a minimum of 10 years before getting an accurate diagnosis. The same study gave some hints about the role that doctors may play in misdiagnosis. Respondents who were misdiagnosed believed the lack of understanding about bipolar disorder among the doctors/professionals consulted was the primary barrier to more timely diagnoses (Hirschfeld et al., 2003). However, it has been also suggested that an excessive campaign against underrecognition, among both doctors and patients, may have been responsible, at times, for a trend to overdiagnose the illness.

Doctors may be sensitive to the marketing message of pharmaceutical companies that many patients deemed to suffer from complex depressive or personality disorders actually could be bipolar and easily responsive to medications such as mood stalibilizers or atypical antipsychotics. This echos the fact that in general clinicians may be inclined to diagnose disorders that they feel more comfortable to treat (Zimmerman et al., 2008). The same campaign may lead a growing number of patients to interpret their symptoms as bipolar, be more informed about the disease, and consult professionals to confirm their own diagnosis.

Nevertheless, in the vast majority of cases, misdiagnosis is likely to be explained by the phenomenological complexity of the disorder itself. Many factors may be relevant in this regard. Age at onset, for example, has been reported as one of the most valid indicator of phenotypic differences among bipolar patients. In a recent study conducted on more than 1,000 bipolar patients, patients with an early onset were found to be more frequently misdiagnosed as suffering from psychotic disorder compared to those with intermediate or late onset. In contrast, late-onset patients received more commonly a previous diagnosis of major depressive or anxiety disorder (Azorin et al., 2013).

First-episode polarity may be also worth mentioning. On the same cohort of patients, it was found that those with a manic polarity at onset were often misdiagnosed as psychotics compared with patients who had a depressive or mixed polarity at onset; patients with a depressive polarity at onset were more frequently diagnosed as major depressives, whereas those with depressive/mixed polarity at onset received more commonly a prior diagnosis of anxious disorder (Azorin, Akiskal, & Hantouche, 2011).

Comorbidity may represent an additional source of diagnostic complexity. Comorbid conditions are multiple in bipolar disorders, including alcohol and substance use disorders, anxiety disorders, eating disorders, ADHD, Axis II personality disorders, as well as medical comorbidities (Krishnan, 2005). Thus a clinician may focus on one of these conditions and miss the presence of an underlying bipolar disorder (Perlis, 2005).

Furthermore, it has been shown that gender is likely to interfere with the aforementioned factors to modify the phenotypic expression of the illness. Differences were reported across gender for predominant polarity, polarity at onset, age at onset, comorbidities, as well as temperament and response to medications (McElroy, Arnold, Altshuler, 2011). Nevertheless, the main problem is probably related to the conception clinicians may have of the disorder itself. If the vast majority of them may be in agreement about the existence of bipolar I disorder, fewer are likely those who recognize the full spectrum of bipolarity.

DIFFERENTIAL DIAGNOSIS

MAJOR DEPRESSIVE DISORDER

As previously mentioned, major depressive disorders represent the main differential diagnosis of bipolar depression. Of course patients with soft bipolar disorders are more frequently misdiagnosed, due to the lack of spontaneous episodes of mania and/or hypomania (Kaye, 2005).

Clinical characteristics of depressive episode may sometimes be of help to orientate the diagnosis. Bipolar depressive patients are likely to be more withdrawn and retarded with tendency for hypersomnia and show more agitation, atypical symptoms of depression, mood lability, and mixicity, as well as psychotic features but less weight loss, anxiety symptoms, somatic complaints, and anger (Singh & Rajput, 2006). Of course, the previously mentioned features related to family history, course of illness, comorbidity, and response to treatment may also help to identify bipolarity (Kaye, 2005). This is well reflected by the criteria proposed by Ghaemi et al. (2002). Mitchell, Goodwin, Johnson, and Hirschfeld (2008) have also suggested a "probabilistic" approach to the diagnosis of bipolar depression in a person experiencing a major depressive episode with no clear prior episodes of mania or hypomania. According to these authors, the greater likelihood of the diagnosis of bipolar depression should be considered if five or more of the following features are present: (a) hypersomnia and/or increased daytime napping, (b) hyperphagia and/or increased weight, (c) other atypical depressive symptoms such as leaden paralysis, psychomotor retardation, psychotic features, and/or pathological guilt, (d) lability of mood/manic symptoms, (e) early onset of first depression (< 25 years), (f) multiple prior episodes of depression (≥ 5 episodes), and (g) positive family history of bipolar disorder. In contrast, the greater likelihood of the diagnosis of unipolar depression should be considered if four or more of the following features are present: (a) initial insomnia/reduced sleep, appetite, and/or weight loss; (b) normal or increased activity levels; (c) somatic complaints; (d) later onset of first depression (> 25 years); (e) long duration of current episode (> 6 months); and (f) negative family history of bipolar disorder.

The differential diagnosis may be particularly difficult if not impossible in patients who experience first episode of major depression in the absence of prior manic or hypomanic episode. This is not a rare situation, as 35% to 60% of patients with bipolar disorders may experience a depressive polarity at onset (Kaye, 2005).

ANXIETY DISORDERS

Frequent misdiagnosis of bipolar disorders with anxiety disorders may be related to their high comorbidity, which may sometimes concern more than 50% of the patients (Perlis, 2005). Moreover some of the features of anxiety and depression or hypomania/mania may overlap; for example, impaired concentration can be associated with all three, as can sleep disruption. Anxious patients, as well as bipolar patients, may report racing thoughts. Therefore, a doctor who stops with a patient's chief complaint of anxiety may miss more subtle symptoms of bipolar disorder (Perlis, 2005).

As in the case of major depression, anxiety disorders have been reported to precede sometimes bipolar disorder, or at least the occurrence of the first manic or hypomanic episode (Perugi, Akiskal, Toni, Simonini, & Gemignani, 2001). The characteristics of the clinical picture may be sometimes of help. For example, bipolar patients comorbid with obsessive-compulsive disorder (OCD), when compared with non-bipolar OCD patients, were shown to have a more gradual onset of their OCD that, nonetheless, pursued a more episodic course with a greater number of concurrent major depressive episodes. Moreover these bipolar OCD patients had significantly higher rates of sexual and religious obsessions and a significantly lower rate of checking rituals. In contrast, unipolar OCD were older, had a more chronic course with hospitalizations and suicide attempts, had greater comorbidity with generalized anxiety disorder and caffeine abuse, and were more likely to have aggressive obsessions and those with a philosophical, superstitious, or bizarre content (Perugi et al., 1997).

In a study comparing the prodromal phase of first-versus multiple-episode mania (Azorin, Kaladjian, Adida, Fakra, Hantouche, et al., 2012), the former was found to be associated with high levels of stressors, suicide attempts, alcohol or substance abuse, and presence of anxiety disorders. This emphasizes the need to look for associated conditions in the presence of an anxiety disorder. Comorbidity with substance abuse disorders, high levels of suicidality, and stress may evoke, in this case, an underlying bipolar disorder.

More generally, it has been suggested that comorbid conditions in bipolar disorder may share the following characteristics: they are multiple (42% patients may have two or more comorbidities), more frequent in women, and associated with an earlier age at onset of illness, a younger age of patients, high rates of suicidality, as well as poor response to treatment and chronicity (McElroy et al., 2001; Krishnan, 2005).

PSYCHOTIC DISORDERS

Bipolar I patients sharing psychotic features are highly likely to be confounded with psychotic disorders. For example, the differential diagnosis may be difficult with schizophrenia and/or schizoaffective disorder when patients present with mood-incongruent psychotic features. In a previous study (Azorin et al., 2006), it was found that manic patients with incongruent psychotic features were characterized by high levels of auditory hallucinations, persecutory delusions, somatic delusions, and delusions of reference, which are common in schizophrenia. These patients were also characterized by their young age at onset (Azorin et al., 2013) and prevalence of female gender (Azorin et al., 2006). Bipolar disorder with mood-incongruent features was shown to be driven by unstable mixed states that may be masked by the presence of psychotic symptoms in the forefront (Azorin et al., 2006). In any event, if the latter occur exclusively during periods of mood disturbance the diagnosis is mood disorder with psychotic features. In schizoaffective disorder, there must be a mood episode that is concurrent with the active phase of symptoms of schizophrenia, mood symptoms must be present for a substantial portion of the total duration of the disturbance, and psychotic features must be present for at least two weeks in the absence of prominent mood symptoms. In contrast, mood symptoms in schizophrenia either have a duration that is brief in relation to the total duration of the disturbance, occur only during the prodromal or residual phases, or do not meet full criteria for a mood episode (American Psychiatric Association, 1994).

In contrast, bipolar patients with mood-congruent psychotic features are more likely to be misdiagnosed as delusional disorder patients (Azorin et al., 2006; Azorin et al., 2013). This may be particularly true in case of patients with severe chronic mania. It has been reported that 13% of hospitalized people with mania pursue a chronic course. Chronic mania may be characterized by euphoric mood and grandiose delusions in presence of lack of neurovegetative, as well as excitatory symptoms (Perugi et al., 1998). In this case too, the distinction depends on the temporal relationship between the mood disturbance and the delusions and on the severity of the mood symptoms (American Psychiatric Association, 1994).

PERSONALITY DISORDERS

The frequency with which bipolar disorder appears to be misdiagnosed with personality disorders is probably linked to the complexity of the relationship of personality to bipolar disorders. In a landmark review, Akiskal, Hirschfeld, and Yerevanian (1983), showed that personality could be an orthogonal dimension to bipolar disorder, a characterologic predisposition to bipolar episodes, a modifier or complication of bipolar episodes, or an attenuated expression of bipolar episodes. The most controversial issues are probably those related to borderline personality disorder. According to Paris, Gunderson, and Weinberg (2007), borderline personality disorder could be an atypical form of bipolar disorder, bipolar disorder could be a phenotypic variant of borderline personality disorder, the two disorders could be independent disorders, or the two disorders could have overlapping etiologies. After reviewing the available evidence, they came to the conclusion that the current

separation of borderline personality disorder from bipolar I was supported, whereas the possibility of shared phenotypes was preserved with bipolar II and the soft spectrum. These conclusions have received support from more recent studies (Angst et al., 2013; Azorin et al., 2013). Borderline personality disorder appeared as a contributory factor to the development of bipolar disorder, which could have favored the progression from unipolar major depression to bipolar disorder, although it could not be excluded that some features of bipolar disorder (especially affective temperaments) may have contributed to the development of borderline personality disorder (Azorin et al., 2013).

Regardless, because the cross-sectional presentation of several personality disorders can be mimicked by an episode of bipolar disorder, the clinician should avoid giving an additional diagnosis of personality disorder based only on cross-sectional presentation without having documented that the pattern of behavior has an early onset and a long-standing course (American Psychiatric Association, 1994).

OTHER ISSUES

The presence of other comorbid conditions may similarly lead to misdiagnoses. This is the case for substance abuse and dependence, which are often present at initial presentation. Alcohol and stimulants can produce symptoms that mimic mood episodes; for patients with ongoing substance use, it can therefore be difficult to discern the presence of an underlying bipolar disorder (Perlis, 2005). As for anxiety disorder, the clinician must rely on the previously mentioned features that may be characteristic of bipolar disorder comorbidity and could therefore facilitate the recognition of bipolarity.

In youth, the main differential diagnosis is ADHD. Mania and ADHD are both characterized by excessive activity, impulsive behaviour, poor judgment, and denial of problems. However, ADHD may be distinguishable by early onset (before seven years), chronic rather than episodic course, lack of relatively clear onsets and offsets, and absence of abnormally expansive or elevated mood. Nonetheless, bipolar disorder may also be comorbid with ADHD: in these cases patients with ADHD plus bipolar disorder have prototypic symptoms of both disorders (American Psychiatric Association, 1994).

In the elderly, bipolar disorder may mimic dementia, presenting therefore as what has been called pseudodementia (Azorin, Kaladjian, Adida, Fakra, Hantouche, et al., 2012). In this case, the clinical picture may be close to that of mixed or agitated depression. Patients present with cognitive, behavioral, and mood symptoms; they display dysphoria, lack of retardation, forgetfulness, vivacious facial expression, spells of weeping, talkativeness, psychic agitation, emotional lability, high levels of anxiety, and suicide attempts. The term "pseudohysterical" behavior has been sometimes used to characterize such excessive reactions and extravagant attitudes patients may develop in response to requests from their close. These patients are usually refractory to antidepressant treatment and/or acetylcholinesterase inhibitors. However, when they are treated as depressive mixed states, they display improvement of mood, behavior, and cognition (Azorin, Kaladjian, Adida, Fakra, Hantouche, et al., 2012). Nevertheless, one must keep in mind that similar pictures are likely to occur in the setting of the early course of dementia, giving rise to what is called bipolar type VI (Akiskal, 2007).

IMPROVING DIAGNOSIS OF BIPOLAR SPECTRUM DISORDERS

Strategies that have been proposed to increase the recognition of bipolar spectrum disorders include use of screening tools, use of diagnostic instruments, and careful interview of patients and other informants (Baldassano, 2005; Kaye, 2005; Perlis, 2005).

SCREENING TOOLS

An ideal tool for routine screening of all depressed patients for bipolar spectrum disorders should be brief and easy to complete by patients themselves without assistance (Baldassano, 2005). One of most popular in this regard is certainly the Mood Disorder Questionnaire (MDQ), which was devised by Hirschfeld et al. (2000). The MDQ is a brief, self-report screening instrument that contains 13 questions plus 2 items assessing symptoms' co-occurrence and the severity of functional impairment caused. It contains questions concerning mood, self-confidence, energy, sociability, interest in sex, and other behaviors. The components of the scale were derived from both *DSM-IV* criteria and clinical experience, and the scale has been validated against the Structured Clinical Interview for *DSM-IV* (SCID; Baldassano, 2005). The screen is judged positive if at least seven symptom items are present and if there is co-occurrence of at least two symptoms and a moderate to severe impairment. Any patient can easily complete this survey in less than five minutes, enabling its integration into a routine office visit, when the patient can fill it out

before seeing the physician (Kaye, 2005). If the specificity was generally found to be good, the sensitivity appeared to be lower: the MDQ could detect bipolar I but was less sensitive for bipolar II. It was speculated that the low sensitivity observed in the general population could have been due to the low sensitivity of the abbreviated version of the SCID used in the population studied (Baldassano, 2005). More probably, the MDQ tends to underdiagnose bipolar II disorder because of its requirement for moderate to severe impairment of functioning, when improved functioning is frequently seen in those with hypomania (Kaye, 2005).

Another widely used screening instrument is the Hypomania Checklist (HCL-32; Angst et al., 2005). The HCL-32 is a 32-item questionnaire that may help identify the hypomanic component of depressive episodes. Individuals with a total score of 14 or higher are considered as potentially bipolar. Factor analyses have consistently shown the presence of two components that correspond to the positive ("sunny") and negative ("dark") aspects of hypomania. The HCL-32 is a screening tool for hypomania but makes no difference between bipolar I and bipolar II disorders. However, it was found to increase the detection rate of both bipolar II and minor bipolar disorders. In a recent study (Gamma et al., 2013) with respect to the discrimination of unipolar from bipolar disorder, the HCL-32 showed sensitivity of 82% with a specificity of 57% when *DSM-IV* criteria for bipolar disorder were used but substantially higher specificity of 73% when bipolarity specifier criteria were applied. The psychometric properties of the HCL-32 have been found to be largely culture independent, and the HCL-32 is currently validated in several countries. The HCL-32 is therefore considered a broadly applicable screening tool for hypomanic features, facilitating the detection of hidden bipolarity in patients with depression, which can then be assessed further in a clinical diagnostic interview (Gamma et al., 2013).

The Bipolar Spectrum Diagnostic Scale (BSDS; Ghaemi et al., 2005) is a self-report questionnaire consisting of a narrative-based scale with a descriptive story that captures subtle features of bipolar symptoms and course. It was originally designed to detect the milder portion of the bipolar spectrum in outpatients. It is composed of two parts. The first part is a paragraph containing 19 positively valenced sentences describing many of the symptoms of bipolar disorder. Each sentence is followed by an underlined space for subjects to place a checkmark if they feel that it applies to them. Each checkmark is worth 1 point. The second part of the BSDS is one simple, multiple-choice question asking subjects to rate how well the story describes them overall. The scoring system gives an indication of the probability of the presence of a bipolar spectrum disorder, with a score of 19 or higher suggesting a high probability, a score of 11 to 18 a modest probability, a score of 6 to 10 a low probability, and a score of < 6 that the presence of a bipolar spectrum disorder is highly unlikely (Baldassano, 2005). The total score on the BSDS can range from zero to 25. The optimum threshold for likelihood of bipolar spectrum disorder is a score ≥ 13.

A head-to-head comparison of the MDQ and the BSDS has shown that the MDQ was better able to identify individuals with bipolar I disorder compared with those with bipolar II or bipolar not otherwise specified (NOS), while the BSDS was equally sensitive in the ability to identify bipolar I and bipolar II/NOS, thus making it useful in detecting subtle subclasses of bipolar illness (Ghaemi et al., 2005). However, the BSDS requires further validation in patient population.

The Hypomanic Personality Scale is another self-report questionnaire that could potentially be used to screen for bipolar disorder (Eckblad & Chapman, 1986). However, its major drawback is the length of time it takes to complete, being comprised of 48 items. It has been validated in the adolescent and student population and appears to be highly predictive for bipolar disorders among patient population. The Hypomanic Personality Scale may be more useful in the psychiatric setting rather than in general practice to identify patients at risk for bipolar disorder (Baldassano, 2005).

The Bipolarity Index is an integrated system of patient profile that considers five dimensions of bipolarity: episode characteristics, age of onset, course of illness, response to treatment, and family history (Sachs, 2004). In this instrument, bipolarity is considered as a continuous dimension construct. The presence of mania or hypomania is only one of the five dimensions. All the other dimensions receive equal weight. Each dimension is worth up 20 points, for a maximum possible score of 100. A theoretical case with the traits most convincing for bipolar disorder on every dimension would score 100 points. A score ≥ 60 is considered as highly suggestive of bipolarity. For example, a patient can receive 60 points even without any history of hypomania or mania: first depression at age 18 (20 points), postpartum depression (5 points), more than three depressive episodes (5 points), agitation while taking an antidepressant (10 points), and a sister with clear bipolar disorder (20 points). Incorporation of this rating system into the initial clinical assessment provides an index of the confidence by considering bipolarity as a continuum dimensional construct and helps to focus evaluation process. The Bipolarity Index

appears particularity suitable to bipolar spectrum disorder but also requires further validation.

The Temperament Evaluation of the Memphis, Pisa, Paris, and San Diego Autoquestionnaire, although not designed to screen for bipolarity, may be useful in clinical practice to assess affective temperaments (Akiskal, Akiskal, Haykal, Manning, & Connor, 2005). The finding of temperaments with hypomanic propensities (e.g., hyperthymic, cyclothymic, and irritable temperaments) can orientate toward a more accurate search for bipolar spectrum disorder, (Akiskal & Pinto, 2000).

Most other instruments have been designed to monitor the longitudinal course of bipolar disorder (Baldassano, 2005). These tools permit to collect the retrospective patient's course of illness, urge patients to continue this on a prospective basis, provide a clear picture of the earlier course of illness (the best predictor of the future episode pattern), clarify pattern of prior medication responsiveness, and encourage the patient's collaboration. Sometimes they may also facilitate the recognition of low-level manic symptoms and therefore help diagnose soft degrees of bipolarity. The National Institute of Mental Meath Life Chart Method (NIMH-LCM) is the most popular among these instruments (Leverich & Post; see http://www.medscape. com). Many individuals with bipolar illness seem to be capable of completing the NIMH-LCM with appropriate training and guidance (Baldassano, 2005).

DIAGNOSTIC INSTRUMENTS

Structured clinical interviews such as the SCID (First, Spitzer, Gibbon, & Williams, 1996) and the Composite International Diagnostic Interview (see http://www.hcp. med.harvard.edu/wmhcidi/about.php) have been widely used for the diagnosis of bipolar disorders. They have shown high validity and reliability in several different populations. However, their reliability may be highest in patients with severe and well-defined symptomatology and lowest among patients whose symptoms are less well defined. Thus they are not very relevant for the diagnosis of soft bipolarity (Baldassano, 2005). The main reason is that certain bipolar symptoms are assessed using a single question and therefore not easily captured (Baldassano, 2005). Semistructured interviews have been proposed to overcome this difficultly (Benazzi, 2003). This is the case for the modified SCID Hypomania Module (SCID-Hba), in which many questions are asked about each symptom to make the question understandable according to each patient (Benazzi & Akiskal, 2009). These instruments emphasize the importance of observable behaviours such as overactivity and have less stringent duration thresholds for the diagnosis of a manic/hypomanic episode.

INTERVIEW OF PATIENTS AND OTHER INFORMANTS

Even though screening tools and diagnostic instruments may be of help in certain cases, for most patients the diagnosis of bipolar disorder relies on clinical interview. Interviews of patients and significant others may focus on current symptoms (mood), illness course (episodes), response to treatment, and family history. There are a number of reasons why it is advisable to attempt to interview the patient's spouse, parent, child, significant other, or close friend. Patients may fail to recall manic or hypomanic symptoms or may have no insight into the impact their symptoms may have had on their functioning. On the other hand, many patients value their heightened activity and energy during hypomanic states and fail to report them as pathologic. Other patients may fear the stigma associated with bipolar disorders. Interviewing someone close to the patient can often provide historical clues to the correct diagnosis. Physical examination, complete medical history, and laboratory evaluations may be necessary to diagnose comorbid medical conditions or substance abuse, as well as to rule out organic disorders that could be responsible for the symptoms observed (Baldassano, 2005; Kaye, 2005).

CONCLUSION

This chapter could be an illustration of what was emphasized 10 years ago by Katzow et al. (2003), that is, that the relative misdiagnosis, underdiagnosis, and overdiagnosis of bipolar disorder is due in a large part to the "soft" symptoms of bipolarity that characterize patients within the bipolar spectrum. To deal with such an issue, an extensive number of screening tools and diagnostic instruments have been devised to help professionals better recognize the manifold manifestations of the subtypes included in this spectrum. If this evolution has made the diagnostic process more complex, it has certainly contributed to improving our knowledge of the disease and its boundaries.

Disclosure statement: Jean-Michel Azorin has received research support and has acted as a consultant and/or served on a speaker's bureau for Bristol-Myers Squibb, Janssen, Lilly, Lundbeck, Roche, and Sanofi-Aventis. Dr. Raoul Belzeaux has no conflicts of interest.

REFERENCES

Akiskal, H. S. (2007). The interface of affective and schizophrenic disorders: A cross between two spectra? In A. Marneros & H. Akiskal (Eds.), *The overlap of affective and schizophrenic spectra* (pp. 277–291). Cambridge, UK: Cambridge University Press.

Akiskal, H. S., Akiskal, K. K., Haykal, R. F., Manning, J. S., & Connor, P. D. (2005). TEMPS-A: Progress towards validation of a self-rated clinical version of the Temperament Evaluation of the Memphis, Pisa, Paris, and San Diego Autoquestionnaire. *Journal of Affective Disorders, 85*, 3–16.

Akiskal, H. S., Hantouche, E. G., & Allilaire, J. F. (2003). Bipolar II with and without cyclothymic temperament: "Clark" and "sunny" expressions of soft bipolarity. *Journal of Affective Disorders, 73*, 49–57.

Akiskal, H. S., Hantouche, E. G., Bourgeois, M. L., Azorin, J. M., Sechter, D., Allilaire, J. F., … Châtenet-Duchêne L. (1998). Gender, temperament, and the clinical picture in dysphoric mixed mania: Findings from a French National Study (EPIMAN). *Journal of Affective Disorders, 50*, 175–186.

Akiskal, H. S., Hirschfeld, R. M., & Yerevanian, B. I. (1983). The relationship of personality to affective disorders. *Archives of General Psychiatry, 40*, 801–810.

Akiskal, H. S., & Pinto, O. (2000). The soft bipolar spectrum: Footnotes to Kraepelin on the interface of hypomania, temperament and depression. In A. Marneros & J. Angst (Eds.), *Bipolar disorders: 100 years after manic-depressive insanity* (pp. 37–62). Dordrecht: Kluwer Academic.

American Psychiatric Association. (1994). *Diagnostic and statistical manual of mental disorders* (4th ed.). Washington, DC: Author.

Angst, J. (1998). The emerging epidemiology of hypomania and bipolar II disorder. *Journal of Affective Disorders, 50*, 143–151.

Angst, J., Adolfsson, R., Benazzi, F., Gamma, A., Hantouche, E., Meyer, T. D., … Scott, J. (2005). The HCL-32: Towards a self-assessment tool for hypomanic symptoms in outpatients. *Journal of Affective Disorders, 88*, 217–233.

Angst, J., Azorin, J. M., Bowden, C. L., Perugi, G., Vieta, E., Gamma, A., & Young, A. H. (2011). Prevalence and characteristics of undiagnosed bipolar disorders in patients with a major depressive episode: The Bridge Study. *Archives of General Psychiatry, 68*, 791–798.

Angst, J., Gamma, A., Benazzi, F., Ajdavic, V., Eich, D., & Rossler, W. (2003a). Diagnostic issues in bipolar disorder. *European Neuropsychopharmacology, 13*(2), 543–550.

Angst, J., Gamma, A., Benazzi, F., Ajdacic, V., Eich, D., & Rössler, W. (2003b). Toward a re-definition of subthreshold bipolarity: Epidemiology and proposed criteria for bipolar II, minor bipolar disorders and hypomania. *Journal of Affective Disorders, 73*, 133–146.

Angst, J., Gamma, A., Bowden, C. L., Azorin, J. M., Perugi, G., Vieta, E., & Young, A. M. (2013). Evidence-based definition of bipolar-I and bipolar-II disorders among 5,635 patients with major depressive episodes in the Bridge Study: Validity and comorbidity. *European Archives of Psychiatry and Clinical Neuroscience, 263*(8), 663–673.

Azorin, J. M., Akiskal, H., & Hantouche, E. (2006). The mood-instability hypothesis in the origin of mood-congruent versus mood-incongruent psychotic distinction in mania: Validation in a French National Study of 1090 patients. *Journal of Affective Disorders, 96*, 215–223.

Azorin, J. M., Bellivier, F., Kaladjian, A., Adida, M., Belzeaux, R., Fakra, E., … Golmard, J. L. (2013). Characteristics and profiles of bipolar I patients according to age-at-onset: Findings from an admixture analysis. *Journal of Affective Disorders, 150*(3), 993–1000.

Azorin, J. M., Kaladjian, A., Adida, M., & Fakra, E. (2012). Late-onset bipolar illness: The geriatric bipolar type VI. *CNS Neurosciences & Therapeutics, 18*, 208–213.

Azorin, J. M., Kaladjian, A., Adida, M., Fakra, E., Hantouche, E., & Lancrenon, S. (2011). Correlates of first episode polarity in a French cohort of 1089 bipolar I disorder patients: Role of temperament and triggering events. *Journal of Affective Disorders, 129*, 39–46.

Azorin, J. M., Kaladjian, A., Adida, M., Fakra, E., Belzeaux, R., Hantouche, E., & Lancrenon, S. (2013). Factors associated with borderline personality disorder in major depressive patients and their relationship to bipolarity. *European Psychiatry, 28*(8), 463–468.

Azorin, J. M., Kaladjian, A., Adida, M., Fakra, E., Hantouche, E, & Lancrenon, S. (2012). Baseline and prodromal characteristics of first-versus multiple-episode mania in a French cohort of bipolar patients. *European Psychiatry, 27*, 557–562.

Baldassano, C. F. (2005). Assessment tools for screening and monitoring bipolar disorder. *Bipolar Disorders, 7*(1), 8–15.

Benazzi, F. (2003). Diagnosis of bipolar II disorder: A comparison of structured versus semistructured interviews. *Progress in Neuro-Psychopharmacology & Biological Psychiatry, 27*, 985–991.

Benazzi, F., & Akiskal, H. S. (2009). The modified SCID Hypomania Module (SCID-Hba): A detailed systematic phenomenologic probing. *Journal of Affective Disorders, 117*, 131–136.

Composite International Diagnostic Interview (CIDI). 2005. Geneva: World Health Organization. http://www.hcp.med.harvard.edu/wmhcidi/

Eckblad, M., & Chapman, L. J. (1986). Development and validation of a scale for hypomanic personality. *Journal of Affective Disorders, 95*, 214–222.

First, M. B., Spitzer, R. L., Gibbon, M., & Williams, J. B. W. (1996). *Structured clinical interview for DSM-IV Axis I disorders: Patient Ed. SCID–P version 2.* New York: Biometrics Research.

Gamma, A., Angst, J., Azorin, J. M., Bowden, C. L., Perugi, G., Vieta, E., & Young, A. H. (2013). Transcultural validity of the Hypomania Checklist–32 (HCL-32) in patients with major depressive episodes. *Bipolar Disorders, 15*(6), 701–712.

Gazalle, F. K., Andreazza, A. C., Cereser, K. M., Hallal, P. C., Santin, A., & Kapczinski, F. (2005). Clinical impact of late diagnose of bipolar disorder. *Journal of Affective Disorders, 86*, 313–316.

Ghaemi, S. N., Ko, J. Y., & Goodwin, F. K. (2002). "Cade's disease" and beyond: Misdiagnosis, antidepressant use, and a proposed definition for bipolar spectrum disorder. *Canadian Journal of Psychiatry, 47*, 125–134.

Ghaemi, S. N., Miller, C. J., Berv, D. A., Klugman, J., Rosenquist, K. J., & Pies, R. W. (2005). Sensitivity and specificity of a new bipolar spectrum diagnostic scale. *Journal of Affective Disorders, 84*, 273–277.

Goodwin, F. K., & Jamison, K. R. (2007). *Manic-depressive illness: Bipolar disorders and recurrent depression* (2nd ed.). New York: Oxford University Press.

Hantouche, E. G., Akiskal, H. S., Azorin, J. M., Châtenet-Duchêne, L., & Lancrenon, S. (2006). Clinical and psychometric characterization of depression in mixed mania: A report from the French National Cohort of 1090 manic patients. *Journal of Affective Disorders, 96*, 225–232.

Hirschfeld, R. M., Lewis, L., & Vornik, L. A. (2003). Perception and impact of bipolar disorder: how far have we really come? Results of the National Depressive and Manic-Depressive Association 2000 survey of individuals with bipolar disorder. *Journal of Clinical Psychiatry, 64*, 161–174.

Hirschfeld, R. M., Williams, J. B., Spitzer, R. L., Calabrese, J. R., Flynn, L., Keck, P. E. Jr., ... Zapecka, J. (2000). Development and validation of a screening instrument for bipolar spectrum disorder: The Mood Disorder Questionnaire. *American Journal of Psychiatry, 157*, 1873–1875.

Judd, L., & Akiskal, H. (2003). The prevalence and disability of bipolar spectrum disorders in the US population: Re-analysis of the ECA database taking into account subthreshold case. *Journal of Affective Disorders, 73*, 123–131.

Kaye, N. S. (2005). Is your depressed patient bipolar? *Journal of the American Board of Family Practice, 18*, 271–281.

Katzow, J. J., Hsu, D. J., & Ghaemi, S. N. (2003). The bipolar spectrum, a clinical perspective. *Bipolar Disorders, 5*, 436–442.

Klerman, G. L. (1981). The spectrum mania. *Comprehensive Psychiatry, 22*, 11–20.

Kraepelin, E. (1921). *Manic depressive insanity and paranoia.* Edinburgh, UK: Livingstone.

Krishnan, K. R. R. (2005). Psychiatric and medical comorbidities of bipolar disorder. *Psychosomatic Medicine, 67*, 1–8.

Leverich, G. S., & Post, R. M. (1998). Charting the course of bipolar illness and its response to treatment. *Medscape Psychiatry & Mental Health, 3*(3). Retrieved from http://www.medscape.com/viewarticle/430628

Lish, J. D., Dime-Menan, S., Whybrow, P. C., Price, R. A., & Hirschfeld, R. M. (1994). The National Depressive and Manic-Depressive Association (DMDA) survey of bipolar members. *Journal of Affective Disorders, 31*, 281–294.

McElroy, S. L., Altshuler, L. L., Suppes, T., Keck, P. E. Jr., Frye, M. A., Denicoff, K. D., ... Post, R. M. (2001). Axis I psychiatric comorbidity and its relationship to historical illness variables in 288 patients with bipolar disorder. *American Journal of Psychiatry, 158*, 420–426.

McElroy, S. L., Arnold, L. M., & Altshuler, L. C. (2011). Bipolarity in women: Therapeutic issues. In H. S. Akiskal & M. Tohen (Eds.), *Bipolar psychopharmacotherapy: Caring for the patient* (2nd ed., pp. 317–350). Chichester, UK: John Wiley.

Mitchell, P. B., Goodwin, G. M., Johnson, G. F., Hirschfeld, R. M. A. (2008). Diagnostic guidelines for bipolar depression: A probabilistic approach. *Bipolar Disorders, 10*, 144–152.

Morselli, P. L., & Elgie, R. (2003). GAMIAN-Europe/BEAM survey I—Global analysis of a patient questionnaire circulated to 3450 members of 12 European advocacy groups operating in the field of mood disorders. *Bipolar Disorders, 5*, 265–278.

Nivoli, A. M. A., Pacchiarotti, I., Rosa, A. R., Popovic, D., Murru, A., Valenti, M., ... Colom, F. (2011). Gender differences in a cohort of 604 bipolar patients: The role of predominant polarity. *Journal of Affective Disorders, 133*, 443–449.

Paris, J., Gunderson, J., & Weinberg, I. (2007). The interface between borderline personality disorder and bipolar spectrum disorders. *Comprehensive Psychiatry, 48*(6), 145–154.

Perlis, R. H. (2005). Misdiagnosis of bipolar disorder. *American Journal of Managed Care, 11*, 5271–5274.

Perugi, G., Akiskal, H. S., Pfanner, C., Presta, S., Gemignani, A., Milanfranchi, A., ... Cassano, G. B. (1997). The clinical impact of bipolar and unipolar affective comorbidity on obsessive-compulsive disorder. *Journal of Affective Disorders, 46*, 15–23.

Perugi, G., Akiskal, H. S., Rossi, L., Paiano, A., Quilici, C., Madaro, D., ... Cassano, G. B. (1998). Chronic mania: Family history, prior course, clinical picture and social consequences. *The British Journal of Psychiatry, 173*, 514–518.

Perugi, G., Akiskal, H. S., Toni, C., Simonini, E., & Gemignani, A. (2001). The temporal relationship between anxiety disorders and (hypo)mania: A retrospective examination of 63 panic, social phobic and obsessive-compulsive patients with comorbid bipolar disorder. *Journal of Affective Disorders, 67*, 199–206.

Regier, D. A., & Kaelber, C. T. (1995). The epidemiologic catchment area (ECA) program: Studying the prevalence and incidence of psychopathology. In M. T. Tsuang, M. Tohen, & G. E. P. Zahner (Eds.), *Textbook in psychiatric epidemiology* (pp. 133–157). New York: John Wiley.

Rouillon, F. (2005). *Epidemiologie des troubles bipolaires.* (L. Suresnes, Ed.).

Ruggero, C. J., Zimmerman, M., Chelminski, I., & Young, D. (2010). Borderline personality disorder and the misdiagnosis of bipolar disorder. *Journal of Psychiatric Research, 44*, 405–408.

Sachs, G. S. (2004). Strategies for improving treatment of bipolar disorder: integration of measurement and management. *Acta Psychiatrica Scandinavica, 110*(422), 7–17.

Singh, T., & Rajput, M. (2006). Misdiagnosis of bipolar disorder. *Psychiatry, 40,* 57–63.

Smith, D. J., Harrison, N., Muir, W., & Blackwood, D. H. (2005). The high prevalence of bipolar spectrum disorders in young adults with recurrent depression: Toward an innovative diagnostic framework. *Journal of Affective Disorders, 84,* 167–178.

Zimmerman, M., Ruggero, C. J., Chelminski, I., & Young, D. (2008). Is bipolar disorder overdiagnosed? *Journal of Clinical Psychiatry, 69,* 935–940.

5.

DIAGNOSING BIPOLAR DISORDER IN CHILDREN AND ADOLESCENTS

Andrew J. Freeman, Kiki Chang, and Eric A. Youngstrom

INTRODUCTION

Pediatric bipolar disorder (PBD) is both more common than conventional wisdom suggests and more rare than popular clinical beliefs in the United States. Meta-analysis of epidemiological studies suggest that a base rate of approximately 2% of the general childhood and adolescent population meet criteria for PBD (Merikangas et al., 2012; Van Meter, Moreira, & Youngstrom, 2011) in contrast to conventional textbook wisdom that suggests PBD occurs rarely or never (e.g., Mash & Barkley, 2003). In the last decade, many have worried about the overdiagnosis of PBD because the diagnostic rate in the community has increased 40-fold (Blader & Carlson, 2007). While the relative risk of diagnosis has increased, the absolute risk, or the overall number, of clinical diagnosis remains very low (Moreno et al., 2007). Additionally, bipolar disorder as diagnosed in the community often serves as a diagnostic label for extreme irritability that may not reflect a mood disorder (Leibenluft, Charney, Towbin, Bhangoo, & Pine, 2003). The purpose of this chapter is to integrate an evidence-based framework for identifying and diagnosing PBD within the structure of a common outpatient office visit.

Evidence-based practice aims to make implicit decisions explicit and to provide clinicians with meaningful tools to do so (Jaeschke, Guyatt, & Sackett, 1994a, 1994b). As humans, clinicians are prone to make errors in thinking due to the efficient, but not always accurate, use of heuristics. To reduce errors, evidence-based decision-making starts with a prior probability that is adjusted by a likelihood ratio to create a new posterior probability using Bayes Theorem. Clinically, this concept translates to an initial index of suspicion (prior probability), testing (likelihood ratios), and an updated index of suspicion (posterior probability). For example, if clinicians use the heuristic that "no children have PBD," then they will underdiagnosis it by definition

because they will have an initial suspicion of 0% that is not adjusted when new information is gathered. If clinicians use the heuristic that "PBD is common and frequently underdiagnosed," then they will likely overdiagnose because they will start with a substantially higher initial suspicion and weight new information too heavily. Clinicians' diagnostic suspicion of PBD shows a range of 100% about both their initial and updated suspicion of PBD when left to interpret data using heuristics (Jenkins, Youngstrom, Washburn, & Youngstrom, 2011). Implementing simple, easy-to-use evidence-based decision-making tools recenters the clinical index of suspicion around the empirical estimate and significantly decreases variability among clinicians (Jenkins et al., 2011).

Here we provide a framework for the implementation of evidence-based decision-making for PBD in the context of the standard office visit. Table 5.1 and Figure 5.1 display the 10 steps for the evidence-based assessment of PBD that can help guide clinical decision-making (Youngstrom, Freeman, & Jenkins, 2009; Youngstrom, Jenkins, Doss, & Youngstrom, 2012). Clinicians make two specific decisions in the assessment process. First, they use a wait-test threshold. Should the risk of PBD be ruled so low that it can be set aside, or should more assessment occur? Second, clinicians have a test-treatment threshold. Should more evidence be gathered, or is there enough evidence to begin treating? Oftentimes these thresholds are implicit and internal to the specific clinician. A family's treatment preference (e.g., tolerance of side effects, beliefs about medication), as well as a clinician's expertise, should be integrated into where these thresholds lie. Some families and clinicians will be more conservative and desire very high levels of suspicion prior to initiating treatment. Integrating the use of explicit decision points should improve the clinical diagnosis of PBD by providing a guidepost as to the next step. A typical office visit

Table 5.1. TEN STEPS FOR THE EVIDENCE-BASED ASSESSMENT OF PEDIATRIC BIPOLAR DISORDER

STEP	RATIONALE	TIME AND COST	WHEN TO ASSESS
A. Know base rate in your setting	Anchors initial index of suspicion	Time: 0 Cost: 0	Prior to visits
B. Information from broad, externalizing scales	Low parent report on Externalizing rules bipolar out High parent report another "red flag" High youth report, teacher report double odds	Time: 10–15 min for family Cost: ~.50	Waiting room
C. Any risk factors?	Risk factors raise "index of suspicion" enough to trigger more assessment	Time: 2–10 min Cost: 0	Interview—family history
D. Add brief screens for hypomania, mania	Parent report screens replace Externalizing score—more specific to bipolar	Time: 5 min for family, 2 min for practitioner Cost: (public domain)	Waiting room or Interview
E. Get multiple perspectives—and plan for differences	Youth and teacher report helpful for measuring pervasiveness and also motivation for treatment	Time: 5 min per informant, 2 min to score Cost: (public domain)	Waiting room or via mail
F. Intensive assessment for bipolar	Clinical interview focusing on mood presentation—FIND and GRAPES mnemonics Semistructured interviews: K-SADS, MINI	Time: 30–120 min Cost: Variable (public domain versus proprietary)	Diagnostic interview
G. Additional assessment for treatment planning	Rule out general medical conditions, other medications; family functioning, quality of life, personality, school adjustment, comorbidities	Time: Variable Cost: Variable (additional checklists or testing)	Diagnostic interview
H. Process monitoring	Life charts, mood, and energy check-ups at each visit, medication monitoring, therapy assignments	Time: < 5 min per day for family, < 5 min per visit for practitioner Cost: –$4 for applications	Waiting room or interview
I. Progress and outcome	Repeat assessment with main severity measures—interview and/or parent report most sensitive to treatment effects	Time: 10–40 min Cost: None	Waiting room or interview
J. Maintenance	Discuss life charting; review triggers, critical events and life transitions	Time: Negligible Cost: None	Waiting room or interview

NOTE: KSADS = Schedule for Affective Disorders and Schizophrenia for School-Age Children; MINI = Mini-International Neuropsychiatric Interview.

consists of checking in, waiting in a waiting room, measuring basic vital signs, waiting in an exam room, and a clinical interview about developmental history, family history, and current symptoms. For families, much of an office visit consists of inefficient waiting, time that could be used efficiently to improve decision-making and treatment monitoring.

GENERAL CLINICAL KNOWLEDGE ABOUT PEDIATRIC BIPOLAR DISORDER AND BASE RATES (STEP A)

The fourth edition (text revision) and fifth edition of the *Diagnostic and Statistical Manual of Mental Disorders* (American Psychiatric Association, 2000, 2013) and International Statistical Classification of Diseases and Related Health Problems (ICD-10; World Health Organization, 1992) all define bipolar disorder as an episodic illness with distinct periods of elevated, expansive, irritable, or hyperenergetic mood along with grandiosity, decreased need for sleep, pressured speech, flight of ideas, racing thoughts, distractibility, increased goal-directed activity, psychomotor agitation, and excessive pleasure-seeking. A classic bipolar disorder prototype exists that consists of the recurrence of distinct, separate depressive and manic episodes with euthymia between episodes. Clinicians typically make diagnoses by comparing the current youth's presentation to this standard model (Garb, 1998). Unfortunately, this prototype poorly matches most adult presentations (Kogan et al., 2004) and youth presentations, which are marked by

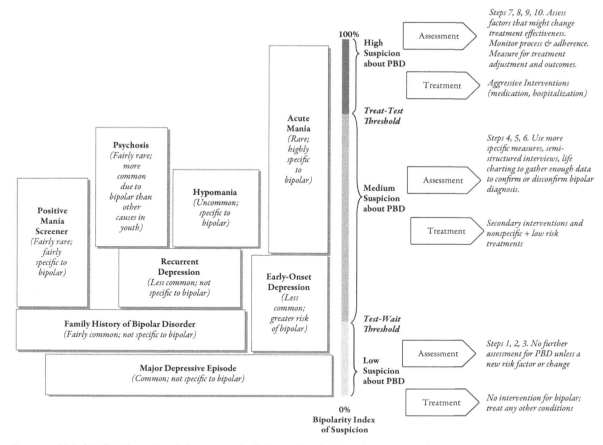

Figure 5.1 Integrated Model of Evidence-Based Assessment for Pediatric Bipolar Disorder.

longer episodes of mixed symptoms and less time spent in euthymia (Geller et al., 2000; Youngstrom, Birmaher, & Findling, 2008a). Additionally, bipolar disorder presents with various phases of illness (e.g., depressed, euthymic, manic, mixed), as well as severity (hypomanic vs. manic), meaning that what is seen during an evaluation period is not necessarily what becomes a final accurate diagnosis. This difficulty likely explains the poor performance of prototype matching in clinical diagnoses of PBD (Biederman, Klein, Pine, & Klein, 1998; Klein, Pine, & Klein, 1998). Therefore, clinicians should be aware that many youth will present with long-duration, mixed episodes, where parents typically describe irritability as the most concerning symptom along with other specific symptoms of mania such as decreased need for sleep.

PBD most notably distinguishes itself from other diagnoses by the presence of specific symptoms and presentation. Decreased need for sleep and elated mood are both specific and sensitive to PBD (Kowatch, Youngstrom, Danielyan, & Findling, 2005). Additionally, PBD is an episodic disorder in that symptoms and severity wax and wane over time. In contrast to the specific symptoms and episodic

nature of PBD, the *Diagnostic and Statistical Manual of Mental Disorders* (fifth edition; American Psychiatric Association, 2013) includes a new diagnosis of disruptive mood dysregulation disorder (DMDD), which was originally proposed to reduce the surmised overdiagnosis of PBD in the general community. DMDD reflects a subset of youth with chronic, severe irritability with moodiness but no other symptoms of mania. When conducting the differential diagnosis between PBD and DMDD, ascertainment of specific mania symptoms, as well as the longitudinal course of the symptoms, should help distinguish PBD from DMDD. DMDD will likely be more common than PBD in both the community and general clinical settings (Axelson et al., 2012; Copeland, Angold, Costello, & Egger, 2013). Additionally, youth with DMDD may typically present as a more severe and "moody" variant of oppositional defiant disorder (Axelson et al., 2012; Copeland et al., 2013). It will be important moving forward to look for other underlying causes of irritability (e.g., anxiety, depression, psychosocial stressors, pervasive developmental disorders) before settling on a DMDD diagnosis, as there are no relevant studies or treatment recommendations for this group of children

Table 5.2. BASE RATES OF PEDIATRIC BIPOLAR DISORDER IN DIFFERENT SETTINGS

SETTING	BASE RATE	POPULATION
General population	2% (4% for spectrum)	Global meta-analysis (Merikangas et al., 2007; Van Meter et al., 2011)
Outpatient or community mental health	5% to 10%	Various (Tillman & Geller, 2007; Youngstrom et al., 2006a)
Specialty outpatient service	15% to 20%	New England, Midwestern USA (Biederman, Faraone, Mick, & Wozniak, 1996)
Incarcerated adolescents	2% to 22%	Chicago and Texas (Pliszka, Sherman, Barrow, & Irick, 2000; Teplin, Abram, McClelland, Dulcan, & Mericle, 2002)
Inpatient and psychiatric hospitalization	25% to 40%	All of United States (record surveillance) (Blader & Carlson, 2007)

(Axelson et al., 2012). Currently, there are no published tests capable of providing evidence-based differentiation between DMDD and other disorders.

In addition to the basic clinical presentation, clinicians should know the base rate of PBD in their setting. In evidence-based medicine, the base rate often serves as the initial index of suspicion. The base rate of PBD varies dramatically across settings, with the rule of thumb that it increases as specialization of services increases. For example, clinicians consulting in schools and screening all individuals would not expect to see many youth with PBD (~2 in 100); however, clinicians working in an adolescent inpatient unit might expect to see many youth with PBD (~25–40 in 100). Table 5.2 provides empirical estimates of base rates in different settings. On the one hand, in low base-rate settings, adding specific screening measures for

Table 5.3. CLINICAL "RED FLAGS" THAT SHOULD TRIGGER MORE EVALUATION OF PBD

RED FLAG	DESCRIPTION	REASON
Family history of bipolar disorder[a]	PBD has genetic contribution Family environment affects treatment adherence and relapse	1st degree relative = 5x–10x 2nd degree relative = 2.5x–5x "Fuzzy" bipolar in relative = 2x (Smoller & Finn, 2003)
Early-onset depression	Onset < 25 years Prepubertal depression	First clinical episode is often depression 20% to 35% of pediatric depressions ultimately show bipolar course (Birmaher et al., 1996)
Antidepressant use	Possibility for manic symptoms while being treated with antidepressants	FDA recommends assessing for hypomania, family history of bipolar before beginning antidepressant "Switch" is often previously undiagnosed PBD (Joseph, Youngstrom, & Soares, 2009)
Episodic mood lability	Rapid switching between depressive and manic symptoms; depressive and manic symptoms at the same time	Common presentation Episodicity more suggestive of mood diagnosis (Youngstrom et al., 2008a)
Episodic aggressive behavior	Episodic; high-energy Not instrumental or planned; reactive	Not specific but common (Youngstrom et al., 2008a)
Psychotic features	True delusions/hallucinations in the context of mood episode	Bipolar more common as source of psychosis than schizophrenia in children (Tillman et al., 2008)
Sleep disturbance	Decreased need for sleep Less sleep but maintains high energy	More specific to bipolar Indicates sleep hygiene component of treatment

NOTE: PBD = pediatric bipolar disorder.

[a] Only family history displays robust empirical evidence.

PBD might not be helpful because low test scores or the lack of risk factors will not add information and high scores or the presence of risk factors will still lead to a situation in which the typical positive screen is a false positive. On the other hand, in high base-rate settings, adding screening procedures can help quickly move many cases above or below common clinical decisions such as whether to assess more thoroughly or whether to treat. Clinically, extremely low base-rate settings would likely not benefit from universal screening for mania symptoms.

THE WAITING ROOM: MAXIMIZING EFFICIENCY (STEP B)

For most clinical visits, the first contact a family has is with a physician extender who completes the check-in process. Questionnaires are widely used in clinical practice. Having the assistant hand parents and/or youth questionnaires to complete while waiting for an exam room or the clinician is an efficient use of time. Widely used broadband measures (e.g., Child Behavior Checklist, Behavior Assessment System for Children, Second Edition) are valuable tools for improving diagnosis because they provide a simple method for assessing many symptoms quickly (Achenbach & Rescorla, 2001; Reynolds & Kamphaus, 1992). These measures are sensitive to PBD, meaning that youth with PBD typically score very high, particularly on Externalizing subscales. However, broadband measures are typically not *specific* to PBD, in that there are many other reasons for a high score (Youngstrom et al., 2004, 2005b). Youth with PBD frequently display a "profile" of elevations on multiple problem behavior scales; this approach adds little to no clinically meaningful information above and beyond the Externalizing subscale (Diler et al., 2009). Table 5.3 provides common cut-scores and likelihood ratios. On broadband measures, low scores on Externalizing (i.e., T score ≤ 60) tend to quickly rule PBD out, clinician can then concentrate on other hypotheses, potentially reducing burden. Clinically elevated scores (i.e., T score ≥ 70) and very elevated scores (i.e., T scores ≥ 81) indicate more clinical screening might be warranted.

THE INTERVIEW—RISK FACTORS? (STEP C)

In addition to positive screens from broadband measures, clinicians should be aware of common risk factors for PBD or clinically meaningful reasons to screen for mania. Table

5.4 lists the common risk factors and reasons for additional screening. First, family history is consistently the most robust risk factor for PBD, and most cases of PBD have a family history of bipolar disorder (Hodgins, Faucher, Zarac, & Ellenbogen, 2002). For example, bipolar disorder in a parent or sibling is linked with a five-fold increase in risk for PBD (Youngstrom, Findling, Youngstrom, &

Table 5.4. SELECTED MEASURES FOR IMPROVING THE DIAGNOSIS OF PEDIATRIC BIPOLAR DISORDER

SCREENING MEASURE	AUC	TEST SCORE	DIAGNOSTIC LIKELIHOOD RATIO
Adolescents (11 to 18)			
Parent General Behavior Inventory—Hypomanic/ Biphasic	.84	<15	.2
		16–24	1.1
		25–39	2.2
		40–48	4.8
		49+	9.2
CBCL Externalizing T Score	.78	<54	.04
		54–56	.5
		65–69	1.3
		70–75	2.1
		76–80	2.7
		81+	4.3
YSR Externalizing T Score	.71	<49	.3
		49–55	.5
		56–69	1.4
		70–76	2.3
		77+	3.0
Adolescent General Behavior Inventory—Hypomanic/ Biphasic	.64	<10	.3
		10–37	1.0
		38–45	2.0
		46+	3.9
Children (5 to 10 years)			
CBCL Externalizing T Score	.82	<58	.1
		58–67	.5
		68–72	1.5
		73+	3.9
Parent General Behavior Inventory—Hypomanic/ Biphasic	.81	<11	.1
		11–20	.5
		21–30	1.3
		31–42	2.3
		43–50	4.9
		51+	6.3

NOTE: AUC = Area Under the Curve; CBCL = Child Behavior Checklist; YSR = Youth Self-Report. Diagnoses based on K-SADS interview by a trained rater combined with review by a clinician. Diagnostic likelihood ratio (DLR) refers to the change in suspicion associated with the test score. Likelihood ratios of 1 indicate no change in suspicion. DLRs larger than 10 or smaller than .10 are frequently clinically decisive; 5 or .2 are helpful, and between 2.0 and .5 are small enough that they rarely result in clinically meaningful changes of suspicion. Data from Youngstrom et al. (2004); Youngstrom et al. (2005b).

Calabrese, 2005a). Second, psychosis in youth is more commonly due to a mood disorder than schizophrenia (Tillman et al., 2008). Third, early-onset depression is present in approximately 1 in 3 cases of PBD at follow-up (Angst, Gamma, Sellaro, Lavori, & Zhang, 2003), and the Food and Drug Administration recommends monitoring all youth prescribed with an antidepressant for side effects, including suicidality and antidepressant-induced mania. Fourth, descriptions of periods where the need for sleep is markedly decreased are likely specific to mania (Kowatch et al., 2005; Murray & Harvey, 2010). Additional clinical presentations that warrant increased attention include bouts of *episodic* aggression (Dickstein & Leibenluft, 2012; Goldstein & Birmaher, 2012) or someone requesting a specific referral to evaluate PBD. Despite the list of many risk factors, family history is the only risk factor that has empirically based weights to change the index of suspicion. All others are clinical considerations that could be PBD but often have different etiologies than PBD.

THE INTERVIEW—COLLECTING MORE INFORMATION (STEPS D AND E)

As the empirical risk of PBD increases, so should the clinical concern. Clinicians should consider adding specific measures of mania to screen more thoroughly. Parents are often the most familiar with a youth's behavior, and their descriptions are typically most valuable—both in terms of clinical information and empirical risk (Youngstrom et al., 2004; Youngstrom, Meyers, Youngstrom, Calabrese, & Findling, 2006a). Questionnaires specific to mania typically outperform broadband measures in discriminating PBD from non-PBD. Broadband measures, which are sensitive to PBD, increase risk mildly, but high scores could reflect many different etiologies. In contrast, high scores on PBD specific measures raise the index of suspicion higher for PBD, and low scores quickly rule out PBD. More important, low scores on mania questionnaires can mitigate increased suspicion due to risk factors such as a positive family history (Youngstrom et al., 2009). Broadband and specific questionnaires are sensitive to PBD. Low scores are more powerful in ruling out PBD than high scores ruling in PBD (Strauss, Glasziou, Richardson, & Haynes, 2010). During an office visit, a parent can complete specific questionnaires while the youth is being interviewed.

Best practices call for clinical information from multiple sources. Expect different information about PBD from each source. Parent-reported manic symptoms show greater diagnostic validity than both youth and teacher report (Youngstrom et al., 2004; Youngstrom, Joseph, & Greene, 2008c). High scores from multiple informants indicate a more severe and impairing condition (Carlson & Youngstrom, 2003; Thuppal, Carlson, Sprafkin, & Gadow, 2002). When considering multiple informants' information, remember that scores that appear to be discrepant might actually be considered in agreement statistically. For example, a parent report of an Externalizing score of 80 compared to a teacher report of a score of 60 not only appears different but the scores also fall in different clinical categories—very elevated versus within typical limits. However, when the difference is benchmarked against typical levels of agreement, these scores reflect higher than average agreement for a group of cases with 80 as the average parent score (Youngstrom, Meyers, Youngstrom, Calabrese, & Findling, 2006b).

Expect informant perspectives to be different about a youth's symptoms, particularly symptoms of mania. Weigh discrepant information more heavily in favor of parents than the youth or teacher. Although youths are believed to be more accurate about reporting depression (Loeber, Green, Lahey, & Stouthamer-Loeber, 1991), parents are more accurate informants about PBD because mania typically compromises insight (Dell'Osso et al., 2002). Teachers do not typically observe hallmark features of mania, such as decreased need for sleep; teachers tend to attribute many problem behaviors to attention deficit hyperactivity disorder (ADHD) or oppositionality (Youngstrom et al., 2008c). Empirical evidence strongly favors parent report in terms of typical diagnostic validity, but factors can influence the credibility of parent report. The less credible that a clinician views a parent's reporting, the less discriminating the parent's reporting is. However, parental stress and parental mood disorder history do not affect credibility in consistent ways (Youngstrom et al., 2011). Therefore when suspicion increases, clinicians should (a) collect mania specific measures, (b) try to always involve the parent, (c) consider other reporters to be informative about overall severity of behavioral and emotional disturbances but not specific about PBD, and (d) remember to use clinical judgment when determining the credibility of parents without discounting information simply because a parent has bipolar disorder or is stressed.

THE INTERVIEW—DETAILED ASSESSMENT (STEP F)

Application of the first five steps should help clinicians determine whether the wait-test threshold has been crossed. If the results indicate low risk to very low risk, they do not cross the wait-test threshold (e.g., low Externalizing scores, no family history); then we can *stop* assessing for PBD. Be aware that Steps A through D are best at ruling out cases of PBD, and these rule-outs will be correct in almost all cases in most settings. After ruling out PBD, clinicians can then treat other conditions such as ADHD or depression with less concern of adverse effects resulting from inappropriate treatment. Additionally, clinicians will be able to document "due diligence."

Even for youth with all these risk factors, the differential diagnosis process is not over because the adjusted index of suspicion is only elevated. Youth with a positive family history of bipolar disorder and high scores on an Externalizing subscale and high scores on a mania questionnaire will have an index of suspicion in the 55th percentile. Clinically, of 10 youth with the same set of risk factors, approximately 5 to 6 out of 10 cases *will* have PBD, and 4 to 5 out of 10 cases *will not* have PBD. Therefore, systematic, intensive assessment of PBD is indicated.

Systematic probing for the presence of mania symptoms occurring in distinct episodes provides the foundation of a diagnosis of PBD. Diagnostic interviewing should include the youth, a collateral informant, and the direct observation of the youth's mental status—particularly in acute care settings. Clinicians typically use unstructured interviewing techniques that could be improved by mixing the FIND criteria (Quinn & Fristad, 2004) and GRAPES mnemonic. The FIND criteria consist of querying the Frequency, Intensity, Number, and Duration of symptoms. The GRAPES mnemonic consists of Grandiosity, Racing thoughts, Activity that is goal-directed, Pressured speech, Elation, and Sleep disturbance—especially decreased need for sleep. Structured or semistructured interviews that cover mania symptoms can aid systematic inquiry about the FIND criteria and GRAPES symptoms. Despite their common use in research, many clinicians are reluctant to use them for many reasons, such as beliefs that clients will dislike structured approaches, that repertoire will be damaged, or that they constrain professional autonomy (Garb, 1998). In contrast to clinicians' beliefs, clients actually prefer structured approaches, and structured approaches do not damage the therapeutic relationship (Suppiger et al., 2009). Semistructured approaches give clinicians more latitude to clinicians because they provide guidance on what to ask but allow clinicians significant leeway in how it is asked. Clinicians should consider administering the mood modules of a semistructured interview (e.g., also Schedule for Affective Disorders and Schizophrenia for School-Age Children [K-SADS]) whenever the index of suspicion is above the wait-test threshold. Comorbidities could be examined through the administration of other modules as necessary or wanted. At the minimum, clinicians should query and document mania-specific symptoms.

Currently, other assessment techniques provide some glimmers of hope both theoretically and empirically. Unfortunately, these approaches cannot be considered evidence-based assessments at this time, due to the lack of controlled studies examining the sensitivity and specificity of these methods. Genetic testing, while promising, currently does not offer such diagnostic specificity. For example, ascertainment of family history by family reporting is more powerful than current genetic tests in determining risk for bipolar disorder (Frey et al., 2013). While structural and functional MRI are starting to show promise in discriminating adults with bipolar disorder from those with other mood disorders (Fournier, Keener, Almeida, Kronhaus, & Phillips, 2013; Rocha-Rego et al., 2013), brain imaging remains a research tool in bipolar disorder, as empirical evidence does not yet exist supporting its use for differential diagnosis in youth or adults. Other assessments such as projective testing (e.g., Rorschach, House-Tree-Person) and even many commercially distributed tests (e.g., Minnesota Multiphasic Personality Inventory–Adolescent) do not have peer-reviewed studies showing predictive validity. When evaluating whether to use these newer techniques, it is prudent to consider whether designs reflective of general clinical populations were used. Designs with fewer exclusion criteria, high rates of depression or ADHD in the comparison groups, and more comorbidity likely reflect clinically generalizable designs (Youngstrom et al., 2006a).

TREATMENT PLANNING (STEP G)

Once the assessment-treat threshold is crossed, then ascertaining more general information that might change treatment choice occurs. Treatment targets for PBD include both symptom reduction and improvement in general functioning (Freeman et al., 2009). Clinicians should consider the youth's current mood episode (i.e., depressed, manic, mixed, or euthymic), common comorbidities such as ADHD (Kowatch et al., 2005), tolerance for specific treatment side effects, current medication or drug use, and prior medication trials. The type of mood episode might change acute intervention (e.g., adjunctive antidepressant or cognitive behavioral therapy for depression) compared to maintenance therapy (e.g., mood stabilizer or family-focused therapy for euthymia). Common comorbidities require monitoring to determine whether they resolve with a change in mood episode or warrant additional treatment (McClellan, Kowatch, & Findling, 2007). Careful reviews of medical history should help rule out whether symptoms are likely due to a general medical condition (e.g., tumor) or a drug side effect (e.g., steroids) or inducement (e.g., cocaine).

With the goal of improving general functioning, clinicians should consider a youth's personality traits, stability of the family, academic functioning, and quality of life. People with bipolar disorder typically display lower levels of conscientiousness, which could lead to forgetting appointments, medication use, or other accidents of omission that might undermine treatment (Barnett et al., 2011). Families affected by PBD display poorer levels of interpersonal functioning, which predicts earlier onset, poor response during treatment, and more rapid relapse (McClellan et al., 2007). Youth with PBD may also have learning needs that the school system can address via individualized education plans. Including each of these areas in a comprehensive treatment plan helps the clinician systematically serve the family. Finally, it is crucial to assess and document potential suicidality because PBD is associated with higher rates of attempts compared to youth with depression (Goldstein et al., 2005; Merikangas et al., 2012).

FUTURE VISITS—IS TREATMENT WORKING? (STEPS H, I, AND J)

During treatment, the role of assessment changes from asking "What is the problem?" and "What are the causes?" to "How bad are your symptoms?" and "Are we making progress toward our goals?" Typically progress is monitored informally by asking questions such as "How are you doing?" By adding a mania questionnaire, clinicians can systematize and standardize the collection of treatment outcomes. Consistently measuring symptom change during treatment is associated with better patient outcomes (Finn & Tonsager, 1997).

Time-consuming assessment (e.g., detailed interviewing) is likely unnecessary and prohibitive; but a brief, valid measure of symptom severity may prove worth repeating as a quick metric of progress. The same questionnaires that aid in establishing the diagnosis of PBD can be used to help monitor improvement in symptoms (Findling et al., 2007; West, Henry, & Pavuluri, 2007; Youngstrom et al., 2013). In principle, longer measures will result in more reliable measurement and earlier detection of treatment response because reliability sets the upper limit on detectable change (Jacobson & Truax, 1991). However,

shortened symptom measures might more accurately detect change because they remove items less specific to mania (Youngstrom, Frazier, Demeter, Calabrese, & Findling, 2008b). Practically, families and clinicians benefit from shorter, specific measures that can be completed in the waiting room, quickly scored, and compared with prior visits. Additionally, parents are more likely to complete these measures, and their reports are often more indicative of change than self-report (Youngstrom et al., 2013).

An alternative to questionnaires for monitoring symptoms is "mood charting" (Denicoff et al., 2002). Mood charting allows families to see treatment response, emergent side effects, and triggering events linked to mood instability (Post et al., 2011). The finer-grained detail provided by mood charting can inform psychotherapy by recording the timing, situation, and behavioral response. Mood charting can note changes in sleep or energy that might be the beginnings of a new mood episode (Sachs, 2004). Currently, mood charting can be done via traditional paper-and-pencil metrics or via free smartphone apps.

Although both questionnaires and mood monitoring provide information about symptom improvement, clinicians should also monitor global change. Adding a simple metric such as the Clinical Global Impressions Scale, scored from 1 (*not impaired*) to 7 (*very impaired*), provides easy documentation of the course of treatment (National Institute of Mental Health, 1985). Using the same impression scale consistently and writing it down provides clinicians with a powerful tool for monitoring complex presentations simply and sensitively (Meehl, 1954; National Institute of Mental Health, 1985). Recording ratings in treatment notes allows one to document change over time.

INTEGRATING THE INFORMATION

Each step outlined in this chapter involves integrating information from distinct sources. A probability nomogram (Figure 5.2) provides a math-free way for clinicians to do this quickly. To use the nomogram, place a mark for the base rate on the left side (initial index of suspicion). Select the first likelihood ratio needed from the table (e.g., high Externalizing score) and place a mark on the likelihood ratio line. Draw a straight line connecting the two dots. The right side gives the updated index of suspicion. This new index of suspicion can be moved back to the left side as new likelihood ratios (e.g., family history) are added (Jenkins et al., 2011).

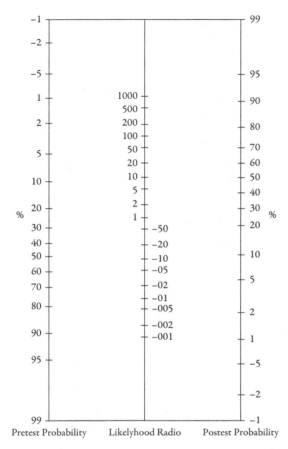

Figure 5.2 Nomogram to Aid in Determining the Index of Suspicion.

This chapter provides guidance about to integrate evidence-based diagnosis of PBD into daily clinical practice. Using each part of the visit efficiently—particularly waiting times—maximizes the benefit to both the family and clinician while minimizing burden on all involved. Actuarial approaches to decision-making are almost always more accurate than clinical decisions for PBD because information is used more consistently (Jenkins et al., 2011). Improving identification should make it easier for clinicians to practice evidence-based treatment, because proper identification of the disorder means that youth are more likely to match existing evidence-based treatments (Chorpita, Bernstein, & Daleiden, 2011).

EVOLUTION OF EVIDENCE-BASED ASSESSMENT

Evidence-based medicine has evolved considerably over the prior two decades, particularly the assessment of PBD. Technology has also evolved dramatically. Twenty years ago, paper and pencil were the primary means for collecting data. Today, computers and smartphones are ubiquitous. Identification of mood episodes via text messaging, online mood charting, and potentially even "listening in" on snippets of the day provide additional avenues for improving diagnosis and treatment outcomes. Imaging techniques and genetics continue to improve and become less expensive, bringing us closer to the goal of being able to use them clinically, as well as having them validated under clinically generalizable conditions. Additionally, a gap exists between which measures researchers are showing to be evidence based (e.g., Child Behavior Checklist, mania specific measures) and which measures clinicians are actually using (e.g., Minnesota Multiphasic Personality Inventory–2; Rorschach; Camara, Nathan, & Puente, 2000). Closing this gap will likely bring the most immediate benefit to families.

Even with the considerable progress in techniques and technology, a skilled clinician remains central to evidence-based diagnosis and treatment. Despite recent advances in evidence that require clinicians to learn new skills such as balancing the quantitative aspects of testing (Strauss et al., 2010), the humanistic, qualitative aspects of interpretation remain crucial to formulating a conceptualization that engages the patient (Finn & Tonsager, 1997). Using evidence-based assessment strategies allow clinicians to quantitatively determine risk, up to a point. Clinicians must always consider the qualitative indicators of psychopathology to confirm or disconfirm the putative quantitative risk, because many youth with multiple risk factors still may not have PBD. Families most appreciate clinicians who value their input and account for their values in treatment planning, something that is only starting to be systematically integrated into quantitative models (Pulleyblank, Chuma, Gilbody, & Thompson, 2013).

Although there remains much room for refinement, evidence-based assessment has grown rapidly from a novel idea to a developed framework for integrating research into clinical decisions about individual patients. The knowledge base about PBD has also expanded geometrically. Combing the clinical data with the principles of evidence-based assessment can deliver better diagnoses and treatment decisions without adding unnecessary time and expense but adding substantial benefit to the families we serve.

Disclosure statement: Dr. Freeman has no conflicts of interest. Dr. Chang is an unpaid consultant for GSK, Lilly, BMS. He is on the DSMB for Sunovion. In the past two years, he has received research support from GSK and Merck. Dr. Youngstrom has consulted with Lundbeck and Otsuka and received grant support from the National Institute of Mental Health.

REFERENCES

Achenbach, T. M., & Rescorla, L. A. (2001). *Manual for the ASEBA School-Age Forms & Profiles*. Burlington: University of Vermont.

Angst, J., Gamma, A., Sellaro, R., Lavori, P. W., & Zhang, H. (2003). Recurrence of bipolar disorders and major depression. A life-long perspective. [Comparative Study]. *European Archives of Psychiatry and Clinical Neuroscience, 253*(5), 236–240.

American Psychiatric Association. (2000). *Diagnostic and statistical manual of mental disorders* (4th ed., text rev.). Washington, DC: Author.

American Psychiatric Association. (2013). *Diagnostic and statistical manual of mental disorders* (5th ed.). Washington, DC: Author.

Axelson, D., Findling, R. L., Fristad, M. A., Kowatch, R. A., Youngstrom, E. A., Horwitz, S. M.,…Birmaher, B. (2012). Examining the proposed disruptive mood dysregulation disorder diagnosis in children in the Longitudinal Assessment of Manic Symptoms study. *Journal of Clinical Psychiatry, 73*(10), 1342–1350.

Barnett, J. H., Huang, J., Perlis, R. H., Young, M. M., Rosenbaum, J. F., Nierenberg, A. A.,…Smoller, J. W. (2011). Personality and bipolar disorder: Dissecting state and trait associations between mood and personality. *Psychological Medicine, 41*(8), 1593–1604.

Biederman, J., Faraone, S., Mick, E., & Wozniak, J. (1996). Attention-deficit hyperactivity disorder and juvenile mania: An overlooked comorbidity? *Journal of the American Academy of Child & Adolescent Psychiatry, 35*(8), 997–1008.

Biederman, J., Klein, R. G., Pine, D. S., & Klein, D. F. (1998). Resolved: Mania is mistaken for ADHD in prepubertal children. *Journal of the American Academy of Child & Adolescent Psychiatry, 37*(10), 1091–1096; discussion 1096–1099.

Birmaher, B., Ryan, N. D., Williamson, D. E., Brent, D. A., Kaufman, J., Dahl, R. E.,…Nelson, B. (1996). Childhood and adolescent depression: A review of the past 10 years: Part I. *Journal of the American Academy of Child & Adolescent Psychiatry, 35*(11), 1427–1439.

Blader, J. C., & Carlson, G. A. (2007). Increased rates of bipolar disorder diagnoses among U.S. child, adolescent, and adult inpatients, 1996–2004. *Biological Psychiatry, 62*(2), 107–114.

Camara, W. J., Nathan, J. S., & Puente, A. E. (2000). Psychological test usage: Implications in professional psychology. *Professional Psychology: Research and Practice, 31*(2), 141–154.

Carlson, G. A., & Youngstrom, E. A. (2003). Clinical implications of pervasive manic symptoms in children. *Biological Psychiatry, 53*(11), 1050–1058.

Chorpita, B. F., Bernstein, A., & Daleiden, E. L. (2011). Empirically guided coordination of multiple evidence-based treatments: An illustration of relevance mapping in children's mental health services. *Journal of Consulting and Clinical Psychology, 79*(4), 470–480.

Copeland, W. E., Angold, A., Costello, E. J., & Egger, H. (2013). Prevalence, comorbidity, and correlates of DSM-5 proposed disruptive mood dysregulation disorder. *The American Journal of Psychiatry, 170*(2), 173–179.

Dell'Osso, L., Pini, S., Cassano, G. B., Mastrocinque, C., Seckinger, R. A., Saettoni, M.,…Amador, X. F. (2002). Insight into illness in patients with mania, mixed mania, bipolar depression and major depression with psychotic features. *Bipolar Disorders, 4*(5), 315–322.

Denicoff, K. D., Ali, O., Sollinger, A. B., Smith-Jackson, E. E., Leverich, G. S., & Post, R. M. (2002). Utility of the daily prospective National Institute of Mental Health-Life Chart Method (NIMH-LCM-P) ratings in clinical trials of bipolar disorder. *Depression and Anxiety, 15*(1), 1–9.

Dickstein, D. P., & Leibenluft, E. (2012). Beyond dogma: From diagnostic controversies to data about pediatric bipolar disorder and children with chronic irritability and mood dysregulation. *Israel Journal of Psychiatry and Related Sciences, 49*(1), 52–61.

Diler, R. S., Birmaher, B., Axelson, D., Goldstein, B., Gill, M., Strober, M.,…Keller, M. B. (2009). The Child Behavior Checklist (CBCL) and the CBCL-bipolar phenotype are not useful in diagnosing pediatric bipolar disorder. *Journal of Child and Adolescent Psychopharmacology, 19*(1), 23–30.

Findling, R. L., Frazier, T. W., Youngstrom, E. A., McNamara, N. K., Stansbrey, R. J., Gracious, B. L.,…Calabrese, J. R. (2007). Double-blind, placebo-controlled trial of divalproex monotherapy in the treatment of symptomatic youth at high risk for developing bipolar disorder. *The Journal of Clinical Psychiatry, 68*(5), 781–788.

Finn, S. E., & Tonsager, M. E. (1997). Information-gathering and therapeutic models of assessment: Complementary paradigms. *Psychological Assessment, 9*(4), 374–385.

Fournier, J. C., Keener, M. T., Almeida, J., Kronhaus, D. M., & Phillips, M. L. (2013). Amygdala and whole-brain activity to emotional faces distinguishes major depressive disorder and bipolar disorder. *Bipolar Disorders 15*(7), 741–752.

Freeman, A. J., Youngstrom, E. A., Michalak, E., Siegel, R., Meyers, O. I., & Findling, R. L. (2009). Quality of life in pediatric bipolar disorder. *Pediatrics, 123*(3), e446–e452.

Frey, B. N., Andreazza, A. C., Houenou, J., Jamain, S., Goldstein, B. I., Frye, M. A.,…Young, L. T. (2013). Biomarkers in bipolar disorder: A positional paper from the International Society for Bipolar Disorders Biomarkers Task Force. *Australian and New Zealand Journal of Psychiatry, 47*(4), 321–332.

Garb, H. N. (1998). Clinical judgment. In *Studying the clinician: Judgment research and psychological assessment* (pp. 173–206). Washington, DC: American Psychological Association.

Geller, B., Zimerman, B., Williams, M., Bolhofner, K., Craney, J. L., Delbello, M. P., & Soutullo, C. A. (2000). Diagnostic characteristics of 93 cases of a prepubertal and early adolescent bipolar disorder phenotype by gender, puberty and comorbid attention deficit hyperactivity disorder. *Journal of Child and Adolescent Psychopharmacology, 10*(3), 157–164.

Goldstein, B. I., & Birmaher, B. (2012). Prevalence, clinical presentation and differential diagnosis of pediatric bipolar disorder. *Israel Journal of Psychiatry and Related Sciences, 49*(1), 3–14.

Goldstein, T. R., Birmaher, B., Axelson, D., Ryan, N. D., Strober, M. A., Gill, M. K.,…Keller, M. (2005). History of suicide attempts in pediatric bipolar disorder: Factors associated with increased risk. *Bipolar Disorders, 7*(6), 525–535.

Hodgins, S., Faucher, B., Zarac, A., & Ellenbogen, M. (2002). Children of parents with bipolar disorder: A population at high risk for major affective disorders. *Child and Adolescent Psychiatric Clinics of North America, 11*(3), 533–554.

Jacobson, N. S., & Truax, P. (1991). Clinical significance: A statistical approach to defining meaningful change in psychotherapy research. *Journal of Consulting and Clinical Psychology, 59*(1), 12–19.

Jaeschke, R., Guyatt, G., & Sackett, D. L. (1994a). Users' guides to the medical literature: III. How to use an article about a diagnostic test: A. Are the results of the study valid? Evidence-Based Medicine Working Group. *Journal of the American Medical Association, 271*(5), 389–391.

Jaeschke, R., Guyatt, G. H., & Sackett, D. L. (1994b). Users' guides to the medical literature: III. How to use an article about a diagnostic test: B. What are the results and will they help me in caring for my patients? Evidence-Based Medicine Working Group. *Journal of the American Medical Association, 271*(9), 703–707.

Jenkins, M. M., Youngstrom, E. A., Washburn, J. J., & Youngstrom, J. K. (2011). Evidence-based strategies improve assessment of pediatric bipolar disorder by community practitioners. *Professional Psychology: Research and Practice, 42*(2), 121–129.

Joseph, M. F., Youngstrom, E. A., & Soares, J. C. (2009). Antidepressant-coincident mania in children and adolescents treated with selective serotonin reuptake inhibitors. *Future Neurology, 4*(1), 87–102.

Klein, R. G., Pine, D. S., & Klein, D. F. (1998). Resolved: Mania is mistaken for ADHD in prepubertal children. *Journal of the*

American Academy of Child & Adolescent Psychiatry, 37(10), 1993–1096.

Kogan, J. N., Otto, M. W., Bauer, M. S., Dennehy, E. B., Miklowitz, D. J., Zhang, H. W.,...Sachs, G. S. (2004). Demographic and diagnostic characteristics of the first 1000 patients enrolled in the Systematic Treatment Enhancement Program for Bipolar Disorder (STEP-BD). *Bipolar Disorders, 6*(6), 460–469.

Kowatch, R. A., Youngstrom, E. A., Danielyan, A., & Findling, R. L. (2005). Review and meta-analysis of the phenomenology and clinical characteristics of mania in children and adolescents. *Bipolar Disorders, 7*(6), 483–496.

Leibenluft, E., Charney, D. S., Towbin, K. E., Bhangoo, R. K., & Pine, D. S. (2003). Defining clinical phenotypes of juvenile mania. *American Journal of Psychiatry, 160*(3), 430–437.

Loeber, R., Green, S. M., Lahey, B. B., & Stouthamer-Loeber, M. (1991). Differences and similarities between children, mothers, and teachers as informants on disruptive child behavior. *Journal of Abnormal Child Psychology, 19*(1), 75–95.

Mash, E. J., & Barkley, R. A. (2003). *Child psychopathology* (2nd ed.). New York: Guilford Press.

McClellan, J., Kowatch, R. A., & Findling, R. L. (2007). Practice parameter for the assessment and treatment of children and adolescents with bipolar disorder. *Journal of the American Academy of Child & Adolescent Psychiatry, 46*(1), 107–125.

Meehl, P. E. (1954). Empirical comparisons of clinical and actuarial prediction. In *Clinical versus statistical prediction: A theoretical analysis and a review of the evidence* (pp. 83–128). Minneapolis: University of Minnesota Press.

Merikangas, K. R., Akiskal, H. S., Angst, J., Greenberg, P. E., Hirschfeld, R. M., Petukhova, M., & Kessler, R. C. (2007). Lifetime and 12-month prevalence of bipolar spectrum disorder in the National Comorbidity Survey Replication. *Archives of General Psychiatry, 64*(5), 543–552.

Merikangas, K. R., Cui, L., Kattan, G., Carlson, G. A., Youngstrom, E. A., & Angst, J. (2012). Mania with and without depression in a community sample of US adolescents. *Archives of General Psychiatry, 69*(9), 943–951.

Moreno, C., Laje, G., Blanco, C., Jiang, H., Schmidt, A. B., & Olfson, M. (2007). National trends in the outpatient diagnosis and treatment of bipolar disorder in youth. *Archives of General Psychiatry, 64*(9), 1032–1039.

Murray, G., & Harvey, A. (2010). Circadian rhythms and sleep in bipolar disorder. *Bipolar Disorders, 12*(5), 459–472.

National Institute of Mental Health. (1985). Rating scales and assessment instruments for use in pediatric psychopharmacology research. *Psychopharmacology Bulletin, 21*(4), 714–1124.

Pliszka, S. R., Sherman, J. O., Barrow, M. V., & Irick, S. (2000). Affective disorder in juvenile offenders: A preliminary study. *American Journal of Psychiatry, 157*(1), 130–132.

Post, R. M., Leverich, G. S., Altshuler, L. L., Frye, M. A., Suppes, T., Keck, P. E.,...Rowe, M. (2011). Differential clinical characteristics, medication usage, and treatment response of bipolar disorder in the US versus The Netherlands and Germany. *International Clinical Psychopharmacology, 26*(2), 96–106.

Pulleyblank, R., Chuma, J., Gilbody, S., & Thompson, C. (2013). Decision curve analysis for assessing the usefulness of tests for making decisions to treat: An application to tests for prodromal psychosis. *Psychological Assessment, 25*(3),730–737.

Quinn, C. A., & Fristad, M. A. (2004). Defining and identifying early onset bipolar spectrum disorder. *Current Psychiatry Reports, 6*(2), 101–107.

Reynolds, C. R., & Kamphaus, R. R. (1992). *Behavior Assessment System for Children: manual*. Circle Pines, MN: American Guidance Service.

Rocha-Rego, V., Jogia, J., Marquand, A. F., Mourao-Miranda, J., Simmons, A., & Frangou, S. (2013). Examination of the predictive value of structural magnetic resonance scans in bipolar disorder: A pattern classification approach. *Psychological Medicine, 44*(3), 519–532.

Sachs, G. S. (2004). Strategies for improving treatment of bipolar disorder: Integration of measurement and management. *Acta Psychiatrica Scandinavica 422* (Supple.), 7–17.

Smoller, J. W., & Finn, C. T. (2003). Family, twin, and adoption studies of bipolar disorder. *American Journal of Medical Genetics, 123C*(1), 48–58.

Strauss, S. E., Glasziou, P., Richardson, W. S., & Haynes, R. B. (2010). *Evidence-based medicine: How to practice and teach it*. London: Churchill Livingstone.

Suppiger, A., In-Albon, T., Hendriksen, S., Hermann, E., Margraf, J., & Schneider, S. (2009). Acceptance of structured diagnostic interviews for mental disorders in clinical practice and research settings. *Behavior Therapy, 40*(3), 272–279.

Teplin, L. A., Abram, K. M., McClelland, G. M., Dulcan, M. K., & Mericle, A. A. (2002). Psychiatric disorders in youth in juvenile detention. *Archives of General Psychiatry, 59*(12), 1133–1143.

Thuppal, M., Carlson, G. A., Sprafkin, J., & Gadow, K. D. (2002). Correspondence between adolescent report, parent report and teacher report of manic symptoms. *Journal of Child and Adolescent Psychopharmacology, 12*(1), 27–35.

Tillman, R., & Geller, B. (2007). Diagnostic characteristics of child bipolar I disorder: Does the "Treatment of Early Age Mania (team)" sample generalize? *Journal of Clinical Psychiatry, 68*(2), 307–314.

Tillman, R., Geller, B., Klages, T., Corrigan, M., Bolhofner, K., & Zimerman, B. (2008). Psychotic phenomena in 257 young children and adolescents with bipolar I disorder: Delusions and hallucinations (benign and pathological). *Bipolar Disorders, 10*(1), 45–55.

Van Meter, A. R., Moreira, A. L., & Youngstrom, E. A. (2011). Meta-analysis of epidemiologic studies of pediatric bipolar disorder. *The Journal of Clinical Psychiatry, 72*(9), 1250–1256.

West, A. E., Henry, D. B., & Pavuluri, M. N. (2007). Maintenance model of integrated psychosocial treatment in pediatric bipolar disorder: A pilot feasibility study. *Journal of the American Academy of Child & Adolescent Psychiatry, 46*(2), 205–12.

World Health Organization. (1992). *ICD-10: International Statistical Classification of Diseases and Related Health Problems*. Geneva: Author.

Youngstrom, E. A., Birmaher, B., & Findling, R. L. (2008a). Pediatric bipolar disorder: Validity, phenomenology, and recommendations for diagnosis. *Bipolar Disorders, 10*(Suppl. 2), 194–214.

Youngstrom, E. A., Findling, R. L., Calabrese, J. R., Gracious, B. L., Demeter, C., Bedoya, D. D., & Price, M. (2004). Comparing the diagnostic accuracy of six potential screening instruments for bipolar disorder in youths aged 5 to 17 years. *Journal of the American Academy of Child & Adolescent Psychiatry, 43*(7), 847–858.

Youngstrom, E. A., Findling, R. L., Youngstrom, J. K., & Calabrese, J. R. (2005a). Toward an evidence-based assessment of pediatric bipolar disorder. *Journal of Clinical Child and Adolescent Psychology, 34*(3), 433–448.

Youngstrom, E. A., Frazier, T. W., Demeter, C., Calabrese, J. R., & Findling, R. L. (2008b). Developing a 10-item Mania Scale from the Parent General Behavior Inventory for Children and Adolescents. *Journal of Clinical Psychiatry, 69*(5), 831–839.

Youngstrom, E. A., Freeman, A. J., & Jenkins, M. M. (2009). The assessment of children and adolescents with bipolar disorder. *Child and Adolescent Psychiatric Clinics of North America, 18*(2), 353–390.

Youngstrom, E. A., Jenkins, M. M., Doss, A. J., & Youngstrom, J. K. (2012). Evidence-based assessment strategies for pediatric bipolar disorder. *Israel Journal of Psychiatry and Related Sciences, 49*(1), 15–27.

Youngstrom, E. A., Joseph, M. F., & Greene, J. (2008c). Comparing the psychometric properties of multiple teacher report instruments as predictors of bipolar disorder in children and adolescents. *Journal of Clinical Psychology, 64*(4), 382–401.

Youngstrom, E. A., Meyers, O., Demeter, C. A., Youngstrom, J. K., Morello, L., Piiparinen, R.,...Findling, R. L. (2005b). Comparing diagnostic checklists for pediatric bipolar disorder in academic and community mental health settings. *Bipolar Disorders, 7*(6), 507–517.

Youngstrom, E. A., Meyers, O., Youngstrom, J. K., Calabrese, J. R., & Findling, R. L. (2006a). Comparing the effects of sampling designs on the diagnostic accuracy of eight promising screening algorithms for pediatric bipolar disorder. *Biological Psychiatry, 60*(9), 1013–1019.

Youngstrom, E. A., Meyers, O., Youngstrom, J. K., Calabrese, J. R., & Findling, R. L. (2006b). Diagnostic and measurement issues in the assessment of pediatric bipolar disorder: Implications for understanding mood disorder across the life cycle. *Development and Psychopathology, 18*(4), 989–1021.

Youngstrom, E. A., Youngstrom, J. K., Freeman, A. J., De Los Reyes, A., Feeny, N. C., & Findling, R. L. (2011). Informants are not all equal: Predictors and correlates of clinician judgments about caregiver and youth credibility. *Journal of Child and Adolescent Psychopharmacology, 21*(5), 407–415.

Youngstrom, E. A., Zhao, J., Mankoski, R., Forbes, R. A., Marcus, R. M., Carson, W.,…Findling, R. L. (2013). Clinical significance of treatment effects with aripiprazole versus placebo in a study of manic or mixed episodes associated with pediatric bipolar I disorder. *Journal of Child and Adolescent Psychopharmacology, 23*(2), 72–79.

6.

EFFECTS OF PUBLIC AWARENESS AND STIGMATIZATION ON ACCURATE AND TIMELY DIAGNOSIS OF BIPOLAR DISORDER

Giampaolo Perna, Tatiana Torti, and Alessandra Alciati

STIGMATIZING ATTITUDES TOWARD MENTAL ILLNESSES

THE DIMENSION OF THE PROBLEM

"Psychiatric stigma" refers to a negative attitude against individuals considered mentally ill. Stigmatizing attitudes have been observed in the general public (Angermeyer & Matschinger, 2003), even at a very young age (O'Driscoll, Heary, Hennessy, & McKeague, 2012), among mental health professionals, (Lauber, Nordt, Braunschweig, & Rössler, 2006) and family caregivers of patients (Gonzalez et al., 2007). A study comparing stereotypes and attitudes toward people with mental illness in mental health professionals and in general public showed that mental health professionals have as many negative stereotypes about people with mental illness as the general public do (Lauber et al., 2006).

Several investigations demonstrate that the majority of people in the United States (Link, Phelan, Bresnahan, Stueve, & Pescosolido, 1999) and in western European countries (Brockington, Hall, Levings, & Murphy, 1993) have stigmatizing attitudes about mental illness. In Asian cultures, stigma against mental illness seems to be less severe. This might be due to the lack of differentiation between psychiatric and nonpsychiatric illness in the non-Western medical conception (Fabrega, 1991).

The 1996 General Social Survey, designed to monitor the public's view about several critical social issues in the United States, reflected a general public negative attitude toward persons with mental health problems who are considered unable to make competent decisions, dangerous to themselves and/or the public, and requiring coerced treatment.

The respondents expressed a less negative reaction to people with depression than those with alcohol and drug dependence but failed to recognize depression as a mental health problem despite widespread formerly implemented (Pescosolido, Monahan, Link., Stueve, & Kikuzawa, 1999). A recent systematic review of all studies examining the time trends of attitudes related to mental illness in the general population published before March 2011 showed a greater mental health literacy, in particular toward a biological model of mental illness but, at the same time, found that attitudes toward persons with mental illness have not changed over the past 20 years but even deteriorated. These results highlight that a biological public understanding of mental illness seems not to reduce the social rejection of mentally ill persons and suggest that education about biological correlates of mental disorders do not seem to improve negative attitudes toward persons with mental illness (Schomerus et al., 2012).

It has also been hypothesized that there have been even unexpected negative consequences of promoting biological models of mental illness. Although greater awareness of the causal role of biological factors decreased negative attributions about personal responsibility for developing a severe mental illness, it is possible that biological models are interpreted as referring to worst outcomes and not effective treatments (Rosen, Walter, & Casey, 2000). Subsequent research supported such concerns, revealing that biogenetic models of mental illness have more negative than positive effects on social acceptance (Rusch, Todd, Bodenhausen, & Corrigan, 2010).

THE STRUCTURE OF STIGMA

Stigma is considered to involve three levels: stereotypes, prejudice, and discrimination. Stereotypes represent a set of believes shared by most of the public toward a group of people. Prejudice endorses the negative stereotypes and produces an emotional reaction that can lead to hostile behaviors such as discrimination (Corrigan & Watson, 2002).

Recent literature emphasizes the distinction between public stigma and personal stigma. The first refers to the endorsement of prejudice and the expression of discrimination against people with mental illness by the general population, (Corrigan & Watson, 2002), whereas the second one includes perceived stigma, experienced stigma, and self-stigma.

The perception/anticipation of stigma refers to beliefs about attitudes toward illness shared by the general population (Lebel, 2008). "Experienced stigma" describes the discrimination actually met by the ill persons. Last, "self-stigma" consists of the internalization and adoption of social stigmatizing attitudes, for which the individual believes that the social stigma is an accurate reflection of him or herself (Livingston & Boyd, 2010).

Measures assessing stigma can be classified into the abovementioned categories as well. In the past 10 years, 79% of stigma research has used a measure of perceived stigma, 46% of experienced stigma, and 33% of self-stigma (Brohan, Slade., Clement, & Thornicroft, 2010).

STIGMA AND BIPOLAR DISORDER

In the past few years the majority of research has focused on stigma against individuals with psychotic disorders, in particular schizophrenia. More recently research has targeted how stigma is experienced by bipolar patients (Hawke, Perikh, & Michalak, 2013). Although it has been shown that the stigmatizing attitudes of public are more negative against schizophrenic persons, individuals with bipolar disorder perceived stigma at strong as individuals with schizophrenia (Day, Edgren, & Eshleman, 2007).

Actually, public attitudes toward bipolar disorder are similar to those toward schizophrenia in terms of visibility of the illness, potential to destroy relationship, efficacy of treatment, and possibility of recovery. The only significant difference in public attitude is related to levels of anxiety that people experience in interpersonal contact, with bipolar patients scoring lower distress than the schizophrenic group (Day et al., 2007).

People with major depressive disorder and bipolar disorder experience similar levels of stigmatizing experiences, as measured by the Stigma Experiences Scale, but individuals with bipolar disorder report significantly greater psychosocial impact of stigma both for themselves and for their

family members (Lazowski, Koller, Stuart, & Milev, 2012). This finding is not surprising, as bipolar disorder is considered more severe when compared to depression and seems to be characterized by a more disruptive behavior, which may elicit heavier stigmatizing attitudes.

In the same way, public attitudes toward depression and mania seem to be different. While manic patients elicit more negative emotional and cognitive reactions than depressed—being considered dangerous, aggressive, and unpredictable—depressed individuals are viewed with more empathy and pity (Wolkenstein & Meyer, 2009).

Personal stigma, in particular self-stigma (i.e., the internalization of social stigmatizing attitudes), has an important negative impact on individuals with bipolar disorder and their family. Qualitative studies of the subjective experience of stigma in bipolar disorder have also consistently shown that patients felt that stigma restricted their opportunities and diminished their value in work, social, and health-care settings (Michalak, Yatham, Maxwell, Hale, & Lam, 2007). A recent qualitative study on occupational functioning showed that bipolar individuals evaluated that stigma had discontinued their working career. Managing self-stigma and making more careful decisions about disclosure may be a useful way to address the problem (Michalak et al., 2011).

The negative impact of self-stigma is amplified by the fact that patients do not consider bipolar disorder as an illness but rather as a sign of weakness and personal failure (Suto et al., 2012). Stigma is perceived also by the family caregivers of persons with diagnoses of bipolar disorder. Factors associated with the caregivers' perceptions of greater illness stigma include higher education (Phelan, Bromet, & Link, 1998), young or older age (Shibre et al., 2001), being the spouse of the person with mental illness, and being female (Phillips, Pearson, Li, Xu, & Yang, 2002). The Family Experience Study, associated with the Systematic Treatment Enhancement Program for Bipolar Disorder study (Gonzalez et al., 2007), showed that caregivers of persons with bipolar disorder with active symptoms perceived as much stigma as caregivers of those with remitted symptoms, revealing that stigma experienced by family members of bipolar individuals did not subside when symptoms remitted.

INCORRECT OR DELAYED DIAGNOSIS IN BIPOLAR DISORDER

Despite the availability of effective pharmacological and psychosocial treatments, individuals with bipolar disorder are often undertreated. This might be due to a delay between symptoms onset, formulation of a correct diagnosis, or prescription of a guideline-defined appropriate intervention.

On some estimates, 40% (Ghaemi, Sachs, Chiou, Pandurangi, & Goodwin, 1999) to 57% (Lish, Dime-Meenan, Whybrow, Price, & Hirschfeld, 1994) of patients with bipolar disorder have initially received an incorrect diagnosis of major depression, and half of them consulted three or more physicians prior to receiving a correct diagnosis.

In the past 25 years, several studies have addressed the issue of delay in or misdiagnosis of bipolar disorder and the consequent latency in appropriate treatment achievement (Hirschfeld & Vornik, 2004). Although studies are difficult to compare directly (some focus on time from early symptoms to diagnosis, others on time from first episode and any treatment, and still others on the delay in prescription of a mood stabilizer), the vast majority of them report a delay in diagnosis or in the introduction of a guideline-defined appropriate treatment between 8 and 10 years (Lish et al., 1994; Wang et al., 2005).

The delay in diagnosis and treatment is significantly longer in bipolar disorder type II patients (Baldessarini, Tondo, & Hennen, 2003). A number of studies report higher rates of undiagnosed hypomania or failure to consider both clinical and treatment implications of the presence of the hypomanic component (Benazzi, 2009). This is a crucial issue because bipolar type II patients may have higher episode frequency, symptoms severity, rapid cycling, and suicidal behavior than bipolar type I patients (Vieta & Suppes, 2008).

A correct diagnosis of bipolar disorder is hampered by the fact that the majority of bipolar patients initiate treatment while depressed. This might be due to a frequent onset of the illness with a comorbid depressive episode (Perugi et al., 2000), dominance of depressive symptoms (Judd et al., 2003), or the subjective suffering associated with the depressed phase.

Patients with bipolar disorder who typically present to physicians reporting depressive symptoms are often hardly distinguishable from those described in unipolar major depressive disorder, even if there is evidence regarding a more precise differential diagnosis between bipolar and unipolar depression. This is so even though the specifiers of atypical, melancholic, and psychotic features are indicated by the *Diagnostic and Statistical Manual of Mental Disorders* (fourth edition; American Psychiatric Association, 1994) as more frequently present in bipolar than in unipolar depression (O'Donovan, Garnham, Hajek, & Alda, 2008).

A correct definition and an accurate detection of mania and hypomania are central to the identification of bipolar disorder. Nevertheless, hypomanic symptoms are underdiagnosed in clinical practice because they are rarely experienced as pathological by the subjects themselves. Moreover, they are often associated with enhanced productivity and masked by the natural diurnal and annual rhythms of mood (Angst et al., 2005).

Accurate and early diagnosis of bipolar disorder may result in improved illness course and long-term functional outcome. On the contrary, misdiagnosis of bipolar disorder may produce both clinical and economic adverse consequences. For example, unrecognized bipolar patients have higher mean monthly medical costs than recognized ones and are less likely to receive a mood stabilizer (Birnbaum et al., 2003). Lithium treatment is associated with a substantial reduction of illness recurrence and suicidal acts in bipolar patients (Baldessarini et al., 2006), and there is evidence that response to lithium is diminished in patients who have already received treatment for several previous depressive or manic episodes (Swann, Bowden, Calabrese, Dilsaver, & Morris, 2000). Delayed initiation of mood stabilizers has also been associated with poorer social functioning, more hospitalizations, and a greater likelihood of attempting suicide (Goldberg & Ernst, 2002).

Contrary to what observed in unipolar depression, treatment with antidepressants alone does not seem to prevent depression among bipolar patients (Ghaemi et al., 2004) and can have a destabilizing effect, which might lead to manic and hypomanic switches (Post et al., 2006). Such findings emphasize the need for early recognition of bipolar disorder in order to maximize treatment response, improve patient functioning, and reduce costs.

The absence of public awareness about bipolar disorder might also play a role in delaying diagnosis; an important factor that might help early detection of this disorder is related to the correct identification of prodromal symptoms (Howes & Falkenberg, 2011). Although the real utility of prodromal symptoms detection is still a matter of debate, some evidence suggests that mood liability, mood swings, and disturbed diurnal rhythm are likely to be the strongest risk factor for subsequent diagnosis of bipolar spectrum disorder (Angst, Gamma, & Endrass, 2003; Zeschel et al., 2013).

EFFECTS OF PUBLIC AND PERSONAL STIGMA ON ACCURATE AND TIMELY DIAGNOSIS OF BIPOLAR DISORDER

We were not able to identify a single study directly addressing the issue of the impact of stigma on accurate and timely diagnosis of bipolar disorder. However, studies that have investigated the role of public and personal stigma on the propensity to seek and maintain treatment and on a patient's global or specific functioning may provide indirect information on the possible interference of stigma on acquisition of a correct and early diagnosis of bipolar disorder. Several investigations have tried to define with quantitative measures the effect of the stigma on different areas of functioning in bipolar disorder patients. Results show that higher levels of self-stigma and stigmatizing experiences are associated with a greater overall functional impairment (Cerit, Filizer, Tural, & Tufan, 2012; Vázquez et al., 2011).

A recent study demonstrated that higher scores of self-perceived stigma were correlated with lower scores of functioning that, in turn, may lead to discrimination. This contributed to higher levels of perceived stigma, highlighting a bidirectional relationship between perceived stigma and functioning (Vázquez et al., 2011).

Since functional impairment among individuals with bipolar disorder is not limited to the affective episode but persists even during remission (Malhi et al., 2007), one of the main targets of treatment of bipolar disorder should be improving general functioning. These findings suggest that interventions that oppose stigmatization may have positive effects on functioning in bipolar patients during the euthymic periods.

Nationwide US epidemiologic studies suggest that 50% to 60% of people who would benefit from treatment do not seek it (Kessler et al., 2001; Regier et al., 1993). It has been hypothesized that stigmatizing attitudes may dissuade people from seeking care probably because they fear being labeled as "mental patients."

An Australian community study also reported that many people would be embarrassed to seek help from professionals if they had depression and believe that other people would judge them negatively if they sought such help. Others expected health professionals to respond negatively to them (Barney, Griffiths, Jorm, & Christensen, 2006). This study showed that self-stigma and perceived stigma about help seeking for depression are prevalent in the community and are associated with a reduced likelihood of seeking help.

Only some dimensions of stigma seemed to be associated with reduced care seeking. In particular, individuals were less likely to consider future care seeking if they viewed people with mental illness as responsible for their disorders. Conversely, viewing people with mental illness as dangerous is unrelated to decreased care seeking (Cooper, Corrigan, & Watson, 2003).

The term "insight" refers to the capacity to recognize that one has an illness that requires treatment, and stigma moderates the associations between insight into one's illness and depression, low quality of life, and negative self-esteem. Patients who have good insight and who also do not perceive much stigmatization have the best outcome on several parameters, while those with poor insight have problems with service engagement and medication compliance. On the other hand, patients with good insight and stigmatizing beliefs are at the highest risk of negative self-esteem, low quality of life, and depressed mood (Staring, Van der Gaag, Van den Berge, Duivenvoorden, & Mulder, 2009). This research suggests that attempts to increase patients' insight into their illness is not enough and must be accompanied by interventions on the perception of stigma.

Few studies have addressed the role of stigma on discontinuation of treatment in depressed individuals, but one study showed that, even if younger patients seemed to perceive higher stigma levels than older patients, stigma predicted treatment discontinuation only in older patients (Sirey et al., 2001a).

Another important obstacle to effective treatment of bipolar disorder is the high rate of nonadherence to prescribed medication regimens. Adherence to antidepressant drug therapy was predicted by higher self-rated severity of illness and lower levels of perceived stigma as reported before beginning pharmacotherapy. High perceived stigma remains a powerful negative predictor of medication adherence even after controlling for perceived severity of illness (Sirey et al, 2001b).

Overall the survey of Wahl (1999) about the experiences of stigma of 1,400 people with mental illness diagnoses provides useful information in identifying the process through which stigma may be an obstacle to the acquisition of an adequate care. Social rejection is one common experience, with respondents reporting that others avoid them more once their psychiatric disorder or treatment is disclosed. Afterward the person is devalued: respondents describe how others no longer place the same value on their opinions or skills and relegate them to more marginal roles at home and work. Strong opinions or emotions are assumed to be manifestations of cognitive impairment or emotional poor control as a consequence of psychiatric illness. In addition, mental illness professionals often discourage patients from pursuing employment or education. Such a protective attitude may convey a message of expected incompetence (Thornicroft, 2006).

We hypothesize that one of the main consequences of encountering the aforementioned stigmatizing attitudes is that people with psychiatric illnesses are less likely to seek needed treatment. To avoid such rejection, people with mental illness will avoid treatment that would expose them to such rejection and devaluation.

CONCLUSION

Several studies we examined agreed that individuals with bipolar disorder perceive stigma at the same quantitative level as that experienced by individuals with schizophrenia. In particular self-stigma (i.e., the internalization of social stigmatizing attitudes) has an important negative impact on the likelihood of help seeking. Overall these studies show that persons with bipolar disorder internalize the devaluing attitudes of society, anticipate rejection by others, and develop coping strategies, such as secrecy about their illness and avoidance of the needed treatment, in an effort to avoid rejection.

This behavior may have dramatic consequences on the long-term outcome of bipolar disorder. Incorrect or late diagnosis has been associated with decreased pharmacological response, poorer functioning, more hospitalizations, and a greater likelihood of attempted suicide.

In the past few years several international programs have been implemented in an effort to raise awareness and to reduce stigma against mental illness. The Global Program to Fight Stigma and Discrimination Because of Schizophrenia, known as "Open-the-Doors" and, in 2005, the World Psychiatric Association's Scientific Section on Stigma and Mental Health are two major undertakings. The initial thrust to the Open-the-Doors program has been fighting stigma and discrimination in schizophrenia. Nonetheless, stigma is still perceived by the general public as a paradigm for mental illness. Raising evidences of a greater impact of stigmatizing attitudes on bipolar disorder individuals suggests extending the program to this diagnostic group.

Disclosure statement: Giampaolo Perna, Tatiana Torti, and Alessandra Alciati have no conflicts of interest to disclose.

REFERENCES

American Psychiatric Association. (1994). *Diagnostic and statistical manual of mental disorders* (4th ed.). Washington, DC: Author.

Angermeyer, M. C., & Matschinger, H. (2003). Public beliefs about schizophrenia and depression: Similarities and differences. *Social Psychiatry and Psychiatric Epidemiology, 38*, 526–534.

Angst, J., Adolfsson, R., Benazzi, F., Gamma, A., Hantouche, E., Meyer, T. D.,...Scott, J. (2005). The HCL-32: Towards a self-assessment tool for hypomanic symptoms in outpatients. *Journal of Affective Disorders, 88*, 217–233.

Angst, J., Gamma, A., & Endrass, J. (2003). Risk factors for the bipolar and depression spectra. *Acta Psychiatrica Scandinavica, 418*, 15–19.

Baldessarini, R. J., Tondo, L., Davis, P., Pompili, M., Goodwin, F. G., & Henned, J. (2006). Decreased risk of suicides and attempts during long-term lithium treatment: a meta-analytic review. *Bipolar Disorder, 8*, 625–639.

Baldessarini, R. J., Tondo, L., & Hennen, J. (2003). Treatment-latency and previous episodes: Relationships to pretreatment morbidity and response to maintenance treatment in bipolar I and II disorders. *Bipolar Disorder, 5*, 169–179.

Barney, L. J., Griffiths, K. M., Jorm, A. F., & Christensen, H. (2006). Stigma about depression and its impact on help-seeking intentions. *Australian and New Zealand Journal of Psychiatry, 40*(1), 51–54.

Benazzi, F. (2009). A prediction rule for diagnosing hypomania. *Progress in Neuropsychopharmacology and Biological Psychiatry, 33*, 317–322.

Birnbaum, H. G., Shi, L., Dial, E. Oster, E. F., Greenberg, P. E., & Mallett, D. A. (2003). Economic consequences of not recognizing bipolar disorder patients: A cross-sectional descriptive analysis. *Journal of Clinical Psychiatry, 64*, 1201–1209.

Brockington, I., Hall, P., Levings, J., & Murphy, C. (1993). The community's tolerance of the mentally ill. *British Journal of Psychiatry, 162*, 93–99.

Brohan, E., Slade, M., Clement, S., Thornicroft G. (2010). Experiences of mental illness stigma, prejudice and discrimination: A review of measures. *BMC Health Services Research, 10*, 80.

Cerit, C., Filizer, A., Tural, U., & Tufan, A. E. (2012). Stigma: A core factor on predicting functionality in bipolar disorder. *Comprehensive Psychiatry, 53*, 484–489.

Cooper, A. E., Corrigan, P. W., & Watson, A. C. (2003). Mental illness stigma and care seeking. *Journal of Nervous and Mental Disease, 191*(5), 339–341.

Corrigan, P. W., & Watson, A. C. (2002). Understanding the impact of stigma on people with mental illness. *World Psychiatry, 1*, 16–20.

Day, E. N., Edgren, K., & Eshleman, A. (2007). Measuring stigma toward mental illness: Development and application of the Mental Illness Stigma scale. *Journal of Applied Social Psychology, 37*, 2191–2219.

Fabrega, H. Jr. (1991). Psychiatric stigma in non-Western societies. *Comprehensive Psychiatry, 32*(6), 534–551.

Ghaemi, S. N., Rosenquist, K. J., Ko, J. Y., Baldassano, C. F., Kontos, N. J., & Baldessarini, R. J. (2004). Antidepressant treatment in bipolar versus unipolar depression. *American Journal of Psychiatry, 161*, 163–165.

Ghaemi, S. N., Sachs, G. S., Chiou, A. M., Pandurangi, A. K., & Goodwin, F. K. (1999). Is bipolar disorder still underdiagnosed? Are antidepressants overutilized? *Journal of Affective Disorders, 52*, 135–144.

Goldberg, J. F., & Ernst, C. L. (2002). Features associated with the delayed initiation of mood stabilizers at illness onset in bipolar disorder. *Journal of Clinical Psychiatry, 63*, 985–991.

Gonzalez, J. M., Perlick, D. A., Miklowitz, D. J., Kaczynski, R., Hernandez, M., Rosen-heck, R. A.,...Bowden, C. L. (2007). Factors associated with stigma among caregivers of patients with bipolar disorder in the STEP-BD study. *Psychiatric Services, 58*, 41–48.

Hawke, L. D., Perikh, S. V., & Michalak, E. E. (2013) Stigma and bipolar disorder: A review of the literature. *Journal of Affective Disorders, 150*, 181–191.

Hirschfeld, R. M., &Vornik, L. A. (2004). Recognition and diagnosis of bipolar disorder. *Journal of Clinical Psychiatry, 65* (Suppl. 15), 5–9.

Howes, O. D., & Falkenberg, I. (2011). Early detection and intervention in bipolar affective disorder: targeting the development of the disorder. *Current Psychiatric Report, 13*, 493–499.

Judd, L. L., Schettler, P. J., Akiskal, H. S., Maser, J., Coryell, W., Solomon, D.,...Keller, M. (2003). Long-term symptomatic status of bipolar I vs. bipolar II disorders. *International Journal of Neuropsychopharmacology, 6*, 127–137.

Kessler, R. C., Berglund, P. A., Bruce, M. L., Koch, J. R., Laska, E. M., Leaf, P. J.,…Wang, P. S. (2001). The prevalence and correlates of untreated serious mental illness. *Health Service Research, 36,* 987–1007.

Lauber, C., Nordt, C., Braunschweig, C., & Rössler, W. (2006). Do mental health professionals stigmatize their patients? *Acta Psychiatrica Scandinavica, 113* (Suppl.), 51–59.

Lazowski, L., Koller, M., Stuart, H., & Milev, R. (2012). Stigma and discrimination in people suffering with a mood disorder: a cross-sectional study. *Depression Research and Treatment, 9,* 724848.

Lebel, T. (2008). Perceptions of and responses to stigma. *Sociology Compass, 2,* 409–432.

Link, B. G., Phelan, J. C., Bresnahan, M., Stueve, A., & Pescosolido, B. A. (1999). Public conceptions of mental illness: Labels, causes, dangerousness, and social distance. *American Journal of Public Health, 89*(9), 1328–1333.

Lish, J. D., Dime-Meenan, S., Whybrow, P. C., Price, R. A., & Hirschfeld, R. M. (1994). The National Depressive and Manic-Depressive Association (DMDA) survey of bipolar members. *Journal of Affective Disorders, 3,* 1281–1294.

Livingston, J. D., & Boyd, J. E. (2010). Correlates and consequences of internalized stigma for people living with mental illness: A systematic review and meta-analysis. *Social Science and Medicine, 71,* 2150–2161.

Michalak, E. E., Livingston, J. D., Hole, R., Suto, M., Hale, S., & Haddock, C. (2011). It's something that I manage but it is not who I am: Reflections on internalized stigma in individuals with bipolar disorder. *Chronic Illness, 7,* 209–224.

Michalak, E. E., Yatham, L. N., Maxwell, V., Hale, S., & Lam, R. W. (2007). The impact of bipolar disorder upon work functioning: a qualitative analysis. *Bipolar Disorder, 9,* 126–143.

Malhi, G. S., Ivanovski, B., Hadzi-Pavlovic, D., Mitchell, P. B., Vieta, E., & Sachdev, P. (2007). Neuropsychological deficits and functional impairment in bipolar depression, hypomania and euthymia. *Bipolar Disorder, 9*(1–2), 114–125.

O'Donovan, C., Garnham, J. S., Hajek, T., & Alda, M. (2008). Antidepressant monotherapy in pre-bipolar depression: Predictive value and inherent risk. *Journal of Affective Disorders, 107,* 293–298.

O'Driscoll, C., Heary, C., Hennessy, E., & McKeague, L. (2012). Explicit and implicit stigma towards peers with mental health problems in childhood and adolescence. *Journal of Child Psychology and Psychiatry, 53,* 1054–1062.

Perugi, C. M., Akiskal, H. S., Madaro, D., Socci, C., Quilici, C., & Musetti, L. (2000). Polarity of the first episode, clinical characteristics, and course of manic depressive illness: A systematic retrospective investigation of 320 bipolar I patients. *Comprehensive Psychiatry, 41,* 13–18.

Pescosolido, B. A., Monahan, J., Link, B. G., Stueve, A., & Kikuzawa, S. (1999). The public's view of the competence, dangerousness, and need for legal coercion of persons with mental health problems. *American Journal of Public Health, 8*(9), 1339–1345.

Phelan, J. C., Bromet, E. J., & Link, B. G. (1998). Psychiatric illness and family stigma. Schizophrenia Bulletin, 24,115–126.

Phillips, M. R., Pearson, V., Li, F., Xu, M., & Yang, L. (2002). Stigma and expressed emotion: A study of people with schizophrenia and their family members in *China. British Journal of Psychiatry, 181,* 488–493.

Post, R. M., Altshuler, L. L., Frye, M. A., Suppes, T., McElroy, S., Keck, P.E. Jr.,…Grunze, H. (2006). New findings from the Bipolar Collaborative Network: clinical implications for therapeutics. *Current Psychiatry Reports, 8,* 489–497.

Regier, D. A., Narrow, W. E., Rae, D. S., Manderscheid, R. W., Locke, B. Z., & Goodwin, F.K. (1993). The de facto US mental and addictive disorders service system: Epidemiological catchment area prospective 1-year prevalence rates of disorders and services. *Archives of General Psychiatry, 50,* 85–94.

Rosen, A., Walter, G., & Casey, D. (2000). Combating psychiatric stigma: An overview of contemporary initiatives. *Australian and New Zealand Journal of Psychiatry, 8,* 19–26.

Rusch, N., Todd, A. R., Bodenhausen, G. V., & Corrigan, P. W. (2010). Biogenetic models of psychopathology, implicit guilt, and mental illness stigma. *Psychiatry Research, 179,* 328–332.

Schomerus, G., Schwahn, C., Holzinger, A., Corrigan, P. W., Grabe, H. J., Carta, M. G., & Angermeyer, M. C. (2012). Evolution of public attitudes about mental illness: a systematic review and meta-analysis. *Acta Psychiatrica Scandinavica, 125*(6), 440–452.

Shibre, T., Negash, A., Kullgren, G., Kebede, D., Alem, A., Fekadu, A.,…Jacobsson, L. (2001). Perception of stigma among family members of individuals with schizophrenia and major affective disorders in rural Ethiopia. *Social Psychiatry and Psychiatric Epidemiology, 58,* 41–48.

Sirey, J. A., Bruce, M. L., Alexopoulos, G. S., Perlick, D. A., Raue, P., Friedman, S. J., & Meyers, B. S. (2001a). Perceived stigma as a predictor of treatment discontinuation in young and older outpatients with depression. *American Journal of Psychiatry, 158,* 479–481.

Sirey, J. A., Bruce, M. L., Alexopoulos, G. S., Perlick, D. A., Friedman, S. J., & Meyers, B. S. (2001b). Stigma as a barrier to recovery: Perceived stigma and patient-rated severity of illness as predictors of antidepressant drug adherence. *Psychiatric Service, 52,* 1615–1620.

Staring, A. B., Van der Gaag, M., Van den Berge, M., Duivenvoorden, H. J., & Mulder, C. L. (2009). Stigma moderates the associations of insight with depressed mood, low self-esteem, and low quality of life in patients with schizophrenia spectrum disorders. *Schizophrenia Research, 115,* 363–369.

Suto, M., Livingston, J. D., Hole, R., Lapsley, S., Hale, S., & Michalak, E. (2012). "Stigma shrinks my Bubble": A qualitative study of understandings and experiences of stigma and bipolar disorder. *Stigma Research and Action, 2,* 85–92.

Swann, A. C., Bowden, C. L., Calabrese, J. R., Dilsaver, S. C., & Morris, D. D. (2000). Mania: differential effects of previous depressive and manic episodes on response to treatment. *Acta Psychiatrica Scandinavica, 101,* 444–451.

Thornicroft, G. (2006). *Shunned: Discrimination against people with mental illness.* Oxford: Oxford University Press

Vázquez, G. H., Kapczinski, F., Magalhaes, P. V., Córdoba, R., Jaramillo, C. L., Rosa, A .R.,…Tohen, M.(2011).Stigma and functioning in patients with bipolar disorder. *Journal of Affective Disorders, 130,* 323–327.

Vieta, E., & Suppes, T. (2008). Bipolar II disorder: arguments for and against a distinct diagnostic entity. *Bipolar Disorder, 10,* 163–178.

Wahl, O. F. (1999). *Telling is risky business: Mental health consumers confront stigma.* Piscataway, NJ: Rutgers University Press.

Wang, P. S., Berglund, P., Olfson, M., Pincus, H. A., Wells, K. B., & Kessler, R. C. (2005). Failure and delay in initial treatment contact after first onset of mental disorders in the National Comorbidity Survey Replication. *Archives of General Psychiatry, 62,* 603–613.

Wolkenstein, L., & Meyer, T. D. (2009).What factors influence attitudes towards people with current depression and current mania? *International Journal of Social Psychiatry, 55,* 124–140.

Zeschel, E., Correll, C. U., Haussleiter, I. S., Krüger-Özgürdal, S., Leopold, K., Pfennig, A.,…Juckel, G. (2013). The bipolar disorder prodrome revisited: Is there a symptomatic pattern? *Journal of Affective Disorders, 151,* 551–560.

SECTION II

INSIGHTS ON PATHOPHYSIOLOGY AND FUTURE TREATMENTS

PART I

MOLECULAR BIOLOGY

7.

OXIDATIVE DAMAGE AND ITS TREATMENT IMPACT

Gislaine Tezza Rezin and Ana Cristina Andreazza

OXIDATIVE STRESS: A BRIEF OVERVIEW

Free radicals are any atom or molecular species able to exist independently that contain one or more unpaired electrons (Halliwell, 1999, 2011; Halliwell & Gutteridge, 2007). Thus they have an extremely high reactivity due to their energetically unstable situation (Maxwell, 1995). These radicals may be formed in both circumstances—physiological and pathological—and they may exert harmful effects on cells and organisms by changing structure and function of lipids, proteins, or deoxyribonucleic acid (DNA). The imbalance between oxidant and antioxidant agents are known as oxidative stress damage (Halliwell, 2011).

Under physiological conditions of aerobic cell metabolism, oxygen is reduced to water formation by tetravalent reduction. However, approximately 5% of the oxygen utilized in the mitochondrial respiratory chain is not fully reduced to water and may be converted into reactive intermediates (Boveris & Chance, 1973). The oxygen molecule remains attached to the Complex IV in the mitochondrial respiratory chain until total oxygen reduction. During this process, partial reduction of oxygen might occur, generating superoxide anion (O_2^-), by receiving only one electron each time. Therefore, adding one more electron to the O_2^-, this is reduced to hydrogen peroxide (H_2O_2); despite not being a free radical, it may react with other O_2^-, or transition metals, forming the hydroxyl radical ($OH^\bullet$), according to the Fenton and Haber-Weiss reactions (Halliwell, 2011). The term "reactive oxygen species" (ROS) include free radicals formed by the reduction of oxygen, such as O_2^- and $OH^\bullet$, as well as some nonradical derivatives of oxygen, such as H_2O_2, and singlet oxygen (Halliwell & Gutteridge, 2007). In addition, the ROS extract electrons from other compounds initiate a chain reaction, with the potential to oxidize biological molecules, including lipids, proteins, and nucleic acids (Maxwell, 1995; Smith, Marks, & Lieberman,

2005). In order to protect the body of consequences of constant production of ROS, the cells have an antioxidant system consisting of enzymatic and nonenzymatic components involved in stopping free radicals damage to biomolecules (i.e., lipids, proteins, and DNA). The antioxidant is any substance that, when present at low concentrations compared to those of an oxidizable substrate, delays or prevents oxidation. The term "oxidizable substrate" includes macromolecules such as lipids, proteins, and nucleic acids. Consequently, the function of antioxidants is to maintain intracellular levels of ROS at low concentrations (Halliwell & Gutteridge, 2007). The main enzymatic defenses include the superoxide dismutase (SOD), catalase (CAT), glutathione S-transferase (GST), and glutathione peroxidase (GPx) enzymes, as well as others that do not directly participate in the process but support the GPx, such as glucose-6-phosphate dehydrogenase and glutathione reductase (Maté & Sánchez-Jiménez, 1999). Also, nonenzymatic defenses are mainly represented by ascorbic acid (vitamin C), α-tocopherol (vitamin E), glutathione, carotenoids, and flavonoids. Importantly, the enzymatic antioxidant defenses act directly on detoxification agents before they cause any damage to biomolecules. The nonenzymatic antioxidants act after the damage has occurred and are responsible for injury repair (Halliwell & Gutteridge, 2007).

The actions of the antioxidant cascade are as follows: (a) the enzyme SOD reduces the O_2^- to H_2O_2 in a dismutation reaction and then (b) the CAT or GPx reduces the H_2O_2 to water (Halliwell & Gutteridge, 2007). The GPx exists as a family of enzymes containing selenium with some differences in their properties and tissue distribution (Smith, Marks, & Lieberman, 2005). GPx eliminates the H_2O_2 by coupling reduced glutathione with water, and consequently oxidizing glutathione, which consists of two reduced glutathione linked by a disulfide bridge. In turn, glutathione reductase can convert oxidized glutathione to reduced glutathione (Halliwell, 2006). Nevertheless, antioxidant defenses

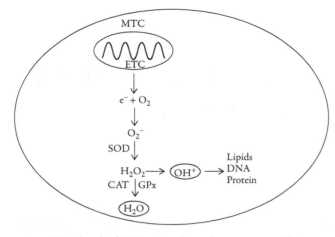

Figure 7.1 Mitochondrial ROS generation and consequent oxidative stress. CAT: Catalase; DNA: Deoxyribonucleic acid; ETC: Electron transport chain; GPx: Glutathione peroxidase; H_2O_2: Hydrogen peroxide; MTC: Mitochondria; O_2^-: Superoxide anion; $OH^\bullet$: Hydroxyl radical; SOD: Superoxide dismutase.

are not 100% effective, since oxidative damage to lipids, proteins, DNA, and other molecules can be demonstrated in living systems in an aerobic environment (Halliwell & Gutteridge, 2007). Indeed, if the antioxidant system fails, the H_2O_2 can react with iron (Fe^{2+}), in a reaction called Fenton and Haber-Weiss to form $OH^\bullet$, which is highly reactive and often causes oxidative damage to lipids, proteins, and DNA (see Figure 7.1; Halliwell & Gutteridge, 2007).

Under physiological conditions, the body is capable of maintaining a balance between oxidant agents and antioxidant defenses, thus preventing oxidative damage (Halliwell & Gutteridge, 2007). If there is augmentation on ROS production, decreased antioxidant defenses, or both, the balance between oxidants and antioxidants is disrupted, leading to a state in the cells called oxidative stress. During mild and transient oxidative stress, the cell can adapt increasing the production of antioxidants. However, during chronic oxidative stress, cells often progress to necrosis or apoptosis due to excess damage to biomolecules structures (Clay, Sillivan, & Konradi, 2010; Halliwell & Gutteridge, 2007; Kato, 2008; Konradi, Sillivan, & Clay, 2012). Of significance, oxidative stress is also a process necessary for the maintenance of normal cellular functions. For example, a variety of stimuli might cause reactive oxygen/nitrogen species to act as signal transducers in signaling pathways, leading to specific cellular phenotypes (D'Autréaux & Toledano, 2007). In this context, cells can respond in several ways to oxidative stress, which depends on the cell type and the severity of oxidative stress. Responses to oxidative stress include (a) increase in proliferation; (b) cell and organism adaptations, by up-regulation of repair systems; (c) cellular damage, by modifying lipids structure from cellular membranes; and (d) senescence or cellular death, by

inducing apoptosis or necrosis for example (Clay, Sillivan, & Konradi, 2010; Halliwell & Gutteridge, 2007; Kato, 2008; Konradi, Sillivan, & Clay, 2012).

SOURCES OF OXIDATIVE STRESS IN BIPOLAR DISORDER

The etiology and pathophysiology of bipolar disorder (BD) involves several biological mechanism; however, evidence postulates that increased oxidative stress; mitochondrial dysfunction; dysfunctional inflammatory response; and alterations in calcium (Ca^{2+}), dopamine, and glutamate signaling are central biological mechanism in BD (for review see Andreazza & Young, 2013). This chapter reviews the implication of these biological systems in BD.

MITOCHONDRIAL DYSFUNCTION, ANTIOXIDANT SYSTEM, AND OXIDATIVE DAMAGE

Preclinical and clinical studies have constantly demonstrated elevated states of oxidative damage, including changes in antioxidant systems or increased oxidative damage to lipids, proteins, or DNA in animal models of mania (Frey, Martins, et al., 2006; Frey, Valvassori, et al., 2006a) and in patients with BD (Andreazza, Cassini, et al., 2007; Andreazza, Frey, et al. 2007, Andreazza et al., 2009; Gergerlioglu et al., 2007; Kapczinski et al., 2011; Kuloglu et al., 2002; Machado-Vieira et al., 2007; Ranjekar et al., 2003; Savas, Gergerlioglu, & Armutcu, 2006; Selek et al., 2008). Studies have suggested an association of mitochondrial dysfunction in the pathophysiology of BD (Andreazza, Shao, Wang, & Young, 2010; Iwamoto, Bundo, & Kato, 2005; Kato & Kato, 2000). More specifically, studies using postmortem brain tissue have demonstrated that mitochondrial genes are down-regulated in the hippocampus (Lieberman, Perkins, & Jarskog, 2007) and dorsolateral prefrontal cortex of patients with BD (Iwamoto, Bundo, & Kato, 2005; Konradi et al., 2004; Sun, Wang, Tseng, & Young, 2006). Konradi and colleagues have shown that messenger ribonucleic acid (mRNA) expression of subunits of complex I-V was significantly reduced in the postmortem hippocampus of patients with BD. Sun et al. also demonstrated a decrease in the levels of mRNA for the NDUFS7 and NDUFS8 subunits of complex I. Additionally, Iwamoto et al. showed a reduction in the levels of mRNA in NDUFS8 and NDUFS1 from patients with BD. Andreazza and colleagues, interestingly, demonstrated that the decreased mRNA levels of NDUFS7 translate to diminished levels of NDUFS7 and affect the activity of complex I in the postmortem brain samples of patients with BD.

Antioxidant enzymes have also been shown to be altered in BD. Benes and colleagues (2006) demonstrated that the expression of genes that encode the major antioxidant enzymes, such as SOD, CAT, GPx, and GST, are also reduced in the hippocampus of patients with BD. Studies also have shown that the SOD activity is increased in BD (Andreazza, Cassini, et al., 2007; Kuloglu et al., 2002; Machado-Vieira et al., 2007; Savas, Gergerlioglu, & Armutcu, 2006). More specifically, Andreazza et al. found an increased in serum SOD activity during the depressive and manic phase but not in patients with BD in the euthymic phase. In support, Gergerlioglu and colleagues (2007) revealed an increase in the levels of SOD in patients with BD during the manic phase. Machado-Vieira et al. demonstrated that naive patients with BD also have increased levels of SOD. However, Savas and colleagues identified increased levels of SOD in patients with BD in the euthymic phase. Other antioxidants enzymes have been evaluated: (a) Andreazza et al. found diminishing serum activity of CAT in patients with BD in the euthymic phase; (b) Machado-Vieira et al. showed an increase in serum CAT activity in patients with BD in the manic phase without treatment, and Kuloglu et al. found decreased levels of CAT in patients with BD (description of which phase patients were when blood was collected were not available); (c) Andreazza et al. showed that patients with BD in the euthymic phase show increased activity of GPx. However, other studies did not found differences in relation to GPx activity when compared to controls (Kuloglu et al., 2002; Ranjekar et al., 2003).

Some studies have demonstrated an increase in lipid peroxidation in patients with BD during manic, depressive, and euthymic phases, as well as in drug-naive patients with BD (Andreazza, Kauer-Sant'Anna, Frey, Bond, et al., 2008; Machado-Vieira et al., 2007). Lipid peroxidation, represented by increased levels of 4-hydroxynonenal, was also observed as increased in the anterior cingulate cortex of patients with BD (Wang, Shao, Sun, & Young, 2009). Andreazza and colleagues (2013) confirmed increased levels of lipid peroxidation in the postmortem prefrontal cortex of patients with BD. Other studies have also shown abnormalities in the anterior cingulate cortex of patients with BD (Beal, 2002; Ji & Bennett, 2003). Studies also report increased levels of nitric oxide (NO) in patients with BD in manic, depressive, and euthymic phases (Gergerlioglu et al., 2007; Savas, Gergerlioglu, & Armutcu, 2006; Selek et al., 2008). Together these findings support the hypothesis of

an important role of oxidative stress in the neurological progression of BD.

INFLAMMATION

Evidence also suggests that inflammatory processes in the periphery and the brain are involved in the pathophysiology of BD (Brietzke et al., 2009; Ortiz-Dominguez et al., 2007; Rao, Harry, Rapoport, & Kim, 2010). Studies have shown altered levels of cytokines in patients with BD depending on the mood state (Brietzke et al., 2009; Kapczinski et al., 2009), as well as staging of the illness (Kapczinski et al., 2008; Kauer-Sant'Anna et al., 2009). More specifically, BD is accompanied by increased peripheral levels of (a) proinflammatory cytokines, such as interleukin-2 (IL-2), interleukin-6 (IL-6), and tumor necrosis factor-α (TNF- α; Brietzke et al., 2009; Kim, Jung, Myint, Kim, & Park, 2007; Ortiz-Dominguez et al., 2007) and (b) anti-inflammatory cytokines including interleukin-1β (IL-1β), nuclear factor κB (NF-κB), and interleukin-1 receptor (IL-1R) antagonist protein (Ortiz-Dominguez et al., 2007; Rao, Harry, Rapoport, & Kim, 2010). mRNA levels of IL-1β, IL-1R, and NF-kB subunits have been also shown to be increased in the postmortem frontal cortex of persons with BD when compared with control subjects (Rao, Harry, Rapoport, & Kim, 2010). Also, increased levels of acute inflammatory response proteins (i.e., haptoglobin and C-reactive protein) have also been demonstrated (Dickerson, Stallings, Origoni, Boronow, & Yolken, 2007; Maes et al., 1997). Complement factors (C3 and C4) have been found as elevated in plasma of patients with BD (Maes et al., 1997; Wadee et al., 2002).

Patients with BD in early (i.e., <3 years of illness) and late (>10 years of illness) stages of illness have been associated with elevated levels of proinflammatory cytokines IL-6 and TNF-α, while interleukin-10 (IL-10), an anti-inflammatory cytokine, was increased only in patients in the early stage of the disorder (Kauer-Sant'Anna et al., 2009). This suggests that anti-inflammatory defense mechanisms are no longer responsive in late-stage BD. Illness progression often results in cumulative effects of oxidative stress, which could result in elevation of antioxidant enzymes (e.g., GST) as a compensatory mechanism among patients with BD, as demonstrated by Andreazza and colleagues (2008). Thus if the compensatory antioxidants mechanisms fail to prevent damage, patients with BD might experience a worse (or faster) progression of the illness. This hypothesis is supported by previous studies that have shown that patients with BD exhibit increased levels of oxidative damage to lipids (Kuloglu et al., 2002; Machado-Vieira et al., 2007), proteins (Andreazza et al., 2009), and DNA (Andreazza, Frey, et al., 2007) and decreased antioxidant enzyme defenses (Savas, Gergerlioglu, & Armutcu, 2006; Selek et al., 2008).

Of significance, a proinflammatory state also activates degradation of tryptophan and serotonin via indoleamine 2,3-dioxygenase, leading to increased consumption of tryptophan (Berk et al., 2011). Stimulation of indoleamine 2,3-dioxygenase and kynurenine monooxygenase by proinflammatory states further results in the production of tryptophan catabolites, including quinolinic acid, which might lead to dysregulation of the neurotransmitter system and mitochondrial energy metabolism (Berk et al., 2011).

CALCIUM

Recent genome-wide association studies using large groups of patients (over 13,000) and controls find out that the alpha 1C subunit of the L-type voltage-gated Ca^{2+} channel (CACNA1C) and ankyrin 3 are strong potential risk genes associated with BD. CACNA1C belongs to the family of L-type Ca^{2+} channels that mediate various Ca^{2+}-dependent processes in neurons. It regulates the dendritic Ca^{2+} influx in response to synaptic activity (Vacher, Mohapatra, & Trimmer, 2008). Ankyrin 3 is a member of a family of ankyrin proteins that plays a role in several cellular signalings, including maintenance of cytoskeleton and membrane domains (Vacher, Mohapatra, & Trimmer, 2008). It is also known to modulate the activity of neuronal sodium channels. The use of genome-wide association studies in very large cohorts has allowed the identification of at least two potential biomarkers of BD: CACNA1C and ankyrin 3. Imaging studies are beginning to unravel the functional correlates and susceptibility mechanisms of these variants (O'Donovan, Craddock, & Owen, 2009; Vacher, Mohapatra, & Trimmer, 2008).

Studies have demonstrated also that BD is associated with the polymorphism of the transient potential receptor melastatin-2 gene, which is involved in the maintenance of intracellular levels of Ca^{2+} and is abundantly expressed in the brain (Perova, Wasserman, Li, & Warsh, 2008; Xu et al., 2009). Moreover, increased intracellular Ca^{2+} levels are a consistent finding in studies of BD (Kato, 2008). Under such conditions, mitochondria are one of organelles responsible for storing Ca^{2+}, while the influx and efflux of Ca^{2+} are mediated by membrane potential, which is generated during the proton gradient of the mitochondrial respiratory chain (Chinopoulos & Adam-Vizi, 2006). Hence, mitochondrial dysfunction may lead to a change in membrane potential, and, consequently, it may reduce

the Ca^{2+} absorption (Wang, 2007). Thus activation of Ca^{2+}-dependent proteins and direct inhibition of the mitochondrial electron transport chain have been shown as an important trigger of oxidative stress (de Gonzalo-Calvo et al., 2010).

NEUROTRANSMITTERS

Another metabolite associated with induction of oxidative stress state in the brain is the dopamine (Berk et al., 2007; Chen et al., 2008; Rees, Florang, Anderson, & Doorn, 2007). Dopamine is metabolized via (a) enzymatic by the monoamine oxidase (MAO), which generates H_2O_2, a ROS, and dihydroxyphenylacetic acid or via (b) autocatalytic by reaction with Fe^{2+} and H_2O_2 forming 6-hydroxydopamine (Berman & Hastings, 1999; Hastings, Lewis, & Zigmond, 1996; Obata, 2002). In vivo, electrochemical analyses have demonstrated that in a few minutes after the administration of 6-hydroxydopamine into the brain, this is converted to p-quinone (Beal, 2002; Obata, 2002). 6-hydroxydopamine can be conjugated, in vivo, with glutathione by the action of GST (Baez, Segura-Aguilar, Widersten, Johansson, & Mannervik, 1997). Importantly, Andreazza and colleagues (2009) demonstrated that patients with BD during the late stages of the illness (over 10 years of illness) have increased levels of glutathione reductase and GST suggesting that patients with BD perhaps are trying to react against the oxidative stress damage by boosting the antioxidant system, which, however, is not sufficient to prevent the full oxidative damage as demonstrated by increased protein oxidation in the same patients. Further studies are indeed necessary to understand how MAO contributes to oxidative damage in BD. Such studies would contribute a crucial piece of information—how oxidative stress modulates neurotransmitter levels.

Studies also have shown that patients with BD have increased levels of NO (Gergerlioglu et al., 2007; Savas et al., 2002; Savas, Gergerlioglu, & Armutcu, 2006). NO is considered a neurotransmitter too. NO may react with the O_2^-, leading to form peroxynitrite, which has the potential to nitrate tyrosine residues of proteins, results in the formation of 3-nitrotyrosine (Ischiropoulos, 2003). Andreazza and colleagues (2009) demonstrated that patients with BD in early or late stages exhibit increased levels of 3-nitrotyrosine. Besides, Ji and Bennett (2003) have shown that GST is activated when exposed to peroxynitrite by nitration of tyrosine residues. Therefore, the activation of GST may avoid a rise in oxidative tissue injury while other antioxidant enzymes, such as SOD (MacMillan-Crow, Crow, & Thompson, 1998) and xanthine oxidase (Lee,

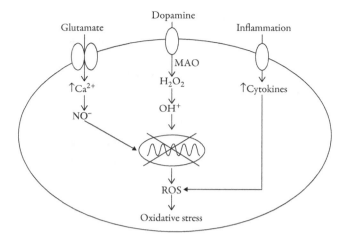

Figure 7.2 Relationship between neurotransmitter, inflammatory system and oxidative stress. Ca2+: Calcium; H2O2: Hydrogen peroxide; MAO: Monoamine oxidase; NO-: Nitric oxide; OH: Hydroxyl radical; ROS: Reactive oxygen species

Liu, & Zweier, 2000) be compromised, due to an excessive formation of peroxynitrite. Considering that the 3-nitrotyrosine may be a marker of the generation of ROS (Hastings, Lewis, & Zigmond, 1996), the nitration process may have an important role in the pathophysiology of BD (Andreazza et al., 2009). Another source of NO is the increase in the release of glutamate. The stimulation of N-methyl D-aspartate (NMDA) by glutamate, allows the passage of Ca^{2+} in the cell, by activating the calcium/calmodulin-dependent protein kinase type IV, which activates nitric oxide synthase increasing the production of NO (Coyle & Puttfarcken, 1993). Remarkably, studies using in vivo proton magnetic resonance spectroscopy have found that patients with BD have higher glutamate levels in discrete subregions of the prefrontal cortex (Frye et al., 2007; Michael et al., 2003).

Here we have reviewed a considerable body of evidence supporting abnormalities in cellular pathways, such as mitochondrial dysfunction, inflammatory response, alteration in Ca^{2+} signaling, and dopamine and glutamate neurotransmission that may result in oxidative stress (Figure 7.2).

HOW CAN WE TREAT OXIDATIVE STRESS?

As discussed previously, growing evidence have suggested that the oxidative stress plays a key role in the pathophysiology of BD (Andreazza, Kauer-Sant'Anna, Frey, Stertz, et al., 2008; Clay, Sillivan, & Konradi, 2010; Machado-Vieira, Manji, & Zarate, 2009); consequently the interest in understanding which antioxidant compounds can be used to treat this illness is indeed growing. We discuss here some

of this clinical and preclinical evidence (Berk et al., 2008; Machado-Vieira et al., 2008; Magalhães et al., 2011).

Some studies have shown that lithium has an important effect on lipid peroxidation (Machado-Vieira et al., 2007; Shao, Young, & Wang, 2005), DNA damage (Shao, Young, & Wang, 2005), and formation of free radicals (Machado-Vieira et al., 2007; Shao, Young, & Wang, 2005), as well as on the antioxidant defense in various models (Machado-Vieira, Manji, & Zarate, 2009). More specifically, studies have demonstrated that lithium has the capacity to diminish the lipid peroxidation in patients with BD (Banerjee, Dasgupta, Rout, & Singh, 2012) and animal models of mania (Frey, Valvassori, et al., 2006b; Macêdo et al., 2012). Lithium also increases the CAT levels and decreases the levels of SOD in patients (Gergerlioglu et al., 2007; Machado-Vieira et al., 2007). Moreover, lithium can balance the SOD/CAT ratio, which diminishes the cellular H_2O_2 concentration and, consequently, the oxidative stress (Machado-Vieira et al., 2007). Another study by Khairova and colleagues (2012) revealed a decrease in the SOD levels in healthy subjects after the use of lithium. However, levels of CAT and thiobarbituric acid reactive substances (TBARS) (a measurement to assess lipid peroxidation) were not altered by the use of this mood stabilizer in healthy subjects (Khairova et al., 2012). Additionally, chronic administration of lithium modifies the affinity of dopamine transporters and therefore decreases the excessive dopaminergic neurotransmission, resulting in the generation of ROS (Carli, Morissette, Hebert, Di Paolo, & Reader, 1997). The mechanism by which lithium reduces the generation of ROS is far from being completely understood, but it can be partially supported by its action on buffering of intracellular Ca^{2+} levels or through the stability of mitochondrial function and oxidative stress (Shao, Young, & Wang, 2005).

Besides the promising effects of lithium, other substances have also been studied in favor of redox balance in BD. N-acetyl cysteine (NAC) is a glutathione precursor, and it contributes to increased levels of antioxidants. Glutathione is a tripeptide containing cysteine, glutamate, and glycine, and it is synthesized by two enzymatic reactions involving glutamate-cysteine ligase and glutathione synthetase. Cysteine is a limiting amino acid for glutathione synthesis (Dringen, Gutterer, & Hirrlinger, 2000). Hence glutathione is the primary antioxidant defense of the organism, and a decrease in glutathione levels in patients with BD has been demonstrated in the postmortem prefrontal cortex of patients with BD (Gawryluk, Wang, Andreazza, Shao, & Young, 2010). Magalhães and colleagues (2011) demonstrated that adjunctive treatment with NAC for patients with BD contributes to improved remission of manic and depressive symptoms. Additionally, the use of NAC leads to an increase in glutathione levels in animal models (Dean et al., 2009). Thus the use of NAC is promising because it increases the levels of glutathione and also reverses the mitochondrial dysfunction present in BD, which leads to the generation of ROS (Andreazza Shao, Wang, & Young, 2010).

Another substance with antioxidant potential is the alpha-lipoic acid. Macêdo and colleagues (2012) found that alpha-lipoic acid is effective in preventing and reversing the locomotor alterations induced by amphetamine in an animal model of mania, which indicates that this acid may be important for the treatment acute episode and maintenance of BD. The alpha-lipoic acid also inhibits the formation of H_2O_2 and $OH^•$, scavenges lipid peroxidation products, chelates redox-activated transition metals (Suzuki, Tsuchiya, & Packer, 1991), and modulates NO levels in the brain (Gross & Wolin, 1995), as well as participates in the recycling of other antioxidants, inducing enzymes associated with glutathione synthesis (Packer, Witt, & Tritschler, 1995). Alpha-lipoic acid has been demonstrated to prevent the inhibition of SOD activity, reverse the decreased levels of glutathione, and ameliorate levels of lipid peroxidation. Thus the increase in glutathione content and SOD activity by the administration of alpha lipoic acid, and the consequent decrease of lipid peroxidation, may characterize the antioxidant effect of this substance (Macêdo et al., 2012).

However, Brennan and colleagues (2013) showed that treatment with acetyl-L-carnitine and alpha lipoic acid does not have antidepressant effects in BD. Their results demonstrated no differences in the Montgomery-Åsberg Depression Rating Scale between patients treated with acetyl-L-carnitine and alpha lipoic acid when compared to a placebo. Nevertheless, their results demonstrated reduced levels of parieto-occipital phosphocreatine in patients who received acetyl-L-carnitine.

Brocardo and colleagues (2010) showed that folic acid prevents (a) an increase TBARS levels, (b) a decrease in GPx activity, and (c) a decrease in the activity of glutathione reductase in a pharmacological animal model of mania using ouabain. The function of GPx is to reduce the H_2O_2 to water while the glutathione reductase is an ancillary enzyme that reduces oxidized glutathione formed by GPx to the thiol form of glutathione (Carlberg & Mannervik, 1985; Wendel, 1981). Thus the use of folic acid may be opportune in the improving glutathione system in BD (Brocardo et al., 2010). Moreover, Bruning, Prigol, Luchese, Pinton, and Nogueira (2012) demonstrated that the diphenyl diselenide (a compound that exhibits similar effects as GPx) was able to prevent the increase of lipid peroxidation, protein carbonyls, and activity of SOD in an animal model of mania induced by ouabain. Diphenyl diselenide has been also shown to decrease the Ca^{2+} influx, which contributes to a reduction in the formation of reactive species (Luchese & Nogueira, 2010; Meotti, Stangherlin, Zeni, Rocha, & Nogueira, 2004). Taken together, the aforementioned findings support that oxidative stress plays a significant role in neurological progression of BD, justifying its importance in the research of new therapeutic targets (see Figure 7.3).

Disclosure statement: Dr. Andreazza and Dr. Rezin have no financial conflicts of interest. Dr. Andreazza has received operating funding from the Canadian Institute of Health Research and Brain and Behavioural Foundation. Dr. Rezin has been supported by the Brazil Without Borders program from CAPES.

REFERENCES

Andreazza, A. C., Cassini, C., Rosa, A. R., Leite, M. C., de Almeida, L. M., Nardin, P., … Gonçalves, C. A. (2007). Serum S100B and antioxidant enzymes in bipolar patients. *Journal of Psychiatric Research, 41*(6), 523–529.

Andreazza, A. C., Frey, B. N., Erdtmann, B., Salvador, M., Goncalves, C. A., & Kapczinski, F. (2007). DNA damage in bipolar disorder. *Psychiatry Research, 153*(1), 27–32.

Andreazza, A. C., Kapczinski, F., Kauer-Sant'Anna, M., Walz, J. C., Bond, D. J., Gonçalves, C. A., … Yatham, L. N. (2009). 3-Nitrotyrosine and glutathione antioxidant system in patients in the early and late stages of bipolar disorder. *Journal of Psychiatry & Neuroscience, 34*(4), 263–271.

Andreazza, A. C., Kauer-Sant'anna, M., Frey, B. N., Bond, D. J., Kapczinski, F., Young, L. T., & Yatham, L. N. (2008). Oxidative stress markers in bipolar disorder: A meta-analysis. *Journal of Affective Disorders, 111*(2–3), 135–144.

Andreazza, A. C., Kauer-Sant'Anna, M., Frey, B. N., Stertz, L., Zanotto, C., Ribeiro, L., … Kapczinski, F. (2008). Effects of mood stabilizers on DNA damage in an animal model of mania. *Journal of Psychiatry & Neuroscience, 33*(6), 516–524.

Andreazza, A. C., Shao, L., Wang, J. F., & Young, L. T. (2010). Mitochondrial complex I activity and oxidative damage to mitochondrial proteins in the prefrontal cortex of patients with bipolar disorder. *Archives of General Psychiatry, 67*(4), 360–368.

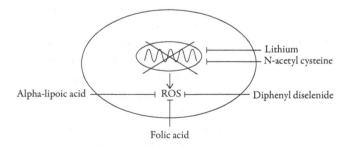

Figure 7.3 Antioxidant effect of lithium, N-acetyl cysteine, alpha lipoic acid, folic acid and diphenyl diselenide on mitochondrial dysfunction and ROS. ROS: Reactive oxygen species.

Andreazza, A. C., & Young, L. T. (2013). The neurobiology of bipolar disorder: Identifying targets for specific agents and synergies for combination treatment. *The International Journal of Neuropsychopharmacology*, *1*, 1–14.

Andreazza, A. C., Wang, J. F., Salmasi, F., Shao, L., & Young, L. T. (2013). Specific subcellular changes in oxidative stress in prefrontal cortex from patients with bipolar disorder. *Journal of Neurochemistry*, *127*(4), 552–561.

Baez, S., Segura-Aguilar, J., Widersten, M., Johansson, A. S., & Mannervik, B. (1997). Glutathione transferases catalyse the detoxication of oxidized metabolites (o-quinones) of catecholamines and may serve as an antioxidant system preventing degenerative cellular processes. *The Biochemical Journal*, *324*(Pt. 1), 25–28.

Banerjee, U., Dasgupta, A., Rout, J. K., & Singh, O. P. (2012). Effects of lithium therapy on Na+–K+-ATPase activity and lipid peroxidation in bipolar disorder. *Progress in Neuro-Psychopharmacology & Biological Psychiatry*, *37*(1), 56–61.

Beal, M. F. (2002). Oxidatively modified proteins in aging and disease. *Free Radical Biology & Medicine*, *32*(9), 797–803.

Benes, F. M., Matzilevich, D., Burke, R. E., & Walsh, J. (2006). The expression of proapoptosis genes is increased in bipolar disorder, but not in schizophrenia. *Molecular Psychiatry*, *11*(3), 241–251.

Berk, M., Copolov, D. L., Dean, O., Lu, K., Jeavons, S., Schapkaitz, I., ... Bush, A. I. (2008). N-acetyl cysteine for depressive symptoms in bipolar disorder: A double-blind randomized placebo-controlled trial. *Biological Psychiatry*, *64*(6), 468–475.

Berk, M., Dodd, S., Kauer-Sant'anna, M., Malhi, G. S., Bourin, M., Kapczinski, F., & Norman, T. (2007). Dopamine dysregulation syndrome: Implications for a dopamine hypothesis of bipolar disorder. *Acta Psychiatrica Scandinavica*, *434*(Suppl.), 41–49.

Berk, M., Kapczinski, F., Andreazza, A. C., Dean, O. M., Giorlando, F., Maes, M., ... Malhi, G. S. (2011). Pathways underlying neuroprogression in bipolar disorder: Focus on inflammation, oxidative stress and neurotrophic factors. *Neuroscience and Biobehavioral Reviews*, *35*(3), 804–817.

Berman, S. B., & Hastings, T. G. (1999). Dopamine oxidation alters mitochondrial respiration and induces permeability transition in brain mitochondria: Implications for Parkinson's disease. *Journal of Neurochemistry*, *73*(3), 1127–1137.

Boveris, A., & Chance, B. (1973). The mitochondrial generation of hydrogen peroxide: General properties and effect of hyperbaric oxygen. *The Biochemical Journal*, *134*(3), 707–716.

Brennan, B. P., Jensen, J. E., Hudson, J. I., Coit, C. E., Beaulieu, A., Pope, H. G. Jr., ... Cohen, B. M. (2013). Placebo-controlled trial of acetyl-L-carnitine and α-lipoic acid in the treatment of bipolar depression. *Journal of Clinical Psychopharmacology*, *33*(5), 627–635.

Brietzke, E., Stertz, L., Fernandes, B. S., Kauer-Sant'anna, M., Mascarenhas, M., Escosteguy Vargas, A., ... Kapczinski, F. (2009). Comparison of cytokine levels in depressed, manic and euthymic patients with bipolar disorder. *Journal of Affective Disorders*, *116*(3), 214–217.

Brocardo, P. S., Budni, J., Pavesi, E., Franco, J. L., Uliano-Silva, M., Trevisan, R., ... Rodrigues, A. L. (2010). Folic acid administration prevents ouabain-induced hyperlocomotion and alterations in oxidative stress markers in the rat brain. *Bipolar Disorders*, *12*(4), 414–424.

Bruning, C. A., Prigol, M., Luchese, C., Pinton, S., & Nogueira, C. W. (2012). Nogueira diphenyl diselenide ameliorates behavioral and oxidative parameters in an animal model of mania induced by ouabain. *Progress in Neuro-Psychopharmacology & Biological Psychiatry*, *38*(2), 168–174.

Carlberg, I., & Mannervik, B. (1985). Glutathione reductase. *Methods in Enzymology*, *113*, 484–489.

Carli, M., Morissette, M., Hebert, C., Di Paolo, T., & Reader, T. A. (1997). Effects of a chronic lithium treatment on central dopamine neurotransporters. *Biochemical Pharmacology*, *54*(3), 391–397.

Chen, L., Ding, Y., Cagniard, B., Van Laar, A. D., Mortimer, A., Chi, W., ... Zhuang, X. (2008). Unregulated cytosolic dopamine causes neurodegeneration associated with oxidative stress in mice. *Journal of Neuroscience*, *28*(2), 425–433.

Chinopoulos, C., & Adam-Vizi, V. (2006). Calcium, mitochondria and oxidative stress in neuronal pathology: Novel aspects of an enduring theme. *The FEBS Journal*, *273*(3), 433–450.

Clay, H. B., Sillivan, S., & Konradi, C. (2010). Mitochondrial dysfunction and pathology in bipolar disorder and schizophrenia. *International Journal of Developmental Neuroscience*, *29*(3), 311–324.

Coyle, J. T., & Puttfarcken, P. (1993). Oxidative stress, glutamate, and neurodegenerative disorders. *Science*, *262*(5134), 689–695.

D'Autréaux, B., & Toledano, M. B. (2007). ROS as signaling molecules: Mechanisms that generate specificity in ROS homeostasis. *Nature Reviews: Molecular Cell Biology*, *8*(10), 813–824.

Dean, O. M., van den Buuse, M., Bush, A. I., Copolov, D. L., Ng, F., Dodd, S., & Berk, M. (2009). A role for glutathione in the pathophysiology of bipolar disorder and schizophrenia: Animal models and relevance to clinical practice. *Current Medicinal Chemistry*, *16*(23), 2965–2976.

de Gonzalo-Calvo, D., Neitzert, K., Fernández, M., Vega-Naredo, I., Caballero, B., García-Macía, M., ... Coto-Montes, A. (2010). Differential inflammatory responses in aging and disease: TNF-alpha and IL-6 as possible biomarkers. *Free Radical Biology & Medicine*, *49*(5), 733–737.

Dickerson, F., Stallings, C., Origoni, A., Boronow, J., & Yolken, R. (2007). Elevated serum levels of C-reactive protein are associated with mania symptoms in outpatients with bipolar disorder. *Progress in Neuro-Psychopharmacology & Biological Psychiatry*, *31*(4), 952–955.

Dringen, R., Gutterer, J. M., & Hirrlinger, J. (2000). Glutathione metabolism in brain metabolic interaction between astrocytes and neurons in the defense against reactive oxygen species. *European Journal of Biochemistry*, *267*(16), 4912–4916.

Frey, B. N., Martins, M. R., Petronilho, F. C., Dal-Pizzol, F., Quevedo, J., & Kapczinski, F. (2006). Increased oxidative stress after repeated amphetamine exposure: Possible relevance as a model of mania. *Bipolar Disorders*, *8*(3), 275–280.

Frey, B. N., Valvassori, S. S., Réus, G. Z., Martins, M. R., Petronilho, F. C., Bardini, K., ... Quevedo, J. (2006a). Changes in antioxidant defense enzymes after d-amphetamine exposure: Implications as an animal model of mania. *Neurochemical Research*, *31*(5), 699–703.

Frey, B. N., Valvassori, S. S., Réus, G. Z., Martins, M. R., Petronilho, F. C., Bardini, K., ... Quevedo, J. (2006b). Effects of lithium and valproate on amphetamine-induced oxidative stress generation in an animal model of mania. *Journal of Psychiatry & Neuroscience*, *31*(5), 326–332.

Frye, M. A., Watzl, J., Banakar, S., O'Neill, J., Mintz, J., Davanzo, P., ... Thomas, M. A. (2007). Increased anterior cingulate/medial prefrontal cortical glutamate and creatine in bipolar depression. *Neuropsychopharmacology*, *32*(12), 2490–2499.

Gawryluk, J. W., Wang, J. F., Andreazza, A. C., Shao, L., & Young, L. T. (2010). Decreased levels of glutathione, the major brain antioxidant, in post-mortem prefrontal cortex from patients with psychiatric disorders. *The International Journal of Neuropsychopharmacology*, *14*(1), 123–130.

Gergerlioglu, H. S., Savas, H. A., Bulbul, F., Selek, S., Uz, E., & Yumru, M. (2007). Changes in nitric oxide level and superoxide dismutase activity during antimanic treatment. *Progress in Neuro-Psychopharmacology & Biological Psychiatry*, *31*(3), 697–702.

Gross, S. S., & Wolin, M. S. (1995). Nitric oxide: Pathophysiological mechanisms. *Annual Review of Physiology*, *57*, 737–769.

Halliwell, B. (1999). Antioxidant defence mechanisms: From the beginning to the end (of the beginning). *Free Radical Research*, *31*(4), 261–272.

Halliwell, B. (2006). Reactive species and antioxidants: Redox biology is a fundamental theme of aerobic life. *Plant Physiology, 141*(2), 312–322.

Halliwell, B. (2011). Free radicals and antioxidants—quo vadis? *Trends in Pharmacological Sciences, 32*(3), 125–130.

Halliwell, B., & Gutteridge, J. M. C. (2007). *Free radical in biology and medicine.* (4th ed.). Oxford: Oxford University Press.

Hastings, T. G., Lewis, D. A., & Zigmond, M. J. (1996). Role of oxidation in the neurotoxic effects of intrastriatal dopamine injections. *Proceedings of the National Academy of Sciences of the United States of America, 93*(5), 1956–1961.

Ischiropoulos, H. (2003). Biological selectivity and functional aspects of protein tyrosine nitration. *Biochemical and Biophysical Research Communications, 305*(3), 776–783.

Iwamoto, K., Bundo, M., & Kato, T. (2005). Altered expression of mitochondria-related genes in postmortem brains of patients with bipolar disorder or schizophrenia, as revealed by large-scale DNA microarray analysis. *Human Molecular Genetics, 14*(2), 241–253.

Ji, Y., & Bennett, B. M. (2003). Activation of microsomal glutathione S-transferase by peroxynitrite. *Molecular Pharmacology, 63*(1), 136–146.

Kapczinski, F., Dal-Pizzol, F., Teixeira, A. L., Magalhaes, P. V., Kauer-Sant'Anna, M., Klamt, F., … Post, R. (2011). Peripheral biomarkers and illness activity in bipolar disorder. *Journal of Psychiatric Research, 45*(2), 156–161.

Kapczinski, F., Dias, V. V., Kauer-Sant'Anna, M., Brietzke, E., Vázquez, G. H., Vieta, E., & Berk, M. (2009). The potential use of biomarkers as an adjunctive tool for staging bipolar disorder. *Progress in Neuro-Psychopharmacology & Biological Psychiatry, 33*(8), 1366–1371.

Kapczinski, F., Frey, B. N., Kauer-Sant'Anna, M., & Grassi-Oliveira, R. (2008). Brain-derived neurotrophic factor and neuroplasticity in bipolar disorder. *Expert Reviews in Neurotherapeutics, 8*(7), 1101–1113.

Kato, T. (2008). Role of mitochondrial DNA in calcium signaling abnormality in bipolar disorder. *Cell Calcium, 44*(1), 92–102.

Kato, T., & Kato, N. (2000). Mitochondrial dysfunction in bipolar disorder. *Bipolar Disorders, 2*(3 Pt. 1), 180–190.

Kauer-Sant'Anna, M., Kapczinski, F., Andreazza, A. C., Bond, D. J., Lam, R. W., Young, L. T., & Yatham, L. N. (2009). Brain-derived neurotrophic factor and inflammatory markers in patients with early- vs. late-stage bipolar disorder. *The International Journal of Neuropsychopharmacology, 12*(4), 447–458.

Khairova, R., Pawar, R., Salvadore, G., Juruena, M. F., de Sousa, R. T., Soeiro-de-Souza, M. G., … Machado-Vieira, R. (2012). Effects of lithium on oxidative stress parameters in healthy subjects. *Molecular Medicine Reports, 5*(3), 680–682.

Kim, Y. K., Jung, H. G., Myint, A. M., Kim, H., & Park, S. H. (2007). Imbalance between pro-inflammatory and anti-inflammatory cytokines in bipolar disorder. *Journal of Affective Disorders, 104*(1–3), 91–95.

Konradi, C., Eaton, M., MacDonald, M. L., Walsh, J., Benes, F. M., & Heckers, S. (2004). Molecular evidence for mitochondrial dysfunction in bipolar disorder. *Archives of General Psychiatry, 61*(3), 300–308.

Konradi, C., Sillivan, S. E., & Clay, H. B. (2012). Mitochondria, oligodendrocytes and inflammation in bipolar disorder: Evidence from transcriptome studies points to intriguing parallels with multiple sclerosis. *Neurobiology of Disease, 45*(1), 37–47.

Kuloglu, M., Ustundag, B., Atmaca, M., Canatan, H., Tezcan, A. E., & Cinkilinc, N. (2002). Lipid peroxidation and antioxidant enzyme levels in patients with schizophrenia and bipolar disorder. *Cell Biochemistry and Function, 20*(2), 171–175.

Lee, C. I., Liu, X., & Zweier, J. (2000). Regulation of xanthine oxidase by nitric oxide and peroxynitrite. *The Journal of Biological Chemistry, 275* (13), 9369–9376.

Lieberman, J. A., Perkins, D. O., & Jarskog, L. F. (2007). Neuroprotection: A therapeutic strategy to prevent deterioration associated with schizophrenia. *CNS Spectrums, 12*(3 Suppl. 4), 1–13.

Luchese, C., & Nogueira, C. W. (2010). Diphenyl diselenide in its selenol form has dehydroascorbate reductase and glutathione S-transferase-like activity dependent on the glutathione content. *Journal of Pharmacy and Pharmacology, 62*(9), 1146–1151.

Macêdo, D. S. Medeiros, C. D., Cordeiro, R. C., Sousa, F. C., Santos, J. V., Morais, T. A., … Carvalho, A. F. (2012). Effects of alpha-lipoic in an animal model of mania induced by D-amphetamine. *Bipolar Disorders, 14*(7), 707–718.

Machado-Vieira, R., Andreazza, A. C., Viale, C. I., Zanatto, V., Cereser, V. Jr., da Silva Vargas, R., … Gentil, V. (2007). Oxidative stress parameters in unmedicated and treated bipolar subjects during initial manic episode: A possible role for lithium antioxidant effects. *Neuroscience Letters, 421*(1), 33–36.

Machado-Vieira, R., Manji, H. K., & Zarate, C. A. Jr. (2009). The role of lithium in the treatment of bipolar disorder: Convergent evidence for neurotrophic effects as a unifying hypothesis. *Bipolar Disorders, 11*(Suppl. 2), 92–109.

Machado-Vieira, R., Soares, J. C., Lara, D. R., Luckenbaugh, D. A., Busnello, J. V., Marca, G., … Kapczinski, F. (2008). A double-blind, randomized, placebo-controlled 4-week study on the efficacy and safety of the purinergic agents allopurinol and dipyridamole adjunctive to lithium in acute bipolar mania. *The Journal of Clinical Psychiatry, 69*(8), 1237–1245.

MacMillan-Crow, L. A., Crow, J. P., & Thompson, J. A. (1998). Peroxynitrite-mediated inactivation of manganese superoxide dismutase involves nitration and oxidation of critical tyrosine residues. *Biochemistry, 37*(6), 1613–1622.

Maes, M., Delange, J., Ranjan, R., Meltzer, H. Y., Desnyder, R., Cooremans, W., & Scharpé, S. (1997). Acute phase proteins in schizophrenia, mania and major depression: Modulation by psychotropic drugs. *Psychiatry Research, 66*(1), 1–11.

Magalhães, P. V., Dean, O. M., Bush, A. I., Copolov, D. L., Malhi, G. S., Kohlmann, K., … Berk, M. (2011). N-acetyl cysteine add-on treatment for bipolar II disorder: A subgroup analysis of a randomized placebo-controlled trial. *Journal of Affective Disorders, 129*(1–3), 317–320.

Maté, J. M., & Sánchez-Jiménez, F. (1999). Antioxidant enzymes and their implications in pathophysiologic processes. *Frontiers in Bioscience: A Journal and Virtual Library, 4*, D339–D345.

Maxwell, S. R. (1995). Prospects for the use of antioxidant therapies. *Drugs, 49*(3), 345–361.

Meotti, F. C., Stangherlin, E. C., Zeni, G., Rocha, J. B. T., & Nogueira, C. W. (2004). Protective role of aryl and alkyl diselenides on lipid peroxidation. *Environmental Research, 94*(3), 276–282.

Michael, N., Erfurth, A., Ohrmann, P., Gössling, M., Arolt, V., Heindel, W., & Pfleiderer, B. (2003). Acute mania is accompanied by elevated glutamate/glutamine levels within the left dorsolateral prefrontal cortex. *Psychopharmacology, 168*(3), 344–346.

Obata, T. (2002). Dopamine efflux by MPTP and hydroxyl radical generation. *Journal of Neural Transmission, 109*(9), 1159–1180.

O'Donovan, M. C., Craddock, N. J., & Owen, M. J. (2009). Genetics of psychosis: Insights from views across the genome. *Human Genetics, 126*(1), 3–12.

Ortiz-Dominguez, A., Hernández, M. E., Berlanga, C., Gutiérrez-Mora, D., Moreno, J., Heinze, G., & Pavón, L. (2007). Immune variations in bipolar disorder: Phasic differences. *Bipolar Disorders, 9*(6), 596–602.

Packer, L., Witt, E. H., & Tritschler, H. J. (1995). Alpha-lipoic acid as a biologic antioxidant. *Free Radical Biology & Medicine, 19*(2), 227–250.

Perova, T., Wasserman, M. J., Li, P. P., & Warsh, J. J. (2008). Hyperactive intracellular calcium dynamics in B lymphoblasts from patients with bipolar I disorder. *The International Journal of Neuropsychopharmacology, 11*(2), 185–196.

Ranjekar, P. K., Hinge, A., Hegde, M. V., Ghate, M., Kale, A., Sitasawad, S., ... Mahadik, S. P. (2003). Decreased antioxidant enzymes and membrane essential polyunsaturated fatty acids in schizophrenic and bipolar mood disorder patients. *Psychiatry Research, 121*(2), 109–122.

Rao, J. S., Harry, G. J., Rapoport, S. I., & Kim, H. W. (2010). Increased excitotoxicity and neuroinflammatory markers in postmortem frontal cortex from bipolar disorder patients. *Molecular Psychiatry, 15*(4), 384–392.

Rees, J. N., Florang, V. R., Anderson, D. G., & Doorn, J. A. (2007). Lipid peroxidation products inhibit dopamine catabolism yielding aberrant levels of a reactive intermediate. *Chemical Research in Toxicology, 20*(10), 1536–1542.

Savas, H. A., Gergerlioglu, H. S., & Armutcu, F. (2006). Elevated serum nitric oxide and superoxide dismutase in euthymic bipolar patients: Impact of past episodes. *The World Journal of Biological Psychiatry, 7*(1), 51–55.

Savas, H. A., Herken, H., Yürekli, M., Uz, E., Tutkun, H., Zoroğlu, S. S., ... Akyol, O. (2002). Possible role of nitric oxide and adrenomedullin in bipolar affective disorder. *Neuropsychobiology, 45*(2), 57–61.

Selek, S., Savas, H. A., Gergerlioglu, H. S., Bulbul, F., Uz, E., & Yumru, M. (2008). The course of nitric oxide and superoxide dismutase during treatment of bipolar depressive episode. *Journal of Affective Disorders, 107*(13), 89–94.

Shao, L., Young, L. T., & Wang, J. F. (2005). Chronic treatment with mood stabilizers lithium and valproate prevents excitotoxicity by inhibiting oxidative stress in rat cerebral cortical cells. *Biological Psychiatry, 58*(11), 879–884.

Smith, C. M., Marks, A. D., & Lieberman, M. A. (2005). *Marks' basic medical biochemistry: A clinical approach* (2nd ed.). Philadelphia: Lippincott Williams & Wilkins.

Sun, X., Wang, J. F., Tseng, M., & Young, L. T. (2006). Downregulation in components of the mitochondrial electron transport chain in the postmortem frontal cortex of subjects with bipolar disorder. *Journal of Psychiatry & Neuroscience, 31*(3), 189–196.

Suzuki, Y. J., Tsuchiya, M., & Packer, L. (1991). Thioctic acid and dihydrolipoic acid are novel antioxidants which interact with reactive oxygen species. *Free Radical Research Communications, 15*(5), 255–263.

Vacher, H., Mohapatra, D. P., & Trimmer, J. S. (2008). Localization and targeting of voltage-dependent ion channels in mammalian central neurons. *Physiological Reviews, 88*(4), 1407–1447.

Wadee, A. A., Kuschke, R. H., Wood, L. A., Berk, M., Ichim, L., & Maes, M. (2002). Serological observations in patients suffering from acute manic episodes. *Human Psychopharmacology, 17*(4), 175–179.

Wang, J. F. (2007). Defects of mitochondrial electron transport chain in bipolar disorder: Implications for mood-stabilizing treatment. *Canadian Journal of Psychiatry, 52*(12), 753–762.

Wang, J. F., Shao, L., Sun, X., & Young, L. T. (2009). Increased oxidative stress in the anterior cingulate cortex of subjects with bipolar disorder and schizophrenia. *Bipolar Disorders, 11*(5), 523–529.

Wendel, A. (1981). Glutathione peroxidase. *Methods in Enzymology, 77*, 325–332.

Xu, C., Li, P. P., Cooke, R. G., Parikh, S. V., Wang, K., Kennedy, J. L., & Warsh, J. J. (2009). TRPM2 variants and bipolar disorder risk: Confirmation in a family-based association study. *Bipolar Disorders, 11*(1), 1–10.

8.

THE ROLE OF SIGNAL TRANSDUCTION SYSTEMS IN THE PATHOPHYSIOLOGY AND TREATMENT OF BIPOLAR DISORDER

Richard S. Jope, Eleonore Beurel, Marta Pardo, Erika Abrial, and Charles B. Nemeroff

INTRODUCTION

Signal transduction systems provide the means for cells to detect changes in the environment and to appropriately respond, which often involves activation of adaptive mechanisms. Abnormalities in these signaling systems can disrupt homeostasis, and in neurons this may lead to maladaptive changes in neural communication mechanisms, disrupting higher processes such as mood and cognition. Assessing the possibility that signal transduction systems may be impaired in bipolar disorder is difficult in the absence of an animal model, leaving imaging approaches and studies of postmortem brain as the major means to directly identify alterations in patients with bipolar disorder. However, these approaches are limited by the structural and functional imaging methods available and the static nature of postmortem measurements. Therefore, many investigators have employed the strategy of examining the effects of lithium and other mood stabilizers on signal transduction systems in cultured cells and in rodents, though this approach suffers to some extent from the lack of a valid animal model of bipolar disorder and the current paucity of methods to confirm in bipolar patients the evidence obtained from such preclinical studies. Nonetheless, this approach has provided a wealth of information about potential abnormal signaling activities that may contribute to bipolar disorder, which are summarized here.

THE PHOSPHOINOSITIDE SIGNAL TRANSDUCTION SYSTEM

The phosphoinositide signal transduction system first became a topic of interest with regard to bipolar disorder with the discovery that lithium inhibits enzymes within this signaling system (reviewed in Agam et al., 2009; Jope & Williams, 1994; O'Brien & Klein, 2009). The central components of the phosphoinositide signal transduction system include a plasma membrane-spanning receptor coupled to a heterotrimeric G-protein of the Gq/11 family. Stimulation of the receptor activates Gq/11, which in turn activates phospholipase C to cleave phosphatidylinositol 4,5-bisphosphate (PIP2). PIP2 cleavage releases two second messengers, diacylglycerol, which activates protein kinase C (PKC), and inositol 1,4,5-trisphosphate (IP3), which stimulates intracellular receptors to induce the release of calcium. IP3 is dephosphorylated by phosphatases, culminating in the action of inositol monophosphatase to produce myo-inositol, which can be reused for the synthesis of PIP2. Lithium inhibits inositol monophosphatase (as well as other phosphatases in this system) with a Ki of 0.8 mM, thus being effective at its therapeutic concentration of 0.5 to 1.2 mM.

The discovery of this inhibitory effect of lithium raised the possibility that lithium may lower the level of free myo-inositol. This may occur because the production of myo-inositol from the sequential dephosphorylation of inositol polyphosphates is reduced by inhibition of inositol monophosphatase, which concomitantly causes the accumulation of inositol monophosphate. This potential block of myo-inositol recycling was hypothesized to consequently deplete PIP2 levels and subsequently decrease the production of IP3 and diacylglycerol upon further stimulation of Gq/11-coupled receptors (Berridge, Downes, & Hanley, 1989). This became known as the inositol depletion hypothesis of the mechanism of action of lithium, which posits that abnormally active phosphoinositide signaling in bipolar disorder is dampened by lithium-induced depletion of myo-inositol and PIP2, thus normalizing this hypothetical hyperactive phosphoinositide signaling.

The inositol depletion hypothesis inspired an intense verification effort in the ensuing decade, which was not entirely successful. We previously reviewed (Jope & Williams, 1994) several early findings that weakened the inositol depletion hypothesis. Although inositol is easily depleted in vitro due to the lack of inositol in the medium of cultured cells or brain slice preparations, in vivo inositol is present in cerebrospinal fluid in millimolar concentrations. This high concentration of inositol made it difficult to detect inositol or PIP2 depletion in vivo after therapeutically relevant lithium administration, thus raising skepticism about the veracity of the inositol depletion hypothesis. This difficulty in verifying depletion of inositol in vivo led to the modification of the hypothesis that perhaps only abnormally active pools of PIP2 may be depleted by lithium, which remains to be established. Further skepticism was raised by discoveries of many other actions of PIP2, such as serving as the precursor for phosphatidylinositol-3,4,5-trisphosphate (PIP3) that is required in many signaling systems, including the signaling response to several neurotrophins and insulin, which would also be expected to be dampened by lithium if PIP2 was depleted. Thus direct studies of the phosphoinositide signaling system have not yet provided clear evidence of whether or not it is abnormally active in bipolar disorder.

Because direct studies with lithium of the inositol depletion hypothesis have been inconclusive, other approaches have been applied to test the inositol depletion theory. Elegant studies with transgenic mice expressing lowered levels of inositol monophosphatase or of an inositol transporter provided mixed results that others have reviewed in detail (Agam et al., 2009; O'Brien & Klein, 2009). Imaging studies designed to detect inositol depletion following lithium administration also have produced mixed results but generally failed to detect inositol depletion (Silverstone & McGrath, 2009; Yildiz-Yesiloglu & Ankerst 2006). Thus the inositol depletion hypothesis remains an attractive explanation for certain actions of lithium, but it has proven difficult to clearly verify or refute. This difficulty may stem from phosphoinositide signaling being hyperactive in discrete circuits in bipolar disorder that are difficult to detect, or it may be that there is sufficient free inositol in the brain to maintain normal levels of PIP2 even if lithium partially inhibits inositol recycling.

PROTEIN KINASE C AND CALCIUM

The potential hyperactivity of phosphoinositide signaling in bipolar disorder raised the possibility that the resultant downstream signaling to induce activation of PKC and release of intracellular calcium may also be elevated in bipolar disorder. PKC refers to a family of serine/threonine kinases that has been subclassified into three families, depending on their structure and specific activators. Conventional PKCs, composed of α, βI, βII, and γ isoforms, need both calcium and diacylglycerol to be activated; novel PKCs (δ, ϵ, η, θ, and μ) require only calcium; and atypical PKCs (ζ and ι/λ) are not activated by calcium or diacylglycerol.

The first evidence of abnormal PKC signaling was obtained in platelets of bipolar patients in the manic state. PKC was found to be hyperactive, and this increase in PKC activity was inhibited by lithium treatment (Friedman, Hoau Yan, Levinson, Connell, & Singh, 1993). PKC hyperactivity was also observed in the frontal cortex of postmortem brains from bipolar subjects (Wang & Friedman, 1996). However, in postmortem studies, it is often difficult to determine the precise mood state of the patient at the time of death and to control the many factors that can alter markers of signaling activity, thus it is currently unknown whether abnormal PKC activation in bipolar disorder is state- or trait-dependent.

Several studies suggest that agents that are therapeutic in bipolar disorder reduce PKC levels and/or activity (Manji & Lenox, 1999). Lithium treatment of cells in vitro or of rodents in vivo decreased the expression of the α and ϵ PKC isoforms and reduced PKC activity, particularly after chronic, rather than subacute, lithium administration (Manji & Lenox, 1999). Examination of the effects of other drugs used therapeutically in bipolar disorder also revealed alterations in PKC. Chronic valproate treatment reduced PKC α and ϵ expression and PKC activity (Manji & Lenox, 1999), and chronic carbamazepine treatment decreased the phosphorylation of PKC substrates in rat brain (Jensen & Mørk, 1997). Investigations on the effects of antidepressants have yielded mixed results, with reports of either increases or decreases in the levels of specific PKC isoforms and PKC activity following chronic treatment with different classes of antidepressants (Szabo et al., 2009). These findings support the possibility that inhibition of PKC activity may be connected with therapeutic effects of drugs used in bipolar disorder.

Behavioral studies have sought to determine if direct blockade of PKC activity may reduce manic-like or depression-like behaviors in rodents. Administration of the PKC inhibitors tamoxifen and chelerythrine attenuated amphetamine-induced locomotor hyperactivity, a widely used model of mania (Abrial et al, 2013; Einat, Yuan, Szabo, Dogra, & Manji, 2007). However, neither of these is adequately specific for PKC to conclude that their actions derive from PKC inhibition; tamoxifen is an estrogen receptor modulator in addition to being a PKC inhibitor, and the potency and specificity of chelerythrine as a selective PKC inhibitor are not well established (Davies, Reddy, Caivano, & Cohen, 2000). PKC inhibitors also have been reported to reduce risk-taking behaviors (Abrial et al., 2013) and hedonic behaviors in response to drugs of abuse (Lai et al., 2008), two distinct facets of mania. Both the amphetamine and sleep deprivation models of manic-like activity increase the phosphorylation of PKC substrates in rat frontal cortex (Szabo et al., 2009). Elsewhere in this volume clinical trials of tamoxifen in bipolar disorder patients that indicate an effective antimanic effect are reviewed. Overall, preclinical data support the hypothesis that PKC may be overactivated in states relevant to mania and that PKC inhibition may produce antimanic-like effects.

In contrast to the evidence that activated PKC is associated with manic-like states, reduced PKC activity, level, or substrate phosphorylation has been consistently found in animal models of depression, such as the chronic mild stress model (Palumbo, Zorrilla Zubilete, Cremaschi, & Genaro, 2009). Furthermore, acute administration of PKC activators produces antidepressant-like effects in rodents (Abrial et al., 2013). Thus the opposite changes in PKC activation in depression and mania might favor an interpretation of state-dependent changes in PKC in bipolar disorder and that PKC inhibitors may be effective in mania but not depression.

Dysregulation of intracellular calcium homeostasis has often been linked to the pathogenesis of bipolar disorder (Bhat et al., 2012; Warsh, Andreopoulos, & Li, 2004). Intracellular calcium is a highly versatile signal, and calcium homeostasis is regulated in a complex manner by a balance between extracellular entry, uptake, and release from internal stores, including endoplasmic/sarcoplasmic reticulum and mitochondria, and binding to calcium-buffering proteins. Increased free calcium in manic patients compared to healthy controls was first reported in platelets (Dubovsky et al., 1989). Since then, there have been consistent findings of elevations in basal and agonist-induced intracellular calcium levels in peripheral blood components of untreated bipolar subjects in either manic or depressive states (Quiroz, Gray, Kato, & Manji, 2008). Moreover, increased agonist-evoked calcium in platelets from untreated bipolar depressed patients is normalized to the control range in lithium-treated euthymic patients (Dubovsky, Lee, Christiano, & Murphy, 1991). Several mechanisms have been suggested to explain how lithium dampens intracellular calcium mobilization, including inhibition of upstream effectors (such as phosphoinositide signaling or cyclic AMP production), regulation of calcium-handling proteins, or modulation of calcium sequestration into mitochondrial or endoplasmic reticulum stores, notably through up-regulation of the intracellular calcium regulator B-cell lymphoma protein 2 (Andreazza & Young, 2014; Distelhorst & Bootman, 2011; ePinton et al., 2000; Warsh et al., 2004).

Because of the possible link of increased intracellular calcium to bipolar disorder, L-type calcium channel (LTCC) antagonists have been investigated for many years as a potential treatment for bipolar disorder. LTCC antagonists, as a class, act primarily by directly binding to various sites on Cav1.2 LTCC, resulting in blockade of the calcium current. Cav1.2 LTCC antagonists, especially dihydropyridine derivatives, have been shown to reduce depression-like behaviors in a variety of rodent models (Bhat et al., 2012). Moreover, CACNA1C heterozygous knockout mice, the gene that codes for the α1C subunit of the Cav1.2 LTCC, display decreased immobility in behavioral despair tests and diminished locomotor response to amphetamine sensitization, indicating that reduced Cav1.2 LTCC expression leads to both antidepressant-like and antimanic-like effects (Bhat et al., 2012). Verapamil has been the most frequently used LTCC blocker in clinical trials, but despite some isolated reports of efficacy, randomized control trials have not demonstrated efficacy of verapamil or other calcium antagonists (Janicak et al., 1998). However, further studies may be warranted because single nucleotide polymorphisms in CACNA1C have consistently been found to be associated with bipolar disorder (Craddock & Sklar, 2013). CACNA1C single nucleotide polymorphisms have also been found to be associated with schizophrenia, major depression, and autism spectrum disorders, suggesting that CACNA1C belongs to a class of shared susceptibility factors. Besides LTCCs, there is also growing interest in a number of other calcium-regulating proteins, such as calcium-permeable transient receptor potential melastatin subtype 2, canonical subtype 3 channels, and mechanisms releasing calcium from intracellular stores in the pathogenesis of bipolar disorder. Overall, dysregulation of calcium dynamics in bipolar disorder is supported by multiple lines of research, suggesting that the development of calcium-targeted interventions merits further investigation.

GLYCOGEN SYNTHASE KINASE-3

Soon after enthusiasm for the inositol depletion hypothesis was waning due to lack of definitive supporting evidence, it was discovered that lithium is a direct inhibitor of glycogen synthase kinase-3 (GSK3; Klein & Melton, 1996; Stambolic, Ruel, & Woodgett, 1996). Although GSK3 was initially named because it was discovered as a kinase that phosphorylates the enzyme glycogen synthase, it is now known to phosphorylate nearly 100 substrates and to regulate many cellular processes, as previously reviewed (Jope & Johnson, 2004; Woodgett, 2001). Thus this discovery raised the concept that lithium's mood-stabilizing actions may arise from inhibiting any of the many cellular actions of GSK3.

GSK3 refers to two paralogs that are commonly referred to as isoforms: GSK3α and GSK3β. GSK3 is predominantly regulated by inhibitory phosphorylation on serine21-GSK3α or serine9-GSK3β, which can be mediated by several kinases, such as Akt. To identify the importance of inhibitory serine-phosphorylation of GSK3, investigators have used GSK3 knockin mice in which the two serines were mutated to alanines to abrogate inhibitory serine phosphorylation of GSK3 (McManus et al., 2005). Besides inhibitory serine-phosphorylation, GSK3 also can be regulated by protein binding partners, which most notably occurs in the Wnt signaling pathway. In this pathway, GSK3 bound to the scaffold protein axin phosphorylates β-catenin, which directs β-catenin to proteasomal degradation. Activation of Wnt signaling disrupts the ability of GSK3 to phosphorylate β-catenin, which allows β-catenin stabilization, accumulation, and transport into the nucleus where it regulates gene expression. Thus direct inhibitors of GSK3, such as lithium, cause increased levels and activation of β-catenin.

Lithium directly inhibits GSK3 with an IC50 of 2 mM, indicating that at therapeutic concentrations lithium is a relatively weak direct inhibitor. However, not only does lithium inhibit GSK3 by directly binding to the enzyme but it also increases the inhibitory serine-phosphorylation of GSK3, which apparently provides a mechanism that amplifies the modest inhibition of 1 mM lithium caused by direct binding (Jope, 2003). The discovery that therapeutically relevant levels of lithium inhibit GSK3 raised the possibility that abnormally active GSK3 contributes to bipolar disorder. However, it is important to consider that abnormalities in GSK3 itself may not be causative in bipolar disorder but that lithium's inhibition of GSK3 may normalize abnormal signaling activities upstream of GSK3 or abnormal actions of substrates of GSK3 that are corrected by lithium-mediated inhibition of GSK3.

As with other signaling factors that may contribute to bipolar disorder, testing the hypothesis that inhibition of GSK3 provides mood stabilization is hampered by the lack of an animal model of bipolar disorder, by the absence of imaging techniques able to detect GSK3-mediated signaling in vivo, and by the inability to detect dynamic signaling activities by measurements using postmortem tissue. Thus this issue has been addressed predominantly by pharmacological and molecular methods in rodent models applied to behaviors that may model depression or manic characteristics. However, it is well recognized that these are merely behavioral assessments, falling short of true models of depression or mania.

Behavioral studies in rodents have provided a wealth of support for the hypothesis that inhibition of GSK3 may bolster mood stabilization, as recently reviewed (Jope, 2011). Depression-like behaviors of rodents are consistently diminished by administration of a variety of GSK3 inhibitors and in mice with reduced expression of GSK3 (O'Brien et al., 2004; O'Brien et al., 2011; Omata et al., 2011; and see references in Beaulieu, Gainetdinov, & Caron, 2009; Jope, 2011). Neuronal overexpression of GSK3 counteracted the behavioral effects of lithium in mice, emphatically verifying that GSK3 is lithium's target for these outcomes (O'Brien et al., 2011). Administration of antidepressants and atypical antipsychotics, which are effective in some bipolar disorder patients, also induce inhibition of GSK3 in rodent brains (Beaulieu et al., 2009; Li et al., 2004; Li, Rosborough, Friedman, Zhu, & Roth, 2007). Inhibition of GSK3 is also evident in mouse brain after administration of ketamine, which is rapidly effective in bipolar depressed patients, and in rodents the inhibition of GSK3 is required for ketamine's antidepressant effect (Beurel, Song, & Jope, 2011). Thus inhibition of GSK3 is induced in rodent brain by drugs that are therapeutic in bipolar disorder, and inhibition of GSK3 consistently alleviates depression-like behaviors in rodents.

Conversely, there is evidence that activation of GSK3 may increase susceptibility to depression. Serotonin and brain-derived neurotrophic factor (BDNF) normally activate signaling pathways that inhibit GSK3, indicating that their postulated deficiencies in patients with mood disorders may contribute to hyperactive GSK3 (Beaulieu et al., 2009; Li et al., 2004; Mai, Jope, & Li, 2002; Sachs et al., 2013). In accordance with this possibility, increased susceptibility to depression-like and manic-like behaviors is exhibited by GSK3 knockin mice that express GSK3 with elevated activity (Polter et al., 2010). Furthermore, mutations in the DISC1 protein that occur in patients with bipolar disorder and other psychiatric diseases reduce its normal inhibition of GSK3 (Mao et al., 2009). Thus studies in rodents have provided substantial evidence that GSK3 promotes depression-like behaviors and therapeutic drugs inhibit GSK3.

The manic phase of bipolar disorder is even more difficult than depression to model in mice. The most widely used model of manic-like behavior is the locomotor hyperactivity induced by amphetamine administration to rodents. Amphetamine administration activates GSK3 in rodent striatum and inhibition or reduced expression of GSK3 attenuates locomotor hyperactivity induced by amphetamine (Beaulieu et al., 2009). Conversely, GSK3 knockin mice with increased GSK3 activity exhibit exaggerated locomotor hyperactivity in response to amphetamine (Polter et al., 2010). Thus within the constraints of this model, there is strong evidence that GSK3 is centrally involved in this manic-like activity.

Human studies of the involvement of GSK3 in bipolar disorder remain meager, limited by the methodologies available. In peripheral blood mononuclear cells, decreased inhibitory serine-phosphorylation of GSK3 was associated with mood disorders and was increased by lithium treatment, verifying that in vivo therapeutic concentrations of lithium inhibit GSK3 in human subjects (Li et al., 2007; Polter et al., 2010). Genetic associations between GSK3 and mood disorders have also been identified (see references in Jope, 2011) but require further tests to determine whether they contribute to bipolar disorder. It is difficult to capture reflections of the state of a signaling system in studies of postmortem brain because of the many antemortem and postmortem factors that can influence dynamic signaling activities. Nonetheless, several studies have reported alterations in the phosphorylation state of GSK3 in postmortem brain regions from patients with mood disorders that are in accordance with the findings in rodents (Karege et al., 2012; Ren, Rizavi, Khan, Dwivedi, & Pandey, 2013).

The concatenation of findings indicates that altered signaling through GSK3 contributes to susceptibility to bipolar disorder. Particularly strong is the evidence that diverse therapeutic drugs effective in bipolar disorder cause inhibition of GSK3. Thus GSK3 is currently a prime candidate signaling molecule that may be abnormally regulated in bipolar disorder.

NEUROTROPHINS AND NEUROGENESIS

Signaling pathways that induce the expression of neurotrophins, such as BDNF, may be impaired in bipolar disorder, leading to neurotrophin deficiencies (Pittenger & Duman, 2008). These neurotrophin deficiencies could affect multiple processes, such as neurogenesis, among others. Furthermore, increasing neurotrophin levels may be an important effect of drugs that are therapeutic in mood disorders.

Neurotrophin deficiencies have been linked to both depression and bipolar disorder. Regarding depression, neurotrophins have often been found to be deficient in animal models of depression and in the serum of patients with depression (Autry & Monteggia, 2012; Duman & Li, 2012). Serum BDNF levels have been reported to be reduced in patients with bipolar disorder and are reduced in rodents by stress or glucocorticoids, both associated with increased susceptibility to mood disorders. Conversely, BDNF levels are elevated in rodents by administration of mood stabilizers. A potential causative function of BDNF deficiency in rodents was established by the demonstration that infusion of BDNF into the hippocampus attenuated depression-like behaviors in rodents (Duric & Duman, 2013). The transcription factor cyclic AMP response element-binding protein (CREB) plays important roles in signaling both upstream and downstream of BDNF. Impairments in pathways activating CREB, such as the production of the second messenger cyclic AMP, have long been implicated in mood disorders, which may contribute to deficiencies in BDNF production. Following its synthesis and release, BDNF activates intracellular signaling by stimulating the plasma membrane TrkB receptor. This action of BDNF affects multiple intracellular signaling molecules, including activation of CREB and inhibition of GSK3, suggesting that BDNF deficiency in mood disorders may contribute to impaired CREB activity and excessive GSK3 activity. There is also increasing evidence that a single nucleotide polymorphism in the BDNF gene, the val66met substitution, affects its signaling activity. Although BDNF has received the greatest attention among the neurotrophins implicated in bipolar disorder, there is also compelling evidence for deficiencies of several others (Duric & Duman, 2013). Thus bipolar disorder may involve impaired signaling systems that are required for sufficient production of a variety of neurotrophins, which in turn control multiple signaling processes that appear to contribute to mood regulation.

One action of BDNF and other neurotrophins is to regulate neurogenesis, the proliferation, migration, and differentiation of neural precursor cells, which occurs in the subventricular zone of the lateral ventricle and the subgranular zone in the hippocampal dentate gyrus in adult mammalian brain. There is much interest in the possibility that hippocampal neurogenesis may be impaired in patients with mood disorders and that increasing neurogenesis is an important component of the therapeutic response to mood stabilizers and antidepressants. However, these links are controversial and remain to be convincingly established or refuted (Hanson, Owens, & Nemeroff, 2011; Samuels & Hen, 2011). The signaling processes that regulate neurogenesis are incompletely understood. Perhaps the best established signaling molecules that regulate neurogenesis are neurotrophins, such as BDNF and vascular endothelial growth factor, which promote neurogenesis (Autry & Monteggia, 2012; Fournier & Duman, 2012). Thus evidence of deficiencies in neurotrophins in patients with mood disorders raises the possibility that such deficiencies may contribute to impaired neurogenesis. Although it remains to be conclusively established whether neurogenesis is impaired in mood disorders, substantial evidence has shown that hippocampal neurogenesis in adult rodents is increased by mood stabilizers and antidepressants, actions that may be mediated by these drugs causing up-regulation of neurotrophins (Chiu, Wang, Hunsberger, & Chuang, 2013; Duric & Duman, 2013; Eisch & Petrik, 2012). In contrast, stressors that can increase susceptibility to depression are known to impair hippocampal neurogenesis (McEwen, 2008). In accordance with evidence that abnormally active GSK3 increases susceptibility to mood disorders, it also impairs neurogenesis (Eom & Jope, 2009). Thus neurotrophins and other signaling molecules that regulate hippocampal neurogenesis may be impaired in patients with bipolar disorder, and neurogenesis may be bolstered by therapeutic drugs, but definitive evidence for these relationships is forthcoming.

INFLAMMATORY AND IMMUNE SIGNALING

Signaling molecules that have traditionally been classified as components of the immune system, particularly inflammatory cytokines, also may be involved in the pathophysiology of bipolar disorder. In addition to being activated by invading pathogens, the inflammatory system responds to "danger" signals (Akira, 2006). The inflammatory molecules produced in response to danger signals appear to be initially involved in the restoration of homeostasis, but severe and/or prolonged cytokine production is often injurious. Inflammatory molecules can be produced by microglia, astrocytes, and even neurons. However, microglia have traditionally been considered to be the major "immune" cells of the brain, acting as sentinels surveying the environment for danger signals that induce an inflammatory response. Microglia are capable of rapidly migrating to accumulate at sites of damage, and both microglia and astrocytes take on characteristic morphological changes when inflammatory systems are activated. The mechanisms

underlying the inflammatory signaling response to danger signals is best understood for pathways utilizing the classical inflammatory receptor, Toll-like receptor 4 (TLR4). First discovered as Toll receptors in *Drosophila*, in mammals TLRs are expressed by microglia, astrocytes, and neurons, as well as by immune cells. Besides being activated by pathogens, TLR4 is also activated by insult-induced endogenous ligands called danger- or damage-associated molecular patterns. These include a wide range of ligands such as high-mobility group box-1 protein, hyaluronan oligosaccharides, heat shock proteins, and others (Akira, 2006). These stress-induced ligands stimulate TLR4 to activate intracellular signaling cascades, including activation of the inflammatory transcription factor NF-κB, to increase the production of a large number of proinflammatory cytokines. It is thought that this pathway underlies the large inflammatory response elicited by psychological stressors that do not involve infections, which may have evolved as a mechanism for surviving infections following injury (Raison & Miller, 2013). Furthermore, activation of NF-κB is necessary for the prodepressive effects of stress (Koo, Russo, Ferguson, Nestler, & Duman, 2010). A remarkable report recently firmly established that a history of autoimmune disease and hospitalization for infection, presumably due to inflammatory activation, are strong risk factors for mood disorders (Benros et al., 2013). Thus immune system activation either by stress or pathogens may increase susceptibility to mood disorders.

Inflammatory signaling molecules are now recognized as having profound influences on many functions in the brain, particularly mood and cognition. Many preclinical and clinical studies have identified links between inflammation and depression, but fewer have specifically examined links between bipolar disorder and inflammation. Several extensive reviews have detailed substantial evidence that activation of the inflammatory response can promote depression in humans and that patients with major depression or bipolar disorder often exhibit markers of inflammatory activation (Dantzer, O'Connor, Freund, Johnson, & Kelley, 2008; Goldstein, Kemp, Soczynska, & McIntyre, 2009; Miller, Maletic, & Raison, 2009; Schiepers, Wichers, & Maes, 2005). For example, measurements of the expression of inflammatory molecules in monocytes from bipolar disorder patients and family members led to the proposal of an inflammatory gene signature as a biomarker (Padmos et al., 2008). Multiple markers of inflammatory activation have also been detected in the postmortem frontal cortex of bipolar disorder patients compared with control subjects (Rao, Harry, Rapoport, & Kim, 2010). A recent meta-analysis found consistent elevations of several inflammatory molecules in 18 studies of bipolar disorder patients (Munkholm, Braüner, Kessing, & Vinberg, 2013). This analysis suggested a macrophage-T cell theory of bipolar disorder, in which bipolar patients display increases in both macrophage-derived cytokines (tumor necrosis factor [TNFα] and soluble interleukin-6 receptor [sIL-6R]) and T cell-derived cytokines (sIL-2R, IL-4) compared to healthy control patients (Munkholm et al., 2013). In addition to inflammatory cytokines, there is also evidence of activation of the inflammatory arachidonic acid signaling cascade in bipolar disorder. Phospholipids in the brain contain a relatively high concentration of the polyunsaturated fatty acid arachidonic acid, which is released when cleaved from phospholipids by phospholipase A2 after it is activated by signaling induced by a wide variety of neurotransmitter receptors. Compared with control subjects, postmortem frontal cortex from bipolar disorder patients exhibited increased expression levels of several enzymes involved in arachidonic acid signaling, including arachidonate-selective cytoplasmic phospholipase A2 (Kim, Rapoport, & Rao, 2011). Notably, mood stabilizers such as lithium reduce markers of arachidonic acid signaling in rodent brain (Rao & Rapoport, 2009). Thus there are certainly increases in inflammatory signaling in bipolar disorder, but it remains to be determined if these are trait- or state-dependent increases and which inflammatory molecules may specifically influence mood regulation.

Testing the hypothesis that inflammatory signaling contributes to bipolar disorder is difficult in patients, but this possibility is supported by studies in rodents. There are no well-validated models of bipolar disorder in rodents, but comprehensive reviews have covered in detail the findings in rodents that depression-like behaviors are often increased by activation of inflammation and by specific inflammatory cytokines (Dantzer et al., 2008; Miller et al., 2009; Schiepers et al., 2005). Conversely, the mood stabilizer lithium effectively produces anti-inflammatory responses in rodents by reducing the production of inflammatory molecules and increasing the production of the anti-inflammatory cytokine IL-10 (Martin, Rehani, Jope, & Michalek, 2005). One would expect to find relationships between different signaling systems that have been implicated in mood disorders, and this is certainly the case with inflammation and GSK3, as GSK3 is profoundly involved in promoting inflammatory responses (Beurel, 2011). GSK3 promotes inflammatory responses by human peripheral immune cells, such as TLR4-mediated production of IL-6, IL-1β, and TNFα (Martin et al., 2005). GSK3 also promotes inflammatory responses of microglia and astrocytes (Beurel & Jope, 2009; Yuskaitis & Jope, 2009).

GSK3 promotes these inflammatory responses in part by contributing to the activation of the key inflammatory transcription factors NF-κB and STAT3 (Beurel & Jope, 2008; Martin et al., 2005). Remarkably, GSK3 inhibits the production of the anti-inflammatory cytokine IL-10 by inhibiting the transcription factor CREB (Martin et al., 2005). Thus one mechanism by which activation of GSK3 may contribute to mood disorder susceptibility is by promotion of inflammatory responses, and GSK3 inhibitors, such as lithium, shift the balance of the inflammatory response from proinflammatory to anti-inflammatory.

The finding that history of an autoimmune disease is a risk factor for mood disorders (Benros et al., 2013) raises the possibility that other components of the immune system in addition to inflammation may contribute to mood disorders. There is some evidence that characteristics of T cells are altered in patients with mood disorders and that mood-relevant behaviors in rodents are influenced by T cells. The Th17 subtype of T cells is particularly implicated in autoimmune diseases, thus it is intriguing that Th17 cells were demonstrated to induce depression-like responses in mice (Beurel, Harrington, & Jope, 2013). This is again linked to GSK3, as GSK3 promotes and lithium blocks the production of the Th17 subtype of T cells (Beurel, Wen-I, Michalek, Harrington, & Jope, 2011). Although these studies are only in their infancy, it appears likely that further signaling activities in the immune system will be found to influence bipolar disorder.

OTHER SIGNALING PATHWAYS

Many additional important signaling pathways have been implicated in bipolar disorder that are too numerous to cover in sufficient detail within the space limitations of this chapter. For example, postmortem studies in tissue from subjects with major depression revealed a large increase in mitogen-activated protein kinase (MAPK) phosphatase-1, a key inhibitory regulator of the MAPK signaling cascade (Duric et al., 2010). This may contribute to earlier observations indicating impaired MAPK signaling in mood disorders (Tanis & Duman, 2007). In addition, previous comprehensive reviews have detailed potential changes in the cyclic AMP signaling system associated with mood disorders (Andreazza & Young, 2014; Tanis & Duman, 2007) and signaling that regulates epigenetic modifications linked to mood disorders (Peter & Akbarian, 2011; Sun, Kennedy, & Nestler, 2013). Additionally, other chapters in this volume focus on signaling pathways involving oxidative stress, neuroprotection and neurodegeneration, circadian rhythms, the hypothalamic-pituitary-adrenal axis, and genetic studies that implicate signaling molecules that may be associated with bipolar disorder.

CONCLUSION

Substantial evidence, although largely indirect, indicates that intracellular signaling pathways are perturbed in bipolar disorder. Discerning which of these is a primary disturbance linked to disease susceptibility and which are secondary events remains to be resolved. Although identifying the targets of mood stabilizers may provide some guidance toward clarifying primary events, their therapeutic actions may just as well be secondary outcomes of modifications of their primary targets. For example, inhibition of GSK3 by lithium and inhibition of histone deacetylases by sodium valproate can easily be envisioned as causing common changes due to altered actions of GSK3 and of modified gene expression. Thus the tremendous effort exerted toward finding a common target of multiple mood stabilizers may be better applied to determine common secondary outcomes that contribute to mood stabilization. Clarification of signaling systems that play a primary role in bipolar disorder would benefit tremendously from the identification of biomarkers that are capable of distinguishing subtypes of the disease, such as may develop from studies of the contributions of inflammation to certain populations of patients with bipolar disorder. A great deal has been learned about how perturbations of signaling pathways can affect mood, but further progress is critical in order to develop improved mood stabilizers that can alleviate the disabling symptoms of bipolar disorder.

ACKNOWLEDGEMENTS

The authors apologize to the many investigators whose work could not be cited due to the limited number of references permitted. Research in the authors' laboratories were supported by National Institutes of Health grants MH038752, MH090236, and MH095380.

Disclosure statement: Richard S. Jope, Eleonore Beurel, Marta Pardo, and Erika Abrial report no financial interests or potential conflicts of interest.

Charles B. Nemeroff reports the following:

Research/Grants:

National Institutes of Health

Speakers Bureau: None

Consulting:

Xhale, Takeda, SK Pharma, Shire, Roche, Lilly, Allergan, Mitsubishi Tanabe Pharma

Development America, Taisho Pharmaceutical Inc., Lundbeck

Stockholder:

CeNeRx BioPharma, PharmaNeuroBoost, Revaax Pharma, Xhale

Other Financial Interests:

CeNeRx BioPharma, PharmaNeuroBoost

Patents:

Method and devices for transdermal delivery of lithium (US 6,375,990B1)

Method of assessing antidepressant drug therapy via transport inhibition of monoamine neurotransmitters by ex vivo assay (US 7,148,027B2)

Scientific Advisory Boards:

American Foundation for Suicide Prevention, CeNeRx BioPharma (2012), National Alliance for Research on Schizophrenia and Depression, Xhale, PharmaNeuroBoost (2012), Anxiety Disorders Association of America, Skyland Trail

Board of Directors:

American Foundation for Suicide Prevention, NovaDel (2011), Skyland Trail, Gratitude America, Anxiety Disorders Association of America

Income sources or equity of $10,000 or more:

PharmaNeuroBoost, CeNeRx BioPharma, NovaDel Pharma, Reevax Pharma, American

Psychiatric Publishing, Xhale

Honoraria:

Various

Royalties:

Various

Expert Witness:

Various

REFERENCES

Abrial, E., Etiévant, A., Bétry, C., Scarna, H., Lucas, G., Haddjeri, N., & Lambás-Señas, L. (2013). Protein kinase C regulates mood-related behaviors and adult hippocampal cell proliferation in rats. *Progress in Neuro-Psychopharmacology & Biological Psychiatry, 43*, 40–48.

Agam, G., Bersudsky, Y., Berry, G. T., Moechars, D., Lavi-Avnon, Y., & Belmaker, R. H. (2009). Knockout mice in understanding the mechanism of action of lithium. *Biochemical Society Transactions, 37*, 1121–1125.

Akira, S. (2006). TLR signaling. *Current Topics in Microbiology and Immunology, 311*, 1–16.

Andreazza A. C., & Young L. T. (2014). The neurobiology of bipolar disorder: Identifying targets for specific agents and synergies for combination treatment. *International Journal of Neuropsychopharmacology, 7*(7), 1039–1052.

Autry, A. E., & Monteggia, L. M. (2012). Brain-derived neurotrophic factor and neuropsychiatric disorders. *Pharmacological Reviews, 64*, 238–258.

Beaulieu, J. M., Gainetdinov, R. R., & Caron, M. G. (2009). Akt/GSK3 signaling in the action of psychotropic drugs. *Annual Review of Pharmacology and Toxicology, 49*, 327–347.

Benros, M. E., Waltoft, B. L., Nordentoft, M., Ostergaard S. D., Eaton W. W., Krogh J., & Mortensen P. B. (2013). Autoimmune diseases and severe infections as risk factors for mood disorders: A nationwide study. *JAMA Psychiatry, 70*, 812–820.

Berridge, M. J., Downes, C. P., & Hanley, M. R. (1989). Neural and developmental actions of lithium: A unifying hypothesis. *Cell, 59*, 411–419, 1989.

Beurel, E. (2011). Regulation by glycogen synthase kinase-3 of inflammation and T cells in the CNS. *Frontiers in Molecular Neuroscience, 4*, 18.

Beurel, E., Harrington, L. E., & Jope, R. S. (2013). Inflammatory Th17 cells promote depression-like behavior in mice. *Biological Psychiatry, 73*, 622–630.

Beurel, E., & Jope, R. S. (2008). Differential regulation of STAT family members by glycogen synthase kinase-3. *The Journal of Biological Chemistry, 283*, 21934–21944.

Beurel, E., & Jope, R. S. (2009). Lipopolysaccharide-induced interleukin-6 production is controlled by glycogen synthase kinase-3 and STAT3 in the brain. *Journal of Neuroinflammation, 6*, 9.

Beurel, E., Song, L., & Jope, R. S. (2011). Inhibition of glycogen synthase kinase-3 is necessary for the rapid antidepressant effect of ketamine in mice. *Molecular Psychiatry, 16*, 1068–1070.

Beurel, E., Wen-I, Y., Michalek, S. M., Harrington, L. E., & Jope R. S. (2011). Glycogen synthase kinase-3 is an early determinant in the differentiation of pathogenic Th17 cells. *Journal of Immunology, 186*, 1391–1398.

Bhat, S., Dao, D. T., Terrillion, C. E., Arad M., Smith R. J., Soldatov N. M., & Gould T. D. (2012). CACNA1C (Cav1.2) in the pathophysiology of psychiatric disease. *Progress in Neurobiology, 99*, 1–14.

Chiu, C., Wang, Z., Hunsberger, J. G., & Chuang D. (2013). Therapeutic potential of mood stabilizers lithium and valproic acid: Beyond bipolar disorder. *Pharmacological Reviews, 65*, 105–142.

Craddock, N., & Sklar, P. (2013). Genetics of bipolar disorder. *Lancet, 381*, 1654–1662.

Dantzer, R., O'Connor, J. C., Freund, G. G., Johnson, R. W., & Kelley, K. W. (2008). From inflammation to sickness and depression: When the immune system subjugates the brain. *Nature Reviews Neuroscience, 9*, 46–56.

Davies, S. P., Reddy, H., Caivano, M., & Cohen, P. (2000). Specificity and mechanism of action of some commonly used protein kinase inhibitors. *Biochemical Journal, 351*, 95–105.

Distelhorst, C. W., & Bootman, M. D. (2011). Bcl-2 interaction with the inositol 1, 4, 5-trisphosphate receptor: Role in Ca(2+) signaling and disease. *Cell Calcium, 50*, 234–241.

Dubovsky, S. L., Christiano, J., Daniell, L. C., Franks, R. D., Murphy, J., Adler, L., Baker, N., & Harris, R. A. (1989). Increased platelet intracellular calcium concentration in patients with bipolar affective disorders. *Archives in General Psychiatry, 46*, 632–638.

Dubovsky, S. L., Lee, C., Christiano, J., & Murphy, J. (1991) Elevated platelet intracellular calcium concentration in bipolar depression. *Biological Psychiatry, 29*, 441–450.

Duman, R. S., & Li, N. (2012). A neurotrophic hypothesis of depression: role of synaptogenesis in the actions of NMDA receptor antagonists. *Philosophical Transactions of the Royal Society of London B: Biological Sciences, 367*, 2475–2484.

Duric, V., Banasr, M., Licznerski, P., Schmidt, H. D., Stockmeier, C. A., Simen, A. A., Newton, S. S., & Duman, R. S. (2010). A negative regulator of MAP kinase causes depressive behavior. *Nature Medicine, 16*, 1328–1332.

Duric, V., & Duman, R. S. (2013). Depression and treatment response: Dynamic interplay of signaling pathways and altered neural processes. *Cellular and Molecular Life Sciences, 70*, 39–53.

Einat, H., Yuan, P., Szabo, S. T., Dogra, S., & Manji, H. K. (2007). Protein kinase C inhibition by tamoxifen antagonizes manic-like behavior in rats: Implications for the development of novel therapeutics for bipolar disorder. *Neuropsychobiology, 55*, 123–131.

Eisch, A. J., & Petrik, D. (2012). Depression and hippocampal neurogenesis: A road to remission? *Science, 338*, 72–75.

Eom, T. Y., & Jope, R. S. (2009). Blocked inhibitory serine-phosphorylation of glycogen synthase kinase-3alpha/beta impairs in vivo neural precursor cell proliferation. *Biological Psychiatry, 66*, 494–502.

Fournier, N. M., & Duman, R. S. (2012). Role of vascular endothelial growth factor in adult hippocampal neurogenesis: Implications for the pathophysiology and treatment of depression. *Behavioural Brain Research, 227*, 440–449.

Friedman, E., Hoau Yan, W., Levinson, D., Connell, T. A., & Singh, H. (1993). Altered platelet protein kinase C activity in bipolar affective disorder, manic episode. *Biological Psychiatry, 33*, 520–525.

Goldstein, B. I., Kemp, D. E., Soczynska, J. K., & McIntyre, R. S. (2009). Inflammation and the phenomenology, pathophysiology, comorbidity, and treatment of bipolar disorder: A systematic review of the literature. *Journal of Clinical Psychiatry, 70*, 1078–1090.

Hanson, N. D., Owens, M. J., & Nemeroff, C. B. (2011). Depression, antidepressants, and neurogenesis: A critical reappraisal. *Neuropsychopharmacology, 36*, 2589–2602.

Janicak, P. G., Sharma, R. P., Pandey, G., & Davis, J. M. (1998). Verapamil for the treatment of acute mania: A double-blind, placebo-controlled trial. *American Journal of Psychiatry, 155*, 972–973.

Jensen, J. B., & Mørk, A. (1997). Altered protein phosphorylation in the rat brain following chronic lithium and carbamazepine treatments. *European Neuropsychopharmacology, 7*, 173–179.

Jope, R. S. (2003). Lithium & GSK3: One inhibitor, two inhibitory actions, multiple outcomes. *Trends in Pharmacological Science, 24*, 441–443.

Jope, R. S. (2011). Glycogen synthase kinase-3 in the etiology and treatment of mood disorders. *Frontiers in Molecular Neuroscience, 4*, 16–26.

Jope, R. S., & Johnson, G. V. W. (2004). The glamour and gloom of glycogen synthase kinase-3 (GSK3). *Trends in Biochemical Science, 29*, 95–102.

Jope, R. S., & Williams M. B. (1994). Lithium and brain signal transduction systems. *Biochemical Pharmacology, 47*, 429–441.

Karege, F., Perroud, N., Burkhardt, S., Fernandez, R., Ballmann, E., La Harpe, R., & Malafosse, A. (2012). Protein levels of β-catenin and activation state of glycogen synthase kinase-3β in major depression: A study with postmortem prefrontal cortex. *Journal of Affective Disorders, 136*, 185–188.

Kim, H. W., Rapoport, S. I., & Rao, J. S. (2011). Altered arachidonic acid cascade enzymes in postmortem brain from bipolar disorder patients. *Molecular Psychiatry. 16*, 419–428.

Klein, P. S., & Melton, D. A. (1996). A molecular mechanism for the effect of lithium on development. *Proceedings of the National Academy of Sciences of the United States of America, 93,* 8455–8459.

Koo, J. W., Russo, S. J., Ferguson, D., Nestler, E. J., & Duman, R. S. (2010). Nuclear factor-kappaB is a critical mediator of stress-impaired neurogenesis and depressive behavior. *Proceedings of the National Academy of Sciences of the United States of America, 107,* 2669–2674.

Lai, Y-T., Fan, H-Y., Cherng, C. G., Chiang, C-Y., Kao, G-S., & Yu, L. (2008). Activation of amygdaloid PKC pathway is necessary for conditioned cues-provoked cocaine memory performance. *Neurobiology of Learning and Memory, 90,* 164–170.

Li, X., Friedman, A. B., Zhu, W., Wang, L., Boswell, S., May, R. S., Davis, L. L., & Jope, R. S. (2007). Lithium regulates glycogen synthase kinase-3β in human peripheral blood mononuclear cells: Implications in the treatment of bipolar disorder. *Biological Psychiatry, 61,* 216–222.

Li, X., Rosborough, K. M., Friedman, A. B., Zhu, W., & Roth, K. A. (2007). Regulation of mouse brain glycogen synthase kinase-3 by atypical antipsychotics. *International Journal of Neuropsychopharmacology, 10,* 7–19.

Li, X., Zhu, W., Roh, M. S., Friedman, A. B., Rosborough, K., & Jope, R. S. (2004). In vivo regulation of glycogen synthase kinase-3β (GSK3β) by serotonergic activity in mouse brain. *Neuropsychopharmacology, 29,* 1426–1431.

Mai, L., Jope, R. S. & Li, X. (2002). BDNF-mediated signal transduction is modulated by GSK3β and mood stabilizing agents. *Journal of Neurochemistry, 82,* 75–83.

Manji, H. K., & Lenox, R. H. (1999). Ziskind-Somerfeld Research Award. Protein kinase C signaling in the brain: Molecular transduction of mood stabilization in the treatment of manic-depressive illness. *Biological Psychiatry, 46,* 1328–1351.

Mao, Y., Ge, X., Frank, C. L., Madison, J. M., Koehler, A. N., Doud, M. K., … Tsai, L. H. (2009). Disrupted in schizophrenia 1 regulates neuronal progenitor proliferation via modulation of GSK3β/β-catenin signaling. *Cell, 136,* 1017–1031.

Martin, M., Rehani, K., Jope, R. S., & Michalek, S. M. (2005). Toll-like receptor-mediated cytokine production is differentially regulated by glycogen synthase kinase 3. *Nature Immunology, 6,* 777–784.

McEwen, B. S. (2008). Central effects of stress hormones in health and disease: Understanding the protective and damaging effects of stress and stress mediators. *European Journal of Pharmacology, 583,* 174–185

McManus, E. J., Sakamoto, K., Armit, L. J., Ronaldson, L., Shpiro, N., Marquez, R., & Alessi, D. R. (2005). Role that phosphorylation of GSK3 plays in insulin and Wnt signalling defined by knockin analysis. *EMBO Journal, 24,* 1571–1583.

Miller, A. H., Maletic, V., & Raison, C. L. (2009). Inflammation and its discontents: The role of cytokines in the pathophysiology of major depression. *Biological Psychiatry, 65,* 732–741.

Munkholm, K., Bräuner, J. V., Kessing, L. V., & Vinberg, M. (2013). Cytokines in bipolar disorder vs. healthy control subjects: A systematic review and meta-analysis. *Journal of Psychiatric Research, 47,* 1119–1133.

O'Brien, W. T., Harper, A. D., Jove, F., Woodgett, J. R., Maretto, S., Piccolo, S., & Klein, P. S. (2004). Glycogen synthase kinase-3β haploinsufficiency mimics the behavioral and molecular effects of lithium. *Journal of Neuroscience, 24,* 6791–6798.

O'Brien, W. T., Haung, J., Buccafusca, R., Garskof, J., Valvezan, A. J., Berry, G. T., & Klein, P. S. (2011). Glycogen synthase kinase-3 is essential for β-arrestin-2 complex formation and lithium-sensitive behaviors in mice. *Journal of Clinical Investigation, 121,* 3756–3762.

O'Brien, W. T., & Klein P. S. (2009). Validating GSK3 as an in vivo target of lithium action. *Biochemical Society Transactions, 37,* 1133–1138.

Omata, N., Chiu, C. T., Moya, P. R., Leng, Y., Wang, Z., Hunsberger, J. G., … Chuang, D. M. (2011). Lentivirally mediated GSK-3β

silencing in the hippocampal dentate gyrus induces antidepressant-like effects in stressed mice. *International Journal of Neuropsychopharmacology, 14,* 711–717.

Padmos, R. C., Hillegers, M. H., Knijff, E. M., Vonk, R., Bouvy, A., Staal, F. J., … Drexhage, H. A. (2008). A discriminating messenger RNA signature for bipolar disorder formed by an aberrant expression of inflammatory genes in monocytes. *Archives of General Psychiatry, 65,* 395–407.

Palumbo, M. L., Zorrilla Zubilete, M. A., Cremaschi, G. A., & Genaro, A. M. (2009). Different effect of chronic stress on learning and memory in BALB/c and C57BL/6 inbred mice: Involvement of hippocampal NO production and PKC activity. *Stress, 12,* 350–361.

Peter, C. J., & Akbarian, S. (2011). Balancing histone methylation activities in psychiatric disorders. *Trends in Molecular Medicine, 17,* 372–379.

Pinton, P., Ferrari, D., Magalhães, P., Schulze-Osthoff, K., Di Virgilio, F., Pozzan, T., & Rizzuto, R. (2000). Reduced loading of intracellular Ca(2+) stores and downregulation of capacitative Ca(2+) influx in Bcl-2-overexpressing cells. *Journal of Cell Biology, 148,* 857–862.

Pittenger, C., & Duman, R. S. (2008). Stress, depression, and neuroplasticity: a convergence of mechanisms. *Neuropsychopharmacology, 33,* 88–109.

Polter, A., Beurel, E., Yang, S., Garner, R., Song, L., Miller, C. A., … Jope, R. S. (2010). Deficiency in the inhibitory serine-phosphorylation of glycogen synthase kinase-3 increases sensitivity to mood disturbances. *Neuropsychopharmacology, 35,* 1761–1774.

Quiroz, J. A., Gray, N. A., Kato, T., & Manji, H. K. (2008). Mitochondrially mediated plasticity in the pathophysiology and treatment of bipolar disorder. *Neuropsychopharmacology, 33,* 2551–2565.

Raison, C. L., & Miller, A. H. (2013). The evolutionary significance of depression in Pathogen Host Defense (PATHOS-D). *Molecular Psychiatry, 18,* 15–37.

Rao, J. S., Harry, G. J., Rapoport, S. I., & Kim, H. W. (2010). Increased excitotoxicity and neuroinflammatory markers in postmortem frontal cortex from bipolar disorder patients. *Molecular Psychiatry, 15,* 384–392.

Rao, J. S., & Rapoport, S. I. (2009). Mood-stabilizers target the brain arachidonic acid cascade. *Current Molecular Pharmacology, 2,* 207–214.

Ren, X., Rizavi, H. S., Khan, M. A., Dwivedi, Y., & Pandey, G. N. (2013). Altered Wnt signalling in the teenage suicide brain: Focus on glycogen synthase kinase-3β and β-catenin. *International Journal of Neuropsychopharmacology, 16,* 945–955.

Sachs, B. D., Rodriguiz, R. M., Siesser, W. B., Kenan, A., Royer, E. L., Jacobsen, J. P., … Caron, M. G. (2013). The effects of brain serotonin deficiency on behavioural disinhibition and anxiety-like behaviour following mild early life stress. *International Journal of Neuropsychopharmacology, 14,* 1–14.

Samuels, B. A., & Hen, R. (2011). Neurogenesis and affective disorders. *European Journal of Neuroscience, 33,* 1152–1159.

Schiepers, O. J., Wichers, M. C., & Maes, M. (2005). Cytokines and major depression. *Progress in Neuro-Psychopharmacology & Biological Psychiatry, 29,* 201–217.

Silverstone, P. H., & McGrath, B. M. (2009). Lithium and valproate and their possible effects on the myo-inositol second messenger system in healthy volunteers and bipolar patients. *International Review of Psychiatry, 21,* 414–423.

Stambolic, V., Ruel, L., & Woodgett, J. R. (1996). Lithium inhibits glycogen synthase kinase-3 activity and mimics wingless signalling in intact cells. *Current Biology, 6,* 1664–1668.

Sun, H., Kennedy, P. J., & Nestler, E. J. (2013). Epigenetics of the depressed brain: Role of histone acetylation and methylation. *Neuropsychopharmacology, 38,* 124–137.

Szabo, S. T., Machado-Vieira, R., Yuan, P., Wang, Y., Wei, Y., Falke, C., … Du, J. (2009). Glutamate receptors as targets of protein kinase C in the pathophysiology and treatment of animal models of mania. *Neuropharmacology, 56,* 47–55.

Tanis, K. Q., & Duman, R. S. (2007). Intracellular signaling pathways pave roads to recovery for mood disorders. *Annuals of Medicine, 39,* 531–544.

Wang, H. Y., & Friedman, E. (1996). Enhanced protein kinase C activity and translocation in bipolar affective disorder brains. *Biological Psychiatry, 40,* 568–575.

Warsh, J. J., Andreopoulos, S., & Li, P. P. (2004). Role of intercellular calcium signaling in the pathophysiology and pharmacotherapy of bipolar disorder: Current status. *Clinical Neuroscience Research, 4,* 201–213.

Woodgett, J. R. (2001). Judging a protein by more than its name: GSK-3. *Science STKE, 100,* re12.

Yildiz-Yesiloglu, A., & Ankerst, D. P. (2006). Neurochemical alterations of the brain in bipolar disorder and their implications for pathophysiology: A systematic review of the in vivo proton magnetic resonance spectroscopy findings. *Progress in Neuro-Psychopharmacology & Biological Psychiatry, 30,* 969–995.

Yuskaitis, C. J., & Jope, R. S. (2009). Glycogen synthase kinase-3 regulates microglial migration, inflammation, and inflammation-induced neurotoxicity. *Cellular Signalling, 21,* 264–273.

9.

CELLULAR RESILIENCE AND NEURODEGENERATION AND THEIR IMPACT ON THE TREATMENT OF BIPOLAR DISORDER

Gabriel Rodrigo Fries and Flávio Kapczinski

INTRODUCTION

Bipolar disorder (BD) is often associated with pronounced cognitive impairments involving executive functions and verbal memory (Martínez-Aran et al., 2000; Robinson et al., 2006). Most notably, these impairments seem to be progressive in nature, increasing with number of episodes and length of illness (Martínez-Aran et al., 2004). Several studies have shown that the cognitive decline observed in BD is associated with neuroanatomical alterations, including gray matter reduction in the dorsolateral prefrontal cortex (Ekman, Lind, Rydén, Ingvar, & Landén, 2010) and enlargement of the lateral ventricles. Notwithstanding, a question has been raised as to whether such alterations are associated with neuroplasticity impairments or neurodegenerative mechanisms (Jakobsson et al., 2013). Even though the exact mechanisms underlying these findings are unknown, cellular resilience and plasticity do seem to play a role in the establishment and progression of BD.

Cellular resilience can be defined as the ability of a given cell to cope with and survive in response to stimuli that would otherwise lead to its death. Resilience mechanisms are constantly activated by cells in response to internal stimuli, such as mitochondrial dysfunction and endoplasmic reticulum (ER) stress, as well as external stimuli, such as activation of certain membrane receptors and excitotoxicity, among others. Moreover, cells can modulate their behavior and connections with other cells in response to stimuli, a process known as cell plasticity. In particular, the so-called neuroplasticity is responsible for the neurons' ability to restore axonal and dendritic connections under specific circumstances, as well as to form new connections in response to environmental stimuli (e.g., stress). Neuroplasticity mechanisms are responsible for

maintaining neuronal networks and cognitive functions, including memory and functioning. As a result, impairments in neuroplasticity can lead to shrinkage of brain structures due to a reduction in the connection between cells or in the complexity of the brain cell network.

As opposed to neuroplasticity impairments, neurodegeneration is defined as neuronal loss of function with an underlying neuropathology and is mostly associated with a cell death outcome. Typical neurodegenerative diseases show markers of protein aggregation and neuronal death/toxicity (e.g., Lewy bodies in Parkinson's disease and beta-amyloid peptides in Alzheimer's disease). Of note, no evidence of Alzheimer-type neurodegeneration (assessed by levels of amyloid precursor protein metabolites in cerebrospinal fluid) was found in patients with BD (Jakobsson et al., 2013). Even so, neuropathological findings strongly support the occurrence of degenerative-like mechanisms in BD, as is discussed over the next sections. This chapter aims to review different findings on neurodegeneration and neuroplasticity in BD and identify the most probable mechanisms underlying BD progression.

NEUROIMAGING AND NEUROPATHOLOGICAL FINDINGS IN BIPOLAR DISORDER

Neuroimaging studies undertaken to better understand BD pathophysiology and progression have suggested that neuroanatomical alterations occur in specific brain regions rather than in the whole brain. One of the neuroanatomical alterations most consistently reported in patients with BD is lateral ventricle enlargement (Kempton, Geddes, Ettinger,

Williams, & Grasby, 2008), which has also been positively correlated with the occurrence of multiple episodes (Brambilla et al., 2001a; Strakowski, Delbello, & Adler, 2002). In fact, several alterations seem to take place with BD progression. For instance, illness duration has been correlated with smaller left putamen and reduced left inferior prefrontal gray matter volume (López-Larson, DelBello, Zimmerman, Schwiers, & Strakowski, 2002), as well as with smaller total brain gray matter volume (Frey et al., 2008). Hippocampal volume has also been reported to progressively decrease as the illness progresses (Javadapour et al., 2010), accompanied by an apparent increase in amygdala volume (Bora, Fornito, Yücel, & Pantelis, 2010). Changes in the shape and volume of the basal ganglia in general and of the striatum in particular have also been described in patients with BD and seem to take place at onset but remain at later stages (Bora et al., 2010; Hwang et al., 2006; Strakowski et al., 1999). In addition, an inverse correlation has been found between age and total gray matter volume in individuals with BD, suggesting faster age-related cortical neuronal loss in BD (Brambilla et al., 2001b). Given that most of the observable cerebral changes in BD involve the gray matter, the occurrence of neurodegenerative processes in association with illness progression has been suggested (Frey et al., 2008). Conversely, no changes in global brain volume have been detected (Hoge, Friedman, & Schulz, 1999; Strakowski et al., 2005).

Neuropathological studies have identified a reduction in glial cell number and density, as well as some alterations in the density and size of specific types of cortical neurons (Rajkowska, 2002). There is also evidence to suggest that both inhibitory and excitatory neurons in the prefrontal and limbic cortical regions are reduced in BD. Finally, postmortem studies have reported reductions in neuronal cell density, apparently more subtle than the corresponding glial alterations (Rajkowska, 2002). It remains to be seen whether most of these changes actually represent a loss of cells or simply a consequence of reduced branching and connections between them.

BIOCHEMICAL EVIDENCE OF CELL DEATH AND LOSS OF CELL RESILIENCE IN BIPOLAR DISORDER

Along with morphometric studies, several biochemical findings suggest the involvement of cell death and loss of resilience in the pathophysiology of BD. For instance, these patients have been shown to present bilateral decreased levels of N-acetyl-aspartate (NAA) in the hippocampus and in the dorsolateral prefrontal cortex (NAA is a molecule found in mature neurons, considered a measure of neuronal as opposed to glial viability, function, and integrity). Patients also present decreased NAA levels in the dorsolateral prefrontal cortex, which may reflect an underdevelopment of dendritic arborizations and synaptic connections (Sassi et al., 2005). Lithium is able to increase NAA levels in the brains of patients with BD (Bertolino et al., 1999; Moore et al., 2000; Winsberg et al., 2000), which further confirms the relevance of this molecule for BD treatment.

A growing body of evidence also points to increased levels of apoptotic factors in BD, including increased apoptotic serum activity (Politi, Brondino, & Emanuele, 2008), DNA damage in peripheral blood (Andreazza et al., 2007), mitochondrial dysfunction (Shao, Sun, Xu, Young, & Wang, 2008), and altered expression of molecules involved in cell survival (Herberth et al., 2011). In fact, a recent study has reported an increased percentage of peripheral blood mononuclear cells (PBMCs) in early apoptosis in patients with BD when compared to controls (Fries et al., 2014), suggesting the relevance of peripheral apoptosis in BD.

With regard to the nervous system, a postmortem study has found signs of apoptosis in olygodendrocytes from the frontal lobe (Broadman Area—BA 10) of brains of patients with BD, including decreased nuclear size, cell shrinkage, and condensation of nuclei and nuclear chromatin (Uranova et al., 2001). Other findings already reported include decreased levels of Bcl-2 and brain-derived neurotrophic factor (BDNF), which can act as an antiapoptotic factor, and increased levels of Bcl-2-associated death promoter, Bcl-2-associated X protein, caspase-9, and caspase-3 in the frontal cortex (BA 9) of patients, all known to induce apoptosis (Gigante et al., 2011; Kim, Rapoport, & Rao, 2010). These results are corroborated by the findings of a microarray study in the hippocampus of patients with BD, in which an up-regulation of 19/44 genes related to apoptosis were identified, along with a down-regulation of antiapoptotic genes (Benes, Matzilevich, Burke, & Walsh, 2006). As a consequence of these alterations, cells from patients with BD are considered to be less resilient to different insults. For instance, cells from the olfactory neuroepithelium of patients with BD have been shown to present an increased vulnerability to cell death (McCurdy et al., 2006), and so have peripheral blood mononuclear cells (Pfaffenseller et al., 2014).

In sum, all of these studies support involvement of cell death in BD and partly explain some of the neuroanatomical findings previously discussed. The mechanisms by which these alterations take place, however, are far from being clearly understood.

POTENTIAL MECHANISMS

A few altered pathways have been consistently reported in patients with BD and seem to play key roles in the modulation of cell death/survival and resilience. In this section, we discuss evidence of biological alterations often found in BD, which could ultimately be involved in these processes, including neurotrophic factors, excitotoxicity, glucocorticoids, mitochondrial dysfunction, and ER stress.

NEUROTROPHIC FACTORS

Neurotrophic factors comprise a family of proteins that are highly abundant in the nervous system and play key roles in the survival, growth, and plasticity of neuronal cells. BDNF is the most abundant neurotrophin in the adult mammalian brain, and it has been shown to be crucial for neuroplasticity and for the mechanisms of action of antidepressants, antipsychotics, and mood stabilizers (Grande, Fries, Kunz, & Kapczinski, 2010). Because of the ability of this neurotrophin to cross the blood-brain barrier, peripheral BDNF levels have been consistently used as a biomarker of disease activity and progression, combined with several clinical variables in patients with BD. For instance, a polymorphism at the *BDNF* gene, which has been reported to decrease the activity-dependent secretion of the protein (Egan et al., 2003), has been associated with impaired cognitive performance on neuropsychological tests measuring prefrontal lobe function in BD patients (Rybakowski, Borkowska, Czerski, Skibińska, & Hauser, 2003), and peripheral BDNF levels have been found to be reduced during acute episodes and to return to normal levels after symptom remission (Fernandes et al., 2011; Tramontina et al., 2009). Moreover, lower BDNF levels have been observed in patients at late stages of illness when compared to early-stage patients and healthy controls (Kauer-Sant'Anna et al., 2009).

Once disrupted, impaired BDNF signaling can lead to decreased dendritic spines and arborization, neuritic dystrophy and degeneration, neuronal atrophy, and reduced neurogenesis (Teixeira, Barbosa, Diniz, & Kummer, 2010). Animal studies have consistently described that these alterations in BDNF can lead to cognitive impairments and depressive behavior, mostly reversible after reestablishment of normal BDNF functions (Teixeira et al., 2010). A scenario of reduced neurotrophic signaling, along with decreased levels of antiapoptotic factors and antioxidant molecules, may partially explain the reduced cell resilience found in BD.

Furthermore, the implication of BDNF in the pathophysiology of BD is strongly supported by studies showing that mood stabilizers are able to increase BDNF levels both in vitro and in vivo (Frey et al., 2006; Yasuda, Liang, Marinova, Yahyavi, & Chuang, 2009; Yoshimura et al., 2006). Interestingly, BDNF alterations in BD seem to be associated with epigenetic changes, as an increased methylation at *BDNF* gene promoter I has been found in PBMCs from patients with BD type II compared with controls. This mechanism may link genetic alterations in BDNF to external stimuli (D'Addario et al., 2012), underscoring the key role of the environment in BD pathophysiology.

CALCIUM, EXCITOTOXICITY, AND ENDOPLASMIC RETICULUM STRESS

The neuroprotective properties of mood stabilizers and antidepressants have been consistently explained, among other mechanisms, by their ability to counteract glutamate-induced excitotoxicity in vitro (Chuang, 2004; Leng, Fessler, & Chuang, 2013). This feature is of great relevance for BD due to the key roles apparently played by glutamate and calcium in the disorder. Increased serum glutamate levels have been reported in patients with BD during mania and depression (Altamura et al., 1993; Hoekstra et al., 2006), and increased glutamate has also been found in the frontal cortex of these patients (Hashimoto, Sawa, & Iyo, 2007). Moreover, individuals with BD have been shown to present increased glutamate and/or glutamine levels in the plasma and cerebrospinal fluid (Zarate et al., 2003), which in turn may explain the increased intracellular calcium levels. Sufficiently high concentrations of calcium can induce excessive cytosolic calcium mobilization and cause overactivity of several calcium-dependent enzymes (Sapolsky, 2000). Finally, this could lead to a scenario of cytoskeletal degradation, protein misfolding, and oxygen-reactive species generation, ultimately leading to cell death. Elevated calcium levels have been found in PBMCs from patients with BD (Perova, Wasserman, Li, & Warsh, 2008), and disturbances of intracellular calcium homeostasis have been consistently reported in BD (Warsh, Andreopoulos, & Li, 2004).

Cells are strictly regulated by several mechanisms to prevent the consequences of increased intracellular calcium levels. Therefore, alterations in intracellular calcium levels, as commonly reported in patients with BD, may be induced by dysfunction of specific cellular organelles (e.g.,

ER and mitochondria, which typically play key roles in intracellular calcium sequestration, buffering, and storage; Warsh et al., 2004). For instance, the ER presents calcium ATPases that pump calcium from the cytosol into the ER lumen, whereas mitochondria may sequester the ion via an electrogenic transporter located on its inner membrane.

ER dysfunction in BD has been suggested by several studies assessing the so-called unfolded protein response (UPR), a mechanism typically activated by the ER to restore its function after the accumulation of unfolded proteins in the lumen. Typically, the ER responds to a transient dysfunction by up-regulating chaperones, which can handle the increasing amount of unfolded proteins, and decreasing overall protein synthesis until homeostasis is restored. Cells from patients with BD have been shown to present an impaired UPR, characterizing ER stress (Pfaffenseller et al., 2014; So, Warsh, & Li, 2007), a scenario that can ultimately lead to the activation of apoptotic pathways. In fact, ER stress has been considered one of the mechanisms against which cells from patients with BD are considered to be the least resilient (Fries et al., 2012). Of note, this mechanism seems to be central for the action of mood stabilizers: chronic valproate and lithium treatment, for example, can increase the expression of ER chaperones in vivo (Chen, Wang, & Young, 2000; Shao et al., 2006) and thus help counteract ER stress.

STRESS, GLUCOCORTICOIDS, AND MITOCHONDRIAL DYSFUNCTION

Several studies have suggested that chronic stress plays a key role in the pathophysiology of BD. Most of the effects of stress are mediated by cortisol, which is released and controlled by the hypothalamus-pituitary-adrenal (HPA) hormonal axis. Typically, high circulating levels of cortisol are able to bind to glucocorticoid receptors in the hypothalamus and repress cortisol release by the adrenal cortex. However, this negative feedback loop can be impaired in some patients, culminating with chronic increased cortisol levels and/or an enhanced cortisol response to stress. Patients with BD have been shown to present impairments in the HPA axis, as seen by the inability of a high number of patients to suppress cortisol release in response to dexamethasone (Daban, Vieta, Mackin, & Young, 2005). Glucocorticoids can also induce regression of dendritic processes in neurons and inhibit neurogenesis (Sapolsky, 2000). Of note, adult neurogenesis has been linked to stress buffering and antidepressant-like behavior (Snyder, Soumier, Brewer, Pickel, & Cameron, 2011). Finally, glucocorticoids can increase glutamate concentrations in hippocampal synapses, potentially contributing to excitotoxic mechanisms, as discussed previously.

In addition, increased cortisol levels may have important long-term consequences at the cellular level. For instance, in vitro and animal studies have shown that chronic stress and chronic exposure to high levels of glucocorticoids can lead to mitochondrial dysfunctions, including reductions in oxygen consumption, mitochondrial membrane potential, and calcium holding capacity (Du et al., 2009). Once dysfunctional, mitochondria can induce the opening of the mitochondrial permeability transition pore, thus releasing cytochrome c from the intermembrane space and inducing apoptotic cascades. Several studies have reported mitochondrial dysfunctions in BD, including impaired energy metabolism, alterations in respiratory chain complex enzymes, and down-regulation of mitochondria-related genes, among others (Quiroz, Brondino, & Emanuele, 2008). Cerebrospinal fluid lactate concentrations have also been shown to be significantly higher in patients with BD than in controls, suggesting increased extra-mitochondrial and anaerobic glucose metabolism (indicators of impaired mitochondrial metabolism; Regenold et al., 2009). In this scenario, the use of "mitochondrial enhancers" as an add-on treatment in the management of BD would be desirable, aiming at preventing mitochondrial dysfunction and thus increasing cellular resilience (Fries & Kapczinski, 2011).

CLINICAL IMPLICATIONS AND TREATMENT IMPACT

Most of the mechanisms described here seem to worsen with illness progression. In other words, neuroprogression in BD seems to be closely associated with a reduction in resilience mechanisms, making patients more vulnerable to new mood episodes and less responsive to medications (Fries et al., 2012; Kapczinski et al., 2008). The type and direction of the association between resilience at the cellular level and stress and coping mechanisms in patients with BD remains to be elucidated; however, considering that neuroprogression is implicated in several of the aforementioned biological mechanisms, one can infer that both scenarios could interfere with each other.

With regard to coping mechanisms, patients with BD are significantly less likely to use adaptive coping strategies and more likely to use maladaptive ones when compared to healthy controls (Fletcher, Parker, & Manicavasagar, 2013). These coping strategies have been hypothesized to be influenced by the neurotoxicity associated with illness progression and allostatic load (Kapczinski et al., 2008), which corroborates our hypothesis of impaired coping mechanisms being caused by reduced cell resilience. A summary of this process is illustrated in Figure 9.1. Briefly, external stimuli can induce cell signaling pathways that need to be dealt with. Depending on the resilience of a given cell, the activated mechanisms can result in cell survival and ultimately lead to a favorable clinical status of coping and cognition. Conversely, in cases of impaired resilience, the same stimuli can lead to cell death and ultimately to clinically observed impairments.

In addition, deficits in neuroplasticity, as suggested by reduced levels of neurotrophic factors, may be directly associated with several of the cognitive impairments reported in patients with BD. These deficits are seen in all mood states (including euthymia) and may include attention, verbal memory, and executive function impairments (Martínez-Arán et al., 2004; Vieta et al., 2013). Some aspects of cognition, (e.g., executive measures) have also been found to be associated with illness duration (Torrent et al., 2012). Among the neurobiological underpinnings of cognition, BDNF has been considered a key mediator of long-term potentiation and other neuroplasticity mechanisms. Therefore, it is possible that the reduction in BDNF levels that takes place with illness progression (Kauer-Sant'Anna et al., 2009) may mediate some of the

cognitive impairments reported in patients. This is a crucial aspect when considering the mechanisms of action of mood stabilizers and antidepressants.

It is currently a consensus that mood stabilizers and other medications used in the treatment of BD improve cell viability, resilience, and plasticity, both in vitro and in vivo (Bachmann, Schloesser, Gould, & Manji, 2005; Paulzen, Veselinovic, & Gründer, 2014). For instance, lithium has the ability to increase the levels of Bcl-2 (an antiapoptotic protein), heat shock protein 70, and BDNF, thus protecting cells against stimuli that would otherwise activate apoptosis. Lithium can also inhibit the enzyme glycogen-synthase kinase 3β, involved in several cellular processes (e.g., inflammation and apoptosis). In this same vein, mood stabilizers have been shown to increase the levels of neurotrophic factors (part of their neuroprotective properties). Finally, by suppressing microglial activation and neuroinflammation, these drugs end up reducing neuronal toxicity and ultimately attenuating neurodegeneration (Yu et al., 2012). Similar protective mechanisms have also been described for other drugs used in BD, such as anticonvulsants, antipsychotics, and antidepressants (Kubera, Obuchowicz, Goehler, Brzeszcz, & Maes, 2011; Paulzen et al., 2014). In summary, the mechanisms of action of drugs used in the treatment of BD, especially of mood stabilizers, seem to counteract most

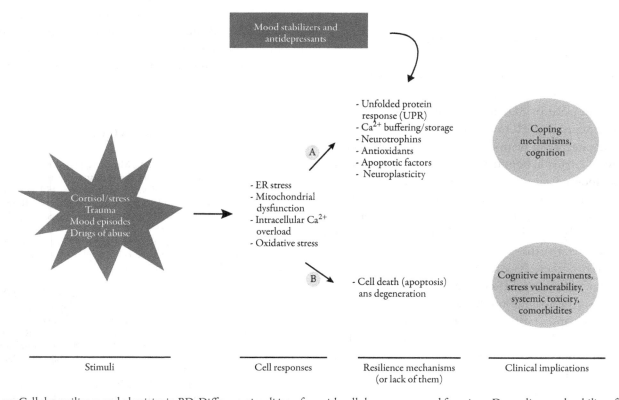

Figure 9.1 Cellular resilience and plasticity in BD. Different stimuli interfere with cellular responses and functions. Depending on the ability of cells to respond to them, they can be resilient (A) or die (B). In the case of neurons, resilience mechanisms can lead to enhanced neuroplasticity and possibly the formation of new dendrites, which have been shown to be induced by the administration of mood stabilizers and antidepressants.

of the loss of neuroplasticity and neurodegenerative-like mechanisms described in patients with BD, which once again underscores the relevance of such alterations for the pathophysiology and treatment of BD.

The fact that illness progression has been associated with reduced responsiveness to treatment (Swann, Bowden, Calabrese, Dilsaver, & Morris, 1999) raises an important question regarding neuroplasticity and neurodegeneration mechanisms in BD. One can hypothesize that epigenetic programming may occur with illness progression, possibly by means of altering DNA methylation at specific genes whose expression would normally be induced by mood stabilizers. Gene methylation is commonly associated with a repression of its expression (e.g., through a reduction of transcription factors' binding) and might account for one of the mechanisms by which some drugs tend to present a reduced treatment efficacy along with illness progression (Swann et al., 1999). In this sense, methylation of neuroprotective genes might reduce the ability of some drugs to induce their expression. As previously mentioned, DNA methylation has been found in BD not only at the *BDNF* promoter (D'Addario et al., 2012) but also at other genes of relevance (Rao, Keleshian, Klein, & Rapoport, 2012; Tamura, Kunugi, Ohashi, & Hohjoh, 2007). Nonetheless, further studies are required to assess the relationship between BD neuroprogression and epigenetic alterations.

CONCLUSION

In summary, there is evidence to suggest that both neuroplasticity impairments and neurodegenerative-like mechanisms take place in BD and are strongly associated with illness progression. However, BD does not seem to fit into the category of neurodegenerative disorders, as is the case with Alzheimer's and Huntington's disease, because the neurodegenerative features observed seem to be more subtle than the neuroplasticity impairments and their consequences. Moreover, BD presents a different pattern of neuronal and glial cell pathology when compared to typical neurodegenerative disorders (Jakobsson et al., 2013).

Some hypotheses have recently been proposed to explain the role of apoptosis and cell death in BD. An interesting approach is the assumption that apoptosis may be engaged locally in synapses rather than in the cell body in a process described as "synaptic apoptosis" (Mattson & Duan, 1999). This would provide a pathophysiological explanation for the apoptotic markers found in postmortem studies in BD, as well as for the synaptic remodeling observed in some brain structures and the reduced plasticity reported in patients.

Of note, lithium has been shown to increase hippocampal dendritic arborization in vivo (Watase et al., 2007), possibly due to its antiapoptotic and neurotrophic properties.

A better understanding of the mechanisms associated with BD neuroprogression, whether involving neurodegeneration or neuroplasticity impairments, may shed light on the mechanisms by which patients become more vulnerable to stress and new mood episodes, thereby establishing a vicious cycle of dysfunction. By enhancing resilience at the cellular level, alterations in neuronal networks and much of the cognitive and functional impairment observed could probably be prevented. Moreover, an increased resilience in peripheral cells would contribute to reducing inflammation and the systemic toxicity reported in patients, ultimately reducing systemic comorbidities (that account for a high clinical burden in patients) and improving their quality of life and life expectancy (Laursen, 2011; Whiteford et al., 2013).

Disclosure statement: Gabriel Rodrigo Fries was supported by a scholarship from the Conselho Nacional de Desenvolvimento Científico e Tecnológico (Brazil) and the German Academic Exchange Service (Germany).

Flávio Kapczinski has received grant/research support from Astra-Zeneca, Eli Lilly, Janssen-Cilag, Servier, Conselho Nacional de Desenvolvimento Científico e Tecnológico, Coordenação de Aperfeiçoamento de Pessoal de Nível Superior, Brain and Behavior Research Foundation, and the Stanley Medical Research Institute; has been a member of speakers' boards for Astra-Zeneca, Eli Lilly, Janssen and Servier; and has served as a consultant for Servier.

REFERENCES

Altamura, C., Mauri, M., Ferrara, A., Moro, A., D'Andrea, G., & Zamberlan, F. (1993). Plasma and platelet excitatory amino acids in psychiatric disorders. *American Journal of Psychiatry, 150*, 1731–1733.

Andreazza, A. C., Frey, B. N., Erdtmann, B., Salvador, M., Rombaldi, F., Santin, A., ... Kapczinski, F. (2007). DNA damage in bipolar disorder. *Psychiatry Research, 153*(1), 27–32.

Bachmann, R. F., Schloesser, R.J., Gould, T. D., & Manji, H. K. (2005). Mood stabilizers target cellular plasticity and resilience cascades: Implications for the development of novel therapeutics. *Molecular Neurobiology, 32*(2), 173–202.

Benes, F. M., Matzilevich, D., Burke, R. E., & Walsh, J. (2006). The expression of proapoptosis genes is increased in bipolar disorder, but not in schizophrenia. *Molecular Psychiatry, 11*(3), 241–251.

Bertolino, A., Frye, M., Callicott, J. H., Mattay, V. S., Rakow, R., Shelton-Repella, J., ... Weinberger, D.R. (1999). Neuronal pathology in the hippocampal area of patients with bipolar disorder. *Biological Psychiatry, 45*, 135S.

Bora, E., Fornito, A., Yücel, M., & Pantelis, C. (2010). Voxelwise meta-analysis of gray matter abnormalities in bipolar disorder. *Biological Psychiatry, 67*(11), 1097–1105.

Brambilla, P., Harenski, K., Nicoletti, M., Mallinger, A. G., Frank, E., Kupfer, D. J., ... Soares, J. C. (2001a). MRI study of posterior fossa structures and brain ventricles in bipolar patients. *Journal of Psychiatric Research*, 35(6), 313–322.

Brambilla, P., Harenski, K., Nicoletti, M., Mallinger, A. G., Frank, E., Kupfer, D. J., ... Soares, J. C. (2001b). Differential effects of age on brain gray matter in bipolar patients and healthy individuals. *Neuropsychobiology*, 43(4), 242–247.

Chen, B., Wang, J. F., & Young, L. T. (2000). Chronic valproate treatment increases expression of endoplasmic reticulum stress proteins in the rat cerebral cortex and hippocampus. *Biological Psychiatry*, 48(7), 658–664.

Chuang, D. M. (2004). Neuroprotective and neurotrophic actions of the mood stabilizer lithium: can it be used to treat neurodegenerative diseases? *Critical Reviews in Neurobiology*, 16(1–2), 83–90.

Daban, C., Vieta, E., Mackin, P., & Young, A. H. (2005). Hypothalamic-pituitary-adrenal axis and bipolar disorder. *Psychiatric Clinics of North America*, 28(2), 469–480.

D'Addario, C., Dell'Osso, B., Palazzo, M. C., Benatti, B., Lietti, L., Cattaneo, E., ... Altamura, A. C. (2012). Selective DNA methylation of BDNF promoter in bipolar disorder: Differences among patients with BDI and BDII. *Neuropsychopharmacology*, 37(7), 1647–1655.

Du, J., Wang, Y., Hunter, R., Wei, Y., Blumenthal, R., Falke, C., ... Manji, H. K. (2009). Dynamic regulation of mitochondrial function by glucocorticoids. *Proceedings of the National Academy of Sciences of the United States of America*, 106(9), 3543–3548.

Egan, M. F., Kojima, M., Callicott, J. H., Goldberg, T. E., Kolachana, B. S., Bertolino, ... Weinberger, D. R. (2003). The BDNF val66met polymorphism affects activity-dependent secretion of BDNF and human memory and hippocampal function. *Cell*, 112(2), 257–269.

Ekman, C. J., Lind, J., Rydén, E., Ingvar, M., & Landén, M. (2010). Manic episodes are associated with grey matter volume reduction—a voxel-based morphometry brain analysis. *Acta Psychiatrica Scandinavica*, 122(6), 507–515.

Fernandes, B. S., Gama, C. S., Ceresér, K. M., Yatham, L.N., Fries, G.R., Colpo, G., ... Kapczinski, F. (2011). Brain-derived neurotrophic factor as a state-marker of mood episodes in bipolar disorders: A systematic review and meta-regression analysis. *Journal of Psychiatric Research*, 45(8):995–1004.

Fletcher, K., Parker, G. B., & Manicavasagar, V. (2013). Coping profiles in bipolar disorder. *Comprehensive Psychiatry*, 54(8), 1177–1184.

Frey, B. N., Andreazza, A. C., Ceresér, K. M., Martins, M. R., Valvassori, S.S., Réus, G.Z., ... Kapczinski, F. (2006). Effects of mood stabilizers on hippocampus BDNF levels in an animal model of mania. *Life Sciences*, 79(3), 281–286.

Frey, B. N., Zunta-Soares, G. B., Caetano, S. C., Nicoletti, M. A., Hatch, J. P., Brambilla, P., ... Soares, J. C. (2008). Illness duration and total brain gray matter in bipolar disorder: evidence for neurodegeneration? *European Neuropsychopharmacology*, 18(10), 717–22.

Fries, G. R., & Kapczinski, F. (2011). N-acetylcysteine as a mitochondrial enhancer: a new class of psychoactive drugs? *Revista Brasileira de Psiquiatria*, 33(4), 321–322.

Fries, G. R., Pfaffenseller. B., Stertz, L., Paz, A. V., Dargél, A. A., Kunz, M., & Kapczinski, F. (2012). Staging and neuroprogression in bipolar disorder. *Current Psychiatry Reports*, 14(6), 667–675.

Fries, G. R., Vasconcelos-Moreno, M. P., Gubert, C., Santos, C., Rosa, A. L. S. T., Eisele, B., ... Kauer-Sant'Anna, M. (2014). Early apoptosis in peripheral blood mononuclear cells from patients with bipolar disorder. *Journal of Affective Disorders* (January), 152–154, 474–477.

Gigante, A. D., Young, L. T., Yatham, L. N., Andreazza, A. C., Nery, F. G., Grinberg, L. T., ... Lafer, B. (2011). Morphometric post-mortem studies in bipolar disorder: Possible association with oxidative stress and apoptosis. *International Journal of Neuropsychopharmacology*, 14(8), 1075–1089.

Grande, I., Fries, G. R., Kunz, M., & Kapczinski, F. (2010). The role of BDNF as a mediator of neuroplasticity in bipolar disorder. *Psychiatry Investigation*, 7(4), 243–250.

Hashimoto, K., Sawa, A., & Iyo, M. (2007). Increased levels of glutamate in brains from patients with mood disorders. *Biological Psychiatry*, 62, 1310–1316.

Herberth, M., Koethe, D., Levin, Y., Schwarz, E., Krzyszton, N. D., Schoeffmann, S., ... Bahn, S. (2011). Peripheral profiling analysis for bipolar disorder reveals markers associated with reduced cell survival. *Proteomics*, 11(1), 94–105.

Hoekstra, R., Fekkes, D., Loonen, A., Pepplinkhuizen, L., Tuinier, S., & Verhoeven, W. (2006). Bipolar mania and plasma amino acids: increased levels of glycine. *European Neuropsychopharmacology*, 16, 71–77.

Hoge, E. A., Friedman, L., & Schulz, S. C. (1999). Meta-analysis of brain size in bipolar disorder. *Schizophrenia Research*, 37(2), 177–181.

Hwang, J., Lyoo, I. K., Dager, S. R., Friedman, S. D., Oh, J. S., Lee, J. Y., ... Renshaw, P. F. (2006). Basal ganglia shape alterations in bipolar disorder. *American Journal of Psychiatry*, 163(2), 276–285.

Jakobsson, J., Zetterberg, H., Blennow, K., Johan Ekman, C., Johansson, A. G., & Landén, M. (2013). Altered concentrations of amyloid precursor protein metabolites in the cerebrospinal fluid of patients with bipolar disorder. *Neuropsychopharmacology*, 38(4), 664–672.

Javadapour, A., Malhi, G.S., Ivanovski, B., Chen, X., Wen, W., & Sachdev, P. (2010). Hippocampal volumes in adults with bipolar disorder. *Journal of Neuropsychiatry and Clinical Neuroscience*, 22(1), 55–62.

Kapczinski, F., Vieta, E., Andreazza, A. C., Frey, B. N., Gomes, F. A., Tramontina, J., ... Post, R. M. (2008). Allostatic load in bipolar disorder: Implications for pathophysiology and treatment. *Neuroscience and Biobehavior Reviews*, 32(4), 675–692.

Kauer-Sant'Anna, M., Kapczinski, F., Andreazza, A. C., Bond, D. J., Lam, R. W., Young, L.T., & Yatham, L. N. (2009). Brain-derived neurotrophic factor and inflammatory markers in patients with early- vs. late-stage bipolar disorder. *International Journal of Neuropsychopharmacology*, 12(4), 447–458.

Kempton, M. J., Geddes, J. R., Ettinger, U., Williams, S. C., & Grasby, P. M. (2008). Meta-analysis, database, and meta-regression of 98 structural imaging studies in bipolar disorder. *Archives of General Psychiatry*, 65(9), 1017–1032.

Kim, H. W., Rapoport, S. I., & Rao, J. S. (2010). Altered expression of apoptotic factors and synaptic markers in postmortem brain from bipolar disorder patients. *Neurobiology of Disease*, 37(3), 596–603.

Kubera, M., Obuchowicz, E., Goehler, L., Brzeszcz, J., & Maes, M. (2011). In animal models, psychosocial stress-induced (neuro) inflammation, apoptosis and reduced neurogenesis are associated with the onset of depression. *Progress in Neuropsychopharmacology and Biological Psychiatry*, 35(3), 744–759.

Laursen, T. M. (2011). Life expectancy among persons with schizophrenia or bipolar affective disorder. *Schizophrenia Research*, 131(1–3), 101–104.

Leng, Y., Fessler, E. B., & Chuang, D. M. (2013). Neuroprotective effects of the mood stabilizer lamotrigine against glutamate excitotoxicity: roles of chromatin remodelling and Bcl-2 induction. *International Journal of Neuropsychopharmacology*, 16(3), 607–620.

López-Larson, M. P., DelBello, M. P., Zimmerman, M. E., Schwiers, M. L., & Strakowski, S. M. (2002). Regional prefrontal gray and white matter abnormalities in bipolar disorder. *Biological Psychiatry*, 52(2), 93–100.

Martínez-Arán, A., Vieta, E., Colom, F., Reinares, M., Benabarre, A., Gastó, C., & Salamero, M. (2000). Cognitive dysfunctions in bipolar disorder: Evidence of neuropsychological disturbances. *Psychotherapy and Psychosomatics*, 69(1), 2–18.

Martínez-Arán, A., Vieta, E., Reinares, M., Colom, F., Torrent, C., Sanchez-Moreno, J., ... Salamero, M. (2004). Cognitive function across manic or hypomanic, depressed, and euthymic states in bipolar disorder. *American Journal of Psychiatry*, 161(2), 262–270.

Mattson, M. P., & Duan, W. (1999). "Apoptotic" biochemical cascades in synaptic compartments: Roles in adaptive plasticity and neurodegenerative disorders. *Journal of Neuroscience Research*, 58(1), 152–166.

McCurdy, R. D., Féron, F., Perry, C., Chant, D. C., McLean, D., Matigian, N., ... Mackay-Sim, A. (2006). Cell cycle alterations in biopsied olfactory neuroepithelium in schizophrenia and bipolar I disorder using cell culture and gene expression analyses. *Schizophrenia Research*, 82(2–3), 163–173.

Moore, G. J., Bebchuk, J. M., Hasanat, K., Chen, G., Seraji-Bozorgzad, N., Wilds, I. B., ... Manji, H. K. (2000). Lithium increases N-acetyl-aspartate in the human brain: In vivo evidence in support of bcl-2's neurotrophic effects? *Biological Psychiatry*, 48(1), 1–8.

Paulzen, M., Veselinovic, T., & Gründer, G. (2014). Effects of psychotropic drugs on brain plasticity in humans. *Restorative Neurology and Neuroscience*, 32(1), 163–181.

Perova, T., Wasserman, M. J., Li, P. P., & Warsh, J. J. (2008). Hyperactive intracellular calcium dynamics in B lymphoblasts from patients with bipolar I disorder. *International Journal of Neuropsychopharmacology*, 11(2), 185–196.

Pfaffenseller, B., Wollenhaupt-Aguiar, B., Fries, G.R., Colpo, G.D., Burque, R.K., Bristot, G., Ferrari, P., Ceresér, K.M., Rosa, A.R., Klamt, F., & Kapczinski, F. (2014). Impaired endoplasmic reticulum stress response in bipolar disorder: cellular evidence of illness progression. *International Journal of Neuropsychopharmacology*, 17(9), 1453–1463.

Politi, P., Brondino, N., & Emanuele, E. (2008). Increased proapoptotic serum activity in patients with chronic mood disorders. *Archives of Medical Research*, 39(2), 242–245.

Quiroz, J. A., Gray, N. A., Kato, T., & Manji, H. K. (2008). Mitochondrially mediated plasticity in the pathophysiology and treatment of bipolar disorder. *Neuropsychopharmacology*, 33(11), 2551–2565.

Rajkowska, G. (2002). Cell pathology in bipolar disorder. *Bipolar Disorders*, 4(2), 105–116.

Rao, J. S., Keleshian, V. L., Klein, S., & Rapoport, S. I. (2012). Epigenetic modifications in frontal cortex from Alzheimer's disease and bipolar disorder patients. *Translational Psychiatry*, 2, e132.

Regenold, W. T., Phatak, P., Marano, C. M., Sassan, A., Conley, R. R., & Kling, M. A. (2009). Elevated cerebrospinal fluid lactate concentrations in patients with bipolar disorder and schizophrenia: Implications for the mitochondrial dysfunction hypothesis. *Biological Psychiatry*, 65(6), 489–494.

Robinson, L. J., Thompson, J. M., Gallagher, P., Goswami, U., Young, A. H., Ferrier, I. N., & Moore, P. B. (2006). A meta-analysis of cognitive deficits in euthymic patients with bipolar disorder. *Journal of Affective Disorders*, 93(1–3), 105–115.

Rybakowski, J. K., Borkowska, A., Czerski, P. M., Skibińska, M., & Hauser, J. (2003). Polymorphism of the brain-derived neurotrophic factor gene and performance on a cognitive prefrontal test in bipolar patients. *Bipolar Disorders*, 5(6), 468–472.

Sapolsky, R. M. (2000). The possibility of neurotoxicity in the hippocampus in major depression: a primer on neuron death. *Biological Psychiatry*, 48(8), 755–765.

Sassi, R. B., Stanley, J. A., Axelson, D., Brambilla, P., Nicoletti, M. A., Keshavan, M. S., ... Soares, J. C. (2005). Reduced NAA levels in the dorsolateral prefrontal cortex of young bipolar patients. *American Journal of Psychiatry*, 162(11), 2109–2015.

Shao, L., Sun, X., Xu, L., Young, L. T., & Wang, J. F. (2006). Mood stabilizing drug lithium increases expression of endoplasmic reticulum stress proteins in primary cultured rat cerebral cortical cells. *Life Sciences*, 78(12), 1317–1323.

Shao, L., Martin, M. V., Watson, S. J., Schatzberg, A., Akil, H., Myers, R. M., ... Vawter, M. P. (2008). Mitochondrial involvement in psychiatric disorders. *Annals of Medicine*, 40(4), 281–295.

Snyder, J. S., Soumier, A., Brewer, M., Pickel, J., & Cameron, H. A. (2011). Adult hippocampal neurogenesis buffers stress responses and depressive behaviour. *Nature*, 476(7361), 458–461.

So, J., Warsh, J. J., & Li, P. P. (2007). Impaired endoplasmic reticulum stress response in B-lymphoblasts from patients with bipolar-I disorder. *Biological Psychiatry*, 62(2), 141–147.

Strakowski, S. M., DelBello, M. P., Sax, K. W., Zimmerman, M. E., Shear, P. K., Hawkins, J. M., & Larson, E. R. (1999). Brain magnetic resonance imaging of structural abnormalities in bipolar disorder. *Archives of General Psychiatry*, 56(3), 254–260.

Strakowski, S. M., DelBello, M. P., Zimmerman, M. E., Getz, G. E., Mills, N. P., Ret, J., ... Adler, C. M. (2002). Ventricular and periventricular structural volumes in first- versus multiple-episode bipolar disorder. *American Journal of Psychiatry*, 159(11), 1841–1847.

Strakowski, S. M., Delbello, M. P., & Adler, C. M. (2005). The functional neuroanatomy of bipolar disorder: a review of neuroimaging findings. *Molecular Psychiatry*, 10(1), 105–116.

Swann, A. C., Bowden, C. L., Calabrese, J. R., Dilsaver, S. C., & Morris, D. D. (1999). Differential effect of number of previous episodes of affective disorder on response to lithium or divalproex in acute mania. *American Journal of Psychiatry*, 156(8), 1264–1266.

Tamura, Y., Kunugi, H., Ohashi, J., & Hohjoh, H. (2007). Epigenetic aberration of the human REELIN gene in psychiatric disorders. *Molecular Psychiatry*, 12(6), 519, 593–600.

Teixeira, A. L., Barbosa, I. G., Diniz, B. S., & Kummer, A. (2010). Circulating levels of brain-derived neurotrophic factor: correlation with mood, cognition and motor function. *Biomarkers in Medicine*, 4(6), 871–887.

Torrent, C., Martínez-Arán, A., del Mar Bonnin, C., Reinares, M., Daban, C., Solé, B., Rosa, A.R., Tabarés-Seisdedos, R., Popovic, D., Salamero, M., Vieta, E. (2012). Long-term outcome of cognitive impairment in bipolar disorder. *Journal of Clinical Psychiatry*, 73(7), e899–e905.

Tramontina, J. F., Andreazza, A. C., Kauer-Sant'anna, M., Stertz, L., Goi, J., Chiarani, F., & Kapczinski, F. (2009). Brain-derived neurotrophic factor serum levels before and after treatment for acute mania. *Neuroscience Letters*, 452(2), 111–113.

Uranova, N., Orlovskaya, D., Vikhreva, A., Zimina, I., Kolomeets, N., Vostrikov, V., & Rachmanova, V. (2001). Electron microscopy of oligodendroglia in severe mental illness. *Brain Research Bulletin*, 55, 597–610.

Vieta, E., Popovic, D., Rosa, A. R., Solé, B., Grande, I., Frey, B. N., ... Kapczinski, F. (2013). The clinical implications of cognitive impairment and allostatic load in bipolar disorder. *European Psychiatry*, 28(1), 21–29.

Warsh, J. J., Andreopoulos, S., & Li, P. P. (2004). Role of intracellular calcium signaling in the pathophysiology and pharmacotherapy of bipolar disorder: current status. *Clinical Neuroscience Research*, 4, 201–213.

Watase, K., Gatchel, J. R., Sun, Y., Emamian, E., Atkinson, R., Richman, R., Mizusawa, H., ... Zoghbi, H. Y. (2007). Lithium therapy improves neurological function and hippocampal dendritic arborization in a spinocerebellar ataxia type 1 mouse model. *PLoS Medicine*, 4(5), e182.

Whiteford, H. A., Degenhardt, L., Rehm, J., Baxter, A. J., Ferrari, A. J., Erskine, H. E., ... Vos, T. (2013). Global burden of disease attributable to mental and substance use disorders: findings from the Global Burden of Disease Study 2010. *Lancet*, 382(9904), 1575–1586.

Winsberg, M. E., Sachs, N., Tate, D. L., Adalsteinsson, E., Spielman, D., & Ketter, T. A. (2000). Decreased dorsolateral prefrontal N-acetyl aspartate in bipolar disorder. *Biological Psychiatry*, 47, 475–481.

Yasuda, S., Liang, M. H., Marinova, Z., Yahyavi, A., & Chuang, D. M. (2009). The mood stabilizers lithium and valproate selectively activate the promoter IV of brain-derived neurotrophic factor in neurons. *Molecular Psychiatry, 14*(1):51–59.

Yoshimura, R., Nakano, Y., Hori, H., Ikenouchi, A., Ueda, N., & Nakamura, J. (2006). Effect of risperidone on plasma catecholamine metabolites and brain-derived neurotrophic factor in patients with bipolar disorders. *Human Psychopharmacology Clinical and Experimental, 21*, 433–438.

Yu, F., Wang, Z., Tchantchou, F., Chiu, C. T., Zhang, Y., & Chuang, D. M. (2012). Lithium ameliorates neurodegeneration, suppresses neuroinflammation, and improves behavioral performance in a mouse model of traumatic brain injury. *Journal of Neurotrauma, 29*(2), 362–374.

Zarate, C. A. Jr., Du, J., Quiroz, J., Gray, N. A., Denicoff, K. D., Singh, J., … Manji, H. K. (2003). Regulation of cellular plasticity cascades in the pathophysiology and treatment of mood disorders: Role of the glutamatergic system. *Annals of the New York Academy of Sciences, 1003*, 273–291.

10.

IMMUNE MECHANISMS AND INFLAMMATION AND THEIR TREATMENT IMPACT

Alice Russell, Carmine M. Pariante, and Valeria Mondelli

INTRODUCTION

Over the past few decades, there has been an increasing body of research supporting the role of inflammation in the pathogenesis of different neuropsychiatric disorders from both preclinical and clinical studies. The most consistent and established findings come from studies in depression, with the macrophage theory of depression having been proposed over 20 years ago (Smith, 1991). Now also known as the malaise or cytokine theory of depression (Miller, Maletic, & Raison, 2009), this hypothesis emphasizes the role of psycho-neuroimmunological dysfunctions where there is activation of the immune system. Indeed, not only is there evidence that patients with affective disorders have elevated levels of biomarkers of inflammation, but it has also been shown that acute administration of cytokines cause sickness behavior, which shares features with depression. Moreover, a large proportion of patients treated therapeutically with cytokines develop depressive symptoms, and mania has also been induced (Raison, Demetrashvili, Capuron, & Miller, 2005; Zunszain, Hepgul, & Pariante, 2013).

The mechanisms through which inflammatory cytokines have been suggested to mediate the onset of depression include interaction with multiple pathways such as monoamine metabolism, neuroendocrine function, and synaptic plasticity (Haroon, Raison, & Miller, 2012). Interestingly, all of these mechanisms are also relevant for the onset and course of bipolar disorder (BD). In recent years, BD too has received a great deal of attention in this respect, with an increasing number of studies building a convincing case for a role of inflammation in the illness (Berk et al., 2011; Goldstein, Kemp, Soczynska, & McIntyre, 2009). However, the precise nature of this role is still unclear.

In line with studies on depression and schizophrenia, perhaps the main focus thus far has been to explore the degree of cytokine abnormalities, a key indicator of immune dysfunction and a proinflammatory state. Though it is now clear that in BD there is also an increase in proinflammatory cytokines, BD has proved somewhat more difficult to study in this regard due to the degree of change in affective states that characterizes this illness. In addition, genetic polymorphisms have been identified that lend further support to the inflammatory hypothesis.

There is also growing support for immunomodulatory effects of existing medications for BD in addition to their effects on the monoaminergic system, suggesting another novel mechanism of action for these psychotropic agents. Interestingly, the effect of psychotropic drugs, such as antidepressants, on inflammation has also been associated with treatment response (Cattaneo et al., 2013) suggesting the immune system as a possible novel therapeutic target. While the results for treatment response to mood stabilizers are less clear, numerous studies have demonstrated existing treatments to reduce inflammation (Goldstein et al., 2009). Furthermore, promising results have been seen in trials of adjuvant anti-inflammatory medications, largely for patients with depression. Their success in improving affective and to some extent cognitive symptoms has resulted in the inclusion of BD patients in larger scale trials both currently and in the near future (Berk et al., 2011).

We discuss evidence for increased inflammation in BD and also consider possible causes of increased inflammation as well as how inflammation might affect the brain. Emerging evidence of the anti-inflammatory action of agents currently used in the treatment of BD, as well as the adjuvant use of anti-inflammatory medications, are also summarized.

EVIDENCE FOR INFLAMMATION IN BIPOLAR DISORDER

CYTOKINE ABNORMALITIES

Several biomarkers of inflammation have been measured in BD using both in vitro and in vivo techniques. Some of the most frequently reported are cytokines produced by innate immune cells, including interleukin-6 (IL-6), and tumor necrosis factor-alpha (TNF-α). However, abnormalities in other inflammatory markers have also been proposed to indicate increased inflammation in BD (for a review see Berk et al. 2011). Indeed, other inflammatory markers, such as the acute phase protein C-reactive protein (CRP), have also been reported to be increased in BD (Goldstein et al., 2009). Also of interest are chemical cytokines, or chemokines, which present chemoattractive properties. Though less studied in this area, there is also evidence to suggest abnormalities, which may be indicative of an inflammatory response (Barbosa et al., 2013).

A recent meta-analysis of 30 studies on cytokine abnormalities in BD concluded that levels of numerous cytokines were elevated in comparison with healthy controls: IL-4, IL-10, soluble interleukin-2 receptor (sIL-2R) and sIL-6R, TNF-α, soluble TNF-receptor 1 (sTNF-R1) and interleukin-1 receptor a (IL-1Ra). Other pro-inflammatory cytokines, namely IL-1β, IL-6, showed a trend for increased levels in BD. Levels of the markers IL-2, INF-γ, and IL-8 were not significantly different from those of healthy volunteers (Modabbernia, Taslimi, Brietzke, & Ashrafi, 2013).

However, research in depression and schizophrenia suggests that some immune markers may be classified as "state" or "trait" markers according to whether these parameters remain stable throughout the illness or increase during acute episodes and normalize during subsequent remission. A similar debate continues in BD, with some markers more consistently associated with acute episodes of illness but others still evident in euthymic states (see Munkholm, Brauner, Kessing, & Vinberg, 2013, for a review). Findings from studies stratified according to affective state, including those following symptomatic patients into remission, are discussed. Additionally, a potential association between cytokine alterations and clinical variables is also explored. Finally, preliminary results from gene expression studies are reviewed.

Mania and depression

One review found evidence for increased proinflammatory markers in mania, with soluble IL-2 receptor (sIL-2R), IL-6, TNF-α, and CRP shown to be relatively consistently high during this affective state (Goldstein et al., 2009). For example, sIL-2R was shown to be increased when compared with healthy volunteers in both in vivo and in vitro studies, as was IL-6, and TNF-α. A recent meta-analysis confirmed the increase in TNF-α and sIL-2R, though increases in IL-6 were not found to be significant when considered overall (Munkholm et al., 2013). This is in contrast to reports that suggest increased levels IL-6 are one of the most consistent findings in BD (Hamdani, Doukhan, Kurtlucan, Tamouza, & Leboyer, 2013).

Other studies supporting an increased inflammatory state during manic phases include findings on soluble TNF-receptor 1 (sTNF-R1), IL1Ra, and CRP. In particular, sTNF-R1 has been found to be increased in patients whose mood was elevated, as well as those who were experiencing acute mania, in comparison to healthy controls and also BD patients experiencing other mood states (Hope et al., 2011; Tsai et al., 2012). In relation to IL1Ra, one study found levels to be significantly higher in manic patients compared to normal controls overall. However, interestingly a third of patients had lower levels than the mean level seen in controls (Tsai et al., 2012). With regard to CRP, this too has been shown to be elevated in mania, as compared with healthy volunteers even after controlling for age. For other proinflammatory markers, results have been less consistent, particularly IL-2, IL-1β, and interferon (IFN)-γ. This is true also for studies looking at anti-inflammatory cytokines in mania, such as IL-4 and IL-10 (Goldstein et al., 2009). In addition, higher levels of the chemokines CCL11 and CXCL-10 and lower levels of CXCL8 were seen in mania as compared to healthy volunteers. No difference in CCL24 was shown (Barbosa et al., 2013).

With regard to bipolar depression, fewer studies have been conducted, though a similar pattern to mania has emerged, with increased levels of IL-6 and TNF-α in depressed patients compared with healthy volunteers (Brietzke et al., 2009), as well as higher levels of sIL-2R (Breunis et al., 2003). Furthermore, CRP has also been shown to be elevated in bipolar depression. However, though results were nearly significant for increased TNF-α in bipolar depressed patients versus controls, in a recent meta-analysis no significant differences between the two groups were found (Munkholm et al., 2013). A more recent study found levels of inflammatory markers in a depressed mood group of BD patients to be similar to those of healthy volunteers and lower than those in the elevated mood group (Hope et al., 2011).

Lower levels of inflammatory markers among bipolar depressed patients when compared with bipolar manic patients may also mean that the differences between bipolar depressed patients and controls exist though are more difficult to identify as a result of the detection limits of current techniques. Nonetheless, it may be possible that levels of inflammation are indeed lower among depressed patients and that more of the inflammation observed occurs during acute mania. To account for this, in line with the interaction between cytokines and catecholamine neurotransmission, it has been proposed that low levels of inflammatory markers in bipolar depressed patients may be related to change in catecholamine neurotransmission, which tends to be low in depression and high in mania (Hope et al., 2011). However, results remain unclear and further clarity is needed.

Euthymia

A limited number of cross-sectional studies have examined cytokine abnormalities in euthymia. They suggest that sIL-2R may be raised in euthymic patients compared with controls (Breunis et al., 2003) and that the anti-inflammatory cytokine IL-4 may be increased (Brietzke et al., 2009), though further studies are required. A recent meta-analysis showed lower levels of TNF-α and sTNFR-1 in euthymic patients compared with those who were manic, with no difference in IL-6 and IL-1RA. However, there were no significant differences in inflammatory markers between depressed and euthymic patients (Munkholm et al., 2013). An additional study found IL-6 to be increased in a neutral mood group of bipolar patients, compared to a control group, though interestingly this result was not evident in symptomatic groups (Hope et al., 2011). A recent study previously mentioned (Barbosa et al., 2013) found that, as in manic patients, levels of the chemokines CCL11, and CXCL-10, were increased in patients with euthymia when compared with healthy volunteers. Additionally, though not significant in mania, levels of CCL24 were also increased in euthymic bipolar patients. There was, however, no difference between the two patient groups, suggesting that these markers are more consistently elevated. On the other hand, Guloksuz et al. (2010) found cytokine levels to have normalized during euthymia but, notably, only if patients were medication-free. Those euthymic patients taking lithium monotherapy showed increased levels of TNF-α and IL-4 compared to healthy volunteers.

Changes after remission/symptomatic improvement

Studies have also been conducted that examine cytokine abnormalities in different stages of remission. Indicating the presence of state markers, levels of certain cytokines appear to change during the course of remission. For example, it has been shown that levels of certain cytokines, specifically TNF-α and IFN-γ, are increased during the immediate remission phase following a depressive episode, as compared to patients who have achieved sustained remission and healthy volunteers (Remlinger-Molenda, Wojciak, Michalak, Karczewski, & Rybakowski, 2012).

In contrast, for patients in immediate remission from a manic episode, higher levels of IL-10 and IL-1RA were observed (Remlinger-Molenda et al., 2012). In addition, a study measuring cytokine levels in the cerebro-spinal fluid, a more direct examination of neuroinflammation, showed IL-1β to be increased in euthymic patients who had recently experienced acute mania or hypomania (Soderlund et al., 2011). A longitudinal study also found IL-1Ra to be elevated in partial remission following mania as compared to healthy controls. Furthermore, while levels remained slightly higher in full remission, this was no longer significant. Within the patient group, compared with the acute manic episode levels were significantly lower in remission (Tsai et al., 2012).

Other studies observed no differences between those patients in sustained remission and healthy volunteers, suggesting that some cytokine abnormalities may resolve after a sufficient period, an effect that may be attributable to treatment (Guloksuz et al., 2010; Remlinger-Molenda et al., 2012). Indeed, Kim, Jung, Myint, Kim, and Park (2007) found that where increased levels of IL-6 were shown among manic patients, these levels had decreased after a period of six weeks. This was also true of increased sIL-2R levels in an acute manic episode, which normalized during remission (Tsai et al., 1999).

Interestingly, for some cytokines an opposite pattern has emerged, with levels appearing to increase during remission. A recent study observed elevated high sensitive CRP levels in patients who had achieved partial remission from a manic episode compared to normal controls. CRP levels remained significantly higher than normal controls even in full remission, even increasing as compared with the partial remission phase. Similarly, levels of sTNF-R1 were significantly higher in partial and full remission compared with healthy volunteers. While in this case levels remained relatively stable from acute mania to full remission, there was a trend for increased levels in full remission as compared to the acute phase (Tsai et al., 2012).

Further research is needed to compare medication-free with treated patients to establish whether reduced inflammation is an effect of medication or the resolution of an inflammatory state associated with the acute episode. In addition, such a design may also shed light on what effect medication might have, if any, on the more stable or increasing levels of other inflammatory markers (Munkholm et al., 2013).

Link with clinical variables

Findings in this regard are still limited and conflicting, with the majority of studies published finding no association between inflammatory markers and clinical or demographic variables, including symptom severity (Goldstein et al., 2009).

However, some studies do suggest a link. For example, Remlinger-Molenda and colleagues (2012) found a positive association between levels of IL-6 and severity of manic symptoms in patients in remission after a manic episode. Furthermore, Tsai and colleagues (1999) and Tsai, Yang, Kuo,Chen, and Leu (2001) also observed a link between a reduction in sIL-2R levels and symptomatic improvement of acute mania, with the two positively correlated. In a less acute sample, STNF-R1 was positively associated with elevated mood among bipolar patients. Osteoprotegerin, a member of the TNF-α superfamily related to inflammation, IL-1Ra and IL-6 were negatively correlated with low mood in the same study (Hope et al., 2011). Increased CRP levels were also shown to be associated with more severe manic symptoms, and levels were shown to be an independent predictor of symptom severity; however, despite the link between CRP and depression there was no association with depressive symptoms among BD patients in this group. Additionally, in a more recent study from the same group, elevated CRP was inversely related to cognitive performance in a group of BD patients. While the cause of this association is not known, the authors propose that they are likely to be related to inflammatory processes occurring within the vasculature of the central nervous system (Dickerson et al., 2013).

Few studies have been conducted that examine clinical markers associated with psychosis in BD patients alongside inflammatory markers. One such study found an association with certain immune markers, even after controlling for numerous confounders: sTNF-R1 was correlated with length of hospital stays and IL-6 with length of hospitalization and a history of psychosis (Hope et al., 2013).

With regard to physical health measures, body mass index (BMI) was found to be positively correlated with levels of IL-1Ra in partial remission. Furthermore, increased plasma sTNF-R1 levels were associated with higher BMI in both acute mania and subsequent partial remission and increased leptin in full remission. The leptin levels were also positively correlated to high sensitive CRP levels but only in full remission (Tsai et al., 2012). In the same study, smoking was associated with increased sTNF-R1 levels in acute mania, though in the same manic phase high sensitive CRP levels were higher in nonsmokers. No other effects of smoking were observed in acute mania, nor did smoking have an effect on cytokine levels in partial or full remission (Tsai et al., 2012). In relation to demographic variables, elevated CRP has been linked with female sex and non-White race. It is important to note that such a lack of evidence for the association between increased inflammation and variables such as gender, smoking, and BMI, may be due to methodological limitations of the studies conducted. For example, common limitations include small sample sizes, heterogeneity in terms of symptoms, or, in some cases, mood state, BD subtype, and concurrent medications (Goldstein et al., 2009).

Gene expression studies

Further evidence for increased inflammation in BD comes from the study of gene expression. A pivotal study has identified a proinflammatory signature in BD, as evidenced in the increased expression of genes relating to different stages of the proinflammatory response. Padmos and colleagues (2008) found that monocytes from BD patients show increased mRNA expression of 19 genes involved directly in inflammation and inflammation-related processes. Specific genes were also shown to be associated with symptom severity; during acute episodes overexpression was further increased, over and above euthymia, in certain cytokines. Furthermore, lithium and antipsychotics, both commonly used in the treatment of BD, were shown to down-regulate the expression of these inflammatory genes (Padmos et al., 2008). A further study by the same group confirmed that BD was most strongly associated with a subgroup of inflammatory-related genes consisting mainly of well-known inflammatory markers, including proinflammatory cytokines and chemokines. However, when examining disease severity, a different cluster of genes was implicated, representing adhesion, motility, and chemotactic factors. As before, such genes were increased in euthymia as compared with healthy controls, with further increases in the expression of specific genes observed during acute phases of illness (Drexhage et al., 2010).

Furthermore, the proinflammatory signature described here has also been shown to be aberrantly expressed in the offspring of patients with BD. The degree of positive matches with the 19 genes identified increased among those offspring who themselves had a mood disorder, as compared with the currently healthy offspring. There was some indication also that the baseline parameters may be used to predict which of the offspring would go on to develop a mood disorder during the follow-up period, and the researchers hope to follow up the healthy offspring for a longer period to establish whether the signature can be used as a long-term predictor of later development of BD (Padmos et al., 2008).

In summary, there is sufficient evidence in the bipolar literature to reveal a dysfunctional immune system, as seen in cytokine abnormalities. While some cytokine levels may vary according to affective state, TNF-α has emerged as consistently high in both manic and depressive phases, supporting the view of this particular cytokine as a state marker (Hamdani et al., 2013). As suggested earlier, further studies are needed that address the methodological limitations apparent in the majority of studies produced to date. Of particular importance is the need for increased sample sizes, control for confounders known to affect inflammation, and standardization of methods used to ascertain cytokines. Furthermore, there have been calls for further studies of younger populations unaffected by age-related inflammation, long treatment duration, and long-term symptom burden (Goldstein et al., 2009). This is in line with the suggestion that the proinflammatory state may differ in early-onset BD as compared with the later stages of the illness, in part due to the cumulative effect of acute episodes. Increasing evidence to support this viewpoint also prompts the need for long-term longitudinal studies (Hamdani et al., 2013).

EFFECTS OF THERAPEUTIC CYTOKINE ADMINISTRATION ON MOOD

Chronic therapeutic administration of interferon-alpha (IFN-α), used in the treatment of viral hepatitis and some cancers, has been shown to lead to depressive symptomatology in up to 50% of patients, who display similar biological alterations as those found in major depression disorder (MDD; Raison et al., 2005). Such evidence has led to IFN-α induced depression being used as a model to identify the specific changes in the immune system that may be involved in instigating the behavioral changes that lead to depression. IFN-α induced mania is less common and therefore less widely studied, though it has been reported in multiple case studies. Some studies have estimated the prevalence rates to be 10% to 20% (Carpiniello, Orru, Baita, Pariante, & Farci, 1998; Raison et al., 2005; Wu, Liao, Peng, Pariante, & Su, 2007). In more severe cases, symptoms include euphoria,

inflated self-esteem, increase in goal-directed behavior, impulsivity, and even psychosis, while more common manifestations include irritability, racing thoughts, distractibility, insomnia, and psychomotor agitation. Indeed, Raison and colleagues stressed the need for clinicians to accurately distinguish between dysphoric mania, characterized by aggression and agitation as opposed to euphoria, and depression in order to ensure patients receive adequate and safe treatment (Raison et al., 2005).

MECHANISMS BEHIND THE INCREASED INFLAMMATION IN BIPOLAR DISORDER

THE ROLE OF GENES

A growing body of research has examined functional polymorphisms in inflammation related genes in an attempt to further explain the cytokine alterations at protein level of those markers implicated in BD.

As shown previously, perhaps one of the most frequently studied cytokines implicated in BD is TNF-α. Production of this cytokine is influenced by a promoter polymorphism, −308G/A, with the mutant A or TNF-2 allele associated with increased TNF-α production. In a Korean sample, BD type I patients were more likely to carry the TNF-2 allele (−308A) compared with healthy volunteers (Pae, Lee, Han, Serretti, & Jun, 2004). Conversely, a Polish study observed that patients with a diagnosis of bipolar affective disorder were more likely to have the G allele of the −308 (G/A) of the gene, compared with healthy volunteers. This same allele was also shown to be associated with a family history of the illness, conferring susceptibility to the disorder (Czerski et al., 2008). An Italian sample also observed that the majority of BD patients studied did not carry the A allele, and indeed none of the BD type II subsample studied did so (Clerici et al., 2009). Still studies have found no association at all, with a study from the United Kingdom showing no link between the polymorphism and BD or puerperal psychosis; nor was an association identified in a Brazilian sample (Meira-Lima et al., 2003; Middle, Jones, Robertson, Lendon, & Craddock, 2000).

Considering the +874 (T/A) polymorphism of the IFN-γ promoter, a Korean study found the T allele, associated with high IFN-γ production, to be significantly more common among BD patients than controls. Interestingly, an association was found between the severity of the manic episode and the genotype, with those carrying the T allele

(T/T or T/A) having significantly higher mania scores than patients with the A/A genotype. Taken together, this suggests that those patients, whose genotype induces a more active inflammatory response, may endure more severe manic symptoms (Yoon & Kim, 2012). In contrast, an Italian study showed bipolar type II patients to be less likely to have the TT genotype or T allele (Clerici et al., 2009).

With regard to IL-1β, increased levels have been observed in postmortem frontal cortex samples, both in protein and mRNA. However, no association was found between BD and variable number of tandem repeats polymorphism of the IL-1RA, a variant of which is said to be associated with enhanced IL-1β production. Nor was an association found between BD and the −511 (C/T) polymorphism in the promoter region of the IL-1β gene (Papiol et al., 2008). In an Italian sample, though no association was found between BD and the 174 (G/C) IL-6 polymorphism, a lower mean age of onset was observed in those patients not carrying the G (high-producer) allele, as compared with those who did carry this SNP. In the same study, no association was found between the −1082 (G/C) IL-10 polymorphism and BD (Clerici et al., 2009). Overall, as compared to the depression and schizophrenia literature, findings are relatively limited and conflicting, and ethnic differences limit the generalizability of some studies.

THE ROLE OF STRESS

Stress has been suggested to play a role in both the onset and the course of BD, as individuals are reported to be more susceptible to the effects of chronic stress. Concomitantly, episodes of stress can induce inflammatory processes. For example, chronic stress, including difficult caregiving and hostile marital relationships, has been associated with increased levels of CRP.

In particular, a stressful childhood seems to produce neuroendocrine and immunological abnormalities that are thought to mediate the development of a proinflammatory phenotype in adulthood. For example, increased reactivity of the hypothalamic-pituitary-adrenal (HPA) axis, one of the main biological systems involved in the stress response, as well as elevated levels of proinflammatory cytokines, have been seen later in life in those individuals who have experienced childhood trauma (Danese et al., 2008; Di Nicola et al., 2013). Furthermore, it has also been demonstrated that such increases may even be predicted by a history of childhood maltreatment. Interestingly, when childhood maltreatment was controlled for, the association between MDD and inflammatory cytokines disappeared (Danese

et al., 2008). Given the high prevalence of childhood maltreatment among patients with BD, early life stress may also be a mediator of the increased inflammation shown in BD (Brietzke, Stabellini, Grassis-Oliveira, & Lafer, 2011).

In general, dysfunction of the HPA axis is consistently seen in BD patients. Hyperactivity of the HPA axis in BD has been demonstrated by increasing circulating cortisol levels and by nonsuppression of cortisol following administration of dexamethasone and dexamethasone/corticotrophin-releasing hormone (CRH), in both acute and euthymic phases of the illness (Watson, Gallagher, Ritchie, Ferrier, & Young, 2004). Interestingly, cortisol levels during the day in patients with BD have been found to be associated with symptom dimensions, in particular as positively associated with the positive psychotic symptoms and excitement and negatively with disorganization (Belvederi Murri et al., 2012). Numerous cytokines are able to activate the HPA axis. Regulation of the HPA axis starts by release of CRH from the paraventricular nucleus of the hypothalamus. CRH leads to the release of adrenocorticotropic hormone in the pituitary, inducing discharge of cortisol from the adrenal cortex. In normal individuals, cortisol binds to two main receptors (glucocorticoid and mineralocorticoid receptors) and exerts a negative feedback mechanism that controls its production by regulating the synthesis of CRH. This feedback mechanism can be altered by cytokines. Acute cytokine administration in humans has been shown to cause both elevated plasma levels of adrenocorticotropic hormone and cortisol and increase CRH release (Pariante & Lightman, 2008; Pariante & Miller, 2001).

When administered chronically, though, cytokines are associated with a flattening of the cortisol response and also increased evening cortisol levels. Inflammatory cytokines can disrupt glucocorticoid receptor (GR) function, while decreasing GR expression (Pace, Hu, & Miller, 2007). For example, cytokines have been found to inhibit GR function in cytokine-releasing immune cells by acting on GR translocation or on GR-mediated gene transcription, resulting in a deregulated production of other proinflammatory cytokines. Mechanisms described include activation of signaling pathways, such as p38 mitogen-activated protein kinase (MAPK), NF-κB, signal transducers, and activators of transcription and cyclooxygenase (Miller, Pariante, & Pearce, 1999; Pariante et al., 1999).

Since communication occurs between the endocrine, immune, and central nervous system, an activation of the inflammatory responses can affect neuroendocrine processes and vice versa (Zunszain, Anacker, Cattaneo, Carvalho, & Pariante, 2011). Several mechanisms may be involved.

A study of peripheral blood monocytes of caregivers of patients with malignant brain cancer supports the idea that chronic stress is accompanied by GR resistance and activation of proinflammatory pathways. These monocytes showed diminished expression of transcripts bearing response elements for glucocorticoids and heightened expression of transcripts with response elements for NF-κB (Hayden, West, & Ghosh, 2006). In relation to an acute stressor, a recent study observed blunted neuroendocrine responses in the form of reduced salivary cortisol and heart rate following exposure to the Trier Social Stress Test in female patients with BD. Furthermore, increased lymphocyte MAPK, p-ERK, and p-NF-κB signaling was observed after the test, as was a relative lymphocyte resistance to dexamethasone (Wieck et al., 2013). These findings suggest that stress produces functional resistance to glucocorticoids, which enables activation of proinflammatory transcription control pathways, even in the absence of decreased GR mRNA expression or excess cortisol production.

This evidence suggests that HPA axis hyperactivity and inflammation might be part of the same pathophysiological process: HPA axis hyperactivity is a marker of glucocorticoid resistance, implying ineffective action of glucocorticoid hormones on target tissues, which could lead to immune activation; equally, inflammation could stimulate HPA axis activity via both a direct action of cytokines on the brain and by inducing glucocorticoid resistance.

CYTOKINE EFFECTS IN THE BRAIN

Other possible mechanisms by which increased inflammation may lead to the onset of BD relate to cytokine effects in the brain. To date, the majority of the research conducted in this area has been in the context of depression, though it may be extended to BD. Cytokine effects on neurotransmission, neurogenesis, plasticity, and degeneration are summarized here, as well as imbalances in the kynurenine pathway.

Cytokines affect the synthesis, release, and reuptake of all neurotransmitters associated with the development and maintenance of affective disorders (Miller et al., 2009). The most studied has been serotonin and, in particular, the function of its transporter, which regulates serotonin uptake into presynaptic neurons. For example, IL-1β has been shown to increase serotonin uptake in the brain, while IFN-α has shown attenuation of the expression of 5HT1A, one of the serotonin receptors. Patients who have been treated with IFN-α, used therapeutically, have shown low levels of serum serotonin, with this effect more pronounced in those who developed depression. Moreover, the severity of the depression correlated with higher cerebral spinal fluid (CSF) levels of IL-6 and lower levels of the serotonin metabolite 5-hydroxyindoleacecetic acid, indicating reduced brain serotonergic activity (Raison et al., 2009).

Also of importance is dopamine. It has been shown that the dopaminergic system is reduced in response to inflammation. Reduced CSF concentrations of homovanillic acid, one of the metabolites of dopamine, have been associated with depressive-like behavior in primates, secondary to IFN-α administration. In rats, administration of IFN-α has also led to decreased concentrations of dopamine in the CSF, in association with increased production of nitric oxide. Finally, effects on norepinephrine have also been observed, with peripheral and central administration of IL-1 or high doses of TNF-α, inducing norepinephrine release in the brain, most markedly in the hypothalamus (Dunn, 2006).

Another route by which cytokines may affect serotonergic neurotransmission is through imbalances in the kynurenine pathway. Several proinflammatory cytokines can induce the enzyme indoleamine 2,3-dioxygenase (IDO), which converts the essential amino acid tryptophan into kynurenine. Kynurenine is a precursor of the bioactive metabolites quinolinic acid (QUIN) and kynurenic acid (KYNA). QUIN is an N-methyl-D-aspartate receptor agonist, potentially neurotoxic and thus potentially contributing to depression, whereas KYNA is an N-methyl-D-aspartate receptor antagonist generally considered neuroprotective. Following IDO activation, both the relative balance between QUIN and KYNA and the reduced peripheral availability of tryptophan (putatively leading to reduced serotonin synthesis in the brain) have been proposed to be of significance in depression and neurodegeneration (Myint & Kim, 2003).

Decreased tryptophan levels, and levels of the kynuerine-dependent tryptophan index, have been shown in bipolar mania (Myint et al., 2007). Furthermore, a postmortem study found increased kynurenine in the anterior cingulated cortex in BD, corresponding to increased density, and intensity of tryptophan 2,3-dioxygenase positive glial cells (Miller, Llenos, Dulay, & Weis, 2006). Therefore it has been proposed that imbalances in this pathway are also implicated in BD (Berk et al., 2011).

Proinflammatory cytokines also influence neuronal functioning through changes in apoptosis, oxidative stress, and metabolic derangement, as well as by impairing processes of synaptic plasticity and neurogenesis (Berk et al., 2011; Mondelli et al., 2011). Such impairments have been proposed to be a central pathophysiological correlate of BD (Brietzke et al., 2011). The proinflammatory cytokines IL-1β and TNF-α have been shown to inhibit long-term potentiation, a form of neuronal plasticity believed to underlie learning and memory, both of which are frequently affected in mood disorders, including BD. IL-1β also decreased hippocampal neurogenesis in both animal and human in vitro models (Zunszain et al., 2012). TNF-α and IFN-γ have shown inhibition of neuronal progenitor cell proliferation. Furthermore, TNF-α induces neuronal cell death through blockade of the glutamate transporter activity, thereby potentiating glutamate neurotoxicity. Indirectly, the detrimental effects of stress on neurogenesis have been reversed by hippocampal transplantation of neural progenitor cells that overexpress IL-1 receptor antagonist or by using IL-1 receptor knockout mice. Concomitantly, this blockade of cytokine action has led to a decrease of depressive symptoms in these models.

MEDICATION

IMMUNOMODULATORY EFFECTS OF CURRENT MEDICATIONS

Existing medications used in the treatment of BD have been shown to have neuroprotective and anti-inflammatory effects (Berk et al., 2011). For example, traditionally used agents such as lithium, valproate, carbamazepine, and lamotrigine have been shown to suppress brain cyclooxygenase (COX)-2 and prostaglandin-2 (Goldstein et al., 2009; Remlinger-Molenda et al., 2012).

Lithium

It has been shown that monocytes from BD patients not currently treated show trends toward low IL-1β and high IL-6 production when stimulated with lipopolysaccharide. However, the effect on IL-1β is reversed by treatment with lithium (Knijff et al., 2007). Lithium has also been shown to normalize sIL-2R and sIL-6R levels. Interestingly, this effect was reversed in healthy controls in whom levels increased (Rapaport, Guylai, & Whybrow, 1999). Furthermore, significantly fewer BD patients taking lithium had elevated CRP levels (Hornig, Goodman, Kamoun, & Amsterdam, 1998). Therapeutic administration of lithium to medication naïve BD patients resulted in a decrease in cytokine production over the three-month course (Boufidou, Nikolaou., Alevizos, Liappas, & Christodoulou, 2004). It has also been demonstrated that lithium down-regulated the expression of inflammatory genes examined, which had been identified as being aberrantly expressed in this bipolar patients (Padmos

et al., 2008). Another relevant point is the finding that, in a subgroup of patients in whom TNF-α remained persistently high, an association was found with nonresponse to lithium (Guloksuz et al., 2012). Insufficient information has made it difficult to conclude the causality of this association, but this is certainly worthy of further attention.

Sodium valproate

Sodium valproate has been found to inhibit TNF-α and IL-6 production in vivo. However, it has previously been shown that while antipsychotic use brought about a decrease in proinflammatory markers in patients with schizophrenia, valproate did not have this effect in manic patients (Maes, Bosmans, Calabrese, Smith, & Meltzer, 1995). Valproate may also decrease the production or activation of NF-κB, which activates the production of proinflammatory cytokines (Remlinger-Molenda et al., 2012). Furthermore, antipsychotics typically used in the treatment of BD, such as olanzapine, have been shown to be associated with a reduction in inflammatory markers (Meyer et al., 2009).

NOVEL USE OF ANTI-INFLAMMATORY AGENTS

COX-1 and COX-2 inhibitors

A nonsteroidal-anti-inflammatory-drug, aspirin is an inhibitor of both COX-1 and -2. It has been shown to reduce inflammatory markers without affecting the negative immunoregulatory cytokines (Berk et al., 2013). The adjunctive use of aspirin in addition to fluoxetine resulted in a greater decrease in markers of oxidative stress as compared with fluoxetine monotherapy (Galecki, Szemraj, Bienkiewicz, Zboralski, & Galecka, 2009). It has also been proposed that aspirin accelerates antidepressant effects by shortening the onset of action (Brunello et al., 2006). More recently, it has been suggested that the beneficial effects may extend to include schizophrenia, with symptomatic reduction after adjuvant use (Mondelli & Pariante, 2010). Furthermore, specifically to BD, an epidemiological study suggested that use of low-dose acetylsalicylic acid reduced the risk of clinical deterioration of patients with BD, as evidenced in a reduced need for dose increases or adjunctive medication (Stolk et al., 2010).

Celecoxib is a selective inhibitor of COX-2. It has been trialed successfully with promising results in MDD. It has been shown to be effective in reducing depressive symptoms when added to either fluoxetine or reboxetine (Haroon et al., 2012). In BD, treatment with celecoxib resulted in a reduction in depressive symptom scores after one week (Nery et al., 2008). It should be noted, however, that cele-coxib is associated with cardiovascular risk (Goldstein et al., 2009).

TNF-α inhibitors

Increases in TNF-α have been observed in the periphery and in the form of transmembrane TNF-α (tm-TNF) in relevant brain regions. Recently there has been a growing interest in the use of drugs targeting the tm-TNF molecule as a result of their effect on affective symptoms (Berk et al., 2011). For example, in the treatment of psoriasis, patients receiving the TNF-α antagonist Etanercept showed an increase in depression scores independent of improvement in their illness (Tyring et al., 2006). Similarly, in the treatment of Crohn's disease, Infliximab has been observed to have a positive impact on affective symptoms (Brietzke et al., 2011). With regard to side effects, the potential to induce mania and a possible risk of lymphoma in children and young adults have been observed (Goldstein et al., 2009). Interestingly, findings from a recent randomized controlled trial with Infliximab in patients with treatment-resistant depression suggest that TNF antagonism does not have generalized efficacy in treatment-resistant depression but may improve depressive symptoms in patients who showed higher inflammation at baseline (Raison et al., 2013). Similarly, it is possible to hypothesize that only bipolar patients who show increased inflammation might benefit from anti-inflammatory treatment.

Omega-3 fatty acids

Polyunsaturated fatty acids (PUFAs) have been shown to play an important role in MDD and have more recently been implicated in BD (Berk et al., 2011), with suggestions that lower levels of ω-3 PUFAs may contribute to these disorders. One possible explanation for the association between depleted levels and mood disturbances is that ω-3 and ω-6 PUFAs modulate immune functions. ω-3 PUFAs, like ethyl-eicosapentanoic acid (EPA), attenuate prosta-glandin E2 synthesis and the production of monocytic and T cell cytokines, including IL-1, 6, TNF-α, and IFN-α (Su, 2009).

Findings regarding the therapeutic benefit of ω-3 PUFAs for BD have been inconsistent: a combination of EPA and docosahexaenoic acid resulted in a significantly longer duration of remission versus placebo, and a second larger study saw an improvement in depressive symptoms after daily administration of ethyl-EPA (Frangou, Lewis, &

McCrone, 2006; Stoll et al., 1999). However, a third study showed no benefit of ethyl-EPA but acknowledged that the dose exceeded the recommended dose as demonstrated successfully in MDD and schizophrenia (Keck et al., 2006). Little benefit, if any, has been seen for manic symptoms thus far, so this treatment may be relevant only for those experiencing depression. One explanation relates to dopamine activity, in that manic and depressive states seem to be accompanied by overactivity and decreased activity, respectively. Regardless, omega-3 fatty acids are relatively side-effect free, and therefore further research is needed to establish clinical benefit.

CONCLUSION

Increasing evidence suggests the presence of a proinflammatory state in patients with BD. While some cytokine levels may vary according to affective state, others have emerged as consistently high in both manic and depressive phases. However, it remains unclear if normalization of inflammatory markers mirrors a clinical response. Studies exploring possible mechanisms behind the presence of a proinflammatory state in BD suggest only a marginal role of a direct genetic predisposition and a possibly stronger effect of environmental factors, such as life stressors. Indeed, future research is needed to better understand causes and specificity of increased inflammatory markers in individuals with BD. Indeed, both studies on the effects of mood stabilizers on inflammation and trials studying the use of add-on treatment with anti-inflammatory agents support inflammation as a potential therapeutic target in BD. As recently suggested for patients with MDD and schizophrenia, it is possible to hypothesize that inflammation plays a critical role in some but not all individuals suffering with BD. Indeed, one of the next challenges for future research will be to clarify which individuals might most benefit from the treatment targeting inflammation.

ACKNOWLEDGMENTS

This work has been supported by the South London and Maudsley National Health Service (NHS) Foundation Trust and Institute of Psychiatry National Institute for Health Research Biomedical Research Centre for Mental Health; a Starter Grant for Clinical Lecturers from the Academy of Medical Sciences, the Wellcome Trust, and the British Heart Foundation to V. Mondelli; and the grant "Persistent Fatigue Induced by Interferon Alpha: A New

Immunological Model for Chronic Fatigue Syndrome" from the Medical Research Council (UK) MR/J002739/1. Additional support has been offered by the Commission of European Communities Seventh Framework Programme (Collaborative Project Grant Agreement no. 22963, Mood Inflame).

Disclosure statement: Carmine M. Pariante has received research funding from pharmaceutical companies interested in the immune system, such as Johnson & Johnson. Professor Pariante and Dr. Mondelli are partly supported by the National Institute for Health Research Biomedical Research Centre at South London and Maudsley NHS Foundation Trust and King's College London. The views expressed are those of the authors and not necessarily those of the NHS, the National Institute for Health Research, or the Department of Health. Alice Russell has no conflicts to disclose.

REFERENCES

Barbosa, I. G., Rocha, N. P., Bauer, M. E., de Miranda, A. S., Huguet, R. B., Reis, H. J.,…Teixeira, A. L. (2013). Chemokines in bipolar disorder: Trait or state? *European Archives of Psychiatry and Clinical Neuroscience*, 263(2), 159–165.

Belvederi Murri, M., Pariante, C. M., Dazzan, P., Hepgul, N., Papadopoulos, A. S., Zunszain, P.,…Mondelli, V. (2012). Hypothalamic-pituitary-adrenal axis and clinical symptoms in first-episode psychosis. *Psychoneuroendocrinology*, 37(5), 629–644.

Berk, M., Dean, O., Drexhage, H., McNeil, J. J., Moylan, S., O'Neil, A.,…Maes, M. (2013). Aspirin: A review of its neurobiological properties and therapeutic potential for mental illness. *BMC Medicine*, 11, 74.

Berk, M., Kapczinski, F., Andreazza, A. C., Dean, O. M., Giorlando, F., Maes, M.,…Malhi, G. S. (2011). Pathways underlying neuroprogression in bipolar disorder: Focus on inflammation, oxidative stress and neurotrophic factors. *Neuroscience and Biobehavioral Reviews*, 35(3), 804–817.

Boufidou, F., Nikolaou, C., Alevizos, B., Liappas, I. A., & Christodoulou, G. N. (2004). Cytokine production in bipolar affective disorder patients under lithium treatment. *Journal of Affective Disorders*, 82(2), 309–313.

Breunis, M. N., Kupka, R. W., Nolen, W. A., Suppes, T., Denicoff, K. D., Leverich, G. S.,…Drexhage, H. A. (2003). High numbers of circulating activated T cells and raised levels of serum IL-2 receptor in bipolar disorder. *Biological Psychiatry*, 53(2), 157–165.

Brietzke, E., Stabellini, R., Grassis-Oliveira, R., & Lafer, B. (2011). Cytokines in bipolar disorder: Recent findings, deleterious effects but promise for future therapeutics. *CNS Spectrums*, 16(7), 157–168.

Brietzke, E., Stertz, L., Fernandes, B. S., Kauer-Sant'anna, M., Mascarenhas, M., Escosteguy Vargas, A.,…Kapczinski, F. (2009). Comparison of cytokine levels in depressed, manic and euthymic patients with bipolar disorder. *Journal of Affective Disorders*, 116(3), 214–217.

Brunello, N., Alboni, S., Capone, G., Benatti, C., Blom, J. M., Tascedda, F.,…Mendlewicz, J. (2006). Acetylsalicylic acid accelerates the antidepressant effect of fluoxetine in the chronic escape deficit model of depression. *International Clinical Psychopharmacology*, 21(4), 219–225.

Carpiniello, B., Orru, M. G., Baita, A., Pariante, C. M., & Farci, G. (1998). Mania induced by withdrawal of treatment with interferon alfa. *Archives of General Psychiatry*, 55(1), 88–89.

Cattaneo, A., Gennarelli, M., Uher, R., Breen, G., Farmer, A., Aitchison, K. J.,…Pariante, C. M. (2013). Candidate genes expression profile associated with antidepressants response in the GENDEP study: Differentiating between baseline "predictors" and longitudinal "targets". *Neuropsychopharmacology*, 38(3), 377–385.

Clerici, M., Arosio, B., Mundo, E., Cattaneo, E., Pozzoli, S., Dell'osso, B.,…Altamura, A. C. (2009). Cytokine polymorphisms in the pathophysiology of mood disorders. *CNS Spectrums*, 14(8), 419–425.

Czerski, P. M., Rybakowski, F., Kapelski, P., Rybakowski, J. K., Dmitrzak-Weglarz, M., Leszczynska-Rodziewicz, A.,…Hauser, J. (2008). Association of tumor necrosis factor -308G/A promoter polymorphism with schizophrenia and bipolar affective disorder in a Polish population. *Neuropsychobiology*, 57(1–2), 88–94.

Danese, A., Moffitt, T. E., Pariante, C. M., Ambler, A., Poulton, R., & Caspi, A. (2008). Elevated inflammation levels in depressed adults with a history of childhood maltreatment. *Archives of General Psychiatry*, 65(4), 409–415.

Di Nicola, M., Cattaneo, A., Hepgul, N., Di Forti, M., Aitchison, K. J., Janiri, L.,…Mondelli, V. (2013). Serum and gene expression profile of cytokines in first-episode psychosis. *Brain, Behavior, and Immunity*, 31, 90–95.

Dickerson, F., Stallings, C., Origoni, A., Vaughan, C., Khushalani, S., & Yolken, R. (2013). Elevated C-reactive protein and cognitive deficits in individuals with bipolar disorder. *Journal of Affective Disorders*, 150(2), 456–459.

Drexhage, R. C., van der Heul-Nieuwenhuijsen, L., Padmos, R. C., van Beveren, N., Cohen, D., Versnel, M. A.,…Drexhage, H. A. (2010). Inflammatory gene expression in monocytes of patients with schizophrenia: Overlap and difference with bipolar disorder. A study in naturalistically treated patients. *International Journal of Neuropsychopharmacology*, 13(10), 1369–1381.

Dunn, A. J. (2006). Effects of cytokines and infections on brain neurochemistry. *Clinical Neuroscience Research*, 6(1–2), 52–68.

Frangou, S., Lewis, M., & McCrone, P. (2006). Efficacy of ethyl-eicosapentaenoic acid in bipolar depression: Randomised double-blind placebo-controlled study. *British Journal of Psychiatry*, 188, 46–50.

Galecki, P., Szemraj, J., Bienkiewicz, M., Zboralski, K., & Galecka, E. (2009). Oxidative stress parameters after combined fluoxetine and acetylsalicylic acid therapy in depressive patients. *Human Psychopharmacology*, 24(4), 277–286.

Goldstein, B. I., Kemp, D. E., Soczynska, J. K., & McIntyre, R. S. (2009). Inflammation and the phenomenology, pathophysiology, comorbidity, and treatment of bipolar disorder: A systematic review of the literature. *Journal of Clinical Psychiatry*, 70(8), 1078–1090.

Guloksuz, S., Altinbas, K., Aktas Cetin, E., Kenis, G., Bilgic Gazioglu, S., Deniz, G.,…van Os, J. (2012). Evidence for an association between tumor necrosis factor-alpha levels and lithium response. *Journal of Affective Disorders*, 143(1–3), 148–152.

Guloksuz, S., Cetin, E. A., Cetin, T., Deniz, G., Oral, E. T., & Nutt, D. J. (2010). Cytokine levels in euthymic bipolar patients. *Journal of Affective Disorders*, 126(3), 458–462.

Hamdani, N., Doukhan, R., Kurtlucan, O., Tamouza, R., & Leboyer, M. (2013). Immunity, inflammation, and bipolar disorder: Diagnostic and therapeutic implications. *Current Psychiatry Reports*, 15(9), 387.

Haroon, E., Raison, C. L., & Miller, A. H. (2012). Psychoneuroimmunology meets neuropsychopharmacology: Translational implications of the impact of inflammation on behavior. *Neuropsychopharmacology*, 37(1), 137–162.

Hayden, M. S., West, A. P., & Ghosh, S. (2006). NF-kappaB and the immune response. *Oncogene*, 25(51), 6758–6780.

Hope, S., Dieset, I., Agartz, I., Steen, N. E., Ueland, T., Melle, I.,...Andreassen, O. A. (2011). Affective symptoms are associated with markers of inflammation and immune activation in bipolar disorders but not in schizophrenia. *Journal of Psychiatric Research*, *45*(12), 1608–1616.

Hope, S., Ueland, T., Steen, N. E., Dieset, I., Lorentzen, S., Berg, A. O.,...Andreassen, O. A. (2013). Interleukin 1 receptor antagonist and soluble tumor necrosis factor receptor 1 are associated with general severity and psychotic symptoms in schizophrenia and bipolar disorder. *Schizophrenia Research*, *145*(1–3), 36–42.

Hornig, M., Goodman, D. B., Kamoun, M., & Amsterdam, J. D. (1998). Positive and negative acute phase proteins in affective subtypes. *Journal of Affective Disorders*, *49*(1), 9–18.

Keck, P. E. Jr., Mintz, J., McElroy, S. L., Freeman, M. P., Suppes, T., Frye, M. A.,...Post, R. M. (2006). Double-blind, randomized, placebo-controlled trials of ethyl-eicosapentanoate in the treatment of bipolar depression and rapid cycling bipolar disorder. *Biological Psychiatry*, *60*(9), 1020–1022.

Kim, Y. K., Jung, H. G., Myint, A. M., Kim, H., & Park, S. H. (2007). Imbalance between pro-inflammatory and anti-inflammatory cytokines in bipolar disorder. *Journal of Affective Disorders*, *104*(1–3), 91–95.

Knijff, E. M., Breunis, M. N., Kupka, R. W., de Wit, H. J., Ruwhof, C., Akkerhuis, G. W.,...Drexhage, H. A. (2007). An imbalance in the production of IL-1beta and IL-6 by monocytes of bipolar patients: Restoration by lithium treatment. *Bipolar Disorders*, *9*(7), 743–753.

Maes, M., Bosmans, E., Calabrese, J., Smith, R., & Meltzer, H. Y. (1995). Interleukin-2 and interleukin-6 in schizophrenia and mania: Effects of neuroleptics and mood stabilizers. *Journal of Psychiatric Research*, *29*(2), 141–152.

Meira-Lima, I. V., Pereira, A. C., Mota, G. F., Floriano, M., Araujo, F., Mansur, A. J.,...Vallada, H. (2003). Analysis of a polymorphism in the promoter region of the tumor necrosis factor alpha gene in schizophrenia and bipolar disorder: Further support for an association with schizophrenia. *Molecular Psychiatry*, *8*(8), 718–720.

Meyer, J. M., McEvoy, J. P., Davis, V. G., Goff, D. C., Nasrallah, H. A., Davis, S. M.,...Lieberman, J. A. (2009). Inflammatory markers in schizophrenia: Comparing antipsychotic effects in phase 1 of the clinical antipsychotic trials of intervention effectiveness study. *Biological Psychiatry*, *66*(11), 1013–1022.

Middle, F., Jones, I., Robertson, E., Lendon, C., & Craddock, N. (2000). Tumour necrosis factor alpha and bipolar affective puerperal psychosis. *Psychiatric Genetics*, *10*(4), 195–198.

Miller, A. H., Maletic, V., & Raison, C. L. (2009). Inflammation and its discontents: The role of cytokines in the pathophysiology of major depression. *Biological Psychiatry*, *65*(9), 732–741.

Miller, A. H., Pariante, C. M., & Pearce, B. D. (1999). Effects of cytokines on glucocorticoid receptor expression and function: Glucocorticoid resistance and relevance to depression. *Advances in Experimental Medicine and Biology*, *461*, 107–116.

Miller, C. L., Llenos, I. C., Dulay, J. R., & Weis, S. (2006). Upregulation of the initiating step of the kynurenine pathway in postmortem anterior cingulate cortex from individuals with schizophrenia and bipolar disorder. *Brain Research*, *1073–1074*, 25–37.

Modabbernia, A., Taslimi, S., Brietzke, E., & Ashrafi, M. (2013). Cytokine alterations in bipolar disorder: A meta-analysis of 30 studies. *Biological Psychiatry*, *74*(1), 15–25.

Mondelli, V., Cattaneo, A., Belvederi Murri, M., Di Forti, M., Handley, R., Hepgul, N.,...Pariante, C. M. (2011). Stress and inflammation reduce brain-derived neurotrophic factor expression in first-episode psychosis: A pathway to smaller hippocampal volume. *Journal of Clinical Psychiatry*, *72*(12), 1677–1684.

Mondelli, V., & Pariante, C. M. (2010). Adding aspirin to antipsychotics reduces psychopathology in adults with schizophrenia spectrum disorders. *Evidence-Based Mental Health*, *13*(4), 122.

Munkholm, K., Brauner, J. V., Kessing, L. V., & Vinberg, M. (2013). Cytokines in bipolar disorder vs. healthy control subjects: A systematic review and meta-analysis. *Journal of Psychiatric Research*, *47*(9), 1119–1133.

Myint, A. M., & Kim, Y. K. (2003). Cytokine-serotonin interaction through IDO: A neurodegeneration hypothesis of depression. *Medical Hypotheses*, *61*(5–6), 519–525.

Myint, A. M., Kim, Y. K., Verkerk, R., Park, S. H., Scharpe, S., Steinbusch, H. W.,...Leonard, B. E. (2007). Tryptophan breakdown pathway in bipolar mania. *Journal of Affective Disorders*, *102*(1–3), 65–72.

Nery, F. G., Monkul, E. S., Hatch, J. P., Fonseca, M., Zunta-Soares, G. B., Frey, B. N.,...Soares, J. C. (2008). Celecoxib as an adjunct in the treatment of depressive or mixed episodes of bipolar disorder: A double-blind, randomized, placebo-controlled study. *Human Psychopharmacology*, *23*(2), 87–94.

Pace, T. W., Hu, F., & Miller, A. H. (2007). Cytokine-effects on glucocorticoid receptor function: Relevance to glucocorticoid resistance and the pathophysiology and treatment of major depression. *Brain, Behavior, and Immunity*, *21*(1), 9–19.

Padmos, R. C., Hillegers, M. H., Knijff, E. M., Vonk, R., Bouvy, A., Staal, F. J.,...Drexhage, H. A. (2008). A discriminating messenger RNA signature for bipolar disorder formed by an aberrant expression of inflammatory genes in monocytes. *Archives of General Psychiatry*, *65*(4), 395–407.

Pae, C. U., Lee, K. U., Han, H., Serretti, A., & Jun, T. Y. (2004). Tumor necrosis factor alpha gene-G308A polymorphism associated with bipolar I disorder in the Korean population. *Psychiatry Research*, *125*(1), 65–68.

Papiol, S., Molina, V., Desco, M., Rosa, A., Reig, S., Sanz, J.,...Fañanás, L. (2008). Gray matter deficits in bipolar disorder are associated with genetic variability at interleukin-1 beta gene (2q13). *Genes, Brain and Behavior*, *7*(7), 796–801.

Pariante, C. M., & Lightman, S. L. (2008). The HPA axis in major depression: Classical theories and new developments. *Trends in Neurosciences*, *31*(9), 464–468.

Pariante, C. M., & Miller, A. H. (2001). Glucocorticoid receptors in major depression: Relevance to pathophysiology and treatment. *Biological Psychiatry*, *49*(5), 391–404.

Pariante, C. M., Pearce, B. D., Pisell, T. L., Sanchez, C. I., Po, C., Su, C.,...Miller, A. H. (1999). The proinflammatory cytokine, interleukin-1alpha, reduces glucocorticoid receptor translocation and function. *Endocrinology*, *140*(9), 4359–4366.

Raison, C. L., Borisov, A. S., Majer, M., Drake, D. F., Pagnoni, G., Woolwine, B. J.,...Miller, A. H. (2009). Activation of central nervous system inflammatory pathways by interferon-alpha: Relationship to monoamines and depression. *Biological Psychiatry*, *65*(4), 296–303.

Raison, C. L., Demetrashvili, M., Capuron, L., & Miller, A. H. (2005). Neuropsychiatric adverse effects of interferon-alpha: Recognition and management. *CNS Drugs*, *19*(2), 105–123.

Raison, C. L., Rutherford, R. E., Woolwine, B. J., Shuo, C., Schettler, P., Drake, D. F.,...Miller, A. H. (2013). A randomized controlled trial of the tumor necrosis factor antagonist infliximab for treatment-resistant depression: The role of baseline inflammatory biomarkers. *JAMA Psychiatry*, *70*(1), 31–41.

Rapaport, M. H., Guylai, L., & Whybrow, P. (1999). Immune parameters in rapid cycling bipolar patients before and after lithium treatment. *Journal of Psychiatric Research*, *33*(4), 335–340.

Remlinger-Molenda, A., Wojciak, P., Michalak, M., Karczewski, J., & Rybakowski, J. K. (2012). Selected cytokine profiles during remission in bipolar patients. *Neuropsychobiology*, *66*(3), 193–198.

Smith, R. S. (1991). The macrophage theory of depression. *Medical Hypotheses*, *35*(4), 298–306.

Soderlund, J., Olsson, S. K., Samuelsson, M., Walther-Jallow, L., Johansson, C., Erhardt, S.,...Engberg, G. (2011). Elevation of cerebrospinal fluid interleukin-1ss in bipolar disorder. *Journal of Psychiatry and Neuroscience*, *36*(2), 114–118.

Stolk, P., Souverein, P. C., Wilting, I., Leufkens, H. G., Klein, D. F., Rapoport, S. I.,...Heerdink, E. R. (2010). Is aspirin useful in patients on lithium? A pharmacoepidemiological study related to bipolar disorder. *Prostaglandins Leukotrienes and Essential Fatty Acids*, *82*(1), 9–14.

Stoll, A. L., Severus, W. E., Freeman, M. P., Rueter, S., Zboyan, H. A., Diamond, E.,...Marangell, L. B. (1999). Omega 3 fatty acids in bipolar disorder: A preliminary double-blind, placebo-controlled trial. *Archives of General Psychiatry*, *56*(5), 407–412.

Su, K. P. (2009). Biological mechanism of antidepressant effect of omega-3 fatty acids: How does fish oil act as a "mind-body interface"? *Neurosignals*, *17*(2), 144–152.

Tsai, S. Y., Chen, K. P., Yang, Y. Y., Chen, C. C., Lee, J. C., Singh, V. K.,...Leu, S. J. (1999). Activation of indices of cell-mediated immunity in bipolar mania. *Biological Psychiatry*, *45*(8), 989–994.

Tsai, S. Y., Chung, K. H., Wu, J. Y., Kuo, C. J., Lee, H. C., & Huang, S. H. (2012). Inflammatory markers and their relationships with leptin and insulin from acute mania to full remission in bipolar disorder. *Journal of Affective Disorders*, *136*(1–2), 110–116.

Tsai, S. Y., Yang, Y. Y., Kuo, C. J., Chen, C. C., & Leu, S. J. (2001). Effects of symptomatic severity on elevation of plasma soluble interleukin-2 receptor in bipolar mania. *Journal of Affective Disorders*, *64*(2–3), 185–193.

Tyring, S., Gottlieb, A., Papp, K., Gordon, K., Leonardi, C., Wang, A.,...Krishnan, R. (2006). Etanercept and clinical outcomes, fatigue, and depression in psoriasis: Double-blind placebo-controlled randomised phase III trial. *Lancet*, *367*(9504), 29–35.

Watson, S., Gallagher, P., Ritchie, J. C., Ferrier, I. N., & Young, A. H. (2004). Hypothalamic-pituitary-adrenal axis function in patients with bipolar disorder. *British Journal of Psychiatry*, *184*, 496–502.

Wieck, A., Grassi-Oliveira, R., do Prado, C. H., Rizzo, L. B., de Oliveira, A. S., Kommers-Molina, J.,...Bauer, M. E. (2013). Differential neuroendocrine and immune responses to acute psychosocial stress in women with type 1 bipolar disorder. *Brain, Behavior, and Immunity*, *34*, 47–55.

Wu, P. L., Liao, K. F., Peng, C. Y., Pariante, C. M., & Su, K. P. (2007). Manic episode associated with citalopram therapy for interferon-induced depression in a patient with chronic hepatitis C infection. *General Hospital Psychiatry*, *29*(4), 374–376.

Yoon, H. K., & Kim, Y. K. (2012). The T allele of the interferon-gamma +874A/T polymorphism is associated with bipolar disorder. *Nordic Journal of Psychiatry*, *66*(1), 14–18.

Zunszain, P. A., Anacker, C., Cattaneo, A., Carvalho, L. A., & Pariante, C. M. (2011). Glucocorticoids, cytokines and brain abnormalities in depression. *Progress in Neuro-Psychopharmacology & Biological Psychiatry*, *35*(3), 722–729.

Zunszain, P. A., Anacker, C., Cattaneo, A., Choudhury, S., Musaelyan, K., Myint, A. M.,...Pariante, C. M. (2012). Interleukin-1beta: A new regulator of the kynurenine pathway affecting human hippocampal neurogenesis. *Neuropsychopharmacology*, *37*(4), 939–949.

Zunszain, P. A., Hepgul, N., & Pariante, C. M. (2013). Inflammation and depression. *Current Topics in Behavioral Neurosciences*, *14*, 135–151.

11

CIRCADIAN RHYTHMS, SLEEP, AND THEIR TREATMENT IMPACT

Joshua Z. Tal and Michelle Primeau

In mania…there is almost complete sleeplessness, at most interrupted a few hours…. In states of depression in spite of great need for sleep, it is for the most part sensibly encroached upon.   E. KRAEPELIN, *1921*

INTRODUCTION

It is well recognized that sleep disruptions are present in many psychiatric conditions, and bipolar disorder is no exception. According to the *Diagnostic and Statistical Manual of Mental Disorders* (fourth edition, text revision [*DSM-IV-TR*]; American Psychiatric Association, 2000), disrupted sleep in some form is a common emanation of both manic and depressed episodes.

SLEEP DISRUPTION AND BIPOLAR DISORDER

The diagnostic criteria for a manic episode includes decreased need for sleep, and the criteria for a depressive episode includes either insomnia or hypersomnia (American Psychiatric Association, 2000). In manic episodes, the characteristic decreased need for sleep aligns well with the clinical presentation. The *DSM-IV-TR* portrays an episode of mania and hypomania through elevated and/or indiscriminate enthusiasm or irritability for a period of time (American Psychiatric Association, 2000). These energetic feelings often lead to goal-oriented behavior, and sleeping is often seen as an impediment to these behaviors. Following this line of thought, the rebounding bipolar depressed mood reflects the descent from mania; bipolar depression is often characterized by hypersomnia (Akiskal et al., 1983; Benazzi & Rihmer, 2000; Benazzi, 2003; Forty et al., 2008; Mitchell et al., 2001). Indeed, a patient's mood can be reflected in his or her sleep disruption. One study employed a mood induction protocol to evaluate effects of mood on sleep in euthymic bipolar subjects (Talbot, Hairston,

Eidelman, Gruber, & Harvey, 2009). The authors found that the induction of sadness led to significantly shorter sleep latencies, relative to controls (Talbot et al., 2009). In addition, they found prompting a happy mood led to significantly longer sleep latencies, akin to the effects of mania (Talbot et al., 2009)

MANIA AND SLEEP

The *DSM-IV-TR* corroborates this presentation by describing the decreased need for sleep as "almost invariably" present in manic episodes. The recent revision of the *DSM-IV-TR* (*Diagnostic and Statistical Manual of Mental Disorders*, fifth edition [*DSM-5*]; American Psychiatric Association, 2013) reinforces the increased energetic qualities of mania by adding in "persistently increased goal-directed activity or energy" into Criterion A of both manic and hypomanic episode criteria. Paired with this depiction, the *DSM-5* describes decreased need for sleep as "one of the most common features" of a manic or hypomanic episode (American Psychiatric Association, 2013). Indeed, one review cited 69% to 99% of surveyed participants experiencing this characteristic decreased need for sleep in manic episodes (Harvey, 2008). The studies included utilized either subjective self-report measures of sleep or polysomnography (PSG), a widely used objective sleep measurement using electroencephalography and other measures (Harvey, 2008; Kushida et al., 2005).

BIPOLAR DEPRESSION AND SLEEP

Disrupted sleep similarly aligns with the characteristic presentation of bipolar depression. Many studies describe hypersomnia as a differentiating feature of bipolar depression when compared to unipolar depression (Akiskal et al., 1983; Benazzi & Rihmer, 2000; Benazzi, 2003; Forty et al., 2008; Mitchell et al., 2001). The desire and ability to increase sleep conforms to feelings of emptiness and sadness, especially following a period of increased energy and lack of sleep (American Psychiatric Association, 2013). Although hypersomnia is very common, insomnia is also seen in bipolar depression, manifested as difficulty falling asleep, difficulty staying asleep, and/or waking up early during depressive episodes (Harvey, 2008).

INTEREPISODE EUTHYMIA AND SLEEP

Beyond the episodes themselves, many studies find interepisode sleep disruption a prevalent issue in bipolar populations. One report analyzing participants in the Systematic Treatment Enhancement Program for Bipolar Disorder (STEP-BD) studies observed 15% of its cohort of 483 euthymic participants reported at least mild sleep disturbance (Sylvia et al., 2012). Harvey, Schmidt, Scarnà, Semler, and Goodwin (2005) observed no significant differences in sleep efficiency and cognitions about sleep in a group of interepisode bipolar subjects compared to nonpolar insomnia subjects. Talbot et al. (2012) found similar sleep efficiency outcomes in a larger group ($n = 49$) of euthymic bipolar subjects relative to insomnia subjects. Multiple investigators have used actigraphy, an objective way of monitoring sleep and activity levels, to confirm interepisode variability in sleep patterns, as well as objective sleep disruption (Jones, Hare, & Evershed, 2005; Millar, Espie, & Scott, 2004; Ritter et al., 2012). Sleep disturbance can be a clinically relevant concern for patients with bipolar disorder even when euthymic.

BIPOLAR DISORDER AND SLEEP DISORDERS

Nights of insomnia, hypersomnia, and reduced need for sleep may not be simply a symptom of the psychiatric condition itself but rather symptomatic of a deeper issue. A sleep disturbance may be a result of a sleep disorder, such as sleep disordered breathing, narcolepsy, periodic limb movement disorder, or even endogenous primary insomnia. Accurate differential diagnosis is critical to accurate and successful treatment. Attended, overnight PSG is considered the current gold standard diagnostic procedure for sleep disordered breathing and periodic limb movement disorder (Kushida et al., 2005). PSG with the addition of a multiple sleep latency test is the primary method of diagnosing

narcolepsy (Kushida et al., 2005). Actigraphy, paired with an in-depth clinical interview, can rule out primary insomnia (Lichstein et al., 2006). If a primary sleep disorder is diagnosed, it will require specific, focused treatment in addition to treatment for the primary mood disorder.

CIRCADIAN RHYTHM

Although not a distinct clinical diagnosis, sleep disturbances in bipolar disorder often reflect a misaligned and abnormal circadian rhythm (Murray & Harvey, 2010). Circadian rhythm refers to the body's biological process for keeping time. The term *circadian* is derived from Latin: *circa* means "around" or "approximately" and *dia* means "day." Thus the term *circadian* refers to the rhythm that undertakes a full cycle approximately the length of one day. The circadian rhythm was proven in humans in 1896, when Patrick and Gilbert discovered that three human subjects displayed predictable patterns of sleepiness following three nights of sleep deprivation in isolation. They realized there must be the presence of an internal, biological, time-keeping mechanism, one that can potentially function outside external stimuli.

ZEITGEBERS AND MELATONIN

Although able to run independently, the circadian rhythm is perpetuated by environmental cues that convey time points, called *zeitgebers* ("timegivers"), which helps individuals' internal rhythms align with their environmental ones (Harvey, 2008). The primary mammalian *zeitgeber* for the human circadian rhythm is the presence of light and its absence, darkness (Roenneberg & Foster, 1997). The human time-keeper resides in the suprachiasmatic nucleus (SCN) of the hypothalamus, and it collects and responds to cues to entrain the body's biological system into accordance with the environment (i.e., sleeping at night, staying awake in the day; Reppert & Weaver, 2002). Melatonin and cortisol are the two hormones that enact the SCN's time-keeping system, by sending time cues to bodily organs with directions for operation (Reppert & Weaver, 2002). Photoreceptors in the eye respond to light by signaling to the SCN to have melatonin synthesized, which aids in causing drowsiness and other biological functions of sleep (Redwine, Hauger, Gillin, & Irwin, 2000). Melatonin not only causes sleep; it gives also insight into the helpful effects of sleep itself. When melatonin is active, it plays a part in initiating immune function, especially seasonal adjustments (Nelson & Drazen,

1999). It similarly displays antioxidant properties (Reiter, Tan, & Maldonado, 2005). Melatonin marshals some of sleep's restorative properties.

MELATONIN, SEROTONIN, AND MOOD

Melatonin is connected to mood disorders. Melatonin is a neurohormonal byproduct of serotonin, a key neurotransmitter underlying the pathology of mood disorders (Lanfumey, Mongeau, & Hamon, 2013). Consequently, mood disorders are one of the primary mental health categories displaying a prominent circadian rhythmicity (Lanfumey et al., 2013). Major depressive disorder is often seen with significant diurnal variations, meaning they get worse or better depending on the time of day. One large sample of 3744 subjects with major depressive disorder from the STEP-BD study found over 20% of the sample displayed diurnal variations (Morris et al., 2007). Other circadian rhythmicity is seen with seasonal affective disorder and bipolar disorder, where environmental factors can also influence mood (Thompson, Stinson, Fernandez, Fine, & Isaacs, 1988).

CIRCADIAN RHYTHM AND BIPOLAR DISORDER

MELATONIN AND BIPOLAR DISORDER

Melatonin and its secretion have become topics of increased interest in understanding bipolar disorder. One study of euthymic bipolar subjects found significantly lower melatonin levels and later peak times for melatonin secretion when compared with unipolar depressed subjects and controls (Nurnberger et al., 2000). Some researchers have suggested that the lower melatonin levels, and thus offset circadian rhythm, may be due to a suppression of melatonin in response to light (Lewy, Wehr, Goodwin, Newsome, & Rosenthal, 1981; Nathan, Burrows, & Norman, 1999). They hoped to prove that this suppression of melatonin response may be the characteristic biomarker of bipolar disorder (Lewy et al., 1981; Nathan et al., 1999). However, Nurnberger et al. (2000) did not find evidence for melatonin suppression in bipolar disorder subjects relative to controls, despite evidence of lowered melatonin levels. Nevertheless, research investigating the effects of commonly used bipolar disorder medications, such as lithium carbonate and sodium valproate, on melatonin suppression found a distinct before and after decrease in melatonin

suppression in light in healthy controls (Hallam, Olver, Horgan, McGrath, & Norman, 2005; Hallam, Olver, & Norman, 2005). Although the mechanism of melatonin's effect on bipolar disorder is mixed, it appears related at least in part to the circadian disturbances observed in bipolar disorder.

LIGHT AND BIPOLAR DISORDER

Some evidence suggests that the potent *zeitgieber* light is of even greater importance for individuals with bipolar disorder. Light exposure may be helpful for resetting offset circadian rhythms. Some studies suggest a hypersensitivity to light in individuals with bipolar disorder (Lewy et al., 1981; Nathan et al., 1999). Sit, Wisner, Hanusa, Stull, and Terman (2007) took a series of nine women with either bipolar I disorder or bipolar II disorder currently experiencing depression and exposed them to bright light therapy either in the morning or midday. With the active morning light condition, three out of four participants developed mixed state, but those provided with midday light sustained a greater response, causing the authors to reason that the bipolar women were more sensitive to morning light (Sit et al., 2007). Other groups have similarly noticed an increase in adverse effects with morning bright light therapy (Kripke, 1991; Liebenluft et al., 1995). However, because light is an important way of normalizing an offset circadian rhythm, the authors suggest brief treatments, such as 15 min., at the midday point instead of early morning (Sit et al., 2007).

EVIDENCE OF A CIRCADIAN RHYTHM DISTURBANCE

When examining objective measures of sleep variables using actigraphy, subjects with bipolar disorder display variable and highly erratic sleep cycles, both during and between episodes, when compared to controls. Jones et al. (2005) utilized actigraphy to compare interepisode bipolar subjects to gender-matched controls for seven days. They found sleep fragmentation and circadian variability to be the only predictor differentiating the bipolar group from controls (Jones et al., 2005). A similar study utilizing actigraphy over five nights also found that circadian variability differentiated from controls, though sleep duration and subjective sleep latency also were nonsignificantly elevated (Millar et al., 2004). More recently, Ritter et al. (2012) confirmed the same actigraphic findings in euthymic bipolar patients. Interestingly, patients at high risk (first- or second-degree relative with the disorder or prior subthreshold symptoms) also had increased sleep disturbance, duration, latency, and variability (Ritter et al., 2012). Further studies verifying abnormal circadian rhythms during and after clinical recovery suggest a trait feature of circadian rhythm abnormalities (Salvatore et al., 2008).

GENETICS

Due to the high prevalence of circadian abnormalities in depressed, manic, interepisode, and recovery state, some researchers have looked to genetics and biomarkers of the connection between circadian rhythm and bipolar disorder (Milhiet, Etain, Boudebesse, & Bellivier, 2011). The hope is the genetic connection may increase understanding of either the etiology or the pathology of bipolar disorder. Indeed, of all the mental disorders, bipolar disorder presents the strongest evidence for associated genetics (Milhiet et al., 2011). Identified circadian single nucleotide polymorphisms *CLOCK, BMAL1, Timeless (TIM), EGR3, PER3,* and *VIP* were all identified in bipolar disorder subjects; however, the varied reproducibility of these studies questions the utility of these identifications (Lamont, Coutu, Cermakian, & Boivin, 2010; Lee et al., 2010; Mansour et al., 2009; Milhiet et al., 2011; Murray & Harvey, 2010; Rocha et al., 2010; Soria et al., 2010). *CLOCK* is one of the main genes responsible for the transcription of circadian promoting processes, thus subjects without the *CLOCK* gene seem to promote delayed sleep latencies and higher eveningness preference scores (Katzenberg et al., 1998). As such, the *CLOCK* gene has one of the most compelling evidence sets linking it to bipolar disorder (Benedetti et al., 2003; Lamont et al., 2010; Lee et al., 2010).

NEUROBIOLOGY

As stated, serotonin's implications may be further evidence of a distinct neurobiological connection. Sleep deprivation's negative effect on mood has been established, and serotonin may provide the link exacerbating normal mood variability into clinical mood disorders (Harvey, Murray, Chandler, & Soehner, 2011). Researchers have supported this idea, finding an association with polymorphisms of the serotonin transporter genes and sleep issues in bipolar disorder (Benedetti, Colombo, Barbini, Campori, & Smeraldi, 1999; Lotrich & Pollock, 2004; Luddington, Mandadapu, Husk, & El-Mallakh, 2009). Benedetti et al. found that bipolar subjects who were heterozygotic and homozygotic for the short variant of a serotonin-linked polymorphic region showed significantly worse mood amelioration

following sleep deprivation. This inability to regulate mood following sleep deprivation underscores the importance of the serotonergic system.

On a neurological level, studies examining sleep deprivation have found decreased medial-prefrontal cortical activity and increased amygdala activation following sleep loss, leading to emotional dysregulation and negative mood (Yoo, Gujar, Hu, Jolesz, & Walker, 2007). Similarly, research examining bipolar disorder subjects have elucidated analogous deficits in prefrontal cortical mediations of emotion (McKenna & Eyler, 2012). Further research is needed to understand the mechanism of sleep loss in people with bipolar disorder.

SLEEP DISRUPTION AS AN INDICATOR OF BIPOLAR DISORDER

SLEEP ARCHITECTURE

As sleep is disrupted in bipolar disorder, investigators have attempted to identify trait markers of the disorder using PSG. PSG is considered to be the "gold standard" in sleep assessment, as it can provide information that cannot be obtained in utilizing self-report or activity monitoring, such as sleep latency, amount of time spent awake after falling asleep, total sleep time, sleep efficiency, and sleep stages. These variables, in turn, may be able to provide a window into underlying neurophysiologic abnormalities.

Classifying the sleep architecture of bipolar disorder presents a unique problem, in that the varied mood states have very different sleep experiences, presumably with differences on PSG. Though limited, more PSG studies have been completed with depressed bipolar patients than with manic bipolar patients, and, interestingly, some differences have been noted between the two states (Harvey, 2008). In the depressed state, patients with bipolar disorder have been found to have both increased and decreased time to the first rapid eye movement (REM) period, as well as increased REM density and REM fragmentation (Harvey, 2008). However, in the manic state, subjects demonstrated reduced total sleep time and seemingly reduced time to the first REM period (Harvey, 2008). Taken together, it is evident that no clear associations have yet been identified in the sleep architecture of patients with bipolar disorder, though some alteration to REM sleep may exist. REM sleep is associated with emotional processing (Walker & van der Helm, 2009), and so alterations to REM sleep may underlie the affective changes noted with each behavioral state.

SLEEP AS A TRIGGER

Just as sleep deprivation leads to deleterious effects on mood, sleep can trigger manic and hypomanic symptoms (Wehr, 1992). When depressed rapid cycling subjects under experimental conditions were made to maintain wakefulness for 40 hours, all either switched out of depression or into mania/hypomania (Wehr, Goodwin, Wirz-Justice, Breitmaier, & Craig, 1982). However, sleep deprivation occurring as a result of medical conditions or work-related deprivation has also been shown to trigger mania (Wehr, 1989, 1992). In fact, prior night's sleep duration is a consistent predictor of hypomanic symptoms the following day, and sleep deprivation occurring in the course of mania has been observed to exacerbate manic symptoms by psychiatric nurse ratings (Barbini, Bertelli, Colombo, & Smeraldi, 1996; Liebenluft, Albert, Rosenthal, & Wehr, 1996).

Consequent to these observations, sleep deprivation has been characterized as the "final common pathway" to the occurrence of mania (Wehr, Sack, & Rosenthal, 1987). In this model, a variety of triggers may precipitate sleep curtailment, which then brings out manic/hypomanic symptoms, which further reinforces the relative reduced amounts of sleep (Figure 11.1). This model has been difficult to test directly due to ethical issues related to inducing manic symptoms in a vulnerable population. However, when sleep deprivation was implemented as a therapeutic intervention for those with bipolar depression, 5% of subjects experiencing bipolar

depression switched to mania or hypomania, regardless of medication status (Colombo, Benedetti, Barbini, Campori, & Smeraldi, 1999). This provides indirect evidence in support of the final common pathway model.

SLEEP AS A PREDICTOR

Because manic symptoms can be induced by sleep deprivation, it therefore follows that sleep disruption may harken the onset of a manic episode. In a systematic review of prodromal symptoms for affective episodes, Jackson, Cavanagh, and Scott (2003) confirmed that sleep disturbance is the most frequently cited prodromal symptom to a manic episode, with 77% of 1,191 subjects in studies reviewed identifying sleep disturbance before the episode. Additionally, sleep disturbance was noted to precede a depressive episode in 24% of individuals (Jackson et al., 2003). Similarly, in children with bipolar disorder (mean age 10.6 years), parents noted sleep disturbance as the initial disturbance 45% of the time and frequently occurring before age 3 (Faedda, Baldessarini, Glovinsky, & Austin, 2004). The early age of onset of sleep disruption and mood symptoms further supports the heritability of bipolar disorder, though family history was not elaborated on in this cohort. Longitudinal work examining the onset of bipolar symptoms in children at high risk for development of bipolar disorders (i.e., offspring of a parent with well-characterized bipolar disorder)

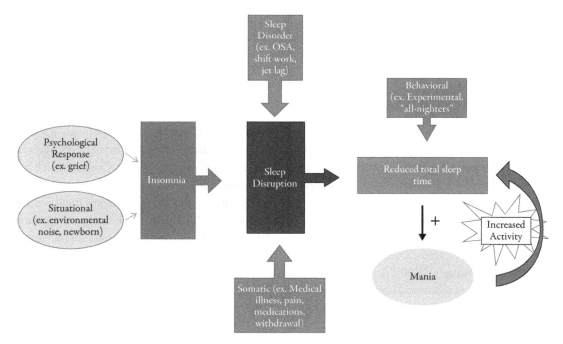

Figure 11.1 Sleep in the final common pathway leading to mania. Sleep disruption (i.e. from sleep disorders, environmental disturbances) or deprivation (i.e. from drugs, stress or external schedule), leads to a reduction in total sleep time that both precipitates and perpetuates the manic state. Adapted from Wehr, 1989.

similarly points to sleep disturbance preceding the manifestation of affective symptoms in adolescence (Duffy, 2010; Duffy, Alda, Crawford, Milin, & Grof, 2007).

Many factors have been purported as triggers of a manic/hypomanic episode, including stressful life events, goal-attainment events, seasonality, and medications (Poudfoot, Doran, Manicavasagar, & Parker, 2011). Additionally, a change in sleep can signal an impending mood episode. Bauer et al. (2006) showed that a change in sleep and time in bed over 3 hours can be a prodromal signal of mood change. They showed that sleep *duration* is more strongly correlated to mood than is the relative timing at which sleep occurs, and, in one cohort, euthymic patients with bipolar disorder demonstrated a mean total sleep time approaching 9 hours (Bauer et al., 2009; Gruber et al., 2011). However, short (less than 6 hours) and long (more than 9 hours) sleep durations are both associated with decreased quality of life in patients with bipolar disorder (Gruber et al., 2011). Sleep *variability* was noted to be associated with increased depression and mania severity but not the presence of mania itself (Gruber et al., 2011).

SLEEP AS A TREATMENT COMPONENT

Manipulations of the sleep–wake cycle have been used to probe the relationship of sleep and bipolar disorder. However, such manipulations have important treatment implications as well. The final section of this chapter reviews the use of sleep-related treatment interventions in bipolar disorder.

SLEEP DEPRIVATION/"WAKE THERAPY"

Sleep deprivation, either total or partial, has been noted to improve the mood of depressed bipolar patients (Wehr, 1992; Barbini et al., 1998; for a review, see Benedetti, 2012). Due to the observation that such mood improvement occurs after a prolonged wake period but is limited by a high rate of relapse after subsequent recovery sleep, some have tested "wake therapy" as a treatment for bipolar disorder (Benedetti, 2012; Wu & Bunney, 1990). A significant limitation of wake therapy is that the mood improvement is not sustained when implemented alone; only 5% of responders to wake therapy sustained the benefit with resumption of normal sleep (Benedetti & Colombo 2011). As such, sleep restriction has been combined with medications such as lithium (Benedetti et al., 1999; Grube & Hartwich,

1990), pindolol (Smeraldi, Benedetti, Barbini, Campori, & Colombo, 1999), and other chronotherapeutics, such as light (Colombo et al., 2000). Wake therapy paired with medications has shown sustained mood improvement, with lower manic relapse rates than antidepressants alone (Benedetti, 2012). Functional MRI studies evaluating the adjunctive use of wake therapy for depression suggests the equivalent neurobiological changes of serotonin in the brain equal to six weeks of conventional antidepressants, paired with up to a 50% reduction in Hamilton Depression Scale Scores (Benedetti & Colombo, 2011).

TIME IN BED EXTENSION/"DARK THERAPY"

Just as curtailed sleep can trigger manic symptoms, enforced extended time in bed has been shown to be somewhat helpful in controlling rapid cycling patients. In one case study, an individual with rapid-cycling bipolar disorder was prescribed extended bed rest (Wirz-Justice et al., 1999). In this instance, her rapid cycling stopped immediately, though she remained depressed until the later addition of bright light therapy. Subsequent work implementing a 14-hour dark period in 16 consecutively admitted manic patients on lithium or valproate successfully hastened recovery from the manic episode and reduced the need for rescue antipsychotics (Barbini et al., 2005). However, benefit was not attained in those with manic symptoms longer than two weeks.

NONPHARMACOLOGICAL TREATMENTS

Cognitive behavioral therapy for insomnia

With all the usual sedating pharmacology and corresponding side effects seen in treating bipolar disorder, additional sleeping medication and its side effects may decrease medication compliance altogether. Cognitive Behavioral Therapy for Insomnia (CBT-I) is an efficacious, nonpharmacological treatment with durable effects in adults with insomnia (Edinger & Means, 2005). The key components of CBT-I are time-in-bed restriction, stimulus control, sleep hygiene, and cognitive restructuring surrounding sleep-related thoughts (Edinger & Means, 2004). Certain instructions inherent to stimulus control, whereby patients are asked to "get into bed only once sleepy" and "get out of bed if not asleep within 20 minutes," may introduce short-term sleep deprivation and theoretically can trigger manic/hypomanic symptoms (Wehr, 1992). In addition, cognitive restructuring may be difficult, as some of bipolar patients' beliefs about their sleep may in fact be true; for example, "If I don't sleep enough, I might become manic." Nevertheless, the significant variability of sleep patterns observed in patients with bipolar disorder (Jones et al., 2005; Millar et al., 2004; Ritter et al., 2012) suggests that CBT-I would be helpful.

It is important, therefore, to modify the treatment protocol somewhat to account for such issues. Recently, Kaplan, and Harvey (2013) examined the treatment efficacy of CBT-I in a group of 15 euthymic bipolar subjects, utilizing modifications for their specific pathology. Setting consistent bedtime and rise times with customized wind-down and wake-up routines, along with individualized modifications of stimulus control, were successful at reducing insomnia severity scores, with only mild elevation in mood rating scales (Kaplan and Harvey, 2013).

While the strongest *zeitgieber* is the exposure to sunlight, other signals, such as social interactions, eating, and physical activity, can also impact the circadian rhythm. Evidence suggests that disrupted social rhythms can precipitate a manic (Malkoff-Schwartz et al., 2000) or depressive (Sylvia et al., 2009) episode. Individuals with bipolar spectrum disorders experience greater social rhythm disruption with positive or negative life events and greater subsequent sleep loss than controls (Boland et al., 2012).

Interpersonal and social rhythms therapy (IPSRT) is based on the premise that, in vulnerable individuals, disrupted social *zeitgebers* leads to circadian disruption, creating somatic symptoms and then perpetuated as a mood episode (Frank, 2007). IPSRT is built on the framework of interpersonal therapy (IPT), with an initial focus on interpersonal relationships and routines, selecting from among the IPT focus areas as may relate to the event that precipitated the individual's mood episodes. The intermediate and maintenance phases of the treatment then focus on modifications for the IPT problem area and the stabilization of social rhythms, even in the face of external disruption (Frank, 2007). Similar to CBT-I, treatment includes work with sleep rhythms, by modification of the patient's time in bed and stabilizing sleep–wake rhythms (Harvey, 2008). IPSRT has been shown to be successful at increasing the time to relapse in patients with bipolar disorder, reducing time to recovery with bipolar depression, and reducing risk of suicide (Frank 2007). It has been successfully implemented in group formats as well (Bouwkamp et al., 2013).

CONCLUSION

Sleep disruption is common to bipolar mania, hypomania, depression, and euthymia. Due to the observed cyclical nature of the disorder, much work has focused on the impact of circadian rhythms, and, taken together, it is evident that sleep–wake variability plays a role in the experience of bipolar disorder. Psychological therapies targeting sleep specifically have been found to be effective in reducing sleep disruption, stabilizing mood, and reducing risk for relapse.

Disclosure statement: Dr. Michelle Primeau has no conflicts of interest. Joshua Z. Tal has no conflicts of interest.

REFERENCES

Akiskal, H. S., Walker, P., Puzantian, V. R., King, D., Rosenthal, T. L., & Dranon, M. (1983). Bipolar outcome in the course of depressive illness. Phenomenologic, familial, and pharmacologic predictors. *Journal of Affective Disorders, 5*(2), 115–128.

American Psychiatric Association. (2000). *Diagnostic and statistical manual of mental disorders* (4th ed., text rev.). Washington, DC: Author.

American Psychiatric Association. (2013). *Diagnostic and statistical manual of mental disorders* (5th ed.). Washington, DC: Author.

Bauer, M., Grof, P., Rasgon, N., Bschor, T., Glenn, T., & Whybrow, P. C. (2006). Temporal relation between sleep and mood in patients with bipolar disorder. *Bipolar Disorders, 8*, 160–167.

Bauer, M., Glenn, T., Grof, P., Rasgon, N., Alda, M., Marsh, W.,…Whybrow, P. C. (2009). Comparison of sleep/wake parameters for self-monitoring bipolar disorder. *Journal of Affective Disorders, 116*, 170–175.

Barbini, B., Benedetti, F., Colombo, C., Dotoli, D., Bernasconi, A., Cigala-Fulgosi, M., … Smeraldi, E. (2005). Dark therapy for mania: A pilot study. *Bipolar Disorder, 7*, 98–101.

Barbini, B., Bertelli, S., Colombo, C., & Smeraldi, E. (1996). Sleep loss, a possible factor in augmenting manic episode. *Psychiatry Research, 65*, 121–125.

Barbini, B., Colombo, C., Benedetti, F., Campori, E., Bellodi, L., & Smeraldi, E. (1998). The unipolar-bipolar dichotomy and the response to sleep deprivation. *Psychiatry Research, 79*, 43–50.

Benazzi, F. (2003). Clinical differences between bipolar II depression and unipolar major depressive disorder: Lack of an effect of age. *Journal of Affective Disorders, 75*(2), 191–195. doi:10.1016/S0165-0327(02)00047-2

Benazzi, F, & Rihmer, Z. (2000). Sensitivity and specificity of *DSM-IV* atypical features for bipolar II disorder diagnosis. *Psychiatry Research, 93*(3), 257–262.

Benedetti, F. (2012). Antidepressant chronotherapeutics for bipolar depression. *Dialogues Clinical Neuroscience, 14*, 401–411.

Benedetti, F., & Colombo, C. (2011). Sleep deprivation in mood disorders. *Neuropsychobiology, 64*(3), 141–151. doi:10.1159/000328947

Benedetti, F., Colombo, C., Barbini, B., Campori, E., & Smeraldi, E. (1999). Ongoing lithium treatment prevents relapse after total sleep deprivation. *Journal of Clinical Psychopharmacology, 19*, 240–245.

Benedetti, F., Serretti, A., Colombo, C., Barbini, B., Lorenzi, C., Campori, E., & Smeraldi, E. (2003). Influence of CLOCK gene polymorphism on circadian mood fluctuation and illness recurrence in bipolar depression. *American Journal of Medical Genetics Part B: Neuropsychiatric Genetics, 123*(1), 23–26. doi:10.1002/ajmg.b.20038

Benedetti, F., Serretti, A., Colombo, C., Campori, E., Barbini, B., di Bella, D., & Smeraldi, E. (1999). Influence of a functional polymorphism within the promoter of the serotonin transporter gene on the effects of total sleep deprivation in bipolar depression. *American Journal of Psychiatry, 156*(9), 1450–1452.

Boland, E. M., Bender, R. E., Alloy, L. B., Conner, B. T., LaBelle, D. R., & Abramson, L. Y. (2012). Life events and social rhtyhms in bipolar spectrum disorders: An examination of social rhythm sensitivity. *Journal of Affective Disorders, 139*, 264–272.

Bouwkamp, C. G., de Kruiff, M. E., van Troost, T. M., Snippe, D., Blom, M. J., de Winter, R. F. P., & Haffmans, M. J. (2013). Interpersonal and social rhythm group therapy for patients with bipolar disorder. *International Journal of Group Psychotherapy, 63*(1), 97–115.

Colombo, C., Benedetti, F., Barbini, B., Campori, E., & Smeraldi, E. (1999). Rate of switch from depression into mania after therapeutic sleep deprivation in bipolar depression. *Psychiatry Research, 86*, 267–270.

Colombo, C., Lucca, A., Benedetti, F., Barbini, B., Campori, E., & Smeraldi, E. (2000). Total sleep deprivation combined with lithium and light therapy in bipolar depression: Replication of main effects and interaction. *Psychiatry Research, 95*, 43–53.

Duffy, A. (2010). The early natural history of bipolar disorder: What we have learned from longitudinal high-risk research. *Canadian Journal of Psychiatry, 55*, 477–485.

Duffy, A., Alda, M., Crawford, L., Milin, R., & Grof, P. (2007). The early manifestations of bipolar disorder: A longitudinal prospective study of the offspring of bipolar parents. *Bipolar Disorder, 9*, 828–838.

Edinger, J. D., & Means, M. K. (2005). Cognitive-behavioral therapy for primary insomnia. *Clinical Psychology Review, 25*, 539–558.

Faedda, G. L., Baldessarini, R. J., Glovinsky, I. P., & Austin, N. B. (2004). Pediatric bipolar disorder: Phenomenology and course of illness. *Bipolar Disorder, 6*, 305–313.

Forty, L., Smith, D., Jones, L., Jones, I., Caesar, S., Cooper, C., ... Craddock, N. (2008). Clinical differences between bipolar and unipolar depression. *British Journal of Psychiatry, 192*(5), 388–389. doi:10.1192/bjp.bp.107.045294

Frank, E. (2007). Interpersonal and social rhythm therapy: A means of improving depression and preventing relapse in bipolar disorder. *Journal of Clinical Psychology: In Session, 63*, 463–473.

Grube, M., & Hartwich, P. (1990). Maintenance of antidepressant effect of sleep deprivation with the help of lithium. *European Archives of Psychiatry and Clinical Neuroscience, 240*, 60–61.

Gruber, J., Miklowitz, D. J., Harvey, A. G., Frank, E., Kupfer, D., Thase, M. E., ... Ketter, T. A. (2011). Sleep matters: Sleep functioning and course of illness in bipolar disorder. *Journal of Affective Disorders. 134*(3), 416–420.

Hallam, K. T., Olver, J. S., Horgan, J. E., McGrath, C., & Norman, T. R. (2005). Low doses of lithium carbonate reduce melatonin light sensitivity in healthy volunteers. *The International Journal of Neuropsychopharmacology, 8*(2), 255–259. doi:10.1017/S1461145704004894

Hallam, K. T., Olver, J. S., & Norman, T. R. (2005). Effect of sodium valproate on nocturnal melatonin sensitivity to light in healthy volunteers. *Neuropsychopharmacology, 30*(7), 1400–1404. doi:10.1038/sj.npp.1300739

Harvey, A. G. (2008). Sleep and circadian rhythms in bipolar disorder: Seeking synchrony, harmony, and regulation. *American Journal of Psychiatry, 165*(7), 820–829. doi:10.1176/appi.ajp.2008.08010098

Harvey, A. G., Murray, G., Chandler, R. A., & Soehner, A. (2011). Sleep disturbance as transdiagnostic: Consideration of neurobiological mechanisms. *Clinical Psychology Review, 31*(2), 225–235. doi:10.1016/j.cpr.2010.04.003

Harvey, A. G., Schmidt, D. A., Scarnà, A., Semler, C. N., & Goodwin, G. M. (2005). Sleep-related functioning in euthymic patients with bipolar disorder, patients with insomnia, and subjects without sleep problems. *American Journal of Psychiatry, 162*(1), 50–57. doi:10.1176/appi.ajp.162.1.50

Jackson. A., Cavanagh, J., & Scott, J. (2003). A systematic review of manic and depressive prodromes. *Journal of Affective Disorders, 74*, 209–217.

Jones, S. H., Hare, D. J., & Evershed, K. (2005). Actigraphic assessment of circadian activity and sleep patterns in bipolar disorder. *Bipolar Disorders, 7*(2), 176–186. doi:10.1111/j.1399-5618.2005.00187.x

Kaplan, K. A. & Harvey, A. G. (2013). Behavioral treatment of insomnia in bipolar disorder. *American Journal of Psychiatry, 170*, 716–720.

Katzenberg, D., Young, T., Finn, L., Lin, L., King, D. P., Takahashi, J. S., & Mignot, E. (1998). A CLOCK polymorphism associated with human diurnal preference. *Sleep: Journal of Sleep Research & Sleep Medicine, 21*(6), 569–576. Retrieved from http://psycnet.apa.org/psycinfo/1998-12423-001

Kraepelin, E. (1921). *Manic depressive insanity and paranoia* (R. M. Barclay Trans.). Edinburgh, UK: Livingstone.

Kripke, D. F. (1991). Timing of phototherapy and occurrence of mania. *Biological Psychiatry, 29*, 1156–1157.

Kushida, C. A., Littner, M. R., Morgenthaler, T., Alessi, C. A., Bailey, D., Coleman J. Jr., ... Kramer, M. (2005). Practice parameters for the indications for polysomnography and related procedures: an update for 2005. *Sleep, 28*(4), 499–521.

Lamont, E. W., Coutu, D. L., Cermakian, N., & Boivin, D. B. (2010). Circadian rhythms and clock genes in psychotic disorders. *The Israel Journal of Psychiatry and Related Sciences, 47*(1), 27–35.

Lanfumey, L., Mongeau, R., & Hamon, M. (2013). Biological rhythms and melatonin in mood disorders and their treatments. *Pharmacology & Therapeutics, 138*(2), 176–184. doi:10.1016/j.pharmthera.2013.01.005

Lee, K. Y., Song, J. Y., Kim, S. H., Kim, S. C., Joo, E.-J., Ahn, Y. M., & Kim, Y. S. (2010). Association between CLOCK 3111T/C and preferred circadian phase in Korean patients with bipolar disorder. *Progress in Neuro-Psychopharmacology & Biological Psychiatry, 34*(7), 1196–1201. doi:10.1016/j.pnpbp.2010.06.010

Lewy, A. J., Wehr, T. A., Goodwin, F. K., Newsome, D. A., & Rosenthal, N. E. (1981). Manic-depressive patients may be supersensitive to light. *Lancet, 1*(8216), 383–384.

Lichstein, K. L., Stone, K. C., Donaldson, J., Nau, S. D., Soeffing, J. P., Murray, D., ... others. (2006). Actigraphy validation with insomnia. *SLEEP 29*(2), 232.

Liebenluft, E., Albert, P. S., Rosenthal, N. E., & Wehr, T. A. (1996). Relationship between sleep and mood in patients with rapid-cycling bipolar disorder. *Psychiatry Research, 63*, 161–168.

Liebenluft, E., Turner, E. H., Feldman-Naim, S., Schwartz, P. J., Wehr, R. A., & Rosenthal. N. E. (1995). Light therapy in patients with rapid cycling bipolar disorder: Preliminary results. *Psychopharmacology Bulletin, 31*, 705–10.

Lotrich, F. E., & Pollock, B. G. (2004). Meta-analysis of serotonin transporter polymorphisms and affective disorders. *Psychiatric Genetics, 14*(3), 121–129.

Luddington, N. S., Mandadapu, A., Husk, M., & El-Mallakh, R. S. (2009). Clinical implications of genetic variation in the serotonin transporter promoter region: A review. *Primary Care Companion to the Journal of Clinical Psychiatry, 11*(3), 93.

Malkoff-Schwartz, S., Frank, E., Anderson, B. P., Hlastala, S. A., Luther, J. F., Sherril, J. T., ... Kupfer, D. J. (2000). Social rhythm disruption and stressful life events in the onset of bipolar and unipolar episodes. *Psychological Medicine, 20*, 1005–1016.

Mansour, H. A., Talkowski, M. E., Wood, J., Chowdari, K. V., McClain, L., Prasad, K., ... Nimgaonkar, V. L. (2009). Association study of 21 circadian genes with bipolar I disorder, schizoaffective disorder, and schizophrenia. *Bipolar Disorders, 11*(7), 701–710. doi:10.1111/j.1399-5618.2009.00756.x

McKenna, B. S., & Eyler, L. T. (2012). Overlapping prefrontal systems involved in cognitive and emotional processing in euthymic bipolar disorder and following sleep deprivation: A review of functional neuroimaging studies. *Clinical Psychology Review, 32*(7), 650–663. doi:10.1016/j.cpr.2012.07.003

Milhiet, V., Etain, B., Boudebesse, C., & Bellivier, F. (2011). Circadian biomarkers, circadian genes and bipolar disorders.

Journal of Physiology, Paris, 105(4–6), 183–189. doi:10.1016/j.jphysparis.2011.07.002

Millar, A., Espie, C. A., & Scott, J. (2004). The sleep of remitted bipolar outpatients: A controlled naturalistic study using actigraphy. *Journal of Affective Disorders, 80*, 145–153.

Mitchell, P. B., Wilhelm, K., Parker, G., Austin, M. P., Rutgers, P., & Malhi, G. S. (2001). The clinical features of bipolar depression: A comparison with matched major depressive disorder patients. *Journal of Clinical Psychiatry, 62*(3), 212–216.

Morris, D. W., Rush, A. J., Jain, S., Fava, M., Wisniewski, S. R., Balasubramani, G. K., Khan, A. Y., & Trivedi, M. H. (2007). Diurnal mood variation in outpatients with major depressive disorder: implications for *DSM-V* from an analysis of the Sequenced Treatment Alternatives to Relieve Depression Study data. *Journal of Clinical Psychiatry, 68*(9), 1339–1347.

Murray, G., & Harvey, A. (2010). Circadian rhythms and sleep in bipolar disorder. *Bipolar Disorders, 12*(5), 459–472. doi:10.1111/j.1399-5618.2010.00843.x

Nathan, P. J., Burrows, G. D., & Norman, T. R. (1999). Melatonin sensitivity to dim white light in affective disorders. *Neuropsychopharmacology, 21*(3), 408–413. doi:10.1016/S0893-133X(99)00018-4

Nelson, R. J., & Drazen, D. L. (1999). Melatonin mediates seasonal adjustments in immune function. *Reproduction Nutrition Development, 39*(3), 383–398. doi:10.1051/rnd:19990310

Nurnberger, J. I. Jr., Adkins, S., Lahiri, D. K., Mayeda, A., Hu, K., Lewy, A., … Davis-Singh, D. (2000). Melatonin suppression by light in euthymic bipolar and unipolar patients. *Archives of General Psychiatry, 57*(6), 572–579.

Patrick, G. T. W., & Gilbert, J. A. (1896). Studies from the psychological laboratory of the University of Iowa: On the effects of loss of sleep. *Psychological Review, 3*(5), 469–483. doi:10.1037/h0075739

Poudfoot, J., Doran, J., Manicavasagar, V., & Parker, G. (2011). The precipitants of manic/hypomanic episodes in the context of bipolar disorder: A review. *Journal of Affective Disorders, 133*, 381–387.

Redwine, L., Hauger, R. L., Gillin, J. C., & Irwin, M. (2000). Effects of sleep and sleep deprivation on interleukin-6, growth hormone, cortisol, and melatonin levels in humans. *Journal of Clinical Endocrinology & Metabolism, 85*(10), 3597–3603.

Reiter, R. J., Tan, D.-X., & Maldonado, M. D. (2005). Melatonin as an antioxidant: Physiology versus pharmacology. *Journal of Pineal Research, 39*(2), 215–216. doi:10.1111/j.1600-079X.2005.00261.x

Reppert, S. M., & Weaver, D. R. (2002). Coordination of circadian timing in mammals. *Nature, 418*(6901), 935–941. doi:10.1038/nature00965

Ritter, P. S., Marx, C., Lewischenko, N., Pfeiffer, S., Leopold, K., Bauer, M., & Pfenning, A. (2012). The characteristics of sleep in patients with manifest bipolar disorder, subjects at high risk of developing the disease and healthy controls. *Journal of Neural Transmission, 119*, 1173–1184.

Rocha, P. M. B., Neves, F. S., Alvarenga, N. B., Hughet, R. B., Barbosa, I. G., & Corrêa, H. (2010). Association of Per3 gene with bipolar disorder: Comment on "Association study of 21 circadian genes with bipolar I disorder, schizoaffective disorder, and schizophrenia." *Bipolar Disorders, 12*(8), 875–876. doi:10.1111/j.1399-5618.2010.00875.x

Roenneberg, T., & Foster, R. G. (1997). Twilight times: Light and the circadian system. *Photochemistry and Photobiology, 66*(5), 549–561. doi:10.1111/j.1751-1097.1997.tb03188.x

Salvatore, P., Ghidini, S., Zita, G., Panfilis, C. D., Lambertino, S., Maggini, C., & Baldessarini, R. J. (2008). Circadian activity rhythm abnormalities in ill and recovered bipolar I disorder patients. *Bipolar Disorders, 10*(2), 256–265. doi:10.1111/j.1399-5618.2007.00505.x

Sit, D., Wisner, K. L., Hanusa, B. H., Stull, S., & Terman, M. (2007). Light therapy for bipolar disorder: A case series in women. *Bipolar Disorders, 9*(8), 918–927. doi:10.1111/j.1399-5618.2007.00451.x

Smeraldi, E., Benedetti, F., Barbini, B., Campori, E., & Colombo, C. (1999). Sustained antidepressant effect of sleep deprivation combined with pindolol in bipolar depression. A placebo-controlled trial. *Neuropsychopharmacology, 20*, 380–385.

Soria, V., Martínez-Amorós, E., Escaramís, G., Valero, J., Pérez-Egea, R., García, C., … Urretavizcaya, M. (2010). Differential association of circadian genes with mood disorders: CRY1 and NPAS2 are associated with unipolar major depression and CLOCK and VIP with bipolar disorder. *Neuropsychopharmacology, 35*(6), 1279–1289. doi:10.1038/npp.2009.230

Sylvia, L. G., Alloy, L. B., Hafner, J. A., Gauger, M. C., Verdon, K., & Abramson, L. Y. (2009). Life events and social rhythms in bipolar spectrum disorders: A prospective study. *Behavior Therapy, 40*, 131–141.

Sylvia, L. G., Dupuy, J. M., Ostacher, M. J., Cowperthwait, C. M., Hay, A. C., Sachs, G. S., … Perlis, R. H. (2012). Sleep disturbance in euthymic bipolar patients. *Journal of Psychopharmacology, 26*(8), 1108–1112. doi:10.1177/0269881111421973

Talbot, L. S., Hairston, I. S., Eidelman, P., Gruber, J., & Harvey, A. G. (2009). The effect of mood on sleep onset latency and REM sleep in interepisode bipolar disorder. *Journal of Abnormal Psychology, 118*(3), 448–458. doi:10.1037/a0016605

Talbot, L. S., Stone, S., Gruber, J., Hairston, I. S., Eidelman, P., & Harvey, A. G. (2012). A test of the bidirectional association between sleep and mood in bipolar disorder and insomnia. *Journal of Abnormal Psychology, 121*(1), 39–50. doi:10.1037/a0024946

Thompson, C., Stinson, D., Fernandez, M., Fine, J., & Isaacs, G. (1988). A comparison of normal, bipolar and seasonal affective disorder subjects using the seasonal pattern assessment questionnaire. *Journal of Affective Disorders, 14*(3), 257–264. doi:10.1016/0165-0327(88)90043-2

Walker, M. P., & van der Helm, E. (2009). Overnight therapy? The role of sleep in emotional brain processing. *Psychological Bulletin, 135*(5), 731–748.

Wehr, T. A. (1989). Sleep loss: A preventable cause of mania and other excitable states. *Journal of Clinical Psychiatry, 50*(Suppl. 12), 8–16.

Wehr, T. A. (1992). Improvement of depression and triggering of mania by sleep deprivation. *JAMA, 267*, 548–551.

Wehr, T. A., Goodwin, F. K., Wirz-Justice, A., Breitmaier, J., & Craig, C. (1982). 48-hour sleep-wake cycles in manic-depressive illness: Naturalistic observations and sleep deprivation experiments. *Archives of General Psychiatry, 39*, 559–565.

Wehr, T. A., Sack, D. A., & Rosenthal, N. E. (1987). Sleep reduction as a final common pathway in the genesis of mania. *American Journal of Psychiatry, 144*, 201–204.

Wirz-Justice, A., Quinto, C., Cajochen, C., Werth, E., & Hock, C. (1999). A rapid-cycling bipolar patient treated with long nights, bedrest and light. *Biological Psychiatry, 45*, 1075–1077.

Wu, J. C., & Bunney, W. E. (1990). The biological basis of an antidepressant response to sleep deprivation and relapse: Review and hypothesis. *American Journal of Psychiatry, 147*, 14–21.

Yoo, S.-S., Gujar, N., Hu, P., Jolesz, F. A., & Walker, M. P. (2007). The human emotional brain without sleep—A prefrontal amygdala disconnect. *Current Biology, 17*(20), R877–R878.

12.

HYPOTHALAMIC-PITUITARY-ADRENAL AXIS AND HYPOTHALAMIC-PITUITARY-THYROID AXIS AND THEIR TREATMENT IMPACT

Michael Bauer and Timothy Dinan

INTRODUCTION

Over the past 30 years numerous studies have been performed examining neuroendocrine aspects of major depression. Far fewer studies have been conducted on patients with bipolar disorder than in patients with unipolar depression. There are several reasons for this, including the fact that unipolar depression is more common, it is difficult to maintain bipolar patients drug-free for any appreciable length of time, and the simplistic but commonly held perception until relatively recently that mania was the biological inverse of depression hampered activity in the field. Over the past decade several important studies have been published examining neuroendocrine aspects of bipolar disorder, and, while some of these studies are limited by the fact that medicated patients were recruited, some investigators have conducted studies in patients who were drug-free for an adequate period. We thus have a body of knowledge regarding hypothalamic-pituitary-adrenal axis (HPA) and hypothalamic-pituitary-thyroid axis (HPT) function in bipolar disorder, and these axes are the primary focus of this chapter.

STRESS BIOLOGY

The HPA is the core endocrine stress system in humans. It not only regulates the body's peripheral functions relating to metabolism and immunity but also has profound effects on the brain by influencing neuronal survival and neurogenesis in structures such as the hippocampus and amygdala, where it plays a pivotal role in memory (Martin, Ressler, Binder, & Nemeroff, 2009). While acute stress activates the sympathoadrenal medullary system, resulting in the components of the "fight or flight" response with a release of catecholamines such as norepinephrine and epinephrine, chronic stress results in alterations of the HPA, which produce a number of adaptive behavioral and physiological changes leading to an increase in the release of cortisol and other steroids from the adrenal cortex (McEwen & Gianaros, 2010).

Under basal conditions, corticotropin releasing hormone (CRH) is produced within the medial paraventricular nucleus of the hypothalamus and is the dominant regulator of the axis, mediating the endocrine response to stress (Lloyd & Nemeroff, 2011). Following any threat to homeostasis, CRH release is triggered. In situations of chronic stress, many parvicellular neurons co-express vasopressin (AVP), which plays an important role in sustaining HPA activation through a synergistic action with CRH (Dinan & Scott, 2005). CRH and AVP act on the anterior pituitary corticotropes to stimulate the release of adrenocorticotropic hormone (ACTH), causing increased synthesis and release of cortisol, the main stress hormone of the axis, from the adrenal glands (see Figure 1.2 for details).

In response to psychological stress, CRH release is controlled by classic central neurotransmitters such as norepinephrine and serotonin. The release of CRH is under excitatory control from the amygdala and inhibitory input from the hippocampus. In response to physical stressors, such as infection, CRH-containing neurones respond to proinflammatory cytokines such as interleukin (IL)-1, IL-6, and tumor necrosis factor (TNF)-α. CRH acts through two different receptors: CRH1 and CRH2 (Bale & Vale, 2004). The former, which is adenyl cyclase linked, mediates the release of ACTH from the anterior pituitary.

The principal mechanism by which cortisol produces its effects is by activation of intracellular receptors that

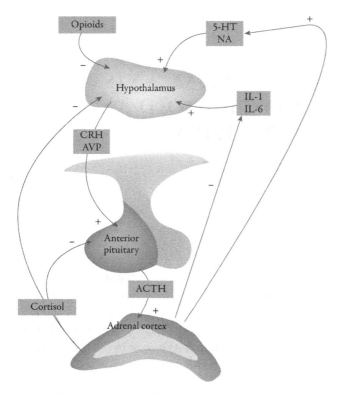

Figure 12.1 Translation and interface from basic and clinical research in bipolar disorder, divided in phase I (translational research per se) e phase II (translational research advances into population benefits and improved health system) (adapted from Machado-Vieira, 2012).

translocate to the nucleus and bind to specific DNA regions, hence modulating gene transcription. Two distinct receptors bind cortisol. The type 1 receptor (MR), which is indistinguishable from the peripheral mineralocorticoid receptor, is distributed principally in the septo-hippocampal region and mediates tonic influences of cortisol or corticosterone monitoring diurnal fluctuations in the steroid; the type 2 or glucocorticoid receptor (GR) has a wider distribution and mediates stress-related changes in cortisol levels (Martocchia, Curto, Toussan, Stefanelli, & Falaschi, 2011). By binding to the GR and the MR, endogenous glucocorticoids serve as potent inhibitory regulators of HPA axis activity. The MR has a 10-fold higher affinity for cortisol than GR does and regulates basal diurnal fluctuation in cortisol, whereas GR becomes progressively occupied only at peaks of cortisol secretion and after a stressful stimulus (De Kloet, 2008). These receptor systems provide negative feedback loops at a limbic, hypothalamic, and pituitary level.

Activity within the HPA is regulated by a balance between forward drive and negative feedback. From a physiological perspective, feedback is defined in terms of speed of response into immediate, intermediate, and delayed. The former is seen within minutes and the latter takes place

over hours. Cortisol feedback takes place at a variety of levels, including the hippocampus, hypothalamus, and anterior pituitary.

Once glucocorticoids are released into the circulation, availability at a cellular level is influenced by various local factors, including corticosteroid binding globulin, multidrug resistance transporter, P-glycoprotein (an efflux pump that decreases intracellular concentrations), and 11β-hydroxysteroid dehydrogenase (11β-HSD, an enzyme with two isoforms (Edwards, 2012). One isoform converts inactive glucocorticoids into their active form (e.g., corticosterone in rodents; cortisol in humans). The second isoform breaks down active glucocorticoids into inactive metabolites. Enhanced corticosteroid binding globulin levels and P-glycoprotein expression, as well as a decrease in 11β-HSD-1 or an increase in 11β-HSD-2, reduce the levels of active glucocorticoids in the cell, contributing to a state of glucocorticoid resistance. Glucocorticoid effects are ultimately determined at the level of the GR. An impaired GR function, whether brought about by reduced expression, binding affinity to its ligand, nuclear translocation, DNA binding, or interaction with other transcription factors (i.e., NF-κB), can also result in a state of glucocorticoid resistance, increasing vulnerability to enhanced inflammatory responses. Thus even when circulating glucocorticoid concentrations are normal, impaired control of immune responses can occur at the cellular and molecular level (Silverman & Sternberg, 2012).

HPA AND BIPOLAR ILLNESS

Mood disorders in general are perceived as stress related. In the case of bipolar disorder, acute episodes can be triggered by environmental stress, especially episodes early in the course of illness. Dysregulation of the HPA in the disorder has been recognized for more than 40 years (Grunze, 2011). Such dysregulation is now perceived as due to an interaction between genetic and environmental factors. Here we review physiological studies exploring axis functioning in the disorder, as well as the potential impact of polymorphisms of key regulatory genes.

HPA POLYMORPHISMS

Two meta-analyses of linkage scans in bipolar disorder report linkage to the 8q region distal to the CRH gene. The more recent study reports genome-wide significance for this locus even when bipolar II disorder patients are included in the analysis (Binder & Nemeroff, 2010). Genome-wide association studies have been published for bipolar disorder and for unipolar depression, but none show convincing association of SNPs within CRF-system loci.

Rare mutations of the *GR* gene have been described, which lead to a generalized cortisol resistance (Charmandari & Kino, 2010). Patients with such mutations present with hypertension and hypokalemic alkalosis indicative of adrenal overproduction of mineralocorticoids and, in females, male pattern baldness, and menstrual irregularities as a consequence of overproduction of adrenal androgens are observed. With defects in the GR, the central negative feedback of cortisol is reduced with increased production by the adrenal gland and with high affinity to the MR. The consequence is hyperactivity of the HPA axis in the absence of a stressor. The mutations that lead to the GC resistance syndrome are principally located in the ligand-binding and DNA-binding domains of the *GR* gene.

The GR is a ligand-dependent transcription factor that belongs to the nuclear hormone receptor super family. There are two principal molecular pathways by which GR controls transcription: (a) it dimerizers and directly binds to positive or negative glucocorticoid response elements in the promoter regions of genes leading to transcriptional increases or decreases and (b) GR monomers indirectly influence the transcription of genes through interactions with other transcription factors (e.g., NF-κB). Mutations leading to cortisol resistance have a low prevalence, and the mental state of those carrying the mutation has not been reported on.

FKBP5 is a co-chaperone of the glucocorticoid receptor. Polymorphisms in the gene encoding this co-chaperone have been shown to be associated with higher FKBP5 leading to increased GR resistance and impaired negative feedback. Binder (2009) indicates a link with bipolar disorder and also presents evidence showing a strong association between antidepressant response and FKBP5 polymorphisms. There is an intriguing possibility that drugs that target FKBP5 have the potential to prevent the long-term effects of trauma on GR responsivity and perhaps restore GR function in mood disorders such as bipolar disorder.

Spijker and van Rossum (2012) found, in a sample of 245 bipolar patients, an association between the 9β polymorphism and reduced risk of hypomania, while Perlis et al. (2010), in a sample of 173 patients with bipolar I depressive episodes, found the response to lamotrigine (used in the treatment of bipolar depression) was associated with the GR polymorphisms rs258,747 and rs6198 (9β).

In addition, genotypes of eight analyzed polymorphisms of GR gene (rs10,052,957, rs6196, rs6198, rs6191, rs258,813, rs33,388, rs6195, rs41,423,247) were investigated in 115

bipolar patients treated with lithium carbonate for 5 to 27 years (Szczepankiewicz, Rybakowski, Suwalska, & Hauser, 2011). Thirty patients were identified as excellent lithium responders, 58 patients as partial responders, and 27 as nonresponders. A significant difference in allele frequencies for BclI polymorphism between patients with different lithium response was observed with C allele associated with excellent lithium response. A strong linkage disequilibrium of five GR polymorphisms (rs6198, rs6191, rs6196, rs258,813, rs33,388), with TAAGA haplotype was prevalent in the group of partial and nonresponders to lithium.

BASAL HPA ACTIVITY IN BIPOLAR DISORDER

Various measurements of cortisol output have been reported in bipolar disorder. These include measurements of cortisol in plasma, saliva, and urine. Few studies have focused on CSF measurements. However, Swann et al. (1992) found elevated CSF cortisol in mania similar to that reported for depression. In a comprehensive study of salivary cortisol secretion, Deshauer et al. (2003) obtained six salivary samples per day for three days in bipolar patients in remission and 28 offspring of bipolar patients. The advantages of measuring salivary cortisol include ease of collection and the fact that salivary cortisol is not protein bound and therefore a reflection of biologically active cortisol. No differences in salivary cortisol levels were observed at any time point. The data indicate that when bipolar patients are in remission, salivary cortisol levels are normal. Furthermore, subjects with a family history of bipolar disorder do not show elevated salivary cortisol levels. These findings are in contrast to those of Wedekind et al. (2007), who examined nocturnal urinary cortisol secretion in bipolar patients who were currently depressed at the beginning and end of inpatient treatment. They found elevations in cortisol, which were especially pronounced in bipolar psychotic patients. They concluded that the HPA overactivity is a trait rather than a state marker.

Increasing evidence suggests that enhanced cortisol response to waking is a robust marker of exaggerated HPA response and has been reported as abnormal in a variety of stress-related conditions. Deshauer et al. (2003) examined the cortisol awakening response in bipolar patients who had responded to lithium. Such patients were found to have an enhanced cortisol response to waking compared with healthy controls. Furthermore, there is now evidence to indicate that the offspring of parents with bipolar disorder have higher mean cortisol levels in the mornings and afternoons than the offspring of parents without mental illness. Similar abnormalities have been reported in schizophrenia in various phases of illness and even in drug-naive patients.

DEXAMETHASONE SUPPRESSION TEST

The low dose (1 mg) dexamethasone suppression test is the most extensively investigated test in the history of biological psychiatry, but its usefulness in a clinical setting is limited due to low sensitivity and specificity. It is fundamentally a test of delayed feedback in the HPA. While this test has been examined primarily in depression, studies in manic patients have also been undertaken. Rates of nonsuppression in mania are in the 40% to 50% range, similar to those reported for depression. However, as in the case of depression, the abnormality usually normalizes with effective treatment.

CRH TEST

The ACTH and free cortisol response to the injection of 100 µg of synthetic human CRH and plasma cortisol-binding globulin levels were measured in 42 lithium-treated patients suffering from Research Diagnostic Criteria bipolar I disorder in remission and 21 age- and sex-matched normal controls (Vieta et al., 1999). A one-year follow-up was conducted to assess any possible relationship between outcome and the hormonal response. Bipolar patients showed higher baseline and peak ACTH concentrations than control subjects. A higher area under ACTH concentration curve after CRH stimulation predicted manic/hypomanic relapse within six months by multiple regression analysis. Bipolar patients in remission showed mild abnormalities in ACTH levels before and after CRH stimulation. Thus CRH challenge may be a potentially good predictor of manic or hypomanic relapse in remitted bipolar patients.

Likewise, in schizophrenia there is only one published study of the CRH test (Roy et al., 1986). While patients were drug-free, ACTH and cortisol response to CRH infusion was similar to that in controls. Treatment with fluphenazine had no effect on response to CRH. This would suggest that patients with bipolar illness and schizophrenia differ in terms of response to CRH. However, there are no studies of adequate sample size comparing both disorders.

DEX/CRH TEST

This test assesses both forward drive and feedback activity in the HPA and is carried out by administering dexamethasone (DEX) the evening prior to the CRH challenge. Subjects usually receive an oral dose of DEX 1.5mg at 11 PM followed by CRH 1 mg/kg. Blood samples are collected at 3:00, 3:15, 3:30, 3:45, 4:00, and 4:15 PM. It is well established that patients with major depression have an enhanced ACTH release relative to healthy controls when CRH is administered after DEX. The reason for this enhancement is not fully understood, though it has been postulated that enhanced vasopressin activity in depression may be involved.

Rybakowski and Twardowska (1999) examined 40 patients with depression, 16 bipolars and 24 unipolars, both during an acute episode of depression and in remission. They found that during depressive episodes bipolar patients had a greater cortisol response to DEX/CRH than unipolar patients and there was a significant correlation between the endocrine response and the severity of depression. Furthermore, this anomaly persisted in the bipolars, even in remission. Schmider et al. (1995) tested acute and remitted manic patients, those in acute depression and healthy controls. ACTH and cortisol release were significantly increased in both manic and depressed patients in comparison to healthy subjects. In remission manic patients had a decreased response but nonetheless a response significantly higher than seen in controls. The data indicate that in either an acute manic episode or in remission, bipolar patients have abnormalities in HPA function. A more comprehensive study of the DEX/CRH test in bipolar patients in remission was carried out by the Newcastle group (Watson, Gallagher, Ritchie, Ferrier, & Young, 2004), which examined 53 bipolar patients, of whom 27 were in remission, and 28 healthy controls. The bipolar patients had an enhanced cortisol response to the DEX/CRH relative to the controls. The authors concluded that the DEX/CRH test is abnormal in both remitted and nonremitted bipolar patients. Patients with a rapid cycling form of bipolar I disorder were investigated. Five patients were sequentially tested with DEX/CRH. The results were stable over time, suggesting that the test yields results that are independent of the mood state in such patients.

For a review of the DEX/CRH test in schizophrenia, see Bradley and Dinan (2010). The most clear-cut study was published by Lammers et al. (1995) who reported on 24 schizophrenia patients and 24 controls. Basal cortisol was statistically significantly greater in patients than in controls, and basal ACTH trended toward being higher in patients. Peak cortisol following DEX and CRH and cortisol AUC 14.00 to 18.00 following DEX, and CRH was significantly greater in schizophrenia patients than controls. There was no evidence for a difference in ACTH AUC following CRH infusion between both groups.

DEX VASOPRESSIN TEST

The release of ACTH from the anterior pituitary is under the joint control of CRH acting through CRH1 receptors and vasopressin acting on V3 (sometimes called V1b) receptors. The latter become more important during chronic stress. Dinan, O'Brien, Lavelle, and Scott (2004) demonstrated increased responsiveness in these receptors in patients with major depression. They used desmopressin to stimulate ACTH release and found that patients with major depression released more ACTH than did healthy subjects. Watson, Gallagher, Ferrier, and Young (2006) examined DEX/negative feedback on AVP release in 64 patients with mood disorder and 21 controls. Forty-one patients were bipolar and the remainder had chronic depressive disorder. Twenty-one of the bipolar patients were in remission, 10 were depressed, and 10 were rapid cycling. All subjects were administered DEX 1.5mgat at 11 PM. On the following afternoon at 3:00 PM, blood was collected for AVP measurement. Post-DEX levels were significantly higher in patients with bipolar illness and chronic depressive than matched healthy controls. It is not clear from the study whether AVP levels were elevated at baseline or whether the AVP emanated from the paraventricular nucleus or the magnocellular nucleus of the hypothalamus. However, it is tempting to speculate that the HPA overactivity seen in patients with bipolar illness may be driven by excess AVP.

PITUITARY VOLUME

Sassi et al. (2001) measured the volumes of the pituitary gland in 23 patients with bipolar disorder and 34 healthy controls. They reported smaller pituitary volumes in bipolar disorder. A more recent MRI study was carried out on 29 remitted patients with bipolar disorder, 49 of their first-degree relatives (of whom 15 had a diagnosis of major depressive disorder), and 52 age- and gender-matched healthy controls (Takahashi et al., 2010). Bipolar patients had a significantly larger pituitary volume compared with their relatives and healthy controls. There is certainly no consensus on this issue.

PHARMACOLOGICAL TARGETING OF THE HPA AXIS

CRF receptor antagonists have shown considerable promise in animal models of stress, but studies in patients have so far proved disappointing. Although there are case reports of patients with bipolar depression responding to treatment with cortisol synthesis inhibitors, most of the research has been focused on the use of glucocorticoid receptor antagonists. Several small studies of the glucocorticoid antagonist RU 486 in patients with bipolar depression and with psychotic depression have been conducted. Evidence of efficacy remains questionable. Some of the data do indicate improvements in cognitive functioning following such treatment. Given the negative effects of high cortisol on hippocampal function, such a positive impact on cognition seems biologically plausible.

DEX has also been proposed as a treatment strategy for bipolar depression. It has long been recognized that glucocorticoids when administered to psychologically healthy subjects can result in elevation of mood. Again, no convincing large-scale studies have been conducted. Also, as in the case of most drugs being developed for treating mood disorders, the bulk of studies with these agents have been conducted in patients with unipolar rather than bipolar depression.

IMPACT

Despite the heterogeneity of outcomes from the studies reviewed here, there is evidence that people with bipolar illness frequently experience periods of heightened cortisol secretion. This hypersecretion may be evident even when patients are normothymic. The variation in results may be explained by varying symptoms of illness, as well as by medication use and exposure to other environmental factors known to influence HPA axis function. It is likely that such hypercortisolism accounts for the increase in cardiovascular disease and poor cognitive outcomes seen in such patients. However, efforts so far aimed at therapeutic targeting of the HPA have proved disappointing. Large-scale prospective studies examining patients in various phases of illness are required.

ORGANIZATION OF THE HPT AXIS

The functionally interrelated hypothamalic-pituitary-thyroid (HPT) axis is a classic endocrine system with a hierarchic organization. The thyroid gland is the largest endocrine organ in the human body. Thyrotropin-releasing hormone (TRH) is a hypothalamic tripeptide synthesized in the paraventricular nucleus and released from the median eminence into the primary plexus of the portal venous system to thus reach the secondary plexus adjacent to anterior pituitary sinusoids. Its synthesis and release are regulated by afferent influences from the limbic forebrain. TRH release is stimulated centrally by α-adrenergic transmission and inhibited by a negative feedback effect of circulating thyroid hormones. It is believed that TRH also functions as a neuro-modulator/neurotransmitter in many regions of the central nervous system (CNS), including the amygdala and hippocampus of humans.

In the pituitary, TRH binds to membrane receptors and induces the production of thyroid-stimulating hormone (TSH). After release into the general circulation, TSH binds to a specific TSH receptor (TSH-R) on the thyroid cell membrane, activating both the G protein-adenylyl cyclase-cAMP and the phospholipase C signaling systems. The activity of the thyroid gland is predominantly regulated by the concentration of TSH. Thus regulation of thyroid function in healthy individuals is to a large extent determined by the factors that regulate the synthesis and secretion of TSH. In the absence of pituitary function, the clinical condition of hypothyroidism occurs.

In healthy individuals, the thyroid gland produces predominantly the prohormone thyroxine (T_4) together with a small amount of the bioactive hormone triiodothyronine (T_3). These two hormones have traditionally been referred to as thyroid hormones. TSH stimulates and regulates the production of thyroid hormones, synthesized from the incorporation of iodide into thyroglobulin. T_4, the major secretion product of the thyroid gland, is converted to its biologically active metabolite, T_3, by widely distributed enzymes called iodothyronine 5' monodeiodinases (deiodinases). Thus T_4 is the precursor for the more potent hormone, T_3. After release into the general circulation, thyroid hormones are necessary for the regulation of various metabolic functions in all body tissues throughout the life span. In addition T_3 and T_4 exert feedback on the thyroid economy at pituitary and hypothalamic levels (review: Santisteban, 2013).

THYROID AND BRAIN

Amazingly, certain clinical facts about the relationship between thyroid hormones and the brain have been known for more than 100 years. Thyroid hormones play an essential role in the development of the human brain, and in the adult brain significant disturbances of the thyroid homeostasis may alter mental function (Bauer et al., 2003; Bauer et al., 2009). Both excess production of thyroid hormones (the clinical condition of hyperthyroidism) and inadequate thyroid hormone production (the clinical syndrome of hypothyroidism) are associated with significant changes in mental functioning, including mood, perception, cognition,

and emotional performance (Bauer, Samuels, & Whybrow, 2013; Schuff, Samuels, Whybrow, & Bauer, 2013). A severe lack of thyroid hormones does mimic melancholic depression and significant impairment in cognitive functioning in most patients suffering hypothyroid conditions (Schuff et al., 2013; Whybrow, Prange, & Treadway, 1969). The fact that disturbed mood and behavior is present in patients who suffer primary thyroid disorders is well established in the scientific literature; so is it possible that changes in the thyroid system play a role in the etiology of mood and other psychiatric disorders? And, if so, might the thyroid hormones have value in the treatment of psychiatric disorders, particularly affective illness?

HPT AXIS IN MOOD DISORDERS

Clinical studies suggest that there may be abnormalities in thyroid hormone metabolism in patients with affective (mood) disorders and that these may not be readily apparent with the standard tests to screen for thyroid disease. In fact, the vast majority of patients with primary affective disorders (greater than 90%) have thyroid hormone blood levels within the euthyroid range (reviewed in O'Connor, Gwirtsman, & Loosen, 2003). However, within that normal range the thyroid hormone economy appears to be predictive of therapeutic response, with growing evidence that thyroid hormone levels in the low–normal range or below-normal range (i.e., thyroid hypofunction) can result in a suboptimal treatment outcome. Frye et al. (1999) have reported that within the "normal" range, a low level of free thyroxin (fT_4) in patients with bipolar disorder is associated with more affective episodes and greater severity of depression during prophylactic lithium treatment. In another study, lower free thyroxin index values and higher TSH values within the normal range were significantly associated with poorer treatment response in bipolar patients during the depressed phase (Cole et al., 2002). Also, a substantial proportion of lithium-treated patients develop thyroid abnormalities, with women having a higher risk than men of developing thyroid disease during lithium treatment (Bauer, Glenn, Pilhatsch, Pfennig, & Whybrow, 2013; Kirov, Tredget, John, Owen, & Lazarus, 2005).

Taken together, these observations suggest that a robust thyroid economy confers an advantage that promotes rapid recovery following treatment. Thus a working hypothesis in seeking to explain these clinical observations is that thyroid hormones modulate the severity and course of depression rather than playing a specific pathogenic role. The hypothesis that thyroid hormones act as modulators in mood disorders is further supported by studies of the relationship between thyroid function and the clinical course of bipolar disorder, especially that of the rapid cycling variant.

THYROID FUNCTION AND RAPID CYCLING

About 10% to 15% of bipolar patients experience rapid cycling; while similar to other bipolar patients nosologically and demographically, they tend to have a longer duration of illness and a more refractory course. Furthermore, there is some evidence that women are disproportionately represented, making up 80% of rapid cycling patients, compared to about 50% of non-rapid cycling patients. A variety of factors may predispose bipolar illness to a rapid cycling course, including treatment with tricyclic antidepressants and monoamine oxidase inhibitors.

It has long been debated whether thyroid axis abnormalities contribute to the development of rapid cycling in patients with bipolar disorder. Several studies have found an association among indices of low thyroid function or clinical hypothyroidism and rapid cycling, while other studies refute this association. For example, one larger study reported that 23% of 30 patients with rapid cycling bipolar disorder had grade I hypothyroidism, while 27% had grade II and 10% had grade III abnormalities (Bauer & Whybrow, 1990). The results from various studies are inconsistent, and the conclusions to be drawn are often limited by their retrospective design and lack of a healthy control comparison group. Most important, many studies included patients who were receiving prophylactic long-term lithium treatment. The adverse effects of lithium on thyroid function do certainly have an impact on thyroid indices. On the other hand, cross-sectional studies of unmedicated patients with rapid cycling bipolar disorder have found no abnormalities in basal TSH and thyroxine levels. It was postulated that patients with rapid cycling may manifest no thyroid abnormalities until physiologically challenged by "antithyroid" stressors. Such stressors may include spontaneously occurring thyroid disease or goiterogenic drugs such as lithium. In a recent controlled study, when previously unmedicated patients with rapid cycling were challenged with therapeutic doses of lithium, a significantly higher delta TSH after thyrotropin-releasing hormone stimulation was found than in age- and gender-matched healthy controls who also received lithium (Gyulai et al., 2003). This finding suggests that a proportion of patients with bipolar disorder has a dysfunction in the HPT axis that remains latent until the axis is challenged by the thyroprivic effect of lithium and that changes in the thyroid economy may play a modulating role in the development of the rapid cycling pattern.

THYROID AUTOIMMUNITY

Some studies have reported a high prevalence for antithyroid antibodies in patients with affective disorders receiving lithium therapy, suggesting that thyroid autoimmunity may mediate the antithyroid effects of lithium. Other studies have not found an increased prevalence of antithyroid antibodies in patients with affective disorders receiving lithium when compared to the general population, normal controls, or controls with psychiatric disorders (Baethge et al., 2005). Furthermore, patients who have thyroid autoimmunity prior to lithium exposure may show a rise in antibody titers and have an increased risk of developing hypothyroidism while receiving lithium therapy. Specifically, thyroid peroxidase (TPO) antibodies were reported to be elevated in bipolar disorder with a prevalence of 28%, while results from other studies were inconsistent with reported rates ranging from 0% to 43%. In community studies, the rates of prevalence of TPO antibodies generally range from about 12% to 18%. The estimate of TPO antibody prevalence varies with the sensitivity and specificity of the testing methodology and is increased in females, in old age, when TSH levels are abnormally high or low, and when individuals with known thyroid disease are included in the population. The impact of increasing age and female gender on the detection of TPO antibodies has also been noted in patients with affective disorders, and elevated thyroid antibodies were reported in some studies of patients with unipolar depression but not in others. It was also hypothesized that autoimmune thyroiditis, with TPO antibody as marker, may be a potential endophenotype for bipolar disorder and is related to the genetic vulnerability to develop bipolar disorder rather than to the disease process itself. While offspring of parents with bipolar disorder were found to have increased vulnerability to develop thyroid autoimmunity as compared to high-school-age controls, this was independent of any psychiatric disorder or symptoms. Thyroid antibody status was also associated with an increased risk for lithium-induced hypothyroidism but not with current or former lithium treatment (Kupka et al., 2002). In a Dutch epidemiological study, the prevalence of a lifetime diagnosis of depression was higher in subjects with positive TPOAb in comparison with participants without TPOAb. Thyroid peroxidase antibodies were positively associated with trait markers of depression, and the authors concluded that the presence of TPOAb may be a vulnerability marker for depression (van de Ven et al., 2012).

THERAPEUTIC USE OF HPT AXIS HORMONES IN MOOD DISORDERS

HISTORICAL PERSPECTIVE

The clinical administration of thyroid axis hormones as a treatment in modern psychiatry has existed since the early 20th century. Norwegian physicians were the first to use hypermetabolic doses of desiccated sheep thyroid gland to successfully treat patients with cyclic mood disorders and periodic catatonia in the 1930s to 1940s. The fact that thyroid hormone deficiency may lead to depression and psychosis ("myxedematous madness") and be reversed by desiccated thyroid administration was demonstrated in a case series by Asher in the late 1940s. Subsequently, with the identification of triiodothyronine (T_3) and thyroxine (T_4) as the natural thyroid hormones in the 1950s, and their subsequent availability as pharmaceutical drugs, as well as the discovery of TRH and TSH, the effects of synthetic hormones of the HPT system (T_3, T_4, TRH, and TSH) alone and in combination with traditional psychotropic drugs have been studied repeatedly in the treatment of affective disorders (reviewed in Bauer & Whybrow, 2002; Bauer et al., 2008).

TREATMENT WITH TRH

Several lines of evidence from experimental animal studies suggest that TRH may produce antidepressant effects. TRH1 receptor knockout mice demonstrated a depressive phenotype, as evidenced by increased immobility in the forced swim test and tail suspension test, common rodent models of depression (Zeng et al., 2007). Soon after the identification and purification of TRH from sheep hypothalami in the late 1960s, two initial reports suggested that administration of 500 μg intravenously produced rapid (within hours) antidepressant effects that persisted up to three days. TRH was previously studied for the treatment of depression in humans but produced unpredictable responses when administered by the oral, intravenous, or subcutaneous routes. This is not surprising given that the peptide is rapidly cleared systemically and availability to the CNS would be limited. To test the hypothesis that TRH has antidepressant properties when given access to the CNS in humans, Marangell and colleagues (1997) administered TRH via an intrathecal injection using a lumbar puncture method. These data provide the most compelling evidence for the rapid antidepressant effects of TRH. Specifically, a single 500 μg bolus dose administered via percutaneous

puncture of the lumbar intrathecal space produced a 50% or greater reduction in the depression rating in the majority (five out of eight) of patients with treatment-resistant depression (some of these patients had bipolar disorder), while producing modest adverse events. An additional study conducted by Callahan et al. (1997), consisting of two of the same patients as the previously mentioned study, demonstrated a repeated positive response to a subsequent intrathecal bolus dose of TRH. Despite some contradictory results, some interesting observations have emerged from these studies suggestive of an increased likelihood of response to TRH infusion in women and in patients with bipolar disorder.

TREATMENT WITH THYROID HORMONES

While thyroid hormone therapy (mono use) has not been established (mostly because not intensively well studied) as adequate treatment for patients with primary mood disorders, since the late 1960s, a series of open and controlled clinical trials have confirmed the therapeutic value of adjunctive treatment with thyroid hormones in these conditions. Specifically, there is evidence that T_3 can accelerate the therapeutic response to tricyclic antidepressants and in treatment-resistant depression, T_3 may augment the response to tricyclic antidepressants, although the results have been inconsistent (reviewed in Bauer et al., 2008).

The hypothesis that suboptimal availability of circulating thyroid hormones may contribute to the high rate of treatment failures in bipolar disorder led researchers to administer thyroid hormones in this condition. In studies of bipolar disorder, the doses of L-T_4 varied broadly from replacement doses (between 50 and 150 μg/d, commonly administered to balance lithium-induced (sub-)clinical hypothyroid conditions) to supraphysiologic doses (250–400 μg/d). Adjunctive L-T_4 at supraphysiologic doses because only such high doses offered promise in previous open-label studies in rapid cycling, prophylaxis-resistant bipolar disorders, and for patients with refractory bipolar depression (Bauer, Berghöfer, et al., 2002; Bauer & Whybrow, 1990; Baumgartner, Bauer, & Hellweg, 1994; Stancer & Persad, 1982). Supraphysiologic L-T_4 may also have immediate therapeutic value in antidepressant-resistant bipolar and unipolar depressed patients during a phase of refractory depression (Bauer et al., 1998; Bauer et al., 2005). In these patients with malignant refractory affective disorder, doses of 250 to 400 μg/d L-T_4 are required to achieve therapeutic effect, much higher than those used in the treatment of primary thyroid disorders (summarized in Table 12.1).

Table 12.1. APPLICATIONS OF ADJUNCTIVE TREATMENT WITH LEVOTHYROXINE (L-T$_4$) IN REFRACTORY MOOD DISORDERS

Clinical indications	• Rapid cycling bipolar disorders • Prophylaxis-resistant mood disorders • Treatment-refractory major depressive episodes (unipolar and bipolar)
Excluding conditions and states	• Thyroid (current hyperthyroidism, previous or current thyroid adenoma) • Cardiac (e.g., history of myocardial infarction, arrhythmia, insufficiency, unstable hypertension) • Pregnancy; breastfeeding; • Postmenopausal women with evidence of osteopenia/osteoporosis and without protection for bone loss • Age > 70 years • Severe organic brain disorder (e.g., dementia)
Pretreatment screening and follow-up investigations[a]	• Psychiatric and medical history and status • Vital signs (blood pressure and pulse) • Body weight • Electrocardiogram[b] • Thyroid function tests (TSH, thyroid hormones[c]) • Routine laboratory evaluations • Optional: • Consultation with endocrinologist or internist[d] • Bone mineral density (dual-energy X-ray absorptiometry—only in patients who receive L-T$_4$ prophylactically > 3 months)
L-T$_4$ dosing regimen[e,f]	• Starting dose: 100 mcg/day • Speed of dose increase: 100 mcg/week • Target dose: 250–300 mcg/day, if no response and good tolerability up to 400 mcg/day

[a] Consider additional radiological investigations in patients with history or suspected thyroid disorder (e.g., sonography of the thyroid gland). [b] Consider 24-h ECG recording if history of arrhythmia. [c] Total T4, free T4, and total T3 levels; optional: free T3 levels and thyroid (TPO) antibodies. [d] Recommended in case of tolerability problems or adverse events. [e] For euthyroid patients only; for patients with overt and subclinical hypothyroidism slower titration. [f] Single morning dose (30 min before breakfast).

A recent controlled study attempted to further understand how thyroid hormones may improve depression in bipolar disorder. The study tested the efficacy of adjunctive treatment with supraphysiologic doses of L-T$_4$ in patients with bipolar depression and the hypothesis that women display a better outcome compared to men in a multicenter, six-week, double-blind, randomized, placebo-controlled fixed-dose (300 μg/day) trial (Stamm et al., 2014). The course of depression scores over time from randomization to Week 6 was significantly different between groups at Week 4 but not at the end of the placebo-controlled phase. The secondary analysis of women revealed a significant difference between groups in mean change of depression scores. High TSH levels, indicating suboptimal levels of circulating thyroid hormones, were predicative for positive treatment outcome in women treated with L-T$_4$. In summary, this controlled study indicated that adjunctive treatment with supraphysiological doses of levothyroxine is a promising strategy to overcome treatment resistance in bipolar depression, especially in women.

Although treatment with supraphysiologic T$_4$ requires close monitoring, the hyperthyroxinemia is tolerated surprisingly well. No serious effects, including loss of bone mineral density, were observed even in patients treated for extended periods (Bauer et al., 2004; Ricken et al., 2012). The low incidence of adverse effects and high tolerability reported by patients with affective disorders who are receiving high-dose thyroid hormone therapy contrasts with that typically seen in patients with primary thyroid disease. For example, patients with thyroid carcinoma treated with high doses of L-T$_4$ to achieve suppression of TSH commonly complain of the symptoms of thyrotoxicosis.

POSSIBLE MECHANISMS OF ACTION

What evidence is there to support this conjecture of a central disturbance of brain-thyroid metabolism in some patients who suffer refractory affective illness? Despite the clinical evidence of a close relationship between thyroid status and behavioral disturbance, metabolic effects of thyroid hormones in the adult mammalian brain have rarely been investigated in vivo. In part this lack of curiosity may be traced to reports in the 1950s and 1960s that suggested that oxygen consumption in the mature human brain did not change with thyroid status. But the absence of a technology capable of direct in vivo measurement of brain thyroid metabolism is also responsible. That still does not exist, but the evaluation of cerebral blood flow and metabolism by functional brain imaging techniques is a starting point, and recent studies have provided promising insights into the thyroid–brain relationship (Bauer et al., 2008; Bauer et al., 2009).

Following the lead of earlier clinical treatment studies (see previous discussion), the effects of adjunctive supraphysiological doses of L-T$_4$ on relative brain activity as a surrogate index of cerebral glucose metabolism were studied in euthyroid women with bipolar depression using PET technology and ^{18}F]-fluorodeoxyglucose as the radiotracer (Bauer et al., 2005). At baseline, pretreatment, bipolar depressed women had functional abnormalities in prefrontal and limbic brain areas compared to healthy controls. Over seven weeks, the treatment with L-T$_4$ (300 μg/d) significantly improved mood and was accompanied by significant changes in relative brain activity. In particular, L-T$_4$ treatment was associated with a widespread relative deactivation of limbic and subcortical structures, including the amygdala, hippocampus, caudate nucleus, ventral striatum, thalamus, and cerebellar vermis. These findings (confirmed in a recent placebo-controlled PET study; Bauer et al., 2015) suggest that in these treatment-resistant patients L-T$_4$ produces mood improvement by actions on the specific limbic and subcortical circuits that have been implicated in the pathophysiology of mood disorders.

Epidemiological studies have documented high rates of comorbidity between bipolar and anxiety disorders. An independent association of comorbid anxiety with greater severity and impairment in bipolar disorder patients and an association of high anxiety levels with poor therapeutic outcome has also been demonstrated. In a secondary analysis of data from the latter study (Bauer et al., 2005), which used FDG and PET, we examined the relationship between parallel changes in anxiety symptoms and in relative regional brain activity among bipolar depressed patients receiving adjunctive high-dose L-T$_4$ treatment. Relationships were assessed between regional brain activity and anxiety symptoms while controlling for depression severity. At baseline, Trait Anxiety Inventory measures covaried positively with relative brain activity bilaterally in the dorsal anterior cingulate, superior temporal gyri, parahippocampal gyri, amygdala, hippocampus, ventral striatum, and right insula; state anxiety showed a similar pattern. After-treatment anxiety was improved significantly, and change in trait anxiety covaried positively with changes in relative activity in the right amygdala and hippocampus. Results from this analysis indicated that comorbid anxiety symptoms have specific regional cerebral metabolic correlates in bipolar depression and cannot only be explained exclusively by the depressive state of the patients (Bauer et al., 2010).

Thyroid hormone receptors are widely distributed in the brain. Many of the limbic system structures where thyroid hormone receptors are prevalent have been implicated in the pathogenesis of mood disorders. However, the cellular and molecular mechanisms underlying these metabolic effects, and the neuropharmacological basis and functional pathways for the modulatory effects of thyroid hormones on mood, are yet to be understood. Interactions of the thyroid and neurotransmitter systems, primarily norepinephrine and serotonin, which are generally believed to play a major role in the regulation of mood and behavior, may contribute to the mechanism of action in the developing and mature brain (Bauer, Heinz, & Whybrow, 2002; Henley & Koehnle, 1997; Whybrow & Prange, 1981). There is robust evidence, particularly from animal studies, that the modulatory effects on the serotonin system may be due to an increase in serotonergic neurotransmission (Bauer, Heinz, et al., 2002). Thyroid hormones also interact with other neurotransmitter systems involved in mood regulation, including dopamine postreceptor and signal transducing processes, as well as gene regulatory mechanisms. Furthermore, within the CNS, the regulatory cascade through which the thyroid hormones, particularly T$_3$, exert their effects is not well understood: deiodinase activity, nuclear binding to genetic loci, and ultimately protein synthesis may all be involved (Bauer et al., 2008).

CONCLUSION

Thyroid hormones have a multitude of effects on the CNS, and it is now widely recognized that disturbances of mood and cognition often emerge in association with putative disturbance of thyroid metabolism in the brain. As knowledge in basic science and appropriate technology evolve, understanding of the role of thyroid hormone function in the adult brain will continue to be refined. Studies of the biology of thyroid hormone action shows that these hormones play an important role in normal brain function and that current laboratory tests of thyroid status may not provide a sufficiently accurate measure of thyroid hormone function within the CNS.

Managing patients with bipolar disorders is a major treatment challenge, and improved therapies will arise only from an increased understanding of the pathophysiology. Part of that increased understanding will involve neuroendocrine investigations. While studies in drug-free and drug-naïve patients are required, the major necessity is for large-scale longitudinal studies of newly diagnosed patients. Only by studying patients prospectively in different phases of their illness can we achieve real understanding of the evolving biology. This may be even more important in female patients, where the hormonal milieu alters not only across the menstrual cycle but from the pre- to postmenopausal stages. The majority of cross-sectional studies currently available have significant limitations. Prospective studies may not only help increase understanding of the disorder but possibly detect new targets for pharmacological intervention.

Disclosure statement: Dr. Michael Bauer has no conflicts of interests in the context of this chapter. Dr. Timothy Dinan has no conflicts of interest.

REFERENCES

Baethge, C., Blumentritt, H., Berghöfer, A., Bschor, T., Glenn, T., Adli, M., … Finke, R. (2005). Long-term lithium treatment and thyroid antibodies: a controlled study. *Journal of Psychiatry and Neuroscience, 30*(6), 423–427.

Bale, T. L. & Vale, W. W. (2004). CRF and CRF receptors: Role in stress responsivity and other behaviors. *Annual Review of Pharmacology and Toxicology, 44*, 525–557.

Bauer, M., Berghöfer, A., Bschor, T., Baumgartner, A., Kiesslinger, U., Hellweg, R., … Müller-Oerlinghausen, B. (2002). Supraphysiological doses of L-thyroxine in the maintenance treatment of prophylaxis-resistant affective disorders. *Neuropsychopharmacology, 27*, 620–628.

Bauer, M., Berman, S., Stamm, T., Plotkin, M., Adli, M., Pilhatsch, M., … Schlagenhauf, F. (2015). Levothyroxine effects on depressive symptoms and limbic glucose metabolism in bipolar disorder: a randomized, placebo-controlled positron emission tomography study. Molecular Psychiatry. Jan 20. doi: 10.1038/mp.2014.186. [Epub ahead of print].

Bauer, M., Berman, S. M., Voytek, B., Rasgon, N., Mandelkern, M. A., Schlagenhauf, F., … London, E. D. (2010). Regional cerebral glucose metabolism and anxiety symptoms in bipolar depression: Effects of levothyroxine. *Psychiatry Research: Neuroimaging, 181*, 71–76.

Bauer, M., Fairbanks, L., Berghöfer, A., Hierholzer, J., Bschor, T., Baethge, C., … Whybrow, P. C. (2004). Bone mineral density during maintenance treatment with supraphysiological doses of levothyroxine in affective disorders: A longitudinal study. *Journal of Affective Disorders, 83*, 183–190.

Bauer, M., Glenn, T., Pilhatsch, M., Pfennig, A., & Whybrow, P. C. (2013). Gender differences in thyroid system function: relevance to bipolar disorder and its treatment. *Bipolar Disorders, 16*(1), 58–71. doi:10.1111/bdi.12150

Bauer, M., Goetz, T., Glenn, T., & Whybrow, P. C. (2008). The thyroid-brain interaction in thyroid disorders and mood disorders. *Journal of Neuroendocrinology, 20*, 1101–1114.

Bauer, M., Heinz, A., & Whybrow, P. C. (2002). Thyroid hormones, serotonin and mood: Of synergy and significance in the adult brain. *Molecular Psychiatry, 7*, 140–156.

Bauer, M., Hellweg, R., Gräf, K. J., & Baumgartner, A. (1998). Treatment of refractory depression with high-dose thyroxine. *Neuropsychopharmacology, 18*, 444–455.

Bauer, M., London, E. D., Rasgon, N., Berman, S. M., Frye, M. A., Altshuler, L. L., … Whybrow, P. C. (2005). Supraphysiological doses of levothyroxine alter regional cerebral metabolism and improve mood in bipolar depression. *Molecular Psychiatry, 10*(5), 456–469.

Bauer, M., Samuels, M. H., & Whybrow, P. C. (2013). Behavioral and psychiatric aspects of thyrotoxicosis. In L. E. Braverman & D. S. Cooper (Eds.), *Werner & Ingbar's the thyroid: A fundamental and clinical text* (10th ed., pp. 475–480). Philadelphia: Lippincott Williams & Wilkins.

Bauer, M., Silverman, D. H. S., Schlagenhauf, F., London, E. D., Geist, C. L., Van Herle, K., … Whybrow, P. C. (2009). Brain glucose metabolism in hypothyroidism: A positron emission tomography study before and after thyroid hormone replacement therapy. *The Journal of Clinical Endocrinology and Metabolism, 94*, 2922–2929.

Bauer, M., Szuba, M. P., & Whybrow, P. C. (2003). Psychiatric and behavioral manifestations of hyper- and hypothyroidism. In O. M. Wolkowitz & T. J. Rothschild (Eds.), *Psychoneuroendocrinology: The scientific basis of clinical practice* (pp. 419–444). Washington, DC: American Psychiatric Press.

Bauer, M., & Whybrow, P. C. (2002). Thyroid hormone, brain and behavior. In D. W. Pfaff, A. P. Arnold, A. M. Etgen, S. E. Fahrbach, & R. T. Rubin (Eds.), *Hormones, brain and behavior* (pp. 239–264). San Diego: Academic Press.

Bauer, M. S., & Whybrow, P. C. (1990). Rapid cycling bipolar affective disorders: II. Treatment of refractory rapid cycling with high-dose levothyroxine: a preliminary study. *Archives of General Psychiatry, 47*, 435–440.

Baumgartner, A., Bauer, M., & Hellweg, R. (1994). Treatment of intractable non-rapid cycling bipolar affective disorder with high-dose thyroxine: An open clinical trial. *Neuropsychopharmacology, 10*, 183–189.

Binder, E. B. (2009). The role of FKBP5, a co-chaperone of the glucocorticoid receptor in the pathogenesis and therapy of affective and anxiety disorders. *Psychoneuronedocrinology, 345*, 5186–5195.

Binder, E. B., & Nemeroff, C. B. (2010). The CRF system, stress, depression and anxiety—Insights from human genetic studies. *Molecular Psychiatry, 15*, 574–588.

Bradley, A. J., & Dinan, T.G. (2010). A systematic review of hypothalamic-pituitary-adrenal axis function in schizophrenia. Implications for mortality. *Journal of Psychopharmacology, 24*(4), 91–118.

Callahan, A. M., Frye, M. A., Marangell, L. B., George, M. S., Ketter, T. A., L'Herrou, T., & Post, R. M. (1997). Comparative antidepressant effects of intravenous and intrathecal thyrotropin-releasing hormone: Confounding effects of tolerance and implications for therapeutics. *Biological Psychiatry, 41*(3), 264–272.

Charmandari, E., & Kino, T. (2010). Chrousos syndrome: A seminal report, a phylogenetic enigma and the clinical implications of glucocorticoid signalling changes. *European Journal of Clinical Investigation, 40*(10), 932–942.

Cole, D. P., Thase, M. E., Mallinger, A. G., Soares, J. C., Luther, J. F., Kupfer, D. J., & Frank, E. (2002). Slower treatment response in bipolar depression predicted by lower pretreatment thyroid function. *American Journal of Psychiatry, 159*, 116–121.

De Kloet, E. R. (2008). About stress hormones and resilience to psychopathology. *Journal of Neuroendocrinology, 20*(6):885–892.

Deshauer, D., Duffy, A., Alda, M., Grof, E., Albuquerque, J., & Grof, P. (2003). The cortisol awakening response in bipolar illness: A pilot study. *Canadian Journal of Psychiatry, 48*(7), 462–466.

Dinan, T. G., O'Brien, S., Lavelle, E., & Scott, L. V. (2004). Further neuroendocrine evidence of enhanced vasopressin V3 receptor responses in melancholic depression. *Psychological Medicine, 34*(1), 169–172.

Dinan, T. G., & Scott, L. V. (2005). Anatomy of melancholia: focus on the hypothalamic-pituitary-adrenal axis overactivation and the role of vasopressin. *Journal of Anatomy, 207*, 259–264.

Edwards, C. (2012). Sixty years after Hench—Corticosteroids and chronic inflammatory disease. *The Journal of Clinical Endocrinology and Metabolism, 97*(5), 1443–1451.

Frye, M. A., Denicoff, K. D., Bryan, A. L., Smith-Jackson, E. E., Ali, S. O., Luckenbaugh, D., … Post, R. M. (1999). Association between lower serum free T4 and greater mood instability and depression in lithium-maintained bipolar patients. *American Journal of Psychiatry*, *156*, 1909–1914.

Grunze, H. (2011). The clinical side of bipolar disorders. *Pharmacopsychiatry*, *44*(1), 43–48.

Gyulai, L., Bauer, M., Bauer, M. S., García-España, F., Cnaan, A., & Whybrow, P. C., (2003). Thyroid hypofunction in patients with rapid cycling bipolar disorder after lithium challenge. *Biological Psychiatry*, *53*, 899–905.

Henley, W. N., & Koehnle, T. J. (1997). Thyroid hormones and the treatment of depression: An examination of basic hormonal actions in the mature mammalian brain. *Synapse*, *27*, 36–44.

Kirov, G., Tredget, J., John, R., Owen, M. J., & Lazarus, J. H. (2005). A cross-sectional and a prospective study of thyroid disorders in lithium-treated patients. *Journal of Affective Disorders*, *87*(2–3), 313–317.

Kupka, R. W., Nolen, W. A., Post, R. M., McElroy, S. L., Altshuler, L. L., Denicoff, K. D., … Drexhage, H. A. (2002). High rate of autoimmune thyroiditis in bipolar disorder: lack of association with lithium exposure. *Biological Psychiatry*, *51*, 305–311.

Lammers, C. H., Garcia-Borreguero, D., Schmider, J., Gotthardt, U., Dettling, M., Holsboer, F., & Heuser, I. J. E. (1995). Combined dexamethasone/corticotropin-releasing hormone test in patients with schizophrenia and in normal controls: II. *Biological Psychiatry*, *38*, 803–807.

Lloyd, R. B., & Nemeroff, C. B. (2011). The role of corticotropin-releasing hormone in the pathophysiology of depression: therapeutic implications. *Current Topics in Medicinal Chemistry*, *11*(6), 609–617.

Marangell, L. B., George, M. S., Callahan, A. M., Ketter, T. A., Pazzaglia, P. J., L'Herrou, T. A., … Post, R. M. (1997). Effects of intrathecal thyrotropin-releasing hormone (protirelin) in refractory depressed patients. *Archives of General Psychiatry*, *54*, 214–222.

Martin, E. I., Ressler, K. J., Binder, E., & Nemeroff, C. B. (2009). The neurobiology of anxiety disorders: Brain imaging, genetics, and sychoneuroendocrinology. *Psychiatric Clinics of North America*, *32*(3), 549–575.

Martocchia, A., Curto, M., Toussan, L., Stefanelli, M., & Falaschi, P. (2011). Pharmacological strategies against glucocorticoid-mediated brain damage during chronic disorders. *Recent Patents on CNS Drug Discovery*, *16*(3), 196–204.

McEwen, B. S., & Gianaros, P. J. (2010). Central role of the brain in stress and adaptation: Links to socioeconomic status, health, and disease. *Annals of the New York Academy of Sciences*, *1186*, 190–222.

O'Connor, D., Gwirtsman, H., & Loosen, P. T. (2003). Thyroid function in psychiatric disorders. In O. M. Wolkowitzv & T. J. Rothschild (Eds.), *Psychoneuroendocrinology: The scientific basis of clinical practice* (pp. 361–418). Washington, DC: American Psychiatric Press.

Perlis, R. H., Adams, D. H., Fijal, B., Sutton, V. K., Farmen, M., Breier, A., & Houston, J. P. (2010). Genetic association study of treatment response with olanzapine/fluoxetine combination or lamotrigine in bipolar 1 depression. *Journal of Clinical Psychiatry*, *71*, 599–605.

Ricken, R., Bermpohl, F., Schlattmann, P., Bschor, T., Adli, M., Mönter, N., & Bauer, M. (2012). Long-term treatment with supraphysiological doses of thyroid hormone in affective disorders—Effects on bone mineral density. *Journal of Affective Disorders*, *136*(1–2), e89–e94.

Roy, A., Pickar, D., Doran, A., Wolkowitz, O., Gallucci, W., Chrousos, G., & Gold, P. (1986). The corticotropin-releasing hormone stimulation test in chronic schizophrenia. *American Journal of Psychiatry*, *143*(11), 1393–1397.

Rybakowski, J. K., & Twardowska, K. (1999). The dexamethasone/corticotropin-releasing hormone test in depression in bipolar and unipolar affective illness. *Journal of Psychiatric Research*, *33*(5), 363–370.

Santisteban, P. (2013). Development of the hypothalamic-pituitary-thyroid axis. In L. E. Braverman & D. S. Cooper (Eds.), *Werner & Ingbar's the thyroid: A fundamental and clinical text* (10th ed., pp. 4–23). Philadelphia: Lippincott Williams & Wilkins.

Sassi, R. B., Nicoletti, M., Brambilla, P., Harenski, K., Mallinger, A. G., Frank, E., … Soares, J. C. (2001). Decreased pituitary volume in patients with bipolar disorder. *Biological Psychiatry*, *50*(4), 271–280.

Schmider, J., Lammers, C. H., Gotthardt, U., Dettling, M., Holsboer, F., & Heuser, I. J. (1995). Combined dexamethasone/corticotropin-releasing hormone test in acute and remitted manic patients, in acute depression, and in normal controls: I. *Biological Psychiatry*, *15*, 38(12), 797–802.

Schuff, K. G., Samuels, M. H., Whybrow, P. C., & Bauer, M. (2013). Psychiatric and cognitive effects of hypothyroidism. In L. E. Braverman & D. S. Cooper (Eds.), *Werner & Ingbar's the thyroid: A fundamental and clinical text* (10th ed., pp. 596–600). Philadelphia: Lippincott Williams & Wilkins.

Silverman, M. N., & Sternberg, E. M. (2012). Glucocorticoid regulation of inflammation and its functional correlates: From HPA axis to glucocorticoid receptor dysfunction. *Annals of the New York Academy of Sciences*, *1261*, 55–63.

Spijker, A. T., & van Rossum, E. F. C. (2012). Glucocorticoid sensitivity in mood disorders. *Neuroendocrinology*, *95*, 179–186.

Stamm, T., Lewitzka, L., Sauer, C., Pilhatsch, M., Smolka, M. N., Koeberle, U., … Bauer, M. (2013). Supraphysiologic doses of levothyroxine as adjunctive therapy in bipolar depression: A randomized, double-blind, placebo-controlled study. *Journal of Clinical Psychiatry*, *75*(2), 162–168.

Stancer, H. C., & Persad, E. (1982). Treatment of intractable rapid-cycling manic-depressive disorder with levothyroxine. *Archives of General Psychiatry*, *39*, 311–312.

Swann, A. C., Stokes, P. E., Casper, R., Secunda, S. K., Bowden, C. L., Berman, N., … Robins, E. (1992). Hypothalamic-pituitary-adrenocortical function in mixed and pure mania. *Acta Psychiatrica Scandinavica*, *85*, 270–274.

Szczepankiewicz, A., Rybakowski, J. K., Suwalska, A., & Hauser, J. (2011). Glucocorticoid receptor polymorphism is associated with lithium response in bipolar patients. *Neuroendocrinology Letters*, *32*(2), 545–551.

Takahashi, T., Walterfang, M., Wood, S. J., Kempton, M. J., Jogia, J., Lorenzetti, V., … Frangou, S. (2010). Pituitary volume in patients with bipolar disorder and their first-degree relatives. *Journal of Affective Disorders*, *124*(3), 256–261.

van de Ven, A. C., Muntjewerff, J. W., Netea-Maier, R. T., de Vegt, F., Ross, H. A., Sweep, F. C., … Janzing, J.G. (2012). Association between thyroid function, thyroid autoimmunity, and state and trait factors of depression. *Acta Psychiatrica Scandinavica*, *126*(5), 377–384.

Vieta, E., Martínez-De-Osaba, M. J., Colom, F., Martínez-Arán, A., Benabarre, A., & Gastó, C. (1999). Enhanced corticotropin response to corticotropin-releasing hormone as a predictor of mania in euthymic bipolar patients. *Psychological Medicine*, *29*(4), 971–978.

Watson, S., Gallagher, P., Ritchie, J. C. Ferrier, I. N., & Young, A. H. (2004). Hypothalamic-pituitary-adrenal axis function in patients with bipolar disorder. *The British Journal of Psychiatry*, *184*, 496–502.

Watson, S., Gallagher, P., Ferrier, N., & Young, A.H. (2006). Post-dexamethasone arginine vasopressin levels in patients with severe mood *disorders. Journal of Psychiatric Research*, *40*, 353–359.

Wedekind, D., Preiss, B., Cohrs, S., Ruether, E., Huether, G., & Adler, L. (2007). Relationship between nocturnal urinary corrtisol excretion and symptom severity in subgroups of patients with depressive disorders. *Neuropsychobiology*, *56*, 119–122.

Whybrow, P. C., & Prange, A. J. Jr. (1981). A hypothesis of thyroid-catecholamine-receptor interaction. *Archives of General Psychiatry*, *38*, 106–113.

Whybrow, P. C., Prange, A. J. Jr., & Treadway, C. R. (1969). Mental changes accompanying thyroid gland dysfunction. *Archives of General Psychiatry*, *20*, 48–63.

Zeng, H., Schimpf, B. A., Rohde, A. D., Pavlova, M. N., Gragerov, A., & Bergmann, J. E. (2007). Thyrotropin releasing hormone receptor 1-deficient mice display increased depression and anxiety-like behavior. *Molecular Endocrinology*, *21*, 2795–2804.

13.

TRANSLATING BIOMARKERS AND BIOMOLECULAR TREATMENTS TO CLINICAL PRACTICE

ASSESSMENT OF HYPOTHESIS-DRIVEN CLINICAL TRIAL DATA

Marcus V. Zanetti, Alexandre Loch, and Rodrigo Machado-Vieira

INTRODUCTION: TRANSLATIONAL MODELS IN BIPOLAR DISORDER

Bipolar disorder (BD) has been associated with a wide range of neurobiological models, but the pathophysiological mechanisms underlying mood regulation and cognitive symptoms are still not fully understood. Nevertheless, recent progress on the understanding about brain processes from structural to molecular mechanisms has provided a new picture on its still complex etiological basis. Also, a considerable number of patients do not benefit from current treatments and present with functional impairment, poor quality of life, severe disability, and increased risk for suicidal behavior. Indeed, despite critical need for new therapeutic targets for BD, we are experiencing a period of less investment in drug development for BD and other psychiatric disorders relative to previous decades. Personalized treatments have become a key goal in BD research, involving the identification of neural circuits implicated in treatment response. Many new tools and technologies have been established but still do not provide more effective therapeutic approaches for the illness; thus more proof-of-concept studies incorporating biological measures to clinical models are required. Such considerations may offer new multifactorial and dimensional models for the pathophysiology of BD, contributing to the development of improved treatments. Surprisingly, so far only lithium has been first approved for the treatment of BD, while all other treatments were first indicated for other neuropsychiatric disorders. Also, there is a critical need to address the role of significant response variability, cognitive functioning, comorbidities, and treatment-resistant cases for the scientific progress and development of new therapeutic agents that may be more effective than the current standard treatments.

In this chapter we present some recent models of the pathophysiology of BD corroborated by proof-of-concept clinical studies. Several new biological targets have shown potential therapeutic relevance in BD using studies focusing on biomarkers and/or Phase I–II clinical studies. Due to space limitation and major emphasis in other chapters, only some candidates associated with neuroprotection and cellular resilience are presented.

TRANSLATING BIOMARKERS AND BIOMOLECULAR TREATMENTS TO CLINICAL PRACTICE: NEW TOOLS AND TECHNOLOGIES

The need for a more specific neurobiologically oriented diagnosis of BD has been emphasized for research purposes. More recently, the possibility of developing medical tools to aid clinicians in improving diagnostic and prognostic accuracy in psychiatric practice have driven the search for biomarkers for BD. Recent development of noninvasive technologies to study human brain structure and function reinforce the relevance for translational investigations in a two-way bridge (back translation), from bench to bedside and vice versa. In this regard, brain imaging, neurocognitive assessment, and the development of the "omics" approaches, such as genomics, proteomics, metabolomics, and others, have been widely employed, and all of these approaches provide important insights into the pathophysiology of BD.

The number of new technologies available for use in psychiatry research today is much higher compared to what we had two or three decades ago. Though we still do not know the exact biological underpinnings of BD, these new tools

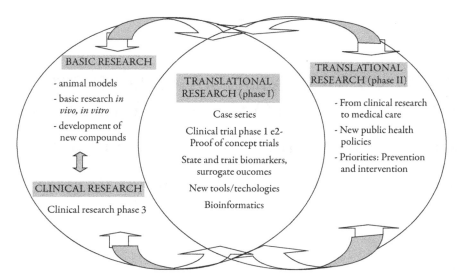

Figure 13.1 Translation and interface from basic and clinical research in bipolar disorder, divided in phase I (translational research per se) e phase II (translational research advances into population benefits and improved health system) (adapted from Machado-Vieira, 2012).

have enabled us to gain a better understanding of disease's pathophysiological processes. As we begin to glimpse what might be happening in the brain of someone with BD, more potential targets for pharmacological intervention become available (see Figure 13.1).

In this "translational" era, all knowledge is merged; efforts are gathered to a common goal, which is the progress of science. Overall, perspectives include improvement in the process of obtaining benefit for patients by transforming scientific discoveries from preclinical research into clinical applications, thus bonding the gap between drug discovery in preclinical models and drug development in humans. This may be possible by providing the identification of more accurate individual treatment through the validation of new biomarkers with potential clinical relevance, including prediction of pharmacological response to a particular treatment and the use of valid surrogate outcomes in BD.

Other challenges to increase effectiveness include the development of new diagnostic tools, score systems for quantitative biomarkers, clinical predictors of response, and surrogate outcomes. Also, small proof-of-concept Phase I trials of novel treatments evaluating surrogate rather than actual populations in clinical trials (e.g., subjects with hyperthymia instead of BD) by employment of certain pharmacological manipulations are able to mimic some of the disease features; such studies in healthy volunteers or special surrogate populations may have a significant impact on the success rates of clinical research in BD at a lower cost and involving less time. In the same context, another model is to design clinical trials that estimate chances of success in initial clinical development, called "quick win, quick kill."

This concept, based on employment of certain biomarkers, focuses on early identification of molecules that will potentially fail or those having the greatest potential for success in Phase I or early Phase II trials.

Another promising issue regarding the elucidation of psychiatric illness pathophysiology and the development of new, improved treatments relies on the recognition of biological signatures at multiple levels (see Figure 13.2). It is nowadays acknowledged that multiple factors with small effects account for the etiology of BD. Consequently, these syndromes would not be recognized by a single biomarker, distinctive of a specific disorder. Instead, a group of biomarkers would constitute a biological signature denoting diverse altered pathological processes underlying the disease (see Table 13.1). If a biological signature for BD is available, biomarker panels could aid in diagnosing BD and possibly also in identifying biological profiles for specific pharmacological interventions. This perspective could bring us one step closer to personalized medicine in psychiatry.

Table 13.1. **BIOMARKERS IN BIPOLAR DISORDER RESEARCH: POTENTIAL UTILITY IN THE CLINICAL PRACTICE AND DEVLOPMENT OF NEW THERAPEUTICS**

- **Diagnostic Tool** *(Trait Marker)*
- **Staging of Disease**
- **Indicator of Disease Prognosis**
- **Prediction and Monitoring of Clinical Response to an Intervention**
- **Phase of the Illness (*State Marker*)**
- **Track Dose-Response**
- **Early Identification of Illness**
- **Mapping of Outcome** *(Natural History Marker)*

CELL ATROPHY AND ILLNESS PROGRESSION

Targets for New Treatments in BD

Levels

NEUROPLASTICITY AND CELLULAR RESILIENCE

BEHAVIORAL COGNITIVE PSYCHOSOCIAL

Treatment-resistant, mood episodes and swings, cognitive deficits, poor social interaction

Mood stabilization (treatment response), fewer episodes, better outcome

MACROSTRUCTURAL

Volume loss (cell death), metabolic syndrome (e.g. HPA axis dysfunction and periphery)

Normal volume in limbic and paralimbic areas, no comorbid conditions)

MACROSTRUCTURAL (MULTIPLE SYNAPSES)

Impaired synaptogenesis/ synaptic loss, decreased synaptic density and connectivity

Strengthen synapses, resilience/adaptability to biological stress, synaptic efficiency

MICROSTRUCTURAL (SINGLE SYNAPSE, CELLULAR LEVEL)

Neuronal and glial atrophy/death

Brain cellular homeostasis

PLASMA MEMBRANE

Receptors dysfunction (monoamines, glutamate, purines..) phospholipases, peroxidation

Normal physicochemical membrane changes

INTRACELLULAR SIGNALING/ SECOND MESSENGERS

Mitochondrial and ER dysfunction, oxidative stress, neurotrophins dysfunction, intracellular signaling, calcium, Bcl2, GSK-3

Multiple functions preservation e.g: energy metabolism, ionic

GENETIC LEVEL

Risk/functional SNPs, altered methylation/RNA expression, epigenetic events, pharmacogenetics, transcriptome changes

DNA integrity

Figure 13.2 Potential therapeutic targets in bipolar disorder at multiple levels (adapted from Machado-Vieira, Soeiro-de-Souza, Richards, Teixeira & Zarate, 2014).

POTENTIAL TARGETS FOR THE DEVELOPMENT OF NEW TREATMENTS FOR BIPOLAR DISORDER

ENERGY METABOLISM AND OXIDATIVE STRESS

Mitochondrial dysfunction

Dysfunction in brain energy metabolism has been considered a key mechanism in the pathophysiology of BD and is supported by different lines of evidence (Quiroz, Gray, Kato, & Manji, 2008). One of the most plausible models to explain this phenomena is the potential occurrence of a subtle mitochondrial dysfunction in BD (Clay, Sillivan, & Konradi, 2011), as corroborated by several lines of investigation. Postmortem studies have found decreased expression of mitochondrial genes encoding the electron transport chain (Konradi et al., 2004; Sun, Wang, Tseng, & Young, 2006), increased upregulation of mitochondria-related genes (Kato, 2007), and abnormal mitochondrial complex I activity (Andreazza, Shao, Wang, & Young, 2010; Andreazza, Wang, Salmasi, Shao, & Young, 2013) in the brain tissue of BD individuals. Also, polymorphisms of mitochondrial DNA have been found to be associated with BD (Kato, Kunugi, Nanko, Kato, 2001; Munakata et al., 2004; Munakata, Iwamoto, Bundo, & Kato, 2005; Xu et al., 2008) and the NDUFAB1 (NADH dehydrogenase [ubiquinone] 1, alpha/beta subcomplex, 1) gene—which encodes a subunit of complex I of the mitochondrial respiratory chain—was encompassed in a region significantly linked to BD by a large case-control genome-wide association (GWA) study (Wellcome Trust Case Control Consortium, 2007).

Mitochondria mainly regulate energy production in the cell, and their dysfunction can result in neuronal damage via multiple mechanisms: decreased adenosine triphosphate (ATP) production, oxidative damage, abnormal calcium sequestration, and apoptosis via activation of caspase proteases. Regarding oxidative damage, under energy stress, mitochondrion generates ATP by anaerobic pathways. These pathways are far less efficient and release only 2 ATPs instead of the 38 of the aerobic pathway. This process also produces lactate, toxic reactive oxygen species and decreases cells' pH levels. In accordance with the theory that BD patients might have impaired cell energy metabolism, magnetic resonance spectroscopy (MRS) studies have documented increased neuronal lactate and lowered pH

levels in BD patients (Dager et al., 2004; Hamakawa et al., 2004). Another sign of compromised mitochondrial energy production are the decreased levels of N-acetyl-aspartate (NAA) seen in BD patients compared to normal controls (Kraguljac et al., 2012). NAA originates in the mitochondria and is a marker of neuronal viability and a proxy for brain energy metabolism. Finally, an elevation of peripheral markers of oxidative stress has been described in BD, which seems to correlate with longer duration of illness and earlier age of onset of BD (Andreazza et al., 2008; Machado-Vieira et al., 2007).

As a consequence of this hypothesis, several substances have been used and are currently being tested as mitochondrial activity modulators: coenzyme Q_{10}, S-Adenosylmethionine, acetyl-L-carnitine, N-acetyl-cysteine, alpha-lipoic acid, creatine monohydrate, and melatonin (Nierenberg et al., 2013). So far, no robust finding regarding these substances has been described. However, some authors argue that combinations of two or more of these candidates for mitochondrial function regulators should be considered for evaluation in rigorous, well-powered clinical trials in patients with BD (Nierenberg et al., 2013).

Arachidonic acid cascade

BD has been associated to increased rates (1.5 to 3 times) of premature death due to medical causes (i.e., unrelated to suicide), higher prevalence of metabolic syndrome (up to 49% of patients in US studies), and greater cardiovascular mortality than that observed in the adult general population (Leboyer et al., 2012). So, besides a possible neurotoxic effect reflected in the worsening of cognitive functioning observed with the disease course, BD also seems to be associated with systemic toxicity. There is also evidence of accelerated aging in BD: individuals with BD exhibit life expectancy reduced by 10 to 13.6 years (Chang et al., 2011; Laursen, 2011) and shortened telomeres (Elvsåshagen et al., 2011; Rizzo et al., 2013) relative to the general population of same age. Moreover, several studies have reported increased peripheral levels of proinflammatory cytokines and decreased levels of regulatory interleukins (such as IL-3, IL-4, and IL-10), suggesting that an imbalance between immune responses Th1 and Th2 might occur at least in the acute phases of BD (for more details, see Chapter 10 on immune mechanisms and inflammation in this volume). As inflammation and increased systemic oxidative stress are known to be linked to atherosclerosis, hypertension, diabetes, and obesity, it has been suggested that inflammatory processes could explain the excess of morbidity and mortality observed in BD and might play a central role in its pathophysiology (Leboyer et al., 2012). Importantly, treatment with mood stabilizers and antipsychotics seem to be protective against premature death and to reduce the excess of cardiovascular mortality observed in BD (Ahrens et al., 1995; Leboyer et al., 2012).

The fact that agents with proven efficacy for the treatment of BD seem to modulate immune-inflammatory activity in patients has been taken as further supportive of a proinflammatory hypothesis in BD. Emerging evidence suggests that antipsychotics and lithium downregulate the expression of inflammatory genes in the monocytes of BD patients (McNamara & Lotrich, 2012; Padmos et al., 2008). Moreover, antipsychotics have been shown to promote inhibition of microglial activity in vitro (Bian et al., 2008; Kato, Monji, Hashioka, & Kanba, 2007). The exact mechanisms by which these agents exert their anti-inflammatory actions are unknown. One hypothesis proposes the arachidonic acid cascade as a potential common target for these medications. Animal studies have revealed that lithium, valproate, and carbamazepine decrease the turnover of arachidonic acid—but not of docosahexaenoic acid—mediated by the calcium-dependent cytosolic isoform of the enzyme phospholipase A2 (cPLA2) in rat brain phospholipids (Rao, Lee, Rapoport, & Bazinet, 2008). This suggests that the therapeutic actions of mood-stabilizer medications are at least partly mediated in part by cyclooxygenase (COX)-2 substrate (arachidonic acid) sequestration in phospholipids and associated reductions in prostaglandin (PG)-E2 production (McNamara & Lotrich, 2012; Rao et al., 2008). Phospholipid-bound arachidonic acid is mobilized via PLA2, and free arachidonic acid is a substrate for COX-mediated biosynthesis of PG, thromboxanes, and prostacyclins, as well as lipoxygenase-mediated biosynthesis of leukotrienes. COX-generated PG-H2 is converted to PG-E2 via PG-E synthase, and PG-E2 stimulates the biosynthesis of downstream proinflammatory cytokines (McNamara & Lotrich, 2012). A small number of trials have investigated the efficacy the anti-inflammatory agents celecoxib (Nery et al., 2008), aspirin (Berk et al., 2013), and long-chain omega-3 fatty acids (Murphy et al., 2012) as adjunctive treatment in BD, with mixed findings.

NEUROPLASTICITY ENHANCERS AND THE GLUTAMATERGIC SYSTEM

Glycogen synthase kinase 3

The enzyme glycogen synthase kinase 3 (GSK3) orchestrates several intracellular pathways, integrating the signaling from neurotransmitters, neurotrophic factors, and hormones (Bartzokis, 2012; Du et al., 2010). GSK3 has nearly 50 substrates in different intracellular compartments and is particularly active in the nucleus and mitochondria, acting as a modulator of several processes related to neuronal function—such as gene expression, neurogenesis, myelination, synaptic plasticity, energy production, inflammation, and neuronal death and survival—through the phosphorylation of other enzymes (Bartzokis, 2012; Li & Jope, 2010; Valvezan & Klein, 2012). The two main isoforms of GSK3, GSK-3α and GSK-3β, are expressed throughout the brain; they are partially active in unstimulated cells and regulated predominantly in an inhibitory manner by similar signaling mechanisms (Li & Jope, 2010). When active, GSK3 blocks myelination (Bartzokis, 2012), progenitor cell proliferation, and neurogenesis (Valvezan & Klein, 2012).

The discovery in 1996 that lithium inhibits GSK3 activity raised the possibility of a link with mood regulation and BD. Since then, different lines of investigation—animal models, in vitro investigation, and clinical studies—suggest that the activity of GSK3 also correlates with mood regulation, although a direct causal or genetic relationship cannot be established (Li & Jope, 2010). Few studies to date have assessed GSK3 activity in the peripheral blood of BD individuals, and the main finding is the reduction of the phosphorylated (inactive) form of the enzyme in patients relative to healthy controls (Li & Jope, 2010). The aforementioned studies have also found that not only lithium but also valproate, antipsychotics, and antidepressants inhibit the GSK3, what could at least partially contribute to its clinical efficacy and suggest that these agents might potentially promote myelination and neurogenesis (Bartzokis, 2012). Consistent with this hypothesis, a recent study of diffusion tensor imaging in bipolar depression have shown that both long-term treatment with lithium and a variant of the GSK-3β promoter gene associated with reduced enzymatic activity were related to increased measures of myelination in key white-matter tracts (Benedetti et al., 2013). There is evidence suggesting that the GSK3 action on mood regulation might be mediated by its effect on glutamatergic transmission (Du et al., 2010) and also by mediating the glucocorticoid-induced inhibition of thyrotropin-releasing hormone (TRH) and TRH-like peptide release in the brain (Pekary, Stevens, Blood, & Sattin, 2010).

Based on these evidences, a number of GSK3 inhibitors have been developed (3-benzofuranyl-4-indolylmaleimides, indirubin, alsterpaullone, TDZD-8, AR-A014418, SB-216763, and SB-627772) and tested in animal models of mania (Gould, Einat, Bhat, & Manji, 2004; Kalinichev & Dawson, 2011; Kozikowski et al., 2007) and depression

(Gould et al., 2004; Ma et al., 2013). Three studies have evaluated the effects of different GSK3 inhibitors in mice with amphetamine-induced hyperactivity and have consistently shown positive results (reduction of activity; Gould et al., 2004; Kalinichev & Dawson, 2011; Kozikowski et al., 2007). The findings of the two studies testing GSK3 inhibitors preclinical models of depression, however, have been mixed. Gould et al. (2004) observed that subacute intraperitoneal injections of AR-A014418 reduced immobility time in rats exposed to the forced swim test. Ma et al. (2013), using a chronic mild stress model in mice, reported that ketamine—but not the GSK3 inhibitor SB216763—significantly attenuated stress (sucrose intake test) and depression (immobility time in the tail suspension test and forced swim test) markers in both stressed and nonstressed (control) groups.

Currently there are no clinical trials testing GSK3 inhibitors in patients with BD. One pilot double-blind, placebo-controlled, randomized trial evaluating the efficacy and safety of the GSK3 inhibitor tideglusib as an add-on treatment in 30 patients with Alzheimer's disease has been recently published (del Ser et al., 2013). A trend toward improvement of cognitive measures was observed in the active group, and tideglusib was associated with a frequency of adverse events similar to that of placebo, with the exception of asymptomatic and transient increases of serum transaminases (del Ser et al., 2013). The fact that a GSK3 inhibitor was generally well tolerated in this preliminary trial suggests that studies investigating the efficacy of these agents in clinical samples of BD patients are feasible in the near future.

Protein kinase C and diacylglycerol

Protein kinase C (PKC) is a group of calcium and phospholipid-dependent enzymes implicated in cell signaling systems with a heterogeneous distribution throughout the body (Hahn & Friedman, 1999; Zarate & Manji, 2009). In the brain, PKC is present in particularly high levels in presynaptic nerve terminals and is thought to play a major role in the regulation of neuronal excitability, neurotransmitters release, and long-term alterations in gene expression and neuroplasticity (Hahn & Friedman, 1999; Zarate & Manji, 2009). Twelve PKC isoforms have been described and are subdivided into three classes (classical/conventional, novel, and atypical) on the basis of activation requirements. Conventional PKC isoforms (α, βI, βII, γ) require calcium and diacylglycerol (DAG) for activation, whereas novel PKC isoforms (δ, ϵ, η, θ, μ), which lack the C2 calcium-binding domain, require only DAG for activation

(Zarate & Manji, 2009). Atypical PKC isoforms (ζ, λ/ι) lack both C2 and DAG-binding C1 domains and, thus are not responsive to calcium or DAG but respond to lipidic mediators such as phosphatidylinositol 3,4,5-triphosphate (Zarate & Manji, 2009). Once activated, PKC translocates from the cytosol to the plasma membrane and other subcellular compartments, which is thought to regulate accessibility to activators and substrates (Hahn & Friedman, 1999; Zarate & Manji, 2009). PKC is activated by such varied upstream signals as G protein-coupled receptors (GPDRs), receptor tyrosine kinases (RTKs), and non-RTKs via DAG activation. Moreover, as alpha-1 adrenergic and 5HT2A receptors are coupled to PKC signaling by GPDRs, norepinephrine and serotonin indirectly activate PKC (Birnbaum et al., 2004), which in turn has been shown to modulate NMDA and AMPA glutamatergic receptor functions through phosphorylation of specific sites (Szabo et al., 2009).

Evidence of different natures have linked BD to abnormalities in PKC signaling and suggest that excessive PKC activation can disrupt prefrontal cortical regulation of thinking and behavior. A number of preclinical studies have demonstrated that (a) lithium and valproate decrease PKC α and γ isoforms in the rat frontal cortex and hippocampus (Birnbaum et al., 2004; Manji et al., 1999); (b) a DAG-like ester, phenylephrine, and a pharmacological stressor were shown to increase PKC α activity in the membrane fraction and decrease acytosolic PKC α activity in prefrontal cortex slices of rats (Birnbaum et al., 2004); (c) when administered to rats and monkeys, these same agents or similar molecules produced a marked impairment of prefrontal cognitive functions; these cognitive deficits were prevented if a PKC inhibitor had been previously administered to the animals (Birnbaum et al., 2004); (d) PKC activity is increased in the prefrontal cortex of animals treated with amphetamine (Szabo et al., 2009), and the use of PKC inhibitors such as tamoxifen has been shown to improve mania-like symptoms (i.e., amphetamine-induced hyperactivity) in animal models (Abrial et al., 2013; Cechinel-Recco et al., 2012; Einat, Yuan, Szabo, Dogra, & Manji, 2007). Abrial et al. also reported that chronic exposure to tamoxifen caused depressive-like behavior in the forced swim test and resulted in a reduction of cell proliferation in the dentate gyrus of the hippocampus, whereas the administration of a PKC activator enhanced risk-taking behavior and induced an antidepressant-like effect in rats.

The results from genetic, postmortem, and clinical investigations also support a role of PKC signaling in the pathophysiology of BD. A polymorphism in the gene encoding phospholipase C, the initial enzyme in the PKC cascade, was identified in a population-based association study of BD patients who were responders to lithium (Turecki et al., 1998). A GWA study of BD in two independent case-control samples of European origin, with a total sample of 1,233 BD type I cases and 1,439 matched controls, found the strongest association signal in the gene encoding DAG kinase eta (DGKH), a key protein for the PKC pathway (Baum et al., 2008). Wang and Friedman (1996), in a postmortem study of BD, observed that cytosolic alpha and membrane-associated gamma and zeta PKC isoforms were elevated in the frontal cortices of BD patients, whereas cytosolic epsilon PKC was found to be reduced, relative to control brain tissue. Finally, increased membrane-associated PKC activity and serotonin-elicited cytosol to membrane PKC translocation have been found in the platelets of BD subjects in acute mania compared to healthy controls, patients with major depression, and patients with schizophrenia (Friedman, Hoau-Yan-Wang, Levinson, Connell, & Singh, 1993; Hahn et al., 2005; Wang, Markowitz, Levinson, Undie, & Friedman, 1999). Interestingly, treatment with lithium or valproate has been shown to reduce both cytosolic and membrane-associated PKC activities and to attenuate PKC translocation (Friedman et al., 1993; Hahn et al., 2005). However, negative (Young, Wang, Woods, & Robb, 1999) and conflicting findings (Pandey et al., 2002; Pandey, Ren, Dwivedi, & Pavuluri, 2008) have also been reported, and more studies are needed to consolidate PKC activity in platelets as a potential clinical biomarker of mania.

While best known for its anti-estrogen properties, tamoxifen is also a potent PKC inhibitor, and its efficacy in acute manic or mixed episodes of BD has been tested by four small clinical trials (Bebchuk et al., 2000; Kulkarni et al., 2006; Yildiz, Guleryuz, Ankerst, Öngür, & Renshaw, 2008; Zarate et al., 2007), all reporting positive results with a rapid onset of action (within five days) and response rates to tamoxifen of up to 63% after three weeks of treatment. In the larger of these studies, Yildiz et al., in a single-agent randomized, double-blind, placebo-controlled (RDBPC) design involving 66 bipolar manic patients (with mean baseline Young Mania Rating Scale [YMRS] scores of 37.9 ± 5.8) found response rates (≥50% improvement in the YMRS) of 48% for tamoxifen and 5% for placebo at Week 3. Importantly, there were no significant between-group differences in adverse effects, and the dropout rates in the placebo group was almost double that of the treatment group with rates of 32% versus 17%, respectively (Yildiz et al., 2008). Also, when only the patients who had been free of any psychotropic medication during the week before randomization were considered, the corresponding rates of responders were 61% with tamoxifen versus 10%

with placebo. Similar responder rates of 63% with tamoxifen versus 13% with placebo was reported in the previous single-agent double-blind study of 16 manic patients conducted at the National Institute of Mental Health (Zarate et al., 2007). Amrollahi et al (2011) conducted a six-week, double-blind, placebo-controlled trial of tamoxifen as an add-on treatment to lithium in 40 inpatients experiencing an acute manic episode and observed that the combination of tamoxifen with lithium was superior to lithium alone for the rapid reduction of manic symptoms.

All the convergent data implicating PKC signaling in the manic phase of BD together with the positive results observed in the clinical trials with tamoxifen are exciting and demonstrate that the development of other compounds targeting PKC inhibition for clinical use is viable. Nevertheless, the efficacy of PKC modulating agents has not been evaluated in other phases of BD or in relapse prevention. Thus more clinical trials with tamoxifen or other PKC inhibitors are needed to address these questions and also to assess long-term safety of PKC inhibitors.

Neurotrophins

Neurotrophins are a group of cellular growth factors also involved in synaptic plasticity and neurogenesis whose effect is partly related to the modulation of activity of the GSK3 (Bartzokis, 2012). The family of neurotrophins is composed of several proteins; the brain-derived neurotrophic factor (BDNF) is the one most extensively studied in BD (Fernandes et al., 2011). One meta-analysis of 13 studies found that the acute phases of BD—both mania and depression—are associated with reduced plasmatic levels of BDNF, whereas euthymic BD patients seem to present similar levels of BDNF to that of healthy controls (Fernandes et al., 2011). Some studies have reported an association between polymorphisms in BDNF promotor gene and vulnerability for the development of BD, and recent works suggest that epistasis and epigenetic alterations affecting this gene are specifically associated with BD type II (D'Addario et al., 2012; Huang et al., 2012; Wang et al., 2012).

Although there are no pharmacological agents specifically targeting the production and/or release of neurotrophins, antidepressants (Molendijk et al., 2014; Shimizu et al., 2003), lithium (Haghighi et al., 2013), electroconvulsive therapy; Haghighi et al., 2013), and the glutamatergic agents ketamine (Duncan et al., 2013; Haile et al., 2014) and memantine (Lu et al., 2012) have been shown to increase peripheral levels of BDNF in patients with major depressive disorder (MDD). Riluzole—another glutamatergic modulator with antidepressant properties (see more details later in the chapter)—has also been demonstrated to increase BDNF levels in patients with Huntington's disease (Squitieri, Ciammola, Colonnese, & Ciarmiello, 2008; Squitieri et al., 2009). However, the results from one recent meta-analysis (Molendijk et al., 2014) and a study evaluating the impact of treatment with venlafaxine and mirtazapine (Deuschle et al., 2013) in serum BDNF concentrations of MDD subjects suggest that neither the association between lower BDNF levels and acute depression nor the effects of different antidepressant agents in BDNF production/release are as consistent as widely accepted. Moreover, while altered levels of neurotrophins in the brain are likely to at least partly contribute to the neurotoxic effects of mood disorders (and underlie the neuroprotective effects of antidepressant and mood stabilizer medications), a direct causal relationship between neurotrophins production and/or release and mood regulation remains to be proven.

Glutamatergic system

The recent reports of a rapid antidepressant action of ketamine—an anesthetic agent that primarily acts as an antagonist of the N-methyl-D-aspartate (NMDA) receptor—in both unipolar and bipolar depression, as well as in cases resistant to other medications and electroconvulsive therapy (Mathews & Zarate, 2013), have brought the attention of the scientific community and pharmaceutical industry to the development of new antidepressants targeting the glutamatergic system.

Glutamate is the most abundant excitatory neurotransmitter in the brain and acts in three different cell compartments—the pre- and postsynaptic neurons and glia—that together characterize the "tripartite glutamatergic synapse." Physiological activity in the glial-neuronal glutamate-glutamine cycle includes the uptake and inactivation of glutamate after its actions as a neurotransmitter have been completed, an effect that aims to prevent toxic effects secondary to overexposure to high glutamate levels (Machado-Vieira, Ibrahim, Henter, & Zarate, 2012).

Glutamate acts through a diversity of ionotropic (ligand-gated cation channels) and metabotropic (G-protein coupled) receptors. The three major types of ionotropic glutamate receptors, which are named after the agonists that were originally identified to activate them selectively, are NMDA (NR1, NR2A, NR2B, NR2C, NR2D, NR3A, and NR3B subunits); α-amino-3-hydroxy-5-methyl-4-isoxazolepropionic (AMPA; GluR1, GluR2, GluR3, GluR4); and kainate (GluR5, GluR6, GluR7, KA1, and KA2). Eight types of the G-protein-coupled metabotropic glutamate receptor family have been identified (mGluR1–8), which have been divided on the basis of sequence homology, second messenger coupling, and pharmacology into three groups: Group I (mGluR1 and 5), Group II (mGluR2 and 3), and Group III (mGluR4, 6, 7, 8; Kew & Kemp, 2005).

Glutamatergic signaling, in particular through ionotropic AMPA and NMDA receptors, plays a crucial role in excitatory neurotransmission, synaptic function, neuroplasticity, and development. Different lines of evidence corroborate the existence of abnormalities in glutamatergic neurotransmission in BD (Machado-Vieira et al., 2012). Postmortem studies have demonstrated downregulation of selected AMPA and NMDA receptor subunits and decreased expression of several glutamate receptors and glutamate transporters in the hippocampus, as well as the frontal and temporal cortex of BD patients (Ginsberg, Hemby, & Smiley, 2012). Importantly, these findings of downregulation/decreased expression of glutamate receptors reported by neuropathological investigations are consistent with the increased levels of brain glutamate (Glx; combination of glutamate plus glutamine) that have been observed in MRS studies (Gigante et al., 2012; Yüksel & Öngür, 2010). The downregulation of both ionotropic and metabotropic glutamate receptors on pyramidal neurons and GABAergic interneurons may have profound downstream effects on excitatory neurotransmission and subsequent behavioral and cognitive implications (Ginsberg et al., 2012). For instance, hypofunction of NMDA receptors in the hippocampus might produce a reduction in the local GABAergic tone, which in turn leads to a disinhibition of hippocampal glutamatergic efferents (overactive pyramidal cells), increased dopamine release in the striatum, and the emergence of psychotic symptoms (Stone et al., 2010). Moreover, animal models suggest that altered NMDA receptor function in the prefrontal cortex may impair GABA neurotransmission, leading to cognitive dysfunction (Lewis & Moghaddam, 2006).

Preclinical and clinical studies have shown that many of the currently available mood stabilizers (lithium, valproate, and lamotrigine) and antidepressants affect the glutamatergic system (Machado-Vieira et al., 2012). Interestingly in this regard, Du et al (2010) have shown that the GSK3 inhibitor AR-A014418 regulated AMPA-induced GluR1 and GluR2 internalization via phosphorylation of kinesin light chain 2 (KLC2)—the key molecule of the kinesin cargo delivery system—providing further evidence of a intercommunication between GSK3 signaling and glutamatergic transmission.

Recently a number of other drugs with known effects on glutamate neurotransmission have been tested for the treatment of depressive disorders, with Riluzole and Ketamine being the most extensively studied. Riluzole (2-amino-6-trifluoromethoxy benzothiazole), which has both neuroprotective and anticonvulsant properties, is a glutamatergic modulator approved by the US Food and Drug Administration for the treatment of amyotrophic lateral sclerosis. Its mechanism of action includes inhibition of voltage-dependent sodium channels in neurons with subsequent inhibition of glutamate release, enhancing AMPA trafficking and membrane insertion of GluR1 and GluR2 and also increasing glutamate reuptake. In the few and small clinical trials conducted to date, riluzole has demonstrated antidepressant efficacy in both unipolar and bipolar depression, including treatment-resistant cases (Machado-Vieira et al., 2012), although two placebo-controlled studies failed to find a significant effect of riluzole for relapse prevention after ketamine infusion (Ibrahim et al., 2012).

Ketamine is a noncompetitive, high-affinity NMDA receptor antagonist. In vitro, ketamine enhances the firing rate of glutamatergic neurons, as well as the presynaptic release of glutamate (Machado-Vieira et al., 2012), which probably relates to the loop with GABA interneurons described earlier. In clinical studies, an initial trial in seven subjects with treatment-resistant MDD found that ketamine improved depressive symptoms within 72 hours after infusion (Berman et al., 2000). Subsequently, a double-blind, placebo-controlled, crossover study showed a fast (first two hours after infusion) and relatively sustained antidepressant effect (one to two weeks) after a single ketamine injection in patients with treatment-resistant MDD (Zarate et al., 2006). More than 70% of patients responded 24 hours after infusion, and 35% showed a sustained response at the end of Week 1. Notably, response rates with ketamine after 24 hours (71%) were similar to those described after six to eight weeks of treatment with traditional monoaminergic-based antidepressants (65%; Machado-Vieira et al., 2012). Since these early pioneer studies were published, several small trials have confirmed the rapid and sustained antidepressant effect of intravenous ketamine in both unipolar and bipolar depression and also in reducing suicidal ideation (Mathews & Zarate, 2013) and, more recently, sublingual administration of ketamine has been tested with promising results (Lara, Bisol, & Munari, 2013). However, larger, "real-world" controlled trials of ketamine in mood disorders are needed before it may be approved for clinical use.

Memantine is a NMDA agent approved for the treatment of dementia that acts as a low-affinity receptor antagonist, with use-voltage dependent effects (Rammes, Danysz, & Parsons, 2008). In clinical trials and in case reports described in the literature, it has been tested as an add-on to mood stabilizers with relatively positive results in both mania (Koukopoulos et al., 2010; Serra, De Chiara, Koukopoulos, & Serra, 2013) and bipolar depression (Stevens, Bies, Shekhar, & Anand, 2013).

A number of novel NMDA antagonists targeting specific subunits of the receptor (mainly NR2A and NR2B) are currently under development in preclinical phases. Moreover, mGluR-modulating agents and AMPA receptors potentiators are also being tested in animal models of mood disorders. Finally, cytoplasmic postsynaptic density–enriched molecules, excitatory amino acid transporters, and vesicular glutamate transporters are also directly involved in synaptic and extra-synaptic glutamate brain levels and represent potential targets for the development of novel pharmacological agents (Machado-Vieira et al., 2012). Other promising targets with ongoing studies are the glycine transporter-1 inhibitors sarcosine and bitopertin and mGluR2/3 modulators such as RO499819 and RO4432717, which have ongoing clinical trials in MDD. Overall, new antidepressants and possibly mood stabilizers based on specific modulation of glutamate neurotransmission are likely to be available for clinical use in the near future.

DOPAMINERGIC SYSTEM

The notion that a dysregulation in the dopaminergic neurotransmission plays an important role in BD pathophysiology is well recognized. Proof of this relationship comes from various levels of evidence.

At the behavioral level, substances that increase dopamine activity are known to produce mania-like clinical presentations (Cousins, Butts, & Young, 2009). Amphetamine, for instance, induces mood elevation and increases goal-directed activities, besides reducing subject's need for sleep. The substance acts by inhibiting dopamine transporter and consequently increasing dopamine at the synapse in the striatum, nucleus accumbens, and frontal cortex. Similarly, the dopamine precursor L-dopa, commonly used in individuals with Parkinson's disease (PD), can induce manic or hypomanic states in such patients. Taking the PD model as an example, this akinetic-rigid syndrome involves loss of dopaminergic neuronal cells. The prevalence of depression among individuals with the disease is higher than that of the general population, ranging from 4% to 70% depending on the screening tool employed (Lieberman, 2006). Nevertheless, depression in PD is qualitatively different from unipolar depression in the way that the former presents with more marked dysphoria, sadness, pessimism, and suicidal ideation than the latter. With progressive increases in dopaminergic therapies, depression in PD eventually progresses to hedonistic homeostatic dysregulation (or dopamine dysregulation syndrome), which mimics BD's mood switch to mania (Berk et al., 2007).

At the biomarker level, it has been observed that levels of homovanillic acid (HVA), a metabolite of dopamine, are decreased in the cerebrospinal fluid of individuals with untreated bipolar depression. On the other hand, HVA are normal or increased in depressed BD subjects taking medication and elevated in unmedicated individuals undergoing a manic state (Zarate et al., 2004).

Regarding dopamine receptors, a few studies have assessed the in vivo availability of dopamine receptor binding by using the single-photon emission computed tomography (SPECT) radiotracer $[^{123}I]$ iodobenzamide. Results are mixed, but a study demonstrated that while D_2 receptor density was normal in all phases of nonpsychotic BD individuals, D_1 receptor binding potentials were reduced in the frontal cortex when compared to healthy controls (Gonul, Coburn, & Kula, 2009).

With compelling evidence pointing toward dopamine as having an important role in BD pathophysiology, atypical antipsychotics are becoming an increasingly frequent prescription for patients with the disease. In a recent RDBPC trial, a group of 343 patients with bipolar depression who received olanzapine monotherapy significantly improved relative to 171 bipolar depression patients receiving a placebo (Tohen et al., 2012). A RDBPC study compared two dosages of quetiapine monotherapy with lithium and with a placebo in 802 individuals with acute bipolar depression. While lithium did not differ significantly from the placebo, quetiapine in 300 or 600 mg daily doses was significantly more effective than both (Young et al., 2010). On the other hand, risperidone (Gopal, Steffens, Kramer, & Olsen, 2005), ziprazidone (Vieta et al., 2010), aripiprazole (Keck et al., 2009), and clozapine (Degner et al., 2000) were seen as effective agents against mania. It has been proposed that these differential effects of atypical antipsychotics involve dopamine regulation. Psychotropics like olanzapine and quetiapine would have specifically increased affinity to block 5-HT_{2A} hetero-receptors located in meso-cortico-limbic dopaminergic neurons. This blockage would increase dopamine release in such neurons, accounting for a better antidepressive profile of both antipsychotics (Brugue & Vieta, 2007). Furthermore, it is also possible that stimulation of 5-HT_{1A} would increase dopamine release in the prefrontal cortex with both quetiapine (Ichikawa, Li, Dai, & Meltzer, 2002) and olanzapine

(Koch, Perry, & Bymaster, 2004) differentially regulating the various components of the dopaminergic projections. For the other atypical agents, dopamine antagonism would account for the main therapeutic effect against mania and hypomania.

An important substance regarding dopamine neurotransmission that has been employed in some proof-of-concept clinical trials is pramipexole. Pramipexole is an aminothiazole derivative, currently approved for Parkinson's disease, which acts as a D_2/D_3 agonist. Data suggest that this medication might have specific D_3 preferring effects, which in theory confers its antidepressant power since D_3 receptor anatomic distribution involves neuronal circuits that have been implicated in depressive states (Zarate et al., 2004). Also, pramipexole has been proven to have neuroprotective effects, since it increases Bcl-2 levels (Inden et al., 2009), an anti-apoptotic protein implicated in bipolar (Shaltiel, Chen, & Manji, 2007) and neurodegenerative disorders (Akhtar, Ness, & Roth, 2004). The first study, published in 2001, enrolled 18 patients with treatment-resistant bipolar II depression receiving either pramipexole or ropinirole (another dopamine agonist) as add-on to their routine treatments. Eight patients were considered as responders, four with pramipexole added on to their normal BD therapeutics (Perugi, Toni, Ruffolo, Frare, & Akiskal, 2001). A study of inpatients with refractory depression enrolled 16 individuals with unipolar depression and 21 individuals with bipolar depression to receive pramipexole added on to their antidepressant treatment. After 16 weeks, 67.7% were considered responders based on reduction on their Montgomery-Åsberg Depression Rating Scale (MADRS) scores (Lattanzi et al., 2002). A first RDBPC trial of pramipexole was conducted in 2004 as add-on therapy for bipolar depression. Twenty-two patients participated in the study. Eight of 12 patients on pramipexole and 2 of 10 patients on a placebo improved significantly as indicated by Hamilton Depression Rating Scale (HAMD) scores (Goldberg, Burdick, & Endick, 2004). This same research group conducted an extended follow-up study with 23 of these patients to assess safety and response. Mean duration of follow-up was 28 weeks. The authors argued that pramipexole was relatively safe and effective in the long term, since 60.9% of the sample encountered sustained remission of their depressive episode (Cassano et al., 2004). Selecting only bipolar II disorder patients in an acute depressive episode, Zarate et al (2004) evaluated 21 patients in a RDBPC study. Sixty percent of pramipexole patients versus 9% placebo patients showed a therapeutic response, as measured by a drop by half in the MADRS scores. A subset of this study's sample was further investigated using PET imaging and [18]FDG as a cerebral metabolism activity radiotracer. Response to pramipexole was associated with a reduction in the regional metabolism of the orbitofrontal, anteromedial, and ventrolateral prefrontal cortex, regions known to have an increased metabolic activity in depressed states. The authors suggest that efficacy of pramipexole augmentation for bipolar depression may have similar mechanisms as other antidepressant therapies (Mah et al., 2011). While targeting cognitive enhancement, Burdick et al (2012) found no significant difference between 24 BD patients receiving a placebo and 21 BD patients receiving pramipexole. Nevertheless, post hoc techniques analyzing only a subset of euthymic BD patients found significant improvement in working memory and processing speed measures. Finally, in another open-label study enrolling 5 BD patients and 12 individuals with unipolar depression, 71% were considered responders (>50% reduction in the HAMD 21-item version) and 59% remitted after 12 weeks of add-on therapy with pramipexole (Hori & Kunugi, 2012).

In sum, pramipexole and other dopaminergic modulators may be considered therapeutic options for bipolar depression, as indicated by proof-of-concept studies. Nevertheless, studies enrolling larger samples are warranted to validate their efficacy and safety.

THE POTENTIAL ROLE OF HORMONES IN BIPOLAR DISORDER: PROOF-OF-CONCEPT STUDIES

As shown in a previous chapter, some core symptoms of depression may be a reflection of primary circadian abnormalities. Circadian rhythms are regulated by the secretion of melatonin by the hypothalamic supra-chiasmatic nucleus (SCN). Regulation occurs mainly by the binding of melatonin to MT1 and MT2 receptors located back in the hypothalamus. Melatonin has a characteristic pattern of secretion, with peaks during the night and valleys during the day, while cortisol is secreted in the opposite way (peaks during the day and valleys at night). The SCN also modulates cognitive performance and cortisol secretion itself, both found altered in mania and in depression (Linkowski et al., 1994).

Pioneering studies linking melatonin to the depression of BD date back 20 years. Decreased overall melatonin levels and clear-cut abnormalities in melatonin secretion pattern have been demonstrated in a number of studies enrolling unipolar and bipolar depressive patients (Lanfumey,

Mongeau, & Hamon, 2013). Conversely, hypercortisolemia is also observed in depressed individuals with a characteristic flattening of circadian variations of cortisol secretion. This finding derives from the classical dexamethasone suppression test (Carroll, Curtis, & Mendels, 1976) and has been replicated over the years. Furthermore, mutant mice deficient in MT1 receptor encoding gene display behavioral abnormalities that resemble some symptoms seen in depression. Melatonin-induced circadian rhythm disturbances can precipitate mood disturbances in a number of ways; for BD regularity of social routines clearly has a protective effect, for instance. At the molecular level, it is plausible that CLOCK genes that are differentially expressed along the day become desynchronized by the disorganization of the circadian cycle.

Consequently, proof-of-concept studies started to focus on this specific neurohormonal target for new pharmacological interventions. Melatonin itself has a well-established hypnotic action and plays a key role in triggering sleep. The substance has been shown to improve sleep disturbances in the context of depression. However, melatonin on its own failed to show any antidepressant efficacy. On the other hand, agomelatine, a MT1 and MT2 agonist but also a 5-HT$_{2C}$ antagonist, demonstrated clear-cut antidepressant activity in animal models of depression. In severely depressed individuals, agomelatine improved sleep–wake rhythms, and treatment with a single dose was capable of restoring sleep architecture. In a study comparing agomelatine with sertraline, the former induced faster improvement than the latter (Kasper & Hamon, 2009). A systematic review carried out by Fornaro, Prestia, Colicchio, and Perugi (2010) stated that agometaline might be an intriguing option for depression. Regarding its use in BD, an open-label study enrolled 21 individuals with bipolar I depression. After receiving agomelatine at 25 mg/day for 6 to 46 weeks, 81% showed marked improvement, with more than 50% reduction in the HAMD scores (Calabrese, Guelfi, Perdrizet-Chevallier, & Agomelatine Bipolar Study Group, 2007).

Other nonpharmacological interventions regarding this neurohormonal system include sleep manipulation/deprivation. The best antidepressive effects were seen in total sleep deprivation or partial sleep deprivation, restricted to the second half of the night. While sleep manipulation still needs to be further investigated regarding its efficacy, its combination with a serotonin specific reuptake inhibitor (SSRI) has been proven to be quite successful, accelerating the improvement of depressive symptoms when compared to SSRI alone. Finally, light therapy has also been proven to be effective against mood disorders, especially for seasonal depression. Here too best results were seen when an antidepressant was combined to the therapeutic regime (Lanfumey et al., 2013).

Besides melatonin, another related hormonal system implicated in mood disorders, also controlled by the hypothalamus, is the hypothalamic–pituitary–adrenal (HPA) axis. The axis functions with the secretion of corticotropin-releasing hormone (CRH) by the hypothalamus; CRH stimulates the release of adrenocorticotropic hormone (ACTH) in the pituitary; and ACTH for its turn enables the secretion of cortisol by the adrenals. Finally, cortisol exerts a negative-feedback effect on the axis when in higher plasma levels.

A study conducting a dexamethasone and CRH test in 28 controls and 53 BD patients showed that the HPA axis function was abnormal in both nonremitted and remitted patients (Watson, Gallagher, Ritchie, Ferrier, & Young, 2004). The authors observed hypersecretion of CRH, blunted corticotropin response to CRH, and both elevated cortisol basal plasma levels and exaggerated cortisol responses to corticotropin (Daban, Vieta, Mackin, & Young, 2005). Changes in CRH secretion may also be detected before a manic or hypomanic episode is clinically evident, constituting a possible trait marker. Consequently, further studies have shown that HPA dysregulation does not seem to be mood specific, being evident in depressed as well as in manic episodes (Daban et al., 2005).

However, severity of depression was correlated with baseline cortisol level in bipolar patients but not in unipolar patients. This suggests a relationship between magnitude of mood episode and intensity of HPA axis dysfunction in BD (Daban et al., 2005). Pharmacological treatment of mood disturbances has also been proven to normalize HPA axis. Tricyclic antidepressants increase glucocorticoid receptor (GR) protein binding and capacity in vivo. This effect was also seen in rats when submitted to lithium therapy or to electroconvulsive therapy. It is supposed that during treatment there might be a gradual reinstatement of appropriate GR function.

As such, one important proof-of-concept substance directed to the HPA axis is mifepristone (RU-486). Paradoxically, mifepristone is a GR antagonist. It is believed that GR antagonists block detrimental effects of hypercortisolism and increase the expression of the receptor itself. In return, this increase would exert more powerful negative feedback on the HPA axis. A double-blind, placebo-controlled crossover study with five patients with psychotic depression found rapid symptomatic improvement following four days of mifepristone (Belanoff, Flores, Kalezhan, Sund, & Schatzberg, 2001). A larger study

replicated this result and also found that higher daily dosages (higher than 600 mg) for short periods might be the optimal treatment (Belanoff et al., 2002). Young et al (2004) enrolled 20 BD patients with depression to receive either mifepristone 600 mg/day or a placebo for six weeks. In the intervention group, neurocognitive measures significantly improved (spatial memory, verbal fluency, spatial recognition memory) and scores on the HAMD significantly decreased. Gallagher, Watson, Elizabeth Dye, Young, and Nicol Ferrier (2008) reported on 19 individuals with BD and 20 individuals with schizophrenia in a seven-day placebo or mifepristone trial. Following mifepristone administration there was a significant increase in cortisol levels from baseline. Nevertheless, at Day 21 of treatment, cortisol levels decreased significantly and fell below the baseline level for both groups. Cortisol levels of individuals on the placebo were unaltered. This reinforces the idea that the substance, acting as a GR antagonist, inhibits the HPA axis in the long term. Finally, in a recent RDBPC trial, Watson et al (2012) evaluated the effect of mifepristone in a lager sample of 60 patients with bipolar depression. The patients received 600 mg/day of mifepristone or placebo as an add-on for seven days and were assessed for their neuropsychological performance. Spatial working memory showed a remarkable improvement, which was sustained seven weeks after cessation of treatment. Magnitude of improvement in spatial working memory was predicted by the magnitude of cortisol response to mifepristone. Nevertheless, no antidepressant effect was observed. Despite this negative result, the authors encourage larger trials with the substance, possibly with higher dosages and plasma levels of mifepristone.

PURINERGIC SYSTEM

The purinergic system dysfunction was indirectly proposed by Kraepelin (1921), who suggested an association between manic symptoms, uric acid excretion, hyperuricemia, and gout. Ten years ago, our group reported the efficacy of an antigout agent and also a purinergic system modulator allopurinol in treatment-resistant mania associated with hyperuricemia (Machado-Vieira, Lara, Souza, & Kapczinski, 2001). The initial report showed improvement of manic symptoms by adding allopurinol to standard treatment, and the observed improvement was associated with a decrease in uric acid levels, which supported an integrative model on the purinergic dysfunction in mania (Machado-Vieira, Lara, Souza, & Kapczinski, 2002). Subsequently, two double-blind, controlled trials supported efficacy of add-on allopurinol in mania (Machado-Vieira et al., 2008, Akhondzadeh et al., 2006). Also, improvement in manic symptoms was associated with a decrease in plasma uric acid levels (Machado-Vieira et al, 2008). A recent systematic review and meta-analysis of randomized controlled trials of adjuvant purinergic modulators in comparison to placebo confirmed their beneficial effects in mania (Hirota & Kishi, 2013).

Also, higher uric acid levels in drug-naive first-episode BD manic patients were recently shown (Salvadore et al., 2010), and the finding seems to be specific for manic episodes (De Berardis et al., 2008). Similarly, subjects with higher uric acid levels presented higher drive, disinhibition, and hyperthymia (Lorenzi et al., 2010). A recent large, nationwide, population-based study with 140,000 subjects displayed an increased risk of gout in subjects with BD (Chung, Huang, & Lin, 2010). Uric acid regulates sleep, motor activity, appetite, cognition, memory, and social interaction (Machado-Vieira et al., 2002). In relevance with the same system, adenosine agonists have shown to be sedative, antiaggressive, anticonvulsant, and antipsychotic, whereas adenosine antagonists, including caffeine, enhance irritability, anxiety, and insomnia (Lara et al., 2006). Importantly, a positive correlation between peripheral and central uric acid levels has been shown (Bowman, Shannon, Frei, Kaye & Quinn, 2010). Finally, recent evidence from genetic studies,

specifically on the P2X7 gene, reinforces involvement of the purinergic system in BD (McQuillin et al., 2009). In conclusion, further research on the purinergic system as a potential therapeutic target in BD is warranted.

IONIC CHANNELS MODULATORS

Increasing evidence suggests that mitochondrial Ca^{2+} sequestration has a key role in modulating the tone of synaptic plasticity in a variety of neuronal circuits. Regulation of mitochondrial function is likely to play important roles in regulating synaptic strength of neuronal circuits mediating complex behaviors (see Figure 13.3).

Intracellular Ca^{2+} concentration is three to four times smaller than extracellular Ca^{2+} concentration. Slight changes in this balance can trigger cell death signaling programs and make neurons escape the capacity of molecular rescue. The endoplasmic reticulum and the mitochondria are critical structures in maintaining this balance through Ca^{2+} sequestration, buffering, and storage and via agonist-activated Ca^{2+} mobilization. Additionally, Ca^{2+} is important in a number of cell-processes, including neurotransmitter synthesis and release, neuronal excitability, synaptogenesis and plasticity, and neuronal cell death.

"...the function or dysfunction of icon channels can have a strong impact on cellular function and cellular signaling."

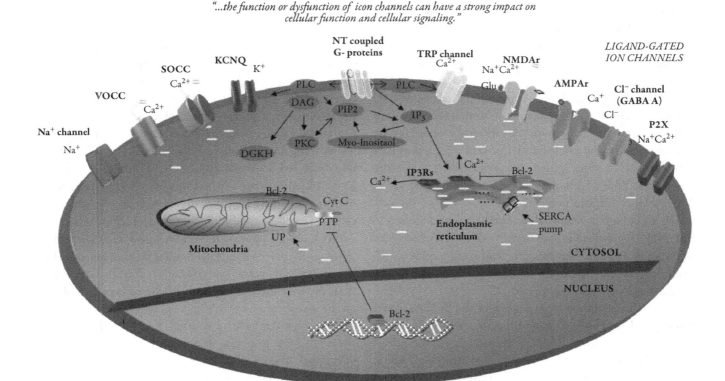

Figure 13.3 Calcium and other ionic channels in the pathophysiology of bipolar disorder: translating biomarkers and bio-molecular treatments.

The first evidence that there might be an impaired Ca^{2+} balance in BD came in 1922, when Weston and Howard observed that Ca^{2+} concentrations in the spinal fluid of individuals with mania were lower than that of depressed individuals. After these findings, a period of controversial results put the theory aside for some decades. The hypothesis of disrupted Ca^{2+} homeostasis in BD began to surface again with findings of higher Ca^{2+} ATPase activity in red blood cells of patients with the disorder compared with controls (Warsh, Andreopoulos, & Li, 2004). Further evidence supported the notion that abnormalities in intracellular Ca^{2+} homeostasis might distinguish BD from MDD patients. It was demonstrated later that intracellular Ca^{2+} was higher in platelets and lymphocytes of BD patients. Also, when Ca^{2+} channels were stimulated, BD displayed an enhanced response to ion-channel agonists in several studies when compared to controls. The question has been raised of whether Ca^{2+} disturbances are trait-specific or state-dependent. However, answering such a question is difficult, since there are several methodological limitations and a variety of confounding factors, such as the effect of pharmacological treatment, for instance. Nevertheless, current evidence is more prone to the hypothesis that Ca^{2+} disturbances are trait-specific (Warsh et al., 2004). Recent studies have pointed to a mitochondrial dysfunction in BD patients, since mitochondria plays a major role in the ion's homeostasis; its dysfunction would possibly contribute to the Ca^{2+} imbalance hypothesis (Clay et al., 2011).

In line with this hypothesis, an increasing body of evidence points to lithium as an important intracellular Ca^{2+} modulator. In animal models, for instance, lithium significantly reduced NMDA receptor-stimulated Ca^{2+} responses. Results were replicated in human subjects, with one observing that lithium inhibits inositol monophosphatase involved in the phosphatidylinositol 4,5-biphosphate turnover (PIP_2), thus influencing intracellular Ca^{2+} concentration (Yildiz, Demopulos, Moore, Renshaw, & Sachs, 2001). Hence lithium prevents entry of Ca^{2+} into the cell, which would affect neuronal excitability, found altered in BD. PIP_2 metabolism is associated with different receptor subtypes (adrenergic, serotonergic, and cholinergic), which would also partly explain the efficacy of lithium in correcting disturbed neurotransmission.

As such, calcium channel antagonists (CCAs) were investigated as potential target-specific treatment candidates for BD. CCAs would act by the mechanisms described previously, but some other hypothetical functions would also be attributed to this class of medications: inactivation of intraneuronal vesicles containing dopamine and attenuation of D_2 receptor sensitization. There are four types of Ca^{2+} channels, but only one is sensitive to CCA in neurons: the slow-gated L channels. Mainly three substances affecting these channels, already used as antihypertensives, were investigated for their action in BD: verapamil, nimodipine, and diltiazem.

One of the first studies of CCAs for BD was carried out with verapamil in the 1980s, which was used in comparison with lithium and a placebo for mania. The two medications had similar antimanic effects, which were significantly more effective than the placebo (Giannini, Houser, Loiselle, Giannini, & Price, 1984). Nevertheless, while early work demonstrated positive results for the drug in the treatment of mania, recent reviews analyzing better-controlled studies have shown inconsistent findings. Keck et al. (2000) pointed out both positive and negative findings for verapamil and suggested that further investigation to establish the effectiveness of the substance was needed. Giannini, Nakoneczie, Melemis, Ventresco, and Condon (2000) observed that verapamil combined with magnesium oxide was more effective than verapamil alone. Janicak, Sharma, Pandey, and Davis (1998) found no benefit of verapamil over a placebo in the treatment of acute mania. In a more recent double-blind study comparing verapamil to lithium, individuals in mania unresponsive to lithium (Phase I) were randomized to verapamil or continuation with lithium (Phase II); those who were still nonresponders were further allocated to a verapamil-lithium combination treatment (Phase III; Mallinger et al., 2008). The authors found that verapamil had some efficacy as a single-agent in mania but had no significant difference when compared to lithium.

Nimodipine was also tested in 30 patients with refractory affective illness (23 with bipolar and 7 with unipolar depression) in a double-blind, placebo-controlled study. One-third of the sample showed a marked response to nimodipine monotherapy. Nonresponders ($n = 14$) further received carbamazepine as an add-on, and 29% achieved remission. The authors noted that individuals with rapid-cycling BD were more prone to respond to the carbamazepine-nimodipine combination (Pazzaglia et al., 1998). Up until now, there have been just a few clinical trials of antihypertensives with modest results, most of them dating back 10 years. Nevertheless, some authors defend that low baseline somatostatin in the cerebro-spinal fluid might predict response to nimodipine (Frye et al., 2003).

Investigators have also tried to establish the effectiveness of diltiazem as an add-on treatment in BD. An open-label, uncontrolled study conducted in 2000 with a very small sample (8 women in either a manic or depressive episode) showed encouraging results. When the six-month time period after the introduction of diltiazem was compared with the same period before the add-on medication, a significant improvement in severity of manic or depressive symptoms was observed (Silverstone & Birkett, 2000). However, as with the other CCAs, studies with better design and recruiting larger samples showed negative findings.

In summary, the potential effects of CCAs on mood regulation have been studied for more than 10 years now. Initial investigations reported some positive results, but these did not endure in the context of more rigorously designed studies. Nevertheless, recent evidence corroborates the occurance of neuronal excitability disturbances in BD, with GWA studies identifying polymorphisms related to ion channel dysfunctions in BD (Craddock & Sklar, 2009). Thus, modulation of Ca^{2+} channels remains a potential target for the development of new pharmacological agents for BD. However, further investigations are still needed in order to improve our understanding on the tole of specific Ca^{2+} channels subtypes in BD, which might also help in the identification of subpopulations of BD patients who would benefit from these agents.

HISTONE DEACETYLASE INHIBITORS

Another potential therapeutic target is protein acetylation. Transcriptional dysregulation of protein acetylation has been involved in the pathophysiology of mood disorders. Histone deacetylase inhibitors (HDAC) are proposed to reverse deficits in molecular brain adaptations, as chromatin remodeling and other epigenetic alterations. These effects increase the ability to produce more "plastic" chromatin, thus strengthening synaptic connections necessary for long-term behavioral changes and mood regulation (Machado-Vieira, Ibrahim, & Zarate, 2011).

Different classes of HDAC inhibitors have been tested, such as Class I and II inhibitors, which include hydroxamates and derivatives of aliphatic acid such as sodium butyrate and valproate. Valproate has been shown to inhibit HDAC activity in vitro in several models, thus suggesting it may play a relevant role in neuroprotection. Due to their potential ability to reverse dysfunctional epigenetic regulation, diverse central nervous system–penetrant HDAC have been proposed for the treatment of affective disorders (Machado-Vieira et al., 2011). For instance, different preclinical studies found that central infusion of an HDAC inhibitor blocked histone deacetylation and induced antidepressant-like effects in rodent models of depression associated with early life stressors (Schroeder et al., 2007, Tsankova et al., 2006; Weaver et al., 20043).

Overall, the active and continuous adaptations of chromatin and the access of gene promoters to transcription factor mechanisms offers solid rationale for the potential therapeutic use of HDAC inhibitors in mood disorders. Limitations include the risk of nonspecific DNA effects and potential side effects. Also, definition of appropriate dose and confirmation that these agents cross the blood-brain barrier are required.

PERSPECTIVES

As discussed in this chapter, a number of molecular systems, neurotransmitters, and cellular signaling circuits are currently under investigation for their role in the pathophysiology of BD and their potential as therapeutic targets for the development of new treatments. It is important to notice that most of these systems (brain energy metabolism, arachidonic acid cascade, GSK3 and PKC signaling pathways, neurotrophins, glutamatergic transmition, and Ca^{2+} channels) interact with each other in a rather complex and imbricated way that is still not fully understood, especially in the living human being. Moreover, we still do not have enough elements to define which of these events would be primary and which would be secondary in the etiological chain of BD neurobiology. The fact that mood stabilizer agents such as lithium and valproate have been shown to modulate most of these targets corroborates this notion.

It is also important to bear in mind that BD is a heterogeneous clinical condition, with high interindividual variability among patients on their clinical manifestations, including the severity and polarity of mood episodes, presence of rapid cycling and cognitive symptoms, and pattern of treatment response. Thus it is unlikely that all of the previously discussed systems would be affected in the same fashion in all subjects with BD and even across the different phases of the illness. For instance, PKC inhibitors (such as tamoxifen) seem to be particularly useful for the treatment of mania but not depression, the inverse occurring with glutamatergic agents (such as ketamine). Also, while relapse prevention is one of the most important aims in the treatment of BD, very little is known about the underlying mechanisms of mood switching. In other words, we have some promising new targets for the treatment of the acute phases of BD but none for sustaining remission over time.

Although the challenges are many, the results of the studies reviewed here suggest that the development of new pharmacological treatments for BD is currently on its way. However, in order to achieve the optimal efficacy and encompass all patients with the full range of clinical manifestations, a great effort is still needed for (a) improving our understanding about the complex mechanisms underlying the full range of manifestations of BD, with special focus on mood switching, and (b) identifying biomarkers of response to specific therapeutic targets in clinical samples of BD individuals ("personalized medicine"). In this sense, multimodal studies combining measures of brain energy metabolism, neurotrophins, GSK3 activity, PKC signaling, and glutamatergic transmission—either through peripheral measures or by using molecular or chemical imaging techniques (i.e., MRS and PET)—in the same subjects are necessary in order to unveil the complex interrelationship between all these factors. Finally, there is also a critical need to "post-translate" results from proof-of-concept clinical research into medical care. In this context, as new technologies allow us to progressively gain a better knowledge of brain functioning, new treatments, aimed at more specific biological targets, will be available for those who need it most.

Disclosure statement: Dr. Rodrigo Machado-Vieira has no conflicts of interest to disclose. Dr. Alexandre Loch has no conflicts of interest to disclose. Dr. Marcus Zanetti has no conflicts of interest to disclose.

REFERENCES

Abrial, E., Etievant, A., Bétry, C., Scarna, H., Lucas, G., Haddjeri, N., & Lambás-Señas, L. (2013). Protein kinase C regulates mood-related behaviors and adult hippocampal cell proliferation in rats. *Progress in Neuro-Psychopharmacology & Biological Psychiatry*, 43, 40–48.

Ahrens, B., Müller-Oerlinghausen, B., Schou, M., Wolf, T., Alda, M., Grof, E., ... Thau K. (1995). Excess cardiovascular and suicide mortality of affective disorders may be reduced by lithium prophylaxis. *Journal of Affective Disorders, 33*(2), 67–75.

Akhondzadeh, S., Milajerdi, M. R., Amini, H., et al. (2006). Allopurinol as an adjunct to lithium and haloperidol for treatment of patients with acute mania: A double-blind, randomized, placebo-controlled trial. *Bipolar Disorders, 8*, 485–489.

Akhtar, R. S., Ness, J. M., & Roth, K. A. (2004). Bcl-2 family regulation of neuronal development and neurodegeneration. *Biochimica et Biophysica Acta, 1644*(2–3), 189–203. doi:10.1016/j.bbamcr.2003.10.013

Amrollahi, Z., Rezaei, F., Salehi, B., Modabbernia, A. H., Maroufi, A., Esfandiari, G. R., ... Akhondzadeh, S. (2011). Double-blind, randomized, placebo-controlled 6-week study on the efficacy and safety of the tamoxifen adjunctive to lithium in acute bipolar mania. *Journal of Affective Disorders, 129*(1–3), 327–331.

Andreazza, A. C., Kauer-Sant'Anna, M., Frey, B. N., Bond, D. J., Kapczinski, F., Young, L. T., & Yatham, L. N. (2008). Oxidative stress markers in bipolar disorder: A meta-analysis. *Journal of Affective Disorders, 111*(2–3), 135–144.

Andreazza, A. C., Shao, L., Wang, J. F., & Young, L. T. (2010). Mitochondrial complex I activity and oxidative damage to mitochondrial proteins in the prefrontal cortex of patients with bipolar disorder. *Archives of General Psychiatry, 67*, 360–368.

Andreazza, A. C., Wang J. F., Salmasi, F., Shao, L., & Young, L. T. (2013). Specific subcellular changes in oxidative stress in prefrontal cortex from patients with bipolar disorder. *Journal of Neurochemistry, 127*(4), 552–561.

Bartzokis, G. (2012). Neuroglialpharmacology: Myelination as a shared mechanism of action of psychotropic treatments. *Neuropharmacology, 62*(7), 2137–2153.

Baum, A. E., Akula, N., Cabanero, M., Cardona, I., Corona, W., Klemens, B., ... McMahon, F. J. (2008). A genome-wide association study implicates diacylglycerol kinase eta (DGKH) and several other genes in the etiology of bipolar disorder. *Molecular Psychiatry, 13*(2), 197–207.

Bebchuk, J. M., Arfken, C. L., Dolan-Manji, S., Murphy, J., Hasanat, K., & Manji, H. K. (2000). A preliminary investigation of a protein kinase C inhibitor in the treatment of acute mania. *Archives of General Psychiatry, 57*(1), 95–97.

Belanoff, J. K., Flores, B. H., Kalezhan, M., Sund, B., & Schatzberg, A. F. (2001). Rapid reversal of psychotic depression using mifepristone. *Journal of Clinical Psychopharmacology, 21*(5), 516–521.

Belanoff, J. K., Rothschild, A. J., Cassidy, F., DeBattista, C., Baulieu, E. E., Schold, C., et al. (2002). An open label trial of C-1073 (mifepristone) for psychotic major depression. *Biological Psychiatry, 52*(5), 386–392.

Benedetti, F., Bollettini, I., et al. (2013). Lithium and GSK3-β promoter gene variants influence white matter microstructure in bipolar disorder. *Neuropsychopharmacology, 38*(2), 313–327.

Berk, M., Dean, O., Drexhage, H., McNeil, J. J., Moylan, S., O'Neil, ... Maes, M. (2013). Aspirin: A review of its neurobiological properties and therapeutic potential for mental illness. *BMC Medicine, 11*, 74.

Berk, M., Dodd, S., Kauer-Sant'Anna, M., Malhi, G. S., Bourin, M., Kapczinski, F., et al. (2007). Dopamine dysregulation syndrome: Implications for a dopamine hypothesis of bipolar disorder. *Acta Psychiatrica Scandinavica, 424*(Suppl.), 41–49.

Berman, R. M., Cappiello, A., Anand, A., Oren, D. A., Heninger, G. R., Charney, D. S., et al. (2000). Antidepressant effects of ketamine in depressed patients. *Biological Psychiatry, 47*, 351–354.

Bian, Q., Kato, T., Monji, A., Hashioka, S., Mizoguchi, Y., Horikawa, H., & Kanba, S. (2008). The effect of atypical antipsychotics, perospirone, ziprasidone and quetiapine on microglial activation induced by interferon-gamma. *Progress in Neuro-Psychopharmacology & Biological Psychiatry, 32*(1), 42–48.

Birnbaum, S. G., Yuan, P. X., Wang, M., Vijayraghavan, S., Bloom, A. K., Davis, D. J., ... Arnsten, A. F. (2004). Protein kinase C overactivity impairs prefrontal cortical regulation of working memory. *Science, 306*(5697), 882–884.

Bowman, G. L., Shannon, J., Frei, B., Kaye, J. A., & Quinn, J. F. (2010). Uric acid as a CNS antioxidant. *Journal of Alzheimers Disease, 19*(4), 1331–1336.

Brugue, E., & Vieta, E. (2007). Atypical antipsychotics in bipolar depression: Neurobiological basis and clinical implications. *Progress in Neuro-Psychopharmacology & Biological Psychiatry, 31*(1), 275–282.

Burdick, K. E., Braga, R. J., Nnadi, C. U., Shaya, Y., Stearns, W. H., Malhotra, A. K. (2012). Placebo-controlled adjunctive trial of pramipexole in patients with bipolar disorder: targeting cognitive dysfunction. *Journal of Clinical Psychiatry, 73*(1), 103–112.

Calabrese, J. R., Guelfi, J. D., Perdrizet-Chevallier, C., & Agomelatine Bipolar Study Group. (2007). Agomelatine adjunctive therapy for acute bipolar depression: preliminary open data. *Bipolar Disorders, 9*(6), 628–635.

Carroll, B. J., Curtis, G. C., & Mendels, J. (1976). Neuroendocrine regulation in depression. I. Limbic system-adrenocortical dysfunction. *Archives of General Psychiatry, 33*(9), 1039–1044.

Cassano, P., Lattanzi, L., Soldani, F., Navari, S., Battistini, G., Gemignani, A., et al. (2004). Pramipexole in treatment-resistant depression: An extended follow-up. *Depression and Anxiety*, *20*(3), 131–138.

Cechinel-Recco, K., Valvassori, S. S., Varela, R. B., Resende, W. R., Arent, C. O., Vitto, M. F., ... Quevedo, J. (2012). Lithium and tamoxifen modulate cellular plasticity cascades in animal model of mania. *Journal of Psychopharmacology*, *26*(12), 1594–1604.

Chang, C. K., Hayes, R. D., Perera, G., Broadbent, M. T., Fernandes, A. C., Lee, W. E., ... Stewart, R. (2011). Life expectancy at birth for people with serious mental illness and other major disorders from a secondary mental health care case register in London. *PLoS One*, *6*(5), e19590.

Chung, K. H., Huang C. C., & Lin, H. C. (2010). Increased risk of gout among patients with bipolar disorder: A nationwide population-based study. *Psychiatry Research*, *180*(2–3), 147–150.

Clay, H. B., Sillivan, S., & Konradi, C. (2011). Mitochondrial dysfunction and pathology in bipolar disorder and schizophrenia. *International Journal of Developmental Neuroscience*, *29*(3), 311–324.

Cousins, D. A., Butts, K., & Young, A. H. (2009). The role of dopamine in bipolar disorder. *Bipolar Disorders*, *11*(8), 787–806.

Craddock, N., & Sklar, P. (2009). Genetics of bipolar disorder: Successful start to a long journey. *Trends in Genetics*, *25*(2), 99–105.

Daban, C., Vieta, E., Mackin, P., & Young, A. H. (2005). Hypothalamic-pituitary-adrenal axis and bipolar disorder. *Psychiatry Clinics of North America*, *28*(2), 469–480.

D'Addario, C., Dell'Osso, B., et al. (2012). Selective DNA methylation of BDNF promoter in bipolar disorder: Differences among patients with BDI and BDII. *Neuropsychopharmacology*, *37*(7), 1647–1655.

Dager, S. R., Friedman, S. D., Parow, A., Demopulos, C., Stoll, A. L., Lyoo, I. K., ... Renshaw, P. F. (2004). Brain metabolic alterations in medication-free patients with bipolar disorder. *Archives of General Psychiatry*, *61*(5), 450–458.

De Berardis, D., Conti, C. M., Campanella, D., et al. (2008). Evaluation of plasma antioxidant levels during different phases of illness in adult patients with bipolar disorder. *Journal of Biological Regulators and Homeostatic Agents*, *22*(3), 195–200.

Degner, D., Bleich, S., Muller, P., Hajak, G., Adler, L., & Ruther, E. (2000). Clozapine in the treatment of mania. *The Journal of Neuropsychiatry and Clinical Neurosciences*, *12*(2), 283.

del Ser, T., Steinwachs, K. C., Gertz, H. J., Andrés, M. V., Gómez-Carrillo, B., Medina, M., ... León, T. (2013). Treatment of Alzheimer's disease with the GSK-3 inhibitor tideglusib: A pilot study. *Journal of Alzheimer's Disease*, *33*(1), 205–215.

Deuschle, M., Gilles, M., Scharnholz, B., Lederbogen, F., Lang, U. E., & Hellweg, R. (2013). Changes of serum concentrations of brain-derived neurotrophic factor (BDNF) during treatment with venlafaxine and mirtazapine: Role of medication and response to treatment. *Pharmacopsychiatry*, *46*(2), 54–58.

Du, J., Wei, Y., Liu, L., Wang, Y., Khairova, R., Blumenthal, R., ... Manji, H. K. (2010). A kinesin signaling complex mediates the ability of GSK-3beta to affect mood-associated behaviors. *Proceedings of the National Academy of Sciences of the United States of America*, *107*(25), 11573–11578.

Duncan, W. C., Sarasso, S., Ferrarelli, F., Selter, J., Riedner, B. A., Hejazi, N. S., ... Zarate, C. A. (2013). Concomitant BDNF and sleep slow wave changes indicate ketamine-induced plasticity in major depressive disorder. *International Journal of Neuropsychopharmacology*, *16*(2), 301–311.

Einat, H., Yuan, P., Szabo, S. T., Dogra, S., & Manji, H. K., (2007). Protein kinase C inhibition by tamoxifen antagonizes manic-like behavior in rats: Implications for the development of novel therapeutics for bipolar disorder. *Neuropsychobiology*, *55*(3–4), 123–131.

Elvsåshagen, T., Vera, E., Bøen, E., Bratlie, J., Andreassen, O. A., Josefsen, D., ... Boye, B. (2011). The load of short telomeres is increased and associated with lifetime number of depressive episodes in bipolar II disorder. *Journal of Affective Disorders*, *135*(1–3), 43–50.

Fernandes, B. S., Gama, C. S., et al. (2011). Brain-derived neurotrophic factor as a state-marker of mood episodes in bipolar disorders: a systematic review and meta-regression analysis. *Journal of Psychiatric Research*, *45*(8), 995–1004.

Fornaro, M., Prestia, D., Colicchio, S., & Perugi, G. (2010). A systematic, updated review on the antidepressant agomelatine focusing on its melatonergic modulation. *Current Neuropharmacology*, *8*(3), 287–304.

Friedman, E., Hoau-Yan-Wang, Levinson, D., Connell, T. A., & Singh, H. (1993). Altered platelet protein kinase C activity in bipolar affective disorder, manic episode. *Biological Psychiatry*, *33*(7), 520–525.

Frye, M. A., Pazzaglia, P. J., George, M. S., Luckenbaugh, D. A., Vanderham, E., Davis, C. L., et al. (2003). Low CSF somatostatin associated with response to nimodipine in patents with affective illness. *Biological Psychiatry*, *53*(2), 180–183.

Gallagher, P., Watson, S., Elizabeth Dye, C., Young, A. H., & Nicol Ferrier, I. (2008). Persistent effects of mifepristone (RU-486) on cortisol levels in bipolar disorder and schizophrenia. *Journal of Psychiatric Research*, *42*(12), 1037–1041.

Giannini, A. J., Houser, W. L. Jr., Loiselle, R. H., Giannini, M. C., & Price, W. A. (1984). Antimanic effects of verapamil. *American Journal of Psychiatry*, *141*(12), 1602–1603.

Giannini, A. J., Nakoneczie, A. M., Melemis, S. M., Ventresco, J., & Condon, M. (2000). Magnesium oxide augmentation of verapamil maintenance therapy in mania. *Psychiatry Research*, *93*(1), 83–87.

Gigante, A. D., Bond, D. J., Lafer, B., Lam, R. W., Young, L. T., & Yatham, L. N. (2012). Brain glutamate levels measured by magnetic resonance spectroscopy in patients with bipolar disorder: A meta-analysis. *Bipolar Disorders*, *14*(5), 478–487.

Ginsberg, S. D., Hemby, S. E., & Smiley, J. F. (2012). Expression profiling in neuropsychiatric disorders: Emphasis on glutamate receptors in bipolar disorder. *Pharmacology Biochemistry & Behavior*, *100*(4), 705–711.

Goldberg, J. F., Burdick, K. E., & Endick, C. J. (2004). Preliminary randomized, double-blind, placebo-controlled trial of pramipexole added to mood stabilizers for treatment-resistant bipolar depression. *American Journal of Psychiatry*, *161*(3), 564–566.

Gonul, A. S., Coburn, K., & Kula, M. (2009). Cerebral blood flow, metabolic, receptor, and transporter changes in bipolar disorder: The role of PET and SPECT studies. *International Review of Psychiatry*, *21*(4), 323–335.

Gopal, S., Steffens, D. C., Kramer, M. L., & Olsen, M. K. (2005). Symptomatic remission in patients with bipolar mania: Results from a double-blind, placebo-controlled trial of risperidone monotherapy. *Journal of Clincial Psychiatry*, *66*(8), 1016–1020.

Gould, T. D., Einat, H., Bhat, R., & Manji, H. K. (2004). AR-A014418, a selective GSK-3 inhibitor, produces antidepressant-like effects in the forced swim test. *International Journal of Neuropsychopharmacology*, *7*(4), 387–390.

Haghighi, M., Salehi, I., Erfani, P., Jahangard, L., Bajoghli, H., Holsboer-Trachsler, E., & Brand, S. (2013). Additional ECT increases BDNF-levels in patients suffering from major depressive disorders compared to patients treated with citalopram only. *Journal of Psychiatric Research*, *47*(7), 908–915.

Hahn, C. G., & Friedman, E. (1999). Abnormalities in protein kinase C signaling and the pathophysiology of bipolar disorder. *Bipolar Disorders*, *1*(2), 81–86.

Hahn, C. G., Umapathy, Wang, H. Y., Koneru, R., Levinson, D. F., & Friedman, E. (2005). Lithium and valproic acid treatments reduce PKC activation and receptor-G protein coupling in platelets of bipolar manic patients. *Journal of Psychiatric Research*, *39*(4), 355–363.

Haile, C. N., Murrough, J. W., Iosifescu, D. V., Chang, L. C., Al Jurdi, R. K., Foulkes, A., ... Mathew, S. J. (2014). Plasma brain derived neurotrophic factor (BDNF) and response to ketamine in treatment-resistant depression. *International Journal of Neuropsychopharmacology, 17*(2), 331–336.

Hamakawa, H., Murashita, J., Yamada, N., et al. (2004). Reduced intracellular pH in the basal ganglia and whole brain measured by P-MRS in bipolar disorder. *Psychiatry Clinical Neuroscience, 58,* 53–59.

Hirota, T., & Kishi, T. (2013. Adenosine hypothesis in schizophrenia and bipolar disorder: a systematic review and meta-analysis of randomized controlled trial of adjuvant purinergic modulators. *Schizophrenia Research, 149*(1–3), 88–95.

Hori, H., & Kunugi, H. (2012). The efficacy of pramipexole, a dopamine receptor agonist, as an adjunctive treatment in treatment-resistant depression: An open-label trial. *ScientificWorldJournal,* 372474.

Huang, C. C., Chang Y. H., et al. (2012). The interaction between BDNF and DRD2 in bipolar II disorder but not in bipolar I disorder. *American Journal of Medical Genetics Part B: Neuropsychiatric Genetics, 159*(5), 501–507.

Ibrahim, L., Diazgranados, N., Franco-Chaves J., Brutsche, N., Henter, I. D., Kronstein, P., … Zarate, C. A. Jr. (2012). Course of improvement in depressive symptoms to a single intravenous infusion of ketamine vs add-on riluzole: results from a 4-week, double-blind, placebo-controlled study. *Neuropsychopharmacology, 37*(6), 1526–1533.

Ichikawa, J., Li, Z, Dai, J., & Meltzer, H. Y. (2002). Atypical antipsychotic drugs, quetiapine, iloperidone, and melperone, preferentially increase dopamine and acetylcholine release in rat medial prefrontal cortex: Role of 5-HT1A receptor agonism. *Brain Research, 956*(2), 349–357.

Inden, M., Kitamura, Y., Tamaki, A., Yanagida, T., Shibaike, T., Yamamoto, A., et al. (2009). Neuroprotective effect of the anti-Parkinsonian drug pramipexole against nigrostriatal dopaminergic degeneration in rotenone-treated mice. *Neurochemistry International, 55*(8), 760–767.

Janicak, P. G., Sharma, R. P., Pandey, G., & Davis, J. M. (1998). Verapamil for the treatment of acute mania: A double-blind, placebo-controlled trial. *American Journal of Psychiatry, 155*(7), 972–973.

Kalinichev, M., & Dawson, L. A. (2011). Evidence for antimanic efficacy of glycogen synthase kinase-3 (GSK3) inhibitors in a strain-specific model of acute mania. *International Journal of Neuropsychopharmacology, 14*(8), 1051–1067.

Kasper, S., & Hamon M. (2009). Beyond the monoaminergic hypothesis: Agomelatine, a new antidepressant with an innovative mechanism of action. *World Journal of Biological Psychiatry, 10*(2), 117–126.

Kato, T. (2007). Mitochondrial dysfunction as the molecular basis of bipolar disorder: Therapeutic implications. *CNS Drugs, 21*(1), 1–11.

Kato, T., Kunugi, H., Nanko, S., & Kato, N. (2001). Mitochondrial DNA polymorphisms in bipolar disorder. *Journal of Affective Disorders, 62,* 151–164.

Kato, T., Monji, A., Hashioka, S., & Kanba, S. (2007). Risperidone significantly inhibits interferon-gamma-induced microglial activation in vitro. *Schizophrenia Research, 92*(1–3), 108–115.

Keck, P. E. Jr., Mendlwicz, J., Calabrese, J. R., Fawcett, J. Suppes T., Vestergaard, P. A., et al. (2000). A review of randomized, controlled clinical trials in acute mania. *Journal of Affective Disorders, 59*(Suppl. 1), S31–S7.

Keck, P. E., Orsulak, P. J., Cutler, A. J., Sanchez, R., Torbeyns, A., Marcus, R. N., et al. (2009). Aripiprazole monotherapy in the treatment of acute bipolar I mania: A randomized, double-blind, placebo- and lithium-controlled study. *Journal of Affective Disorders, 112*(1–3), 36–49.

Kew, J. N., & Kemp, J. A. (2005). Ionotropic and metabotropic glutamate receptor structure and pharmacology. *Psychopharmacology (Berlin), 179*(1), 4–29.

Koch, S., Perry, K. W., & Bymaster, F. P. (2004). Brain region and dose effects of an olanzapine/fluoxetine combination on extracellular monoamine concentrations in the rat. *Neuropharmacology, 46*(2), 232–242.

Konradi, C., Eaton, M., MacDonald, M. L., Walsh, J., Benes, F. M., & Heckers, S. (2004). Molecular evidence for mitochondrial dysfunction in bipolar disorder. *Archives of General Psychiatry, 61,* 300–308.

Koukopoulos, A., Reginaldi, D., Serra, G., Koukopoulos, A., Sani, G., & Serra, G. (2010). Antimanic and mood-stabilizing effect of memantine as an augmenting agent in treatment-resistant bipolar disorder. *Bipolar Disorders, 12*(3), 348–349.

Kozikowski, A. P., Gaisina, I. N., Yuan, H., Petukhov, P. A., Blond, S. Y., Fedolak, A., … McGonigle P. (2007). Structure-based design leads to the identification of lithium mimetics that block mania-like effects in rodents: Possible new GSK-3 beta therapies for bipolar disorders. *Journal of the American Chemical Society, 129*(26), 8328–8332.

Kraepelin, E. (1921). *Manic-depressive insanity and paranoia.* Edinburgh, UK: E&S Livingstone.

Kraguljac, N. V., Reid, M., White, D., Jones, R., den Hollander, J., Lowman, D., & Lahti, A. C., (2012). Neurometabolites in schizophrenia and bipolar disorder—A systematic review and meta-analysis. *Psychiatry Research, 203*(2–3), 111–125.

Kulkarni, J., Garland, K. A., Scaffidi, A., Headey, B., Anderson, R., de Castella, A., … Davis, S. R. (2006). A pilot study of hormone modulation as a new treatment for mania in women with bipolar affective disorder. *Psychoneuroendocrinology, 31*(4), 543–547.

Lanfumey, L., Mongeau, R., & Hamon, M. (2013). Biological rhythms and melatonin in mood disorders and their treatments. *Pharmacological Therapy, 138*(2), 176–184.

Lara, D. R., Bisol, L. W., & Munari, L. R. (2013). Antidepressant, mood stabilizing and procognitive effects of very low dose sublingual ketamine in refractory unipolar and bipolar depression. *International Journal of Neuropsychopharmacology, 16*(9), 2111–2117.

Lara, D. R., Dall'Igna, O. P., Ghisolfi, E. S., et al. (2006). Involvement of adenosine in the neurobiology of schizophrenia and its therapeutic implications. *Progress in Neuro-Psychopharmacology & Biological Psychiatry, 30*(4), 617–629.

Lattanzi, L., Dell'Osso, L., Cassano, P., Pini, S., Rucci, P., Houck, P. R., et al. (2002). Pramipexole in treatment-resistant depression: a 16-week naturalistic study. *Bipolar Disorders, 4*(5), 307–314.

Laursen, T. M. (2011). Life expectancy among persons with schizophrenia or bipolar affective disorder. *Schizophrenia Research, 131*(1–3), 101–104.

Leboyer, M., Soreca, I., Scott, J., Frye, M., Henry, C., Tamouza, R., & Kupfer, D. J. (2012). Can bipolar disorder be viewed as a multi-system inflammatory disease? *Journal of Affective Disorders, 141*(1), 1–10.

Lewis, D. A., & Moghaddam, B. (2006). Cognitive dysfunction in schizophrenia: Convergence of gamma-aminobutyric acid and glutamate alterations. *Archives of Neurology, 63*(10), 1372–1376.

Li, X., & Jope, R. S. (2010). Is glycogen synthase kinase-3 a central modulator in mood regulation? *Neuropsychopharmacology, 35*(11), 2143–2154.

Lieberman, A. (2006). Depression in Parkinson's disease—A review. *Acta Psychiatrica Scandinavica, 113*(1), 1–8.

Linkowski, P., Kerkhofs, M., Van Onderbergen, A., Hubain, P., Copinschi, G., L'Hermite-Baleriaux, M., et al. (1994). The 24-hour profiles of cortisol, prolactin, and growth hormone secretion in mania. *Archives of General Psychiatry, 51*(8), 616–624.

Lorenzi, T. M., Borba. D. L., Dutra, G., et al. (2010). Association of serum uric acid levels with emotional and affective temperaments. *Journal of Affective Disorders, 121*(1–2), 161–164.

Lu, R. B., Chen, S. L., Lee, S. Y., Chang, Y. H., Chen, S. H., Chu, C. H., et al. (2012). Neuroprotective and neurogenesis agent for treating bipolar II disorder: Add-on memantine to mood stabilizer works. *Medical Hypotheses, 79*(2), 280–283.

Ma, X. C., Dang, Y. H., Jia, M., Ma, R., Wang, F., Wu, J., … Hashimoto, K. (2013). Long-lasting antidepressant action of ketamine, but not glycogen synthase kinase-3 inhibitor SB216763, in the chronic mild stress model of mice. *PLoS One, 8*(2), e56053.

Machado-Vieira, R., Andreazza, A. C., Viale, C. I., Zanatto, V., Cereser, V. Jr., da Silva Vargas, R., ... Gentil, V. (2007). Oxidative stress parameters in unmedicated and treated bipolar subjects during initial manic episode: A possible role for lithium antioxidant effects. *Neuroscience Letters, 421*(1), 33–36.

Machado-Vieira, R., Ibrahim, L., Henter, I. D., & Zarate, C. A. Jr. (2012). Novel glutamatergic agents for major depressive disorder and bipolar disorder. *Pharmacology Biochemistry & Behavior, 100*(4), 678–687.

Machado-Vieira, R., Ibrahim, L., & Zarate, C. A. Jr. (2011). Histone deacetylases and mood disorders: Epigenetic programming in gene-environment interactions. *CNS Neuroscience Therapy, 17*(6), 699–704.

Machado-Vieira, R., Lara, D. R., Souza, D. O., & Kapczinski, F. (2001). Therapeutic efficacy of allopurinol in mania associated with hyperuricemia. . *Journal of Clinical Psychopharmacology, 21*(6), 621–622.

Machado-Vieira, R., Lara, D. R., Souza, D. O., & Kapczinski, F. (2002). Purinergic dysfunction in mania: An integrative model. *Medical Hypotheses, 58*(4), 297–304.

Machado-Vieira, R., Soares, J. C., Lara, D. R., Luckenbaugh, D. A., Busnello, J. V., Marca, G., . . . Kapczinski, F. (2008). A double-blind, randomized, placebo-controlled 4-week study on the efficacy and safety of the puriniergicagents allopurinol and dipyridamole adjunctive to lithium in acute bipolar mania. *Journal of Clinical Psychiatry, 69*(8), 1237–1245.

Machado-Vieira, R., Soeiro-De-Souza, M. G., Richards, E. M., Teixeira, A. L., & Zarate, C. A. Jr. (2014). Multiple levels of impaired neural plasticity and cellular resilience in bipolar disorder: developing treatments using an integrated translational approach. *World Journal of Biological Psychiatry, 15*(2), 84–95.

Machado-Vieira, R. (2012). Tracking the impact of translational research in psychiatry: state of the art and perspectives. *Journal of Translational Medicine, 10*, 175.

Mah, L., Zarate, C. A. Jr., Nugent, A. C., Singh, J. B., Manji, H. K., & Drevets, W. C. (2011). Neural mechanisms of antidepressant efficacy of the dopamine receptor agonist pramipexole in treatment of bipolar depression. *International Journal of Neuropsychopharmacology, 14*(4), 545–551.

Mallinger, A. G., Thase, M. E., Haskett, R., Buttenfield, J., Luckenbaugh, D. A., & Frank, E., et al. (2008). Verapamil augmentation of lithium treatment improves outcome in mania unresponsive to lithium alone: Preliminary findings and a discussion of therapeutic mechanisms. *Bipolar Disorders, 10*(8), 856–866.

Manji, H. K., Bebchuk, J. M., Moore, G. J., Glitz, D., Hasanat, K. A., & Chen, G. (1999). Modulation of CNS signal transduction pathways and gene expression by mood-stabilizing agents: Therapeutic implications. *Journal of Clinical Psychiatry, 60*(Suppl. 2), 27–39.

Mathews, D. C., & Zarate, C. A. Jr. (2013). Current status of ketamine and related compounds for depression. *Journal of Clincial Psychiatry, 74*(5), 516–517.

McNamara, R. K., & Lotrich, F. E. (2012). Elevated immune-inflammatory signaling in mood disorders: A new therapeutic target? *Expert Review of Neurotherapeutics, 12*(9), 1143–1161.

McQuillin, A., Bass, N. J., Choudhury, K., et al. (2009). Case-control studies show that a non-conservative amino-acid change from a glutamine to arginine in the P2RX7 purinergic receptor protein is associated with both bipolar- and unipolar-affective disorders. *Molecular Psychiatry, 14*(6), 614–620.

Munakata, K., Iwamoto, K., Bundo, M., & Kato, T. (2005). Mitochondrial DNA 3243A>G mutation and increased expression of LARS2 gene in the brains of patients with bipolar disorder and schizophrenia. *Biological Psychiatry, 57*(5), 525–532.

Munakata, K., Tanaka, M., Mori, K., Washizuka, S., Yoneda, M., Tajima, O., ... Kato, T. (2004). Mitochondrial DNA 3644T→C mutation associated with bipolar disorder. *Genomics, 84*, 1041–1050.

Murphy, B. L., Stoll, A. L., Harris, P. Q., Ravichandran, C., Babb, S. M., Carlezon, W. A. Jr., & Cohen, B. M. (2012). Omega-3 fatty acid treatment, with or without cytidine, fails to show therapeutic properties in bipolar disorder: A double-blind, randomized add-on clinical trial. *Journal of Clinical Psychopharmacology, 32*(5), 699–703.

Nery, F. G., Monkul, E. S., Hatch, J. P., Fonseca, M., Zunta-Soares, G. B., Frey, B. N., ... Soares, J. C. (2008). Celecoxib as an adjunct in the treatment of depressive or mixed episodes of bipolar disorder: A double-blind, randomized, placebo-controlled study. *Human Psychopharmacology, 23*(2), 87–94.

Nierenberg, A. A., Kansky, C., Brennan, B. P., Shelton, R. C., Perlis, R., & Iosifescu, D. V. (2013). Mitochondrial modulators for bipolar disorder: A pathophysiologically informed paradigm for new drug development. *Australian & New Zealand Journal of Psychiatry, 47*(1), 26–42.

Padmos, R. C., Hillegers, M. H., Knijff, E. M., Vonk, R., Bouvy, A., Staal, F. J., ... Drexhage, H. A. (2008). A discriminating messenger RNA signature for bipolar disorder formed by an aberrant expression of inflammatory genes in monocytes. *Archives of General Psychiatry, 65*(4), 395–407.

Pandey, G. N., Dwivedi, Y., SridharaRao, J., Ren, X., Janicak, P. G., & Sharma, R. (2002). Protein kinase C and phospholipase C activity and expression of their specific isozymes is decreased and expression of MARCKS is increased in platelets of bipolar but not in unipolar patients. *Neuropsychopharmacology, 26*(2), 216–228.

Pandey, G. N., Ren, X., Dwivedi, Y., & Pavuluri, M. N. (2008). Decreased protein kinase C (PKC) in platelets of pediatric bipolar patients: Effect of treatment with mood stabilizing drugs. *Journal of Psychiatric Research, 42*(2), 106–116.

Pazzaglia, P. J., Post, R. M., Ketter, T. A., Callahan, A. M., Marangell, L. B., Frye, M. A., et al. (1998). Nimodipine monotherapy and carbamazepine augmentation in patients with refractory recurrent affective illness. *Journal of Clinical Psychopharmacology, 18*(5), 404–413.

Pekary, A. E., Stevens, S. A., Blood, J. D., & Sattin, A. (2010). Rapid modulation of TRH and TRH-like peptide release in rat brain, pancreas, and testis by a GSK-3beta inhibitor. *Peptides, 31*(6), 1083–1093.

Perugi, G., Toni, C., Ruffolo, G., Frare, F., & Akiskal, H. (2001). Adjunctive dopamine agonists in treatment-resistant bipolar II depression: an open case series. *Pharmacopsychiatry, 34*(4), 137–141.

Quiroz, J. A., Gray, N. A., Kato, T., & Manji, H. K. (2008). Mitochondrially mediated plasticity in the pathophysiology and treatment of bipolar disorder. *Neuropsychopharmacology, 33*(11), 2551–2565.

Rammes, G., Danysz, W., & Parsons, C. G. (2008). Pharmacodynamics of memantine: An update. *Current Neuropharmacology, 6*(1), 55–78.

Rao, J. S., Lee, H. J., Rapoport, S. I., & Bazinet, R. P. (2008). Mode of action of mood stabilizers: Is the arachidonic acid cascade a common target? *Molecular Psychiatry, 13*(6), 585–596.

Rizzo, L. B., Do Prado, C. H., Grassi-Oliveira, R., Wieck, A., Correa, B. L., Teixeira, A. L., & Bauer, M. E. (2013). Immunosenescence is associated with human cytomegalovirus and shortened telomeres in type I bipolar disorder. *Bipolar Disorders, 15*(8), 832–838.

Salvadore, G., Viale, C. I., Luckenbaugh, D. A., et al. (2010). Increased uric acid levels in drug-naïve subjects with bipolar disorder during a first manic episode. *Progress in Neuro-Psychopharmacology & Biological Psychiatry, 34*(6), 819–821.

Schroeder, F. A., Lin, C. L., Crusio, W. E., et al. (2007). Antidepressant-like effects of the histone deacetylase inhibitor, sodium butyrate, in the mouse. *Biological Psychiatry, 62*, 55–64.

Serra, G., De Chiara, L., Koukopoulos, A., & Serra, G. (2013). Antimanic and long-lasting mood stabilizing effect of memantine in bipolar I mood disorder: Two case reports. *Journal of Clinical Psychopharmacology, 33*(5), 715–717.

Shaltiel, G., Chen, G., & Manji, H. K. (2007). Neurotrophic signaling cascades in the pathophysiology and treatment of bipolar disorder. *Current Opinions in Pharmacology, 7*(1), 22–26.

Shimizu, E., Hashimoto, K., Okamura, N., Koike, K., Komatsu, N., Kumakiri, C., … Iyo, M. (2003). Alterations of serum levels of brain-derived neurotrophic factor (BDNF) in depressed patients with or without antidepressants. *Biological Psychiatry, 54*(1), 70–75.

Silverstone, P. H., & Birkett, L. (2000). Diltiazem as augmentation therapy in patients with treatment-resistant bipolar disorder: A retrospective study. *Journal of Psychiatry & Neuroscience, 25*(3), 276–280.

Squitieri, F., Ciammola, A., Colonnese, C., & Ciarmiello, A. (2008). Neuroprotective effects of riluzole in Huntington's disease. *European Journal of Nuclear Medicine and Molecular Imaging, 35*(1), 221–222.

Squitieri, F., Orobello, S., Cannella, M., Martino, T., Romanelli, P., Giovacchini, G., et al. (2009). Riluzole protects Huntington disease patients from brain glucose hypometabolism and grey matter volume loss and increases production of neurotrophins. *European Journal of Nuclear Medicine and Molecular Imaging, 36*(7), 1113–1120.

Stevens, J., Bies, R. R., Shekhar, A., & Anand, A. (2013). Bayesian model of Hamilton Depression Rating Score (HDRS) with memantine augmentation in bipolar depression. *British Journal of Clinical Psychopharmacology, 75*(3), 791–798.

Stone, J. M., Howes, O. D., Egerton, A., Kambeitz, J., Allen, P., Lythgoe, D. J., … McGuire, P. (2010). Altered relationship between hippocampal glutamate levels and striatal dopamine function in subjects at ultra high risk of psychosis. *Biological Psychiatry, 68*(7), 599–602.

Sun, X., Wang, J. F., Tseng, M., & Young, L. T. (2006). Downregulation in components of the mitochondrial electron transport chain in the postmortem frontal cortex of subjects with bipolar disorder. *Journal of Psychiatry & Neuroscience, 31*, 189–196.

Szabo, S. T., Machado-Vieira, R., Yuan, P., Wang, Y., Wei, Y., Falke, C., … Du, J. (2009). Glutamate receptors as targets of protein kinase C in the pathophysiology and treatment of animal models of mania. *Neuropharmacology, 56*(1), 47–55.

Tohen, M., McDonnell, D. P., Case, M., Kanba, S., Ha, K., Fang, Y. R., et al. (2012). Randomised, double-blind, placebo-controlled study of olanzapine in patients with bipolar I depression. *British Journal of Psychiatry, 201*(5), 376–382.

Tsankova, N. M., Berton, O., Renthal, W., et al. (2006). Sustained hippocampal chromatin regulation in a mouse model of depression and antidepressant action. *Nature Neuroscience, 9*, 519–525.

Turecki, G., Grof, P., Cavazzoni, P., Duffy, A., Grof, E., Ahrens, B., … Alda, M. (1998). Evidence for a role of phospholipase C-gamma1 in the pathogenesis of bipolar disorder. *Molecular Psychiatry, 3*(6), 534–538.

Valvezan, A. J., & Klein, P. S. (2012). GSK-3 and Wnt signaling in neurogenesis and bipolar disorders. *Frontiers in Molecular Neuroscience, 5*, 1.

Vieta, E., Ramey, T., Keller, D., English, P. A., Loebel, A. D., & Miceli, J. (2010). Ziprasidone in the treatment of acute mania: A 12-week, placebo-controlled, haloperidol-referenced study. *Journal of Psychopharmacology, 24*(4), 547–558.

Wang, H. Y., & Friedman, E. (1996). Enhanced protein kinase C activity and translocation in bipolar affective disorder brains. *Biological Psychiatry, 40*(7), 568–575.

Wang, H. Y., Markowitz, P., Levinson, D., Undie, A. S., & Friedman E. (1999). Increased membrane-associated protein kinase C activity and translocation in blood platelets from bipolar affective disorder patients. *Journal of Psychiatric Research, 33*(2), 171–179.

Wang, Z., Li, Z., et al. (2012). Association of BDNF gene polymorphism with bipolar disorders in Han Chinese population. *Genes, Brain and Behavior, 11*(5), 524–528.

Warsh, J. J., Andreopoulos, S., & Li, P. P. (2004). Role of intracellular calcium signaling in the pathophysiology and pharmacotherapy of bipolar disorder: current status. *Clinical Neuroscience Research, 4*(3–4), 201–213.

Watson, S., Gallagher P., Porter R. J., Smith, M. S., Herron, L. J., Bulmer, S., et al. (2012). A randomized trial to examine the effect of mifepristone on neuropsychological performance and mood in patients with bipolar depression. *Biological Psychiatry, 72*(11), 943–949.

Watson, S., Gallagher, P., Ritchie, J. C., Ferrier, I. N., & Young A. H. (2004). Hypothalamic-pituitary-adrenal axis function in patients with bipolar disorder. *British Journal of Psychiatry, 184*, 496–502.

Weaver, I. C., Cervoni, N., Champagne, F. A., et al. (2004). Epigenetic programming by maternal behavior. *Nature Neuroscience, 7*, 847–854.

Wellcome Trust Case Control Consortium. (2007). Genome-wide association study of 14,000 cases of seven common diseases and 3,000 shared controls. *Nature, 447*(7145), 661–678.

Weston, P. G., & Howard, M. Q. (1992). The determination of sodium, potassium, calcium and magnesium in the blood and spinal fluid of patients suffering from manic-depressive insanity. *Archives of Neurology & Psychiatry, 8*(2), 179–183.

Xu, C., Li, P. P., Kennedy, J. L., Green, M., Hughes, B., Cooke, R. G., … Warsh J. J. (2008). Further support for association of the mitochondrial complex I subunit gene NDUFV2 with bipolar disorder. *Bipolar Disorders, 10*, 105–110.

Yildiz, A., Demopulos, C. M., Moore, C. M., Renshaw, P. F., & Sachs, G. S. (2001). Effect of lithium on phosphoinositide metabolism in human brain: A proton-decoupled 31P MRS Study. *Biological Psychiatry, 50*(1), 3–7.

Yildiz, A., Guleryuz, S., Ankerst, D. P., Öngür, D., & Renshaw, P. F. (2008). Protein kinase C inhibition in the treatment of mania: A double-blind, placebo-controlled trial of tamoxifen. *Archives of General Psychiatry, 65*(3), 255–263.

Young, A. H., Gallagher, P., Watson, S., Del-Estal, D., Owen, B. M., & Ferrier, I. N. (2004). Improvements in neurocognitive function and mood following adjunctive treatment with mifepristone (RU-486) in bipolar disorder. *Neuropsychopharmacology, 29*(8), 1538–1545.

Young, A. H., McElroy, S. L., Bauer, M., Philips, N., Chang, W., Olausson, B., et al. (2010). A double-blind, placebo-controlled study of quetiapine and lithium monotherapy in adults in the acute phase of bipolar depression (EMBOLDEN I). *Journal of Clincial Psychiatry, 71*(2), 150–162.

Young, L. T., Wang J. F., Woods, C. M., & Robb, J. C. (1999). Platelet protein kinase C alpha levels in drug-free and lithium-treated subjects with bipolar disorder. *Neuropsychobiology, 40*(2), 63–66.

Yüksel, C., & Öngür, D. (2010). Magnetic resonance spectroscopy studies of glutamate-related abnormalities in mood disorders. *Biological Psychiatry, 68*(9), 785–794.

Zarate, C. A. Jr., Singh, J. B., Carlson, P. J., Quiroz, J., Jolkovsky, L., Luckenbaugh, D. A., & Manji, H. K. (2007). Efficacy of a protein kinase C inhibitor (tamoxifen) in the treatment of acute mania: a pilot study. *Bipolar Disorders, 9*(6), 561–570.

Zarate, C. A. Jr., Payne, J. L., Singh, J., Quiroz, J. A., Luckenbaugh, D. A., Denicoff, K. D., et al. (2004). Pramipexole for bipolar II depression: a placebo-controlled proof of concept study. *Biological Psychiatry, 56*(1), 54–60.

Zarate, C. A. Jr., Singh, J. B., Carlson, P. J., Brutsche, N. E., Ameli, R., Luckenbaugh, D. A., et al. (2006). A randomized trial of an N-methyl-D-aspartate antagonist in treatment-resistant major depression. *Archives of General Psychiatry, 63*, 856–864.

Zarate, C. A., & Manji, H. K. (2009). Protein kinase C inhibitors: Rationale for use and potential in the treatment of bipolar disorder. *CNS Drugs, 23*(7), 569–582.

PART II

GENETIC

14.

THE APPLE AND THE TREE

WHAT FAMILY AND OFFSPRING STUDIES OF BIPOLAR DISORDER SHOW ABOUT MECHANISMS OF RISK AND PREVENTION

Guillermo Perez Algorta, Anna Van Meter, and Eric A. Youngstrom

INTRODUCTION

Being a parent is a challenging and often emotionally charged life role. Suffering from a mental illness, such as bipolar disorder (BD), adds complications to one's role as a parent and can result in unexpected outcomes. Though conventional perspectives focus on the ways in which parents influence and mold their children—through genes, parenting practices, and environment—children have a significant impact on their parents as well. Parenting is a dynamic phenomenon determined by the child's characteristics, contextual sources of stress and support, and parent personality (Belsky, 1984). For people with BD, becoming a parent can be protective, by providing new motivation for better self-care with the goal of remaining healthy and present as a parent, but having a child can also be a risk factor due to significant time and energy expenditures associated with parenting (Ehlers, Frank, & Kupfer, 1988). Our goal is to review the role that heritability plays in families with BD and to extend the discussion beyond genes and biology to include the reciprocal social and behavioral influences parents and offspring have on one another.

BIPOLAR FAMILIES: THE ROLE OF GENES AND BIOLOGY

Bipolar disorder is highly heritable (Smoller & Finn, 2003). Among youth with one parent with BD, the rate of BD is 5% to 15% (Birmaher et al., 2009; Lapalme et al., 1997; Singh et al., 2007). Among those youth who have two parents with BD, the rate is as high as 30% (Goodwin & Jamison, 2007; Gottesman, Laursen, Bertelsen, & Mortensen, 2010). This is a risk of 5 to 10 times higher than expected in the

general population (Merikangas et al., 2010; Van Meter, Moreira, & Youngstrom, 2011). The concordance rate for BD in monozygotic twins is 50% to 60% and 13% to 23% in dizygotic twins and non-twin siblings (Goodwin & Jamison, 2007), further increasing the likelihood of multiple cases of BD within a family. Greater familial loading is associated with earlier illness onset (Lapalme et al., 1997; Pauls, 1992), which often leads to a more difficult illness course (James, 2011). Like other youth with BD, those who have a family history tend to have an index mood episode of depression, followed by a high rate of recurrence and/or chronic mood lability (Duffy, Alda, Hajek, & Grof, 2009).

The heritability of BD may vary as a function of the type of bipolar or the severity of illness in the parent. In one study, the odds ratio of meeting criteria for an Axis I disorder for BD offspring was 15.0 when a parent had BD with a lifetime history of psychotic symptoms versus 3.3 when a parent had bipolar II disorder (Garcia-Amador et al., 2013). In the same study, half of BD offspring met the diagnostic criteria for at least one Axis I disorder, the most common being attention deficit hyperactivity disorder (30%), anxiety disorders (14%), and other affective disorders (10%; Garcia-Amador et al., 2013), indicating that bipolar family history is a risk factor for a wide range of pathology and not specifically for BD.

In addition to BD, other affective disorders and anxiety are the most common Axis I disorders among BD offspring (Lapalme, Hodgins, & LaRoche, 1997; Vandeleur et al., 2012), with BD offspring being about three times more likely to develop a non-BD Axis I disorder than healthy controls, on average. However, some studies have found rates of Axis I disorders as high as 72% among BD offspring (Mesman, Nolen, Reichart, Wals, & Hillegers, 2013). In addition to increased risk of BD, bilineal BD history is associated with greater severity of symptoms such as depressed and irritable mood, lack of mood reactivity, and rejection sensitivity. In families parented by someone with BD, the likelihood of the offspring having BD or another Axis I disorder is high, which further impacts the family dynamic and functioning.

Conversely, better functioning in biological co-parents is associated with a significantly lower frequency of Axis I disorder in BD offspring (Garcia-Amador et al., 2013), suggesting that genes are not fate; parent behavior and environment play an important role too. Family members' behavior can affect the illness course, and the illness reciprocally impacts family functioning (Lytton, 1990a, 1990b).

Children's reaction to their family environment further influences the likelihood of Axis I pathology. Consistent with the diathesis-stress model (Zuckerman, 1999), a genetic vulnerability, plus individual differences in biological reactivity to stress, may increase susceptibility for developing a mental illness. One mechanism proposed to explain the intergenerational transmission of risk for psychopathology and other negative health outcomes in the offspring of depressed parents is dysregulation of the hypothalamic-pituitary-adrenal (HPA) axis, one of the body's major stress-response systems (Goodman & Gotlib, 1999). Specifically, heightened HPA axis reactivity to environmental stressors has been posited to play a role in the process linking stress to illness (Holsboer, 2000).

Both genetics and experience play a role in the stress response. Cortisol reactivity is moderately heritable (Steptoe, van Jaarsveld, Semmler, Plomin, & Wardle, 2009), and individual traits, such as temperament and behavior, are linked to cortisol response to stress (Gunnar & Vazquez, 2006). Furthermore, environmental influences, such as stress, adversity, and parental psychopathology, are linked to poor HPA functioning in youth, but a positive family environment can moderate the relation between early adversity and offspring neuroendocrine functioning (Essex et al., 2011; Luecken & Appelhans, 2006). These effects can be long-lasting, with exposure to maternal psychopathology in childhood associated with dysregulated basal cortisol into the offspring's adolescence (Essex et al., 2011). The effects can also be additive; offspring exposed to both parental depression and hostile parenting behaviors during early childhood displayed high cortisol levels in response to a laboratory stressor (Dougherty, Tolep, Smith, & Rose, 2013). Other studies have found high levels of cortisol in depressed adolescents and adults, suggesting that increased stress sensitivity, due to early dysregulation of the HPA axis, may render high-risk offspring more vulnerable

to the depressogenic effects of stress later in life (Dougherty et al., 2013).

Certain temperamental styles are thought to represent a genetic risk factor for the development of affective disorders (Evans et al., 2008; Gonda et al., 2006; Greenwood, Akiskal, Akiskal, & Kelsoe, 2012), and it has been proposed that temperament may be the primary route by which genetic risk for BD is passed on (Evans et al., 2005; Yuan et al., 2012). Even before meeting criteria for a psychiatric illness, children of BD parents often show temperamental characteristics thought to precede clinical symptoms in many cases. These include high motor activity, low frustration tolerance, and emotional sensitivity, which may be evident very early in a child's life, reflecting innate characteristics (Chang, Steiner, & Ketter, 2000). These traits increase the propensity to have exaggerated or inappropriate emotional reactions to negative life events and stressors, along with poor affective regulation (Duffy et al., 2007). BD offspring tend toward greater mood lability and irritability than other children (Birmaher et al., 2013), increasing the risk for, and intensity of, conflict with both parents and other individuals. There also is a tendency for bipolar offspring to experience heightened distress in response to conflict and to react in suboptimal ways to psychosocial stressors. This situation may develop into a positive feedback loop for both the child and the parent, whereby each exacerbates the other's mood symptoms through heightened reactivity and conflict. These strong, negative responses can create a chain reaction, making it difficult for children with BD to socialize appropriately (Bella et al., 2011; Chang, Steiner, & Ketter, 2003). Some will act aggressively or otherwise alienate peers and family members, limiting social support and increasing the risk for affective psychopathology above and beyond the genetic risk conferred.

BIDIRECTIONALITY

The default message communicated by family studies of BD is that parents with BD confer great risk of psychiatric illness on their children. However, children also create risk for their parents. Even if they do not meet criteria for any psychiatric illness, children require a great amount of time and energy. They test their parents' patience and are often associated with increased stress, sleep deprivation, and poor self-care—all risk factors for the onset of a mood episode.

Social *zeitgeber* theory suggests that genetically vulnerable individuals may be at high risk for a mood episode when they experience a disruption of their routine. Other people, obligations, and even the seasons act as *zeitgebers*, imposing structure on individuals and helping them to maintain regular moods. If a *zeitgeber* is disturbed, or if a *zeitstörer*, an external rhythm disrupter, appears, the regularity of routine is threatened and mood episodes are more likely to occur (Frank, Swartz, & Kupfer, 2000).

Children exert powerful influences on parents' schedules. Once they begin attending school and have regular routines themselves, they may become *zeitgebers*, imposing structure on their parents with positive effects. However, as new babies, children are undoubtedly *zeitstörers*, making routine very difficult with irregular and important demands. This is likely a factor in the development of postpartum pathology.

Though the birth of a child is usually a happy event, the incidence of psychiatric disturbance among parents—both mothers and fathers—increases in the perinatal and postpartum periods (Davenport & Adland, 1982). Perinatal factors increase risk of BD specifically (Sharma, 2012). Some mothers with diagnosed BD may choose or be advised by their doctor to discontinue some medications to reduce risk to the fetus, which increases the likelihood of a mood episode (Davenport & Adland, 1982). Hormonal changes may affect a woman's mood (Meinhard, 2013). Extreme changes to either parent's sleep–wake cycle or schedule are risk factors, as is the potential for discord in the marital relationship (Marks, 1992; Murray, 2010). Finally, the transitional period around the addition of a child is often very emotional; for people at risk for BD or who already have affective pathology, heightened emotional responses—and an inability to successfully regulate these responses—can result in a mood episode (Davenport & Adland, 1982).

Emotion-regulation deficits are common among both youth and adults with BD (Green, Cahill, & Malhi, 2007; Townsend, 2012). According to Hodgins et al.'s (2002) model, children born with a genetic predisposition to depression or BD inherit "a tendency to react emotionally to stressors and daily hassles" and are likely to have parent(s) who also tend to react strongly. This combination of high reactivity from both child and parents leads to higher levels of stress and conflict within the family.

Such emotionally labile environments may provoke the onset, or serve to maintain, mood episodes. A child with a short emotional fuse may also have a parent prone to strong emotional responses, which creates a family environment where parent and child repeatedly trigger strong emotional exchanges. Additionally, a child with a parent who reacts strongly has fewer opportunities to learn how to regulate his or her emotions, making it more likely that emotionally-intense interactions will occur frequently—both with family members and others.

An emotionally charged family environment may also serve as a method of transmission, whereby the behavior of a parent (or child) experiencing a mood episode triggers a mood episode in the other family member (Lytton, 1990a). Behavioral geneticists describe this as an "extended phenotype," where the genes of risk in the child also are present in the parent, conveying not only biological risk but also changing the environment in a way that further amplifies effects (Plomin, 1995). Factors such as expressed emotion and family environment are important to the onset and maintenance of both mood episodes and periods of euthymic mood (Calam, 2012; Miklowitz, 2004; Miklowitz & Johnson, 2009), and many of the empirically supported treatments for BD focus on reducing expressed emotion and building stable family environments in order to reduce mood episode frequency and intensity. When multiple members experience mood disruptions, families are less likely to achieve the type of structure and stability that promotes good mental health.

THE APPLE: LIFE FOR THE CHILDREN OF PARENTS WITH BIPOLAR DISORDER

Reports on the psychosocial effects of having a parent with BD are inconsistent (Jones & Bentall, 2008). Offspring of parents with BD often show aggressive behavior that is strongly influenced by deficient parenting (Chang et al., 2003). Parent behavior, and the associated psychosocial disturbance in the family, likely confers as much if not more risk than genes (Rutter & Quinton, 1984). But some healthy offspring of BD parents perceive their mothers as less rejecting, more emotionally warm, and less overprotective than offspring of healthy parents (Reichart et al., 2007). Interestingly, the same study found that offspring with BD reported more rejection by their fathers and mothers compared with offspring with other diagnoses or without diagnosis. Perhaps the offspring's disorder has a greater impact on the child-rearing practices of the parents than the BD of the parents, or perhaps the child's experience of the parents is filtered by the child's psychopathology.

Offspring with BD may be more sensitive to cues from their parents, particularly negative ones. Studies of emotion perception find that youth with BD tend to interpret neutral faces as more hostile and fear provoking (Dickstein et al., 2007; Rich et al., 2005). These negative perceptual biases in social interactions may then evoke more extreme emotional responses (Green et al., 2007).

Children of BD parents face multiple challenges. During manic episodes, parents are overactive, aggressive, unpredictable, or destructive. During depressive episodes, they are inactive, absent, or even suicidal. The consequences—painful emotions, anger, anxiety, concern, and ambivalence—take a toll on the offspring (Hinshaw, 2008; Sturges, 1977). Compared to depressed or healthy mothers, mothers with BD can be more negative in their interactions with their children (Inoff-Germain, Nottelmann, & Radke-Yarrow, 1992). The toddler and preschool years may be a neurodevelopmental period particularly sensitive to negative environmental exposures, producing lasting perturbations to offspring stress physiology (Melhem, Walker, Moritz, & Brent, 2008). From as early as infancy and preschool, children of parents with mood disorders exhibit psychosocial, emotional, and behavioral problems (Brennan et al., 2000; Hammen, 2009), likely related to the fact that mood disorders are associated with negative, hostile child-rearing behaviors (Lovejoy, Graczyk, O'Hare, & Neuman, 2000).

Later events also have detrimental effects, as children gain awareness of their situation. Older children start to see the effects of medication on a parent; in one study a child described his mother as being "doped up to the hilt" (Maybery, Ling, Szakacs, & Reupert, 2005). A parent's decision to stop taking medication, or to make some other change in his or her life, can result in declining mental health and an unnerving or frightening situation for the child (Spiegelhoff & Ahia, 2011).

Children often do not know the specifics of their parent's illness, though they are attuned to changing parental behavior due to mental illness. Not having an explanation for why a parent is acting erratically is more upsetting than when behavior changes can be attributed to mental illness (Mordoch & Hall, 2008). Parents often try to comfort children, rather than answering their questions or talking with them openly about the situation, which can further confuse and scare children (Sturges, 1977). Lack of knowledge, or lack of conversation, about the illness may also leave the child feeling as though something is "wrong" or that there is a shameful family secret.

Children also experience negative emotions, including fear and anxiety, when a parent must be hospitalized (Mordoch & Hall, 2008; Sturges, 1977). A lack of openness about the situation can compound these fears, as worries about the parent dying or otherwise not returning home arise (Riebschleger, 2004). Children also may feel guilt related to parent hospitalization, perhaps due to questions about what their role was in the hospitalization or to having to rely on others during a parent's absence. When the

parent returns home, children may have ambivalent feelings about the parent (Sturges, 1977). Fear and uncertainty can also interfere with the child's relationship with his or her parent, leading children to keep a distance in an effort to protect themselves (Mordoch & Hall, 2008). Children may also take on "adult" responsibilities, feeling that they cannot count on a parent to provide for them (Handley, Farrell, Josephs, Hanke, & Hazelton, 2001; Maybery et al., 2005). These extra responsibilities can contribute to poor coping. Children report withdrawing, not attending school, and keeping feelings to themselves when faced with adversity at home (Maybery et al., 2005). Although there is likely to be greater responsibility placed on BD offspring than other youth, in many cases they may be unable to meet these demands. Children and adolescents with BP experience significant functional impairment across multiple domains, including academic, interpersonal, and overall measures of functioning (Freeman et al., 2009; Goldstein et al., 2009).

Unfortunately, when a parent is ill, the children are often neglected—at least from a mental health perspective. Parent hospitalization is a stressful event, associated with odds ratios of 3.3 for a child first episode of mania (Kessing, Agerbo, & Mortensen, 2004), and there are few resources available to help children cope in these situations (Handley et al., 2001; Maybery et al., 2005). There is limited coordination between mental health services and child protective services in most communities, and institutions are often unaware that a hospitalized patient has children at home, adding to the challenge of marshalling good childcare while the parent is receiving mental health services (Park, Solomon, & Mandell, 2006).

Additionally, assortative mating increases the likelihood that the remaining parent may also have a psychiatric illness (Melhem et al., 2008), introducing other complications (Sands, Koppelman, & Solomon, 2004). A child in this situation may be sent to stay with unfamiliar people during a period of parental illness or may stay and observe negative behavior changes in a remaining parent. Most mothers with mental illness are single parents, and children from single-parent homes will very likely find themselves in unfamiliar, stressful circumstances when a parent has a mood episode (Sands et al., 2004).

Parental psychiatric hospitalization doubles the risk of the family's involvement with child protective services and triples likelihood of children being removed from the home (Park et al., 2006). Children of mothers with mental illness are more likely to become foster children, and their parents are then put in the position of having to defend their parental fitness, rather than the burden of proof falling on the state (Spiegelhoff & Ahia, 2011). Neglect and participation in foster/residential care are both associated with increased suicide risk for youth (Christoffersen, Poulsen, & Nielsen, 2003).

Research suggests that the amount of stress due to parental mental illness on a child may be greater than the stress attached to a death or divorce (Sturges, 1977). Sadly, children of people with BD may experience both; these youth are at heightened risk of losing a parent to suicide (Gould, Greenberg, Velting, & Shaffer, 2003; Ljung et al., 2013). This can become a cascade. Death of one parent by suicide increases the risk of mental illness in the remaining parent (Melhem et al., 2008), leading to even more stress in the household (Kuramoto, Brent, & Wilcox, 2009). The effects of parental suicide on the child can be long-lasting and include depressive symptoms, interpersonal problems, stigma, guilt, and anger. Parental death by suicide is also associated with the development of BD in the offspring (Tsuchiya, Agerbo, & Mortensen, 2005), with an odds ratio of between 4 and 5, depending on the age at death (Mortensen, Pedersen, Melbye, Mors, & Ewald, 2003). Parental death by suicide before age 11 has also been associated with more frequent suicide attempts by the offspring (Goodwin, Beautrais, & Fergusson, 2004).

THE TREE: HOW PARENTHOOD AFFECTS PEOPLE WITH BIPOLAR DISORDER

Adults with BD who are able to manage their symptoms effectively have better outcomes. Unfortunately, during the age range when most people start families, many people with BD are undiagnosed and not receiving optimal treatment. Parenting responsibilities often interfere with adults seeking mental health services for themselves (Knight & Wallace, 2003). Drancourt et al. (2013) report that, on average, the first full syndromal mood episode occurs at 25.3 years, and the mean age at first recorded treatment with a mood stabilizer is 34.9, giving a mean of duration of untreated BD of 9.6 years. Longer duration of untreated BD correlates with negative outcomes, including suicide attempts, more major mood episodes, greater mood instability, and more frequent mixed episodes. At the time when young children might be drawing most heavily on a parent's internal resources, the likelihood that bipolar symptoms would be unrecognized or untreated is high. Substance abuse frequently occurs with BD, and it often contributes to delays in diagnosis and treatment, making it more difficult

for a parent to meet his or her obligations (Spiegelhoff & Ahia, 2011). Extreme mood variability, suicidality, and frequent mood episodes will threaten the parent's ability to form a healthy attachment with the child, adding to worse outcomes for both the parent and child.

Difficulty connecting with one's child may trigger negative feelings in the parent. Parents with BD rate themselves in a more critical light than control parents (Spitzer, 2002). Many of the psychosocial difficulties associated with BD may also create extra challenges for parents. People with BD experience declines in job status and income, failure to marry, interpersonal relationship deficits, lower enjoyment of recreational activities, and overall diminished contentment compared with controls (Calabrese et al., 2003; Coryell, Scheftner, Keller, Endicott, & al, 1993; Maybery et al., 2005; Spiegelhoff & Ahia, 2011), all of which have the potential to increase the sense of burden associated with parenting.

Parents with BD report having both considerable personal difficulties and difficulties in rearing their children (Livesley, 1995). Parents with mental illness also report higher levels of stress related to parenting and lower levels of satisfaction in the relationships with their children than other parents (Park et al., 2006). They also report that their children have greater adjustment difficulties and higher levels of behavior problems than other youth. Parents with BD judge their families as less cohesive, less organized, and more conflicted than other parents (Chang, Blasey, Ketter, & Steiner, 2001). Though the offspring of a parent with BD often have behavioral and mood problems, parents may also perceive the behaviors as being even worse due to their own stress and compromised coping (De Los Reyes, Goodman, Kliewer, & Reid-Quinones, 2008; Youngstrom, Loeber, & Stouthamer-Loeber, 2000). Child characteristics, parent characteristics, and parenting situations influence functioning and stress in the dyadic system (Abidin, 1992). Typically, reports about parenting and mental illness focus on risks to children when a parent has a mental illness (Rutter & Quinton, 1984), but this understates the impact of child psychopathology on the parent's behavior. At the extreme, child behavior problems can exacerbate the risk of suicide in parents with BD (Cerel, Fristad, Weller, & Weller, 1999).

Risk for hospitalization worsens parents' self-critical, negative feelings as it keeps them from their children for extended periods of time. Parents facing hospitalization can have difficulty asking for help from others (Handley et al., 2001), increasing the likelihood of negative circumstances befalling their children. Even short hospital stays are challenging, as parents are more likely to remain symptomatic and may not be able to return to their responsibilities effectively once discharged (Thomas & Kalucy, 2003).

Parents report a scarcity of professional support for their children during their hospitalization, and they also are uncertain about what and how much to tell their children about their mental illness (Maybery et al., 2005), heightening the sense of secrecy and burden. Rates of women with mental health problems having children are increasing, a change from the past when mentally ill people were often hospitalized long term, but mental health and family services have not kept up (Sands et al., 2004). Because professional services are lacking, welfare often becomes the default support for women with mental illness and their families. Women and their children are often separated at the point of hospitalization or due to disruptive behavior during a mood episode (Sands et al., 2004). Mothers with mental illness are also more likely to lose custody of their children than other mothers (Park et al., 2006). In one study, 25% of women with mental illness had involvement with child welfare services versus only 4% of women without mental illness (Park et al., 2006). Mothers often report poor communication regarding their children's status, as well as confusion as to whether custodial arrangements made while they were ill are permanent (Sands et al., 2004). Due to worries about losing custody, parents with mental illness are often reluctant to disclose that they have children; however, this also limits professionals' ability to help the children or to offer parenting resources (Spiegelhoff & Ahia, 2011).

If mental health services are available for offspring, parents may still be resistant to their children seeing a therapist (Sturges, 1977). Parents with mental illness often worry about "passing on" their mental illness to their children and may feel guilty about any emotional or behavioral problems their children demonstrate (Goodwin & Jamison, 1990). The suggestion that a child see a therapist, whether due to his or her mental state or to a situation brought on by the parent's illness, may activate feelings of defensiveness or denial.

NURTURE CHANGING NATURE: HOW TO INTERVENE EFFECTIVELY TO HELP FAMILIES WITH BIPOLAR DISORDER

There are multiple ways that biology and environment transact with each other. The complexity of the relations offers multiple points for intervention in the family system, both to reduce the negative effects and to promote positive functioning.

ASSESSMENT FOR BETTER DETECTION AND EARLIER INTERVENTION

The first steps in intervening are identifying the problem, gauging how far it has progressed, and then defining intervention targets. We argue that the unit of assessment should be the family and not just the identified patient: Family-level factors play key roles in illness transmission and moderate illness progression; they also have similar roles in efficacious treatments. Assessing the family provides more contextual information about the individual case, but it also can enhance chances of treatment success. There is huge unmet need: More than 50% of people suffering BD are receiving *no* treatment in the United States (Wang et al., 2005). The global burden of BD appears similarly high around the world, and the chances of obtaining adequate assessment and treatment are yet lower in countries with less developed mental health service systems.

One strategy for improving detection would be to routinely assess family history for every case seeking treatment for BD. This approach would branch out from the identified patient to identify other affected and high-risk individuals in the family tree. Primary care is another setting where many people come who would not otherwise consider mental health services (Mitchell, Vaze, & Rao, 2009). School-based services provide a third opportunity to provide education about mental health services and BD in particular, as well as a potential additional setting for deployment of mental health services (Weist, Nabors, Myers, & Armbruster, 2000).

The challenge is finding balanced ways to detect more cases of BD without having an offsetting number of false positive diagnoses. Early enthusiasm for screening programs for many other disorders—including breast and prostate cancer—has been tempered by high rates of false alarms and poor predictive power in many settings (Gigerenzer, 2002). No single risk factor or positive result on a screening test is discriminating enough to confirm a diagnosis of BD in isolation (Zimmerman, 2012). Instead, evidence-based assessment recommends using a series of tools and risk factors in sequence, starting with low-cost tools (e.g., Algorta et al., 2013) and following up with additional, in-depth evaluation when multiple findings raise the index of suspicion for bipolarity (Youngstrom, Jenkins, Jensen-Doss, & Youngstrom, 2012). Goals for the evaluation process should include understanding what strengths and unmet service needs each family member might have and then formulating a plan to maximize benefits while avoiding possible treatment-sabotaging dynamics.

From a pharmacological perspective, family assessment is crucial to discern (a) who would benefit from medication, (b) who can help with medication management, (c) what family processes might interfere with a sense of congruence between treatment recommendations and personal beliefs, and (d) what behaviors might directly complicate treatment. For young children, it may be essential to have the parent manage the medication; for teenagers or spouses, having the collateral person involved with the medications could be a source of conflict. A patient might decide to stop taking medication, or to overdose, as a result of high expressed negative emotion. On the positive side, supportive and empathic family members promote engagement with treatment, and relatives who have done well on medication provide successful role models as well as clues about choice of intervention, inasmuch as there may be a genetic basis to individual differences in treatment response (Alda, Grof, Rouleau, Turecki, & Young, 2005).

From a psychosocial perspective, family engagement increases the chances of success for any intervention. High expressed emotion and conflict predict earlier age of onset, worse treatment response, and higher rates of relapse. Psychoeducational interventions not only increase family member's understanding of the illness but also improve engagement, enhance family processes, and mediate better outcomes for pharmacological interventions (Fristad & Macpherson, 2014). Psychosocial interventions focusing on the individual are still likely to benefit from a thorough understanding of the family. There is growing evidence that family therapy also directly improves communication, reduces conflict, and leads to more durable improvements than pharmacological treatment alone (Miklowitz et al., 2008; Miklowitz & Scott, 2009), but much work is needed in terms of dissemination of these approaches. Family assessment also enhances prospects for early intervention and prevention programs in at-risk youths (Pfennig et al., 2013).

Family intervention should not focus only on symptom reduction. Family members and caregivers report a lack of information about how to deal with the person's illness, and about the changes and losses that commonly ensue, and report feeling isolated, alone, and unsupported (Pirkis et al., 2010; Rowe, 2012). Health professionals do not always have time to provide information for caregivers, and confidentiality concerns compound the difficulty of implementing collaborative family-friendly models (Peters, Pontin, Lobban, & Morriss, 2011; Wilkinson & McAndrew, 2008; Wynaden & Orb, 2005). Despite these obstacles, it is valuable to pursue engagement, education, and support of the family system. People with BD have commented on the valuable role close family or friends can play in helping them to manage their illness and maintain a good quality of life, but caregivers need information about ways to do this without jeopardizing their own health (Michalak, Yatham, Kolesar, & Lam, 2006; Russell & Browne, 2005). Acknowledging each family member's needs and setting some limits defining tolerable behaviors will also reduce resentment and anger. Mental health literacy is not simply a matter of having knowledge; it links knowledge to the possibility of action that benefits family members' mental health (Jorm, 2012).

CONCLUSION

It is well established that BD is a highly heritable illness. A large part of the heritability is due to genetic factors, although these have proven far more complex and less tractable than initially hoped. The field has also learned that it is not a question of nature or nurture but rather a matter of understanding how the two are intertwined. The parent has effects on the child through biological, environmental, and social pathways that also interact with each other. Genes of risk in the parent can lead to behaviors that disrupt parenting, further altering the home environment and amplifying the genetic effects.

But children are not passive recipients of these influences. In addition to any inherited biology, they also learn from their parents, absorbing meta-rules for emotions and relationships the same way they absorb language—another construct that runs in families without a biological basis for transmission. The child sometimes withdraws, sometimes pushes back against the parent, and both the parent and child provoke powerful responses in each other that activate biological as well as cognitive systems. Decades of research show how family factors convey risk and mediate some illness processes as well as worsening the course over time. More recent work is illuminating ways that understanding family processes, and helping families make sense of BD, can establish virtuous cycles that promote treatment engagement, remission, and positive functioning.

Disclosure statement: Anna Van Meter and Guillermo Perez Algorta have no conflicts to disclose. Dr. Eric Youngstrom has consulted with Lundbeck and Otsuka and received grant support from the National Institute of Mental Health.

REFERENCES

Abidin, R. R. (1992). The determinants of parenting behavior. *Journal of Clinical Child Psychology, 21,* 407–412.

Alda, M., Grof, P., Rouleau, G. A., Turecki, G., & Young, L. T. (2005). Investigating responders to lithium prophylaxis as a strategy for mapping susceptibility genes for bipolar disorder. *Progress in Neuro-psychopharmacology & Biological Psychiatry, 29,* 1038–1045.

Algorta, G. P., Youngstrom, E. A., Phelps, J., Jenkins, M. M., Youngstrom, J. K., & Findling, R. L. (2013). An inexpensive family index of risk for mood issues improves identification of pediatric bipolar disorder. *Psychological Assessment, 25,* 12–22.

Bella, T., Goldstein, T., Axelson, D., Obreja, M., Monk, K., Hickey, M. B., … Birmaher, B. (2011). Psychosocial functioning in offspring of parents with bipolar disorder. *Journal of Affective Disorders, 133,* 204–211.

Belsky, J. (1984). The determinants of parenting: a process model. *Child Development, 55,* 83–96.

Birmaher, B., Axelson, D., Monk, K., Kalas, C., Goldstein, B., Hickey, M. B., … Brent, D. (2009). Lifetime psychiatric disorders in school-aged offspring of parents with bipolar disorder: the Pittsburgh Bipolar Offspring study. *Arch Gen Psychiatry, 66*(3), 287–296.

Birmaher, B., Goldstein, B. I., Axelson, D. A., Monk, K., Hickey, M. B., Fan, J., … Kupfer, D. J. (2013). Mood lability among offspring of parents with bipolar disorder and community controls. *Bipolar Disorders, 15,* 253–263.

Brennan, P. A., Hammen, C., Andersen, M. J., Bor, W., Najman, J. M., & Williams, G. M. (2000). Chronicity, severity, and timing of maternal depressive symptoms: Relationships with child outcomes at age 5. *Developmental Psychology, 36,* 759–766.

Calabrese, J. R., Hirschfeld, R., Reed, M., Davies, M. A., Frye, M. A., Keck, P. E. J., … Wagner, K. D. (2003). Impact of bipolar disorder on a U.S. community sample. *The Journal of Clinical Psychiatry, 64,* 425–432.

Calam, R. (2012). Parenting and the emotional and behavioural adjustment of young children in families with a parent with bipolar disorder. *Behavioural and Cognitive Psychotherapy, 40,* 425–437.

Cerel, J., Fristad, M. A., Weller, E. B., & Weller, R. A. (1999). Suicide-bereaved children and adolescents: A controlled longitudinal examination. *Journal of the American Academy of Child & Adolescent Psychiatry, 38,* 672–679.

Chang, K., Steiner, H., & Ketter, T. (2003). Studies of offspring of parents with bipolar disorder. *American Journal of Medical Genetics, 123C,* 26–35.

Chang, K. D., Blasey, C., Ketter, T. A., & Steiner, H. (2001). Family environment of children and adolescents with bipolar parents. *Bipolar Disorders, 3,* 73–78.

Chang, K. D., Steiner, H., & Ketter, T. A. (2000). Psychiatric phenomenology of child and adolescent bipolar offspring. *Journal of the American Academy of Child & Adolescent Psychiatry, 39,* 453–460.

Christoffersen, M. N., Poulsen, H. D., & Nielsen, A. (2003). Attempted suicide among young people: Risk factors in a prospective register based study of Danish children born in 1966. *Acta Psychiatrica Scandinavica, 108,* 350–358.

Coryell, W., Scheftner, W., Keller, M., Endicott, J., Maser, J., & Klerman, G. L. (1993). The enduring psychosocial consequences of mania and depression. *American Journal of Psychiatry, 150,* 720–727.

Davenport, Y. B., & Adland, M. L. (1982). Postpartum psychoses in female and male bipolar manic-depressive patients. *American Journal of Orthopsychiatry, 52,* 288–297.

De Los Reyes, A., Goodman, K. L., Kliewer, W., & Reid-Quinones, K. (2008). Whose depression relates to discrepancies? Testing relations between informant characteristics and informant discrepancies from both informants' perspectives. *Psychological Assessment, 20,* 139–149.

Dickstein, D., Rich, B., Roberson-Nay, R., Berghorst, L., Vinton, D., Pine, D., & Leibenluft, E. (2007). Neural activation during encoding of emotional faces in pediatric bipolar disorder. *Bipolar Disorders, 9,* 679–692.

Dougherty, L. R., Tolep, M. R., Smith, V. C., & Rose, S. (2013). Early exposure to parental depression and parenting: Associations with young offspring's stress physiology and oppositional behavior. *Journal of Abnormal Child Psychology, 41*(8), 1299–1310.

Drancourt, N., Etain, B., Lajnef, M., Henry, C., Raust, A., Cochet, B., … Bellivier, F. (2013). Duration of untreated bipolar disorder: Missed opportunities on the long road to optimal treatment. *Acta Psychiatrica Scandinavica, 127,* 136–144.

Duffy, A., Alda, M., Hajek, T., & Grof, P. (2009). Early course of bipolar disorder in high-risk offspring: Prospective study. *British Journal of Psychiatry, 195,* 457–458.

Duffy, A., Alda, M., Trinneer, A., Demidenko, N., Grof, P., & Goodyer, I. M. (2007). Temperament, life events, and psychopathology among the offspring of bipolar parents. *European Child & Adolescent Psychiatry, 16,* 222–228.

Ehlers, C. L., Frank, E., & Kupfer, D. J. (1988). Social zeitgebers and biological rhythms: A unified approach to understanding the etiology of depression. *Archives of General Psychiatry, 45,* 948–952.

Essex, M. J., Shirtcliff, E. A., Burk, L. R., Ruttle, P. L., Klein, M. H., Slattery, M. J., … Armstrong, J. M. (2011). Influence of early life stress on later hypothalamic-pituitary-adrenal axis functioning and its covariation with mental health symptoms: A study of the allostatic process from childhood into adolescence. *Development and Psychopathology, 23,* 1039–1058.

Evans, L., Akiskal, H., Keck, P., McElroy, S., Sadovnick, A. D., Remick, R., & Kelsoe, J. (2005). Familiality of temperament in bipolar disorder: support for a genetic spectrum. *Journal of Affective Disorders, 85,* 153–168.

Evans, L. M., Akiskal, H. S., Greenwood, T. A., Nievergelt, C. M., Keck, P. E., McElroy, S. L., … Kelsoe, J. R. (2008). Suggestive linkage of a chromosomal locus on 18p11 to cyclothymic temperament in bipolar disorder families. *American Journal of Medical Genetics, 147B,* 326–332.

Frank, E., Swartz, H. A., & Kupfer, D. J. (2000). Interpersonal and social rhythm therapy: Managing the chaos of bipolar disorder. *Biological Psychiatry, 48,* 593–604.

Freeman, A. J., Youngstrom, E. A., Michalak, E., Siegel, R., Meyers, O. I., & Findling, R. L. (2009). Quality of life in pediatric bipolar disorder. *Pediatrics, 123,* e446–e452.

Fristad, M. A., & Macpherson, H. A. (2014). Evidence-based psychosocial treatments for child and adolescent bipolar spectrum disorders. *Journal of Clinical Child & Adolescent Psychology, 43*(3), 339–355.

Garcia-Amador, M., de la Serna, E., Vila, M., Romero, S., Valenti, M., Sanchez-Gistau, V., … Castro-Fornieles, J. (2013). Parents with bipolar disorder: Are disease characteristics good predictors of psychopathology in offspring? *European Psychiatry, 28,* 240–246.

Gigerenzer, G. (2002). *Calculated risks: How to know when numbers deceive you.* New York: Simon & Schuster.

Goldstein, T. R., Birmaher, B., Axelson, D., Goldstein, B. I., Gill, M. K., Esposito-Smythers, C., . . . Keller, M. (2009). Psychosocial functioning among bipolar youth. *Journal of Affective Disorders, 114,* 174–183.

Gonda, X., Rihmer, Z., Zsombok, T., Bagdy, G., Akiskal, K. K., & Akiskal, H. S. (2006). The 5HTTLPR polymorphism of the serotonin transporter gene is associated with affective temperaments as measured by TEMPS-A. *Journal of Affective Disorders, 91,* 125–131.

Goodman, S. H., & Gotlib, I. H. (1999). Risk for psychopathology in the children of depressed mothers: A developmental model for understanding mechanisms of transmission. *Psychological Review, 106,* 458–490.

Goodwin, F., & Jamison, K. (1990). *Manic-depressive illness* (1st ed.). New York: Oxford University Press.

Goodwin, F. K., & Jamison, K. R. (2007). *Manic-depressive illness* (2nd ed.). New York: Oxford University Press.

Goodwin, R. D., Beautrais, A. L., & Fergusson, D. M. (2004). Familial transmission of suicidal ideation and suicide attempts: Evidence from a general population sample. *Psychiatry Research, 126,* 159–165.

Gottesman, I. I., Laursen, T. M., Bertelsen, A., & Mortensen, P. B. (2010). Severe mental disorders in offspring with 2 psychiatrically ill parents. *Archives of General Psychiatry, 67,* 252–257.

Gould, M., Greenberg, T., Velting, D., & Shaffer, D. (2003). Youth suicide risk and preventive interventions: A review of the past 10 years. *Journal of the American Academy of Child & Adolescent Psychiatry, 42,* 386–405.

Green, M. J., Cahill, C. M., & Malhi, G. S. (2007). The cognitive and neurophysiological basis of emotion dysregulation in bipolar disorder. *Journal of Affective Disorders, 103,* 29–42.

Greenwood, T. A., Akiskal, H. S., Akiskal, K. K., & Kelsoe, J. R. (2012). Genome-wide association study of temperament in bipolar disorder reveals significant associations with three novel loci. *Biological Psychiatry, 72,* 303–310.

Gunnar, M. R., & Vazquez, D. (2006). Stress neurobiology and developmental psychopathology. In D. Cicchetti & D. J. Cohen (Eds.), *Developmental psychopathology: Developmental neuroscience* (2nd ed., Vol. 2, pp. 533–577). Hoboken, NJ: John Wiley.

Hammen, C. (2009). Adolescent depression: Stressful interpersonal contexts and risk for recurrence. *Current Directions in Psychological Science, 18,* 200–204.

Handley, C., Farrell, G. A., Josephs, A., Hanke, A., & Hazelton, M. (2001). The Tasmanian children's project: The needs of children with a parent/carer with a mental illness. *Australian & New Zealand Journal of Mental Health Nursing, 10,* 221–228.

Hinshaw, S. P. (Ed.). (2008). *Breaking the silence.* New York: Oxford University Press.

Hodgins, S., Faucher, B., Zarac, A., & Ellenbogen, M. (2002). Children of parents with bipolar disorder: A population at high risk for major affective disorders. *Child & Adolescent Psychiatric Clinics of North America, 11,* 533–553.

Holsboer, F. (2000). The corticosteroid receptor hypothesis of depression. *Neuropsychopharmacology, 23,* 477–501.

Inoff-Germain, G., Nottelmann, E. D., & Radke-Yarrow, M. (1992). Evaluative communications between affectively ill and well mothers and their children. *Journal of Abnormal Child Psychology, 20,* 189–212.

James, A. (2011). Early-onset bipolar disorder. In *Child psychology and psychiatry* (pp. 210–216). Hoboken, NJ: John Wiley.

Janet Kuramoto, S., Brent, D. A., & Wilcox, H. C. (2009). The impact of parental suicide on child and adolescent offspring. *Suicide & Life Threatening Behaviors, 39,* 137–151.

Jones, S. H., & Bentall, R. P. (2008). A review of potential cognitive and environmental risk markers in children of bipolar parents. *Clinical Psychology Review, 28,* 1083–1095.

Jorm, A. F. (2012). Mental health literacy: Empowering the community to take action for better mental health. *American Psychologist, 67,* 231–243.

Kessing, L. V., Agerbo, E., & Mortensen, P. B. (2004). Major stressful life events and other risk factors for first admission with mania. *Bipolar Disorders, 6,* 122–129.

Knight, D. K., & Wallace, G. (2003). Where are the children? An examination of children's living arrangements when mothers enter residential drug treatment. *Journal of Drug Issues, 33,* 305–324.

Lapalme, M., Hodgins, S., & LaRoche, C. (1997). Children of parents with bipolar disorder: A metaanalysis of risk for mental disorders. *Canadian Journal of Psychiatry, 42,* 623–631.

Livesley, W. J. (1995). *The DSM-IV personality disorders.* New York: Guilford Press.

Ljung, T., Lichtenstein, P., Sandin, S., D'Onofrio, B., Runeson, B., Långström, N., & Larsson, H. (2013). Parental schizophrenia and increased offspring suicide risk: Exploring the causal hypothesis using cousin comparisons. *Psychological Medicine, 43,* 581–590.

Lovejoy, M. C., Graczyk, P. A., O'Hare, E., & Neuman, G. (2000). Maternal depression and parenting behavior: A meta-analytic review. *Clinical Psychology Review, 20,* 561–592.

Luecken, L. J., & Appelhans, B. M. (2006). Early parental loss and salivary cortisol in young adulthood: The moderating role of family environment. *Development and Psychopathology, 18,* 295–308.

Lytton, H. (1990a). Child and parent effects in boys' conduct disorder: A reinterpretation. *Developmental Psychology, 26,* 683–697.

Lytton, H. (1990b). Child effects—Still unwelcome? Response to Dodge and Wahler. *Developmental Psychology, 26,* 705–709.

Marks, M. N. (1992). Contribution of psychological and social factors to psychotic and non-psychotic relapse after childbirth in women with previous histories of affective disorder. *Journal of Affective Disorders, 24,* 253–263.

Maybery, D., Ling, L., Szakacs, E., & Reupert, A. (2005). Children of a parent with a mental illness: Perspectives on need. *Advances in Mental Health, 4,* 78–88.

Meinhard, N. (2013). The role of estrogen in bipolar disorder: A review. *Nordic Journal of Psychiatry,* 1–7.

Melhem, N. M., Walker, M., Moritz, G., & Brent, D. A. (2008). Antecedents and sequelae of sudden parental death in offspring and surviving caregivers. *Archives of Pediatrics & Adolescent Medicine, 162,* 403–410.

Merikangas, K., He, J., Burstein, M., Swanson, S., Avenevoli, S., Cui, L., . . . Swendsen, J. (2010). Lifetime prevalence of mental disorders in U.S. adolescents: Results from the National Comorbidity Survey Replication–Adolescent Supplement (NCS-A). *Journal of the American Academy of Child & Adolescent Psychiatry, 49,* 980–989.

Mesman, E., Nolen, W. A., Reichart, C. G., Wals, M., & Hillegers, M. H. (2013). The Dutch Bipolar Offspring Study: 12-year follow-up. *American Journal of Psychiatry, 170,* 542–549.

Michalak, E. E., Yatham, L. N., Kolesar, S., & Lam, R. W. (2006). Bipolar disorder and quality of life: A patient-centered perspective. *Quality of Life Research, 15,* 25–37.

Miklowitz, D. J. (2004). The role of family systems in severe and recurrent psychiatric disorders: A developmental psychopathology view. *Development and Psychopathology, 16,* 667–688.

Miklowitz, D., & Johnson, B. (2009). Social and familial factors in the course of bipolar disorder: Basic processes and relevant interventions. *Clinical Psychology: Science and Practice, 16,* 281–296.

Miklowitz, D. J., Axelson, D. A., Birmaher, B., George, E. L., Taylor, D. O., Schneck, C. D., . . . Brent, D. A. (2008). Family-focused treatment for adolescents with bipolar disorder: Results of a 2-year randomized trial. *Archives of General Psychiatry, 65,* 1053–1061.

Miklowitz, D. J., & Scott, J. (2009). Psychosocial treatments for bipolar disorder: Cost-effectiveness, mediating mechanisms, and future directions. *Bipolar Disorders, 11,* 110–122.

Mitchell, A. J., Vaze, A., & Rao, S. (2009). Clinical diagnosis of depression in primary care: A meta-analysis. *Lancet, 374,* 609–619.

Mordoch, E., & Hall, W. A. (2008). Children's perceptions of living with a parent with a mental illness: Finding the rhythm and maintaining the frame. *Qualitative Health Research, 18,* 1127–1144.

Mortensen, P. B., Pedersen, C. B., Melbye, M., Mors, O., & Ewald, H. (2003). Individual and familial risk factors for bipolar affective disorders in Denmark. *Archives of General Psychiatry, 60,* 1209–1215.

Murray, G. (2010). Circadian rhythms and sleep in bipolar disorder. *Bipolar disorders, 12,* 459–472.

Park, J. M., Solomon, P., & Mandell, D. S. (2006). Involvement in the child welfare system among mothers with serious mental illness. *Psychiatric Services, 57,* 493–497.

Pauls, D. L., Morton, L. A., & Egeland, J. A. (1992). Risks of affective illness among first-degree relatives of bipolar I old-order Amish probands. *Arch Gen Psychiatry, 49*(9), 703–708.

Peters, S., Pontin, E., Lobban, F., & Morriss, R. (2011). Involving relatives in relapse prevention for bipolar disorder: A multi-perspective qualitative study of value and barriers. *BMC Psychiatry, 11,* 172.

Pfennig, A., Correll, C. U., Marx, C., Rottmann-Wolf, M., Meyer, T. D., Bauer, M., & Leopold, K. (2013). Psychotherapeutic interventions in individuals at risk of developing bipolar disorder: A systematic review. *Early Intervention Psychiatry, 8*(1), 3-11.

Pirkis, J., Burgess, P., Hardy, J., Harris, M., Slade, T., & Johnston, A. (2010). Who cares? A profile of people who care for relatives with a mental disorder. *Australian & New Zealand Journal of Psychiatry, 44*, 929–937.

Plomin, R. (1995). Genetics and children's experiences in the family. *Journal of Child Psychology and Psychiatry, 36*, 33–68.

Reichart, C. G., van der Ende, J., Hillegers, M. H., Wals, M., Bongers, I. L., Nolen, W. A., . . . Verhulst, F. C. (2007). Perceived parental rearing of bipolar offspring. *Acta Psychiatrica Scandinavica, 115*, 21–28.

Rich, B. A., Schmajuk, M., Perez-Edgar, K. E., Pine, D. S., Fox, N. A., & Leibenluft, E. (2005). The impact of reward, punishment, and frustration on attention in pediatric bipolar disorder. *Biological Psychiatry, 58*, 532–539.

Riebschleger, J. (2004). Good days and bad days: The experiences of children of a parent with a psychiatric disability. *Psychiatric Rehabilitation Journal, 28*, 25–31.

Rowe, J. (2012). Great expectations: A systematic review of the literature on the role of family carers in severe mental illness, and their relationships and engagement with professionals. *Journal of Psychiatric Mental Health Nursing, 19*, 70–82.

Russell, S. J., & Browne, J. L. (2005). Staying well with bipolar disorder. *Australian & New Zealand Journal of Psychiatry, 39*, 187–193.

Rutter, M., & Quinton, D. (1984). Parental psychiatric disorder: Effects on children. *Psychological Medicine, 14*, 853–880.

Sands, R. G., Koppelman, N., & Solomon, P. (2004). Maternal custody status and living arrangements of children of women with severe mental illness. *Health & Social Work, 29*, 317–325.

Sharma, V. (2012). Pregnancy and bipolar disorder: A systematic review. *Journal of Clinical Psychiatry, 73*, 1447–1455.

Singh, M. K., DelBello, M. P., Stanford, K. E., Soutullo, C., McDonough-Ryan, P., McElroy, S. L., & Strakowski, S. M. (2007). Psychopathology in children of bipolar parents. *J Affect Disord, 102*(1–3), 131–136.

Smoller, J. W., & Finn, C. T. (2003). Family, twin, and adoption studies of bipolar disorder. *American Journal of Medical Genetics, 123C*, 48–58.

Spiegelhoff, S. F., & Ahia, C. E. (2011). Impact of parental severe mental illness: Ethical and clinical issues for counselors. *The Family Journal, 19*, 389–395.

Spitzer, R. L. (2002). *DSM-IV-TR casebook: A learning companion to the* Diagnostic and Statistical Manual of Mental Disorders, *fourth edition, text revision* (1st ed.). Washington, DC: American Psychiatric Publishing

Steptoe, A., van Jaarsveld, C. H., Semmler, C., Plomin, R., & Wardle, J. (2009). Heritability of daytime cortisol levels and cortisol reactivity in children. *Psychoneuroendocrinology, 34*, 273–280.

Sturges, J. S. (1977). Talking with children about mental illness in the family. *Health & Social Work, 2*, 87–109.

Thomas, L., & Kalucy, R. (2003). Parents with mental illness: Lacking motivation to parent. *International Journal of Mental Health Nursing, 12*, 153–157.

Townsend, J. (2012). Emotion processing and regulation in bipolar disorder: A review. *Bipolar Disorders, 14*, 326–339.

Tsuchiya, K. J., Agerbo, E., & Mortensen, P. B. (2005). Parental death and bipolar disorder: A robust association was found in early maternal suicide. *Journal of Affective Disorders, 86*, 151–159.

Van Meter, A., Moreira, A., & Youngstrom, E. (2011). Meta-analysis of epidemiologic studies of pediatric bipolar disorder. *Journal of Clinical Psychiatry, 72*, 1250–1256.

Vandeleur, C., Rothen, S., Gholam-Rezaee, M., Castelao, E., Vidal, S., Favre, S., . . . Preisig, M. (2012). Mental disorders in offspring of parents with bipolar and major depressive disorders. *Bipolar Disorders, 14*, 641–653.

Wang, P. S., Lane, M., Olfson, M., Pincus, H. A., Wells, K. B., & Kessler, R. C. (2005). Twelve-month use of mental health services in the United States: Results from the National Comorbidity Survey Replication. *Archives of General Psychiatry, 62*, 629–640.

Weist, M. D., Nabors, L. A., Myers, C. P., & Armbruster, P. (2000). Evaluation of expanded school mental health programs. *Community Mental Health Journal, 36*, 395–411.

Wilkinson, C., & McAndrew, S. (2008). "I'm not an outsider, I'm his mother!" A phenomenological enquiry into carer experiences of exclusion from acute psychiatric settings. *International Journal of Mental Health Nursing, 17*, 392–401.

Wynaden, D., & Orb, A. (2005). Impact of patient confidentiality on carers of people who have a mental disorder. *International Journal of Mental Health Nursing, 14*, 166–171.

Youngstrom, E. A., Jenkins, M. M., Jensen-Doss, A., & Youngstrom, J. K. (2012). Evidence-based assessment strategies for pediatric bipolar disorder. *Israel Journal of Psychiatry & Related Sciences, 49*, 15–27.

Youngstrom, E. A., Loeber, R., & Stouthamer-Loeber, M. (2000). Patterns and correlates of agreement between parent, teacher, and male adolescent ratings of externalizing and internalizing problems. *Journal of Consulting and Clinical Psychology, 68*, 1038–1050.

Yuan, C., Yu, S. Y., Li, Z., Huang, J., Qian, Y., & Fang, Y. (2012). P-222—The 5HTTLPR is associated with bipolar disorder and affective temperaments as measured by TEMPS-A in Chinese population. *European Psychiatry, 27*(Suppl. 1), 1.

Zimmerman, M. (2012). Misuse of the Mood Disorders Questionnaire as a case-finding measure and a critique of the concept of using a screening scale for bipolar disorder in psychiatric practice. *Bipolar Disorders, 14*, 127–134.

Zuckerman, M. (1999). *Vulnerability to psychopathology: A biosocial model.* Washington, DC: American Psychological Association.

15.

THE EMERGING GENETICS OF BIPOLAR DISORDER

Roy H. Perlis

INTRODUCTION

Bipolar disorder often recurs within families. This observation, familiar to most clinicians and dating back many decades, prompted aggressive efforts to identify the specific genetic variations that may confer risk for this disorder. These efforts have begun to bear fruit, with at least five distinct regions of the genome demonstrated to contribute to bipolar disorder liability and evidence that hundreds more await discovery. While these discoveries have immediate implications for investigating the neurobiology of bipolar disorder, they have not yet reached the point of being clinically actionable.

FAMILY AND TWIN STUDIES OF BIPOLAR DISORDER

The standard approach to estimating how much bipolar disorder runs in families examines constellations of family members—at minimum, a child and a parent but often extended pedigrees over multiple generations. These data allow an estimate of recurrence risk based on family distance from an affected individual. For example, lambda's refers to the recurrence risk for a sibling, with whom an individual will share (on average) ~50% of DNA.

Initial estimates supported a lambda's of ~8—that is, if a parent has bipolar disorder, the child's relative risk of bipolar disorder is eight-fold greater than average for that population (Lichtenstein et al., 2009; Smoller & Finn; 2003). In lieu of the laborious task of identifying and interviewing each family member, a recent investigation made use of health registry data collected in Sweden to derive specific risks for each family relationship. Notably, these values are not identical for each first-degree relationship. When one parent has bipolar disorder, the child's relative risk for bipolar is ~6.4 (95% confidence interval [CI] 5.9–7.1);

when a sibling has bipolar disorder, the other sibling's relative risk is ~7.9 (95% CI 7.1–8.8).

Several other characteristics of bipolar disorder familiality are apparent in studies with these designs. First and foremost, bipolar disorder does not appear to follow a Mendelian pattern of inheritance, like recessive or dominant transmission. At minimum, this suggests incomplete penetrance—unlike some rare genetic diseases, knowing parental status does not allow reliable prediction of offspring status. Analysis of pedigrees, in conjunction with additional phenotypic data, also strongly suggests that other recognized inheritance patterns are not present in most bipolar disorder pedigrees. For example, there is not strong evidence of genetic anticipation, as observed in Huntington's disease and other trinucleotide repeat disorders, in which age at onset tends to decrease with subsequent generations; likewise, there is not strong evidence of maternal inheritance as is observed in mitochondrial diseases. In general, mathematical modeling was useful in excluding certain genetic models of disease (Craddock, Khodel, Van Eerdewegh, & Reich, 1995).

Second, in addition to increasing the risk for bipolar disorder, a bipolar disorder family member increases the risk for other psychiatric illness, including major depressive disorder and schizophrenia (Lichtenstein et al., 2009). For example, risk for schizophrenia is elevated in offspring of individuals with bipolar disorder, with relative risk estimated to be 2.4 (95% CI 2.1–2.6). Table 15.1 illustrates the relative risk to first-degree relatives (offspring or siblings) of individuals affected with bipolar disorder or schizophrenia. Importantly, a first-degree family member of a patient with bipolar disorder is more likely to have a diagnosis of major depression than bipolar disorder. While the *relative* risk for bipolar disorder is greater than that for major depressive disorder, because the prevalence of major depressive disorder is so much greater (~15% vs. 5%), the absolute risk for major depression exceeds that of bipolar disorder. This

Table 15.1. RECURRENCE RISKS FOR SCHIZOPHRENIA AND BIPOLAR DISORDER AND CO-MORBIDITY IN PARENT-OFFSPRING AND SIBLINGS

PROBAND	RELATION TO PROBAND	RISK FOR SCHIZOPHRENIA WHEN PROBAND HAS SCHIZOPHRENIA		RISK FOR BIPOLAR DISORDER WHEN PROBAND HAS BIPOLAR DISORDER		RISK FOR SCHIZOPHRENIA WHEN PROBAND HAS BIPOLAR DISORDER		RISK FOR BIPOLAR DISORDER WHEN PROBAND HAS SCHIZOPHRENIA	
		RELATIVE RISK	95% CI	RELATIVE RISK	95% CI	RELATIVE RISK	95% CI	RELATIVE RISK	95% CI
Parent	Offspring	9.9	8.5–11.6	6.4	5.9–7.1	2.4	2.1–2.6	5.2	4.4–6.2
Sibling	Sibling	9	8.1–9.9	7.9	7.1–8.8	3.9	3.4–4.4	3.7	3.2–4.2
Sibling	Maternal half-sibling	3.6	2.3–5.5	4.5	2.7–7.4	1.4	0.7–2.6	1.2	0.6–2.4
Sibling	Paternal half-sibling	2.7	1.9–3.8	2.4	1.4–4.1	1.6	1.0–2.7	2.2	1.3–3.8
Adoptive relationships									
Biological parent	Adopted away offspring	13.7	6.1–30.8	4.3	2.0–9.5	4.5	1.8–10.9	6	2.3–15.2
Sibling	Adopted away biological sibling	7.6	0.7–87.8	—		3.9	0.2–63.3	5	0.3–79.9
Adoptive parent	Adoptee	—		1.3	0.5–3.6	1.5	0.7–3.5	—	
Sibling	Non-biological sibling	1.3	0.1–15.1	—		—	—	2	0.1–37.8

crucial point is often missed in clinical practice, where a report of family history of bipolar disorder biases the clinician to diagnose bipolar disorder (Perlis, 2005).

Another key point to emerge from population and cohort studies of bipolar disorder is that despite the familiality, *most* cases of disease are sporadic. That is, most individuals with bipolar disorder will not have a first-degree family member with bipolar disorder (Perlis, Dennehy, et al., 2009).

It should also be noted that some family studies also suggest cotransmission of risk with other medical disorders. For example, one study indicated that migraine may segregate with affective illness in some families (Merikangas, Merikangas, & Angst, 1993). Another report suggested a similar effect for panic disorder. The evidence for such cotransmission is not strong and is not consistent across studies. Still, these investigations provide hypotheses about the pleiotropic effects of bipolar disorder risk genes that may be investigated as specific risk variants are identified. Given the large number of brain genes also expressed elsewhere, it would not be surprising to find subtle non-brain manifestations of bipolar disorder in some individuals.

Taken together, studies of families with bipolar disorder probands strongly indicate the familiality of this disease.

However, familial is not the same as genetic—specific characteristics may be run in families but not be based on inherited genetic variation. A prime example is wealth: parental wealth is predictive of wealth in offspring, but no genetic predisposition to wealth has yet been identified.

To understand the extent to which risk is a result of shared genetic variation, the twin-pair design has been applied. This strategy takes advantage of the difference between monozygotic twins, who share nearly all of their DNA, and dizygotic twins, who share on average 50% like any other pair of siblings. By contrasting the concordance for disease between monozygotic and dizygotic twins, one can partition out the shared genetic risk from, for example, environmental risk.

In large twin-pair studies, when one monozygotic twin has bipolar disorder, the other has approximately a 40% to 70% likelihood of having that illness (Craddock & Jones, 1999). (As family studies would predict, the co-twin also has an elevated likelihood of other disorders.) For dizygotic twins, the likelihood is approximately 5% to 10%. These data allow estimates that up to ~90% of the risk for bipolar disorder is heritable. For example, a large registry-based study of more than 19,000 twin pairs in Finland reported a heritability of 93% (Kieseppa, Partonen, Haukka, Kaprio, &

Lonnqvist, 2004). Using an alternative non-twin methodology, heritability was estimated at 62%, similar to that of schizophrenia (67%) and roughly twice that of major depressive disorder (32%; Wray & Gottesman, 2012).

Another approach to heritability examines circumstances where twins are adopted and thus exposed to different environmental risk. These studies also support the heritability of bipolar disorder—illness in the biological parent, but not the adoptive parent, is predictive of bipolar risk (Lichtenstein et al., 2009).

An underappreciated aspect of bipolar studies such as these is the implication for the bipolar disorder phenotype itself. Despite loud critiques of the *Diagnostic and Statistical Manual of Mental Disorders* and structured interviews in general, the fact remains that these criteria identify a strongly familial disorder with heritability similar to or greater than many nonpsychiatric disorders. Thus the predictive validity of these diagnostic criteria actually compares quite favorably to criteria used for other diseases.

COMMON VARIANT ASSOCIATION STUDIES

Buoyed by strong evidence of heritability, initial investigations of bipolar disorder focused on so-called candidate genes, primarily genes coding for proteins implicated in hypothesized models of bipolar disorder liability. Beginning with neurotransmitter genes, which had known functional variants that were inexpensive to genotype, such studies proceeded to more creative candidate genes, including those related to circadian rhythms and those related to the putative mechanisms of action of lithium, a gold-standard treatment for this disorder.

Unfortunately, such studies failed to converge on convincing evidence of association for any of these loci (Seifuddin et al., 2012). In hindsight, this lack of success is perhaps not surprising, given the limited understanding of the biology of this disease that motivated such studies, the relatively modest ability to capture genetic variation in these studies, and the limited statistical power to detect smaller effects. In essence, such investigations looked for lost keys under the lightpost, focusing on genes that were well studied and straightforward to characterize.

Advances in genotyping technology facilitated a new generation of investigations, which sought to examine common variation across the genome rather than simply in particular genes of interest. Such studies had the substantial advantage of being unbiased—that is, they opened the door to truly new discoveries rather than being constrained

to focus on a small subset of genes with strong prior probabilities. This advantage was also a substantial disadvantage, however: with anywhere from 300,000 to as many as 2.5 million single nucleotide polymorphisms on an array, the multiple testing problem became acute. A rigorous approach to such multiple testing mandated correction for 1 million tests, a p value of 5×10^{-8}, as a threshold for so-called genome-wide significance.

While initial single-cohort studies using genome-wide approaches did not identify bipolar disorder risk genes at a genome-wide level of significance, investigators quickly recognized the need to combine cohorts to improve statistical power to detect association. Under the aegis of the Psychiatric Genomics Consortium, the size of such studies has rapidly grown.

Among the first bipolar disorder liability genes was the L-type calcium channel subunit, *CACNA1C* (Ferreira et al., 2008). This association has persisted as sample sizes have increased, while another initial association with ANK3 has been less consistently supported (Green, Hamshere, et al., 2013).

By late 2012, at least five loci associated with bipolar disorder had been reported (Green, Hamshere, et al., 2013; Psychiatric GWAS Consortium Bipolar Disorder Working Group, 2011). In addition to *CACNA1C*, these included variants in *ODZ4, NCAN*[14], and *SYNE1* (Green, Grozeva, et al., 2013). As sample sizes continue to grow, additional loci are likely to emerge; for example, a recent report of nearly 25,000 bipolar cases included genome-wide evidence for *ADCY2* and an intergenic region on 6q16.1 (Muhleisen et al., 2014).

With progress in identifying individual loci, there have been efforts to integrate these loci into pathways that might facilitate biological investigations and therapeutic development (Holmans et al., 2009). In particular, such analyses strongly implicate other calcium channel subunit genes in bipolar disorder risk. In addition, a recent analysis of genome-wide data suggested involvement of diverse signaling pathways related to corticotropin-releasing hormone, beta-adrenergic function, phospholipase C, and glutamate receptors, as well as endothelin 1 and cardiac hypertrophy (Nurnberger et al., 2014). Notably, some genes in these pathways were differentially expressed in dorsolateral prefrontal cortex, one brain region suggested to be affected in bipolar disorder. Pathway analysis has also been applied directly to try to identify critical cell types associated with illness; for example, an analysis of genome-wide association study data suggested involvement of oligodendrocytes in schizophrenia, while multiple glial pathways were associated with bipolar disorder (Duncan et al., 2014). Still, such analyses must be regarded as hypothesis-generating, indicating pathways or brain regions to be prioritized for further study.

In fact, experience with *CACNA1C* underscores the key point that even if individual genetic variations are not clinically actionable because of modest effect sizes, they may still point the way to important neurobiological investigation. In general, much is known about the physiology of calcium channels; Figure 15.1 illustrates the subunit structure of voltage-gated calcium channels. The functional implications of individual *CACNA1C* common variants have not been established—that is, they do not obviously or consistently impact expression levels, truncate the protein prematurely, or change 3-dimensional protein structure, for example. In other words, are the resulting L-type calcium channels underexpressed, overexpressed, or expressed at normal levels but with some gain or loss of function? As the implications of CACNA1C variants are studied at a molecular level, a growing number of studies investigate the functional implications of these variants in vivo. For example, one study suggested differences in processing facial expressions in individuals with bipolar disorder carrying a risk variant (Dima et al., 2013). Building on a long history of investigation of calcium channel antagonists primarily in bipolar mania (Casamassima, Hay, Benedetti, Lattanzi, Cassano, & Perlis, 2010), which might correct a gain of function, a pilot study suggested efficacy for the calcium channel antagonist isradipine in bipolar depression (Ostacher et al., 2014).

More generally, as a growing number of genetic variations are associated with bipolar disorder liability, more efficient means of understanding the impact of these variants at a molecular level will be required. These strategies may include examining patterns of expression in brain regions or cell types relevant to bipolar disorder as these are identified—keeping in mind that expression may change during development, so important effects may require examining specific stages of neurodevelopment. Emerging approaches that allow specific genetic variants to be introduced into cells should accelerate efforts to study the impact of a given variant.

RARE VARIANT ASSOCIATION STUDIES

An alternate hypothesis, albeit not one mutually exclusive from the common-variant model, suggests that bipolar disorder is the result of rare genetic variation that may be more likely to have large effects and thus be highly penetrant. Such variants might be particularly apparent from the study of trios—offspring with two unaffected parents—if the variants are de novo (i.e., not present in the parents).

One form of rare variation is referred to as copy-number variation (CNV). This includes deletions or duplications of specific regions of chromosome, ranging from relatively small to quite large. These variations can be detected by some genotyping arrays, particularly more recent ones that are designed with probes to detect the number of copies of a particular region present in a sample; they can also be identified using whole-genome or whole-exome sequencing approaches, discussed in more detail later.

Copy-number variations have advantages in that their functional implications are clearer than many common variants. Deleting an entire gene is likely to decrease expression of that gene's product; deleting an exon or group of exons may cause expression of an altered, dysfunctional protein. Conversely, duplicating a gene may cause increase in expression. Thus extrapolating from a variation to a potential deleterious effect is more straightforward than with most common single-nucleotide polymorphisms. On the other hand, all apparently healthy individuals carry some CNVs, and in fact many proteins are entirely normal despite being hemizygous (i.e., individuals carrying only one copy of the functional gene).

In some neuropsychiatric disorders, including autism and schizophrenia, a growing body of evidence suggests that the overall burden of CNV—that is, the number of CNV's carried by an individual—is increased. In bipolar disorder, however, the data regarding CNV burden is less clear. Some studies suggest an increase in overall CNV burden (Malhotra et al., 2011), while others do not (Bergen et al., 2012).

While CNV studies in bipolar disorder remain a work in progress, there is evidence that certain recognized syndromes involving deletions may be associated with bipolar

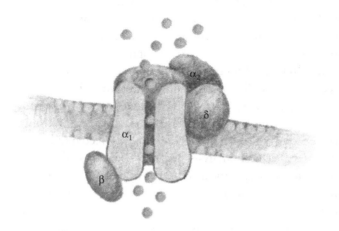

Figure 15.1 Structure of voltage-gated calcium channels

symptomatology, or even frank bipolar disorder. Perhaps the best example to date is a deletion of 22q11.2, so-called velocardiofacial syndrome (VCFS), which has been associated with bipolar spectrum features (Papolos et al., 1996). Individuals with VCFS may have a variety of congenital anomalies, including cardiac and renal abnormalities, cleft lip/palate, hearing loss, intellectual disability, and immune dysfunction. While there is a characteristic facial appearance involving small mouth and ears 'and smaller, squared-off ears, these features may be quite subtle, and the systemic manifestations may also be missed when mild. To date, the prevalence of individuals with VCFS in genetic association studies of bipolar disorder appears to be extremely low, suggesting rates of missed diagnosis may be low, or that these individuals may be more often characterized as having psychiatric disorders other than bipolar. However, the actual prevalence of VCFS among clinical populations with bipolar disorder has not been determined.

In addition to CNVs, the role of rare single nucleotide variation has also begun to be examined in bipolar disorder. (By convention, "rare" variants are generally considered to be those with a frequency of less than 1%, although this threshold reflects genotyping platform design rather than any particular discontinuity between common and rare variation.) Investigations of rare variants generally utilize sequencing methodologies—that is, reading every base pair. While technology exists for sequencing an entire genome, a more cost-effective strategy is sequencing only expressed (transcribed) regions of the genome, so-called whole-exome sequencing. More recently, in an effort to make genotyping of rare variants more cost-effective, arrays have been developed to genotype panels of rare variants.

The challenge in such studies, as with investigations of CNV, is that all individuals carry rare variants, the majority of which have no apparent functional implications whatsoever. To date, definitive results from sequencing studies in bipolar disorder have not been reported. An intriguing case report describes an individual with Timothy Syndrome, an autism-like syndrome with multiple congenital anomalies that has been shown to arise as a result of rare functional variants (mutations) in *CACNA1C*, who developed bipolar disorder in adulthood (Gershon et al., 2013).

POLYGENIC STUDIES

As a complement to studies of individual loci, it is also possible to examine the cumulative burden of potential risk variants in an individual. This strategy was demonstrated to be sensitive even to common variants that have not yet reached a threshold for being considered genome-wide significant (International Schizophrenia Consortium et al., 2009). These aggregate risk scores, sometimes referred to as polygene scores because they integrate data from a large number of genetic loci, have multiple applications. First, they may be used to examine the relationship between individual disorders by estimating the extent to which risk (loading) for one disease predicts risk for another. One initial application demonstrated that schizophrenia loading predicted bipolar disorder risk (but not risk for multiple non-psychiatric disorders), helping to refine psychiatric nosology and highlighting the overlap between disorders at a genetic level (International Schizophrenia Consortium et al., 2009). The most recent estimates of polygenic effect suggest that loading for schizophrenia can explain a substantial proportion of genetic risk for bipolar disorder, highlighting this overlap. A second application simply summarizes the extent to which genome-wide studies have succeeded in identifying risk loci. That is, polygenic scores can be used to summarize how much risk for a given disorder is explained by a set of common variants. Finally, polygene scores may serve as a useful summary measure for how much loading for common risk variants a given individual carries. The potential application of such scores is addressed in more detail in the clinical section later in this chapter.

SUBPHENOTYPES

In an effort to speed the identification of risk variants in bipolar disorder, a number of groups have tried to refine the bipolar disorder phenotype to identify more strongly heritable forms of illness (Potash et al., 2007). Some twin studies suggest similar heritability across bipolar I and II, for example (Edvardsen et al., 2008), even though the latter group is often excluded from bipolar disorder association studies. Other phenotypes have been investigated that cross diagnostic boundaries. One example is suicide attempt, for which risk is increased up to 20-fold in individuals with mood disorders (Osby, Brandt,Correia, Ekbom, & Sparen, 2001). To date, efforts to identify risk genes for suicide have not yielded results at a genome-wide level of significance (Perlis, Huang, et al., 2010; Willour et al., 2012), although efforts to understand this subphenotype in larger cohorts are ongoing.

Treatment response in bipolar disorder represents a particularly appealing subphenotype, as it might provide convergent support for particular loci or pathways in bipolar disorder. That is, genes that influence response to bipolar pharmacotherapies might overlap with those influencing disease pathophysiology. There are a relative paucity of cohorts with prospectively-derived treatment response data—that is, investigations that do not rely on retrospective report of benefit. Such retrospective reports by patients have been shown in electronic health records to be frequently discordant from actual outcomes (Simon, Rutter, Stewart, Pabiniak, & Wehnes, 2012).

The first genome-wide association study of lithium response (Perlis, Smoller, et al., 2009) failed to identify any loci at a level of genome-wide significance. However, looking across two distinct cohorts, it did identify five loci with suggestive evidence in both, most notably a variant in the gene coding for the glutamate/alpha-amino-3-hydroxy-5-methyl-4-isoxazolpropionate receptor *GRIA2*. A subsequent study among 294 Han Chinese individuals associated common variation in the glutamic acid decarboxylase-like 1 gene with differential response, with a minimum p value of 5.50×10^{-37} (Chen et al., 2014). Of note, despite the gene name, it does not appear to play a role in glutamatergic synapses, and so the two sets of genome-wide association study results do not necessarily implicate similar pathways. Moreover, multiple other replication efforts, including one by a consortium of groups studying lithium response genetics, provided no support for this locus (Schulze et al., 2010).

To date, no genome-wide studies of response to other pharmacotherapies have been reported. A modest number of candidate-gene studies have been reported (e.g., with the combination of olanzapine and fluoxetine; Perlis, Adams, et al., 2010), but none have yet been replicated. Efforts are also ongoing to establish larger lithium-response cohorts that rely on retrospective determination of response using a standardized measure referred to as the Alda scale (Grof et al., 2001). A preliminary report suggested reasonable interrater reliability for the efficacy ("A domain") aspect of this measure (Manchia et al., 2013).

NEW DIRECTIONS

As main effects are reliably identified for individual loci, the possibility of detecting gene-by-environment interactions becomes more plausible. Even for monozygotic twin pairs in which one twin is affected, the risk is only ~50% that the co-twin is affected, which argues for such effects. More generally, based on the twin studies addressed earlier in this chapter, it is clear that environmental risk (either independently or through interactions with genetic variation) should account for one-third to one-half of overall bipolar disorder risk.

Unfortunately, characterizing such environmental risks is challenging because of the sheer breadth of such potential risks and the paucity of appropriate data sets. One area of focus has been early adversity—major traumas occurring during childhood—in part because data on such environmental risk exists and has been associated with major depressive disorder. One investigation suggests that early adversity is also associated with bipolar disorder risk, as has been observed with major depressive disorder, consistent with prior, smaller studies (Gilman, Dupuy, & Perlis, 2012). In particular, childhood physical abuse and sexual maltreatment have been associated with later risk for bipolar disorder and may sensitize individuals to subsequent stressors, such that these later stressors are more apt to precipitate mania (Gilman et al., 2014).

An obstacle to understanding gene-by-environment interactions is the need for even larger cohorts to achieve adequate power to detect such interactions, particularly cohorts in which a range of potential environmental risk is assessed. Similar challenges apply to efforts to identify epistatic effects (i.e., gene-by-gene interactions, where individual effects are not merely additive).

CLINICAL APPLICATIONS

At present, there is no genetic diagnostic tool with clinical utility in bipolar disorder. While investigations of common and rare variation explain a growing proportion of bipolar risk, in absolute terms this quantity remains modest—the variant in *CACNA1C* of largest effect increases bipolar risk by ~18% (Craddock & Sklar, 2013). Still, there is substantial reason to expect that, perhaps in combination with clinical risk factors, the emerging genetics of bipolar disorder will begin to contribute to longitudinal intervention studies of high-risk individuals, biomarker-stratified clinical trials, and ultimately truly novel diagnostic and therapeutic tools.

Disclosure statement: Dr. Roy Perlis has served on scientific advisory boards or consulted to Genomind, Healthrageous, Perfect Health, Psybrain, and RID Ventures.

REFERENCES

Bergen, S. E., O'Dushlaine, C. T., Ripke, S., Lee, P. H., Ruderfer, D. M., Akterin, S., … Sullivan, P. F. (2012). Genome-wide association study in a Swedish population yields support for greater CNV and MHC involvement in schizophrenia compared with bipolar disorder. *Molecular Psychiatry, 17*, 880–886.

Casamassima, F., Hay, A. C., Benedetti, A., Lattanzi, L., Cassano, G. B., & Perlis, R. H. (2010). L-type calcium channels and psychiatric disorders: A brief review. *American Journal of Medical Genetics: Part B, Neuropsychiatric Genetics, 153*, 1373–1390.

Chen, C. H., Lee, C. S., Lee, M. T., Ouyang, W. C., Chen, C. C., Chong, M. Y.,... Cheng, A. T. (2014). Variant GADL1 and response to lithium therapy in bipolar I disorder. *The New England Journal of Medicine, 370*, 119–128.

Cichon, S., Muhleisen, T. W., Degenhardt, F. A., Mattheisen, M., Miró, X., Strohmaier, J.,... Nöthen, M. M. (2011). Genome-wide association study identifies genetic variation in neurocan as a susceptibility factor for bipolar disorder. *American Journal of Human Genetics, 88*, 372–381.

Craddock, N., & Jones, I. (1999). Genetics of bipolar disorder. *Journal of Medical Genetics, 36*, 585–594.

Craddock, N., & Sklar, P. (2013). Genetics of bipolar disorder. *Lancet, 381*, 1654–1662.

Craddock, N., Khodel, V., Van Eerdewegh, P., & Reich, T. (1995). Mathematical limits of multilocus models: The genetic transmission of bipolar disorder. *American Journal of Human Genetics,; 57*, 690–702.

Dima, D., Jogia, J., Collier, D., Vassos, E., Burdick, K. E., & Frangou, S. (2013). Independent modulation of engagement and connectivity of the facial network during affect processing by CACNA1C and ANK3 risk genes for bipolar disorder. *JAMA Psychiatry, 70*, 1303–1311.

Duncan, L. E., Holmans, P. A., Lee, P. H., O'Dushlaine, C. T., Kirby, A. W., Smoller, J. W.,... Cohen, B. M. (2014). Pathway analyses implicate glial cells in schizophrenia. *PLoS One, 9*, e89441.

Edvardsen, J., Torgersen, S., Roysamb, E., Lygren, S., Skre, I., Onstad, S., & Oien, P. A. (2008). Heritability of bipolar spectrum disorders. Unity or heterogeneity? *Journal of Affective Disorders, 106*, 229–240.

Ferreira, M. A., O'Donovan, M. C., Meng, Y. A., Jones, I. R., Ruderfer D. M., Jones, L.,... Craddock, N. (2008). Collaborative genome-wide association analysis supports a role for ANK3 and CACNA1C in bipolar disorder. *Nature Genetics, 40*, 1056–1058.

Gershon, E. S., Grennan, K., Busnello, J., Badner, J. A., Ovsiew, F., Memon S.,... Liu, C. (2013). A rare mutation of CACNA1C in a patient with bipolar disorder, and decreased gene expression associated with a bipolar-associated common SNP of CACNA1C in brain. *Molecular Psychiatry 2013*.

Gilman, S. E., Dupuy, J. M., & Perlis, R. H. (2012). Risks for the transition from major depressive disorder to bipolar disorder in the National Epidemiologic Survey on Alcohol and Related Conditions. *The Journal of Clinical Psychiatry, 73*, 829–836.

Gilman, S. E., Ni, M. Y., Dunn, E. C., Breslau, J., McLaughlin, K. A., Smoller, J. W., & Perlis, R. H. (2014). Contributions of the social environment to first-onset and recurrent mania. *Molecular Psychiatry*. Advance online publication. doi:10.1038/mp.2014.36.

Green, E. K., Grozeva, D., Forty, L., Gordon-Smith, K., Russell, E., Farmer, A.,... Craddock, N. (2013). Association at SYNE1 in both bipolar disorder and recurrent major depression. *Molecular Psychiatry, 18*, 614–617.

Green, E. K., Hamshere, M., Forty, L., Gordon-Smith, K., Fraser, C., Russell, E.,... Craddock, N. (2013). Replication of bipolar disorder susceptibility alleles and identification of two novel genome-wide significant associations in a new bipolar disorder case-control sample. *Molecular Psychiatry, 18*, 1302–1307.

Grof, P., Duffy, A., Cavazzoni, P., Grof, E., Garnham, J., MacDougall, M.,... Alda, M. (2002). Is response to prophylactic lithium a familial trait? *Journal of Clinical Psychiatry, 63*, 942–947.

Holmans, P., Green, E. K., Pahwa, J. S., Ferreira, M. A., Purcell, S. M., Sklar, P.,... Craddock, N. (2009). Gene ontology analysis of GWA study data sets provides insights into the biology of bipolar disorder. *American Journal of Human Genetics, 85*, 13–24.

International Schizophrenia Consortium, Purcell, S. M., Wray, N. R., Stone, J. L., Visscher, P. M., O'Donovan, M. C.,... Sklar, P. (2009). Common polygenic variation contributes to risk of schizophrenia and bipolar disorder. *Nature, 460*, 748–752.

Kieseppa, T., Partonen, T., Haukka, J., Kaprio, J., & Lonnqvist, J. (2004). High concordance of bipolar I disorder in a nationwide sample of twins. *The American Journal of Psychiatry, 161*, 1814–1821.

Lichtenstein, P., Yip, B. H., Bjork, C., Pawitan Y., Cannon T. D., Sullivan P. F., & Hultman C. M. (2009). Common genetic determinants of schizophrenia and bipolar disorder in Swedish families: A population-based study. *Lancet, 373*, 234–239.

Malhotra, D., McCarthy, S., Michaelson, J. J., Vacic, V., Burdick, K. E., Yoon, S.,... Sebat, J. (2011). High frequencies of de novo CNVs in bipolar disorder and schizophrenia. *Neuron, 72*, 951–963.

Manchia, M., Adli, M., Akula, N., Ardau, R., Aubry, J. M., Backlund, L.,... Alda, M. (2013). Assessment of Response to lithium maintenance treatment in bipolar disorder: A Consortium on Lithium Genetics (ConLiGen) Report. *PLoS One, 8*, e65636.

Merikangas, K. R., Merikangas, J. R., & Angst, J. (1993). Headache syndromes and psychiatric disorders: Association and familial transmission. *Journal of Psychiatric Research, 27*, 197–210.

Muhleisen, T. W., Leber, M., Schulze, T. G., Strohmaier, J., Degenhardt, F., Treutlein, J.,... Cichon, S. (2014). Genome-wide association study reveals two new risk loci for bipolar disorder. *Nature Communications, 5*, 3339.

Nurnberger, J. I. Jr., Koller, D. L., Jung, J., Edenberg, H. J., Foroud, T., Guella I.,... Kelsoe, J. R. (2014). Identification of pathways for bipolar disorder: A meta-analysis. *JAMA Psychiatry, 71*(6), 657–664.

Osby, U., Brandt, L., Correia, N., Ekbom, A., & Sparen, P. (2001). Excess mortality in bipolar and unipolar disorder in Sweden. *Archives of General Psychiatry, 58*, 844–850.

Ostacher, M. J., Iosifescu, D. V., Hay, A., Blumenthal, S. R., Sklar, P., & Perlis, R. H. (2014). Pilot investigation of isradipine in the treatment of bipolar depression motivated by genome-wide association. *Bipolar Disorders, 16*, 199–203.

Papolos, D. F., Faedda, G. L., Veit, S., Goldberg, R., Morrow, B., Kucherlapati, R., & Shprintzen, R. J. (1996). Bipolar spectrum disorders in patients diagnosed with velo-cardio-facial syndrome: Does a hemizygous deletion of chromosome 22q11 result in bipolar affective disorder? *The American Journal of Psychiatry, 153*, 1541–1547.

Perlis, R. H. (2005). Misdiagnosis of bipolar disorder. *American Journal of Managed Care, 11*, S271–S274.

Perlis, R. H., Adams, D. H., Fijal, B., Sutton, V. K., Farmen, M., Breier, A., & Houston, J. P. (2010). Genetic association study of treatment response with olanzapine/fluoxetine combination or lamotrigine in bipolar I depression. *The Journal of Clinical Psychiatry, 71*, 599–605.

Perlis, R. H., Dennehy, E. B., Miklowitz, D. J., Delbello, M. P., Ostacher, M., Calabrese, J. R.,... Sachs, G. (2009). Retrospective age at onset of bipolar disorder and outcome during two-year follow-up: Results from the STEP-BD study. *Bipolar Disorders, 11*, 391–400.

Perlis, R. H., Huang, J., & Purcell, S., Fava, M., Rush, A. J., Sullivan, P. F.,... Smoller, J. W. (2010). Genome-wide association study of suicide attempts in mood disorder patients. *The American Journal of Psychiatry, 167*, 1499–1507.

Perlis, R. H., Smoller, J. W., Ferreira, M. A., McQuillin, A., Bass, N., Lawrence, J.,... Purcell, S. (2009). A genomewide association study of response to lithium for prevention of recurrence in bipolar disorder. *The American Journal of Psychiatry, 166*, 718–725.

Potash, J. B., Toolan, J., Steele, J., Miller, E. B., Pearl, J., Zandi, P. P.,... McMahon, F. J. (2007). The bipolar disorder phenome database: a resource for genetic studies. *The American Journal of Psychiatry, 164*, 1229–1237.

Psychiatric GWAS Consortium Bipolar Disorder Working Group. (2011). Large-scale genome-wide association analysis of bipolar disorder identifies a new susceptibility locus near ODZ4. *Nature Genetics, 43*, 977–983.

Schulze, T. G., Alda, M., Adli, M., Akula, N., Ardau, R., Bui, E. T.,... McMahon, F. J. (2010). The International Consortium on Lithium Genetics (ConLiGen): an initiative by the NIMH and

IGSLI to study the genetic basis of response to lithium treatment. *Neuropsychobiology, 62,* 72–78.

Seifuddin, F., Mahon, P. B., Judy, J., Pirooznia, M., Jancic, D., Taylor, J.,...Zandi, P. P. (2012). Meta-analysis of genetic association studies on bipolar disorder. *American Journal of Medical Genetics: Part B, Neuropsychiatric Genetics;159,* 508–518.

Simon, G. E., Rutter, C. M., Stewart, C., Pabiniak, C., & Wehnes, L. (2012). Response to past depression treatments is not accurately recalled: Comparison of structured recall and patient health questionnaire scores in medical records. *The Journal of Clinical Psychiatry, 73,* 1503–1508.

Smoller, J. W., & Finn, C. T. (2003). Family, twin, and adoption studies of bipolar disorder. *American Journal of Medical Genetics, Part C: Seminars in Medical Genetics, 123,* 48–58.

Willour, V. L., Seifuddin, F., Mahon, P. B., Jancic, D., Pirooznia, M., Steele, J.,...(2012). A genome-wide association study of attempted suicide. *Molecular Psychiatry, 17,* 433–444.

Wray, N. R., & Gottesman, I. I. (2012). Using summary data from the Danish national registers to estimate heritabilities for schizophrenia, bipolar disorder, and major depressive disorder. *Frontiers in Genetics, 3,* 118.

PART III

COGNITION

16.

COGNITIVE IMPAIRMENTS AND EVERYDAY DISABILITY IN BIPOLAR ILLNESS

Colin A. Depp, Alexandrea L. Harmell, and Philip D. Harvey

INTRODUCTION

Bipolar disorder (BD), by any measure, produces substantial disability. Historical depictions of BD as a relapsing illness with inter-episode recovery of function now appear to be inaccurate for most patients. Longitudinal data suggests that the majority of patients spend most of their time experiencing some amount of disability. Even though up to 90% of patients recover from a first episode of mania, only one-third experience a return to premorbid functioning (Tohen et al., 2003). Globally, according to the World Health Organization's worldwide burden of disease study, BD is the seventh leading cause of years of life lost to disability among all illnesses. These functional impairments translate to massive indirect costs, such as from lost productivity and absenteeism, which were estimated in 2009 to total $150 million in the United States per year (Dilsaver, 2011). This cost estimate is about double that of schizophrenia, possibly because of the higher levels of functioning of employed patients with bipolar illness. Historically, much of the focus on the cause of these functional deficits has been on the affective symptoms experienced by patients. However, more recent work has suggested that cognitive impairments play a substantial role in producing disability, perhaps even more so than affective symptoms over the long term.

The intersection of cognitive ability and functional disability has been better documented in other psychiatric illnesses, particularly in schizophrenia (Bowie & Harvey, 2005). Coordinated and federally funded efforts such as the MATRICS initiative (Nuechterlein et al., 2008) and VALERO (Leifker, Patterson, Heaton, & Harvey, 2011) have delineated the impact and measurement issues in functional outcome in schizophrenia. There is now a strong evidence base in schizophrenia guiding data collection strategies and modalities on functional measurement and the role of such measures in gauging the impact of new treatments.

A number of lessons can be drawn from these efforts as they apply to BD (Harvey, Wingo, Burdick, & Baldessarini, 2010), yet there are several unique aspects of BD that necessitate bipolar-specific data. In particular, cognitive impairments in BD are less common and severe than among patients with schizophrenia, with a meta-analysis of 24 studies estimating that BD is associated with approximately a 0.5 standard deviation better performance on neuropsychological testing than schizophrenia (Krabbendam, Arts, Van Os, & Aleman, 2005). Bipolar patients additionally appear to have higher levels of premorbid functioning than do people with schizophrenia (Reichenberg et al., 2002), and, unlike the generalized neurocognitive deficits seen in schizophrenia, the deficits associated with BD are thought to be more selective (Goldberg & Chengappa, 2009). Such heterogeneity in level and domain of impairment also appears to be present in the realm of disability. In this chapter, we draw from lessons learned in schizophrenia research, as well as the accumulating data in bipolar samples on the impact of cognitive impairments on functional abilities. We also provide directions for future research and discuss implications for cognitive and functional rehabilitation.

RATES OF FUNCTIONAL IMPAIRMENT IN BIPOLAR DISORDER

Functional outcome is a multidimensional construct with no single indicator, spanning the impact of illness on physical, emotional, social, and productive life domains. Moreover, there is considerable variation in the measurement strategies used to quantify disability. Research on functional impairment in BD has largely focused on measuring the impact of the illness on vocational outcomes and subjective quality of life, with relatively less work on social, residential, and independent living skills. We summarize briefly the prevalence of disability across measurement strategies in BD, prior to describing the impact of cognitive ability on these disabilities.

MILESTONES

We refer to lifespan achievements such as the attainment of employment, residential independence, or marriage as functional milestones, which can be differentiated from functional outcome measures that typically involve summative clinician or patient ratings on standardized instruments that also address "subthreshold" achievements, such as seeking work. In regard to employment, a recent quantitative review indicated that about 40% to 60% of patients were currently participating in paid employment. Followed over time, over 50% of patients experienced a downward change in the level of employment (Marwaha, Durrani, & Singh, 2013). At the population level, patients with BD experienced 1.7 disability days per month, higher than most physical disorders, and 50 days of lost work due to illness per year (Dean, Gerner, & Gerner, 2004). Half of patients with BD reported missing at least one week of work in the past month (Stang, Frank, Ulcickas Yood, Wells, & Burch, 2007). In a Norwegian sample, 48% of patients were receiving disability compensation associated with work dysfunction (Schoeyen et al., 2011). In regard to marriage, in a multinational survey, patients with BD were reported to be 1.6 times more likely to be divorced compared to population controls (Breslau et al., 2011). As far as residential independence, in a relatively high-functioning sample, 18% of patients were not independently residing (i.e., residing in sheltered housing; Depp, Mausbach, Bowie, et al., 2012). Finally, incarceration is a different sort of milestone, and in a large sample of persons who were serving criminal sentences, BD was associated with a three-fold higher risk of four of more incarcerations. This elevated level of risk of repeated incarcerations was higher than that associated with any other mental illness and may also be associated with additional comorbidities such as substance abuse.

Two somewhat divergent conclusions can be drawn from these figures. On the one hand, BD produces remarkable global burden, second only to schizophrenia among mental illnesses per person affected. On the other hand, it is apparent that a substantial proportion of people with BD are married, employed, and residing independently. Thus understanding the factors that account for heterogeneity in

disability in BD is highly important, perhaps more so than in schizophrenia.

STANDARDIZED CLINICIAN RATED MEASURES OF FUNCTIONING AND QUALITY OF LIFE

A range of clinical and self-reported measures have been used to assess functional outcome in BD. Nonetheless, general (e.g., Medical Outcomes Study), psychiatric-illness focused (e.g., Specific Level of Functioning Scale; Schneider & Struening, 1983), and disease-specific (e.g., Functional Assessment Short Test) instruments have been used to assess functioning and quality of life and patients with BD evidence global impairments of approximately 0.5 standard deviations below age-matched comparison subjects. Examples of common functional outcome instruments are provided in Box 16.1. Of note, it is clear from work in schizophrenia that these scales frequently suffer from suspect validity when indexed to neurocognitive ability or even to functional milestones. It is also apparent that a considerable proportion of patients over- or underestimate their own functioning (Bowie et al., 2007), with cognitive impairments and poor levels of functioning often associated with overestimation (Sabbag et al., 2011) and significant depression associated with underestimation (Bowie et al., 2007). Interestingly, mild to moderate levels of depression are associated with accurate assessment of current functioning (Sabbag et al., 2012). It is not known whether these same biases are evident in BD, although there is reason to suspect that such problems may exist. This is likely to be important, given findings suggesting that many patients with bipolar illness experience stable mild depression (Judd & Akiskal, 2003; Judd et al., 2012) in the context of fluctuations between depression and euphoria. Thus fluctuations in the ability to evaluate current functioning may have a changeable course, much like everyday functioning, in response to mood states.

Box 16.1. FUNCTIONAL OUTCOME
INSTRUMENTS USED IN BIPOLAR
DISORDER

Medical Outcomes Study (SF-36)
Specific Level of Functioning Scale (SLOF)
Multidimensional Scale for Independent Functioning (MSIF)
Functional Assessment Short Test (FAST)
Social Adjustment Scale (SAS)
LIFE Range of Impaired Functioning Tool (LIFE-RIFT)

Moreover, a key consideration is the extent to which these impairments are state-dependent (e.g., exacerbated during manic or depressive episodes). The general finding is that quality of life is diminished during both manic and depressive episodes but is also considerably diminished compared to healthy controls during euthymic periods. As such, functional impairment is likely to be both a state and a trait in BD. In addition, mood state may produce biases in the self-evaluation of functioning, which may be particularly evident in BD and are discussed later in this chapter.

FUNCTIONAL CAPACITY

Only recently have objective performance-based measures of functional capacity been used to quantify functional impairment in BD. These instruments, which have become commonplace as proximal or secondary measures in schizophrenia treatment trials, typically involve observed performance on ecologically valid real-world tasks such as managing medication dosing schedules or navigating public transportation. In the few studies that have employed performance based measures, such as the UCSD Performance-Based Skills Assessment, Social Skills Performance Assessment, Performance Assessment of Self-Care Skills, and Medication Management Ability Assessment, patients with BD evidence impairment compared to normal controls on independent living skills, medication management ability, and social competence (Depp et al., 2009; Gildengers et al., 2013). Patients across clinical states perform worse than healthy comparators, with relatively little influence of symptom severity on performance on these measures. Moreover, performance on the Performance-Based Skills Assessment predicts real-world performance in employment and residential status in outpatients with BD. Thus disability in BD may arise from skill deficits, which are more stable and closely linked to cognitive abilities than to mood symptoms.

IMPACT OF COGNITIVE FUNCTIONING ON DISABILITY

META-ANALYSIS OF THE IMPACT OF COGNITIVE IMPAIRMENT ON DISABILITY

The recognition of cognitive impairments in BD is relatively recent in the literature, as is the persistence of disability across mood states. Nonetheless, a number of cross-sectional studies have examined the impact of cognitive ability on various indicators of functioning. Our recent meta-analysis of 22 studies estimated the aggregate strength of association between specific neurocognitive abilities and everyday functioning by examining the pooled correlation coefficient reported in these studies. The modal study was cross-sectional, small (mean $n = 61$, $SD = 23$) and used a convenience clinical sample of outpatients. One of the key limitations of this meta-analysis was the measurement of disability, as the majority of studies (14 out of 22) measured functional outcome with the Global Assessment of Functioning (Endicott, Spitzer, Fleiss, & Cohen, 1976; Jones, Thornicroft, Coffey, & Dunn, 1995), a single-item clinical rating that is confounded with symptom severity(Soderberg, Tungstrom, & Armelius, 2005).

Notwithstanding the limitations of this body of research, in regard to the estimated impact of cognitive ability on functioning, the mean correlation coefficient was $r = 0.22$, which is identical to that found in a similar meta-analysis in schizophrenia by Fett and colleagues (2011). Notably, there were no moderating influences of the mean age of the sample or sample size. There were also no moderating influences of whether or not the sample was restricted to euthymic patients. As such, even though the average cognitive performance in BD is substantially better than that in schizophrenia, the proportion of variation in predicting functional outcome is the same. The significant association between cognitive and functional measures seemed to be fairly robust across unique samples with varying restrictions based on demographic characteristics of symptom severity.

LONGITUDINAL STUDIES OF THE IMPACT OF COGNITIVE IMPAIRMENT ON DISABILITY

A smaller number of longitudinal studies have examined the long-term impact of cognitive impairment on functional outcome. Specifically, in a group of recently diagnosed patients with BD I, Torres et al. (2011) found a significant association between memory and six-month functional outcome using the Multidimensional Scale of Independent Functioning, even after partialing out the effects of mood symptomatology. Another study examined a sample of euthymic patients with BD and found that impairments in the areas of attention, executive function, and verbal memory at baseline independently predicted level of functional outcome one year later (as assessed by Global Assessment of Functioning scores and scores on the Functioning Assessment Short Test). Significant associations have also been reported between cognitive impairment and functional outcomes at 2- (Gildengers et al., 2013), 6- (Mora, Portella, Forcada, Vieta, & Mur, 2013), and 15-year follow-up visits (Burdick, Goldberg, & Harrow, 2010). Despite the fact that there has been very little research exploring whether or not cognitive functioning predicts future functional outcomes, of the studies that do evaluate this relationship, there appear to be robust findings showing that cognitive impairment among patients with BD is significantly associated with poorer long-term functioning.

EVIDENCE FOR SPECIFICITY IN COGNITIVE DOMAINS AND DISABILITY MEASURES

A number of individual studies have implicated impaired executive functioning in particular as a predictor of functional deficits in BD (Bonnin et al., 2010). Other studies have identified selective impact of attention and verbal memory deficits (Andreou & Bozikas, 2013; Martino et al., 2009) or processing speed (Burdick et al., 2010; Mur, Portella, Martinez-Aran, Pifarre, & Vieta, 2008) as being among the most significant predictors of functional outcomes. In the more developed literature in schizophrenia, there does not appear to be substantial evidence that any one cognitive domain is associated with greater functional impairment (Dickinson & Harvey, 2009; Jabben, Arts, van Os, & Krabbendam, 2010); To help evaluate whether or not a similar global versus specific pattern of cognitive impairment is representative in BD, individual cognitive domains were assessed for their mean correlation with functional outcome in the meta-analysis described previously (Depp, Mausbach, Harmell, et al., 2012). The proportion of variance accounted for by cognition in predicting various measures of functioning was significant for all cognitive domains measured (lowest correlation was $r = 0.21$ for Visual Learning and Memory domain and the highest was $r = 0.29$ for Working Memory). There was no statistical evidence for significant variation among these domains. Thus there does not appear to be compelling evidence that any one cognitive domain produces more disability than others, combining evidence from the meta-analysis, individual studies, and the larger body of literature in schizophrenia.

In contrast, there may be greater variation in the correlation between cognition and outcomes depending on the method by which disability is measured. As in schizophrenia, there does seem to be a discrepancy with performance-based measurements of functional capacity being more convergent with performance-based assessments of cognitive ability than clinician or self-reports. The strongest correlations, pooling effects across cognitive domains, were seen with Performance-Based ($r = 0.32$) and Functional Milestone ($r = 0.33$) measures of functioning. Weaker correlations were evident in Clinician-Reported ($r = 0.23$) and Self-Reported Functioning ($r = 0.20$). It is likely that functional capacity measures are more apt to assess what patients "can do," which is more specifically determined by cognitive ability, rather than ratings on functional outcome measures, which also reflect motivation and social-environmental opportunities. Moreover, Zarate, Tohen, Land, and Cavanagh (2000) concluded that individuals with BD may perform well in one area of functioning but poorly in others. In examining the relative determination of functional outcome domains using multivariate models, Bowie et al. (2010) found that cognitive ability accounted for a higher proportion of variation in predicting instrumental activities than interpersonal functioning, with work skills being an intermediate of the two.

COMPARISON OF FINDINGS TO SCHIZOPHRENIA

In addition to having a similar strength of association between cognitive and functional domains as schizophrenia, the structure of the association between cognition, functional capacity, and functional outcome is quite similar. Indeed, Bowie et al. (2010) found that the same structural relationships were evident in BD, with objective functional capacity measures mediating cognitive-functional outcome associations in work abilities, interpersonal functioning, and independent living abilities. However, there were more subtle but potentially important differences. First, direct and unmediated associations with functional outcome were evident with depressive and manic symptoms, whereas symptoms had little direct impact in schizophrenia. As such, the contributors to disability in BD are possibly more complex than in schizophrenia, driven additionally by dynamic mood symptoms. Second, a greater proportion of functional outcome in BD is (currently) unexplained—the prediction of work, social, and instrumental outcomes was roughly two-thirds ($R^2 = .30 - .46$) of that seen in schizophrenia ($R^2 = .40 - .55$). In Table 16.1 we summarize some of the challenges in extrapolating functional assessment methods from schizophrenia to BD, along with potential solutions.

Table 16.1. CHALLENGES IN EXTRAPOLATING FUNCTIONAL OUTCOME RESEARCH FROM SCHIZOPHRENIA TO BIPOLAR DISORDER

BIPOLAR DISORDER IN COMPARISON TO SCHIZOPHRENIA	PSYCHOMETRIC CHALLENGES	METHODOLOGICAL SOLUTIONS
1. More subtle and selective deficits in cognition and functioning	• Possible ceiling effects	• Use of more difficult tests of functional capacity
2. Greater cross-sectional impact of symptoms, particularly depression, on ability and real world (RW) functioning	• Relationship between neuropsychological (NP) and functioning may differ by mood states • Self-assessment may diverge from observation and both may be affected by current mood state	• Longitudinal analysis of impact of depression construct validity • Measure divergence between observer and patient reports • Inclusion of measures of social cognitive deficits
3. Greater between- and within-person variability	• Instability of estimates • Practice effects	Use of within-subjects analyses to quantify stability across phases
4. Higher rates of achievement of functional milestones	Capacity measures and rating scales may not be sensitive to milestones	Validation against functional milestones such as employment and independence

COMPARISON OF FINDINGS TO UNIPOLAR DEPRESSION

Although both patients with unipolar depression and patients with BD have been reported to perform below the level of nonpsychiatric controls on cognitive tasks, when the two groups are directly compared to one another, BD has been shown to be related to worse overall performance in areas such as delayed memory, executive functioning, language, and visuomotor abilities (Gildengers et al., 2012). Moreover, in a separate study investigating BD versus depression-specific markers of affective disorders, impaired sustained attention was shown to be more specific to BD (irrespective of euthymic or depressive state), and executive functioning was reported to be a potential marker more specific to depression as a whole (as this domain was found to be impaired in both unipolar depression and depressed BD patients; Maalouf et al., 2010). Among patients with jobs, BD has also been associated with twice the absenteeism as unipolar depression (Laxman, Lovibond, & Hassan, 2008). One study assessing work impairment over 15 years, reported that BD-I patients were unable to carry out work-role functions during 30% of assessed months, a value significantly higher than patients with unipolar depression (21%; Judd et al., 2008). Therefore, although both affective disorders have wide-ranging clinical and economic implications, there are key features that distinguish them from one another in that BD appears to be associated with more persistent and pronounced patterns of cognitive and functional impairment.

COGNITIVE ABILITY AND ITS ASSOCIATION WITH RISK FACTORS FOR DISABILITY

BIOLOGICAL MECHANISMS OF BIPOLAR DISORDER

Although it is becoming increasingly recognized that cognitive impairment is a core feature of BD, the exact etiology of this impairment has not been well defined. Different mechanisms have been hypothesized as potential origins including, but not limited to, dysregulation of dopaminergic and glutamatergic systems, the presence of mitochondrial dysfunction and oxidative stress, and inflammation of cytokines and neurotrophins (Berk et al., 2010). Individuals experiencing recurrent episodes have also been shown to have progressive ventricular enlargement (Strakowski et al., 2002) and loss of grey-matter thickness (Lyoo et al., 2006), both of which may contribute to similarly progressive changes in neurocognition. Compounding the difficulty in finding specific causes of cognitive impairment is the fact that circumscribed cognitive deficits may have iatrogenic origins, as many of the medications used to treat BD may have secondary effects on cognition and functioning.

ACCELERATED AGING

In the small number of samples restricted to older adults with BD, the association between cognitive ability and functional outcome appears to be somewhat stronger. Normal aging is, of course, associated with decreased cognitive performance and reduced everyday functional abilities. There is some short-term evidence that cognitive impairments worsen at a faster rate in middle-aged and older patients with BD than age-matched healthy comparators (Dhingra & Rabins, 1991; Gildengers et al., 2009), with a number of authors describing BD as akin to a neurodegenerative illness. Because of the design of these studies, it is unclear whether functional deficits accumulate at a faster rate than in normal aging. Concurrently, there is also evidence that the severity and frequency of manic symptoms are diminished in older patients with BD, and there is also strong indication that substance abuse comorbidity is about half as common as among younger adults. Thus, given the lessening of some of the other risk factors for functional impairment with aging, limited evidence suggests that older age may be associated with a stronger link between cognitive impairment and functional outcome in BD.

MOOD AND PSYCHOTIC SYMPTOMS

The National Institute of Mental Health Collaborative Depression Study and others have shown that at least 40% of patients' time is spent experiencing depressive symptoms and that these symptoms are a stronger driver of functional impairments than are manic symptoms (which are present only 10% of the time; Judd et al., 2005). There is somewhat inconsistent evidence that cognitive impairments are worsened during depressive phases of the illnesses, with perhaps more evidence for impairment in selected domains during the manic phase.

A key question is whether the impact of cognition and affective symptoms are additive or interactive; few studies are available to help address this question. Our group has previously shown by using multivariate path analytic models that depression appears to exert an independent unmediated effect on interpersonal and work skills. In addition, the relative impact of these associations may not be monotonic. For example, in a sample of outpatients with BD, neurocognitive ability was the strongest predictor of obtaining any work, whereas depression was most associated with poor work performance among those who do work (Depp, Mausbach, Bowie et al., 2012). The implication of this finding is that cognitive enhancement would not improve work performance and reducing depression would not increase the likelihood of finding work. Additional symptom and comorbidity drivers of functional impairment include comorbidities such as anxiety (lifetime diagnosis ~55%; Simon et al., 2004), substance abuse (lifetime diagnosis ~50%; Cassidy, Ahearn, & Carroll, 2001), and psychotic features (lifetime diagnosis ~50%; Keck, 2003). Given that 90% of patients with BD have at least one other Axis I diagnosis, it is particularly challenging to determine the extent to which any one cluster of symptoms interacts with functional outcome.

MEDICAL COMORBIDITY

In BD, the presence of comorbid medical illnesses that may affect cognition are ubiquitous, yet is often underrecognized. The strong connection between BD and medical comorbidity can largely be attributed to common risk factors inherent to both, such as insufficient access to health care, lower socioeconomic status, poor medical adherence, higher rates of smoking and substance abuse, lack of exercise, and poor diet. As such, the prevalence of chronic fatigue syndrome, migraines, asthma, chronic bronchitis, hypertension, and gastric ulcer have all been reported to be significantly higher in BD groups and have also been shown to have deleterious and reciprocal effects on functional outcomes, including less successful employment, greater dependency on others for assistance, and higher utilization of mental health care services (McIntyre et al., 2006). Additional common medical conditions found in patients with BD include hyperlipidemia (23%), type 2 diabetes (17%), obesity (12%), and infectious diseases such as hepatitis C (6%; Kilbourne et al., 2004). The interactions between medical comorbidity, decrements in cognition, and functional domain trajectories will continue to be an important area of further investigation, as there is currently a large gap in studies that specifically examine the reciprocal relationships among these three closely related factors.

LIMITATIONS OF EXTANT RESEARCH AND SUGGESTIONS

SAMPLE SIZE AND RESEARCH DESIGN

Most of the extant knowledge on cognitive ability and functioning in BD derives from cross-sectional studies with a modest sample size (n ~60). As such, there is currently limited information about moderators, such as diagnostic heterogeneity or comorbid factors. There is also little known about the short- or long-term trajectories of cognitive impairment and functional disability or the mechanisms by which cognitive abilities impact functioning. Study designs that model dynamic interactions between symptoms and cognitive impairments may account for greater variation in functioning (Bowie et al. 2010).

STANDARDIZATION OF
COGNITIVE ASSESSMENT

Improvement in the measures used to quantify cognitive impairment and everyday functioning would also contribute to this literature. Unlike in schizophrenia and the MATRICS battery, there is no corollary consistent battery of cognitive tests for BD. Recent data and consensus has indicated that the MATRICS Consensus Cognitive Battery is largely appropriate for BD, with possible inclusion of additional executive functioning tasks and the use of the more challenging California Verbal Learning Test. In addition, the inclusion of instruments that bridge cognitive and affective domains (e.g., impulsivity, theory of mind) may predict greater proportion of variation in everyday functioning, although there are considerable reservations about the measurement properties of many of these measures (Pinkham et al., 2013).

EMERGING DIRECTIONS IN THE
MEASUREMENT OF DISABILITY

There are a number of advances in the measurement of everyday functioning that have been introduced initially in research on aging and other severe mental illnesses such as schizophrenia. These include considerations of the validity of different reports of functioning, such as self-reports and the reports of other informants such as caregivers. In addition, remote assessment has advanced to a considerable extent in these other areas, including both Internet- and smartphone-based assessments. These areas of investigation are just beginning to develop in bipolar illness, and some preliminary research has suggested that some of the same factors are operative in BD.

IMPAIRED SELF-ASSESSMENT

Neuropsychiatric conditions accompanied by impairments on performance-based cognitive assessments also appear to include substantial deficits in the ability to accurately evaluate current levels of functioning. These impairments include self-assessments of cognitive abilities (Burdick, Endick, & Goldberg, 2005; Keefe, Poe, Walker, Kang, & Harvey, 2006) and everyday functional skills. For instance, in a recent study of patients with schizophrenia, individuals who had never worked in any type of employment at any time in their lives rated themselves as more competent at vocational skills than people with schizophrenia with current full-time employment (Gould, Sabbag, Durand, Patterson, & Harvey, 2013). At the same time, these life-long unemployed patients performed significantly more poorly than the employed patients on direct assessments of cognitive and functional skills, suggesting that their inflated self-assessments may be related to cognitive impairments.

In fact, in other neuropsychiatric conditions, poor scores on the index of interest, either everyday functioning or performance-based measures, is typically the best predictor of overestimation of functioning. Individuals with disinhibition syndromes in multiple sclerosis report that they are more capable in domains of cognitive functioning as compared to their actual functioning (Carone, Benedict, Munschauer, Fishman, & Weinstock-Guttman, 2005), with similar findings in traumatic brain injury (Spikman & van der Naalt, 2010). This is a potentially trivial finding, in that if performance is very poor, the only error in estimation that can be made is overestimation. However, multiple other predictive factors have emerged. In particular, both psychotic and negative symptoms predict overestimation of functioning in people with schizophrenia (Sabbag et al., 2012). Across all of these conditions, and particularly relevant to bipolar illness, the presence of symptoms of depression has a substantial role in the accuracy of self-assessment of abilities and potential across an array of neuropsychiatric conditions and in the healthy population.

Healthy people routinely overestimate their capabilities and the likelihood of positive outcomes in ambiguous situations, referred to as the "optimistic" bias (Ehrlinger & Dunning, 2003). In contrast, the presence of mild depression is associated with increased accuracy of self assessment, with this phenomenon referred to as "depressive realism" (Dunning & Story, 1991). In healthy people, deflating feedback increases the extent to which self-assessments become more congruent with objective reality (Ehrlinger, Johnson, Banner, Dunning, & Kruger, 2008). Bipolar disorder is perhaps the condition most likely to see variable ability to perform adequate self-assessments across the course of illness, as individuals with both BD I and II experience mood shifts ranging from elevated to depressed mood.

Although there has been little research on this topic, the results in patients with BD seem quite consistent with results from other conditions. Burdick et al. (2005) evaluated 37 BD patients using three different ratings of cognitive impairment by patient self-report, as well as a short objective battery of neuropsychological tests. Patients' self-reports correlated poorly with objectively measured cognitive deficits, and, although not statistically significant, there was a clear trend toward mood-state effect on self-report measures. Specifically, depression ratings were positively correlated with cognitive complaints while mania ratings coincided with fewer deficits by patient report, suggesting a possible affective bias in self-reports. Another study of 60 euthymic BD subjects found that a subset of BD patients were able to accurately identify their cognitive problems by self-report and that these patients who had better insight into their deficits had higher levels of subsyndromal depression, with an increased number of prior episodes and an earlier age of onset as compared with the BD patients who were unaware of their objective impairment (Martinez-Aran et al., 2005). Consistent with this, BD patients' own assessment of functional capacity and quality of life may also be influenced by their affective state. In 90 BD subjects, Piccinni et al. (2007) reported that partially remitted manic patients reported a significantly better quality of life across all domains of function compared with the partially remitted BD depressed group, despite nearly identical clinician-based ratings of global functioning. These cross-sectional studies suggest that the changes in mood state that are associated with the lifetime course of BD may not only influence real-world functioning but also may influence the accuracy of self-assessments of current functioning, highlighting the importance of formal evaluation.

COMPUTERIZED ASSESSMENT AND ECOLOGICAL MOMENTARY ASSESSMENT

Given the questions raised about the validity of self-reports of cognitive functioning and disability, it is clearly important to utilize direct assessments of ability to accurately estimate future potential. At the same time, even performance-based assessments may have limitations. Neuropsychological tests have been shown in BD to be indirectly related to real-world functioning when functional capacity measures are also collected (Bowie et al., 2010; Mausbach et al., 2010). This may not be surprising because neuropsychological tests measure relatively general skills that may be required for the performance of skilled acts in the environment, although not specifically overlapping with the content of those skills. Even current functional capacity measures have some limitations. For instance, given the rapid development of technology, many of the tasks in commonly used functional capacity measures are now less commonly performed. For instance, the UCSD Performance-Based Skills Assessment has a subtest that measures the ability to write a check, and the Advanced Finances subtest of the Everyday functioning battery requires wiring checks, making bank deposits with a deposit slip, and maintaining a balance. With the changes in banking technology in the past decade, there are individuals who have never written a check or completed a deposit slip who are actually quite skilled at banking through the use of ATMs, computerized account management, and even smartphone banking apps.

A solution to the problem of outdated and indirect assessments is the development of realistic simulations of functionally skilled tasks. Such simulations have been used previously for both assessment, such as to examine the ability of older healthy people to manage ATM and Internet technology, and for treatment, such as through the development of virtual reality simulations of classrooms and combat situations. These simulations have the advantages of often being a complete replica of real-world demands such as in banking, telephone voice menus, or Internet bill-paying scenarios. They can be placed into the homes of individuals who do not have a computer of their own, and they can be administered in laboratory settings. The disadvantages of the method are that some individuals may have never had computer interactions, meaning that the results may not be applicable for individuals who have avoided computer interaction to date. This concern may be somewhat overstated, as survey results indicated that 91% of individuals under 50 and 53% of individuals over 65 were regular Internet users as of 2012. In individuals over age 65, regular Internet use increased from 10% in 2000 to the current level in 2012 (Zickuhr & Madden, 2012). Thus use of realistic simulation technology to assess functional capacity in people with bipolar illness is clearly on the horizon.

Ecological momentary assessment (EMA) is an additional technology with high potential. EMA technology currently employs smartphones, which can contact the participant, obtain answers to a series of questions, and directly transmit the information to a central database. In contrast to older monitoring strategies, such as diaries, the EMA technology allows for time stamping of information and delivery of reminders to increase adherence. Current smartphones also have GPS features, which allow for monitoring of activity. These technologies can also be used to collect multidimensional information, including mood state, current activity, others present, and level of assistance being received or provided. As a result, their direct and momentary information far surpasses self-reported information, particularly over extended periods such as the typical one-month period between clinical visits.

EMA assessment is feasible, in that in our previous research we found that more than 75% of bipolar patients already had a smartphone. Moreover, adherence to monitoring requests was in the 90% range, and smartphones provided to research participants were returned over 95% of the time.

FUNCTIONAL AND COGNITIVE REHABILITATION

From these facts it stands to reason that cognitive deficits are a potential treatment target for functional rehabilitation in BD (Green, 2006; Harvey et al., 2010). It is also clear that functional outcome should be a secondary outcome in efforts to improve cognitive functioning. In schizophrenia, the Food and Drug Administration (Buchanan et al., 2010) has provided strong guidance that functional outcome should be an end-point in clinical trials of agents targeting cognitive enhancement; it is likely that people with BD will be provided cognitive enhancing medications approved for schizophrenia, and it will be essential to determine if the benefits of these extend to functional outcome in BD.

There have been few attempts at improving cognitive functioning in BD. One of the few studies implementing cognitive remediation treatment in an effort to improve neurocognitive abilities (i.e., difficulties with organization, planning attention, and memory), as well as simultaneously treat residual depressive symptoms in BD, found decreased residual symptoms and increased occupational and overall psychosocial functioning following treatment and at three-month follow-up (Deckersbach et al., 2010). Another study looking within patients with BD in the depressive phase of the disorder found similar improvements in depression and reports of less difficulty in everyday coping following an eight-week computer-based online cognitive training program (Preiss, Shatil, Cermakova, Cimermanova, & Ram, 2013). Consistent with these results, a large multicenter, randomized, rater-blind clinical trial comparing a novel functional remediation intervention with psychoeducation and treatment as usual found that the functional remediation intervention showed superiority over treatment as usual in improving both occupational and interpersonal functioning (Torrent et al., 2013). Given these promising findings supporting the connection between improved cognition and functional outcomes, efforts to continue to develop and test functional and cognitive rehabilitation programs are very much warranted.

CONCLUSION

Bipolar disorder is a highly disabling illness for most patients, and it is becoming clear that cognitive impairments are a major source of this disability. Even though BD produces less disability, on average, than schizophrenia, many findings of the more established body of literature on cognition as a determinant of functional outcome can be transported from schizophrenia to BD. As in schizophrenia, there does not appear to be strong evidence that any one cognitive domain causes greater impairment, functional measurement with objective performance-based measure appears to more strongly associated with cognition than other measurement modalities, and cognitive rehabilitation may have a distal positive impact on functioning. However, the influence of self-assessment, mood symptoms, and comorbidities add to the complexity of cognitive and functional impairments in BD, and so it is clear that longitudinal research would be needed to understand the dynamic and lifespan influences among cognitive and functional markers. Finally, it does not seem premature to develop and evaluate cognitive remediation strategies in order to improve functional outcome in BD. Ultimately, these adjunctive therapies targeting neurocognitive impairment may lead to long-lasting improvements in the everyday functioning and quality of life for the millions of people suffering from BD.

Disclosure statement: Alexandrea Harmell has no conflicts of interest. Over the past three years Dr. Harvey has served as a consultant to Abbvie, Boeheringer-Ingelheim, Forest Labs, Forum (Formerly En Vivo), Genentech, Lundbeck, Otsuka America, Roche Pharma, Sunovion, Takeda, and Teva Pharma. He received contract research support from Genentech. Dr. Colin A. Depp has not disclosed any conflicts of interest.

REFERENCES

Andreou, C., & Bozikas, V. P. (2013). The predictive significance of neurocognitive factors for functional outcome in bipolar disorder. *Current Opinions in Psychiatry, 26*(1), 54–59.

Berk, M., Conus, P., Kapczinski, F., Andreazza, A. C., Yucel, M., Wood, S. J.,…McGorry, P. D. (2010). From neuroprogression to neuroprotection: implications for clinical care. *Medical Journal of Australia, 193*(4 Suppl.), S36–S40.

Bonnin, C. M., Martinez-Aran, A., Torrent, C., Pacchiarotti, I., Rosa, A. R., Franco, C.,…Vieta, E. (2010). Clinical and neurocognitive predictors of functional outcome in bipolar euthymic patients: A long-term, follow-up study. *Journal of Affective Disorders, 121*(1–2), 156–160.

Bowie, C. R., Depp, C., McGrath, J. A., Wolyniec, P., Mausbach, B. T., Thornquist, M. H.,…Pulver, A. E. (2010). Prediction of real-world functional disability in chronic mental disorders: A comparison of schizophrenia and bipolar disorder. *American Journal of Psychiatry, 167*(9), 1116–1124.

Bowie, C. R., & Harvey, P. D. (2005). Cognition in schizophrenia: Impairments, determinants, and functional importance. *Psychiatric Clinics of North America, 28*(3), 613–633, 626.

Bowie, C. R., Twamley, E. W., Anderson, H., Halpern, B., Patterson, T. L., & Harvey, P. D. (2007). Self-assessment of functional status in schizophrenia. *Journal of Psychiatric Research, 41*(12), 1012–1018. doi:10.1016/j.jpsychires.2006.08.003

Breslau, J., Miller, E., Jin, R., Sampson, N. A., Alonso, J., Andrade, L. H.,...Kessler, R. C. (2011). A multinational study of mental disorders, marriage, and divorce. *Acta Psychiatrica Scandinavica*, *124*(6), 474–486.

Buchanan, R. W., Keefe, R. S., Umbricht, D., Green, M. F., Laughren, T., & Marder, S. R. (2010). The FDA-NIMH-MATRICS guidelines for clinical trial design of cognitive-enhancing drugs: What do we know 5 years later? *Schizophrenia Bulletin, 37*(6), 1209–1217. doi:10.1093/schbul/sbq038

Burdick, K. E., Endick, C. J., & Goldberg, J. F. (2005). Assessing cognitive deficits in bipolar disorder: Are self-reports valid? *Psychiatry Research, 136*(1), 43–50.

Burdick, K. E., Goldberg, J. F., & Harrow, M. (2010). Neurocognitive dysfunction and psychosocial outcome in patients with bipolar I disorder at 15-year follow-up. *Acta Psychiatrica Scandinavica, 122*(6), 499–506.

Carone, D. A., Benedict, R. H., Munschauer, F. E. III, Fishman, I., & Weinstock-Guttman, B. (2005). Interpreting patient/informant discrepancies of reported cognitive symptoms in MS. *Journal of the International Neuropsychological Society, 11*(5), 574–583.

Cassidy, F., Ahearn, E. P., & Carroll, B. J. (2001). Substance abuse in bipolar disorder. *Bipolar Disorders, 3*(4), 181–188.

Dean, B. B., Gerner, D, & Gerner, R. H. (2004). A systematic review evaluating health-related quality of life, work impairment, and healthcare costs and utilization in bipolar disorder. *Current Medical Research and Opinion, 20*, 139–154.

Deckersbach, T., Nierenberg, A. A., Kessler, R., Lund, H. G., Ametrano, R. M., Sachs, G.,...Dougherty, D. (2010). RESEARCH: Cognitive rehabilitation for bipolar disorder: An open trial for employed patients with residual depressive symptoms. *CNS Neuroscience & Therapeutics, 16*(5), 298–307.

Depp, C. A., Mausbach, B. T., Bowie, C., Wolyniec, P., Thornquist, M. H., Luke, J. R.,...Patterson, T. L. (2012). Determinants of occupational and residential functioning in bipolar disorder. *Journal of Affective Disorders, 136*(3), 812–818.

Depp, C. A., Mausbach, B. T., Eyler, L. T., Palmer, B. W., Cain, A. E., Lebowitz, B. D.,...Jeste, D. V. (2009). Performance-based and subjective measures of functioning in middle-aged and older adults with bipolar disorder. *Journal of Nervous and Mental Disease, 197*(7), 471–475.

Depp, C. A., Mausbach, B. T., Harmell, A. L., Savla, G. N., Bowie, C. R., Harvey, P. D., & Patterson, T. L. (2012). Meta-analysis of the association between cognitive abilities and everyday functioning in bipolar disorder. *Bipolar Disorders, 14*(3), 217–226. doi:10.1111/j.1399-5618.2012.01011.x

Dhingra, U., & Rabins, P. V. (1991). Mania in the elderly: A 5-7 year follow-up. *Journal of the American Geriatrics Society, 39*(6), 581–583.

Dickinson, D., & Harvey, P. D. (2009). Systemic hypotheses for generalized cognitive deficits in schizophrenia: A new take on an old problem. *Schizophrenia Bulletin, 35*(2), 403–414.

Dilsaver, S. C. (2011). An estimate of the minimum economic burden of bipolar I and II disorders in the United States: 2009. *Journal of Affective Disorders, 129*(1–3), 79–83. doi:10.1016/j.jad.2010.08.030

Dunning, D., & Story, A. L. (1991). Depression, realism, and the overconfidence effect: Are the sadder wiser when predicting future actions and events? *Journal of Personality and Social Psychology, 61*(4), 521–532.

Ehrlinger, J., & Dunning, D. (2003). How chronic self-views influence (and potentially mislead) estimates of performance. *Journal of Personality and Social Psychology, 84*(1), 5–17.

Ehrlinger, J., Johnson, K., Banner, M., Dunning, D., & Kruger, J. (2008). Why the unskilled are unaware: Further explorations of (absent) self-insight among the incompetent. *Organizational Behavior and Human Decision Processes, 105*(1), 98–121.

Endicott, J., Spitzer, R. L., Fleiss, J. L., & Cohen, J. (1976). The Global Assessment Scale: A procedure for measuring overall severity of psychiatric disturbance. *Archives of General Psychiatry, 33*(6), 766.

Fett, A. K., Viechtbauer, W., Dominguez, M. D., Penn, D. L., van Os, J., & Krabbendam, L. (2011). The relationship between neurocognition and social cognition with functional outcomes in schizophrenia: A meta-analysis. *Neuroscience and Biobehavioral Reviews, 35*(3), 573–588. doi:S0149-7634(10)00114-4 [pii] 10.1016/j.neubiorev.2010.07.001

Gildengers, A. G., Butters, M. A., Chisholm, D., Anderson, S. J., Begley, A., Holm, M.,...Mulsant, B. H. (2012). Cognition in older adults with bipolar disorder versus major depressive disorder. *Bipolar Disorders, 14*(2), 198–205.

Gildengers, A. G., Chisholm, D., Butters, M. A., Anderson, S. J., Begley, A., Holm, M.,...Mulsant, B. H. (2013). Two-year course of cognitive function and instrumental activities of daily living in older adults with bipolar disorder: evidence for neuroprogression? *Psychological Medicine, 43*(4), 801–811.

Gildengers, A. G., Mulsant, B. H., Begley, A., Mazumdar, S., Hyams, A. V., Reynolds Iii, C. F.,...Butters, M. A. (2009). The longitudinal course of cognition in older adults with bipolar disorder. *Bipolar Disorders, 11*(7), 744–752.

Goldberg, J. F., & Chengappa, K. N. (2009). Identifying and treating cognitive impairment in bipolar disorder. *Bipolar Disorders, 2*, 123–137.

Gould, F., Sabbag, S., Durand, D., Patterson, T. L., & Harvey, P. D. (2013). Self-assessment of functional ability in schizophrenia: milestone achievement and its relationship to accuracy of self-evaluation. *Psychiatry Research, 207*(1–2), 19–24.

Green, M. F. (2006). Cognitive impairment and functional outcome in schizophrenia and bipolar disorder. *Journal of Clinical Psychiatry, 67*(10), e12.

Harvey, P. D., Wingo, A. P., Burdick, K. E., & Baldessarini, R. J. (2010). Cognition and disability in bipolar disorder: lessons from schizophrenia research. *Bipolar Disorders, 12*(4), 364–375.

Jabben, N., Arts, B., van Os, J., & Krabbendam, L. (2010). Neurocognitive functioning as intermediary phenotype and predictor of psychosocial functioning across the psychosis continuum: Studies in schizophrenia and bipolar disorder. *Journal of Clinical Psychiatry, 71*(6), 764–774.

Jones, S. H., Thornicroft, G., Coffey, M., & Dunn, G. (1995). A brief mental health outcome scale—Reliability and validity of the Global Assessment of Functioning (GAF). *The British Journal of Psychiatry, 166*(5), 654.

Judd, L. L., & Akiskal, H. S. (2003). Depressive episodes and symptoms dominate the longitudinal course of bipolar disorder. *Current Psychiatry Reports, 5*(6), 417–418.

Judd, L. L., Akiskal, H. S., Schettler, P. J., Endicott, J., Leon, A. C., Solomon, D. A.,...Keller, M. B. (2005). Psychosocial disability in the course of bipolar I and II disorders: A prospective, comparative, longitudinal study. *Archives of General Psychiatry, 62*(12), 1322–1330.

Judd, L. L., Schettler, P. J., Akiskal, H., Coryell, W., Fawcett, J., Fiedorowicz, J. G.,...Keller, M. B. (2012). Prevalence and clinical significance of subsyndromal manic symptoms, including irritability and psychomotor agitation, during bipolar major depressive episodes. *Journal of Affective Disorders, 138*(3), 440–448.

Judd, L. L., Schettler, P. J., Solomon, D. A., Maser, J. D., Coryell, W., Endicott, J., & Akiskal, H. S. (2008). Psychosocial disability and work role function compared across the long-term course of bipolar I, bipolar II and unipolar major depressive disorders. *Journal of Affective Disorders, 108*(1–2), 49–58.

Keck, P. E. (2003). Psychosis in bipolar disorder: Phenomenology and impact on morbidity and course of illness. *Comprehensive Psychiatry, 44*(4), 263–269.

Keefe, R. S., Poe, M., Walker, T. M., Kang, J. W., & Harvey, P. D. (2006). The Schizophrenia Cognition Rating Scale: An interview-based assessment and its relationship to cognition, real-world functioning, and functional capacity. *American Journal of Psychiatry, 163*(3), 426–432.

Kilbourne, A. M., Cornelius, J. R., Han, X., Pincus, H. A., Shad, M., Salloum, I.,...Haas, G. L. (2004). Burden of general medical conditions among individuals with bipolar disorder. *Bipolar Disorders*, *6*(5), 368–373.

Krabbendam, L., Arts, B. M., Van Os, J., & Aleman, A. (2005). Cognitive functioning in patients with schizophrenia and bipolar disorder: A quantitative review. *Schizophrenia Research*, *80*(2–3), 137–149.

Laxman, K. E., Lovibond, K. S., & Hassan, M. K. (2008). Impact of bipolar disorder in employed populations. *American Journal of Managed Care*, *14*(11), 757–764.

Leifker, F. R., Patterson, T. L., Heaton, R. K., & Harvey, P. D. (2011). Validating measures of real-world outcome: The results of the VALERO expert survey and RAND panel. *Schizophrenia Bulletin*, *37*(2), 334–343. doi:10.1093/schbul/sbp044

Lyoo, I. K., Sung, Y. H., Dager, S. R., Friedman, S. D., Lee, J. Y., Kim, S. J.,...Renshaw, P. F. (2006). Regional cerebral cortical thinning in bipolar disorder. *Bipolar Disorders*, *8*(1), 65–74.

Maalouf, F. T., Klein, C., Clark, L., Sahakian, B. J., Labarbara, E. J., Versace, A.,...Phillips, M. L. (2010). Impaired sustained attention and executive dysfunction: bipolar disorder versus depression-specific markers of affective disorders. *Neuropsychologia*, *48*(6), 1862–1868.

Martinez-Aran, A., Vieta, E., Colom, F., Torrent, C., Reinares, M., Goikolea, J. M.,...Sanchez-Moreno, J. (2005). Do cognitive complaints in euthymic bipolar patients reflect objective cognitive impairment? *Psychotherapy and Psychosomatics*, *74*(5), 295–302.

Martino, D. J., Marengo, E., Igoa, A., Scapola, M., Ais, E. D., Perinot, L., & Strejilevich, S. A. (2009). Neurocognitive and symptomatic predictors of functional outcome in bipolar disorders: A prospective 1 year follow-up study. *Journal of Affective Disorders*, *116*(1–2), 37–42.

Marwaha, S., Durrani, A., & Singh, S. (2013). Employment outcomes in people with bipolar disorder: A systematic review. *Acta Psychiatrica Scandinavica*, *4*(10), 12087.

Mausbach, B. T., Harvey, P. D., Pulver, A. E., Depp, C. A., Wolyniec, P. S., Thornquist, M. H.,...Patterson, T. L. (2010). Relationship of the Brief UCSD Performance-based Skills Assessment (UPSA-B) to multiple indicators of functioning in people with schizophrenia and bipolar disorder. *Bipolar Disorders*, *12*(1), 45–55.

McIntyre, R. S., Konarski, J. Z., Soczynska, J. K., Wilkins, K., Panjwani, G., Bouffard, B.,...Kennedy, S. H. (2006). Medical comorbidity in bipolar disorder: Implications for functional outcomes and health service utilization. *Psychiatric Services*, *57*(8), 1140–1144.

Mora, E., Portella, M. J., Forcada, I., Vieta, E., & Mur, M. (2013). Persistence of cognitive impairment and its negative impact on psychosocial functioning in lithium-treated, euthymic bipolar patients: A 6-year follow-up study. *Psychological Medicine*, *43*(6), 1187–1196.

Mur, M., Portella, M. J., Martinez-Aran, A., Pifarre, J., & Vieta, E. (2008). Long-term stability of cognitive impairment in bipolar disorder: A 2-year follow-up study of lithium-treated euthymic bipolar patients. *Journal of Clinical Psychiatry*, *69*(5), 712–719.

Nuechterlein, K. H., Green, M. F., Kern, R. S., Baade, L. E., Barch, D. M., Cohen, J. D.,...Marder, S. R. (2008). The MATRICS Consensus Cognitive Battery, Part 1: Test selection, reliability, and validity. *American Journal of Psychiatry*, *165*(2), 203–213.

Piccinni, A., Catena, M., Del Debbio, A., Marazziti, D., Monje, C., Schiavi, E.,...Dell'Osso, L. (2007). Health-related quality of life and functioning in remitted bipolar I outpatients. *Comprehensive Psychiatry*, *48*(4), 323–328.

Pinkham, A. E., Penn, D. L., Green, M. F., Buck, B., Healey, K., & Harvey, P. D. (2013). The Social Cognition Psychometric Evaluation Study: Results of the expert survey and RAND panel. *Schizophrenia Bulletin*, *31*, 31.

Preiss, M., Shatil, E., Cermakova, R., Cimermanova, D., & Ram, I. (2013). Personalized cognitive training in unipolar and bipolar disorder: A study of cognitive functioning. *Frontiers in Human Neuroscience*, *7*, 108.

Reichenberg, A., Weiser, M., Rabinowitz, J., Caspi, A., Schmeidler, J., Mark, M.,...Davidson, M. (2002). A population-based cohort study of premorbid intellectual, language, and behavioral functioning in patients with schizophrenia, schizoaffective disorder, and nonpsychotic bipolar disorder. *American Journal of Psychiatry*, *159*(12), 2027–2035. doi:10.1176/appi.ajp.159.12.2027

Sabbag, S., Twamley, E. M., Vella, L., Heaton, R. K., Patterson, T. L., & Harvey, P. D. (2011). Assessing everyday functioning in schizophrenia: Not all informants seem equally informative. *Schizophrenia Research*, *131*(1–3), 250–255.

Sabbag, S., Twamley, E. W., Vella, L., Heaton, R. K., Patterson, T. L., & Harvey, P. D. (2012). Predictors of the accuracy of self assessment of everyday functioning in people with schizophrenia. *Schizophrenia Research*, *137*(1–3), 190–195. doi:10.1016/j.schres.2012.02.002

Schneider, L. C., & Struening, E. L. (1983). SLOF: A behavioral rating scale for assessing the mentally ill. *Social Work Research and Abstracts*, *19*(3), 9–21.

Schoeyen, H. K., Birkenaes, A. B., Vaaler, A. E., Auestad, B. H., Malt, U. F., Andreassen, O. A., & Morken, G. (2011). Bipolar disorder patients have similar levels of education but lower socio-economic status than the general population. *Journal of Affective Disorders*, *129*(1–3), 68–74. doi:10.1016/j.jad.2010.08.012

Simon, N. M., Otto, M. W., Wisniewski, S. R., Fossey, M., Sagduyu, K., Frank, E.,...Pollack, M. H. (2004). Anxiety disorder comorbidity in bipolar disorder patients: Data from the first 500 participants in the Systematic Treatment Enhancement Program for Bipolar Disorder (STEP-BD). *The American Journal of Psychiatry*, *161*(12), 2222.

Soderberg, P., Tungstrom, S., & Armelius, B. A. (2005). Special section on the GAF: Reliability of Global Assessment of Functioning ratings made by clinical psychiatric staff. *Psychiatric Services*, *56*(4), 434–438. doi:10.1176/appi.ps.56.4.434

Spikman, J. M., & van der Naalt, J. (2010). Indices of impaired self-awareness in traumatic brain injury patients with focal frontal lesions and executive deficits: Implications for outcome measurement. *Journal of Neurotrauma*, *27*(7), 1195–1202.

Stang, P., Frank, C., Ulcickas Yood, M., Wells, K., & Burch, S. (2007). Impact of bipolar disorder: Results from a screening study. *Primary Care Companion to the Journal of Clinical Psychiatry*, *9*(1), 42–47.

Strakowski, S. M., DelBello, M. P., Zimmerman, M. E., Getz, G. E., Mills, N. P., Ret, J.,...Adler, C. M. (2002). Ventricular and periventricular structural volumes in first- versus multiple-episode bipolar disorder. *The American Journal of Psychiatry*, *159*(11), 1841–1847.

Tohen, M., Zarate, C. A. Jr., Hennen, J., Khalsa, H. M., Strakowski, S. M., Gebre-Medhin, P.,...Baldessarini, R. J. (2003). The McLean-Harvard First-Episode Mania Study: Prediction of recovery and first recurrence. *The American Journal of Psychiatry*, *160*(12), 2099–2107.

Torrent, C., Del Mar Bonnin, C., Martinez-Aran, A., Valle, J., Amann, B. L., Gonzalez-Pinto, A.,...Vieta, E. (2013). Efficacy of functional remediation in bipolar disorder: A multicenter randomized controlled study. *The American Journal of Psychiatry*, *20*(10), 12070971.

Torres, I. J., DeFreitas, C. M., DeFreitas, V. G., Bond, D. J., Kunz, M., Honer, W. G.,...Yatham, L. N. (2011). Relationship between cognitive functioning and 6-month clinical and functional outcome in patients with first manic episode bipolar I disorder. *Psychological Medicine*, *41*(5), 971–982.

Zarate, C. A. Jr., Tohen, M., Land, M., & Cavanagh, S. (2000). Functional impairment and cognition in bipolar disorder. *Psychiatric Quarterly*, *71*(4), 309–329.

Zickuhr, K., & Madden, M. (June 6, 2012). Older adults and Internet use. Retrieved from http://www.pewinternet.org/Reports/2012/Older-adults-and-internet-use.aspx

PART IV

NEUROIMAGING

17.

STRUCTURAL AND FUNCTIONAL MAGNETIC RESONANCE IMAGING FINDINGS AND THEIR TREATMENT IMPACT

Marguerite Reid Schneider, David E. Fleck, James C. Eliassen,

and Stephen M. Strakowski

INTRODUCTION

Magnetic resonance imaging (MRI) has been instrumental in helping to define the neuropathology of bipolar disorder at the level of brain networks. This work has provided potential biological markers to potentially predict the onset of disease, disease chronicity, and the likelihood of treatment response. Moreover, new MRI-based imaging techniques, including diffusion tensor imaging (DTI), and new analysis approaches, such as functional connectivity (FC), promise to further characterize bipolar neuropathology in the interest of informing treatment. However, the validity of neuroimaging effects identified in bipolar disorder to date is almost universally compromised by confounding factors such as medication exposure. Untangling the independent influences of genetics, symptomatology, and medication exposure on brain structure and function is a primary goal of psychiatric imaging research at the beginning of this new millennium. Toward this end, this chapter reviews MRI techniques, approaches to image analysis, current structural and functional findings, treatment effects, and predictors of treatment response as they relate to bipolar disorder at the beginning of the 21st century. It is hoped that this information will provide a solid foundation for rapid neuroimaging-based medical advances in the years to come, including a more definitive diagnosis of bipolar disorder, a better understanding of its development and progression, identification of clinically useful biological treatment targets, and more successful evaluation of treatment effects.

STRUCTURAL MAGNETIC RESONANCE IMAGING APPROACHES

Structural MRI (sMRI) consists of a set of techniques to examine the anatomy of the body, including the brain. Unlike computed tomography (CT), sMRI does not use ionizing radiation. Instead it relies on the different magnetic properties of various tissue types to generate a three-dimensional static image. There are two primary approaches to analyzing sMRI images of the brain: region of interest (ROI) and voxel based morphometry (VBM), although others are being developed (Fleck et al., 2008). The use of an ROI or VBM approach depends, in part, on the research question at hand, the study design, and the inherent advantages and disadvantages of each approach.

Region of interest analysis

Historically, sMRI image processing involved isolating macroscopic brain morphology (specific brain regions or structures of interest) by manually "tracing" them on the computer screen. The measurements are obtained by manually tracing each region/structure in consecutive image "slices" based on anatomical landmarks and then averaging voxels (volumetric pixels). The total volume of each ROI is then calculated and compared among different experimental groups or across baseline and treatment conditions. As one might imagine, manual ROI analysis is very time consuming and painstaking and, as such, can generally be used only to examine a relatively few a priori defined brain regions. In addition to time constraints for tracing each ROI manually, the number of regions examined is further constrained by the time and training required to obtain acceptable inter- and intrarater reliability for all ROI tracings. More recently, technological advances allow semi- or fully automated computer algorithms in sMRI measurements. The use of these newer automated tracing procedures bypasses many time and training limitations but is restricted to structures with highly demarcated edge lines that are easily detected and, as such, is not applicable to all possible ROIs. As an artifact of manual and automated tracing limitations, ROI analysis is typically employed as a hypothesis-driven technique in which brain regions are prespecified and hypothesized to increase or decrease in volume as a group or treatment effect.

ROI approaches offer the advantage of construct and face validity because they are directly linked to neuroanatomy and provide absolute volumes as outcome measures. Generally, ROI assessments can be conducted accurately and provide robust results. The primary drawback of this approach is the substantial time, effort, and cost required to insure reliable and valid measurement as discussed. Other limitations include variability in how regions are anatomically defined (subregions of frontal cortex, for instance that are better defined functionally than anatomically), tracer drift (which requires periodic recalibration training), and individual heterogeneity of brain structures, especially in individuals with neuropathology such as in bipolar disorder.

Voxel-based morphometry analysis

Unlike ROI analysis, VBM examines sMRI images on a voxel-by-voxel basis for differences in signal intensity, volume, and shape across the whole brain. The newer VBM approach to data processing requires that every voxel in a brain image be examined through an automated process. This technique detects volume differences throughout the brain very rapidly, despite the large quantity of data input. Unlike the hypothesis-driven approach of ROI analysis, VBM is an exploratory, hypothesis-generating technique for examining each voxel in a data array and allowing comparisons among corresponding voxels. Rather than generating absolute volumes, as in ROI analysis, the VBM approach requires data be "normalized" into stereotactic space, and, as such, between-group differences represent relative volumes within each voxel.

The VBM approach has a number of distinct advantages and disadvantages relative to ROI analysis. Its most important advantage is the objective and rapid measurements of whole-brain structure. It also requires relatively little experimenter effort since it is highly automated (e.g., image segmentation that distinguishes gray matter, white matter,

cerebrospinal fluid, and non-brain tissues). Recently, segmentation algorithms have been combined with metods for intersubject alignment (normalization) and averaging to create new approaches, including volume- and shape-based morphometry methods (e.g., mesh mapping). Surface-based approaches also exist in which surface-of-interest or point-by-point comparisons can be made among individuals on measures such as gray matter thickness. These automated techniques provide high throughput in a single experiment, but they may assess features of the MRI signal that have an inexact correspondence with specific structural quantities such as tissue volume or thickness. They also rely heavily on the accuracy of the digital image processing technique employed and on intersubject comparisons for validity. Indeed, a primary disadvantage of VBM is that it is subject to errors based on the assumption that all brains can be similarly transformed into stereotactic space. For instance, overall brain size differences identified in bipolar samples suggest that the removal of overall brain size information during normalization may be an invalid assumption. Another disadvantage is that this method is potentially less sensitive to regional differences in small subcortical structures relative to ROI analysis.

Diffusion tensor imaging

Diffusion tensor imaging (DTI) is an MRI-based anatomical connectivity technique that uses measurements of in vivo water diffusion to examine white matter integrity. Water diffusion within white matter tracts is strongly influenced by specific structural features including the myelin sheath and the tightly packed nature of axonal bundles. In the absence of any constraints on diffusion, the volume over which water molecules diffuse is isotropic; that is, it forms a sphere. The structure of normal white matter, however, results in a more rapid diffusion along the axis of the tract. This relative freedom of movement in only one direction gives rise to a nonisotropic (anisotropic) diffusion pattern, upon which various DTI measurements are built.

Fractional anisotropy (FA) is one DTI measure derived from the ratio between water molecule movements parallel with and perpendicular to the axonal tract; this approach has been widely used by bipolar disorder researchers. Decreased FA may represent axonal pathology such as neuropathic changes, a loss of bundle coherence (i.e., less tightly packed fibers), or a disruption in axonal organization (Foong et al., 2002). Mean diffusivity is another measure derived from DTI of white matter tracts that has been widely employed. Increased diffusivity is thought to reflect a loss of impediments to water movement in and around white matter tracts that has been observed with edema and axonal demyelization and loss (Beaulieu, 2002).

Diffusion weighted imaging techniques, such as DTI, have limited spatial resolution but are useful as whole brain in vivo markers of temporal changes in fiber tracts. The physical pattern of anatomical connections is relatively stable over short time periods (seconds to hours). Over longer periods (days to weeks), structural connectivity patterns are likely subject to morphological change and plasticity, which may make DTI useful in treatment monitoring.

FUNCTIONAL MAGNETIC RESONANCE IMAGING APPROACHES

In contrast to structural brain imaging techniques, functional imaging allows examinations of online brain activity. Functional MRI (fMRI) builds on the basic principles of sMRI and adds a step allowing brain activation to be inferred from changes in the blood-oxygenation-level dependent (BOLD) response. The BOLD response occurs because the magnetic properties of hemoglobin differ depending on whether the molecule is oxygenated or deoxygenated. Because active brain regions have an increased rate of neural firing, they recruit more blood flow, which is detected by the BOLD response.

Functional MRI has the advantage over positron emission tomography (PET) and single photon emission computed tomography (SPECT) of not requiring the use of ionizing radiation. Functional MRI also provides better spatial resolution than PET and SPECT. An additional advantage is that fMRI requires little special equipment beyond a standard MRI console as used to perform structural scans. Disadvantages of fMRI include a slow temporal resolution, on the order of seconds, and a potential loss of signal along air/tissue interfaces such as the sinuses. Similar to sMRI, fMRI data can also be analyzed using either ROI or voxel-wise (whole brain) approaches. However, brain network approaches to fMRI analysis (e.g., FC) have recently become especially popular due to their ability to identify functional relationships between brain structures. Other network-based approaches also exist, such as effective connectivity, which examines information flow and can be compared and contrasted with the FC approach. However, for the illustrative rather than technical purposes of this chapter we restrict the current exposition to a brief overview of FC analysis and direct the reader to Eickhoff and Grefkes (2011) and Ramnani et al. (2004) for comprehensive reviews of FC and effective connectivity analyses (Eickhoff & Grefkes, 2011; Ramnani, Behrens, Penny, & Matthews, 2004).

Functional connectivity analysis

Functional connectivity is a type of fMRI analysis that looks at statistical associations between BOLD intensity time series for different brain regions. The FC approach is useful to explore the brain's functional organization and to determine if it is altered in brain disorders such as bipolar disorder. The term "functional connectivity" refers to connections among brain regions that share functional properties. More specifically, it can be defined as temporal correlations between spatially remote neurophysiological events (fMRI brain activation in this case) expressed as a deviation from statistical independence across these events (Biswal, Van Kylen, & Hyde, 1997). FC analysis is conducted with fMRI data collected while an individual is either actively performing a task (an event-related or blocked working memory task for instance) or in a resting state to evaluate regional brain interactions that occur when not actively engaged in an explicit task. Because brain activity is present even in the absence of external stimuli, in resting state FC, any brain region can have seemingly spontaneous fluctuations in the BOLD response that may represent aspects of the individual's internal state (mood, future planning, daydreaming, etc.).

Resting-state FC research has revealed a number of networks with patterns of synchronous activity that are consistently found in healthy individuals. The default mode network (DMN) is a network that is active when an individual is awake and at rest. The DMN is an anatomically defined brain system that preferentially activates when one's focus is on internal experiences such as daydreaming, planning, or memory retrieval. It is negatively correlated with brain systems responsible for external visual or auditory signal processing and is one of the most studied networks of resting state brain activity, and one of the most easily visualized. Depending on the method of resting state analysis, FC researchers have reported a number of neural networks that appear to be functionally connected during rest. The key networks include, but are not limited to, the DMN, a sensory/motor component, an executive control component, numerous visual components, frontal/parietal components, an auditory component, and a temporal/parietal component.

OVERVIEW OF sMRI FINDINGS IN BIPOLAR DISORDER

The neural substrates of bipolar disorder are incompletely defined. However, sMRI provides a detailed in vivo examination of neuroanatomy that is beginning to differentiate individuals with bipolar disorder from other psychiatric groups and from healthy individuals. Structural MRI studies have been useful not only to define the neural substrates of bipolar disorder but also in guiding fMRI and neurochemical studies using magnetic resonance spectroscopy (discussed in Chapter 18).

WHITE MATTER ABNORMALITIES

White matter hyperintensities

One of the most replicated anatomic abnormalities in bipolar disorder is a greater incidence of T2-signal hyperintensities in white matter tracts relative to healthy and psychiatric comparison samples (Altshuler et al., 1995). These small lesions appear on T2-weighted MRI scans as areas of higher signal intensity relative to surrounding tissue. It should be noted that white matter hyperintensities are likely only secondarily related to bipolar disorder, with primary relations to cardiovascular risk factors, which are more common in individuals with bipolar disorder and due to advancing age and to a positive treatment history. The etiology of these hyperintense lesions, and their specificity to bipolar disorder, is an issue that has yet to be resolved. It has been speculated that they adversely affect signaling between frontosubcortical and limbic structures, thereby influencing mood and cognition (Norris, Krishnan, & Ahearn, 1997; Strakowski, DelBello, Adler, Cecil, & Sax, 2000). This possibility is consistent with DTI studies implicating abnormalities in white matter tract composition in bipolar disorder.

Diffusion tensor imaging

Diffusion tensor imaging has only been used to examine white matter tracts in individuals with bipolar disorder for approximately a decade, and findings have been mixed. For the most part, bipolar disorder research has been concerned with white matter tracts within and connecting to frontal cortex. Elsewhere in the brain, DTI findings have been either inconsistent or lack replication. One exception is the corpus callosum, in which Wang, Kalmar, et al. (2008) identified reduced FA in the anterior corpus callosum in adults with bipolar disorder. This finding is consistent with another report of reduced corpus callosum FA in adult patients, possibly indicating altered interhemispheric connectivity (Yurgelun-Todd, Silveri, Gruber, Rohan, & Pimentel, 2007). Additionally, reduced FA has been reported in temporal cortex (Bruno, Cercignani, & Ron,

2008), posterior cingulate (Wang, Jackowski, et al., 2008), and subcortical white matter (Haznedar et al., 2005). By contrast, mean diffusivity changes have not been widely identified outside of frontosubcortical white matter tracts (Beyer et al., 2005; Houenou et al., 2007; Yurgelun-Todd et al., 2007). In general, the greater reliability of frontosubcortical DTI findings, and the neurodevelopmental implication that frontosubcortical white matter abnormalities underlie a behavioral "disconnection syndrome" involving disinhibition and risk-taking behaviors, has driven the focus on these circuits in bipolar disorder.

Some investigators have reported reduced FA in anterior prefrontal white matter tracts, suggesting neuropathic changes (Adler et al., 2004; Wang, Jackowski, et al., 2008), while others have reported either a lack of FA differences in prefrontal white matter (Beyer et al., 2005; Bruno et al., 2008; Haznedar et al., 2005; Yurgelun-Todd et al., 2007) or increased FA (Versace et al., 2008). The areas involved, however, do not entirely overlap, and it is still unclear to what extent discrepant findings between studies reflect methodological differences. Similarly, frontosubcortical diffusivity has been found to be both increased (the direction of pathology) or unchanged in adult patients with bipolar disorder (Adler et al., 2004; Beyer et al., 2005; Bruno et al., 2008; Yurgelun-Todd et al., 2007). Nonetheless, a pattern of structural frontosubcortical network disruption is the most consistent finding in adults with bipolar disorder.

Only a few DTI studies have been conducted examining children and adolescents with bipolar disorder, and findings here have also been inconsistent. Adler et al. (2006) studied a small group of bipolar and healthy youth ranging from 10 to 18 years of age. Individuals with bipolar disorder were experiencing their first manic or mixed episode when they were scanned. Findings mirrored the results obtained in older patients; FA was reduced in anterior white matter tracts while diffusivity was unchanged. In an additional analysis of posterior white matter tracts, no between-group differences in either FA or mean diffusivity were found (Adler et al., 2006). Frazier et al. (2007) examined a somewhat younger group of bipolar children. Decreased FA was again observed in superior-frontal white matter tracts in addition to orbitofrontal white matter and corpus callosum. Moreover, FA values did not correlate with age. They extended their study to include a group of high-risk children that showed similar but smaller differences in FA compared with healthy individuals (Frazier et al., 2007). The combination of reduced FA values in acute and at-risk children independent of age suggests that these findings are risk markers for bipolar disorder rather than developmental in nature. The combination of reduced FA without changes in mean diffusivity suggests that frontal white matter abnormalities in youth with bipolar disorder may represent axonal disorganization rather than frank axonal loss (Adler et al., 2006). However, these findings are not pathognomonic for bipolar disorder. Changes in anisotropy and diffusivity have also been observed in patients with other affective and psychotic disorders, including major depressive disorder and schizophrenia (Kyriakopoulos, Bargiotas, Barker, & Frangou, 2008). Many of these changes suggest similar pathology in frontosubcortical tracts consistent with elements of overlapping symptomatology observed among bipolar disorder, major depressive disorder, and schizophrenia.

VENTRICULAR SYSTEM CHANGES

Despite the fact that DTI, and white matter hyperintensity counts and confluence ratings, indicate white matter pathology in bipolar disorder, brain tissue segmentation (into white matter, gray matter, and cerebral spinal fluid) studies often demonstrate little loss of white matter volume (e.g., Haldane & Frangou, 2004). This conclusion stands in contrast to tissue segmentation and postmortem studies involving the ventricular system in which abnormalities are readily apparent. Indeed, one of the earliest and most replicated findings in the psychiatric literature in general is ventricular enlargement in schizophrenia (e.g., see Shenton, Dickey, Frumin, & McCarley, 2001, for a review). Although enlargement of the lateral and third ventricles is less consistently observed in bipolar disorder (Norris et al., 1997), ventricular enlargement in bipolar disorder, when present, may represent underdevelopment or degeneration of periventricular structures rather than a ventricular abnormality per se (Strakowski, DelBello, et al., 2002; Strakowski et al., 1993). This suggestion is supported by a large literature reporting both periventricular and other regional gray matter abnormalities in bipolar disorder.

REGIONAL GRAY MATTER ABNORMALITIES

Advances in MRI resolution have made research into regional brain volumes common and increasingly accurate. ROI analysis and VBM are the state-of-the-art image analysis techniques most often used today, although newer approaches such as cortical thickness analysis and deformation based morphometry are continually being developed. Consistent with findings in major depressive disorder (Coffey et al., 1993; Husain et al., 1991; Krishnan et al., 1992; Kumar, Bilker, Jin, & Udupa, 2000), sMRI studies

suggest that brain abnormalities in bipolar disorder are primarily regional, as global measures of total cerebral volumes, and gray and white matter volumes are frequently unaffected (Haldane & Frangou, 2004). This contention is supported by meta-analyses (Hallahan et al., 2011; Hoge, Friedman, & Schulz, 1999; McDonald et al., 2004). Consistent with findings in major depressive disorder, Hoge et al. concluded that there are no cerebral volume differences in bipolar disorder based on a meta-analysis. In a larger meta-analysis, McDonald et al. also found no difference in total brain volume. However, despite a lack of significant group differences in this regard, Hallahan et al. found that cerebral volume reduction was associated with longer illness durations in individuals with bipolar disorder. In light of often-reported null mean effects for global cerebral volume, many investigators have chosen to focus on volume changes in specific brain regions related to mood and cognitive regulation, primarily structures within frontosubcortical networks and their intersection with medial temporal circuits.

Frontal cortex

Although abnormalities in cerebral brain regions are reported inconsistently in bipolar disorder, when present they typically consist of decreased frontal or prefrontal cortical volumes (Strakowski, Adler, & DelBello, 2002). Such findings are consistent with histological reports of glial and neuronal cell loss in prefrontal and anterior cingulate cortex in patients with bipolar disorder. Decreased volumes have been observed particularly in cortical regions encompassing ventrolateral and dorsolateral prefrontal cortex (Harvey, Persaud, Ron, Baker, & Murray, 1994; Strakowski et al., 1993), which help regulate emotion and cognition. For instance, Sax et al. (1999) noted that decreased prefrontal volume correlated with decrements in sustained attention on a continuous performance task. Drevets et al. (1997) specifically examined the subgenual prefrontal cortex and noted that not only was the volume decreased in individuals with bipolar disorder but the decrease was also associated with decreased metabolic activity as well (Drevets et al., 1997). However, McDonald et al. (2004), who examined prefrontal and subgenual prefrontal cortex in a meta-analysis, found no volume differences in these brain regions, thereby highlighting the inconsistency of sMRI findings in frontal cortex. Measurements of cortical thickness, on the other hand, have consistently demonstrated thinning of prefrontal cortex in bipolar I (Foland-Ross et al., 2011; Lyoo et al., 2006; Rimol et al., 2010) and bipolar II disorder (Elvsashagen et al., 2013); similar findings have been reported in other cortical regions including temporal (Elvsashagen et al., 2013; Rimol et al., 2010) and anterior cingulate cortex (Foland-Ross et al., 2011; Lyoo et al., 2006). Unlike cortical thinning, however, cortical surface area may not be affected in bipolar I or II disorders (Elvsashagen et al., 2013; Rimol et al., 2012).

Medial temporal structure: Amygdala

In addition to frontal lobe volume deficits, medial temporal lobe structures may also be abnormal in bipolar disorder (Schlaepfer et al., 1994). Many prior research studies identified volume changes in the amygdala (Altshuler et al., 2000; Altshuler, Bartzokis, Grieder, Curran, & Mintz, 1998; Pearlson et al., 1997; Strakowski et al., 1999). Strakowski et al. found bilaterally increased amygdala volume in bipolar relative to health individuals, and Altshuler et al. found increased amygdala volumes in individuals with bipolar disorder relative to both schizophrenic and healthy individuals. Pearlson et al., however, reported that individuals with bipolar disorder had decreased left amygdala volumes relative to healthy individuals and no volume differences relative to individuals with schizophrenia.

Indeed, one of the most important neurodevelopmental distinctions in the sMRI literature to date has been the finding of reduced amygdala volume in bipolar youth relative to normal or enlarged amygdala volume in adults with bipolar disorder (Fleck et al., 2008; Pfeifer, Welge, Strakowski, Adler, & DelBello, 2008). In studies involving pediatric bipolar samples, reduced amygdala volume has been the most consistent neuroanatomical finding (Blumberg, Kaufman, et al., 2003; Chen et al., 2004; DelBello, Zimmerman, Mills, Getz, & Strakowski, 2004; Dickstein et al., 2005; Frazier et al., 2005). In contrast, studies of individuals with adult-onset bipolar disorder have found either increased (Altshuler et al., 2000; Brambilla et al., 2003; Frangou, Donaldson, Hadjulis, Landau, & Goldstein, 2005; Sax et al., 1999; Strakowski et al., 1999) or normal (Strakowski, DelBello, et al., 2002; Swayze, Andreasen, Alliger, Yuh, & Ehrhardt, 1992) amygdala volumes relative to healthy individuals. Smaller amygdala volumes have even been reported in first-episode bipolar samples (Rosso et al., 2007), suggesting that amygdala volume deficits are apparent early in the illness course and might be useful as an illness biomarker. Smaller amygdala volumes have also been noted in bipolar youth who have a parent with bipolar disorder (Chang et al., 2005), but studies of children at familial risk for developing bipolar disorder do not always demonstrate a significant decrease in amygdala volume (Blumberg, Kaufman, et al., 2003; Chen et al., 2004; Singh, Delbello, Adler, Stanford, &

Strakowski, 2008), so the use of reduced amygdala size as a risk biomarker of incipient mania prior to illness onset is still tenuous. However, despite a lack of mean group volumetric differences, Chen et al. observed that amygdala size was positively correlated with age in bipolar adolescents but negatively correlated with age in healthy adolescents, suggesting abnormal amygdala development in at-risk individuals. This result provides an indication that the developmental trajectory of the amygdala is different in bipolar disorder than healthy individuals, consistent with a recent finding that adolescents experiencing a first manic episode do not show increases in amygdala volume over 12 months seen in healthy adolescents and adolescents with attention deficit hyperactivity disorder (Bitter, Mills, Adler, Strakowski, & DelBello, 2011). Indeed, reduced amygdala volumes may represent a disease-specific finding, as this effect has not been associated with other childhood-onset disorders such as attention deficit hyperactivity disorder and autism (Filipek et al., 1997; Schumann et al., 2004).

Medial temporal structure: Hippocampus

Unlike amygdala changes, and contrary to findings in major depression, there appears to be little change in hippocampal volume in bipolar disorder. Videbech and Ravnkilde (2004) combined data from six studies reporting hippocampal volumes in bipolar relative to healthy individuals, only one of which showed changes in bipolar disorder. No differences in hippocampal volume were identified in the resulting meta-analysis either, consistent with a separate meta-analysis by McDonald et al. (2004) conducted in the same year. Based on such findings, Strakowski, Adler, et al. (2002) suggested that affective illness may involve underdeveloped or atrophied prefrontal regions that lead to a loss of cortical modulation of emotional circuits involving the amygdala. Possible reasons for a preferential impact on amygdala volume, to a greater degree than hippocampal volume, are unclear considering the functional and anatomical proximity of these structures and the fact that bipolar disorder is characterized by declarative memory deficits in addition to mood dysregulation.

Bearden et al., (2008), demonstrated that total hippocampal volume was significantly smaller in adolescents with bipolar disorder relative to healthy individuals. Using a mesh mapping approach, the authors were able to identify localized deformations in the head and tail of the left hippocampus in adolescents with bipolar disorder relative to their healthy counterparts, suggesting that by probing the microstructure of common ROIs new insights regarding the impact of bipolar disorder on brain structure are possible. Additionally, in the same study, there was a significant positive correlation between hippocampal size and age in individuals with bipolar disorder, whereas healthy adolescents showed an inverse relation; associations similar to those previously demonstrated for the amygdala in bipolar and healthy adolescents, respectively (Chen et al., 2004).

Basal ganglia and thalamus

Several studies reported morphological differences between bipolar and healthy individuals in the basal ganglia (Aylward et al., 1994; Strakowski et al., 1999), as well as the thalamus (McIntosh et al., 2004; Strakowski et al., 1999). Consistent with the field as a whole, however, sMRI studies of the basal ganglia and thalamus have been mixed in bipolar disorder, with most showing no differences compared with healthy individuals (Dupont, Jernigan, et al., 1995; Harvey et al., 1994; Sax et al., 1999; Strakowski et al., 1993; Swayze et al., 1992). However, Strakowski et al. (1999) found bilaterally increased striatal volumes in individuals with bipolar disorder and Aylward et al. (1994) also found increased basal ganglia volumes but in males with bipolar disorder only. Similarly, although certain investigators report no abnormalities in thalamic volume in bipolar disorder (Caetano et al., 2001; Dupont, Jernigan, et al., 1995; Sax et al., 1999; Strakowski et al., 1993), Strakowski et al. and Dupont, Butters, et al. (1995) found increased thalamic volumes.

OVERVIEW OF fMRI FINDINGS IN BIPOLAR DISORDER

Bipolar disorder has long been considered primarily a disorder of mood regulation. While abnormal emotional processing is a core feature of the illness, neuropsychological research has demonstrated that individuals with bipolar disorder also demonstrate deficits in a number of cognitive domains, including attention, executive function, and verbal memory (Fleck et al., 2009). These deficits are reviewed in detail in Chapter 16. Functional MRI studies in bipolar disorder can be largely divided along these emotional-cognitive lines. The majority of fMRI studies of the bipolar brain have attempted to detect functional abnormalities associated with emotional processing and regulation. However, there is also a significant body of research that has sought to assess the functional alterations associated with purely cognitive tasks and executive function in bipolar disorder. Similar to sMRI studies, fMRI research in bipolar disorder is complicated by

numerous factors, most significantly the episodic nature of the illness and the effects of medications. In adults, the majority of functional studies have used euthymic patients, and only a smaller body of research explores functional activation patterns during episodes of depression or mania, despite the fact that mania is the defining feature of the illness. In addition, the majority of functional imaging studies are confounded by current or prior psychotropic medication exposure among participants, with only a small minority of studies assessing medication naïve individuals.

EMOTIONAL PROCESSING STUDIES

Emotional processing studies in bipolar disorder have employed a variety of behavioral paradigms, including both implicit and explicit emotional processing and regulation. The brain regions most commonly studied in emotional processing and regulation paradigms overlap significantly with those that have been the focus of sMRI studies in bipolar individuals and include the amygdala, the anterior cingulate cortex, and the medial and ventrolateral prefrontal cortices. In healthy individuals, these regions interact as a network that functions to identify and process emotional stimuli and to regulate emotional responses. In this model, the amygdala functions to detect and signal the salience of potentially emotional stimuli. Amygdala activation in response to such stimuli triggers physiological and behavioral responses via connections between this region and both the autonomic nervous system and the hypothalamic-pituitary-adrenal axis. The prefrontal regions in this network are thought to play a regulatory or inhibitory role through reciprocal connections with amygdala and other limbic regions. For example, the medial prefrontal cortex and the ventrolateral prefrontal cortex may act to dampen response to threatening stimuli both by reducing the activation of amygdala and via inhibitory connections between the ventrolateral prefrontal cortex and the autonomic nervous system. In tasks involving healthy participants, successful emotional regulation is often associated with increased activation of ventrolateral and medial prefrontal cortices and reductions in amygdala activation. The anterior cingulate cortex is thought to function in healthy individuals to manage attentional processing, in part by modulating attentional commitment to emotional stimuli. The anterior cingulate may also be involved in regulation of reciprocal interactions between emotional and cognitive processing systems (Yamasaki, LaBar, & McCarthy, 2002). For more through reviews of healthy human circuitry for emotional perception and regulation see Ochsner and Gross (2005) or Phillips, Drevets, Rauch, and Lane (2003).

As might be expected, given the prominence of emotional dysregulation in individuals with bipolar disorder, studies of emotional processing in this population have often found altered patterns of functional activation in this emotional processing network. The abnormalities detected align with the hypothesis that bipolar disorder is associated with heightened emotional reactivity and decreased emotional regulation. The most frequently replicated findings in both youth and adults are hyperactivation of the amygdala and hypoactivation in ventrolateral prefrontal cortex, although the striatum is also frequently involved (Townsend & Altshuler, 2012). A recent meta-analysis found that during emotional processing tasks, individuals with bipolar disorder show an overall pattern of increased activation in the medial temporal lobe, including the amygdala, hippocampus, and parahippocampal gyrus, and in putamen, along with decreased activation in the inferior frontal gyrus (Chen, Suckling, Lennox, Ooi, & Bullmore, 2011). Interestingly, in bipolar youth hyperactivity of the amygdala in response to emotional stimuli has been found to correlate with decreases in volume (Kalmar et al., 2009). The degree of hyperactivity of amygdala during emotional tasks has also been found to correlate with symptom severity as measured by the Young Mania Rating Scale (Bermpohl et al., 2009).

A comprehensive understanding of emotional processing in bipolar disorder is complicated by the multiple mood states that bipolar individuals experience over the course of their illness. While the majority of imaging studies in adults have included only subjects that were euthymic at the time of the scan, several studies have included individuals during manic or depressive episodes. When these studies are considered together, there is evidence that the functional alterations associated with emotional processing in bipolar disorder have both state- and trait-related components. Specifically, amygdala hyperactivation during the processing of emotional stimuli is seen in the majority of studies performed with participants in the manic state and is less frequently replicated in depressed or euthymic samples (Townsend & Altshuler, 2012). Therefore, amygdala hyperactivity, at least in response to emotional stimuli, may be a state-related finding exclusive to mania. In contrast, hypoactivation in the ventrolateral prefrontal cortex has been detected in the majority of studies of emotional processing in bipolar disorder, regardless of mood state, suggesting that altered function in that region may be a trait abnormality in bipolar disorder (Townsend & Altshuler, 2012). Given the ventrolateral prefrontal cortex's role in

emotional regulation, hypoactivation in this region may contribute to the increased emotional reactivity seen in bipolar patients, even those not currently experiencing an acute mood episode. Further research in this area is needed, as very few fMRI studies have directly compared the functional correlates of emotional processing in bipolar individuals in different mood states, and even fewer have done so by following the same patients longitudinally.

COGNITIVE PROCESSING STUDIES

While emotional processing alterations are core features of bipolar disorder, these individuals also demonstrate significant deficits in purely cognitive tasks, particularly those associated with domains of executive function. Understanding the functional underpinnings of these deficits is essential because executive function deficits are associated with significant functional impairment and poor outcomes in both youth and adults with bipolar disorder (Biederman et al., 2011; Pavuluri et al., 2006). Studies of functional correlates of cognitive tasks in individuals with bipolar disorder have employed a variety of behavioral paradigms, including sustained attention, response inhibition, interference control, and working-memory tasks. This diversity of paradigms generally means that relatively few studies have been conducted for each executive function domain. However, there are some commonalities across studies of cognitive processing in bipolar disorder.

In the past, cognitive and emotional processing systems were thought of as separate, both anatomically and functionally. In such models, cognitive processing was thought to be "top-down," primarily involving dorsal regions of the prefrontal cortex, while emotional systems were more "bottom-up," relying on limbic system and ventral prefrontal regions. Such hypotheses separating emotion from cognition have largely fallen out of favor, as recent findings suggest that the classically "cognitive" brain regions, including the anterior cingulate and dorsolateral prefrontal cortex, and classically "emotional" regions interact significantly across a variety of tasks. Some of these interactions reflect the idea of reciprocal interactions between emotional and cognitive processing. That is to say, "purely cognitive" processing involves suppression of emotional networks, whereas strong emotional activation interferes with cognitive processing (Yamasaki et al., 2002). For a review of the literature on the interactions between cognitive and emotional processing systems in healthy individuals, see Pessoa (2008).

It is not surprising, then, that the alterations seen in fMRI studies of cognitive processing paradigms in individuals with bipolar disorder often involve the same regions found to be dysfunctional in tasks of emotional processing. In a meta-analysis, the performance of purely cognitive tasks by individuals with bipolar disorder across multiple studies was associated with decreased activation in the inferior frontal gyrus, the lingual gyrus, and the putamen (Chen et al., 2011). Dysregulation in regions of the ventrolateral prefrontal cortex has been detected during sustained attention, response inhibition, and interference control in individuals with bipolar disorder (Altshuler et al., 2005; Blumberg, Leung, et al., 2003; Schneider et al., 2012). Indeed, a recent meta-analysis of functional imaging studies in bipolar disorder reported decreased activation in the inferior frontal gyrus during cognitive processing tasks (Chen et al., 2011). Similarly, hyperactivation of the amygdala has been detected in cognitive paradigms, even in the absence of emotionally valenced stimuli (Fleck et al., 2012). However, limbic hyperactivation is less reliably detected in purely cognitive tasks than in tasks using emotionally valenced stimuli (Chen et al., 2011). In addition, striatal, parietal, and cingulate abnormalities appear to be more prominent during tasks requiring cognitive processing than during emotional processing, and dorsal prefrontal alterations have been detected, most prominently in studies employing memory paradigms (Kupferschmidt & Zakzanis, 2011). Interestingly, alterations in dorsal prefrontal regions include both hypoactivity and hyperactivity. It is possible that, in some situations, processing is impaired by insufficient recruitment of dorsal prefrontal regions, while in others the dorsolateral prefrontal cortex is disproportionally recruited, perhaps as a compensatory control.

THE ROLE OF GENETICS

Recently, several studies have explored relationships among single nucleotide polymorphisms in genes associated with bipolar disorder and MRI findings. While genetic associations with structural alterations have been rare, several studies in both healthy and bipolar samples have found an association between the risk alleles at several gene loci, including CACNA1C, ANK3, and ODZ4, and activation patterns associated with bipolar disorder, especially limbic hyperactivity during emotional and reward tasks (Dima et al., 2013; Heinrich et al., 2013; Jogia et al., 2011; Tesli et al., 2013). However, several of these studies also suggest a complicated picture, with significant gene-by-diagnosis interactions, such that individuals with bipolar disorder show an opposite pattern of activation change associated with risk allele load than healthy subjects (Dima et al., 2013; Jogia et al., 2011). More research in this area is needed

to clarify relationships between genes associated with bipolar disorder and functional alterations.

MEDICATION EFFECTS IN IMAGING STUDIES OF BIPOLAR DISORDER

Bipolar disorder is a serious psychiatric illness that is most often treated with psychotropic medications, including atypical antipsychotics, lithium, and other mood stabilizers. As ethical limitations prevent delaying or terminating effective treatment for the purpose of research, the majority of MRI studies in bipolar patients are confounded by the potential effects of medications on brain structure and function. Very limited research has attempted to directly assess the effects of medication on the brains of bipolar individuals. Rather, the majority of studies that explore the effects of medications on imaging findings do so as a secondary analysis, for the most part in an attempt to identify the influence of medication exposure as a confound on the interpretation of results. The majority of studies that have taken this approach have found either no significant effects of medication on either brain structure or function in bipolar individuals or have found medication exposure to have a normalizing effect. This pattern suggests that medication exposure confounds may be increasing risk of type II error but not introducing spurious findings not associated with the pathophysiology of the disease.

LITHIUM

The medication most frequently associated with significant volumetric changes is lithium; therefore, the effect of lithium on brain volume has received considerable attention relative to other mood stabilizers. An early study demonstrated that increases in T1-weighted signal values in frontal white matter normalized with lithium treatment (Rangel-Guerra et al., 1983). More recently, Brambilla, et al., (2001) found no effect of lithium on total brain volume in individuals with bipolar disorder, but most extant studies suggest an effect. For instance, Moore et al. (2000) found increased total brain volume in bipolar disorder after four weeks of lithium treatment. Drevets (2000) found that individuals taking either lithium or valproic acid do not exhibit the same reductions in subgenual prefrontal cortex volumes seen in those not taking these medications.

The preponderance of evidence points to lithium's influence on the amygdala-hippocampal complex in particular, in both pediatric and adult bipolar samples. It was reported that amygdala size is negatively associated with antidepressant exposure and duration of illness (DelBello et al., 2004), but positively associated with lithium or divalproex exposure in pediatric samples (Chang et al., 2005), possibly indicating that antidepressants (and increased illness duration) potentate the risk of amygdala reductions, while lithium and mood stabilizers protect against volume loss in pediatric bipolar disorder.

Foland et al. (2008) assessed whether lithium treatment was associated with volume differences in the amygdala and hippocampus in adults with bipolar disorder using tensor-based morphometry, which derives volumes from the amount of warping required to match structures to a common template. Group comparisons of deformation maps showed that lithium-treated individuals exhibited significantly increased volumes of amygdala and hippocampus compared with individuals not receiving lithium. Bearden et al., (2008) also reported that total hippocampal volumes were significantly larger in lithium-treated individuals with bipolar disorder compared with healthy and unmedicated individuals with bipolar disorder, indicating that the greater volume reflects a neurotropic effect of lithium. As can be seen in Figure 17.1, mesh mapping results from this study revealed localized increases in regions of the hippocampus in lithium-treated individuals with bipolar disorder compared with healthy individuals. Observed reductions in subregions of the hippocampus in unmedicated bipolar disorder were proposed as a possible neural correlate of the declarative memory deficits reported in the illness. (Bearden et al., 2008). Beyond the possible impact of these results on treatment models of bipolar disorder, they also highlight the ability of sMRI to probe the microstructure of even small brain volumes. Finally, in a recent meta-analysis of 321 individuals with bipolar I disorder and 442 healthy individuals, Hallahan et al. (2011) demonstrated that bipolar disorder is characterized by increased right lateral ventricular, left temporal lobe, and right putamen volumes. More important, individuals treated with lithium displayed significantly increased hippocampal and amygdala volumes compared with untreated and healthy individuals. Therefore lithium exposure appears to be a source of considerable heterogeneity in sMRI results and to have a possible neuroprotective effect, as suggested by its association with increased amygdala-hippocampal complex volumes (Hallahan et al., 2011).

A small prospective study by Selek and colleagues (2013) directly assessed the impact of lithium treatment

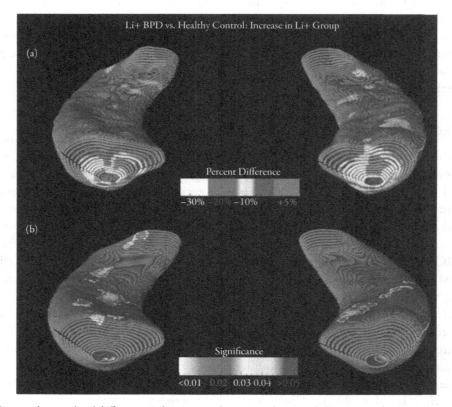

Figure 17.1 Statistical 3-D maps showing local differences in hippocampal structures between lithium-treated participants with bipolar disorder and healthy comparison participants in terms of percent difference (a) and statistical significance (b). The right hippocampus is on the left side of the figure (from Bearden et al., 2008).

on brain volumes in bipolar individuals longitudinally over a four-week treatment period. This study used automated ROI techniques to test treatment effects on volume of the hippocampus, amygdala, anterior cingulate, and dorsolateral prefrontal cortex, as well as prefrontal cortex overall. The results suggested that the neurotropic effects of lithium on brain volumes may be region-specific and related to the level of treatment response. Specifically, individuals who responded to lithium treatment showed increased volumes with treatment in left dorsolateral prefrontal cortex and prefrontal cortex overall that was not seen in those who did not respond to treatment. Those who did not respond to lithium showed volume decreases in the left hippocampus and the right anterior cingulate. Healthy controls not treated with medications and bipolar individuals who were euthymic at baseline showed no volumetric changes (Selek et al., 2013). Interpretation of these results, particularly for the nonresponder group, is limited by the very small sample size, as only six individuals failed to respond. However, complex interactions between treatment response and volumetric effects may explain some of the heterogeneity in correlational analyses. Interestingly, this study also found that those who did not respond to lithium had smaller right amygdala volumes at baseline, suggesting that regional volumes may also be useful in predicting response prior to the onset of treatment. Despite the fact that lithium effects on sMRI findings have frequently been explored, fMRI effects have been explored only as secondary analyses attempting to control for medication effects. Longitudinal studies exploring the functional effects of lithium treatment are needed to determine if the structural changes seen in patients treated with lithium are associated with functional normalization in the same regions.

ANTIPSYCHOTICS

Even short-term treatment with conventional antipsychotics has been associated with increased basal ganglia volumes, especially caudate volume, and a variety of decreased cortical gray matter volumes. By contrast, atypical antipsychotics seem to have little influence on the caudate, possibly consistent with their relative lack of extrapyramidal side effects, and have been related to increased cortical gray matter volume (Kumari & Cooke, 2006; Scherk & Falkai, 2004), suggesting that atypicals may ameliorate structural changes produced by psychopathology and/or typical antipsychotic use. In fact, switching from typical to atypical antipsychotics may reduce basal ganglia volumes to values comparable to healthy individuals (Scherk & Falkai, 2006).

PROSPECTIVE MEDICATION STUDIES

A much smaller body of research has prospectively assessed the effects of medication directly through repeated structural or functional scanning of individuals before and after specific medication regimens. The majority of these studies were conducted in youth with bipolar disorder. Some significant limitations are common to much of the published research in this area. First, these studies have almost universally employed treatment courses of 14 weeks or less and in some cases as few as 4 weeks. Second, due in part to the ethical issues associated with withholding treatment from acutely ill individuals for research purposes, the majority of studies do not include a placebo group and instead employ only healthy youth as comparison subjects. To date, only one published report has included a placebo-treated group of youth with bipolar disorder followed longitudinally to control for activation changes associated with untreated disease course (Schneider et al., 2012). Third, these studies employed a variety of different cognitive tasks, which complicates interpretation of results across studies. Finally, the majority of studies included only youth in manic, hypomanic, or mixed states. Only two prospective studies explored treatment effects in the depressed phase of illness, one using lamotrigine monotherapy (Chang, Wagner, Garrett, Howe, & Reiss, 2008) and another using a naturalistic treatment protocol (Diler et al., 2013). Despite these limitations, published research in this area has significant potential to inform our understanding of the neurofunctional correlates of treatment and response in individuals with bipolar disorder.

Two published studies prospectively looked at treatment effects in adults with bipolar disorder. Both employed a 12-week course of lamotrigine in adults who were stable at baseline. In an emotional processing task (sad affect recognition), lamotrigine treatment was associated with increases in activation, including both dorsomedial and ventrolateral prefrontal cortex. These increases were interpreted as normalizing, as bipolar individuals showed decreased activation relative to healthy subjects at baseline prior to lamotrigine treatment (Jogia, Haldane, Cobb, Kumari, & Frangou, 2008). Another study employed both emotional (angry affect recognition) and cognitive (n-back working memory) tasks. In this study, treatment with lamotrigine was associated with increased activation in bilateral superior frontal and cingulate cortices during the n-back task and increased activation in the right middle frontal gyrus and left medial frontal cortex (Haldane et al., 2008). As this study did not employ a comparison group of healthy participants, it is difficult to determine if these changes were normalizing. One significant limitation of these studies is that they included only participants who were stable at baseline, and participants showed little change in symptom severity with treatment. Given that there are state-related differences in functional activation patterns in individuals with bipolar disorder, these findings might not extend to individuals experiencing manic or depressive episodes.

Longitudinal studies of medication effects have been more common in youth with bipolar disorder. In particular, several medications have been studied longitudinally using functional imaging paradigms in manic youth, including lamotrigine, risperidone, divalproex, and ziprasidone. Lamotrigine treatment has been associated with normalization of prefrontal activation patterns in several cognitive tasks, and this change in activation in several key regions is correlated with treatment response. During a response inhibition task, youth with bipolar disorder showed decreased activation in ventral prefrontal regions relative to healthy subjects. Activation increased with lamotrigine treatment, and the increased activation in the ventrolateral prefrontal cortex was correlated with improvements in manic symptoms (Pavuluri, Passarotti, Harral, & Sweeney, 2010). In an affective color-matching task, prior to treatment bipolar individuals showed increased activation in both dorsolateral and medial prefrontal regions relative to healthy subjects. Following lamotrigine treatment, activity in both of these regions normalized, and the increase in medial prefrontal cortex activity was correlated with a decrease in manic symptoms. Similar results of prefrontal normalization with lamotrigine treatment correlating with symptomatic improvement were obtained in an affective working-memory task. However, for the affective working-memory task, significant amygdala hyperactivation relative to healthy youth was detected at baseline, and while there was some decrease in activation with treatment, the amygdala remained hyperactive at the end of the study period (Passarotti, Sweeney, & Pavuluri, 2011). Unfortunately, none of the studies of lamotrigine treatment employed a placebo-treated control group. As these studies all had a very high response rate, it is difficult to determine if the activation changes detected are associated with lamotrigine treatment specifically or with symptomatic improvement more broadly.

The functional effects of risperidone and divalproex on functional activity in manic youth with bipolar disorder have been studied in six-week, double-blind, randomized studies. In these studies participants were randomized to treatment with either risperidone or divalproex, and treatment groups were compared to assess directly how medication effects may differ between treatments. While symptoms improved for individuals in both treatment groups, the two medications differed in their effects on activation during emotional working memory, affective color matching, and response inhibition (Pavuluri, Ellis, Wegbreit, Passarotti, & Stevens, 2012; Pavuluri, Passarotti, Fitzgerald, Wegbreit, & Sweeney, 2012; Pavuluri, Passarotti, Lu, Carbray, & Sweeney, 2011). For example, in an emotional working-memory task, risperidone was associated with increases in activation in the anterior cingulate and striatal regions, while divalproex was associated with increased activation in the inferior frontal gyrus (Pavuluri, Passarotti, et al., 2012). In a response-inhibition task, the medications were also found to have differential effects on FC patterns, with risperidone showing greater increases in FC of the insula in an affective circuit, while divalproex was associated with increases in subgenual cingulate connectivity (Pavuluri, Ellis, et al., 2012). The difference in findings between treatment groups supports the hypothesis that the functional effects were related to the actions of the medications themselves as opposed to treatment response, despite the absence of a placebo control groups.

To date, the only placebo-controlled study of the neurofunctional correlates of pharmacological treatment in manic youth with bipolar disorder employed ziprasidone in a four-week, randomized, double-blind trial, which employed a sustained attention task. Treatment with ziprasidone was associated with greater increases in activation in the right ventral prefrontal cortex. In addition, individuals with lower baseline activation in right BA 47 were more likely to respond to ziprasidone treatment, and baseline activation in this region was significantly correlated with symptomatic improvement as measured by reduction in Young Mania Rating Scale scores (Schneider et al., 2012).

Only a single, small study has explored the effects of a specific medication on functional activation patterns in youth during the depressed phase of bipolar illness. Chang and colleagues (2008) scanned eight depressed bipolar youth during an emotional stimulus rating task before and after eight weeks of lamotrigine therapy. Analysis focused on ROIs in the dorsolateral prefrontal cortex and amygdala bilaterally. All patients responded to treatment, and decreases in right amygdala activation between baseline and endpoint were significantly correlated with symptomatic improvement, as measured by the Children's Depression Rating Scale, Revised (Chang et al., 2008). A more recent study looked at treatment effects more generally, scanning 10 depressed adolescents with bipolar disorder on a purely cognitive go/no-go task before and after six weeks of naturalistic treatment, which included psychotherapy and either medication changes or dose increases for most participants. When posttreatment scans were compared to baseline, increased activation was seen in the right hippocampus and left thalamus, and the decrease in depression scores was correlated with the increase in left thalamus activity in the six individuals who responded to the treatment regimens. Interestingly, the treatment effects in this study do not appear to reflect normalization, as both of these regions of increased activation were hyperactive relative to healthy subjects. Additionally, abnormally increased activation in ventrolateral prefrontal cortex relative to healthy subjects persisted following treatment. The small sample and complicated treatment protocol, including uncontrolled psychotherapy, make it difficult to interpret these findings in the context of specific medication effects.

The limitation of almost all prospective studies is that they assess the effects of monotherapy over a very brief timeframe—14 weeks or less—in a small number of subjects. In contrast, individuals with bipolar disorder often remain on medication regimens for years, and many are treated with multiple medications and combinations of medications over the course of their illness. One recent study, by Yang and colleagues (2013), looked at the longer term effects of treatment in a small pediatric bipolar disorder sample. In this study, unmedicated youth were scanned at baseline during the performance of the pediatric affective color-matching task. Individuals were then treated following a standard treatment algorithm and underwent follow-up scans at both 16 weeks and 3 years. A comparison group of typically developing youth was scanned at the same time points. The results demonstrate that youth with bipolar disorder showed abnormal hyperactivation of right dorsolateral prefrontal cortex, striatum, amygdala, and anterior cingulate and that the activation in these regions normalized over the three-year course of treatment. Interestingly, the right dorsolateral prefrontal cortex had significantly normalized by 16 weeks, while the other regions took longer to do so, suggesting that cognitive circuitry may recover more quickly with symptom resolution than limbic areas. There are significant limitations to this study: the large span between the 16-week and three-year time points prevented pinpointing the time to recovery in later recovering regions; moreover, the subjects did not all receive the same treatment but were treated using a flexible protocol that allowed for multiple treatment options, medication changes, and medication combinations. Finally, the sample size was small, with only 13 youth in the bipolar group and 10 healthy subjects. Nonetheless, the study is significant in that it is the first to explore prospectively treatment effects over the long courses of medication exposure typically used

in bipolar disorder. Further research is needed to better assess the long-term effects of treatment with specific medications on both structure and function of the brain in both pediatric and adult samples of bipolar disorder patients.

Interestingly, it appears that nonpharmacological interventions for bipolar disorder may also have effects on functional activation patterns. In a small study, Ives-Delperi and colleagues (2013) scanned 16 bipolar individuals who were mildly symptomatic at enrollment before and after eight weeks of mindfulness-based cognitive therapy (MBCT). A comparison group of 7 bipolar individuals who were wait-listed for the mindfulness training and 10 healthy subjects were scanned at the same intervals. Following the MBCT program, participants reported increased emotional regulation and decreased anxiety and showed improved performance on neurocognitive testing. Relative to healthy subjects, bipolar individuals overall showed decreased activation in the medial prefrontal cortex, a region associated with emotional regulation. Treatment with MBCT was associated with an increase in activation in this region, as well as the right posterior cingulate. Among those who underwent the treatment, the change in activation in the medial prefrontal cortex was correlated with self-reported increases in mindfulness (Ives-Delperi, Howells, Stein, Meintjes, & Horn, 2013). The cognitive task used in this study was a block design mindfulness meditation task. It is not clear if this functional normalization extends to emotional regulation in other contexts. However, mindfulness strategies have been shown to be effective in attenuating emotional responsiveness, although the mechanism may differ between beginning and very experienced meditators (Taylor et al., 2011).

CONCLUSION

Structural MRI has been instrumental in uncovering patterns of brain abnormalities in bipolar disorder. Although global volumetrics are often unaffected, it is now clear that bipolar disorder is characterized by regional changes in both white and gray matter. Increased numbers of white matter hyperintensities have been observed (Aylward et al., 1994; Bearden, Hoffman, & Cannon, 2001; Norris et al., 1997), and, although DTI data are still sparse, results suggest that white matter pathology in frontosubcortical tracts and the corpus callosum is present across bipolar age groups (Adler et al., 2004; Agarwal, Port, Bazzocchi, & Renshaw, 2010; Wang, Kalmar, et al., 2008). Furthermore, white matter abnormalities in these pathways may be intrinsic to bipolar disorder and result in changes to the neurodevelopmental trajectory of networked structures (Bruno et al., 2008; Frazier et al., 2007).

The most consistent regionally defined structural abnormalities identified in bipolar studies to date have been in the prefrontal cortex (Drevets et al., 1997; Strakowski, Adler, et al., 2002), subgenual anterior cingulate cortex (Agarwal et al., 2010), basal ganglia (Aylward et al., 1994; Strakowski et al., 1999), thalamus (McIntosh et al., 2004; Strakowski et al., 1999), and especially the amygdala (Altshuler et al., 2000; Pearlson et al., 1997; Strakowski et al., 1999). As noted, although hypothesis-driven ROI studies are often limited to frontosubcortical regions based on the behavioral manifestation of bipolar disorder (calling into question the regional specificity of ROI results), brain-wide VBM results have helped confirm the important role that these regions play in the neuropathology of bipolar disorder.

With respect to brain function, bipolar disorder is often thought of as resulting from a disruption in emotional processing systems. This hypothesis is supported by the frequent replication of functional alterations in regions associated with emotional processing when participants with bipolar are exposed to emotionally valenced stimuli. Some alterations may be specific to mood state, for example, amygdala hyperactivation appears to be most prominent during mania, while other functional abnormalities, in particular ventral prefrontal hypoactivation, may be associated with bipolar disorder across all mood presentations (Townsend & Altshuler, 2012). Abnormal interactions among these ventral prefrontal–limbic emotional networks and more dorsal cognitive processing systems may be partially responsible for the neurocognitive deficits associated with bipolar disorder.

A growing body of research has combined structural and functional imaging techniques within the same study (e.g., DTI and fMRI) to distinguish bipolar disorder from other common psychiatric illnesses that have significant symptomatic overlap with bipolar disorder, including depression and schizophrenia. For reviews of these direct comparison studies, see Whalley et al. (2012) and Cardaso de Almeida and Phillips (2013). These studies found both distinct and overlapping patterns of structural and functional alterations associated with these illnesses. This approach of combining structural and functional techniques will likely prove essential to future progress in the field. Other methodological and technical advances have come from advances in computer science. Very recent studies have shown that computer analysis algorithms that use imaging parameters may be useful in distinguishing individuals with bipolar disorder from healthy individuals and those with depression or schizophrenia on an individual level, with varying accuracy (Grotegerd et al., 2013; Rocha-Rego et al., 2013; Schnack et al., 2013). The practicality and clinical utility of such techniques remain to be seen but offer promise.

Recent reviews of treatment effects indicate that psychotropic medications have a primary influence on brain volumetrics, possibly to a greater extent than DTI and fMRI, in both child and adolescent (Singh & Chang, 2012) and adult samples (Hafeman, Chang, Garrett, Sanders, & Phillips, 2012). Studies suggest that lithium, in particular, is neuroprotective and is associated with increased volumes in corticolimbic regions subserving mood regulation (Hafeman et al., 2012), including the amygdala/hippocampal complex (Hallahan et al., 2011). In general, psychotropic medications appear to either normalize or have no effect on sMRI indices, suggesting that they likely do not explain MRI findings in bipolar disorder. Similarly, the effects of medication on functional activation appear to be primarily normalizing. However, different pharmacological treatments appear to be associated with disparate functional effects, although the absence of a placebo control group complicates the interpretation of most prospective medication studies using fMRI.

Since measures of symptomatic improvement often correlate with changes in activation patterns, these studies suggest that there may be promise for functional imaging patterns as predictors of treatment response; however, far more research is needed in this area before this suggestion could yield clinically actionable results. Finally, almost all of the prospective studies that explore the effects of medication have been conducted in pediatric samples. It is likely that early-onset bipolar disorder differs from adult-onset presentations, and therefore those results might not extend to adults.

Several factors need to be considered when attempting to differentiate patients with mood disorders on the basis of MRI. First, volume and activation changes may occur only as a cumulative effect in proportion to the number of affective episodes (DelBello, Strakowski, Zimmerman, Hawkins, & Sax, 1999; Mills, Delbello, Adler, & Strakowski, 2005). Alternatively, these changes may reflect the cumulative effects of medications or illness severity may influence measurements. An understanding of these, and other, caveats with respect to the use of MRI in bipolar disorder will be essential to move the field forward. However, MRI findings may be useful to predict and monitor treatment response. In the future, the use of serial MRI to measure the rate of brain changes might provide a method for quantifying not only disease progression but also treatment efficacy in bipolar disorder. Structural MRI studies are already being used to predict treatment response in major depressive disorder (Videbech & Ravnkilde, 2004). In one prospective study, Chen et al. (2007) correlated sMRI findings with treatment in depressed individuals before eight weeks of fluoxetine treatment. Individuals with increased volume of the anterior cingulate cortex, insula, and right temporoparietal cortex showed faster rates of recovery from depression (Chen et al., 2007). In bipolar disorder, Schneider and colleagues (2012) reported that youth with lower activity in right Brodmann area 47 at baseline were more likely to respond to ziprasidone treatment for mania. These findings support the extended use of MRI to help assign treatment for bipolar disorder in the future.

On the technological front, the ongoing development and more routine use of higher field-strength magnets and multicoil receivers will continue to advance the field. With all other variables being equal (e.g., gradient strength), high field magnets allow superior quality of neuroanatomical images with resolution in the submillimeter range by delivering images with improved contrast-to-noise ratio.

This resolution provides superior boundary demarcation between gray and white matter, which will be essential for continued improvement in automatic VBM gray/white segmentation algorithms. The use of multicoil receivers can also improve resolution and/or reduce imaging time to allow visualization of more and more subtle structural changes, reduce costs, and improve patient comfort. This technology will allow a more fine-grained analysis of the microstructure of the brain using newer mesh mapping techniques. On the macroscopic level, newer analysis techniques, such as FC analysis, have provided insight into network function and dysfunction in bipolar disorder, setting the stage for examining connections among multiple regions using density mapping, an example of which is depicted in Figure 17.2, structural equation modeling, and graph theory approaches.

The ability of any single brain region to predict or track the development of bipolar disorder with diagnostic

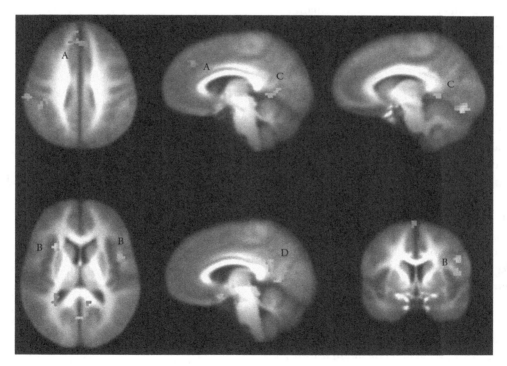

Figure 17.2 These images show local and remote functional connectivity density (LFCD/RFCD) mapping results conducted as reported by Dardo Tomasi and Nora D. Volkow [Functional connectivity density mapping, PNAS 2010; 107:9885-9890.] using the fMRI data from a single run of an attentional task. Working successively through all voxels in the brain and beginning with the data from one subject, the number of functional connections between a given voxel and all other voxels was computed. Using a voxel's time series as the regressor of interest, we calculated the correlation between that voxel and all other brain voxels. This image was then thresholded at r > 0.5 and the number significant voxels that were direct neighbors of the given voxel or its significant neighbors, i.e, the number of "local connections," were counted. This count was then placed into a new dataset at the same location, and the whole process was repeated for each voxel. The resulting dataset contained the number of local connections (significant correlations) for each voxel, a LFCD map. We also counted the number of remote connections, i.e., non-neighboring significant "remote connections" and placed that count into an RFCD map. In total we included the data from 31 manic patients and 28 healthy comparison subjects. The FCD maps were compared between groups using a t-test with a p-threshold of p < 0.01 and 25 or more voxels in a cluster for LFCD (Top Row) and RFCD (bottom row). The regions that exhibited significantly greater LFCD in manic patients than healthy subjects included (A) right medial superior frontal gyrus, BA 8, 6, and 9, and (C) Left Lingual Gyrus, BA 30. The regions that exhibited significantly greater RFCD in manic patients that healthy subjects included (B) bilateral insula, BA 13, and (D) bilateral posterior cingulate cortex, BA 23.

reliability remains fairly limited and has led to the suggestion that deterioration in interregional communication processes (i.e., connectivity) may underlie the development of adolescent bipolar disorder (Rich et al., 2008). Basic seed-region FC methods have been used since the very earliest days of functional MRI (Biswal, Yetkin, Haughton, & Hyde, 1995) and can identify interregional low-frequency BOLD correlations. As imaging research broadened to include psychiatry, these methods have been implemented to understand FC in mental illness. Seed-region FC suffers from the problem inherent in many imaging studies of mental illnesses, namely that the correct region must be chosen in order to identify meaningful connectivity differences. Characterization of multiple seed regions might address this concern, but few studies examine a large set of regions. Also, the results of seed-region FC analyses provide a fairly limited assessment of connectivity, only between a single brain region and elsewhere (i.e., first-order connections). The relationships among the other brain regions (i.e., second-order connections to the seed region) remain completely undescribed by this method. As a result, seed-region FC does not provide a quantitative view of complex network structure in the brain.

Graph theory methods have been adapted over the past decade or so to the study of brain network organization (Bullmore & Sporns, 2009). These methods rely on seed-region FC calculations as the starting point for assessing network structure. Unlike seed-region FC, interregional correlations are calculated among every pair of regions (or sometimes voxels). This approach allows for characterization of a wide variety of network measures, such as node degree (the number of "significant" connections to a seed region or seed voxel, i.e., node, but now calculated for every node). Other network characteristics include degree distribution (variation in degree from node to node), clustering coefficients (the amount of connectivity among nearest neighbors of a particular node, which is a characteristic of second-order connections to a node), and path length and its inverse, efficiency (average distance between two nodes). These measures allow for characterization of whole-brain features of a network. Recent research has found that connection density (the spatial clustering of high-degree nodes) is predictive of intelligence. The extensive and largely untapped possibilities for examining whole-network connectivity in bipolar disorder and the successful identification of relationships among behavior and connectivity measures (e.g., IQ; van den Heuvel, Stam, Kahn, & Hulshoff Pol, 2009) suggests that graph theory approaches could significantly advance understanding of the effects of bipolar disorder on brain structure and function (Guye, Bettus, Bartolomei, & Cozzone, 2010).

Disclosure statement: Dr. Strakowski serves as data-safety and monitoring board chair for Sunovion, Inc. and Novartis, Inc. He is an EAP consultant to Procter & Gamble and has performed grant reviews for the National Institutes of Health. He has previously published with Oxford University Press.

REFERENCES

Adler, C. M., Adams, J., DelBello, M. P., Holland, S. K., Schmithorst, V., Levine, A.,…Strakowski, S. M. (2006). Evidence of white matter pathology in bipolar disorder adolescents experiencing their first episode of mania: A diffusion tensor imaging study. *American Journal of Psychiatry, 163*(2), 322–324. doi:10.1176/appi.ajp.163.2.322

Adler, C. M., Holland, S. K., Schmithorst, V., Wilke, M., Weiss, K. L., Pan, H., & Strakowski, S. M. (2004). Abnormal frontal white matter tracts in bipolar disorder: A diffusion tensor imaging study. *Bipolar Disorders, 6*(3), 197–203. doi:10.1111/j.1399-56004.00108.x

Agarwal, N., Port, J. D., Bazzocchi, M., & Renshaw, P. F. (2010). Update on the use of MR for assessment and diagnosis of psychiatric diseases. *Radiology, 255*(1), 23–41. doi:10.1148/radiol.09090339

Altshuler, L. L., Bartzokis, G., Grieder, T., Curran, J., Jimenez, T., Leight, K.,…Mintz, J. (2000). An MRI study of temporal lobe structures in men with bipolar disorder or schizophrenia. *Biological Psychiatry, 48*(2), 147–162.

Altshuler, L. L., Bartzokis, G., Grieder, T., Curran, J., & Mintz, J. (1998). Amygdala enlargement in bipolar disorder and hippocampal reduction in schizophrenia: An MRI study demonstrating neuroanatomic specificity. *Archives of General Psychiatry, 55*(7), 663–664.

Altshuler, L. L., Bookheimer, S. Y., Townsend, J., Proenza, M. A., Eisenberger, N., Sabb, F.,…Cohen, M. S. (2005). Blunted activation in orbitofrontal cortex during mania: A functional magnetic resonance imaging study. *Biological Psychiatry, 58*(10), 763–769. doi:10.1016/j.biopsych.2005.09.012

Altshuler, L. L., Curran, J. G., Hauser, P., Mintz, J., Denicoff, K., & Post, R. (1995). T2 hyperintensities in bipolar disorder: Magnetic resonance imaging comparison and literature meta-analysis. *American Journal of Psychiatry, 152*(8), 1139–1144.

Aylward, E. H., Roberts-Twillie, J. V., Barta, P. E., Kumar, A. J., Harris, G. J., Geer, M.,…Pearlson, G. D. (1994). Basal ganglia volumes and white matter hyperintensities in patients with bipolar disorder. *American Journal of Psychiatry, 151*(5), 687–693.

Bearden, C. E., Hoffman, K. M., & Cannon, T. D. (2001). The neuropsychology and neuroanatomy of bipolar affective disorder: a critical review. *Bipolar Disorders, 3*(3), 106–150; discussion 151–103.

Bearden, C. E., Soares, J. C., Klunder, A. D., Nicoletti, M., Dierschke, N., Hayashi, K. M.,…Thompson, P. M. (2008). Three-dimensional mapping of hippocampal anatomy in adolescents with bipolar disorder. *Journal of the American Child & Adolescent Psychiatry, 47*(5), 515–525. doi:10.1097/CHI.0b013e31816765ab

Beaulieu, C. (2002). The basis of anisotropic water diffusion in the nervous system—A technical review. *NMR in Biomedicine, 15*(7–8), 435–455. doi:10.1002/nbm.782

Bermpohl, F., Dalanay, U., Kahnt, T., Sajonz, B., Heimann, H., Ricken, R.,…Bauer, M. (2009). A preliminary study of increased amygdala activation to positive affective stimuli in mania. *Bipolar Disorders, 11*(1), 70–75. doi:10.1111/j.1399-5618.2008.00648.x

Beyer, J. L., Taylor, W. D., MacFall, J. R., Kuchibhatla, M., Payne, M. E., Provenzale, J. M.,…Krishnan, K. R. (2005). Cortical white matter microstructural abnormalities in bipolar disorder. *Neuropsychopharmacology, 30*(12), 2225–2229. doi:10.1038/sj.npp.1300802

Biederman, J., Petty, C. R., Wozniak, J., Wilens, T. E., Fried, R., Doyle, A.,…Faraone, S. V. (2011). Impact of executive function deficits in youth with bipolar I disorder: A controlled study. *Psychiatry Research, 186*(1), 58–64. doi:10.1016/j.psychres.2010.08.029

Biswal, B. B., Van Kylen, J., & Hyde, J. S. (1997). Simultaneous assessment of flow and BOLD signals in resting-state functional connectivity maps. *NMR Biomedicine, 10*(4–5), 165–170.

Biswal, B., Yetkin, F. Z., Haughton, V. M., & Hyde, J. S. (1995). Functional connectivity in the motor cortex of resting human brain using echo-planar MRI. *Journal of Magnetic Resonance Imaging, 34*(4), 537–541.

Bitter, S. M., Mills, N. P., Adler, C. M., Strakowski, S. M., & DelBello, M. P. (2011). Progression of amygdala volumetric abnormalities in adolescents after their first manic episode. *Journal of the American Child & Adolescent Psychiatry, 50*(10), 1017–1026. doi:10.1016/j.jaac.2011.07.001

Blumberg, H. P., Kaufman, J., Martin, A., Whiteman, R., Zhang, J. H., Gore, J. C.,…Peterson, B. S. (2003). Amygdala and hippocampal volumes in adolescents and adults with bipolar disorder. *Archives of General Psychiatry, 60*(12), 1201–1208. doi:10.1001/archpsyc.60.12.1201

Blumberg, H. P., Leung, H. C., Skudlarski, P., Lacadie, C. M., Fredericks, C. A., Harris, B. C.,…Peterson, B. S. (2003). A functional magnetic resonance imaging study of bipolar disorder: State- and trait-related dysfunction in ventral prefrontal cortices. *Archives of General Psychiatry, 60*(6), 601–609. doi:10.1001/archpsyc.60.6.601

Brambilla, P., Harenski, K., Nicoletti, M., Mallinger, A. G., Frank, E., Kupfer, D. J.,…Soares, J. C. (2001). MRI study of posterior fossa structures and brain ventricles in bipolar patients. *Journal of Psychiatric Research, 35*(6), 313–322.

Brambilla, P., Harenski, K., Nicoletti, M., Sassi, R. B., Mallinger, A. G., Frank, E.,…Soares, J. C. (2003). MRI investigation of temporal lobe structures in bipolar patients. *Journal of Psychiatric Research, 37*(4), 287–295.

Bruno, S., Cercignani, M., & Ron, M. A. (2008). White matter abnormalities in bipolar disorder: A voxel-based diffusion tensor imaging study. *Bipolar Disorders, 10*(4), 460–468. doi:10.1111/j.1399-5618.2007.00552.x

Bullmore, E., & Sporns, O. (2009). Complex brain networks: graph theoretical analysis of structural and functional systems. *Nature Reviews Neuroscience, 10*(3), 186–198. doi:10.1038/nrn2575

Caetano, S. C., Sassi, R., Brambilla, P., Harenski, K., Nicoletti, M., Mallinger, A. G.,…Soares, J. C. (2001). MRI study of thalamic volumes in bipolar and unipolar patients and healthy individuals. *Psychiatry Research, 108*(3), 161–168.

Cardaso de Almeida, J. R., & Phillips M. L. (2013). Distinguishing between unipolar depression and bipolar depression: Current and future clinical and neuroimaging perspectives. *Biological Psychiatry, 73*(2), 111–118. doi:10.1016/j.biopsych.2012.06.010.

Chang, K., Karchemskiy, A., Barnea-Goraly, N., Garrett, A., Simeonova, D. I., & Reiss, A. (2005). Reduced amygdalar gray matter volume in familial pediatric bipolar disorder. *Journal of the American Child & Adolescent Psychiatry, 44*(6), 565–573. doi:10.1097/01.chi.0000159948.75136.0d

Chang, K. D., Wagner, C., Garrett, A., Howe, M., & Reiss, A. (2008). A preliminary functional magnetic resonance imaging study of prefrontal-amygdalar activation changes in adolescents with bipolar depression treated with lamotrigine. *Bipolar Disorders, 10*(3), 426–431. doi:10.1111/j.1399-5618.2007.00576.x

Chen, C. H., Ridler, K., Suckling, J., Williams, S., Fu, C. H., Merlo-Pich, E., & Bullmore, E. (2007). Brain imaging correlates of depressive symptom severity and predictors of symptom improvement after antidepressant treatment. *Biological Psychiatry, 62*(5), 407–414. doi:10.1016/j.biopsych.2006.09.018

Chen, B. K., Sassi, R., Axelson, D., Hatch, J. P., Sanches, M., Nicoletti, M.,…Soares, J. C. (2004). Cross-sectional study of abnormal amygdala development in adolescents and young adults with bipolar disorder. *Biological Psychiatry, 56*(6), 399–405. doi:10.1016/j.biopsych.2004.06.024

Chen, C. H., Suckling, J., Lennox, B. R., Ooi, C., & Bullmore, E. T. (2011). A quantitative meta-analysis of fMRI studies in bipolar disorder. *Bipolar Disorders, 13*(1), 1–15. doi:10.1111/j.1399-5618.2011.00893.x

Coffey, C. E., Wilkinson, W. E., Weiner, R. D., Parashos, I. A., Djang, W. T., Webb, M. C.,…Spritzer, C. E. (1993). Quantitative cerebral anatomy in depression: A controlled magnetic resonance imaging study. *Archives of General Psychiatry, 50*(1), 7–16.

DelBello, M. P., Strakowski, S. M., Zimmerman, M. E., Hawkins, J. M., & Sax, K. W. (1999). MRI analysis of the cerebellum in bipolar disorder: a pilot study. *Neuropsychopharmacology, 21*(1), 63–68. doi:10.1016/S0893-133X(99)00026-3

DelBello, M. P., Zimmerman, M. E., Mills, N. P., Getz, G. E., & Strakowski, S. M. (2004). Magnetic resonance imaging analysis of amygdala and other subcortical brain regions in adolescents with bipolar disorder. *Bipolar Disorders, 6*(1), 43–52.

Dickstein, D. P., Milham, M. P., Nugent, A. C., Drevets, W. C., Charney, D. S., Pine, D. S., & Leibenluft, E. (2005). Frontotemporal alterations in pediatric bipolar disorder: Results of a voxel-based morphometry study. *Archives of General Psychiatry, 62*(7), 734–741. doi:10.1001/archpsyc.62.7.734

Diler, R. S., Segreti, A. M., Ladouceur, C. D., Almeida, J. R., Birmaher, B., Axelson, D. A.,…Pan, L. (2013). Neural correlates of treatment in adolescents with bipolar depression during response inhibition. *Journal of Child and Adolescent Psychopharmacology, 23*(3), 214–221. doi:10.1089/cap.2012.0054

Dima, D., Jogia, J., Collier, D., Vassos, E., Burdick, K. E., & Frangou, S. (2013). Independent modulation of engagement and connectivity of the facial network during affect processing by CACNA1C and ANK3 risk genes for bipolar disorder. *JAMA Psychiatry, 70*(12), 1303–1311. doi:10.1001/jamapsychiatry.2013.2099

Drevets, W. C. (2000). Neuroimaging studies of mood disorders. *Biological Psychiatry, 48*(8), 813–829.

Drevets, W. C., Price, J. L., Simpson, J. R., Jr., Todd, R. D., Reich, T., Vannier, M., & Raichle, M. E. (1997). Subgenual prefrontal cortex abnormalities in mood disorders. *Nature, 386*(6627), 824–827. doi:10.1038/386824a0

Dupont, R. M., Butters, N., Schafer, K., Wilson, T., Hesselink, J., & Gillin, J. C. (1995). Diagnostic specificity of focal white matter abnormalities in bipolar and unipolar mood disorder. *Biological Psychiatry, 38*(7), 482–486.

Dupont, R. M., Jernigan, T. L., Heindel, W., Butters, N., Shafer, K., Wilson, T.,…Gillin, J. C. (1995). Magnetic resonance imaging and mood disorders. Localization of white matter and other subcortical abnormalities. *Archives of General Psychiatry, 52*(9), 747–755.

Eickhoff, S. B., & Grefkes, C. (2011). Approaches for the integrated analysis of structure, function and connectivity of the human brain. *Clinical EEG Neuroscience, 42*(2), 107–121.

Elvsashagen, T., Westlye, L. T., Boen, E., Hol, P. K., Andreassen, O. A., Boye, B., & Malt, U. F. (2013). Bipolar II disorder is associated with thinning of prefrontal and temporal cortices involved in affect regulation. *Bipolar Disorders, 15*(8), 855–864. doi:10.1111/bdi.12117

Filipek, P. A., Semrud-Clikeman, M., Steingard, R. J., Renshaw, P. F., Kennedy, D. N., & Biederman, J. (1997). Volumetric MRI analysis comparing subjects having attention-deficit hyperactivity disorder with normal controls. *Neurology, 48*(3), 589–601.

Fleck, D. E., Eliassen, J. C., Durling, M., Lamy, M., Adler, C. M., DelBello, M. P.,…Strakowski, S. M. (2012). Functional MRI of sustained attention in bipolar mania. *Molecular Psychiatry, 17*(3), 325–336. doi:10.1038/mp.2010.108

Fleck, D. E., Nandagopal, J., Cerullo, M. A., Eliassen, J. C., DelBello, M. P., & Adler, C. M., & Strakowski, S. M. (2008). Morphometric magnetic resonance imaging in psychiatry.

Topics in Magnetic Resonance Imaging, 19(2), 131–142. doi:10.1097/RMR.0b013e3181808152

Fleck, D. E., Shear, P. K., & Strakowski, S. M. (2009). Manic distractibility and processing efficiency in bipolar disorder. In S. J. Woods, N. B. Allen, & C. Pantelis (Eds.), *The neuropsychology of mental illness*. New York: Cambridge University Press.

Foland, L. C., Altshuler, L. L., Sugar, C. A., Lee, A. D., Leow, A. D., Townsend, J.,…Thompson, P. M. (2008). Increased volume of the amygdala and hippocampus in bipolar patients treated with lithium. *Neuroreport, 19*(2), 221–224.

Foland-Ross, L. C., Thompson, P. M., Sugar, C. A., Madsen, S. K., Shen, J. K., Penfold, C.,…Altshuler, L. L. (2011). Investigation of cortical thickness abnormalities in lithium-free adults with bipolar I disorder using cortical pattern matching. *American Journal of Psychiatry, 168*(5), 530–539. doi:10.1176/appi.ajp.2010.10060896

Foong, J., Symms, M. R., Barker, G. J., Maier, M., Miller, D. H., & Ron, M. A. (2002). Investigating regional white matter in schizophrenia using diffusion tensor imaging. *NeuroReport, 13*(3), 333–336.

Frangou, S., Donaldson, S., Hadjulis, M., Landau, S., & Goldstein, L. H. (2005). The Maudsley Bipolar Disorder Project: Executive dysfunction in bipolar disorder I and its clinical correlates. *Biological Psychiatry, 58*(11), 859–864. doi:10.1016/j.biopsych.2005.04.056

Frazier, J. A., Breeze, J. L., Papadimitriou, G., Kennedy, D. N., Hodge, S. M., Moore, C. M.,…Makris, N. (2007). White matter abnormalities in children with and at risk for bipolar disorder. *Bipolar Disorders, 9*(8), 799–809. doi:10.1111/j.1399-5618.2007.00482.x

Frazier, J. A., Chiu, S., Breeze, J. L., Makris, N., Lange, N., Kennedy, D. N.,…Biederman, J. (2005). Structural brain magnetic resonance imaging of limbic and thalamic volumes in pediatric bipolar disorder. *American Journal of Psychiatry, 162*(7), 1256–1265. doi:10.1176/appi.ajp.162.7.1256

Grotegerd, D., Suslow, T., Bauer, J., Ohrmann, P., Arolt, V., Stuhrmann, A.,…Dannlowski, U. (2013). Discriminating unipolar and bipolar depression by means of fMRI and pattern classification: a pilot study. *European Archives of Psychiatry and Clinical Neuroscience, 263*(2), 119–131. doi:10.1007/s00406-012-0329-4

Guye, M., Bettus, G., Bartolomei, F., & Cozzone, P. J. (2010). Graph theoretical analysis of structural and functional connectivity MRI in normal and pathological brain networks. *MAGMA, 23*(5–6), 409–421. doi:10.1007/s10334-010-0205-z

Hafeman, D. M., Chang, K. D., Garrett, A. S., Sanders, E. M., & Phillips, M. L. (2012). Effects of medication on neuroimaging findings in bipolar disorder: An updated review. *Bipolar Disorders, 14*(4), 375–410. doi:10.1111/j.1399-5618.2012.01023.x

Haldane, M., & Frangou, S. (2004). New insights help define the pathophysiology of bipolar affective disorder: neuroimaging and neuropathology findings. *Progress in Neuro-Psychopharmacology & Biological Psychiatry, 28*(6), 943–960. doi:10.1016/j.pnpbp.2004.05.040

Haldane, M., Jogia, J., Cobb, A., Kozuch, E., Kumari, V., & Frangou, S. (2008). Changes in brain activation during working memory and facial recognition tasks in patients with bipolar disorder with Lamotrigine monotherapy. *European Neuropsychopharmacology, 18*(1), 48–54. doi:10.1016/j.euroneuro.2007.05.009

Hallahan, B., Newell, J., Soares, J. C., Brambilla, P., Strakowski, S. M., Fleck, D. E.,…McDonald, C. (2011). Structural magnetic resonance imaging in bipolar disorder: An international collaborative mega-analysis of individual adult patient data. *Biological Psychiatry, 69*(4), 326–335. doi:10.1016/j.biopsych.2010.08.029

Harvey, I., Persaud, R., Ron, M. A., Baker, G., & Murray, R. M. (1994). Volumetric MRI measurements in bipolars compared with schizophrenics and healthy controls. *Psychological Medicine, 24*(3), 689–699.

Haznedar, M. M., Roversi, F., Pallanti, S., Baldini-Rossi, N., Schnur, D. B., Licalzi, E. M.,…Buchsbaum, M. S. (2005). Fronto-thalamo-striatal gray and white matter volumes and anisotropy of their connections in bipolar spectrum illnesses.

Biological Psychiatry, 57(7), 733–742. doi:10.1016/j.biopsych.2005.01.002

Heinrich, A., Lourdusamy, A., Tzschoppe, J., Vollstadt-Klein, S., Buhler, M., Steiner, S.,…Nees, F. (2013). The risk variant in ODZ4 for bipolar disorder impacts on amygdala activation during reward processing. *Bipolar Disorders, 15*(4), 440–445. doi:10.1111/bdi.12068

Hoge, E. A., Friedman, L., & Schulz, S. C. (1999). Meta-analysis of brain size in bipolar disorder. *Schizophrenia Research, 37*(2), 177–181.

Houenou, J., Wessa, M., Douaud, G., Leboyer, M., Chanraud, S., Perrin, M.,…Paillere-Martinot, M. L. (2007). Increased white matter connectivity in euthymic bipolar patients: diffusion tensor tractography between the subgenual cingulate and the amygdalo-hippocampal complex. *Molecular Psychiatry, 12*(11), 1001–1010. doi:10.1038/sj.mp.4002010

Husain, M. M., McDonald, W. M., Doraiswamy, P. M., Figiel, G. S., Na, C., Escalona, P. R.,…Krishnan, K. R. (1991). A magnetic resonance imaging study of putamen nuclei in major depression. *Psychiatry Research, 40*(2), 95–99.

Ives-Deliperi, V. L., Howells, F., Stein, D. J., Meintjes, E. M., & Horn, N. (2013). The effects of mindfulness-based cognitive therapy in patients with bipolar disorder: A controlled functional MRI investigation. *Journal of Affective Disorders, 150*(3), 1152–1157. doi:10.1016/j.jad.2013.05.074

Jogia, J., Haldane, M., Cobb, A., Kumari, V., & Frangou, S. (2008). Pilot investigation of the changes in cortical activation during facial affect recognition with lamotrigine monotherapy in bipolar disorder. *British Journal of Psychiatry, 192*(3), 197–201. doi:10.1192/bjp.bp.107.037960

Jogia, J., Ruberto, G., Lelli-Chiesa, G., Vassos, E., Maieru, M., Tatarelli, R.,…Frangou, S. (2011). The impact of the CACNA1C gene polymorphism on frontolimbic function in bipolar disorder. *Molecular Psychiatry, 16*(11), 1070–1071. doi:10.1038/mp.2011.49

Kalmar, J. H., Wang, F., Chepenik, L. G., Womer, F. Y., Jones, M. M., Pittman, B.,…Blumberg, H. P. (2009). Relation between amygdala structure and function in adolescents with bipolar disorder. *Journal of Academy of Child & Adolescent Psychiatry, 48*(6), 636–642. doi:10.1097/CHI.0b013e31819f6fbc

Krishnan, K. R., McDonald, W. M., Escalona, P. R., Doraiswamy, P. M., Na, C., Husain, M. M.,…Nemeroff, C. B. (1992). Magnetic resonance imaging of the caudate nuclei in depression: Preliminary observations. *Archives of General Psychiatry, 49*(7), 553–557.

Kumar, A., Bilker, W., Jin, Z., & Udupa, J. (2000). Atrophy and high intensity lesions: Complementary neurobiological mechanisms in late-life major depression. *Neuropsychopharmacology, 22*(3), 264–274. doi:10.1016/S0893-133X(99)00124-4

Kumari, V., & Cooke, M. (2006). Use of magnetic resonance imaging in tracking the course and treatment of schizophrenia. *Expert Review Neurotherapy, 6*(7), 1005–1016.

Kupferschmidt, D. A., & Zakzanis, K. K. (2011). Toward a functional neuroanatomical signature of bipolar disorder: Quantitative evidence from the neuroimaging literature. *Psychiatry Research, 193*(2), 71–79. doi:10.1016/j.pscychresns.2011.02.011

Kyriakopoulos, M., Bargiotas, T., Barker, G. J., & Frangou, S. (2008). Diffusion tensor imaging in schizophrenia. *European Psychiatry, 23*(4), 255–273. doi:10.1016/j.eurpsy.2007.12.004

Lyoo, I. K., Sung, Y. H., Dager, S. R., Friedman, S. D., Lee, J. Y., Kim, S. J.,…Renshaw, P. F. (2006). Regional cerebral cortical thinning in bipolar disorder. *Bipolar Disorders, 8*(1), 65–74. doi:10.1111/j.1399-5618.2006.00284.x

McDonald, C., Zanelli, J., Rabe-Hesketh, S., Ellison-Wright, I., Sham, P., Kalidindi, S.,…Kennedy, N. (2004). Meta-analysis of magnetic resonance imaging brain morphometry studies in bipolar disorder. *Biological Psychiatry, 56*(6), 411–417. doi:10.1016/j.biopsych.2004.06.021

McIntosh, A. M., Job, D. E., Moorhead, T. W., Harrison, L. K., Forrester, K., Lawrie, S. M., & Johnstone, E. C. (2004). Voxel-based morphometry of patients with schizophrenia or bipolar disorder and their unaffected relatives. *Biological Psychiatry, 56*(8), 544–552. doi:10.1016/j.biopsych.2004.07.020

Mills, N. P., Delbello, M. P., Adler, C. M., & Strakowski, S. M. (2005). MRI analysis of cerebellar vermal abnormalities in bipolar disorder. *American Journal of Psychiatry, 162*(8), 1530–1532. doi:10.1176/appi.ajp.162.8.1530

Moore, G. J., Bebchuk, J. M., Wilds, I. B., Chen, G., & Manji, H. K. (2000). Lithium-induced increase in human brain grey matter. *Lancet, 356*(9237), 1241–1242.

Norris, S. D., Krishnan, K. R., & Ahearn, E. (1997). Structural changes in the brain of patients with bipolar affective disorder by MRI: A review of the literature. *Progress in Neuro-Psychopharmacology & Biological Psychiatry, 21*(8), 1323–1337.

Ochsner, K. N., & Gross, J. J. (2005). The cognitive control of emotion. *Trends in Cognitive Science, 9*(5), 242–249. doi:10.1016/j.tics.2005.03.010

Passarotti, A. M., Sweeney, J. A., & Pavuluri, M. N. (2011). Fronto-limbic dysfunction in mania pre-treatment and persistent amygdala over-activity post-treatment in pediatric bipolar disorder. *Psychopharmacology (Berlin), 216*(4), 485–499. doi:10.1007/s00213-011-2243-2

Pavuluri, M. N., Ellis, J. A., Wegbreit, E., Passarotti, A. M., & Stevens, M. C. (2012). Pharmacotherapy impacts functional connectivity among affective circuits during response inhibition in pediatric mania. *Behavioural Brain Research, 226*(2), 493–503. doi:10.1016/j.bbr.2011.10.003

Pavuluri, M. N., Passarotti, A. M., Fitzgerald, J. M., Wegbreit, E., & Sweeney, J. A. (2012). Risperidone and divalproex differentially engage the fronto-striato-temporal circuitry in pediatric mania: A pharmacological functional magnetic resonance imaging study. *Journal of Academy of Child & Adolescent Psychiatry, 51*(2), 157–170. doi:10.1016/j.jaac.2011.10.019

Pavuluri, M. N., Passarotti, A. M., Harral, E. M., & Sweeney, J. A. (2010). Enhanced prefrontal function with pharmacotherapy on a response inhibition task in adolescent bipolar disorder. *Journal of Clinical Psychiatry, 71*(11), 1526–1534. doi:10.4088/JCP.09m05504yel

Pavuluri, M. N., Passarotti, A. M., Lu, L. H., Carbray, J. A., & Sweeney, J. A. (2011). Double-blind randomized trial of risperidone versus divalproex in pediatric bipolar disorder: fMRI outcomes. *Psychiatry Research, 193*(1), 28–37. doi:10.1016/j.pscychresns.2011.01.005

Pavuluri, M. N., Schenkel, L. S., Aryal, S., Harral, E. M., Hill, S. K., Herbener, E. S., & Sweeney, J. A. (2006). Neurocognitive function in unmedicated manic and medicated euthymic pediatric bipolar patients. *American Journal of Psychiatry, 163*(2), 286–293. doi:10.1176/appi.ajp.163.2.286

Pearlson, G. D., Barta, P. E., Powers, R. E., Menon, R. R., Richards, S. S., Aylward, E. H.,…Tien, A. Y. (1997). Ziskind-Somerfeld Research Award 1996: Medial and superior temporal gyral volumes and cerebral asymmetry in schizophrenia versus bipolar disorder. *Biological Psychiatry, 41*(1), 1–14.

Pessoa, L. (2008). On the relationship between emotion and cognition. *Nature Reviews Neuroscience, 9*(2), 148–158. doi:10.1038/nrn2317

Pfeifer, J. C., Welge, J., Strakowski, S. M., Adler, C. M., & DelBello, M. P. (2008). Meta-analysis of amygdala volumes in children and adolescents with bipolar disorder. *Journal of Academy of Child & Adolescent Psychiatry, 47*(11), 1289–1298. doi:10.1097/CHI.0b013e318185d299

Phillips, M. L., Drevets, W. C., Rauch, S. L., & Lane, R. (2003). Neurobiology of emotion perception: I. The neural basis of normal emotion perception. *Biological Psychiatry, 54*(5), 504–514.

Ramnani, N., Behrens, T. E., Penny, W., & Matthews, P. M. (2004). New approaches for exploring anatomical and functional connectivity in the human brain. *Biological Psychiatry, 56*(9), 613–619. doi:10.1016/j.biopsych.2004.02.004

Rangel-Guerra, R. A., Perez-Payan, H., Minkoff, L., & Todd, L. E. (1983). Nuclear magnetic resonance in bipolar affective disorders. *AJNR American Journal of Neuroradiology, 4*(3), 229–231.

Rich, B. A., Fromm, S. J., Berghorst, L. H., Dickstein, D. P., Brotman, M. A., Pine, D. S., & Leibenluft, E. (2008). Neural connectivity in children with bipolar disorder: Impairment in the face emotion processing circuit. *Journal of Child Psychology and Psychiatry, 49*(1), 88–96. doi:10.1111/j.1469-7610.2007.01819.x

Rimol, L. M., Hartberg, C. B., Nesvag, R., Fennema-Notestine, C., Hagler, D. J., Jr., Pung, C. J.,…Agartz, I. (2010). Cortical thickness and subcortical volumes in schizophrenia and bipolar disorder. *Biological Psychiatry, 68*(1), 41–50. doi:10.1016/j.biopsych.2010.03.036

Rimol, L. M., Nesvag, R., Hagler, D. J., Jr., Bergmann, O., Fennema-Notestine, C., Hartberg, C. B.,…Dale, A. M. (2012). Cortical volume, surface area, and thickness in schizophrenia and bipolar disorder. *Biological Psychiatry, 71*(6), 552–560. doi:10.1016/j.biopsych.2011.11.026

Rocha-Rego, V., Jogia, J., Marquand, A. F., Mourao-Miranda, J., Simmons, A., & Frangou, S. (2013). Examination of the predictive value of structural magnetic resonance scans in bipolar disorder: A pattern classification approach. *Psychological Medicine, 44*(3), 519–532. doi:10.1017/s0033291713001013

Rosso, I. M., Killgore, W. D., Cintron, C. M., Gruber, S. A., Tohen, M., & Yurgelun-Todd, D. A. (2007). Reduced amygdala volumes in first-episode bipolar disorder and correlation with cerebral white matter. *Biological Psychiatry, 61*(6), 743–749. doi:10.1016/j.biopsych.2006.07.035

Sax, K. W., Strakowski, S. M., Zimmerman, M. E., DelBello, M. P., Keck, P. E. Jr., & Hawkins, J. M. (1999). Frontosubcortical neuroanatomy and the continuous performance test in mania. *American Journal of Psychiatry, 156*(1), 139–141.

Scherk, H., & Falkai, P. (2004). Changes in brain structure caused by neuroleptic medication. *Nervenarzt, 75*(11), 1112–1117.

Scherk, H., & Falkai, P. (2006). Effects of antipsychotics on brain structure. *Current Opinion in Psychiatry, 19*(2), 145–150.

Schlaepfer, T. E., Harris, G. J., Tien, A. Y., Peng, L. W., Lee, S., Federman, E. B.,…Pearlson, G. D. (1994). Decreased regional cortical gray matter volume in schizophrenia. *American Journal of Psychiatry, 151*(6), 842–848.

Schnack, H. G., Nieuwenhuis, M., van Haren, N. E., Abramovic, L., Scheewe, T. W., Brouwer, R. M.,…Kahn, R. S. (2013). Can structural MRI aid in clinical classification? A machine learning study in two independent samples of patients with schizophrenia, bipolar disorder and healthy subjects. *Neuroimage, 84c*, 299–306. doi:10.1016/j.neuroimage.2013.08.053

Schneider, M. R., Adler, C. M., Whitsel, R., Weber, W., Mills, N. P., Bitter, S. M.,…Delbello, M. P. (2012). The effects of ziprasidone on prefrontal and amygdalar activation in manic youth with bipolar disorder. *The Israel Journal of Psychiatry and Related Sciences, 49*(2), 112–120.

Schumann, C. M., Hamstra, J., Goodlin-Jones, B. L., Lotspeich, L. J., Kwon, H., Buonocore, M. H.,…Amaral, D. G. (2004). The amygdala is enlarged in children but not adolescents with autism: The hippocampus is enlarged at all ages. *Journal of Neuroscience, 24*(28), 6392–6401. doi:10.1523/JNEUROSCI.1297-04.2004

Selek, S., Nicoletti, M., Zunta-Soares, G. B., Hatch, J. P., Nery, F. G., Matsuo, K.,…Soares, J. C. (2013). A longitudinal study of fronto-limbic brain structures in patients with bipolar I disorder during lithium treatment. *Journal of Affective Disorders, 150*(2), 629–633. doi:10.1016/j.jad.2013.04.020

Shenton, M. E., Dickey, C. C., Frumin, M., & McCarley, R. W. (2001). A review of MRI findings in schizophrenia. *Schizophrenic Research, 49*(1–2), 1–52.

Singh, M. K., & Chang, K. D. (2012). The neural effects of psychotropic medications in children and adolescents. *Adolescent Psychiatric Clinics of North America., 21*(4), 753–771. doi:10.1016/j.chc.2012.07.010

Singh, M. K., Delbello, M. P., Adler, C. M., Stanford, K. E., & Strakowski, S. M. (2008). Neuroanatomical characterization of child offspring of bipolar parents. *J Am Journal of American Academy of Child & Adolescent Psychiatry*, *47*(5), 526–531. doi:10.1097/CHI.0b013e318167655a

Strakowski, S. M., Adler, C. M., & DelBello, M. P. (2002). Volumetric MRI studies of mood disorders: Do they distinguish unipolar and bipolar disorder? *Bipolar Disorders*, *4*(2), 80–88.

Strakowski, S. M., DelBello, M. P., Adler, C., Cecil, D. M., & Sax, K. W. (2000). Neuroimaging in bipolar disorder. *Bipolar Disorders*, *2*(3 Pt. 1), 148–164.

Strakowski, S. M., DelBello, M. P., Sax, K. W., Zimmerman, M. E., Shear, P. K., Hawkins, J. M., & Larson, E. R. (1999). Brain magnetic resonance imaging of structural abnormalities in bipolar disorder. *Arch Gen Psychiatry*, *56*(3), 254–260.

Strakowski, S. M., DelBello, M. P., Zimmerman, M. E., Getz, G. E., Mills, N. P., Ret, J.,...Adler, C. M. (2002). Ventricular and periventricular structural volumes in first- versus multiple-episode bipolar disorder. *American Journal of Psychiatry*, *159*(11), 1841–1847.

Strakowski, S. M., Wilson, D. R., Tohen, M., Woods, B. T., Douglass, A. W., & Stoll, A. L. (1993). Structural brain abnormalities in first-episode mania. *Biological Psychiatry*, *33*(8–9), 602–609.

Swayze, V. W. II, Andreasen, N. C., Alliger, R. J., Yuh, W. T., & Ehrhardt, J. C. (1992). Subcortical and temporal structures in affective disorder and schizophrenia: A magnetic resonance imaging study. *Biological Psychiatry*, *31*(3), 221–240.

Taylor, V. A., Grant, J., Daneault, V., Scavone, G., Breton, E., Roffe-Vidal, S.,...Beauregard, M. (2011). Impact of mindfulness on the neural responses to emotional pictures in experienced and beginner meditators. *Neuroimage*, *57*(4), 1524–1533. doi:10.1016/j.neuroimage.2011.06.001

Tesli, M., Skatun, K. C., Ousdal, O. T., Brown, A. A., Thoresen, C., Agartz, I.,...Andreassen, O. A. (2013). CACNA1C risk variant and amygdala activity in bipolar disorder, schizophrenia and healthy controls. *PLoS One*, *8*(2), e56970. doi:10.1371/journal.pone.0056970

Townsend, J., & Altshuler, L. L. (2012). Emotion processing and regulation in bipolar disorder: A review. *Bipolar Disorders*, *14*(4), 326–339. doi:10.1111/j.1399-5618.2012.01021.x

van den Heuvel, M. P., Stam, C. J., Kahn, R. S., & Hulshoff Pol, H. E. (2009). Efficiency of functional brain networks and intellectual performance. *Journal of Neuroscience*, *29*(23), 7619–7624. doi:10.1523/JNEUROSCI.1443-09.2009

Versace, A., Almeida, J. R., Hassel, S., Walsh, N. D., Novelli, M., Klein, C. R.,...Phillips, M. L. (2008). Elevated left and reduced right orbitomedial prefrontal fractional anisotropy in adults with bipolar disorder revealed by tract-based spatial statistics. *Archives of General Psychiatry*, *65*(9), 1041–1052. doi:10.1001/archpsyc.65.9.1041

Videbech, P., & Ravnkilde, B. (2004). Hippocampal volume and depression: A meta-analysis of MRI studies. *American Journal of Psychiatry*, *161*(11), 1957–1966. doi:10.1176/appi.ajp.161.11.1957

Wang, F., Jackowski, M., Kalmar, J. H., Chepenik, L. G., Tie, K., Qiu, M.,...Blumberg, H. P. (2008). Abnormal anterior cingulum integrity in bipolar disorder determined through diffusion tensor imaging. *British Journal of Psychiatry*, *193*(2), 126–129. doi:10.1192/bjp.bp.107.048793

Wang, F., Kalmar, J. H., Edmiston, E., Chepenik, L. G., Bhagwagar, Z., Spencer, L.,...Blumberg, H. P. (2008). Abnormal corpus callosum integrity in bipolar disorder: A diffusion tensor imaging study. *Biological Psychiatry*, *64*(8), 730–733. doi:10.1016/j.biopsych.2008.06.001

Whalley, H. C., Papmeyer, M., Sprooten, E., Lawrie, S. M., Sussmann, J. E., & McIntosh, A. M. (2012). Review of functional magnetic resonance imaging studies comparing bipolar disorder and schizophrenia. *Bipolar Disorders*, *14*(4), 411–431. doi:10.1111/j.1399-5618.2012.01016.x

Yamasaki, H., LaBar, K. S., & McCarthy, G. (2002). Dissociable prefrontal brain systems for attention and emotion. *Proceedings of the American Academy of Sciences USA*, *99*(17), 11447–11451. doi:10.1073/pnas.182176499

Yang, H., Lu, L. H., Wu, M., Stevens, M., Wegbreit, E., Fitzgerald, J.,...Pavuluri, M. N. (2013). Time course of recovery showing initial prefrontal cortex changes at 16 weeks, extending to subcortical changes by 3 years in pediatric bipolar disorder. *Journal of Affective Disorders*, *150*(2), 571–577. doi:10.1016/j.jad.2013.02.007

Yurgelun-Todd, D. A., Silveri, M. M., Gruber, S. A., Rohan, M. L., & Pimentel, P. J. (2007). White matter abnormalities observed in bipolar disorder: A diffusion tensor imaging study. *Bipolar Disorders*, *9*(5), 504–512. doi:10.1111/j.1399-5618.2007.00395.x

18.

MAGNETIC RESONANCE SPECTROSCOPY FINDINGS AND THEIR TREATMENT IMPACT

Marsal Sanches, Frank K. Hu, and Jair C. Soares

INTRODUCTION

Bipolar disorder (BD) is a chronic and potentially severe psychiatric condition that affects up to 4% of the population (Merikangas & Lamers, 2012). In addition to its considerable impact on the psychological well-being and functional impact on patients, BD is associated with high rates of suicide and is currently listed as one of the leading causes of disability worldwide (Zimmerman, 2010).

Since the description of the therapeutic effects of lithium in the late 1940s, treatment of BD has undergone countless progress. In addition to mood stabilizers, the advent of atypical antipsychotics revolutionized the pharmacological management of this condition (Sanches, Newberg, & Soares, 2010). Yet available evidence demonstrates that lack of adequate treatment response is common among bipolar patients. Prospective studies have shown that residual depressive symptoms, frequent cycling, and chronic cognitive impairment seem to be the rule rather than the exception in BD (Miklowitz, 2011; Vieta, Reinares, & Rosa, 2011). Longitudinal results from the STEP-BD study indicate that, over a two-year period of follow-up, 48.5% of bipolar patients experienced recurrence of mood symptoms. Moreover, among patients who were symptomatic at the time of inclusion in the study, just 58.5% achieved recovery (Perlis et al., 2006).

Over the past two decades, neuroimaging studies have provided valuable advances in the understanding of the brain circuits involved in the pathophysiology of BD (Brambilla, Glahn, Balestrieri, & Soares, 2005; Brambilla, Hatch, & Soares, 2008; Soares & Mann, 1997). More recently, emphasis has been placed on the clinical implication of these findings, with the ultimate goal of advancing the diagnosis and management of this illness (Phillips, Travis, Fagiolini, & Kupfer, 2008; Soares, 2002).

This chapter comprises a critical analysis of the current evidence on the potential role of magnetic resonance spectroscopy (MRS), one of the currently available brain imaging approaches, in the treatment of BD. It begins with basic concepts of MRS techniques, followed by a review of the most consistent MRS findings in BD. Next, MRS results that seem to reflect the effects of medications on the brain are described, as well as findings associated with clinical response to certain treatments. Finally, some perspectives regarding the potential applications of MRS for the treatment of BD are discussed.

BASIC CONCEPTS OF MRS IMAGING

MRS is a neurochemical imaging technique that allows measurement of different molecules in the living brain, including metabolites and some medications (Figure 18.1). It is based on the same principle as magnetic resonance imaging (MRI) and utilizes a strong magnetic field and a radio frequency current, allowing detection of the magnetic signal of certain isotopes present in different neurochemicals. A chemical spectra, containing different peaks, is then obtained (Figure 18.2). The area under each peak reflects the concentration of the measured chemical in the brain (Sassi & Soares, 2003).

For example, proton spectroscopy (Table 18.1) enables the measurement of neurotransmitters such as gamma amino butyric acid (GABA), glutamate, and glutamine, as well as myo-inositol, choline, and N-acetylaspartate, an indicator of neuronal viability (Stanley, 2002). On the other hand, 31-phosphorus spectroscopy allows the measurement of neurochemicals involved in the neuronal membrane phospholipid turnover, including adenosine triphosphate,

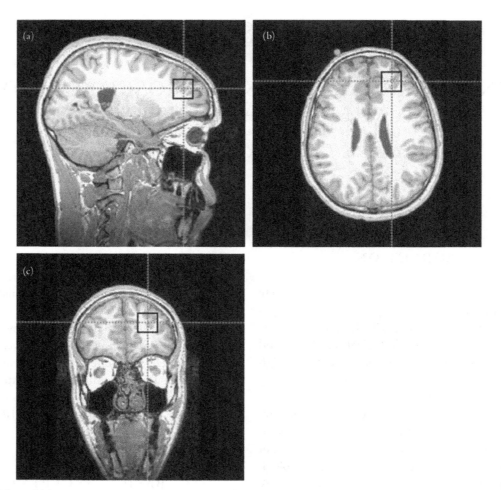

Figure 18.1 Sagittal (a), axial (b), and coronal (c) views of 1H spectroscopy images showing the location of the 8 cm3 voxel in the left dorsolateral prefrontal cortex (Reproduced from Nery et al., 2009, with permission)

phosphocreatine, and phosphodiesters. Different imaging protocols allow the measurement of these metabolites in distinct brain areas. Furthermore, spectroscopy can be valuable in the assessment of the pharmacokinetic properties of psychotropic drugs that contain isotopes such as 7Li and 19F, whose brain concentration can be detected through MRS (Soares, Boada, & Keshavan, 2000).

This technique soon became widely used for the assessment of brain neurochemicals across the lifespan in different psychiatric conditions, including BD. Since MRS utilizes no ionizing radiation, it allows the performance of repeated imaging assessments, which makes MRS well suited for the identification of neurochemical differences among bipolar patients across the different phases of the illness (Sassi & Soares, 2003). It also facilitates the search for treatment effects through the performance of imaging studies pre- and posttreatment, allowing the identification of possible correlations between the levels of certain neurochemicals and the clinical response to the treatment in question. Nevertheless, the appropriate implementation of a MRS acquisition protocol may be technically complex

and usually requires the participation of a magnetic resonance physicist (Drost, Riddle, Clarke, & AAPM MR Task Group #9, 2002). Among other issues, the strength of the magnetic field is a particularly critical feature, which impacts the spatial resolution and the signal-to-noise ratio (Dager, Corrigan, Richards, & Posse, 2008). Lower strengths also implicate in prolonged acquisition time, which can be troublesome when assessing certain groups of subjects, such as children, patients in acute mania, and claustrophobic subjects, who are supposed to remain motionless during the entire duration of the scan.

OVERVIEW OF MRS FINDINGS IN BIPOLAR DISORDER

PROTON MRS

Available evidence suggests that N-acetylaspartate (NAA) levels are decreased in the dorsolateral prefrontal cortex (DLPC), anterior cingulate gyrus, hippocampus, and

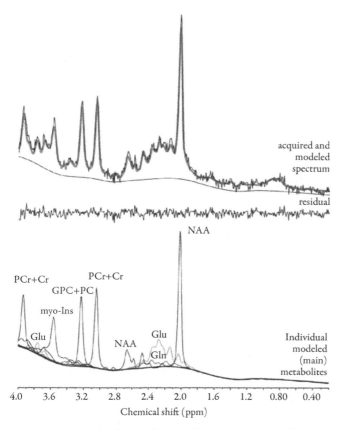

Figure 18.2 An example of quantifying a 1H spectrum acquired from the dorsolateral prefrontal cortex. The modeled spectrum (thick line) is superimposed on the acquired spectrum, and the residuals and the individual modeled curves of the main metabolites are shown below. NAA = N-acetyl-aspartate, Glu = glutamate, Gln = glutamine, PCr + Cr = phosphocreatine plus creatine, GPC + PC = choline-containing compounds, myo-Ins = myo-inositol. (Reproduced from Nery et al., 2009, with permission).

possibly the basal ganglia of patients with BD (Yildiz & Ankerst, 2006). NAA is synthesized in the mitochondria from the amino-acid aspartic acid. It is considered a marker of neuronal viability, reflecting neuronal metabolism and also mitochondrial function (Clark, 1998).

Although these findings regarding NAA levels in the bipolar brain seem to be mood state-independent, it is unclear, at this point, whether the changes in NAA levels among bipolar patients are mediated by genetic or environmental factors. Decreased NAA in the DLPC and cerebellar vermis seems to be a consistent finding among children with BD (Yildiz & Ankerst, 2006), suggesting that these changes occur early in the course of illness. On the other hand, a more recent study (Gallelli et al., 2005) addressed specifically the potential role of decreased NAA as an endophenotype for BD. In that study, 60 offspring (children and adolescents) of bipolar patients underwent MRS, aiming at the measurement of NAA levels in the DLPC. No statistically significant differences between offspring and controls were found in regard to NAA levels. The authors concluded that NAA levels in the DLPC might not be used as a marker of vulnerability for BD and that decreases in NAA among bipolar patients possibly take place later in the course of illness. However, we should note that how many of these children will develop BD is yet unknown; a longitudinal MRS investigation in thee subgroups with manifestation of BD would be much informative. In addition, despite some negative studies, it is well established that lithium use is associated with increases in the NAA levels in several brain regions (see "Medication Effects in MRS Studies" section).

Table 18.1. PATHOPHYSIOLOGICAL RELEVANCE OF MAIN BRAIN METABOLITES QUANTIFIED THROUGH PROTON MAGNETIC RESONANCE SPECTROSCOPY[a]

METABOLITE	RELEVANCE
N-acetylaspartate	Synthesized in the mitochondria from the amino-acid aspartic acid. Considered a marker of neuronal viability, reflecting neuronal metabolism and also mitochondrial function
Myo-inositol	Results from the dephosphorylation of inositol monophosphates by the enzyme inositol monophosphatase. Involved in maintenance of calcium homeostasis and activity of protein kinase C, with eventual effects on neuronal cytoskeletal restructuring
Glutamate	The main excitatory neurotransmitter in the central nervous system. Increased glutamatergic activity seems to produce neurotoxicity. Due to technical issues and overlapping between the glutamate, GABA, and glutamine peaks, glutamine is often adopted as a common description of these three combined metabolites.
Creatine/phosphocreatine	The creatine/phosphocreatine system works as a storage and transportation mechanism for high-energy phosphate bonds. Usually adopted as a standard for comparison, due to its relatively stability
Choline	Reflects density of cell membranes, as well as membrane and myelin turnover
Gamma aminobutyric acid	The most important inhibitory neurotransmitter in the brain. Results from glutamate decarboxylation by the enzyme glutamic acid decarboxylase

[a] Based on Stanley (2002); Sassi and Soares (2003); Maddock and Buonocore (in press).

On the other hand, in a more recent meta-analysis, 43 studies on MRS findings among BD patients were pooled (Kraguljac et al., 2012). Analyses of NAA, creatine, and choline in the frontal lobe (anterior cingulate cortex and DLPFC), hippocampus, and basal ganglia were performed. Results indicated that decreased NAA levels in the basal ganglia were the most consistent MRS finding among BD patients. Interestingly, the analysis showed increased NAA levels in the DLPC of bipolar patients compared to healthy controls. The authors suggest that their findings are consistent with evidence describing direct correlations between glutamate and NAA levels among healthy volunteers (Waddell et al., 2011) and point to the possibility that NAA, rather than just an indicator of neuronal viability, might also be involved in other pathophysiological processes still poorly understood. However, the authors of the meta-analysis in question were not able to carry out subgroup analysis taking into account possible medication effects, which could explain the discrepant findings mentioned earlier.

Moreover, myo-inositol levels seem to be abnormal in the frontal lobes, temporal lobes, cingulate gyrus, and basal ganglia of bipolar patients during the depressive and manic phases. While manic patients seem to have increased myo-inositol levels when compared to controls, results among patients with bipolar depression are less consistent, with reports of increased and decreased myo-inositol concentrations (Silverstone, McGrath, & Kim, 2005). Myo-inositol is a downstream product of the phosphatidylinositol cycle and results from the dephosphorylation of inositol monophosphates by the enzyme inositol monophosphatase. Dysfunctions in this cycle may affect calcium homeostasis and produce abnormal activity of protein kinase C, with eventual disruptions in neuronal cytoskeletal restructuring (Machado-Vieira, Manji, & Zarate, 2009). Lithium is an inhibitor of inositol monophosphatase (Yildiz, Demopulos, Moore, Renshaw, & Sachs, 2001), and its therapeutic effect in the treatment of BD led to the so-called inositol depletion hypothesis of BD. A critical appraisal of this hypothesis in light of available evidence is discussed in the next section.

Studies also suggest that glutamate levels are increased in several brain regions (including the parietal area, DLPFC, and basal ganglia) among BD patients independently of mood state or treatment status (Yildiz & Ankerst, 2006). Glutamate is the main excitatory neurotransmitter in the central nervous system, and increased glutamatergic activity seems to be the result in neurotoxicity. A recent meta-analysis (Gigante et al., 2012) reviewed 17 studies describing glutamate findings among BD patients and found increased levels of glutamate plus glutamine in bipolar patients compared to healthy subjects when all brain areas were combined and also when results on the frontal brain areas were analyzed separately. The authors argue that the contribution of glutamine to the glutamate plus glutamine signal is relatively small and that their findings are consistent with increased glutamine in the bipolar brain. However, when whole-brain glutamate was specifically analyzed, just a statistical trend toward higher levels of glutamate among patients was found.

The creatine/phosphocreatine ratio has also been assessed among patients with BD. The creatine/phosphocreatine system works as a storage and transportation mechanism for high-energy phosphate bonds (Maddock & Buonocore, 2012). It is usually adopted as a standard for comparison due to its relatively stability. Some studies have found significant differences in the levels of creatine in different brain areas among bipolar patients compared to controls, but the results are inconsistent in regard to the relationship between these findings and the different phases of illness, the brain areas where these findings seem to be more prominent (hippocampus, thalamus, frontal lobe), and their actual meaning under a pathophysiological point of view (Yildiz & Ankerst, 2006).

Finally, there is evidence suggesting increased brain choline levels among BD patients. Patients with bipolar depression seem to have higher choline levels in the basal ganglia and anterior cingulate cortex when compared to healthy controls. The choline levels are regarded as a measure of membrane phospholipids metabolism, since it seems to reflect not only the density of cell membranes but also cell membrane and myelin turnover (Maddock & Buonocore, 2012). Of note, lithium treatment seems to have a decreasing effect on choline (see "Medication Effects in MRS Studies" section).

PHOSPHORUS MRS

Through phosphorus magnetic resonance spectroscopy, it is possible to separate metabolites containing the 31-phosphorous nucleus into different peaks, which reflect phospholipid anabolism (phosphomonoesters, such as phosphocholine and phosphoethanolamine), catabolism (phosphodiesters, like glycerophosphocholine and glycerophosphoethanolamine), neuronal pH (inorganic phosphate), as well as phosphocreatine and adenosine triphosphate. Phospholipids are major constituents of cell membranes, and alterations in membrane phospholipid composition may be related to the cognitive impairment found in different conditions, including BD (Agarwal, Port, Bazzocchi, & Renshaw, 2010).

Moreover, state-dependent alterations in membrane phospholipids have been reported among bipolar patients (Yildiz, Sachs, Dorer, & Renshaw, 2001). Euthymic patients with BD seem to have lower phosphomonoester (PME) levels in the frontal lobe and possibly the temporal lobe when compared to healthy controls, as well as lower whole-brain pH. On the other hand, patients acutely depressed or manic have higher pH and PME levels compared to euthymic patients. No differences seem to be present between bipolar patients and controls in regard to phosphodiesters levels (for a review, see Yildiz, Sachs, et al., 2001). These findings suggest that trait- and state-dependent disruptions in membrane phospholipid metabolism seem to be involved in the pathophysiology of BD.

MEDICATION EFFECTS IN MRS STUDIES: THE BIOLOGICAL BASIS OF RECOVERY IN BIPOLAR DISORDER

The putative effect of treatment status on neuroimaging findings in psychiatric disorders, including BD, has traditionally been regarded as a potential confounding factor. Consequently, the inclusion of patients currently treated with psychotropics in neuroimaging studies is usually listed as a methodological limitation, often evoked as a possible explanation for negative findings in cross-sectional studies. Nevertheless, in recent years this position has been revisited, not only due to difficulties in studying unmedicated patients but also to the fact that including medicated subjects can provide valuable information about the mechanism of action of psychotropics, medications currently available for the treatment of mental disorders (Table 18.2). Furthermore, prospective designs allow the direct evaluation of medication effects on the brain through the performance of repeated imaging assessments, allowing the comparison of pre- versus posttreatment imaging findings. In this sense, the comparison of MRS findings in treated versus untreated patients seems to be particularly attractive, given the relatively safety of this technique and its high sensitivity in the detection of overtime changes.

LITHIUM

One of the most effective medications for the treatment of BD, lithium seems to have markedly neuroprotective effects. MRS findings among lithium-treated bipolar patients might be able to fill this gap, contributing to a better understanding of the mechanisms involved in the mood-stabilizing effect of this medication.

For instance, some studies found no differences between lithium-treated BD patients and healthy controls in terms of NAA levels in the anterior cingulate cortex, prefrontal cortex, and DLPC. Since evidence from studies with untreated patients overall point to decreased levels of NAA in BD, these findings may reflect a possible normalizing effect of lithium treatment on NAA (Yildiz & Ankerst, 2006). This hypothesis is supported by other cross-sectional studies that describe increased NAA levels in the temporal lobe and basal ganglia of lithium-treated bipolar subjects. Similarly, Hajek et al. (2012) showed significant lower DLPFC NAA levels among untreated BD patients compared to healthy controls, whose NAA levels were similar to those of lithium-treated bipolar patients. On the other hand, several different cross-sectional studies failed to demonstrate significant differences between lithium-treated bipolar patients and controls in regard to NAA levels in different brain regions, including the anterior cingulate cortex and the basal ganglia (DelBello & Strakowski, 2004).

Table 18.2. OVERVIEW OF EVIDENCE ON MEDICATION EFFECTS IN MAGNETIC RESONANCE SPECTROSCOPY STUDIES AMONG BIPOLAR PATIENTS

MEDICATIONS	POSSIBLE EFFECT ON METABOLITES (DIFFERENT REGIONS OF INTEREST)				
	↑ IN NAA	↓ IN MYO-INOSITOL	↓ IN GLUTAMATE	↑ IN GABA	↓ IN CHOLINE
Lithium	+++[a]	+[b]	+	−	+
VPA	−	+	+	+	−
Lamotrigine	−	−	+	−	−
Atypical antipsychotics	+	−	+	−	+

NOTE: NAA = N-acetylaspartate; GABA = gamma-aminobutyric acid; VPA = valproic acid.

[a] Positive results regarding mainly the dorsolateral prefrontal cortex, anterior cingulate, and prefrontal cortex; may represent a disease-specific effect (not found among controls medicated with lithium).

[b] Results are overall inconsistent; one study shows increases in myo-inositol levels among lithium-treated patients (Sharma et al., 1992).

Other studies analyzed the longitudinal effect of lithium treatment on MRS findings. Again, results seem to be inconsistent. At least two studies described positive results changes in NAA levels associated with lithium treatment. In one of these studies (Moore et al., 2000), 12 medication-free BD patients and 9 healthy controls underwent MRS at baseline and after four weeks of lithium administration. Results indicated statistically significant increases in NAA levels in all brain areas analyzed, including the frontal, temporal, and occipital lobes. In contrary, another study, which analyzed adolescents with bipolar depression, described decreases in ventral prefrontal NAA levels after six weeks of lithium treatment (Patel et al., 2008). Also utilizing a prospective design, our group (Brambilla et al., 2004) failed to demonstrate any increases in the DLPFC NAA levels among healthy controls after four weeks of lithium treatment. These results suggest that increases in NAA may be a specific effect of lithium on the brain of bipolar patients, not found among patients who are in depressive phase of the illness or do not suffer from that disorder.

Further, given the putative effect of lithium on the phosphatidylinositol cycle (see previous section), the possible impact of lithium treatment on myo-inositol levels is of high interest (Yildiz, Demopulos, et al., 2001). However, most studies have failed to demonstrate significant differences between lithium-treated bipolar patients and controls in regard to myo-inositol levels in different brain areas. Sharma, Venkatasubramanian, Bárány, and Davis (1992) found increased levels of myo-inositol in the basal ganglia among lithium-treated patients. In another study (Forester et al., 2008), utilizing a different design, nine geriatric patients with BD type I underwent proton MRS and lithium spectroscopy. Results indicated direct correlations between lithium levels and brain NAA and myo-inositol levels. Yet in a recent review of available evidence, it was proposed that, regardless of the promising evidence regarding the effect of lithium on inositol monophosphatase, it is unlikely that lithium might produce a persistent reduction in myo-inositol levels and phosphatidylinositol cycle turnover (Silverstone et al., 2005).

With respect to other metabolites, a recent study described significantly higher glutamine/glutamate ratio in the anterior cingulate cortex and parieto-occipital cortex among BD patients in acute mania compared to controls (Ongür et al., 2008). No differences were found between unmedicated patients and those receiving lithium, anticonvulsants, or benzodiazepines. These findings suggest that while increased glutamatergic activity seems to be involved in the pathophysiology of acute manic states, currently available mood stabilizers, including lithium, apparently do not play a significant role in the modulation of the glutamatergic system. Alternatively, technical limitations on obtaining individual peaks for glutamate, glutamine, and GABA, enabling their individual concentration estimates in the commonly used lower field magnets might have masked disease- or treatment-induced alterations in glutamate. In contrast, another study demonstrated decreases in the glutamine and glutamate plus glutamine levels in the basal ganglia of bipolar patients following two weeks of lithium administration (Shibuya-Tayoshi et al., 2008). GABA levels, on the contrary, did not show any significant changes associated with lithium administration.

Another study (Colla et al., 2009) attempted to address the possible role of lithium in modulating and counterbalancing the effects of hypothalamic–pituitary–adrenal axis hyperactivity on the hippocampus among bipolar patients. In that study, 21 euthymic patients with BD type I on chronic lithium maintenance treatment underwent proton MRS of the left and right hippocampus, as well as measurement of salivary cortisol. While absolute concentrations of NAA, choline, and creatine were similar among patients and controls, hippocampal glutamate concentrations were higher among patients. Further, patients and controls displayed inverse correlations between salivary cortisol levels and not only hippocampal NAA values but also glutamate levels. These results suggest that the neurotropic effects of lithium, which may counterbalance the toxic effects of increased hypothalamic–pituitary–adrenal activity on the hippocampus, seem to take place through mechanisms distinct from decreasing the glutamatergic activity.

Overall, results pointing to the effects of lithium treatment on MRS findings are only partially consistent. Several methodological limitations may account for these heterogeneous results, including variable duration of lithium treatment, different lithium doses, and distinct history of previous lithium exposure. One of the studies mentioned previously (Hajek et al., 2012) suggested that duration of illness and illness burden might affect the brain response to lithium, and these factors should be controlled when assessing the neurochemical changes associated with lithium treatment.

VALPROIC ACID

Valproic acid (VPA) is widely used for the treatment of BD, particularly manic states. It has strong GABAergic effects, which seem to account, at least in part, for its mood stabilizer properties. To date, very few studies have focused specifically on MRS findings associated with use of VPA.

In several studies, bipolar patients on VPA were included in the same pool as patients receiving lithium or other anticonvulsants, making the identification of VPA-specific effects rather difficult. For example, in one study euthymic bipolar patients on divalproex and gabapentin were found to have increased occipital and medial prefrontal GABA levels when compared to healthy controls (Wang et al., 2002).

It has been suggested that VPA may share the same putative normalizing effect on some brain metabolites as lithium. For instance, in Silverstone et al.'s (2002) study, patients on VPA were found to have myo-inositol and PME levels similar to lithium treated patients and healthy controls. In another study (O'Donnell et al., 2003), rats showed statistically significant increases in the concentration of inositol monophosphates and decreases in the levels of myo-inositol following lithium treatment. Administration of VPA produced similar results. The authors concluded that lithium and VPA might share similar effects on the phosphatidylinositol cycle, which is probably related to their mood stabilizer effect.

In contrast, other studies point to differences between lithium and VPA-treated patients in regard to MRS findings. Silverstone et al. (2003) described elevated concentrations of NAA among euthymic BD patients treated with lithium but not with VPA. These results are partially in agreement with another study (Cecil, DelBello, Morey, & Strakowski, 2002), which described negative correlations between NAA concentration in the orbitofrontal cortex and duration of VPA treatment among bipolar patients in mania. In another study (Friedman et al., 2004), patients on lithium were found to have decreased glutamate-glutamine and increased myo-inositol compared to controls, whereas subjects on VPA failed to display any significant differences.

Similarly, another group compared patients on lithium and VPA in regard to their choline levels measured through MRS (Wu et al., 2004). When euthymic BD patients on either lithium or VPA were pooled together and compared to healthy controls, significantly lower temporal lobe choline/creatine ratios were found among patients. On the other hand, when only VPA-treated patients were compared to healthy controls, no differences on choline levels were identified.

Finally, one study utilized proton MRS for the postmortem assessment of the DLPFC among patients with a history of BD (Lan et al., 2009). Findings were then compared to MRS findings in the brain of rats following administration of mood stabilizers (lithium or VPA). The brains of BD subjects displayed higher levels of glutamate, myo-inositol, and creatine when compared to controls,

and no differences were found between medicated versus unmedicated subjects. Interestingly, the previously mentioned findings mirrored the results obtained in rodents medicated with mood stabilizers, which displayed decreases in the levels of myo-inositol and creatine (with lithium and VPA ministration), increases in glutamine levels with consequent decreases in the glutamate/glutamine ratio (with VPA only), and increases in GABA (with lithium only). Furthermore, in rodent studies, no changes in the NAA levels were found in association with the administration of mood stabilizers. The authors suggested that the lack of differences between medicated and unmedicated subjects is most likely secondary to methodological issues, since it is not possible to ascertain the patients' compliance with their medications. The fact that some of the medicated patients had committed suicide may indicate that they had been noncompliant with the mood stabilizers or, alternatively, that the medications had not been clinically effective. The mirroring effect between the postmortem findings and the results among medicated rats supports the hypothesis of a normalizing effect of mood stabilizers on the levels of the metabolites in question. Finally, the lack of increases in NAA levels in response to the administration of mood stabilizers in rats is mentioned as an argument in favor of the hypothesis that increases in NAA in response to mood stabilizers may be a disease-specific finding, present only among bipolar patients.

In summary, these findings are heterogeneous and suggest that, while lithium and VPA might share some common mechanisms in regard to their mood stabilizer properties, they might have distinct profiles regarding their neuroprotective effects.

LAMOTRIGINE

An anticonvulsant, lamotrigine is Food and Drug Administration approved for the maintenance treatment of bipolar I disorder, although there is evidence suggesting it might also be effective for the treatment of acute bipolar depression. Its mechanism of action is complex and involves blockage of voltage-sensitive sodium channels, as well as some possible neuroprotective effects through glutamatergic modulation (Sanches & Soares, 2011). However, scant evidence is currently available regarding brain metabolites and lamotrigine. In rats, the administration of anticonvulsants (including lamotrigine) did not seem to be associated with increases in myo-inositol levels, contrary to the administration of lithium (McGrath, Greenshaw, McKay, Slupsky, & Silverstone, 2007).

On the other hand, in the only longitudinal study to assess the possible impact of lamotrigine use on MRS findings (Frye et al., 2007), 23 unmedicated depressed BD patients were compared to 12 controls in regard to MRS findings. After 12 weeks of treatment with lamotrigine, patients underwent a new MRS study. At baseline, patients displayed lower levels of glutamate, glutamate plus glutamine, and creatine plus phosphocreatine when compared to controls. Results after 12 weeks of treatment showed a strong interaction with treatment response, with significantly lower levels of glutamine among responders compared to nonresponders.

ATYPICAL ANTIPSYCHOTICS

Atypical antipsychotics are becoming increasingly popular for the treatment of BD, although marked differences seem to be present in regard to their efficacy across the different phases of the illness (Sanches & Soares, 2011). Over the past few years, several MRS studies have addressed possible brain neurochemical changes associated with their use. In some of these studies, atypical antipsychotics were combined with mood stabilizers.

For example, Atmaca, Yildirim, Ozdemir, Ogur, and Tezcan (2007) hippocampal MRS findings were compared across four different groups: medication-free BD patient, VPA-treated BD patients, VPA plus quetiapine treated–BD patients, and healthy controls. Untreated patients showed statistically significant lower NAA/creatine and NAA/choline ratios compared to both groups of treated patients, as well as to healthy controls. On the other hand, patients on VPA plus quetiapine showed higher NAA/choline ratios compared to bipolar patients treated only with VPA. These findings suggest that augmentation of VPA with quetiapine may produce additional neuroprotection compared to VPA monotherapy.

In another cross-sectional study (Shahana et al., 2011), MRS findings on the caudate among unmedicated bipolar patients, medicated patients (most of whom receiving atypical antipsychotics), and healthy controls were compared. Bipolar patients receiving atypical antipsychotics displayed statistically significantly higher creatine/choline ratios when compared to controls and unmedicated bipolar patients, as well as significantly lower choline/NAA ratios when compared to unmedicated BD patients. These findings suggest that atypical antipsychotics may cause decreases in the choline levels in the caudate of bipolar patients, a finding that may reflect a curing effect on the putative oxidative injury (as well as some possible neuroprotective effect) associated with atypical antipsychotic

treatment. However, some patients included in the analysis were receiving mood stabilizers, limiting the generalization of the findings.

Moore et al. (2007) compared MRS findings among unmedicated children with BD and bipolar children medicated with risperidone. Unmedicated patients showed lower glutamate plus glutamine/creatine ratios in the anterior cingulate cortex compared to risperidone-medicated children. Of note, all unmedicated patients were manic at the time of the scan, while medicated patients were euthymic. The authors argue that these findings suggest decreased metabolism in the anterior cingulate cortex of bipolar children in mania, which could be reversed by the treatment with risperidone. However, confounding by combined concentration estimates of three different metabolites of glutamate, glutamine, and GABA is a concern.

Finally, one longitudinal study analyzed the impact of treatment with olanzapine on MRS findings among first episode manic adolescents (DelBello, Cecil, Adler, Daniels, & Strakowski, 2006). Overall, olanzapine seemed to produce significant increases in ventral prefrontal choline levels, but not in NAA. However, remitters and nonremitters seemed to display distinct patterns of changes in NAA concentrations. These and other results involving prediction of response will be discussed at the next section of the present chapter.

CAN MAGNETIC RESONANCE SPECTROSCOPY FINDINGS PREDICT RESPONSE TO TREATMENT IN BIPOLAR PATIENTS?

The identification of specific features able to predict the clinical response to certain therapeutic interventions for BD is possibly one of the most fascinating potential practical applications of neuroimaging techniques. However, despite some promising results, evidence in that regard is still preliminary.

PROTON MRS FINDINGS

Some studies have attempted to identify predictors of future response to lithium through the performance of repeated MRS scans over the course of the treatment. In one (Moore et al., 1999), depressed bipolar patients underwent MRS at baseline (when off medications for at least two weeks), after five to seven days on lithium and after three to four weeks of lithium treatment. Results indicated rapid decreases in the myo-inositol levels in the right frontal lobe at the time of the second MRS assessment, which persisted until the time of the third imaging study. The authors concluded that although lithium seems to induce decreases in the myo-inositol levels, these changes do not seem to be correlated with clinical improvement in the depressive symptoms, since they seem to occur early in the course of the treatment with lithium, before the onset of its therapeutic effect. Alternatively, decreases in myo-inositol may represent the first step of a sequence of lithium-induced neurochemical changes, which are eventually responsible for its therapeutic effect.

These results are in contrast those from Davanzo et al. (2001), in which 11 children with BD underwent MRS scans at baseline and after seven days of lithium treatment. Differently from nonresponders, lithium responders displayed a statistically significant decrease in the myo-inositol/creatine ratio in the anterior cingulate cortex from baseline to follow-up.

Adopting a similar design, DelBello et al. (2006) utilized repeated proton MRS studies to search for brain neurochemical changes associated with olanzapine monotherapy treatment among bipolar adolescents with a first manic or mixed episode. Patients who achieved remission after four weeks of treatment displayed different patterns of change in their NAA levels in the medial ventral prefrontal cortex compared to nonremitters. While among remitters the NAA levels increased from baseline to endpoint, the opposite happened among nonremitters. Further, NAA levels among remitters showed a direct correlation with decreases in the Young Mania Rating Scale scores. Finally, although choline levels increased in response to treatment among remitters and nonremitters, baseline (pretreatment) levels of choline at the medial ventral prefrontal cortex were higher among remitters than nonremitters. These findings suggest that response to olanzapine may be associated with possible neurotropic effects of this medication or with normalization of abnormal mitochondrial metabolism, reflected by the increases in NAA levels. The authors also suggested that the increase in choline levels induced by olanzapine may contribute to its therapeutic effect through putative inhibition of hyperactive second-messenger systems by choline and downstream inhibition of cell membrane breakdown. This hypothesis would explain why patients with higher baseline concentrations of choline would be more likely to respond to the treatment with olanzapine.

Similarly, 25 adolescent bipolar patients in manic/mixed states on treatment with divalproex underwent serial MRS scans to assess the possible impact of that medication on the glutamatergic system (Strawn et al., 2012). No differences were found in the glutamate and glutamate plus glutamine levels at the different brain regions analyzed (anterior cingulate cortex and left and right ventrolateral prefrontal cortex) when patients and controls were compared at baseline. Among patients, those who achieved remission after four weeks of treatment displayed lower glutamate plus glutamine concentrations at the left ventrolateral prefrontal cortex compared to nonremitters. Moreover, decreases in glutamate concentrations at the left ventrolateral prefrontal cortex showed direct correlations with changes in the Young Mania Rating Scale scores among remitters. The authors concluded that response to treatment with divalproex is most likely related to modulation of the glutamatergic system induced by that mood stabilizer.

Finally, Change et al. (2012) performed serial MRS scans to analyze the impact of monotherapy treatment with quetiapine on the neurochemical aspects of bipolar adolescents in the depressive phase. Patients were randomized to receive either quetiapine or placebo, and scans were performed at baseline and after eight weeks of treatment. No differences were observed between the medication and the placebo groups in regard to changes in the NAA levels at the DLPF and anterior cingulate cortex. As previously, no baseline differences were found when responders were compared with nonresponders regarding the levels of any metabolites. However, responders showed statistically significantly lower concentrations of myo-inositol in the anterior cingulate cortex when compared to nonresponders. These findings point to the possibility that, similarly to lithium, quetiapine might also display effects on the phosphatidylinositol cycle, which may be correlated with its clinical efficacy.

PHOSPHORUS MRS

In one of the few studies that utilized phosphorus MRS (P MRS) in an attempt to identify predictors of response to lithium, 32 patients with BD type I underwent serial P MRS scans (Kato, Inubushi, & Kato, 2000). Responders were found to have lower brain intracellular pH when compared to nonresponders. The authors hypothesized that the decreased pH might reflect differences in the pathophysiology of BD between responders and nonresponders, although the actual meaning of these findings remains unclear.

Murashita, Kato, Shioiri, Inubushi, and Kato (2000) also compared lithium-responsive, lithium-resistant, and healthy controls utilizing serial 31 P MRS scans. The subjects underwent photic stimulation, and scans were performed at baseline and at two different endpoints during the photic stimulation treatment. Lithium-resistant patients, differently from controls and lithium responders, showed lower levels of phosphocreatine levels at the two follow-up scans than at the pretreatment scan. The authors concluded that mitochondrial dysfunction might be involved in lithium resistance in BD.

LITHIUM MRS FINDINGS

Lithium MRS (^{7}Li MRS) enables measurement of lithium levels in the living human brain, allowing not only the acquisition of pharmacokinetic data and regional differences in lithium levels at the brain but also the search for possible correlations for the brain lithium levels and response to lithium treatment in BD (Lyoo & Renshaw, 2003; Sanches, Brambilla, & Soares, 2006; Soares et al., 2000). Nevertheless, while several studies over the past two decades have addressed lithium pharmacokinetics, little research has analyzed brain lithium concentrations as a predictor of response.

Overall, studies point to a positive correlation between brain and serum lithium levels among bipolar patients. However, the strength of this correlation seems to decrease when a narrower range of serum lithium levels is considered (Sachs et al., 1995). These results suggest that, within the usual therapeutic range adopted in clinical practice in regard to serum lithium levels, the correlation with brain lithium levels might not be as strong as usually assumed (for a review see DelBello & Strakowski, 2004).

Some studies have attempted to identify a minimal brain concentration of lithium necessary for clinical response to lithium. In Kushnir et al. (1993), no statistically significant differences between lithium responders and nonresponders were identified among patients whose serum concentration ranged from 0.28 to 0.86 mEq/L. In Kato et al. (1994), poor response was significantly correlated with brain levels of lithium below 0.2 mEq/L. In the same study, brain lithium concentration was strongly correlated with improvement in manic symptoms. While improvement was also correlated with the brain/serum lithium ratio, it was not correlated with serum concentration per se. Finally, in regard to side effects, patients who experience lithium-related hand tremor seem to have significantly higher brain concentrations of lithium than those who do not display that side effect (Kato, Fujii, Shioiri, Inubushi, & Takahashi, 1996).

Moreover, in a more recent study (Forester et al., 2009), younger and older bipolar patients were found to have distinct patterns of association between brain lithium levels and clinical features. Among older (>50 years) BD patients, lithium levels showed a direct association with frontal cognitive impairment and higher scores on the Hamilton Depression Rating Scale. The authors argue that, among older patients, lower brain levels of lithium might be more appropriate, since younger patients had similar brain concentrations but did not display the associations in question.

Thus in regard to ^{7}Li MRS studies trying to predict treatment response, results have mostly been inconclusive, largely due to poor anatomical resolution of the technique (voxels are generally very large), as well as pronounced variability in brain lithium concentration across different anatomical regions. It is unclear whether this might be a way forward in trying to understand lithium's mechanisms of action or predicting and monitoring treatment response.

PERSPECTIVES ON MRS AND ITS IMPACT ON THE TREATMENT OF BIPOLAR DISORDER

Despite the growing number of MRS studies in BD and some promising results regarding its potential role in improving the treatment of this condition, currently available evidence is still in a preliminary phase. Relatively few studies have addressed predictors of response to treatment, and overall MRS results on medication effects are not very consistent.

Several methodological factors may account for these heterogeneous results. Some of them are methodological in nature, including

1. Variability regarding the choice of the areas of interest. Current evidence suggests that the areas that most consistently display positive findings in MRS studies of BD are the DLPFC, the anterior cingulate cortex, the prefrontal cortex, the hippocampus, and the basal ganglia. Due to technical issues regarding the acquisition of MRS data and the long period of time to complete an MRS sequence when using scans with lower field strength, most of the currently available studies seem to prioritize just some of these areas. The growing availability of scans with higher field strength should allow the performance of more comprehensive spectroscopy studies, allowing the comparison of results across different groups regarding the possible impact of treatment on different brain regions. Similarly, technical improvements should allow the

acquisition of ^{31}P MRS and ^3Li MRS data with better spatial resolution and greater reliability.

2. The longitudinal and changeable nature of BD. While some of the currently available results come from samples comprised of euthymic patients, others were obtained from patients in acute mania or during depressive episodes. Given the cyclical course of BD, it is expected that distinct MRS patterns are associated with response to treatment across the different phases of the disease. Cross-sectional studies aiming at treatment effects, although easy to implement, provide very limited information in a condition like BD due to the potential presence of confounders and large variability in terms of duration of illness, severity of mood symptoms, degree of functional impact, and previous treatment history. Longitudinal studies examining the same patients across different phases of the disease should progressively become the rule rather than the exception when addressing treatment effects in MRS.

3. The excessive focus on BD as a categorical construct. Virtually all studies to address treatment effects in MRS among bipolar patients adopt categorical conceptualizations not only for the diagnosis of the illness but also for characterization of mood states. It is well established, however, that subsyndromical mood symptoms may implicate in important psychopathological and functional burden, yet patients are often characterized as remitted when experiencing such symptoms. Moreover, growing evidence suggests that a dimensional approach for BD may be more appropriate than the currently adopted categorical view. Future MRS studies on treatment effect and predictors of response should include a dimensional measure in the characterization of the sample, as well as take into consideration the possible presence of subsyndromic symptoms when full criteria for an acute mood episode are not met.

In addition, other difficulties in the identification of treatment effects in MRS studies result from the relatively lack of knowledge, in light of available evidence, in regard to which neurochemical changes should be targeted as possible indicators of medication effect or response to treatment. The current approach is usually based on assumptions regarding the mechanism of action of these medications. Often these assumptions result from preclinical information on the agents in question. However, some of the currently available results suggest that many of the medication-related changes detected through MRS seem to be disease-specific and not necessarily associated with clinical improvement in a timely manner. It is possible that the current MRS, although sound, are not sensitive enough to detect more subtle neurochemical changes in different metabolites that could take place downstream and might be more directly associated with clinical response. The constant improvement in the technical aspects of MRS should be able to address these issues in the near future.

CONCLUSION

After two decades of research utilizing these techniques in the field of psychiatry, MRS has served as a valuable research tool, but it has yet to yield much that can be translated clinically. This is not unique to MRS as a technique and corroborates the complexity of the diseases we study, illustrating ongoing challenges in the understanding of the inner workings of the living brain and the neurobiological basis of major mental illnesses. Nonetheless, primarily as resolution improves and the field of psychiatry continues to make progress in further refining our diagnoses and target phenotypes, MRS continues to be a promising imaging approach for the study of in vivo brain mechanisms and the identification of treatment effects and predictors of clinical response in BD. Future research should focus on longitudinal studies, which should include serial MRS scans over the course of the treatment, enabling the better characterization of neurochemical findings among responders and nonresponders, as well as the identification of pretreatment neurochemical profiles that can anticipate the response to specific pharmacological approaches.

ACKNOWLEDGEMENTS

This work was partly funded by the Pat Rutherford Jr. Chair in Psychiatry (UTHealth) and National Institutes of Health grant 1R01MH085667

REFERENCES

Agarwal N., Port, J. D., Bazzocchi, M., & Renshaw, P. F. (2010). Update on the use of MR for assessment and diagnosis of psychiatric diseases. *Radiology*, 255(1), 23–41.

Atmaca, M., Yildirim, H., Ozdemir, H., Ogur, E., & Tezcan, E. (2007). Hippocampal 1H MRS in patients with bipolar disorder taking valproate versus valproate plus quetiapine. *Psychological Medicine*, 37(1), 121–129.

Brambilla, P., Hatch, J. P., & Soares, J. C. (2008). Limbic changes identified by imaging in bipolar patients. *Current Psychiatry Reports*, 10(6), 505–509.

Brambilla, P., Glahn, D. C., Balestrieri, M., & Soares, J. C. (2005). Magnetic resonance findings in bipolar disorder. *Psychiatric Clinics of North America*, 28(2), 443–467.

Brambilla, P., Stanley, J. A., Sassi, R. B., Nicoletti, M. A., Mallinger, A. G., Keshavan M. S., & Soares, J. C. (2004). 1H MRS study of dorsolateral prefrontal cortex in healthy individuals before and after lithium administration. *Neuropsychopharmacology*, 29(10), 1918–1924.

Cecil, K. M., DelBello, M. P., Morey, R., & Strakowski, S. M. (2002). Frontal lobe differences in bipolar disorder as determined by proton MR spectroscopy. *Bipolar Disorders*, 4(6), 357–365.

Chang, K., Delbello, M., Chu, W. J., Garrett, A., Kelley, R., Mills, N., ... Strakowski, S. M. (2012). Neurometabolite effects of response to quetiapine and placebo in adolescents with bipolar depression. *Journal of Child and Adolescent Psychopharmacology*, 22(4), 261–268.

Clark, J. B. (1998). N-acetyl aspartate: A marker for neuronal loss or mitochondrial dysfunction. *Developmental Neuroscience*, 20(4–5), 271–276.

Colla, M., Schubert, F., Bubner, M., Heidenreich, J. O., Bajbouj, M., Seifert, F., ... Kronenberg G. (2009). Glutamate as a spectroscopic marker of hippocampal structural plasticity is elevated in long-term euthymic bipolar patients on chronic lithium therapy and correlates inversely with diurnal cortisol. *Molecular Psychiatry*, 14(7), 696–704, 647.

Dager, S. R., Corrigan, N. M., Richards, T. L., & Posse, S. (2008). Research applications of magnetic resonance spectroscopy to investigate psychiatric disorders. *Topics in Magnetic Resonance Imaging*, 19(2), 81–96.

Davanzo, P., Thomas, M. A., Yue, K., Oshiro, T., Belin, T., Strober, M., McCracken, J. (2001). Decreased anterior cingulate myo-inositol/creatine spectroscopy resonance with lithium treatment in children with bipolar disorder. *Neuropsychopharmacology*, 24(4), 359–369.

DelBello M. P., Cecil, K. M., Adler, C. M., Daniels, J. P., & Strakowski, S. M. (2006). Neurochemical effects of olanzapine in first-hospitalization manic adolescents: A proton magnetic resonance spectroscopy study. *Neuropsychopharmacology*, 31(6), 1264–1273.

Delbello, M. P., & Strakowski, S. M. (2004). Neurochemical predictors of response to pharmacologic treatments for bipolar disorder. *Current Psychiatry Reports*, 6(6), 466–472.

Drost, D. J., Riddle, W. R., Clarke, G. D., & AAPM MR Task Group #9. (2002). Proton magnetic resonance spectroscopy in the brain: Report of AAPM MR Task Group #9. *Medical Physics*, 29(9), 2177–2197.

Forester, B. P., Finn, C. T., Berlow, Y. A., Wardrop, M., Renshaw, P. F., & Moore, C. M. (2008). Brain lithium, N-acetyl aspartate and myo-inositol levels in older adults with bipolar disorder treated with lithium: A lithium-7 and proton magnetic resonance spectroscopy study. *Bipolar Disorders*, 10(6), 691–700.

Forester, B. P., Streeter, C. C., Berlow, Y. A., Tian, H., Wardrop, M., Finn, C T., .. Moore, C. M. (2009). Brain lithium levels and effects on cognition and mood in geriatric bipolar disorder: A lithium-7 magnetic resonance spectroscopy study. *American Journal of Geriatric Psychiatry*, 17(1), 13–23.

Friedman, S. D., Dager, S. R., Parow, A., Hirashima, F., Demopulos, C., ... Renshaw P. F. (2004). Lithium and valproic acid treatment effects on brain chemistry in bipolar disorder. *Biological Psychiatry*, 56(5), 340–348.

Frye, M. A., Watzl, J., Banakar, S., O'Neill, J., Mintz, J., Davanzo, P., ... Thomas, M. A. (2007). Increased anterior cingulate/medial prefrontal cortical glutamate and creatine in bipolar depression. *Neuropsychopharmacology*, 32(12), 2490–2499.

Gallelli, K. A., Wagner, C. M., Karchemskiy, A., Howe, M., Spielman, D., Reiss, A., & Chang, K. D. (2005). N-acetylaspartate levels in bipolar offspring with and at high-risk for bipolar disorder. *Bipolar Disorders*, 7(6), 589–597.

Gigante, A. D., Bond, D. J., Lafer, B., Lam, R. W., Young. L. T., & Yatham, L. N. (2012). Brain glutamate levels measured by magnetic resonance spectroscopy in patients with bipolar disorder: a meta-analysis. *Bipolar Disorders*, 14(5), 478–487.

Hajek, T., Bauer, M., Pfennig, A., Cullis, J., Ploch, J., O'Donovan, C., ... Alda, M. (2012). Large positive effect of lithium on prefrontal cortex N-acetylaspartate in patients with bipolar disorder: 2-centre study. *Journal of Psychiatry & Neuroscience*, 37(3), 185–192.

Kato, T., Fujii, K., Shioiri, T., Inubushi, T., & Takahashi, S. (1996). Lithium side effects in relation to brain lithium concentration measured by lithium-7 magnetic resonance spectroscopy. *Progress in Neuro-Psychopharmacology & Biological Psychiatry*, 20(1), 87–97.

Kato, T., Inubushi, T., & Kato, N. (2000). Prediction of lithium response by 31P-MRS in bipolar disorder. *International Journal of Neuropsychopharmacology*, 3(1), 83–85.

Kato, T., Inubushi, T., & Takahashi, S. (1994). Relationship of lithium concentrations in the brain measured by lithium-7 magnetic resonance spectroscopy to treatment response in mania. *Journal of Clinical Psychopharmacology*, 14(5), 330–335.

Kraguljac, N. V., Reid, M., White, D., Jones, R., den Hollander, J., Lowman, D., & Lahti, A. C. (2012). Neurometabolites in schizophrenia and bipolar disorder—A systematic review and meta-analysis. *Psychiatry Research*, 203(2–3), 111–125.

Kushnir, T., Itzchak, Y., Valevski, A., Lask, M., Modai, I., & Navon, G. (1993). Relaxation times and concentrations of 7Li in the brain of patients receiving lithium therapy. *NMR in Biomedicine*, 6(1), 39–42.

Lan, M. J., McLoughlin, G. A., Griffin, J. L., Tsang, T. M., Huang, J. T., Yuan, P., ... Bahn, S. (2009). Metabonomic analysis identifies molecular changes associated with the pathophysiology and drug treatment of bipolar disorder. *Molecular Psychiatry*, 14(3), 269–279.

Lyoo, I. K., & Renshaw, P. F. (2003). Magnetic spectroscopy as a tool for psychopharmacological studies. In J. C. Soares (Ed.), *Brain imaging in affective disorders* (pp. 245–282). New York: Marcel Dekker.

Machado-Vieira, R., Manji, H. K., & Zarate, C. A. Jr. (2009). The role of lithium in the treatment of bipolar disorder: Convergent evidence for neurotrophic effects as a unifying hypothesis. *Bipolar Disorders*, 11(Suppl. 2), 92–109.

Maddock, R. J., & Buonocore, M. H. (2012). MR spectroscopic studies of the brain in psychiatric disorders. *Current Topics in Behavioral Neurosciences, 11*, 199–251.

McGrath, B. M., Greenshaw, A. J., McKay, R., Slupsky, C. M., & Silverstone, P. H. (2007). Unlike lithium, anticonvulsants and antidepressants do not alter rat brain myo-inositol. *NeuroReport*, 18(15), 1595–1598.

Merikangas, K. R., & Lamers, F. (2012). The "true" prevalence of bipolar II disorder. *Current Opinions in Psychiatry*, 25(1), 19–23.

Miklowitz, D. J. (2011). Functional impairment, stress, and psychosocial intervention in bipolar disorder. *Current Psychiatry Reports*, 13(6), 504–512.

Moore, C. M., Biederman, J., Wozniak, J., Mick, E., Aleardi, M., Wardrop, M., ... Renshaw, P. F. (2007). Mania, glutamate/glutamine and risperidone in pediatric bipolar disorder: A proton magnetic resonance spectroscopy study of the anterior cingulate cortex. *Journal of Affective Disorders*, 99(1–3), 19–25.

Moore, G. J., Bebchuk, J. M., Hasanat, K., Chen, G., Seraji-Bozorgzad, N., Wilds, I. B., ... Manji, H. K. (2000). Lithium increases N-acetyl-aspartate in the human brain: in vivo evidence in support of bcl-2's neurotrophic effects? *Biological Psychiatry;* 48(1), 1–8.

Moore, G. J., Bebchuk, J. M., Parrish, J. K., Faulk, M. W., Arfken, C. L., Strahl-Bevacqua, J., & Manji, H. K. (1999). Temporal dissociation between lithium-induced changes in frontal lobe myo-inositol and clinical response in manic-depressive illness. *The American Journal of Psychiatry*, 156(12), 1902–1908.

Murashita, J., Kato, T., Shioiri, T., Inubushi, T., & Kato, N. (2000). Altered brain energy metabolism in lithium-resistant bipolar disorder detected by photic stimulated 31P-MR spectroscopy. *Psychological Medicine, 30*(1), 107–115.

Nery, F. G., Stanley, J. A., Chen, H. H., Hatch, J. P., Nicoletti, M. A., Monkul, E. S.,...Soares, J. C. (2009). Normal metabolite levels in the left dorsolateral prefrontal cortex of unmedicated major depressive disorder patients: A single voxel (1)H spectroscopy study. *Psychiatry Research, 174*(3), 177–183.

O'Donnell, T., Rotzinger, S., Nakashima, T. T., Hanstock, C. C., Ulrich, M., & Silverstone, P. H. (2003). Chronic lithium and sodium valproate both decrease the concentration of myoinositol and increase the concentration of inositol monophosphates in rat brain. *European Journal of Neuropsychopharmacology, 13*(3), 199–207.

Ongür, D., Jensen, J. E., Prescot, A. P., Stork, C., Lundy, M., Cohen, B. M., & Renshaw, P. F. (2008). Abnormal glutamatergic neurotransmission and neuronal-glial interactions in acute mania. *Biological Psychiatry, 64*(8), 718–726.

Patel, N. C., Cecil, K. M., Strakowski, S. M., Adler, C. M., & DelBello, M. P. (2008). Neurochemical alterations in adolescent bipolar depression: a proton magnetic resonance spectroscopy pilot study of the prefrontal cortex. *Journal of Child and Adolescent Psychopharmacology, 18*(6), 623–627.

Perlis, R. H., Ostacher, M. J., Patel, J. K., Marangell, L. B., Zhang, H., Wisniewski, S. R.,...Thase, M. E. (2006). Predictors of recurrence in bipolar disorder: Primary outcomes from the Systematic Treatment Enhancement Program for Bipolar Disorder (STEP-BD). *The American Journal of Psychiatry, 163*, 217–224.

Phillips, M. L., Travis, M. J., Fagiolini, A., & Kupfer, D. J. (2008). Medication effects in neuroimaging studies of bipolar disorder. *The American Journal of Psychiatry, 165*(3), 313–320.

Sachs, G. S., Renshaw, P. F., Lafer, B., Stoll, A. L., Guimarães, A. R., Rosenbaum, J. F., Gonzalez, R. G. (1995). Variability of brain lithium levels during maintenance treatment: a magnetic resonance spectroscopy study. *Biological Psychiatry, 1, 38*(7), 422–428.

Sanches, M., & Soares, J. C. (2011). New drugs for bipolar disorder. *Current Psychiatry Reports, 13*(6), 513–521

Sanches, M., Brambilla, P., & Soares, J. C. (2006). The role of imaging techniques in the development and clinical use of psychotropic drugs. In F. López-Muñoz & C. Alamo (Eds.), *Historia de la psicofarmacología* (pp. 479–494). Barcelona: Editorial Medica Panamericana.

Sanches, M., Newberg, A. R., & Soares, J. C. (2010). Emerging drugs for bipolar disorder. *Expert Opinion on Emerging Drugs, 15*(3), 453–466.

Sassi, R., & Soares, J. C. (2003). Brain imaging methods in neuropsychiatry. In J. C. Soares (Ed.), *Brain imaging in affective disorders* (pp. 1–17). New York: Marcel Dekker.

Shahana, N., Delbello, M., Chu, W. J., Jarvis, K., Fleck, D., Welge, J.,...Adler, C. (2011). Neurochemical alteration in the caudate: Implications for the pathophysiology of bipolar disorder. *Psychiatry Research, 193*(2), 107–112.

Sharma, R., Venkatasubramanian, P. N., Bárány, M., & Davis, J. M. (1992). Proton magnetic resonance spectroscopy of the brain in schizophrenic and affective patients. *Schizophrenia Research, 8*(1), 43–49.

Shibuya-Tayoshi, S., Tayoshi, S., Sumitani, S., Ueno, S., Harada, M., & Ohmori, T. (2008). Lithium effects on brain glutamatergic and GABAergic systems of healthy volunteers as measured by proton magnetic resonance spectroscopy. *Progress in Neuro-Psychopharmacology & Biological Psychiatry, 32*(1), 249–256.

Silverstone, P. H., McGrath, B. M., & Kim, H. (2005). Bipolar disorder and myo-inositol: A review of the magnetic resonance spectroscopy findings. *Bipolar Disorders, 7*(1), 1–10.

Silverstone, P. H., Wu, R. H., O'Donnell, T., Ulrich, M., Asghar, S. J., & Hanstock, C. C. (2002). Chronic treatment with both lithium and sodium valproate may normalize phosphoinositol cycle activity in bipolar patients. *Human Psychopharmacology, 17*(7), 321–327.

Silverstone, P. H., Wu, R. H., O'Donnell, T., Ulrich, M., Asghar, S. J., & Hanstock, C. C. (2003). Chronic treatment with lithium, but not sodium valproate, increases cortical N-acetyl-aspartate concentrations in euthymic bipolar patients. *International Clinical Psychopharmacology, 18*(2), 73–79.

Soares, J. C. (2002). Can brain-imaging studies provide a "mood stabilizer signature?" *Molecular Psychiatry, 7*(Suppl. 1), S64–S70.

Soares, J. C., Boada, F., & Keshavan, M. S. (2000). Brain lithium measurements with (7)Li magnetic resonance spectroscopy (MRS): A literature review. *European Neuropsychopharmacology, 10*(3), 151–158.

Soares, J. C., & Mann, J. J. (1997). The anatomy of mood disorders—review of structural neuroimaging studies. *Biological Psychiatry, 41*(1), 86–106.

Stanley, J. A. (2002). In vivo magnetic resonance spectroscopy and its application to neuropsychiatric disorders. *Canadian Journal of Psychiatry, 47*(4), 315–326.

Strawn, J. R., Patel, N. C., Chu, W. J., Lee, J. H., Adler, C. M., Kim, M. J.,...DelBello, M. P. (2012). Glutamatergic effects of divalproex in adolescents with mania: A proton magnetic resonance spectroscopy study. *Journal of the American Academy of Child & Adolescent Psychiatry, 51*(6), 642–651.

Vieta, E., Reinares, M., & Rosa, A. R. (2011). Staging bipolar disorder. *Neurotoxicity Research, 19*(2), 279–285.

Waddell, K. W., Zanjanipour, P., Pradhan, S., Xu, L., Welch, E. B., Joers, J. M.,...Gore, J. C. (2011). Anterior cingulate and cerebellar GABA and Glu correlations measured by ¹H J-difference spectroscopy. *Magnetic Resonance Imaging, 29*(1), 19–24.

Wang, P. W., Dieckmann, N., Sailasuta, N., Adalsteinsson, E., Spielman, D. & Ketter, T. A. (2002). *3 Tesla 1H-magnetic resonance spectroscopic measurements of prefrontal cortical gamma-aminobutyric acid (GABA) levels in bipolar disorder patients and healthy volunteers.* Paper presented at the 57th Annual Convention and Scientific Program of the Society of Biological Psychiatry. Philadelphia.

Wu, R. H., O'Donnell, T., Ulrich, M., Asghar, S. J., Hanstock, C. C., & Silverstone, P. H. (2004). Brain choline concentrations may not be altered in euthymic bipolar disorder patients chronically treated with either lithium or sodium valproate. *Annals of General Psychiatry, 3*(1), 13.

Yildiz, A., Demopulos, C. M., Moore, C. M., Renshaw, P. F., & Sachs, G. S. (2001). Effect of lithium on phosphoinositide metabolism in human brain: A proton-decoupled 31P MRS study. *Biological Psychiatry, 50*(1), 3–7.

Yildiz, A., Sachs, G. S., Dorer, D. J., & Renshaw, P. F. (2001). 31P Nuclear magnetic resonance spectroscopy findings in bipolar illness: A meta-analysis. *Psychiatry Research, 106*(3), 181–191.

Yildiz-Yesiloglu, A., & Ankerst, D. P. (2006). Neurochemical alterations of the brain in bipolar disorder and their implications for pathophysiology: A systematic review of the in vivo proton magnetic resonance spectroscopy findings. *Progress in Neuro-Psychopharmacology & Biological Psychiatry, 30*(6), 969–995.

Zimmerman, M. (2010). Problems diagnosing bipolar disorder in clinical practice. *Expert Review of Neurotherapeutics, 10*(7), 1019–1021.

19.

THE USE OF MOLECULAR IMAGING TO INVESTIGATE BIPOLAR DISORDER

FINDINGS AND TREATMENT IMPLICATIONS

Allison Greene, Christopher Bailey, and Alexander Neumeister

INTRODUCTION

Like many psychiatric illnesses, bipolar disorder (BD) remains incompletely understood. However, advances in structural and functional neuroimaging have provided researchers with the tools to investigate its pathophysiology more closely. Molecular imaging modalities such as positron emission tomography (PET) and single photon emission computed tomography (SPECT) allow researchers to examine various measures of neuronal functioning in vivo such as cerebral blood flow, glucose metabolism, and relative densities of specific neurochemical receptors and transporters within the brain (Gonul, Coburn, & Kula, 2009). By exploring how these features differ between individuals with and without BD, researchers have been able to identify specific abnormalities associated with this complex disease. Specifically, PET and SPECT research over the past three decades has revealed regional dysfunction in brain metabolism and altered transporter and receptor densities in patients with BD. In this chapter, we review seminal work within these two broad categories and discuss their current and future treatment implications.

EARLY FINDINGS

Some of the first molecular imaging investigations of BD date back to the mid-1980s. This work was facilitated by the advent of [18F]-deoxyglucose in the late 1970s, which allowed researchers to measure neuronal activity in psychiatric patients by tracing glucose metabolism in the brain (Buchsbaum et al., 1982; Metter, Hanson, Wasterlain, Kuhl, & Phelps, 1979). Many early psychiatric studies that implemented this technique grouped illnesses such as schizophrenia, BD, and unipolar depression into broad diagnostic categories and thus offered limited information on BD specifically. However, such investigations revealed a relationship between metabolic abnormalities and affective pathology and thus created a strong foundation for future imaging work in BD.

In 1984 Buchsbaum and colleagues explored glucose metabolism in a cohort of patients with schizophrenia and unipolar or bipolar depression. Patients and healthy controls exhibited an anteroposterior gradient in glucose metabolism, with greater glucose utilization toward frontal regions of the brain. Notably, this gradient was diminished in the patient group. Based on this observation, the authors suggested that goal-planning behaviors, which are disrupted in schizophrenia, are localized toward frontal areas of the brain. This hypothesized link between symptomology and reduced frontal glucose metabolism was a key addition to a growing body of research on neural abnormalities in affective disease processes.

Two years later, Buchsbaum et al. (1986) group repeated their study with a greater focus on unipolar and bipolar depression. The authors found that the anteroposterior metabolic gradient was diminished in bipolar depressed patients but amplified in unipolar depressed patients compared to healthy controls. Not only did these results highlight the presence of metabolic abnormalities in BD, but they also revealed a discrete pathophysiological difference between unipolar and bipolar depression.

During the same time period, Baxter et al. (1985) measured glucose metabolism in BD and unipolar depression during resting-state conditions. The authors found that bipolar depression and bipolar mixed-states were characterized by diminished whole-brain metabolism relative to euthymic, manic, and healthy comparison groups.

Perhaps the more significant finding from this study was that whole-brain metabolism progressively increased from depressive to euthymic to manic patient groups, offering preliminary evidence that mood changes may be associated with metabolic fluctuations (Schwartz, Baxter, Mazziotta, Gerner, & Phelps, 1987).

As the 1980s proceeded, psychiatric researchers continued to use molecular imaging to explore differences between depressive subtypes (e.g., Kishimoto et al., 1987; Phelps, Mazziotta, Baxter, & Gerner, 1984; Schwartz et al., 1987). In fact, this question remains an area of active research (see Hosokawa, Momose, & Kasai, 2009). As the unipolar–bipolar dichotomy became more clearly understood, there was a gradual shift in psychiatric imaging research away from studies on "affective pathology" toward studies on specific affective diagnoses. Refinements in neuroimaging techniques have also allowed researchers to explore specific brain regions more closely.

CONTEMPORARY PERSPECTIVES: REGIONAL ABNORMALITIES IN BIPOLAR DEPRESSION

PREFRONTAL CORTEX

As mentioned, Buchsbaum et al. (1984, 1986) found a diminished anteroposterior gradient in glucose metabolism, or hypofrontal glucose utilization, in individuals with affective disorders including bipolar depression. Over time, this observation has been largely supported (Baxter et al., 1989; Hosokawa et al., 2009; Ketter et al., 2001). On the other hand, one investigation reported no differences in metabolism between BD patients and healthy individuals (Tutus et al., 1998). A small number of studies have also reported increased metabolism in certain areas of the prefrontal cortex (PFC; reviewed in Ketter et al., 2001).

Reduced prefrontal metabolism has also been observed in patients with primary and secondary unipolar depression (Drevets, 1999), suggesting that there might be a common neural pathway underlying depressive symptoms that is independent of subtype or etiology (Ketter et al., 2001). However, we are gradually learning that hypofrontal metabolic patterns may manifest differently in unipolar and bipolar depression. Ketter et al. found increased cerebello-posterior metabolism in bipolar depression only, indicating that this abnormality may be unique to the bipolar subtype. Furthermore, Hosokawa et al. (2009) found reduced right anterior cingulate metabolism in bipolar depression only and a reduced right temporal gyrus, right insula, and left posterior cingulate metabolism in unipolar depression only, further highlighting the differences between these two illnesses.

In the 1980s we were just beginning to understand the role of the frontal and PFCs in the regulation of cognition and executive function (e.g., see Coffman, Bornstein, Olson, Schwarzkopf, & Nasrallah, 1990; Morice, 1990; Stuss & Benson, 1984). As a result, we were able to develop preliminary hypotheses linking the cognitive symptoms of BD to the prefrontal metabolic abnormalities revealed by novel neuroimaging techniques. For instance, Buchsbaum et al. (1986) suggested that the hypofrontality observed in bipolar depression might reflect the "nonspecific cognitive deficits" associated with some psychiatric illnesses. Over the past 30 years, our understanding of the relationship between prefrontal metabolic alterations and cognitive symptomology in BD has increased dramatically.

In 2005 Benabarre and colleagues used a battery of neuropsychological assessments in conjunction with SPECT imaging to explore the relationship between cerebral flood flow and cognitive dysfunction in BD. Deficits in executive function, logical memory, and verbal learning were associated with reduced frontal perfusion; poor performance in executive function and psychomotor function was associated with anterior temporal hyperperfusion; and poor performance in memory, executive function, and attention was associated with striate hyperperfusion. Not only do these associations contribute to our understanding of the pathophysiology of BD, but they are also an important step in the development of comprehensive psychological treatments.

Most recently, Li et al. (2012) explored executive function and glucose metabolism in remitted BD type I (BD-I) and type II (BD-II) patients. Compared to BD-II patients and healthy controls, BD-I patients performed significantly worse on the Wisconsin Card Sorting Test, a measure of executive function and mental flexibility. BD-I patients also demonstrated reduced metabolism in several regions, including the insula, striatum, and part of the PFC. These observations suggest that prefrontal glucose metabolism and cognitive processing are differentially related in BD-I and BD-II.

SUBGENUAL ANTERIOR CINGULATE CORTEX

Over the past 15 years, PET imaging in BD has focused largely on the subgenual region of the PFC, which has been implicated in the regulation of mood and emotion (Baggio et al., 2012; Kim et al., 2012; Kohn et al., 2013).

Drevets et al. (1997) first noted the significance of this region to BD when they reported a 39% left-lateralized, mood state-independent reduction in cortical volume and decreased metabolism in the PFC ventral to the genu of the corpus callosum in familial bipolar depression. This volumetric reduction was associated with a reduction in glial cells without neuronal loss (Ongür, Drevets, & Price, 1998).

Drevets and colleagues (1999) later used computer simulations to correct for the effects of grey matter reduction and found that metabolism in the remaining subgenual PFC tissue was actually increased in bipolar depression rather than decreased. Many lines of investigation support this observation. By 2008, Drevets, Savitz, and Trimble had more specifically localized the subgenual PFC significant in BD pathophysiology as the subgenual anterior cingulate cortex (sgACC), including Brodmann area 24 and parts of 25.

Several lines of evidence have found left-lateralized volumetric reductions in sgACC in familial adult, adolescent, and pediatric BD (Baloch et al., 2010; Hirayasu et al., 1999; Singh et al., 2012; Wilke, Kowatch, DelBello, Mills, & Holland, 2004), as well as unaffected individuals with a familial history of mood disorders (Boes, McCormick, Coryell, & Nopoulos, 2008). One study reported a right-lateralized sgACC reduction in familial and nonfamilial BD (Sharma et al., 2003), and several studies have found no volumetric abnormalities in BD (Brambilla et al., 2002; Hajek et al., 2010, Sanches et al., 2005; Zimmerman, DelBello, Getz., Shear, & Strakowski, 2006) or at-risk children (Singh, Delbello, Adler, Stanford, & Strakowski, 2008).

Drevets et al. (1999) attribute this variability within the literature to technical issues such as low spatial resolution during image acquisition and/or image blurring prior to analysis. Another contributing factor may be the neuroprogressive nature of BD itself. Several studies have suggested that the natural course of the disease may result in a progressive loss of PFC grey matter volume over time (reviewed in Lim et al., 2013). Therefore, inconsistencies among studies on the sgACC in BD may reflect the possibility that this region progressively changes throughout the course of the BD illness. Furthermore, medications such as lithium have been shown to attenuate gray matter reductions in the sgACC in adults (Bora, Fornito, Yücel, & Pantelis, 2010; Moore et al., 2009) and children (Mitsunaga et al., 2011). Thus it may also be important to consider medication history when interpreting sgACC imaging data.

In addition to volumetric abnormalities, there have also been several reports of metabolic alterations in the sgACC in BD. As previously mentioned, Drevets et al. (1999) found increased activity in this region in a group of familial bipolar depressed patients. These results were replicated in a group of depressed bipolar women (Bauer et al., 2005) and a group of unmedicated BD-II patients (Mah et al., 2007). Other studies have found trending but insignificant metabolic increases in this region (Brooks et al., 2009; Krüger, Seminowicz, Goldapple, Kennedy, & Mayberg, 2003), while a few investigations have shown no metabolic alterations (Brooks et al., 2006) or reduced metabolism relative to healthy controls (Brooks et al., 2009).

Just as medical treatments may affect sgACC volume, they may also affect glucose metabolism in this region. Bauer et al. (2005) found that following treatment with the synthetic thyroid hormone levothyroxine, a group of euthyroid bipolar depressed women demonstrated metabolic reductions in the right sgACC as well as improved mood. Interestingly, Mah et al. (2007) found that BD-II patients undergoing treatment with lithium or divalproex maintained elevated metabolism in the right sgPFC, suggesting that these medications may not produce the same metabolic effects as hormone-modulating therapies. Bauer and colleagues (2003) noted that several limbic structures that are involved in the pathophysiology of mood disorders also have high densities of thyroid hormone receptors. The relationship between thyroid function and BD and the treatment implications of this association remain targets of active research (Krishna et al., 2013; Pompili et al., 2012).

There have also been studies on the relationship between cognition and sgACC metabolism in BD. Brooks et al. (2006) explored glucose metabolism in BD during a continuous performance task and found no difference in metabolism or performance between the bipolar group and healthy individuals. However, the authors did observe that reduced metabolism in the sgACC was associated with a slower hit rate reaction time and more omission errors in the bipolar group only. Once again, we see that cognitive function and cortical activation are abnormally related in BD.

LATERAL PREFRONTAL CORTEX

Abnormalities in the lateral PFC have also been indicated in bipolar depression. This region of the brain is involved in cognitive processes such as working memory, causal reasoning, decision-making, and inhibitory control (Brandt, Bergström, Buda, Henson, & Simons, 2013; Brooks et al., 2006; Christakou et al., 2013; Zhang, Yao, Zhang, Long, & Zhao, 2013). Subdivisions of this region, namely the dorsolateral, ventrolateral, and anterolateral PFC, may play discrete roles in the modulation of these processes (Akaishi, Ueda, & Sakai, 2013; Barbey & Patterson, 2011).

Baxter and colleagues (1985, 1989) first reported alterations in the lateral PFC, noting that unipolar and bipolar depressed patients demonstrated reduced metabolic activity in the left anterolateral PFC. The authors also found an inverse relationship between hypometabolism and patients' score on the Hamilton Depression Rating Scale, suggesting that the degree of metabolic reduction is directly related to symptom severity. Since these early discoveries, metabolic reductions in this area of the brain have been among the least disputed neural abnormalities in bipolar depression.

Most of the supporting research throughout the 1990s focused specifically on the dorsolateral PFC (al-Mousawi et al., 1996; reviewed in Drevets, 2000, and Gonul et al., 2009). Several lines of evidence from the 1990s also support the idea that degree of metabolic reduction is correlated positively with symptom severity (reviewed in Benson et al., 2008; Drevets et al., 1992).

Over the past decade, researchers have expanded on this literature to elucidate more detailed information regarding dorsolateral PFC function. In 2003, Kruger and colleagues induced transient sadness in a group of euthymic and depressed bipolar patients to explore the brain regions that may underlie the emotional sensitivity that persists during symptom remission. Both BD patient groups demonstrated dorsolateral PFC hypoperfusion at resting state, but only the depression group exhibited hypoperfusion during emotional stress. This discrepancy suggests that pathways involving the dorsolateral PFC may be preserved during symptom remission (Krüger et al., 2003). In 2006, Krüger et al. repeated the emotional challenge paradigm in a group of lithium-responsive patients and compared their results to a previously studied cohort of valproate-responders. Interestingly, the valproate-responders exhibited PFC hypoperfusion, but the lithium-responders did not. This discrepancy suggests that neural processes involving the dorsolateral PFC may be preserved during emotional stress in the latter group (Krüger et al., 2006). However, the authors stress that it is difficult to determine if lithium is responsible for the stabilization of this region or if this region remains intact inherently in this patient group.

It also appears that BD patients may demonstrate abnormal patters of associativity between the dorsolateral PFC and other brain regions during specific cognitive tasks. Benson et al. (2008) administered an auditory continuous performance task to a cohort of 30 individuals with treatment-refractory BD and assessed interregional cerebral metabolic activity. Bipolar patients had more positive and fewer negative correlations between the left dorsolateral PFC and other brain regions and lacked the "normal inverse relationship between the dorsolateral PFC and the cerebellum" and limbic regions such as the anterior cingulate cortex (ACC; Benson et al., 2008). This study was one of the first to explore the discrete functional connectivity of the brain regions implicated in the pathophysiology of BD and offered important insight into the systematic dysregulation of these regions during cognitive activation.

LIMBIC SYSTEM

The limbic system is a series of brain structures including the amygdala, hippocampus, and parahippocampus that are involved in the regulation of mood, emotion, memory, learning, and fear (LeDoux, 1998). Because of their roles in mood and emotion, limbic structures have been an important target of investigation in BD research over the past 30 years.

Early studies from the late 1980s and early 1990s reported decreased limbic perfusion in bipolar depression patients (e.g., see Ito et al., 1996), but many of these studies were limited by low signal quality (Gonul et al., 2009). In contrast, more recent investigations have largely reported increased metabolism in limbic regions. For example, Drevets et al. (2002) observed increased amygdala activity in both unipolar and bipolar depressed patients relative to controls. Mah et al. (2007) later focused specifically on BD-II patients and again reported increased metabolism in the amygdala.

Interestingly, Li and colleagues (2012) observed differential limbic function between BD-I and BD-II patients. Specifically, the authors found decreased activity in the ACC, insula, striatum, and PFC and increased activity in the parahippocampus in BD-I patients relative to BD-II and healthy controls. These observations are consistent with the lower levels of executive function seen in BD-I. With respect to the manic state, early investigations into limbic function have yielded findings of both decreased glucose metabolism and increased regional cerebral blood flow in limbic regions (al Mousawi et al., 1996; reviewed in Gonul et al., 2009).

METABOLIC ABNORMALITIES IN BIPOLAR MANIA

While there is a robust body of literature on neuroimaging in bipolar depression, there are relatively few studies that focus primarily on mania. As a result, our understanding of this state remains somewhat limited. However, we have made important observations over the past 20 years that provide significant insight into mania's underlying pathophysiology.

Several investigations have revealed a relationship between mood state and metabolic fluctuations. In particular, the metabolic reductions found in bipolar depression tend to normalize as depressive symptoms improve such that global metabolism is greater in the euthymic and manic states than in the depressive state (Baxter et al., 1985; Ketter et al., 2001). However, Goodwin and colleagues (1997) made the important observation that the neural correlates of mania may not necessarily be the reverse of those found in depression, even though "depression is conceptually at the opposite end of bipolar illness." In fact, there appear to be several neural abnormalities that are common to both depression and mania, including volumetric reductions in the left sgACC and increased activity in the remaining sgACC tissue (Brooks, Hoblyn, & Ketter, 2010; Drevets et al., 1997). Al-Mousawi et al. (1996) also found that acute mania, like bipolar depression, is characterized by hypofrontal metabolism, specifically in the dorsolateral PFC. These observations suggest that there may be an abnormal pattern of brain development or an effect of recurrent illness that persists throughout the different mood states of BD (Drevets et al., 1997).

On the other hand, there are neural correlates of BD that appear to be unique to the manic state, particularly in the cingulate cortex (reviewed in Gonul et al., 2009). Specifically, mania has been associated with increased activity in the cingulate cortex (Benabarre et al., 2005; Brooks et al., 2010) and more specifically in the left dorsal cingulate cortex (Blumberg et al., 2000; Rubinsztein et al., 2001) during both resting state and cognitive activation. Conversely, depression is commonly associated with increased activity in the ventral cingulate cortex (Diler et al., 2013). Based on these observations, Gonul et al. (2009) suggest that dorsal and ventral divisions of the cingulate cortex might play differential roles in the pathophophysiology of mania and depression.

Limbic dysregulation has also been implicated in the manic state. Blumberg and colleagues (2000) found heightened activity in the left caudate nucleus during resting state and decreased right rostral and bilateral orbital prefrontal perfusion during a word-generation task (Blumberg et al., 1999). Similarly, Brooks, Hoblyn, and Ketter (2010) noted heightened activity in the parahippocampal complex and ACC and decreased activity in dorsal PFC. These studies support Brooks et al.'s model of "simultaneous resting limbic/paralimbic hypermatabolism and prefrontal hypometabolism" in mania.

Interestingly, al-Mousawi et al. (1996) found metabolic reductions in limbic regions including the left amygdala and increases in activity in the right temporal cortex in mania,

though the authors were unsure if these effects were linked to medication use within their patient group. To explore this possibility, Goodwin et al. (1997) investigated cortical perfusion in manic bipolar patients before and after lithium withdrawal. Withdrawal was associated with increased anxiety and worsening executive function coupled with decreases in perfusion in limbic areas, including the ACC. It was unclear, however, whether the observed results were directly related to lithium withdrawal or the appearance of manic symptoms. The impact of mediation use on neural activity in BD remains an area of active investigation.

A MODEL OF FUNCTIONAL NEUROCIRCUITRY IN BIPOLAR DISORDER

In the following section, we propose a general hypothesis of the emotion dysregulation seen in BD based on the information presented in the previous sections. In the depressed and manic mood state, emotion and cognitive processing are impaired in a fronto-striatal-limbic circuit leading to depressive or manic symptomology. At the center of this circuit is the amygdala, which is responsible for emotion regulation and fear. The existing body of literature has, for the most part, consistently reported increased baseline amygdala activation in depressed BD patients (reviewed in Strakowski et al., 2012).

Based on the function of the amygdala, it has been postulated that increased amygdala activation may underlie anxious symptomology in the depressed state or agitation in the manic state (reviewed in Savitz & Drevets, 2009). However, it is essential to remember that the amygdala receives connections from many other regions that shape its function (Strakowski et al., 2012). Regions of the PFC, specifically the ventromedial and orbitofrontal cortex, modulate amygdala activation. Since the PFC modulates amygdala activation, decreased activation within prefrontal brain regions in BD may lead to disinhibited amygdala activation leading to emotional extremes such as depression, mania, and excessive anxiety (Blond, Fredericks, & Blumberg, 2012; Strakowski et al., 2012).

The striatum is responsible for reward and goal-directed behavior. Currently, there are no strong consensus striatal findings within the BD neuroimaging literature. Conceivably, striatal dysfunction could be related to the anhedonic symptomology commonly seen in depressed patients or the agitated phenotype in manic patients (Savitz & Drevets, 2009). A representation of this hypothesis is presented in Figure 19.1. It is important to note that this

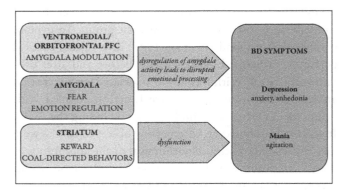

Figure 19.1 A proposed model of dysfunctional neurocircuitry in bipolar depression.

explanation represents a simplified model of neuronal dysfunction and may not include all brain regions involved in the pathophysiology of BD.

RECEPTOR AND TRANSPORTER IMAGING

PET imaging studies on glucose metabolism have yielded an enormous amount of information on the pathophysiology of BD. While the paradigms we outlined earlier will continue to be an indispensible component of BD research, we believe the next generation of PET imaging work will most likely involve in vivo investigations of receptor and transporter expression. Currently, PET receptor imaging studies in mood disorders such as BD have focused largely on the dopaminergic and serotonergic systems (reviewed extensively in Savitz & Drevets, 2013). In this section, we highlight the critical PET receptor imaging findings dopamine in serotonin systems produced over the past two decades.

Summaries of findings for dopaminergic and serotonergic imaging are presented in Figures 19.2 and 19.3, respectively.

DOPAMINE

The dopaminergic system has been implicated in the pathophysiology of BD. Evidence that supports this system's role comes primarily from pharmacological studies and clinical observation of mood state changes with a variety of drugs that modulate dopamine (Anand et al., 2011). Currently, PET studies that investigate dopaminergic function in BD have focused on the dopamine D1 and D2 receptors and the dopamine transporter (DAT), which is responsible for the reuptake of dopamine into the presynaptic neuron (Camardese et al., 2014).

In 1992 Suhara and colleagues utilized the D1-selective radioligand [11C]-SCH23390 to investigate receptor binding—a measure of receptor availability or density—in a small cohort of BD patients in different mood states. The authors found that, relative to healthy controls, the BD patients had significantly lower D1 binding in the frontal cortex but not in the striatum. Moreover, the authors did not find any differences in binding between symptomatic and asymptomatic BD patients. The authors proposed that these results reflected differing neural networks in the frontal cortex and striatum. Though this study was limited by the debated selectivity of [11C]-SCH23390 and small sample size, it was the first quantitative PET study of the D1 receptor in BD and thus an important contribution to a nascent body of research on dopamine function BD (Suhara et al., 1992).

The earliest studies on the dopamine D2 receptor in BD reported increased caudate D2 receptor signal in

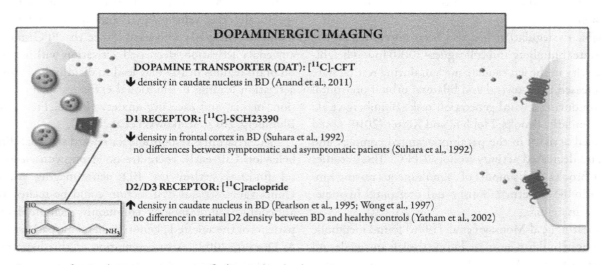

Figure 19.2 Summary of major dopaminergic imaging findings in bipolar depression.

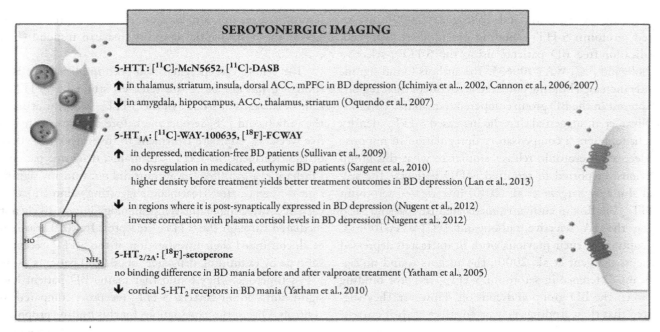

Figure 19.3 Summary of major serotonergic imaging findings in bipolar depression.

BD patients (Pearlson et al., 1995; Wong et al., 1997). In 2002, Yatham and colleagues employed PET and the selective D2/D3 receptor ligand [11C]-raclopride to examine D2 binding in 13 nonpsychotic, manic BD patients. The authors found no significant differences in D2 receptor density in the striatum between patients and matched healthy controls. In addition, [11C]-raclopride scans were repeated in 10 mood-stabilized naïve patients from the BD group following two to six weeks of treatment with divalproex sodium. Once again, the authors found no significant effects on D2 receptor density (Yatham et al., 2002).

Anand and colleagues (2011) continued the discussion of dopaminergic transmission in the striatum. Using the DAT-selective ligand [11C]-CFT, they investigated the function of the DAT in unmediated euthymic and depressed BD patients. The authors found that there was significantly less DAT availability in the caudate of the BD group compared to healthy controls, with no differences between the depressed and euthymic groups. The authors proposed the possibilities that BD patients simply possess fewer DATs or that there are post-transcriptional modifications of the DAT that affect its availability. Importantly, they warned that interpretation of their results should be done after a solid animal model of BD is developed, so that dopaminergic signaling could be investigated thoroughly and comprehensively. Despite this precaution, Anand et al. provided important evidence for abnormal dopaminergic signaling in BD.

Due to the paucity of imaging studies investigating dopamine in BD thus far and the variable function of dopamine receptors and transporters across brain regions, it is difficult to derive a convincing model for dopamine's contribution to the pathophysiology BD (Savitz & Drevets, 2013). It is clear, however, that altered dopaminergic transmission plays a key role in the pathophysiology of BD. Further investigation of this system is certainly warranted and will likely yield exciting results in the upcoming years.

SEROTONIN

The serotonergic system is perhaps the most widely studied neurochemical system in the exploration of mood disorders. Dysfunctional serotonergic transmission has been linked to depressive and manic symptomology through animal models, large-scale clinical trials, and clinical practice (Greene, Bailey, & Neumeister, 2013). The most convincing evidence linking serotonergic function to BD symptomology comes from clinical experience of drugs that increase intrasynaptic serotonin (SSRIs and SNRIs) and their efficacy in depressed individuals with BD and major depressive disorder (MDD) (Baldessarini, Vieta, Calabrese, Tohen, & Bowden, 2010). PET receptor imaging studies in BD have explored the serotonin 5-HT$_{1A}$ and 5-HT$_{2A}$ receptor subtypes and the serotonin transporter (5-HTT; Savitz & Drevets, 2013).

Two groundbreaking studies on the serotonin 1A receptor were published between 2009 and 2010. The first study by Sullivan and colleagues (2009) investigated serotonin 5-HT$_{1A}$ binding potential in depressed, medication-free BD patients using the 5-HT$_{1A}$-selective radioligand [^{11}C]-WAY-100635. The authors found significantly increased binding potential across all of their regions of interest in the BD group compared to matched controls. Sullivan et al. suggested that the increased 5-HT$_{1A}$ density might represent a compensatory upregulation in response to decreased serotonin release, similar to what this group previously reported in remitted MDD patients. The second study by Sargent et al. (2010) investigated serotonin 5-HT$_{1A}$ binding in euthymic, medicated BD patients, also using the 1A selective radioligand [^{11}C]-WAY-100635. In contrast to their previous work in untreated depressed patients (Sargent et al., 2000), the authors found no significant difference in serotonin 5-HT$_{1A}$ receptor binding between the BD group and controls. However, they suggested that these findings may be an effect of their current antidepressant medications or reflect the possibility that decreased 5-HT$_{1A}$ is characteristic of only the depressant mood state (Sargent et al., 2010).

In 2012 Nugent and colleagues continued to explore serotonin 5-HT$_{1A}$ expression by utilizing the highly selective radioligand [^{18}F]-FCWAY in unmedicated, depressed BD patients. They found that serotonin 5-HT$_{1A}$ biding potential was significantly decreased in regions where the receptor primarily is postsynaptically expressed (i.e., mesotemporal cortex). The authors also reported an inverse correlation with plasma cortisol levels, suggesting that high cortisol levels attenuate the expression of serotonin 5-HT1A receptors, an effect that has frequently been reported in other mood and anxiety disorders (Nugent et al., 2013).

Most recently, Sullivan et al., (2009), who had reported increased 5-HT$_{1A}$ receptor binding in BD, explored pre-medication treatment levels of 5-HT$_{1A}$ to determine whether high baseline 5-HT$_{1A}$ predicted better treatment outcomes. Using [^{11}C]-WAY-100635 once again, the investigators imaged medication-free, depressed BD patients before beginning antidepressant treatment. Three months following treatment, the authors split their sample into remitters and nonremitters based on an accepted clinical rating scale of depressive symptomology. Remarkably, they found that the remitted group had significantly higher global 5-HT$_{1A}$ pretreatment binding compared with non-remitters, suggesting that higher pretreatment 5-HT$_{1A}$ is associated with better treatment outcomes. One hypothesis offered by the authors suggests that greater compensatory upregulation in response to low endogenous serotonin levels allows for a more robust response to pharmacologic

serotonin upregulation because there is a greater density of the postsynaptic receptors that can respond (Lan et al., 2013).

The 5-HT$_{2A}$ receptor has also been implicated in BD, though it has not been as extensively studied as 5-HT$_{1A}$. One of the earliest studies of the 5-HT$_{2A}$ receptor utilized the radioligand [^{18}F]-setoperone before and after three to five weeks of valproate treatment to investigate the effect of the treatment on 5-HT$_{2A}$ in manic, drug-free patients (Yatham et al., 2005). The authors did not find any significant difference after treatment, suggesting valproate's efficacy in controlling manic symptomology is most likely not mediated through the 5-HT$_{2A}$ receptor. In 2010, Yatham et al. continued their investigation of the 5-HT$_2$ receptor subtype by examining drug-free, manic BD patients using [^{18}F]-setoperone. They found that manic BD patient had significantly lower cortical 5-HT$_2$ receptors compared to controls. One of the explanations for this finding proposed by the authors is that downregulation of 5-HT$_2$ receptors can cause/predispose one to manic symptoms based on our understanding that antidepressant medications can worsen mania through the downregulation of 5-HT$_2$ receptors (Yatham et al., 2010).

The serotonin transporter 5-HTT is responsible for the reuptake of serotonin into the presynaptic neuron. Recently, several studies have investigated this transporter system in BD. The first evidence of 5-HTT dysregulation in BD came from a study that included both MDD and BD patients, which investigated this transporter using the radioligand [^{11}C]-McN5652 (Ichimiya et al., 2002). The authors noted that in a combined MDD and BD patient group, there was significantly higher binding in the thalamus relative to matched controls. Though this study was not specific to BD, it laid the groundwork for following studies.

The first landmark study of 5-HTT specifically in BD utilized the [^{11}C]-DASB radioligand to investigate the binding potential of 5-HTT in a cohort of unmedicated, depressed BD patients and matched controls. Compared to controls, the BD group demonstrated increased 5-HTT binding potential in the thalamus, dorsal ACC, mPFC, and insula and decreased 5-HTT binding in the brainstem compared to the control group. Of note, anxiety ratings were positively correlated with the cortical findings (Cannon et al., 2006). Cannon et al. (2007) continued their investigation with a follow-up study that aimed to characterize differential 5-HTT binding potential in BD in comparison to both MDD and healthy controls. Again the authors employed the [^{11}C]-DASB radioligand. Compared to the control group, both MDD and BD demonstrated increased binding in the thalamus, striatum, and insula, similar to their previous report. However, the BD group demonstrated significantly reduced binding in the pontine raphe nucleus compared to the other groups. This finding was very important because it was one of the few findings from the PET receptor imaging literature that provided evidence for differential pathophysiology between MDD and BD. In addition, the findings were largely consistent with the animal literature, which showed that stressed animals with a depressed phenotype have increased 5-HTT and greater serotonin turnover in the mPFC, striatum, and limbic regions, similar to the regions with significantly increased 5-HTT in both studies.

Oquendo and colleagues (2007) investigated 5-HTT receptor binding potential in unmedicated, depressed patients using the [^{11}C]-McN5652 radioligand. In contrast to the aforementioned studies, the authors found significantly decreased binding potential in the amygdala, hippocampus, ACC, thalamus, and striatum. One of their explanations for this finding was that low intrasynaptic serotonin in BD leads to 5-HTT internalization (Oquendo et al., 2007).

CONCLUSION AND FUTURE DIRECTIONS

After almost three decades of use, PET imaging data has transformed the way investigators view and approach the neurobiological investigation of BD. While many of the findings discussed here are incompletely understood, the rich array of data generated from these investigations has triggered paradigm shifts in our understanding of BD and has taken researchers in several new and promising directions. The next generation of BD studies are likely to heavily utilize receptor imaging techniques with novel radioligands that can probe a variety of neurochemical systems, in vivo, implicated in mood and anxiety disorders such as serotonin 1B receptor subtypes and the endogenous cannabinoid system (Bailey & Neumeister, 2011; Murrough et al., 2011). Future PET findings will continue to provide us with a clearer understanding of neuronal dysfunction in BD and perhaps will lead to development of new evidence-oriented, target-, and state-specific treatments.

Disclosure statement: Dr. Christopher Bailey has not disclosed any conflicts of interest. Dr. Neumeister has received grant support from the National Institute of Mental Health, the Department of Defense, and the Department of Veterans Affairs, as well as Eli Lilly, Inc. He has also received consulting fees from Pfizer, Inc. All of these activities are unrelated to his contribution to this book chapter. Allison Greene has not disclosed any conflicts of interest.

REFERENCES

Akaishi, R., Ueda, N., & Sakai, K. (2013). Task-related modulation of effective connectivity during perceptual decision making: dissociation between dorsal and ventral prefrontal cortex. *Frontiers in Human Neuroscience, 7,* 365.

al-Mousawi, A. H., Evans, N., Ebmeier, K. P., Roeda, D., Chaloner, F., & Ashcroft, G. W. (1996). Limbic dysfunction in schizophrenia and mania: A study using 18F-labelled fluorodeoxyglucose and positron emission tomography. *The British Journal of Psychiatry, 169*(4), 509–516.

Anand, A., Barkay, G., Dzemidzic, M., Albrecht, D., Karne, H., Zheng, Q.-H., & Yoder, K. K. (2011). Striatal dopamine transporter availability in unmedicated bipolar disorder. *Bipolar Disorders, 13*(4), 406–413.

Baggio, H. C., Segura, B., Ibarretxe-Bilbao, N., Valldeoriola, F., Marti, M. J., Compta, Y., & Junqué, C. (2012). Structural correlates of facial emotion recognition deficits in Parkinson's disease patients. *Neuropsychologia, 50*(8), 2121–2128.

Bailey, C. R., & Neumeister, A. (2011). Cb1 receptor-mediated signaling emerges as a novel lead to evidence-based treatment development for stress-related psychopathology. *Neuroscience Letters, 502*(1), 1–4.

Baldessarini, R. J., Vieta, E., Calabrese, J. R., Tohen, M., & Bowden, C. L. (2010). Bipolar depression: Overview and commentary. *Harvard Review of Psychiatry, 18,* 143–157.

Baloch, H. A., Hatch, J. P., Olvera, R. L., Nicoletti, M., Caetano, S. C., Zunta-Soares, G. B., & Soares, J. C. (2010). Morphology of the subgenual prefrontal cortex in pediatric bipolar disorder. *Journal of Psychiatric Research, 44*(15), 1106–1110.

Barbey, A. K., & Patterson, R. (2011). Architecture of explanatory inference in the human prefrontal cortex. *Frontiers in Psychology, 2,* 162.

Bauer, M., London, E. D., Rasgon, N., Berman, S. M., Frye, M. A., Altshuler, L. L., & Whybrow, P. C. (2005). Supraphysiological doses of levothyroxine alter regional cerebral metabolism and improve mood in bipolar depression. *Molecular Psychiatry, 10*(5), 456–469.

Bauer, M., London, E. D., Silverman, D. H., Rasgon, N., Kirchheiner, J., & Whybrow, P. C. (2003). Thyroid, brain and mood modulation in affective disorder: Insights from molecular research and functional brain imaging. *Pharmacopsychiatry, 36*(Suppl. 3), S215–S221.

Baxter, L. R. Jr., Schwartz, J. M., Phelps, M. E., Mazziotta, J. C., Guze, B. H., Selin, C. E., ... Sumida, R. M. (1989). Reduction of prefrontal cortex glucose metabolism common to three types of depression. *Archives of General Psychiatry, 46*(3), 243–250.

Baxter, L. R. Jr., Phelps, M. E., Mazziotta, J. C., Schwartz, J. M., Gerner, R. H., Selin, C. E., & Sumida, R. M. (1985). Cerebral metabolic rates for glucose in mood disorders: Studies with positron emission tomography and fluorodeoxyglucose F 18. *Archives of General Psychiatry, 42*(5), 441–447.

Benabarre, A., Vieta, E., Martínez-Arán, A., Garcia-Garcia, M., Martín, F., Lomeña, F., ... Valdés, M. (2005). Neuropsychological disturbances and cerebral blood flow in bipolar disorder. *The Australian and New Zealand Journal of Psychiatry, 39*(4), 227–234.

Benson, B. E., Willis, M. W., Ketter, T. A., Speer, A., Kimbrell, T. A., George, M. S., & Post, R. M. (2008). Interregional cerebral metabolic associativity during a continuous performance task: Part II. Differential alterations in bipolar and unipolar disorders. *Psychiatry Research, 164*(1), 30–47.

Blond, B. N., Fredericks, C. A., & Blumberg, H. P. (2012). Functional neuroanatomy of bipolar disorder: Structure, function, and connectivity in an amygdala-anterior paralimbic neural system. *Bipolar Disorders, 14*(4), 340–355.

Blumberg, H. P., Stern, E., Martinez, D., Ricketts, S., de Asis, J., White, T., & Silbersweig, D. A. (2000). Increased anterior cingulate and caudate activity in bipolar mania. *Biological Psychiatry, 48*(11), 1045–1052.

Boes, A. D., McCormick, L. M., Coryell, W. H., & Nopoulos, P. (2008). Rostral anterior cingulate cortex volume correlates with depressed mood in normal healthy children. *Biological Psychiatry, 63*(4), 391–397.

Bora, E., Fornito, A., Yücel, M., & Pantelis, C. (2010). Voxelwise meta-analysis of gray matter abnormalities in bipolar disorder. *Biological Psychiatry, 67*(11), 1097–1105.

Brambilla, P., Nicoletti, M. A., Harenski, K., Sassi, R. B., Mallinger, A. G., Frank, E., & Soares, J. C. (2002). Anatomical MRI study of subgenual prefrontal cortex in bipolar and unipolar subjects. *Neuropsychopharmacology, 27*(5), 792–799.

Brandt, V. C., Bergström, Z. M., Buda, M., Henson, R. N. A., & Simons, J. S. (2013). Did I turn off the gas? Reality monitoring of everyday actions. *Cognitive, Affective and Behavioral Neuroscience, 14*(1), 209–219.

Brooks, J. O. III, Hoblyn, J. C., & Ketter, T. A. (2010). Metabolic evidence of corticolimbic dysregulation in bipolar mania. *Psychiatry Research, 181*(2), 136–140.

Brooks, J. O. III, Wang, P. W., Bonner, J. C., Rosen, A. C., Hoblyn, J. C., Hill, S. J., & Ketter, T. A. (2009). Decreased prefrontal, anterior cingulate, insula, and ventral striatal metabolism in medication-free depressed outpatients with bipolar disorder. *Journal of Psychiatric Research, 43*(3), 181–188.

Brooks, J. O. III, Wang, P. W., Strong, C., Sachs, N., Hoblyn, J. C., Fenn, R., & Ketter, T. A. (2006). Preliminary evidence of differential relations between prefrontal cortex metabolism and sustained attention in depressed adults with bipolar disorder and healthy controls. *Bipolar Disorders, 8*(3), 248–254.

Buchsbaum, M. S., DeLisi, L. E., Holcomb, H. H., Cappelletti, J., King, A. C., Johnson, J., & Morihisa, J. (1984). Anteroposterior gradients in cerebral glucose use in schizophrenia and affective disorders. *Archives of General Psychiatry, 41*(12), 1159–1166.

Buchsbaum, M. S., Ingvar, D. H., Kessler, R., Waters, R. N., Cappelletti, J., van Kammen, D. P., & Sokoloff, L. (1982). Cerebral glucography with positron tomography: Use in normal subjects and in patients with schizophrenia. *Archives of General Psychiatry, 39*(3), 251–259.

Buchsbaum, M. S., Wu, J., DeLisi, L. E., Holcomb, H., Kessler, R., Johnson, J., & Post, R. M. (1986). Frontal cortex and basal ganglia metabolic rates assessed by positron emission tomography with [18F]2-deoxyglucose in affective illness. *Journal of Affective Disorders, 10*(2), 137–152.

Camardese, G., Di Giuda, D., Di Nicola, M., Cocciolillo, F., Giordano, A., Janiri, L., & Guglielmo, R. (2014). Imaging studies on dopamine transporter and depression: A review of literature and suggestions for future research. *Journal of Psychiatric Research, 51C*, 7–18.

Cannon, D. M., Ichise, M., Fromm, S. J., Nugent, A. C., Rollis, D., Gandhi, S. K., & Drevets, W. C. (2006). Serotonin transporter binding in bipolar disorder assessed using [11C]DASB and positron emission tomography. *Biological Psychiatry, 60*(3), 207–217.

Cannon, D. M., Ichise, M., Rollis, D., Klaver, J. M., Gandhi, S. K., Charney, D. S.,…Drevets, W. C. (2007). Elevated serotonin transporter binding in major depressive disorder assessed using positron emission tomography and [11C]DASB; comparison with bipolar disorder. *Biological Psychiatry, 62*(8), 870–877.

Christakou, A., Gershman, S. J., Niv, Y., Simmons, A., Brammer, M., & Rubia, K. (2013). Neural and psychological maturation of decision-making in adolescence and young adulthood. *Journal of Cognitive Neuroscience, 25*(11), 1807–1823.

Coffman, J. A., Bornstein, R. A., Olson, S. C., Schwarzkopf, S. B., & Nasrallah, H. A. (1990). Cognitive impairment and cerebral structure by MRI in bipolar disorder. *Biological Psychiatry, 27*(11), 1188–1196.

Diler, R. S., Ladouceur, C. D., Segreti, A., Almeida, J. R. C., Birmaher, B., Axelson, D. A.,…Pan, L. A. (2013). Neural correlates of treatment response in depressed bipolar adolescents during emotion processing. *Brain Imaging and Behavior, 7*(2), 227–235.

Drevets, W. C. (1999). Prefrontal cortical-amygdalar metabolism in major depression. *Annals of the New York Academy of Sciences, 877*, 614–637.

Drevets, W. C. (2000). Neuroimaging studies of mood disorders. *Biological Psychiatry, 48*(8), 813–829.

Drevets, W. C., Price, J. L., Bardgett, M. E., Reich, T., Todd, R. D., & Raichle, M. E. (2002). Glucose metabolism in the amygdala in depression: Relationship to diagnostic subtype and plasma cortisol levels. *Pharmacology, Biochemistry, and Behavior, 71*(3), 431–447.

Drevets, W. C., Price, J. L., Simpson, J. R. Jr., Todd, R. D., Reich, T., Vannier, M., & Raichle, M. E. (1997). Subgenual prefrontal cortex abnormalities in mood disorders. *Nature, 386*(6627), 824–827.

Drevets, W. C., Savitz, J., & Trimble, M. (2008). The subgenual anterior cingulate cortex in mood disorders. *CNS Spectrums, 13*(8), 663–681.

Drevets, W. C., Videen, T. O., Price, J. L., Preskorn, S. H., Carmichael, S. T., & Raichle, M. E. (1992). A functional anatomical study of unipolar depression. *The Journal of Neuroscience, 12*(9), 3628–3641.

Gonul, A. S., Coburn, K., & Kula, M. (2009). Cerebral blood flow, metabolic, receptor, and transporter changes in bipolar disorder: The role of PET and SPECT studies. *International Review of Psychiatry, 21*(4), 323–335.

Goodwin, G. M., Cavanagh, T. O., Glabus, M. F., Kehoe, R. F., O'Carroll, R. E., & Ebmeier, K. P. (1997). Uptake of 99mTc-exametazime shown by single photon emission computed tomography before and after lithium withdrawal in bipolar patients: associations with mania. *The British Journal of Psychiatry, 179*, 426–430.

Greene, A., Bailey, C., & Neumeister, A. (2013). A biopsychosocial approach to anxiety. In S. Stahl & B. Moore (Eds.), *Anxiety disorders: A guide for integrating psychopharmacology and psychotherapy*. New York: Routledge.

Hajek, T., Novak, T., Kopecek, M., Gunde, E., Alda, M., & Höschl, C. (2010). Subgenual cingulate volumes in offspring of bipolar parents and in sporadic bipolar patients. *European Archives of Psychiatry and Clinical Neuroscience, 260*(4), 297–304.

Hirayasu, Y., Shenton, M. E., Salisbury, D. F., Kwon, J. S., Wible, C. G., Fischer, I. A., & McCarley, R. W. (1999). Subgenual cingulate cortex volume in first-episode psychosis. *The American Journal of Psychiatry, 156*(7), 1091–1093.

Hosokawa, T., Momose, T., & Kasai, K. (2009). Brain glucose metabolism difference between bipolar and unipolar mood disorders in depressed and euthymic states. *Progress in Neuro-Psychopharmacology & Biological Psychiatry, 33*(2), 243–250.

Ichimiya, T., Suhara, T., Sudo, Y., Okubo, Y., Nakayama, K., Nankai, M., & Shibuya, H. (2002). Serotonin transporter binding in patients with mood disorders: A PET study with [11C](+)McN5652. *Biological Psychiatry, 51*(9), 715–722.

Ito, H., Kawashima, R., Awata, S., Ono, S., Sato, K., Goto, R., & Fukuda, H. (1996). Hypoperfusion in the limbic system and prefrontal cortex in depression: SPECT with anatomic standardization technique. *Journal of Nuclear Medicine, 37*(3), 410–414.

Ketter, T. A., Kimbrell, T. A., George, M. S., Dunn, R. T., Speer, A. M., Benson, B. E., & Post, R. M. (2001). Effects of mood and subtype on cerebral glucose metabolism in treatment-resistant bipolar disorder. *Biological Psychiatry, 49*(2), 97–109.

Kim, P., Jenkins, S. E., Connolly, M. E., Deveney, C. M., Fromm, S. J., Brotman, M. A., & Leibenluft, E. (2012). Neural correlates of cognitive flexibility in children at risk for bipolar disorder. *Journal of Psychiatric Research, 46*(1), 22–30.

Kishimoto, H., Takazu, O., Ohno, S., Yamaguchi, T., Fujita, H., Kuwahara, H., & Iio, M. (1987). 11C-glucose metabolism in manic and depressed patients. *Psychiatry Research, 22*(1), 81–88.

Kohn, N., Falkenberg, I., Kellermann, T., Eickhoff, S. B., Gur, R. C., & Habel, U. (2013). Neural correlates of effective and ineffective mood induction. *Social Cognitive and Affective Neuroscience, 9*(6), 864–872.

Krishna, V. N., Thunga, R., Unnikrishnan, B., Kanchan, T., Bukelo, M. J., Mehta, R. K., & Venugopal, A. (2013). Association between bipolar affective disorder and thyroid dysfunction. *Asian Journal of Psychiatry, 6*(1), 42–45. doi:10.1016/j.ajp.2012.08.003

Krüger, S., Alda, M., Young, L. T., Goldapple, K., Parikh, S., & Mayberg, H. S. (2006). Risk and resilience markers in bipolar disorder: Brain responses to emotional challenge in bipolar patients and their healthy siblings. *The American Journal of Psychiatry, 163*(2), 257–264.

Krüger, S., Seminowicz, D., Goldapple, K., Kennedy, S. H., & Mayberg, H. S. (2003). State and trait influences on mood regulation in bipolar disorder: Blood flow differences with an acute mood challenge. *Biological Psychiatry, 54*(11), 1274–1283.

Lan, M. J., Hesselgrave, N., Ciarleglio, A., Ogden, R. T., Sullivan, G. M., Mann, J. J., & Parsey, R. V. (2013). Higher pretreatment 5-HT1A receptor binding potential in bipolar disorder depression is associated with treatment remission: A naturalistic treatment pilot PET study. *Synapse, 67*(11), 773–778.

LeDoux, J. (1998). Fear and the brain: Where have we been, and where are we going? *Biological Psychiatry, 44*(12), 1229–1238.

Li, C.-T., Hsieh, J.-C., Wang, S.-J., Yang, B.-H., Bai, Y.-M., Lin, W.-C., & Su, T.-P. (2012). Differential relations between fronto-limbic metabolism and executive function in patients with remitted bipolar I and bipolar II disorder. *Bipolar Disorders, 14*(8), 831–842.

Lim, C. S., Baldessarini, R. J., Vieta, E., Yucel, M., Bora, E., & Sim, K. (2013). Longitudinal neuroimaging and neuropsychological changes in bipolar disorder patients: Review of the evidence. *Neuroscience and Biobehavioral Reviews, 37*(3), 418–435.

Mah, L., Zarate, C. A. Jr., Singh, J., Duan, Y.-F., Luckenbaugh, D. A., Manji, H. K., & Drevets, W. C. (2007). Regional cerebral glucose metabolic abnormalities in bipolar II depression. *Biological Psychiatry, 61*(6), 765–775.

Metter, E. J., Hanson, W., Wasterlain, C. G., Kuhl, D. E., & Phelps, M. (1979). Usefulness of [18F]-deoxyglucose local metabolic rates in aphasia. *Transactions of the American Neurological Association, 104*, 200–203.

Mitsunaga, M. M., Garrett, A., Howe, M., Karchemskiy, A., Reiss, A., & Chang, K. (2011). Increased subgenual cingulate cortex volume in pediatric bipolar disorder associated with mood stabilizer exposure. *Journal of Child and Adolescent Psychopharmacology, 21*(2), 149–155.

Moore, G. J., Cortese, B. M., Glitz, D. A., Zajac-Benitez, C., Quiroz, J. A., Uhde, T. W., & Manji, H. K. (2009). A longitudinal study of the effects of lithium treatment on prefrontal and subgenual prefrontal gray matter volume in treatment-responsive bipolar disorder patients. *Journal of Clinical Psychiatry, 70*(5), 699–705.

Morice, R. (1990). Cognitive inflexibility and pre-frontal dysfunction in schizophrenia and mania. *The British Journal of Psychiatry, 157*, 50–54.

Murrough, J. W., Czermak, C., Henry, S., Nabulsi, N., Gallezot, J.-D., Gueorguieva, R.,…Neumeister, A. (2011). The effect of early trauma exposure on serotonin type 1B receptor expression revealed by reduced selective radioligand binding. *Archives of General Psychiatry, 68*(9), 892–900.

Nugent, A. C., Bain, E. E., Carlson, P. J., Neumeister, A., Bonne, O., Carson, R. E., & Drevets, W. C. (2013). Reduced post-synaptic serotonin type 1A receptor binding in bipolar depression. *European Neuropsychopharmacology, 23*(8), 822–829.

Ongür, D., Drevets, W. C., & Price, J. L. (1998). Glial reduction in the subgenual prefrontal cortex in mood disorders. *Proceedings of the National Academy of Sciences of the United States of America, 95*(22), 13290–13295.

Oquendo, M. A., Hastings, R. S., Huang, Y.-Y., Simpson, N., Ogden, R. T., Hu, X.-Z., & Parsey, R. V. (2007). Brain serotonin transporter binding in depressed patients with bipolar disorder using positron emission tomography. *Archives of General Psychiatry, 64*(2), 201–208. doi:10.1001/archpsyc.64.2.201

Pearlson, G. D., Wong, D. F., Tune, L. E., Ross, C. A., Chase, G. A., Links, J. M., & Wagner, H. N. Jr. (1995). In vivo D2 dopamine receptor density in psychotic and nonpsychotic patients with bipolar disorder. *Archives of General Psychiatry, 52*(6), 471–477.

Phelps, M. E., Mazziotta, J. C., Baxter, L., & Gerner, R. (1984). Positron emission tomographic study of affective disorders: Problems and strategies. *Annals of Neurology, 15*(Suppl.), S149–156.

Pompili, M., Gibiino, S., Innamorati, M., Serafini, G., Del Casale, A., De Risio, L.,…Girardi, P. (2012). Prolactin and thyroid hormone levels are associated with suicide attempts in psychiatric patients. *Psychiatry Research, 200*(2–3), 389–394.

Rubinsztein, J. S., Fletcher, P. C., Rogers, R. D., Ho, L. W., Aigbirhio, F. I., Paykel, E. S.,…Sahakian, B. J. (2001). Decision-making in mania: A PET study. *Brain, 124*(Pt. 12), 2550–2563.

Sanches, M., Sassi, R. B., Axelson, D., Nicoletti, M., Brambilla, P., Hatch, J. P., & Soares, J. C. (2005). Subgenual prefrontal cortex of child and adolescent bipolar patients: A morphometric magnetic resonance imaging study. *Psychiatry Research, 138*(1), 43–49.

Sargent, P. A., Kjaer, K. H., Bench, C. J., Rabiner, E. A., Messa, C., Meyer, J.,…Cowen, P. J. (2000). Brain serotonin1A receptor binding measured by positron emission tomography with [11C] WAY-100635: Effects of depression and antidepressant treatment. *Archives of General Psychiatry, 57*, 174–180.

Sargent, P. A., Rabiner, E. A., Bhagwagar, Z., Clark, L., Cowen, P., Goodwin, G. M., & Grasby, P. M. (2010). 5-HT(1A) receptor binding in euthymic bipolar patients using positron emission tomography with [carbonyl-(11)C]WAY-100635. *Journal of Affective Disorders, 123*(1–3), 77–80.

Savitz, J. B., & Drevets, W. C. (2013). Neuroreceptor imaging in depression. *Neurobiology of Disease, 52*, 49–65.

Savitz, J., & Drevets, W. C. (2009). Bipolar and major depressive disorder: neuroimaging the developmental-degenerative divide. *Neuroscience and Biobehavioral Reviews, 33*(5), 699–771.

Schwartz, J. M., Baxter, L. R. Jr., Mazziotta, J. C., Gerner, R. H., & Phelps, M. E. (1987). The differential diagnosis of depression. Relevance of positron emission tomography studies of cerebral glucose metabolism to the bipolar-unipolar dichotomy. *JAMA, 258*(10), 1368–1374.

Sharma, V., Menon, R., Carr, T. J., Densmore, M., Mazmanian, D., & Williamson, P. C. (2003). An MRI study of subgenual prefrontal cortex in patients with familial and non-familial bipolar I disorder. *Journal of Affective Disorders, 77*(2), 167–171.

Singh, M. K., Chang, K. D., Chen, M. C., Kelley, R. G., Garrett, A., Mitsunaga, M. M., & Gotlib, I. H. (2012). Volumetric reductions in the subgenual anterior cingulate cortex in adolescents with bipolar I disorder. *Bipolar Disorders, 14*(6), 585–596.

Singh, M. K., Delbello, M. P., Adler, C. M., Stanford, K. E., & Strakowski, S. M. (2008). Neuroanatomical characterization of child offspring of bipolar parents. *Journal of the American Academy of Child & Adolescent Psychiatry, 47*(5), 526–531.

Strakowski, S. M., Adler, C. M., Almeida, J., Altshuler, L. L., Blumberg, H. P., Chang, K. D., & Townsend, J. D. (2012). The functional neuroanatomy of bipolar disorder: A consensus model. *Bipolar Disorders, 14*(4), 313–325.

Stuss, D. T., & Benson, D. F. (1984). Neuropsychological studies of the frontal lobes. *Psychological Bulletin, 95*(1), 3–28.

Suhara, T., Nakayama, K., Inoue, O., Fukuda, H., Shimizu, M., Mori, A., & Tateno, Y. (1992). D1 dopamine receptor binding in mood disorders measured by positron emission tomography. *Psychopharmacology, 106*(1), 14–18.

Sullivan, G. M., Ogden, R. T., Oquendo, M. A., Kumar, J. S. D., Simpson, N., Huang, Y., & Parsey, R. V. (2009). Positron emission tomography quantification of serotonin-1A receptor binding in medication-free bipolar depression. *Biological Psychiatry, 66*(3), 223–230.

Tutus, A., Simsek, A., Sofuoglu, S., Nardali, M., Kugu, N., Karaaslan, F., & Gönül, A. S. (1998). Changes in regional cerebral blood flow demonstrated by single photon emission computed tomography in depressive disorders: Comparison of unipolar vs. bipolar subtypes. *Psychiatry Research, 83*(3), 169–177.

Wilke, M., Kowatch, R. A., DelBello, M. P., Mills, N. P., & Holland, S. K. (2004). Voxel-based morphometry in adolescents with bipolar disorder: first results. *Psychiatry Research, 131*(1), 57–69.

Wong, D. F., Pearlson, G. D., Tune, L. E., Young, L. T., Meltzer, C. C., Dannals, R. F., & Gjedde, A. (1997). Quantification of neuroreceptors in the living human brain: IV. Effect of aging and elevations of D2-like receptors in schizophrenia and bipolar illness. *Journal of Cerebral Blood Flow and Metabolism, 17*(3), 331–342.

Yatham, L. N., Liddle, P. F., Erez, J., Kauer-Sant'Anna, M., Lam, R. W., Imperial, M., & Ruth, T. J. (2010). Brain serotonin-2 receptors in acute mania. *The British Journal of Psychiatry, 196*(1), 47–51.

Yatham, L. N., Liddle, P. F., Lam, R. W., Adam, M. J., Solomons, K., Chinnapalli, M., & Ruth, T. J. (2005). A positron emission tomography study of the effects of treatment with valproate on brain 5-HT2A receptors in acute mania. *Bipolar Disorders, 7*(Suppl. 5), 53–57.

Yatham, L. N., Liddle, P. F., Lam, R. W., Shiah, I.-S., Lane, C., Stoessl, A. J., & Ruth, T. J. (2002). PET study of the effects of valproate on dopamine D(2) receptors in neuroleptic- and mood-stabilizer-naive patients with nonpsychotic mania. *The American Journal of Psychiatry, 159*(10), 1718–1723.

Zhang, G., Yao, L., Zhang, H., Long, Z., & Zhao, X. (2013). Improved working memory performance through self-regulation of dorsal lateral prefrontal cortex activation using real-time fMRI. *PloS One, 8*(8), e73735.

Zimmerman, M. E., DelBello, M. P., Getz, G. E., Shear, P. K., & Strakowski, S. M. (2006). Anterior cingulate subregion volumes and executive function in bipolar disorder. *Bipolar Disorders, 8*(3), 281–288.

PART V

POSTMORTEM STUDIES

20

POSTMORTEM FINDINGS IN BIPOLAR DISORDER

Dost Öngür

INTRODUCTION

It is now widely accepted that mood disorders, including bipolar disorder (BD), are associated with significant abnormalities in the cellular composition of brain areas involved in processing emotional stimuli and setting mood (Banasr, Dwyer, & Duman, 2011; Harrison, 2002). These abnormalities include altered densities of neurons and glial cells (Cotter, Pariante, & Everall, 2001; Rajkowska & Miguel-Hidalgo, 2007). The term *glia* is derived from the Greek word for "glue," which reflects the now-classic conceptualization of the primary role of these cells in the brain as supportive (Golgi, 1989). We now know that glia play an active role as partners to neurons in normal brain function, as well as in the pathophysiology and treatment of psychiatric illness.

The notion that functions of specific cellular elements in the brain are abnormal in BD and that treatments target these abnormalities was established largely thanks to postmortem brain research. Despite the recent excitement in the field, there are many unanswered questions regarding the relationship between specific anomalies and the pathophysiology of BD. In this chapter, I start by offering some perspective on the contributions of postmortem research, then provide an overview of the evidence for cellular abnormalities in BD derived from postmortem studies. Next I discuss the pathophysiological implications of these findings and then link these findings to recent efforts at treatment development in BD. For a more detailed picture of postmortem research in BD, the reader is referred to other work on the topic (Cotter, Hudson, & Landau, 2005; Harrison, 2002; Rajkowska, 2002; Rajkowska & Miguel-Hidalgo, 2007).

CHALLENGES OF POSTMORTEM RESEARCH

Postmortem brain research in psychiatry was long considered a fruitless endeavor. This arose from the fact that psychiatric disorders, unlike neurological ones, were not associated with gross abnormalities in brain appearance at autopsy and did not show any microscopic abnormalities with casual pathological examination. However, starting in the 1980s, the development of modern cellular and molecular staining tools opened a whole new window onto brain abnormalities in psychiatric disorders. Armed with immunohistochemistry and several other techniques, investigators were able to examine specific cellular processes that were not previously amenable to study in major psychiatric conditions. This development led to the emergence of a large literature on postmortem brain research in psychiatry. For the first time, we could probe specific cell types or the expression of specific proteins in a spatially specific manner, for example across different cortical layers or within pre- or postsynaptic cellular structures.

The promise of this line of research does nothing short of reveal the cellular basis of mental disorders. The advances described in this chapter provide evidence that significant insights can indeed be obtained from this work. On the other hand, a word of caution is required to temper the excitement and place postmortem findings in perspective. The limitations of postmortem research in psychiatry come from two main sources: the small sample sizes and unavoidable confounds. Since this research relies on brain donations, brain banks often take years to accumulate samples from sufficient numbers of patients. The largest postmortem research publications have 15 or so brains in each diagnostic category. These numbers are often not sufficient to explore the impact of clinical and demographic factors on any disease-related finding. This issue has limited excitement around postmortem studies since the early days. The second limitation has to do with unavoidable confounds. Because brain samples can only be obtained after death, researchers cannot control the circumstances prior to donation. Variable agonal periods and postmortem intervals introduce significant variability into the quality of the brain tissue available for research. In addition, since researchers often have access to a relatively small number of brains from individuals with and without the disorder of interest, they have to accept the fact that some of these individuals may have abused substances; had comorbid psychiatric, neurological, or medical conditions; or have been exposed to an unknown number and variety of toxins, environmental stressors, head injuries, and the like. In essence, postmortem findings integrate over a lifetime of uncontrolled exposures, and this has to be weighed in the interpretation of any significant findings associated with the disorder of interest.

Taken together, the foregoing discussion captures both the excitement and promise of this line of research, as well as the cautionary note that the findings need to be evaluated carefully and corroborated with convergent evidence from other modalities. What follows is an overview of what we have learned about BD from postmortem studies, keeping these issues in mind.

NEURONS

Studies of brain tissue from patients with BD were not widely reported until the last decade. Improved brain collection and preservation techniques have now provided opportunities that were not available previously. Most early attention was understandably on neurons. As the "business end" of the brain, their critical involvement in information processing made neurons clear candidates for discovering abnormalities. There have indeed been reports of abnormal neuronal packing density (Harrison, 2002) as well as neuronal cell body size (Cotter et al., 2005) in parts of the prefrontal cortex and in the amygdala (Berretta, Pantazopoulos, & Lange, 2007). These findings are also commonly reported in major depressive disorder and schizophrenia, suggesting they may characterize most major psychiatric conditions and are not specifically related to the pathophysiology of BD. There are other reports of abnormalities in GABAergic interneuron subtypes that may have some mechanistic significance. There is a reduction in the density of calbindin containing

GABAergic interneurons in the anterior cingulate cortex in BD, as well as abnormal spatial clustering of parvalbumin containing GABAergic interneurons (Cotter, Landau, et al., 2002). BD-specific abnormalities have also been reported in the hippocampus in parvalbumin and somatostatin containing GABAergic interneurons, including in cell size, packing density, and mRNA levels of key proteins in these neurons (Heckers et al., 2002; Konradi et al., 2011; Wang et al., 2011). These findings have been interpreted as reflecting abnormal GABAergic inhibition in BD and may have pathophysiologic significance (Benes & Berretta, 2001).

A different line of postmortem research suggests that neurons in BD are under oxidative stress and that this stress impacts mitochondrial function negatively (Andreazza et al., 2009; Andreazza et al., 2008; Andreazza, Shao, Wang, & Young, 2010; Andreazza, Wang, Salmasi, Shao, & Young, 2013; Andreazza & Young, 2014). Indeed, bioenergetic abnormalities secondary to mitochondrial dysfunction have long been suggested in BD (Stork & Renshaw, 2005). Although this research has consistently found abnormalities, it is not clear what these mean for neuronal activity and information processing in the brain.

GLIAL CELLS

Recent work has also provided consistent evidence for reductions in the density and number of glial cells in areas of the prefrontal cortex and in the amygdala in BD (Bowley, Drevets, Ongur, & Price, 2002; Cotter, Mackay, et al., 2002; Cotter, Mackay, Landau, Kerwin, & Everall, 2001; Harrison, 2002; Öngür, Drevets, & Price, 1998; Rajkowska, Halaris, & Selemon, 2001). In one study, researchers attempted to subtype glial cells in BD and concluded that oligodendrocytes were selectively reduced in the amygdala (Hamidi, Drevets, & Price, 2004). Similar reductions in glial number were not seen in somatosensory area 3b, an area not implicated in emotional processing selected as a control region (Öngür et al., 1998). Gene expression studies in postmortem brains have led to findings that suggest glial abnormalities, including reduced expression of oligodendrocyte related transcripts in BD (Tkachev et al., 2003). Postmortem studies have also found reductions in glial number in the hippocampus (Korbo, 1999) and dorsolateral prefrontal cortex in alcoholism, with and without comorbid mood disorder (Miguel-Hidalgo & Rajkowska, 2003).

Why are these findings relevant? There are three subtypes of glia: astrocytes, oligodendrocytes, and microglia. Astrocytes are enriched in the grey matter and are metabolically and morphologically activated by a variety of signals (Pekny & Nilsson, 2005). These cells are important for numerous brain processes, including but not limited to gliotic response to brain injury (Sofroniew, 2005), coupling neuronal activity with cerebral metabolism (Kasischke, Vishwasrao, Fisher, Zipfel, & Webb, 2004; Magistretti & Pellerin, 1999), and ion channel and neurotransmitter transporter synthesis (Gallo & Ghiani, 2000). Astrocytes ensheathe synapses in the CNS, and they modulate neurotransmission by taking up glutamate and GABA from the synaptic cleft (Araque, Sanzgiri, Parpura, & Haydon, 1999). This close apposition led to the term *tripartite synapse*, acknowledging the astrocyte as an essential part of the synapse along with the presynaptic and postsynaptic neurons (Araque, Parpura, Sanzgiri, & Haydon, 1999). Astrocytes also modulate synapse numbers in cell culture, perhaps playing a role in inducing and stabilizing synapses (Ullian, Sapperstein, Christopherson, & Barres, 2001). Notably, astrocytes synthesize a number of neuromodulators, including d-serine, a partial agonist at the N-methyl-D-aspartate glutamate receptor site (Boehning & Snyder, 2003); adenosine, a tonic suppressor of synaptic transmission (Halassa, Fellin, & Haydon, 2009; Halassa, Florian, et al., 2009; Pascual et al., 2005); and glutathione, the main antioxidant in the brain (Dringen, Gutterer, & Hirrlinger, 2000).

Oligodendrocytes are smaller, enriched in the white matter, and responsible for myelin synthesis. The interaction between oligodendrocytes and axons is complex; these glia can help generate sprouting of axons, while axonal signals are needed in turn for oligodendrocyte survival (Miller, 2002). Abnormalities specific to oligodendrocytes have been reported in BD (Bowley et al., 2002; Edgar & Sibille, 2012).

Microglia are derived from peripheral blood macrophages and mediate the brain's inflammatory response (Schwartz, 2003). Although they have been implicated in a variety of neuropsychiatric conditions, including Alzheimer's disease (Aguzzi, Barres, & Bennett, 2013), autism spectrum disorders (Hughes, 2012), and AIDS-related dementia, they have not yet been the focus of study in mood disorders.

IMPLICATIONS FOR PATHOPHYSIOLOGY AND TREATMENT DEVELOPMENT

Postmortem findings in BD have specific pathophysiologic implications since neuronal and glial cell subtypes have differing functions. For example, reports highlighting GABAergic interneurons in the cortex and hippocampus suggest abnormal inhibitory circuit activity in BD. This is consistent with the GABAergic activity of many commonly used mood-stabilizing medications (Li, Ketter, & Frye, 2002), as well as electroconvulsive therapy (Kato, 2009), a highly effective treatment for mood disorders. Among glial cells, abnormalities are seen in astrocytes and oligodendrocytes but not yet microglia, suggesting that synaptic function (see also Lopez de Lara et al., 2010) and white matter integrity are impacted, but immune monitoring and inflammatory response may not be. Astrocytes play a major role in handling glutamate released into the synaptic cleft (Figure 20.1), and they release glutamate receptor modulators. Therefore abnormalities in astrocytes implicate abnormal glutamatergic neurotransmission in BD. This is consistent with abnormalities reported in expression of genes involved in glutamate signaling as well (Beneyto, Kristiansen, Oni-Orisan, McCullumsmith, & Meador-Woodruff, 2007).

How can we reconcile the GABAergic and glutamatergic findings in BD postmortem? These two are the major inhibitory and excitatory systems in the brain, respectively. There is an intricate balance between inhibition and excitation in the brain, and disruption of one system is sure to impact the other. For example, in schizophrenia abnormalities in N-methyl-D-aspartate receptors localized on GABAergic, interneurons are thought to drive circuit-wide disruptions in information processing (Coyle, 2004; Lisman et al., 2008). Although the evidence base is not as developed in BD as in schizophrenia, it is not surprising to find concurrent abnormalities in glutamate and GABA in this condition. Therefore the picture in BD is likely to be one of generalized abnormalities in the brain's ability to regulate excitation–inhibition balance in its circuitry (related concepts are discussed in Uhlhaas & Singer, 2012).

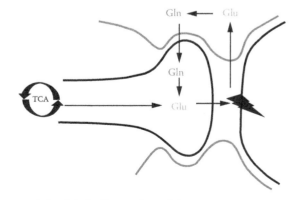

Figure 20.1 Role of glial cells in cycling of glutamate at the synapse. Glutamate (Glu) can be synthesized de novo from the tricyclic acid (TCA) cycle. Once it is released into the synapse, it is taken up by glial cells (red profiles) and converted to glutamine (Gln). Gln is then free to diffuse back to neurons where it is converted back to Glu.

This discussion also suggests that treatment interventions that regulate the excitation–inhibition balance or modify activity at glutamatergic and GABAergic synapses may be salutary in BD. The most recent example of such an approach is ketamine, which has antidepressant properties in BD (Diazgranados et al., 2010). Ketamine has a strikingly rapid onset of antidepressant action, suggesting that it may act at nodes that are critical for the setting of mood. This is unlike currently used antidepressant medications, which take full effect over four to six weeks and likely act in distant sites upstream from these critical nodes. The postmortem literature strongly supports the recent emergence of interest in glutamatergic and GABAergic pharmacotherapies in BD. It is hoped that ketamine is only the first example of novel mood disorder therapeutics with high efficacy and rapid onset of action.

The other biological system that is highlighted by postmortem findings in BD is the white matter. Information processing in the human brain depends critically on white matter integrity (Nave, 2010). Abnormalities in this system, such as those seen in BD, would have major consequences for brain function. These findings are also consistent with the in vivo human neuroimaging literature in this condition (Heng, Song, & Sim, 2010). It is not clear what kind of disruption in information processing will arise from the specific white matter changes seen in BD, and more work is needed to elucidate this issue (Figure 20.2). Nonetheless, treatments that might improve white matter health, and especially oligodendrocyte function, may prove beneficial in this condition. This is a relatively understudied area and a suggested area of future focus.

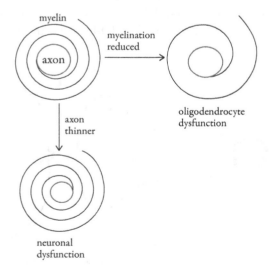

Figure 20.2 Potential mechanisms of white matter abnormalities in bipolar disorder, demonstrating the role of neuronal or oligodendrocyte dysfunction. Note that these two mechanisms are not mutually exclusive and in fact likely occur in concert in any potential pathology.

FUTURE DIRECTIONS

Postmortem research has highlighted glutamate and GABA mechanisms as well as white matter integrity as relevant to the pathophysiology of BD. Multiple questions still need to be answered before these insights can be translated into diagnostic and therapeutic advances for those already suffering and to measures to prevent BD in those at risk. However, the impetus provided by postmortem studies has already generated useful advances and offered hope for future developments in our field.

Disclosure statement: Dr. Dost Öngür was on the Scientific Advisory Board for Lilly in 2013.

REFERENCES

Aguzzi, A., Barres, B. A., & Bennett, M. L. (2013). Microglia: scapegoat, saboteur, or something else? *Science, 339*(6116), 156–161. doi: 10.1126/science.1227901

Andreazza, A. C., Kapczinski, F., Kauer-Sant'Anna, M., Walz, J. C., Bond, D. J., Goncalves, C. A., . . . Yatham, L. N. (2009). 3-Nitrotyrosine and glutathione antioxidant system in patients in the early and late stages of bipolar disorder. *Journal of Psychiatry Neuroscience, 34*(4), 263–271.

Andreazza, A. C., Kauer-Sant'Anna, M., Frey, B. N., Bond, D. J., Kapczinski, F., Young, L. T., & Yatham, L. N. (2008). Oxidative stress markers in bipolar disorder: A meta-analysis. *Journal of Affective Disorders, 111*(2–3), 135–144. doi:10.1016/j.jad.2008.04.013

Andreazza, A. C., Shao, L., Wang, J. F., & Young, L. T. (2010). Mitochondrial complex I activity and oxidative damage to mitochondrial proteins in the prefrontal cortex of patients with bipolar disorder. *Archives of General Psychiatry, 67*(4), 360–368. doi:10.1001/archgenpsychiatry.2010.22

Andreazza, A. C., Wang, J. F., Salmasi, F., Shao, L., & Young, L. T. (2013). Specific subcellular changes in oxidative stress in prefrontal cortex from patients with bipolar disorder. *Journal of Neurochemistry, 127*(4), 552–561. doi:10.1111/jnc.12316

Andreazza, A. C., & Young, L. T. (2014). The neurobiology of bipolar disorder: Identifying targets for specific agents and synergies for combination treatment. *International Journal of Neuropsychopharmacology, 17*(7), 1039–1052. doi:10.1017/S1461145713000096

Araque, A., Parpura, V., Sanzgiri, R. P., & Haydon, P. G. (1999). Tripartite synapses: Glia, the unacknowledged partner. *Trends in Neuroscience, 22*(5), 208–215.

Araque, A., Sanzgiri, R. P., Parpura, V., & Haydon, P. G. (1999). Astrocyte-induced modulation of synaptic transmission. *Canadian Journal of Physiology and Pharmacology, 77*(9), 699–706.

Banasr, M., Dwyer, J. M., & Duman, R. S. (2011). Cell atrophy and loss in depression: Reversal by antidepressant treatment [Review]. *Current Opinions in Cell Biology, 23*(6), 730–737. doi:10.1016/j.ceb.2011.09.002

Benes, F. M., & Berretta, S. (2001). Gabaergic interneurons: Implications for understanding schizophrenia and bipolar disorder. *Neuropsychopharmacology, 25*, 1–27.

Beneyto, M., Kristiansen, L. V., Oni-Orisan, A., McCullumsmith, R. E., & Meador-Woodruff, J. H. (2007). Abnormal glutamate receptor expression in the medial temporal lobe in schizophrenia and mood disorders. *Neuropsychopharmacology, 32*(9), 1888–1902. doi:10.1038/sj.npp.1301312

Berretta, S., Pantazopoulos, H., & Lange, N. (2007). Neuron numbers and volume of the amygdala in subjects diagnosed with bipolar disorder or schizophrenia. *Biological Psychiatry*, *62*(8), 884–893.

Boehning, D., & Snyder, S. H. (2003). Novel neural modulators. *Annual Reviews of Neuroscience*, *26*, 105–131.

Bowley, M. P., Drevets, W. C., Ongur, D., & Price, J. L. (2002). Low glial numbers in the amygdala in major depressive disorder. *Biological Psychiatry*, *52*(5), 404–412.

Cotter, D., Hudson, L., & Landau, S. (2005). Evidence for orbitofrontal pathology in bipolar disorder and major depression, but not in schizophrenia. *Bipolar Disorders*, *7*(4), 358–369. doi:10.1111/j.1399-5618.2005.00230.x

Cotter, D., Landau, S., Beasley, C., Stevenson, R., Chana, G., MacMillan, L., & Everall, I. (2002). The density and spatial distribution of GABAergic neurons, labelled using calcium binding proteins, in the anterior cingulate cortex in major depressive disorder, bipolar disorder, and schizophrenia. *Biological Psychiatry*, *51*(5), 377–386.

Cotter, D., Mackay, D., Chana, G., Beasley, C., Landau, S., & Everall, I. P. (2002). Reduced neuronal size and glial cell density in area 9 of the dorsolateral prefrontal cortex in subjects with major depressive disorder. *Cerebral Cortex*, *12*(4), 386–394.

Cotter, D., Mackay, D., Landau, S., Kerwin, R., & Everall, I. (2001). Reduced glial cell density and neuronal size in the anterior cingulate cortex in major depressive disorder. *Archives of General Psychiatry*, *58*(6), 545–553.

Cotter, D. R., Pariante, C. M., & Everall, I. P. (2001). Glial cell abnormalities in major psychiatric disorders: the evidence and implications. *Brain Research Bulletin*, *55*(5), 585–595.

Coyle, J. T. (2004). The GABA-glutamate connection in schizophrenia: Which is the proximate cause? *Biochemical Pharmacology*, *68*(8), 1507–1514.

Diazgranados, N., Ibrahim, L., Brutsche, N. E., Newberg, A., Kronstein, P., Khalife, S., . . . Zarate, C. A., Jr. (2010). A randomized add-on trial of an N-methyl-D-aspartate antagonist in treatment-resistant bipolar depression. *Archives of General Psychiatry*, *67*(8), 793–802. doi:10.1001/archgenpsychiatry.2010.90

Dringen, R., Gutterer, J. M., & Hirrlinger, J. (2000). Glutathione metabolism in brain metabolic interaction between astrocytes and neurons in the defense against reactive oxygen species. *European Journal of Biochemistry*, *267*(16), 4912–4916.

Edgar, N., & Sibille, E. (2012). A putative functional role for oligodendrocytes in mood regulation. *Transl Psychiatry*, *2*, e109. doi:10.1038/tp.2012.34

Gallo, V., & Ghiani, C. A. (2000). Glutamate receptors in glia: new cells, new inputs and new functions. *Trends in Pharmacological Sciences*, *21*(7), 252–258.

Golgi, C. (1989). On the structure of nerve cells. *Journal of Microsociology*, *155*(Pt. 1), 3–7.

Halassa, M. M., Fellin, T., & Haydon, P. G. (2009). Tripartite synapses: roles for astrocytic purines in the control of synaptic physiology and behavior [Review]. *Neuropharmacology*, *57*(4), 343–346. doi:10.1016/j.neuropharm.2009.06.031

Halassa, M. M., Florian, C., Fellin, T., Munoz, J. R., Lee, S. Y., Abel, T., . . . Frank, M. G. (2009). Astrocytic modulation of sleep homeostasis and cognitive consequences of sleep loss. *Neuron*, *61*(2), 213–219. doi:10.1016/j.neuron.2008.11.024

Hamidi, M., Drevets, W. C., & Price, J. L. (2004). Glial reduction in amygdala in major depressive disorder is due to oligodendrocytes. *Biological Psychiatry*, *55*(6), 563–569.

Harrison, P. J. (2002). The neuropathology of primary mood disorder. *Brain*, *125*(Pt. 7), 1428–1449.

Heckers, S., Stone, D., Walsh, J., Shick, J., Koul, P., & Benes, F. M. (2002). Differential hippocampal expression of glutamic acid decarboxylase 65 and 67 messenger RNA in bipolar disorder and schizophrenia. *Archives in General Psychiatry*, *59*(6), 521–529.

Heng, S., Song, A. W., & Sim, K. (2010). White matter abnormalities in bipolar disorder: Insights from diffusion tensor imaging studies. *Journal of Neural Transmission*, *117*(5), 639–654. doi:10.1007/s00702-010-0368-9

Hughes, V. (2012). Microglia: The constant gardeners. *Nature*, *485*(7400), 570–572. doi:10.1038/485570a

Kasischke, K. A., Vishwasrao, H. D., Fisher, P. J., Zipfel, W. R., & Webb, W. W. (2004). Neural activity triggers neuronal oxidative metabolism followed by astrocytic glycolysis. *Science*, *305*(5680), 99–103.

Kato, N. (2009). Neurophysiological mechanisms of electroconvulsive therapy for depression. *Neuroscience Research*, *64*(1), 3–11. doi:10.1016/j.neures.2009.01.014

Konradi, C., Zimmerman, E. I., Yang, C. K., Lohmann, K. M., Gresch, P., Pantazopoulos, H., . . . Heckers, S. (2011). Hippocampal interneurons in bipolar disorder. *Archives of General Psychiatry*, *68*(4), 340–350. doi:10.1001/archgenpsychiatry.2010.175

Korbo, L. (1999). Glial cell loss in the hippocampus of alcoholics. *Alcoholism: Clinical and Experimental Research*, *23*(1), 164–168.

Li, X., Ketter, T. A., & Frye, M. A. (2002). Synaptic, intracellular, and neuroprotective mechanisms of anticonvulsants: Are they relevant for the treatment and course of bipolar disorders? [Review]. *Journal of Affective Disorders*, *69*(1–3), 1–14.

Lisman, J. E., Coyle, J. T., Green, R. W., Javitt, D. C., Benes, F. M., Heckers, S., & Grace, A. A. (2008). Circuit-based framework for understanding neurotransmitter and risk gene interactions in schizophrenia. *Trends in Neuroscience*, *31*(5), 234–242.

Lopez de Lara, C., Jaitovich-Groisman, I., Cruceanu, C., Mamdani, F., Lebel, V., Yerko, V., . . . Turecki, G. (2010). Implication of synapse-related genes in bipolar disorder by linkage and gene expression analyses. *International Journal of Neuropsychopharmacology*, *13*(10), 1397–1410. doi:10.1017/S1461145710000714

Magistretti, P. J., & Pellerin, L. (1999). Astrocytes couple synaptic activity to glucose utilization in the brain. *News in Physiological Sciences*, *14*, 177–182.

Miguel-Hidalgo, J. J., & Rajkowska, G. (2003). Comparison of prefrontal cell pathology between depression and alcohol dependence. *Journal of Psychiatry Research*, *37*(5), 411–420.

Miller, R. H. (2002). Regulation of oligodendrocyte development in the vertebrate CNS. *Progress in Neurobiology*, *67*(6), 451–467.

Nave, K. A. (2010). Myelination and the trophic support of long axons. *Nature Reviews Neuroscience*, *11*(4), 275–283. doi:10.1038/nrn2797

Öngür, D., Drevets, W. C., & Price, J. L. (1998). Glial reduction in the subgenual prefrontal cortex in mood disorders. *Proceedings of the National Academy of Sciences of the United States of America*, *95*(22), 13290–13295.

Pascual, O., Casper, K. B., Kubera, C., Zhang, J., Revilla-Sanchez, R., Sul, J. Y., . . . Haydon, P. G. (2005). Astrocytic purinergic signaling coordinates synaptic networks. *Science*, *310*(5745), 113–116.

Pekny, M., & Nilsson, M. (2005). Astrocyte activation and reactive gliosis. *Glia*, *50*(4), 427–434.

Rajkowska, G. (2002). Cell pathology in bipolar disorder. *Bipolar Disorders*, *4*(2), 105–116.

Rajkowska, G., Halaris, A., & Selemon, L. D. (2001). Reductions in neuronal and glial density characterize the dorsolateral prefrontal cortex in bipolar disorder. *Biological Psychiatry*, *49*(9), 741–752.

Rajkowska, G., & Miguel-Hidalgo, J. J. (2007). Gliogenesis and glial pathology in depression. *CNS Neurological Disorder Drug Targets*, *6*(3), 219–233.

Schwartz, M. (2003). Macrophages and microglia in central nervous system injury: are they helpful or harmful? *Journal of Cerebral Blood Flow & Metabolism*, *23*(4), 385–394.

Sofroniew, M. V. (2005). Reactive astrocytes in neural repair and protection. *Neuroscientist*, *11*(5), 400–407.

Stork, C., & Renshaw, P. F. (2005). Mitochondrial dysfunction in bipolar disorder: evidence from magnetic resonance spectroscopy research. *Molecular Psychiatry, 10*(10), 900–919.

Tkachev, D., Mimmack, M. L., Ryan, M. M., Wayland, M., Freeman, T., Jones, P. B., . . . Bahn, S. (2003). Oligodendrocyte dysfunction in schizophrenia and bipolar disorder. *Lancet, 362*(9386), 798–805.

Uhlhaas, P. J., & Singer, W. (2012). Neuronal dynamics and neuropsychiatric disorders: Toward a translational paradigm for dysfunctional large-scale networks. *Neuron, 75*(6), 963–980. doi:10.1016/j.neuron.2012.09.004

Ullian, E. M., Sapperstein, S. K., Christopherson, K. S., & Barres, B. A. (2001). Control of synapse number by glia. *Science, 291*(5504), 657–661.

Wang, A. Y., Lohmann, K. M., Yang, C. K., Zimmerman, E. I., Pantazopoulos, H., Herring, N., . . . Konradi, C. (2011). Bipolar disorder type 1 and schizophrenia are accompanied by decreased density of parvalbumin- and somatostatin-positive interneurons in the parahippocampal region. *Acta Neuropathologica, 122*(5), 615–626. doi:10.1007/s00401-011-0881-4

SECTION III

CURRENT TREATMENTS

PART I

PHARMACOLOGICAL TREATMENTS

21.

TREATMENT OF MANIA

Paul E. Keck, Susan L. McElroy, and Ayşegül Yildiz

INTRODUCTION

Manic episodes occurring during the course of bipolar disorder are characterized by severe disturbances in mood, activity, perception, and cognition often constituting medical emergencies and hospitalization to ensure safety and an optimal environment for treatment (Keck & McElroy, 2009). The diagnostic criteria for manic episodes and manic or depressive epsides with mixed features are presented in the Diagnostic and Statistical Manual of Mental Disorders (fifth edition; American Psychiatric Association, 2013; see "Summary of DSM-5 Criteria for Mood Episodes Occurring in Bipolar Disorders," pp. 123–154). Looking beyond these criteria, a majority of patients experiencing manic episodes have accompanying psychotic symptoms, and manic or depressive epsides with mixed features may pose an increased risk of suicidal ideation compared with pure manic presentations (Keck & McElroy, 2009). Moreover, patients in manic or mixed states often have prominent symptoms of anxiety, impulsivity, recklessness, elevated libido, poor insight, inattention, and sensory hyperacuity (Keck & McElroy, 2009).

Fortunately, the treatment of manic episodes has been the target of a substantial body of scientific scrutiny over the past 25 years, leading to the development of a number of agents with demonstrated efficacy in rigorous, randomized controlled clinical trials, as well as intriguing pilot studies of potentially new therapeutic approaches. Here we review the evidence-based treatment of acute manic episodes in patients with bipolar disorder.

SETTING AND TREATMENT GOALS

The goal of treatment of individuals experiencing a manic episode is to provide rapid symptom amelioration toward full remission in a setting that provides for patient safety. Although patients experiencing mild symptoms may be effectively treated on an outpatient basis, for most patients displaying moderate or more severe symptoms, a hospital level of care is usually required.

Patients may be considered to have severe symptoms if they display suicidal, homicidal, or aggressive ideation or behavior; psychotic features; or impaired judgment that places themselves or others at imminent risk of harm. Psychological approaches to patients experiencing manic or mixed episodes focus primarily on deescalation of symptoms, reassurance, establishing a treatment alliance, and ensuring structure and safety in the treatment environment. As symptoms improve, subsequent goals include patient and family education, emphasis on treatment adherence, avoidance of alcohol and substance abuse, and identification of precipitants and prodromal signs of relapse. Pharmacotherapy is the cornerstone of treatment of manic episodes. Essentials of a basic diagnostic evaluation include consideration of possible medical, medicine, or substance-induced causes of manic or mixed symptoms and medical history and physical examination to assess for co-occurring conditions (both psychiatry and medical) that may affect treatment recommendations. Since bipolar disorder is a recurrent and lifelong illness for the vast majority of individuals, the treatment of acute manic episodes also provides a "portal of entry" to establish a foundation of treatment for subsequent maintenance and relapse prevention. Thus treatment considerations may include whether a particular agent with established efficacy in ameliorating manic or mixed symptoms is also an agent that can be successfully maintained beyond remission of the acute index episode. Recommendations regarding acute treatment can be made with an eye toward the efficacy, safety, and tolerability of that treatment in longer term illness management.

EVIDENCE REVIEW: MONOTHERAPY

LITHIUM

Lithium has been an established treatment for acute mania for nearly 60 years. Lithium has demonstrated superior efficacy in numerous randomized controlled trials (RCTs) compared with placebo and comparable efficacy when compared with other antimanic agents, including divalproex, carbamazepine, risperidone, olanzapine, quetiapine, and aripiprazole, as well as first-generation antipsychotic (FGA) agents (Yatham et al., 2013). Patients with psychosis in these trials displayed improvement in tandem with improvement in other manic symptoms. There is some evidence to suggest that patients with manic (rather than mixed) symptoms and relatively few lifetime mood episodes may have a better response to lithium compared to patients who have mixed episodes, recent rapid cycling course of illness, and numerous prior mood episodes (Bowden, 1995).

Response to lithium varies in relationship to plasma concentrations, with high response rates but increased side effects at the upper end of the therapeutic range (1.0–1.4 mmol/L; Keck & McElroy, 2009). Plasma concentrations may be lowered to improve tolerability toward maintenance treatment following remission of symptoms. Improvement in RCTs was usually evident by Day 7 to 14 in patients displaying a response, assuming a gradual titration to therapeutic levels (Keck & McElroy, 2009). The rate of response may be accelerated by more rapid titration (Goldberg, Garno, Leon, Kocsis, & Portera, 1998). Common side effects associated with lithium include nausea, vomiting, tremor, somnolence, weight gain, and cognitive slowing.

VALPROATE (DIVALPROEX, DIVALPROEX ER)

Divalproex (and related formulations of valproic acid) was superior to placebo in seven of eight placebo-controlled trials (Yatham et al., 2013). In the only negative trial, suboptimal dosing and a high drop-out rate may have posed methodological limitations on the results (Hirschfeld, Bowden, Vigna, Wozniak, & Collins, 2010). In one of few studies in ambulatory patients with milder manic symptoms, divalproex was superior to placebo in the reduction of hypomanic and mild to moderate symptoms (McElroy et al., 2010). In trials involving active comparator agents, divalproex had comparable efficacy with lithium, haloperidol, and olanzapine, with one other trial finding superior efficacy for olanzapine. In the olanzapine comparison

trials, differences in starting dose and sample size may have contributed to the mixed results. Response to divalproex does not appear to be predicted by the presence of absence of psychosis or whether patients are displaying manic or mixed symptoms (Yatham et al., 2013).

Divalproex may be administered in a loading dose strategy (20–30 mg/kg/day) designed to produce therapeutic plasma concentrations (50–125 mg/L) within 24 hours and accelerate treatment response (Keck & McElroy, 2009). As with lithium, plasma concentrations at the higher end of the therapeutic range for divalproex may be associated with greater response (Keck & McElroy, 2009).

Common side effects of divalproex reported in trials in patients with acute manic or mixed episodes include somnolence, nausea, vomiting, tremor, weight gain, and cognitive slowing. Rare serious side effects reported with divalproex and related formulations include significant hepatic transaminase elevations, hepatic failure, pancreatitis, thrombocytopenia, hyperammonemicencephalopathy in patients with urea cycle dysfunction, and polycystic ovarian syndrome.

CARBAMAZEPINE

The largest and most definitive controlled trials establishing the efficacy of carbamazepine for the treatment of manic and mixed episodes were studies that showed the superiority of the extended release formulation over placebo (Yatham et al., 2013). One of these two trials found comparable efficacy for carbamazepine in manic and mixed patients whereas the other found greater efficacy in manic patients (although this subgroup analysis was limited by the small number of patients with mixed episodes in the study). In comparison trials, likely limited by small sample sizes, carbamazepine exerted comparable antimanic efficacy with lithium and chlorpromazine (Keck, McElroy, & Nemeroff, 1992).

Therapeutic plasma concentrations of carbamazepine in the treatment of acute mania have not been reliably established, but the range used for the treatment of epilepsy (4–12 mcg/mL) is commonly used as a guide (Keck & McElroy, 2009). Carbamazepine is a potent inducer of cytochrome P450 enzymes, leading to autoinduction of its own metabolism (and subsequent need for dosage adjustment upward in many patients), as well as induction of the metabolism of other agents whose degradation follows through this system.

Common side effects associated with carbamazepine in these studies were somnolence, fatigue, nausea, diplopia, blurred vision, and ataxia. Less common side effects include rash, mild leukopenia, thrombocytopenia, and hyponatremia. Rare serious side effects are agranulocytosis, aplastic anemia, thrombocytopenia, pancreatitis, hepatic failure, Stevens-Johnson syndrome, and toxic epidermal necrolysis. These latter reactions appear to be more common during the early phases of treatment and in individuals with the HLA-B*1502 allele, which is prevalent in Asian populations, including South Asian Indians (Hung et al., 2006). In the Unites States, the Food and Drug Administration recommends screening for the presence of this allele in patients from these higher risk ethnic groups (Yatham et al., 2013).

ANTIPSYCHOTIC AGENTS

Typical (first-generation) antipsychotics

Chlorpromazine was the first antipsychotic (AP) shown to be efficacious in the treatment of acute mania in a randomized, placebo-controlled trial (Klein, 1967). Haloperidol has demonstrated efficacy in the treatment of acute mania in numerous clinical trials, both as a target of study and as an active comparator in trials of other agents (Yatham et al., 2013). In addition to the drawbacks of neurological and neuroendocrinological side effects of these agents, FGAs also appear to increase the risk of postmanic depressive symptoms and episodes (Keck & McElroy, 2009).

ATYPICAL (SECOND-GENERATION) ANTIPSYCHOTICS

Risperidone and paliperidone

RCTs of risperidone monotherapy have demonstrated superior efficacy of risperidone compared with placebo and comparable efficacy compared with olanzapine, haloperidol, and lithium (Yatham et al., 2013). In these trials, risperidone exerted similar therapeutic efficacy in patients with manic or mixed presentations and in patients with or without psychosis. Extrapyramidal side effects were low when risperidone was administered at doses of less than 4 mg/day but not when administered at doses of 6 mg/day (Keck & McElroy, 2009). Other side effects associated with risperidone treatment were akathisia, somnolence, dyspepsia, nausea, and prolactin elevation. Paliperidone (9-hydroxyrisperidone), an active metabolite of risperidone, was superior to placebo in reduction of manic symptoms in 2 placebo-controlled trials (Yatham et al., 2013).

Olanzapine

In monotherapy trials, olanzapine was superior to placebo and comparable to divalproex, haloperidol, and risperidone in mean reduction of manic symptoms (Yatham et al., 2013). Olanzapine was superior to divalproex in one comparison trial, but this may have been due to disparities in dosing and rate of titration (Tohen, Baker, et al., 2002). In studies with an initial starting dose of 15 mg/day, the rate of improvement in manic symptoms was faster than in trials with an initial starting dose of 10 mg/day (Keck & McElroy, 2009). Olanzapine exerted comparable therapeutic effects in patients with manic and mixed symptoms and in patients with or without psychosis. In these short-term trials (three to six weeks in duration), common side effects associated with olanzapine included somnolence, constipation, increased appetite, weight gain, dry mouth, and orthostatic hypotension.

Quetiapine

Quetiapine was superior to placebo and comparable in efficacy to lithium and haloperidol in RCTs of up to 12 weeks duration in patients with acute mania (Yatham et al., 2013). Patients with mixed episodes were excluded from several of these trials, so the efficacy of quetiapine in patients with mixed episodes has not been thoroughly addressed. The mean modal of quetiapine among responders in these trials was 600 mg/day (Keck & McElroy, 2009). Common quetiapine side effects were somnolence, constipation, weight gain, headache, dry mouth, and dizziness.

Ziprasidone

The efficacy of ziprasidone in the treatment of acute manic and mixed episodes has been established as superior efficacy compared with placebo and comparable efficacy compared with haloperidol (Yatham et al., 2013). Ziprasidone was equally effective in patients with and without psychosis. Mean dose associated with response in these trials was 120 mg/day. Common side effects associated with ziprasidone were dizziness, akathisia, extrapyramidal signs, somnolence, and headache. There were no significant adverse effects on appetite or weight gain.

Aripiprazole

Aripiprazole was superior to placebo in three 3-week RCTs and comparable to haloperidol in two 12-week comparison trials (Yatham et al., 2013), one of which included a placebo arm with both aripiprazole and haloperidol demonstrating superiority (Young et al., 2009). Response to aripiprazole was comparable for patients with manic and mixed episodes and with or without psychosis. The mean modal dose of aripiprazole in these studies was 23 mg/day. Aripiprazole-associated side effects were headache, nausea, vomiting, constipation, insomnia, and akathisia.

Asenapine

Asenapine was superior to placebo in improvement in manic and mixed symptoms in two placebo-controlled trials (Yatham et al., 2013). Olanzapine was included as an active comparator in each trial and was superior in efficacy to both placebo and asenapine. The presence of absence of psychosis did not predict response to asenapine. Common side effects associated with asenapine in these trials included somnolence, insomnia, extrapyramidal signs, headache, akathisia, dizziness, weight gain, and elevated triglycerides.

Cariprazine

Cariprazine, an investigational agent in late-phase development at the time of this writing, and a partial D_2/D_3 agonist, was superior to placebo in three 3-week placebo-controlled trials in patient with acute bipolar manic and mixed episodes (Keck et al., 2013). Cariprazine was efficacious in patients with manic and mixed episodes and with or without psychosis at a mean dose of 7.4 mg/day and modal dose of 12 mg/day. Side effects associated with cariprazine were headache, nausea, vomiting, constipation, insomnia, and akathisia.

Other agents

Several positive placebo-controlled pilot studies of the protein kinase C inhibitor tamoxifen (Yildiz, Guleryuz, Ankerst, Ongur, & Renshaw, 2008; Zarate et al., 2007) suggest a promising role for this agent but require replication in larger, RCTs and further data regarding optimal dosing and duration of treatment.

In addition to the positive studies of monotherapies, it is important to review the agents that have not demonstrated efficacy in the treatment of acute manic and mixed episodes. In replicated placebo-controlled trials, gabapentin, topiramate, and verapamil were not superior to placebo in antimanic efficacy (Keck & McElroy, 2009). Moreover, studies of several agents including lamotrigine, oxcarbazepine, tiagabine, and levetiracetam have yielded mixed results or insufficient evidence of antimanic efficacy to date (Keck & McElroy, 2009).

EVIDENCE-REVIEW: COMBINATION THERAPY

The evidence reviewed here is important in establishing the efficacy of agents as monotherapy in acute manic and mixed episodes. In general, absolute response rates (defined as 50% or greater reduction in manic symptoms, unadjusted for placebo response rates) to monotherapy in placebo-controlled three- to four-week trials converge at 50% across most studies, with remission rates of 20% to 25% (again unadjusted for placebo remission rates; Ketter, 2008). Response rates to combination therapy with two antimanic agents are typically higher than with monotherapy, ranging from 65% to 70%, and rate of response is usually accelerated (Suppes et al., 2005). Patients with moderate to severe manic or mixed episodes or with psychosis are particular candidates for combination treatment (Keck & McElroy, 2009).

RCTs of combination (or adjunctive) treatment in patients with manic or mixed episodes have typically examined the efficacy of lithium or divalproex in combination with an AP (first- or second-generation) agent.

VALPROATE ADJUNCTIVE TO FIRST-GENERATION ANTIPSYCHOTICS

Although most trials of combination therapy begin with lithium, divalproex, or carbamazepine in one trial, with the adjunctive treatment arm consisting of an AP, one study examined the addition of valproate to ongoing treatment of patients with mania with an FGA agent (Müller-Oerlinghausen, Retzow, Henn, Giedke, & Walden, 1999). In this three-week study, patients receiving an FGA for a manic episode were randomized to valproate or placebo. Significantly more patients receiving valproate compared with placebo displayed a decrease in the need for AP medications, the study outcome measure.

SECOND-GENERATION ANTIPSYCHOTICS ADJUNCT TO LITHIUM, VALPROATE, OR CARBAMAZEPINE

Risperidone and paliperidone

Adjunctive risperidone was superior to placebo and comparable to haloperidol when added to lithium or divalproex in one trial (Sachs, Grossman, Ghaemi, Okamoto, & Bowden, 2002). In a second adjunctive treatment trial, risperidone was not superior to placebo in combination with lithium, divalproex, or carbamazepine (Yatham,

Grossman, Augustyns, Vieta, & Ravindran, 2003). It is possible that there were significant reductions in risperidone plasma concentrations in patients receiving carbamazepine in this study, which may have affected the results. One placebo-controlled study examined the efficacy of adjunctive paliperidone to lithium or valproate in patients with an inadequate response to these latter agents as monotherapy (Berwaerts et al., 2011). There were so significant differences in measure of improvement between adjunctive paliperidone and placebo in this study.

Olanzapine

Addition of olanzapine to patients who had not displayed an adequate response to lithium or divalproex monotherapy for two weeks was superior to addition of placebo in reduction of manic symptoms (Tohen, Chengappa, et al., 2002).

Quetiapine

Adjunctive quetiapine was superior to adjunctive placebo in two RCTs in combination with lithium or divalproex (Sachs et al., 2004; Yatham, Paulsson, Mullen, & Vagaro, 2004).

Ziprasidone

Ziprasidone did not separate from placebo in efficacy in an adjunctive treatment trial designed to show superior onset by Day 14 of treatment (Weisler, Dunn, & English, 2003). Patients receiving ziprasidone displayed greater improvement earlier in the trial, however, with greater efficacy over placebo in combination with lithium by Day 4. Nevertheless, in a second placebo-controlled trial, with efficacy determined by mean reduction in manic symptoms by three weeks of treatment, adjunctive ziprasidone was not superior to placebo when added to lithium or divalproex (Sachs, Vanderburg, et al., 2012). In an instructive post hoc analysis, this trial appears to have been compromised by enrollment of a substantial proportion of patients who did not meet eligibility criteria (Sachs, Vanderburg, et al., 2012).

Aripiprazole

Adjunctive aripiprazole was superior to placebo in a six-week trial in bipolar manic patients who had an inadequate response to monotherapy with lithium or divalproex (Vieta et al., 2008). Efficacy of adjunctive aripiprazole over placebo was evident by the end of Week 1 in this trial.

Asenapine

Adjunctive asenapine was superior to adjunctive placebo in combination with lithium or divalproex in a 12-week randomized trial (Szegedi et al., 2012).

Other agents

Several positive placebo-controlled pilot studies of allopurinol (Akhondzadeh, Milajerdi, Amini, & Tehrani-Doost, 2006; Machado-Vieira et al., 2008) suggest a promising role for this agent but require replication in larger, RCTs and further data regarding optimal dosing and duration of treatment.

The 5-HT$_2$ antagonist ritanserin was examined versus placebo as adjunctive treatment to lithium and haloperidol in 45 patients with bipolar mania (Akhondzadeh, Mohajari, Reza, & Amini, 2003).

EVIDENCE-SYNTHESIS RESULTS: EFFECT SIZES OF ANTIMANIC TREATMENTS

RCTs starting from similar baseline risks, with adequate statistical power when designed and conducted as unbiased and blind, should provide optimal evidence pertaining to clinical efficacy (Piantadosi, 1997). However, most of available evidence, especially with active comparators, suffers from inadequate power, and conflicting results on similar interventions are not infrequent. Consequently, meta-analytic evidence synthesis approaches are often employed for determining clinical practice guidelines, as well as reimbursement strategies (Becker, 2007). Indeed, evidence review overall provides information in a wider range, particularly on unquantifiable measures. However, evidence synthesis approaches principally grounded on quantifiable measures offer concrete information as point estimates on competing interventions; as such they provide insights on the dimension of effect rather than simpler statements on effectiveness [please refer to the Chapter 45: Traditional and Novel Research Synthesis Approaches to Support Evidence-Based Treatment Decisions]. Several standard pair-wise meta-analysis (SPM) to date have reported on the dimension of antimanic treatments' effects as relative to placebo (Tamayo, Zarate, Vieta, & Vázquez, 2010; Tarr, Herbison, Leon de la Barra, & Glue, 2011; Yildiz, Vieta, Leucht, & Baldessarini, 2011). Among these, the most recent and comprehensive one pooled data from 56 drug-placebo comparisons of 17 agents involving 10,800 patients with acute bipolar I mania. This SPM reported a pooled standardized mean difference as Hedges' g (SMD) based on manic symptom improvements of 0.42 (95% confidence intervals [CI]: 0.36–0.48); pooled responder rate based risk-ratio of 1.52 (95% CI: 1.42–1.62); and pooled responder-rate difference of 17% (drug: 48%, placebo: 31%), yielding an estimated number-needed-to-treat of 6 (all p < .0001) for the 13 effective antimanic treatments (Yildiz et al., 2011). In several direct comparisons, responses to various APs were reported as somewhat greater or more rapid than lithium, valproate, or carbamazepine; lithium did not differ from valproate, nor did second-generation antipsychotics (SAGs) differ from haloperidol (Yildiz et al., 2011).

In comparisons by class effect, another SPM involving 41 RCTs of APs, mood stabilizers (MSs), and combinations of these agents against placebo indicated greater mean reductions in the manic symptom ratings by the Young Mania Rating Scale for all three active treatment arms: 4.7 95% CI: 3 to 6.4 for MSs; 5.9 95% CI: 4.2 to 7.6 for APs; and 8.3 95% CI: 6.4 to 10.2 for combined MSs/APs (Tarr, Herbison, Leon de la Barra, & Glue, 2011). Within the active treatment arms, the rank ordering of change in the Young Mania Rating Scale scores was for combination treatment > APs > MSs, with approximately 2 points between each group (Tarr et al., 2011). The SPM, involving only single-agent trials in a data set involving 56 drug versus placebo, and 33 drug versus drug comparisons of antimanic treatments indicated an SMD as Hedges' g of 0.40 (95% CI: 0.32–0.47) for the SGAs; 0.54 (95% CI: 0.34–0.74) for the FGA, haloperidol, and 0.38 (95% CI: 0.26–0.50) for the MSs (lithium, valproate, carbamazepine) against placebo, all with p < .0001 (Yildiz et al., 2011). Direct head-to-head comparisons of SGAs as a group yielded greater effect size than MSs (in eight trials with 1,464 patients, SMD = 0.17, 95% CI: 0.07–0.28, p = .001). Similarly, comparison of MSs versus APs (SGAs or haloperidol) also favored the APs (SMD = 0.18, 95% CI: 0.08–0.28 in 10 trials with 1,530 subjects, p < .0001), and SGAs did not differ from haloperidol (Hedges' g = −0.001, 95% CI: −0.24 to +0.24 in six trials with 1,536 subjects, p = .99; Yildiz et al., 2011).

Reported SPM-based effect sizes for the antimanic treatments individually or by drug class were based on artificial groups created by effectiveness or by class, as direct comparisons involving exact same treatments are only a few per drug (see Tables 21.1 and 21.2). Even by consideration of artificial groups, the SPM is limited by the availability of direct evidence and cannot integrate all evidence from several comparators and many available drugs, which have not been compared head to head. Another meta-analytic evidence synthesis approach, called the network or multiple-treatments meta-analysis (MTM), enables indirect comparisons among competing interventions by combining findings from separate trials involving a common comparator, even when they have not been compared directly in the same trial (Salanti, Higgins, Ades, & Ioannidis, 2008). Two recent reports employing the MTM approach within the Bayesian framework evaluated comparative efficacy and acceptability of antimanic treatments (Cipriani et al., 2011; Yildiz, Nikodem, Vieta, Correll, & Baldessarini, 2014). The first MTM considered all RCTs against placebo or other treatments as monotherapy (N = 51) but also included trials involving add-on and combination designs (N = 15), involving 14 active antimanic treatments and placebo in 16,073 patients with bipolar acute mania (Cipriani et al., 2011).The latter recently updated network consists of 57 single-agent studies, yielding 95 direct comparisons in a total of 14,256 manic patients randomized to one of 18 active treatments or placebo (Tables 21.1 and 21.2; Yildiz, Nikodem, et al., 2014). Effectiveness of 13 antimanic treatments—aripiprazole, asenapine, carbamazepine, cariprazine, haloperidol, lithium, olanzapine, paliperdone, quetiapine, risperidone, tamoxifen, valproate, and ziprasidone—against placebo are confirmed by the two MTM (Cipriani et al., 2011; Yildiz, Nikodem, et al., 2014).

The most updated and recent MTM indicated SMD-based point estimates changing from 0.32 to 0.66 for the 12 effective antimanic drugs, which are on clinical use, with no indication of superiority of one to another but risperidone versus aripiprazole (0.27, 95% credible interval [CrI]: 0.01–0.54) and valproate (0.33, 95% CrI: 0.06–0.58; Table 21.3; Yildiz, Nikodem, et al., 2014). According to the Cohen's d, an SMD of 0.2 is small, 0.5 is medium, and 0.8 is large; as such, the range of SMDs established for the effective antimanic treatments overall indicate a medium effect size (Leucht, Hierl, Kissling, Dold, & Davis, 2012). However, Cohen described this only as a rule of thumb, and the interpretation depends on the clinical context (please see the Chapter 42. Strategies for Improving Randomized Trial Evidence for Treatment of Bipolar Disorder in this book). The SMD-based point estimates computed as relative to placebo in the recent network were compatible with the previous network (Cipriani et al., 2011) and with the SPM conducted by the Bayesian and frequentist approaches (Table 21.3; Yildiz, Nikodem, et al., 2014; Yildiz et al., 2011). However, numerous disagreements between the present and prior MTM were detected on the ranking by efficacy as well as the SMD-based effect size estimates between the competing interventions. In the preceding MTM, haloperidol was found superior to seven (aripiprazole, asenapine,

Table 21.1. CHARACTERISTICS OF INCLUDED RANDOMIZED, PLACEBO-CONTROLLED SINGLE-AGENT TRIALS OF ACUTE MANIA[A]

SOURCE	DRUG	DOSE (MG/DAY, MEQ/L)	PATIENTS (N, ITT)	MANIA RATING SCALE	BASELINE MANIA (MEAN ± SD)		MANIA SCORE CHANGE (MEAN ± SD)		CHANGE (%)		RESPONSE (%)	
					RX	PBO	RX	PBO	RX	PBO	RX	PBO
Keck et al., 2003a	Aripiprazole	15–30	243	YMRS	28.2 ± 5.0	29.7 ± 5.0	8.2 ± 12.0	3.4 ± 12.0	29.1	11.4	39.8	19.2
Sachs et al., 2006	Aripiprazole	15–30	268	YMRS	28.8 ± 4.9	28.5 ± 4.9	12.5 ± 11.0	7.2 ± 11.0	43.4	25.3	52.9	32.6
Keck et al 2009	Aripiprazole	15–30	317	YMRS	28.5 ± 5.6	28.9 ± 5.9	12.6 ± 10.0	9.0 ± 10.0	44.4	31.2	46.8	34.4
Young et al., 2009	Aripiprazole	15–30	318	YMRS	28.0 ± 5.8	28.3 ± 5.8	12.0 ± 10.0	9.7 ± 10.0	42.8	34.3	47.0	38.2
El Mallakh et al., 2010	Aripiprazole	15	257	YMRS	27.9 ± 5.4	28.3 ± 5.4	10.0 ± 11.0	10.1 ± 11.0	35.8	35.8	40.9	37.7
El Mallakh et al., 2010	Aripiprazole	30	259	YMRS	27.8 ± 5.5	28.3 ± 5.4	10.8 ± 11.0	10.1 ± 11.0	38.8	35.8	45.0	37.7
McIntyre, et al., 2009	Asenapine	18.2 ± 3.1	292	YMRS	28.3 ± 5.5	29.0 ± 6.1	13.1 ± 11.3	7.4 ± 11.6	46.3	25.5	42.3	25.2
McIntyre et al., 2010	Asenapine	18.4 ± 2.7	277	YMRS	29.4 ± 6.7	28.3 ± 6.3	11.5 ± 10.8	7.8 ± 10.7	39.1	27.6	42.6	34.0
Weisler et al., 2004	Carbamazepine	756	192	YMRS	26.6 ± 5.5	27.3 ± 5.3	8.7 ± 11.0	5.2 ± 9.4	32.8	18.9	40.4	21.4
Weisler et al., 2005	Carbamazepine	643	235	YMRS	28.5 ± 4.4	27.9 ± 4.9	15.1 ± 9.6	7.1 ± 9.2	53.0	25.5	60.8	28.7
Knesevich et al., 2009	Cariprazine	3–12	236	YMRS	30.6 ± 5.4	30.2 ± 5.4	13.3 ± 12.0	7.2 ± 11.9	43.5	23.8	48.3	24.8
Bose et al., 2012	Cariprazine	3–12	310	YMRS	32.3 ± 5.8	32.1 ± 5.6	17.3 ± 12.2	12.8 ± 11.7	53.6	39.9	58.9	44.1
Calabrese et al., 2013	Cariprazine	3–6	327	YMRS	33.2 ± 5.6	32.6 ± 5.8	17.5 ± 11.2	11.3 ± 11.7	52.7	34.7	60.6	37.5
Calabrese et al., 2013	Cariprazine	6–12	325	YMRS	32.9 ± 4.7	32.6 ± 5.8	16.8 ± 10.4	11.3 ± 11.7	51.1	34.7	59.3	37.5
McIntyre et al., 2005	Haloperidol	2–8	198	YMRS	32.3 ± 6.0	33.1 ± 6.6	15.7 ± 13.0	8.3 ± 13.0	48.6	25.1	56.1	35.0
Smulevich et al., 2005	Haloperidol	2–12	282	YMRS	32.1 ± 6.9	31.5 ± 6.7	15.1 ± 10.0	9.4 ± 11.0	47.0	29.8	47.7	33.3
Young et al., 2009	Haloperidol	5–15	313	YMRS	27.6 ± 5.6	28.3 ± 5.8	12.8 ± 10.0	9.7 ± 10.0	46.5	34.3	49.7	38.2
Vieta et al., 2010b	Haloperidol	8–30	258	MRS	30.7 ± 7.4	31.3 ± 7.7	15.9 ± 10.6	6.1 ± 9.9	51.9	19.5	54.7	20.5
Katagiri et al., 2012	Haloperidol	2.5–10	117	YMRS	26.6 ± 4.5	26.9 ± 5.6	14.3 ± 11.4	6.8 ± 14	53.8	25.3	65.0	44.3
Bowden et al., 2000	Lamotrigine	25–200	151	MRS	29.6 ± 7.8	295 ± 7.0	11.6 ± 14.0	11.4 ± 12.3	39.2	38.6	55.4	39.0
Goldsmith et al., 2003	Lamotrigine	50	179	MRS	26.4 ± 6.5	25.9 ± 6.1	9.3 ± 11.0	9.5 ± 11.0	35.2	36.7	44.0	46.3
CLIC477D2301, 2007	Licarbazepine	1,000–2,000	313	YMRS	27.5 ± 5.2	27.4 ± 5.3	9.2 ± 10.3	8.3 ± 9.3	33.5	30.3	35.5	34.8
Bowden et al., 1994	Lithium	≥1,200	107	MRS	27.1 ± 7.4	28.1 ± 6.3	9.3 ± 16.0	4.1 ± 11.0	34.3	14.4	48.6	25.0

(continued)

Table 21.1. CONTINUED

SOURCE	DRUG	DOSE (MG / DAY, MEQ/L)	PATIENTS (N, ITT)	MANIA RATING SCALE	BASELINE MANIA (MEAN ± SD)		MANIA SCORE CHANGE (MEAN ± SD)		CHANGE (%)		RESPONSE (%)	
					RX	PBO	RX	PBO	RX	PBO	RX	PBO
Bowden et al., 2000	Lithium	0.7–1.3	154	MRS	28.7 ± 6.9	29.5 ± 7.0	15.6 ± 13.0	11.4 ± 12.3	54.4	38.6	62.3	39.0
Goldsmith et al., 2003	Lithium	0.8–1.3	131	MRS	26.2 ± 5.9	25.9 ± 6.1	10.7 ± 12.0	9.5 ± 11.0	40.8	36.7	41.7	46.3
Bowden et al., 2005	Lithium	900	193	YMRS	33.3 ± 7.1	34.0 ± 6.9	15.2 ± 15.0	6.7 ± 15.0	45.6	19.7	53.1	27.4
Kushner et al., 2006	Lithium	1,500	224	YMRS	30.1 ± 7.4	30.0 ± 6.3	12.9 ± 12.0	7.7 ± 12.0	42.9	25.7	46.0	28.0
Kushner et al., 2006	Lithium	1,500	226	YMRS	30.7 ± 75	31.7 ± 7.3	13.8 ± 12.0	8.4 ± 12.0	45.0	26.5	46.0	28.0
Keck et al., 2009	Lithium	900–1,500	318	YMRS	29.4 ± 5.9	28.9 ± 5.9	12.0 ± 10.0	9.0 ± 10.0	40.9	31.2	45.8	34.4
Tohen et al., 1999	Olanzapine	5–20	136	YMRS	28.7 ± 6.7	27.7 ± 6.5	10.3 ± 13.0	4.9 ± 12.0	35.8	17.6	48.6	24.2
Tohen et al., 2000	Olanzapine	5–20	110	YMRS	28.8 ± 6.7	29.4 ± 6.8	14.8 ± 13.0	8.1 ± 13.0	51.4	27.6	64.8	42.9
Tohen et al., 2008	Olanzapine	11.4 ± 2.5	300	YMRS	23.8 ± 2.8	23.5 ± 2.5	9.4 ± 8.5	7.4 ± 8.0	39.5	31.5	40.8	31.3
McIntyre et al., 2009	Olanzapine	15.8 ± 2.3	291	YMRS	28.6 ± 5.9	29.0 ± 6.1	13.9 ± 10.7	7.4 ± 11.6	48.6	25.5	50.0	25.2
McIntyre et al., 2010	Olanzapine	15.9 ± 2.5	297	YMRS	29.7 ± 6.6	28.3 ± 6.3	14.6 ± 11.4	7.8 ± 10.7	49.2	27.6	54.7	34.0
Katagiri et al., 2012	Olanzapine	5–20	201	YMRS	27.7 ± 5.9	26.9 ± 5.6	12.6 ± 10.0	6.8 ± 14.0	45.5	25.3	51.0	44.3
Vieta et al., 2010a	Paliperidone	6–12	294	YMRS	27.3 ± 5.0	26.5 ± 5.0	13.2 ± 8.7	7.4 ± 10.7	48.4	27.9	44.2	34.6
Berwaerts et al., 2012	Paliperidone	12	224	YMRS	28.2 ± 5.0	28.7 ± 5.2	13.5 ± 9.2	10.1 ± 10.2	47.9	35.2	51.0	43.0
Berwaerts et al., 2012	Paliperidone	6	227	YMRS	28.0 ± 5.6	28.7 ± 5.2	11.4 ± 10	10.1 ± 10.2	40.7	35.2	43.0	43.0
Berwaerts et al., 2012	Paliperidone	3	222	YMRS	28.7 ± 6.3	28.7 ± 5.2	9.1 ± 11.2	10.1 ± 10.2	31.7	35.2	36.0	43.0
Bowden et al., 2005	Quetiapine	600–800	202	YMRS	32.7 ± 6.5	34.0 ± 6.9	14.6 ± 16.0	6.7 ± 15.0	44.7	19.7	53.3	27.4
McIntyre et al., 2005	Quetiapine	600–800	201	YMRS	34.0 ± 6.1	33.1 ± 6.6	12.3 ± 14.0	8.3 ± 13.0	36.1	25.1	42.6	35.0
Vieta et al., 2010a	Quetiapine	100–800	296	YMRS	27.6 ± 5.1	26.5 ± 5.0	11.7 ± 9.3	7.4 ± 10.7	42.4	27.9	49.0	34.6
Cutler et al., 2011	Quetiapine	400–800	308	YMRS	28.8 ± 5.4	28.4 ± 5.1	14.3 ± 11.0	10.5 ± 11.0	49.8	37.0	55.0	33.3
Hirschfeld et al., 2004	Risperidone	1–6	246	YMRS	29.1 ± 5.1	29.2 ± 5.5	10.6 ± 9.5	4.8 ± 9.5	36.4	16.4	43.3	24.4
Khanna et al., 2005	Risperidone	1–6	286	YMRS	37.1 ± 8.5	37.5 ± 8.4	22.7 ± 13.0	10.5 ± 16.0	61.2	28.0	74.3	36.6
Smulevich et al., 2005	Risperidone	1–6	291	YMRS	31.3 ± 6.5	31.5 ± 6.7	13.9 ± 10.0	9.4 ± 11.0	44.4	29.8	47.2	33.3
Zarate et al., 2007	Tamoxifen	20–140	16	YMRS	30.3 ± 7.0	24.3 ± 5.3	18.3 ± 4.3	−4.7 ± 4.1	60.4	−19.2	62.5	12.5

Study	Drug	Dose	N	Scale								
Yildiz et al., 2008	Tamoxifen	80	58	YMRS	38.6 ± 5.0	37.2 ± 6.6	16.6 ± 12.0	-4.8 ± 9.1	43.0	-12.9	43.8	3.8
Kushner et al., 2006	Topiramate	200+400	326	YMRS	30.5 ± 7.5	30.0 ± 6.3	6.0 ± 12	7.7 ± 12.0	19.7	25.7	27.0	28.0
Kushner et al., 2006	Topiramate	400+600	308	YMRS	29.2 ± 5.7	28.3 ± 5.8	8.1 ± 11	7.7 ± 10.0	27.6	27.2	27.0	28.0
Kushner et al., 2006	Topiramate	400	213	YMRS	30.4 ± 7.3	29.5 ± 5.7	5.1 ± 10	6.4 ± 10.0	16.8	21.7	27.0	28.0
Kushner et al., 2006	Topiramate	400	227	YMRS	30.8 ± 6.8	31.7 ± 7.3	8.2 ± 12	8.4 ± 12.0	26.6	26.5	27.0	28.0
Pope et al., 1991	Valproate	≥750	36	YMRS	28.2 ± 5.8	28.6 ± 6.9	11.4 ± 10.0	0.2 ± 9.9	40.5	0.6	52.9	10.5
Bowden et al., 1994	Valproate	≥1,000	139	MRS	27.2 ± 7.6	28.1 ± 6.3	9.2 ± 12.0	4.1 ± 11.0	34.0	14.4	47.8	25.0
Bowden et al., 2006	Valproate	3,057	364	MRS	26.6 ± 5.6	26.6 ± 5.6	11.9 ± 11.0	9.0 ± 11.0	44.7	33.8	48.1	33.9
Tohen et al., 2008	Valproate	848 ± 136	285	YMRS	23.9 ± 2.8	23.5 ± 2.5	8.2 ± 8.5	7.4 ± 8.0	34.3	31.5	40.3	31.3
Hirschfeld et al., 2010	Valproate	500–2500	222	MRS	32.9 ± 5.8	33.0 ± 6.7	10.1 ± 10.8	8.5 ± 12	30.7	25.8	—	—
Janicak et al., 1998	Verapamil	480	20	MRS	29.0 ± 9.0	26.0 ± 7.0	1.1 ± 11	1.3 ± 13.0	3.8	5.0	37.5	16.7
Keck et al., 2003b	Ziprasidone	130 ± 34	197	MRS	27.0 ± 3.8	26.7 ± 7.0	12.4 ± 12	7.8 ± 13.0	45.9	29.2	50.4	34.8
Potkin et al., 2005	Ziprasidone	126	202	MRS	26.2 ± 7.2	26.4 ± 7.5	11.1 ± 12	5.6 ± 9.6	42.4	21.3	46.7	29.2
Vieta et al., 2010b	Ziprasidone	116	264	MRS	29.6 ± 8.0	31.3 ± 7.7	10.4 ± 11.1	6.1 ± 9.9	35.2	19.5	36.9	20.5

NOTE: SD = standard deviation; Rx = treated with study drug; PBO = placebo. YMRS = Young Mania Rating Scale; MRS = Mania Rating Scale. Test drugs are listed alphabetically.

In studies where actual site numbers are not reported, they are estimated as twice the reported number of countries.

Ratings and changes are based on mania ratings by YMRS (11 items, range 0–60) or MRS (11 items, range 0–53) from the Schedule for Affective Disorders and Schizophrenia–Change Version. Response is defined as ≥ 50% improvement in the mania rating scale used relative to baseline.

Adapted from Yildiz, Nikodem, et al., 2014.

[a] 61 comparisons from 41 studies.

Table 21.2. CHARACTERISTICS OF RANDOMIZED, SINGLE-AGENT TRIALS COMPARING TWO ACTIVE DRUGS FOR TREATMENT OF ACUTE MANIA[a]

DESIGN	DRUGS (RX) RX1	DRUGS (RX) RX2	PATIENTS (N, ITT) RX1	PATIENTS (N, ITT) RX2	MANIA RATING/TRIAL WEEKS	BASELINE MANIA (MEAN ± SD) RX1	BASELINE MANIA (MEAN ± SD) RX2	SEVERITY (% OF MAX) RX1	SEVERITY (% OF MAX) RX2	CHANGE (%) RX1	CHANGE (%) RX2	RESPONSE (%) RX1	RESPONSE (%) RX2	SOURCE
RDB	Li	LTG	15	15	MRS / 4	31.6	34.4	59.6	64.9	58.2	58.4	60.0	53.3	Ichim et al., 2000[b]
RDB	Li	LTG	77	74	MRS / 6	28.7 ± 6.9	29.6 ± 7.8	54.2	55.9	54.4	39.2	62.3	55.4	Bowden et al., 2000[c]
RDB	Li	LTG	36	84	MRS / 3	26.2 ± 5.9	26.4 ± 6.5	49.4	49.8	40.8	35.2	41.7	44.1	Goldsmith et al., 2003[c]
RDB	Li	TPM	113	215	YMRS / 3	30.1 ± 7.4	30.5 ± 7.5	50.2	50.8	42.9	19.7	46.0[e]	27.0[e]	Kushner et al., 2006[c]
RDB	Li	TPM	114	115	YMRS / 3	30.7 ± 7.5	30.8 ± 6.8	51.2	51.3	45.0	26.6	46.0[e]	27.0[e]	Kushner et al., 2006[c]
RDB	Li	CBZ	24	24	YMRS / 8	30.3	30.9	50.5	51.5	32.0	27.5	33.3[e]	33.3[e]	Small et al., 1991
RDB	Li	VPA	13	14	MRS[f] / 3	43.4 ± 20.3	52.9 ± 12.3	—	—	76.5	48.8	92.3	64.3	Freeman et al., 1992[g]
RDB	Li	VPA	35	67	MRS / 3	27.1 ± 7.4	27.2 ± 7.6	51.1	51.3	34.3	34.0	48.6	47.8	Bowden et al., 1994[c]
RDB	Li	APZ	155	154	YMRS / 3	29.4 ± 5.9	28.5 ± 5.6	49.0	46.7	40.9	44.4	45.8	46.8	Keck et al., 2009[c]
RDB	Li	HAL	15	15	YMRS / 4	28.4	24.8	47.3	41.3	55.3	41.1	—	—	Segal et al., 1998[h]
RDB	Li	OLZ	15	15	MRS / 4	31.6	31.7	59.6	59.8	58.2	67.8	—	—	Berk et al., 1999[b]
RDB	Li	OLZ	71	69	YMRS / 4	32.4 ± 7.2	34 ± 6.8	54.0	56.7	62.2	72.4	73.2	87.0	Niufan et al., 2008
RDB	Li	OLZ	20	20	MSRS / 3	79.2 ± 9.6	80.3 ± 8.7	60.9	61.8	17.3	6.8	25	15	Shafti, 2010[g]
RDB	Li	QTP	98	107	YMRS / 3	33.3 ± 7.1	32.7 ± 6.5	55.5	62.9	45.7	44.7	53.1	53.3	Bowden et al., 2005[c]
RDB	Li	QTP	77	77	YMRS / 4	29.8 ± 5.7	29.3 ± 5.8	49.7	48.8	—	—	59.7	77.9	Li et al., 2008
RDB	Li	RSP	15	15	YMRS / 4	28.4	28.6	47.3	47.7	55.3	43.4	—	—	Segal et al., 1998[h]
RDB	VPA	CBZ	15	15	YMRS / 4	43.5 ± 8.1	41.3 ± 6.5	72.5	68.8	75.4	50.4	73.3	53.3	Vasudev et al., 2000
RDB	VPA	OxCBZ	30	30	YMRS / 3 (12)[j]	34.6 ± 6.5	33.8 ± 5.4	57.7	56.3	28.8	29.4	90.0[i]	80.0[i]	Kakkar et al., 2009
RSB	VPA	HAL	21	15	YMRS / 1	36.1 ± 11	37.2 ± 8.8	60.2	62.0	42.7	34.7	47.6	33.3	McElroy et al., 1996
RDB	VPA	OLZ	123	125	YMRS / 3	27.9 ± 6.6	27.4 ± 5.2	46.5	45.7	37.3	48.9	42.3	54.4	Tohen et al., 2002
RDB	VPA	OLZ	60	55	MRS / 3	30.8	32.3	58.1	60.9	48.1	53.3	—	—	Zajecka et al., 2002
RDB	VPA	OLZ	186	201	YMRS / 3	23.9 ± 2.8	23.8 ± 2.8	39.8	39.7	34.3	39.5	40.3	40.8	Tohen et al., 2008[c]
RDB	APZ	HAL	173	164	YMRS / 3 (12)	31.1 ± 6.6	31.5 ± 7.9	51.8	52.5	50.5	49.8	50.9	42.6	Vieta et al., 2005

	Drug 1	Drug 2	N1	N2	Scale/sites	Baseline 1	Baseline 2							Study
RDB	APZ	HAL	166	161	YMRS / 3	28 ± 5.8	27.6 ± 5.6	46.7	46.0	42.8	46.5	47.0	49.7	Young et al., 2009c
RDB	OLZ	ASN	188	189	YMRS / 3	28.6 ± 5.9	28.3 ± 5.5	47.7	47.2	48.6	46.3	50.0	42.3	McIntyre et al., 2009c
RDB	OLZ	ASN	203	183	YMRS / 3	29.7 ± 6.6	29.4 ± 6.7	49.5	49.0	49.2	39.1	54.7	42.6	McIntyre et al., 2010c
RDB	OLZ	HAL	231	213	YMRS / 6 (12)	31.1 ± 7.6	30.6 ± 7.7	51.8	51.0	—	—	55.0j	62.0j	Tohen et al., 2003
RDB	OLZ	HAL	104	20	YMRS / 3	27.7 ± 5.9	26.6 ± 4.5	46.2	44.3	45.5	53.8	51.0	65.0	Katagiri et al., 2012c
RDB	OLZ	RSP	164	164	YMRS / 3	26.6 ± 5.0	26.7 ± 5	44.3	44.5	56.5	62.3	62.1	59.5	Perlis et al., 2006
RDB	QTP	HAL	101	98	YMRS / 3	34 ± 6.1	32.3 ± 6	56.7	53.8	36.2	48.6	42.6	56.1	McIntyre et al., 2005c
RDB	QTP	PPD	192	190	YMRS / 3	27.6 ± 5.1	27.3 ± 5	46.0	45.5	42.4	48.4	49.0	44.2	Vieta et al., 2010ac
RDB	RSP	HAL	15	15	YMRS / 4	28.6	24.8	47.7	41.3	43.4	41.1	—	—	Segal et al., 1998h
RDB	RSP	HAL	153	144	YMRS / 3	32.1 ± 6.9	31.3 ± 6.5	53.5	52.2	47.0	44.4	47.7	47.2	Smulevich et al., 2005c
RDB	ZPS	HAL	176	170	MRS / 3	29.6 ± 8.0	30.7 ± 7.4	55.9	57.9	35.2	51.9	36.9	54.7	Vieta et al., 2010bc

NOTE: Studies listed based on comparisons. SD = standard deviation; Rx = treated with study drug; RDB = randomized double blind; RO = randomized open; YMRS = Young Mania Rating Scale; MRS = Mania Rating Scale; APZ = aripiprazole; ASN = asenapine; CBZ = carbamazepine; HAL = haloperidol; Li = lithium; OLZ = olanzapine; OxCBZ = oxcarbazepine; PPD = paliperidone; QTP = quetiapine; RSP = risperidone; TPM = topiramate; VPA = valproate; ZPS = ziprasidone.

Ratings and changes are based on mania ratings by YMRS (11 items, range 0–60) or MRS (11 items, range 0–53) from the Schedule for Affective Disorders and Schizophrenia–Change Version or Beigel-Murphy Manic State Rating Scale (26 items, range 0–130).

In studies where actual site numbers are not reported, they are estimated as twice the reported number of countries.

Unless otherwise specified, response is defined as ≥ 50% improvement in the mania rating scale scores administered as relative to baseline.

a 34 comparisons; 16 from three-armed placebo controlled trials. b Lithium arm from the same study with two active controls published separately. c Indicates results from placebo-controlled studies with two active treatment arms. d Indicates pooled results. e Response is defined as moderate improvement with Clinical Global Impressions Scale. f Freeman et al. (1992) used a software system that unit normalized the MRS scores. g Actual score at the endpoint; note that smaller score at the endpoint reflects larger improvement. h Same study tabulated three times as it has three comparisons between three active drugs. j Mania score change results are at three weeks, and response indicates rate of remission (defined as YMRS of ≤12) at 12 weeks.

Adapted from Yildiz, Nikodem, et al., 2014.

Table 21.3. DIFFERENCES IN EFFECT SIZE ESTIMATIONS BETWEEN COMPETING INTERVENTIONS AS DETECTED BY EMPLOYMENT OF DIFFERENT NETWORKS OR ANALYTIC APPROACHES

COMPARISON	MULTIPLE-TREATMENTS META-ANALYSES (MTM) (SMD AS HEDGES' G (CRI))		STANDARD PAIR-WISE META-ANALYSES (SPM) (SMD AS HEDGES' G)	
	YILDIZ ET AL. (IN PRESS) SINGLE AGENT TRIALS ONLY	CIPRIANI ET AL. (2011) SINGLE AGENT AND ADD-ON TRIALS	YILDIZ ET AL. (IN PRESS) SINGLE AGENT TRIALS ONLY BY BAYESIAN APPROACH (CRI)[a]	CIPRIANI ET AL. (2011) SINGLE AGENT AND ADD-ON TRIALS BY FREQUENTIST APPROACH (CI)
Aripiprazole vs Placebo	−0.37 [−0.55 to −0.20]*	−0.37 [−0.51 to −0.23]*	−0.34 [−0.52 to −0.15]*	−0.31 [−0.42 to −0.20]*
Asenapine vs Placebo	−0.36 [−0.63 to −0.08]*	−0.30 [−0.53 to −0.07]*	−0.43 [−0.84 to −0.02]*	−0.42 [−0.59 to −0.24]*
Carbamazepine vs Placebo	−0.44 [−0.71 to −0.15]*	−0.36 [−0.60 to −0.11]**	−0.61 [−0.93 to −0.28]*	−0.50 [−0.69 to −0.30]*
Cariprazine vs Placebo	−0.47 [−0.73 to −0.22]*	—	−0.47 [−0.72 to −0.22]*	—
Haloperidol vs Placebo	−0.54 [−0.70 to −0.38]*	−0.56 [−0.68 to −0.43]*	−0.58 [−0.77 to −0.40]*	−0.58 [−0.77 to −0.39]*
Lithium vs Placebo	−0.45 [−0.61 to −0.30]*	−0.37 [−0.50 to −0.25]*	−0.37 [−0.54 to −0.20]*	−0.40 [−0.54 to −0.26]*
Olanzapine vs Placebo	−0.48 [−0.62 to −0.34]*	−0.43 [−0.54 to −0.32]*	−0.40 [−0.57 to −0.24]*	−0.44 [−0.56 to −0.32]*
Paliperdone vs Placebo	−0.37 [−0.66 to −0.08]*	−0.50 [−0.63 to −0.38]**	−0.37 [−0.66 to −0.08]*	−0.50 [−0.67 to −0.33]**
Quetiapine vs Placebo	−0.35 [−0.56 to −0.14]*	−0.37 [−0.51 to −0.23]*	−0.35 [−0.55 to −0.14]*	−0.37 [−0.51 to −0.24]*
Risperidone vs Placebo	−0.65 [−0.85 to −0.44]*	−0.50 [−0.63 to −0.38]**	−0.69 [−0.93 to −0.45]*	−0.50 [−0.67 to −0.33]**
Tamoxifen vs Placebo	−2.92 [−3.48 to −2.38]*	—	−2.92 [−3.48 to −2.38]*	—
Valproate vs Placebo	−0.32 [−0.50 to −0.15]*	−0.20 [−0.37 to −0.04]*	−0.30 [−0.51 to −0.10]*	−0.16 [−0.30 to −0.03]*
Ziprasidone vs Placebo	−0.33 [−0.59 to −0.08]*	−0.19 [−0.37 to −0.03]*	−0.34 [−0.60 to −0.09]*	−0.24 [−0.49 to −0.01]*
Aripiprazole vs Risperidone	−0.27 [−0.54 to −0.01]*	−0.13 [−0.31 to 0.05]	—	—
Aripiprazole vs Haloperidol	−0.17 [−0.37 to 0.04]	−0.19 [−0.36 to −0.02]*	−0.04 [−0.34 to 0.26]	−0.05 [−0.20 to 0.10]
Asenapine vs Haloperidol	−0.18 [−0.49 to 0.13]	−0.26 [−0.52 to −0.01]*	—	—
Asenapine vs Olanzapine	−0.12 [−0.39 to 0.15]	−0.14 [−0.36 to 0.10]	−0.18 [−0.47 to 0.12]	−0.22 [−0.37 to −0.08]*
Carbamazepine vs Haloperidol	−0.10 [−0.43 to 0.21]	−0.20 [−0.36 to −0.01]*	−0.09 [−0.56 to 0.38]	−0.09 [−0.56 to 0.38]
Lithium vs Haloperidol	−0.09 [−0.29 to 0.13]	−0.19 [−0.36 to −0.01]*	0.51 [−0.29 to 1.30]	−1.11 [−1.89 to −0.33]*

Quetiapine vs Haloperidol	−0.19 [−0.43 to 0.07]	−0.19 [−0.37 to −0.01]*	—	−0.42 [−0.71 to −0.14]*
Valproate vs Haloperidol	−0.22 [−0.43 to 0.02]	−0.36 [−0.56 to −0.15]*	0.23 [−0.52 to 0.99]	—
Valproate vs Lithium	−0.13 [−0.34 to 0.09]	−0.10 [−0.41 to 0.23]	−0.36 [−0.85 to 0.12]	−1.01 [−1.82 to −0.20]*
Valproate vs Olanzapine	−0.16 [−0.34 to 0.04]	−0.23 [−0.40 to −0.06]*	−0.22 [−0.48 to 0.04]	−0.20 [−0.34 to −0.05]*
Valproate vs Risperidone	−0.33 [−0.58 to −0.06]*	−0.30 [−0.50 to −0.10]*	—	—
Ziprasidone vs Haloperidol	−0.21 [−0.48 to 0.08]	−0.36 [−0.56 to −0.15]*	−0.52 [−0.94 to −0.08]*	−0.51 [−0.72 to −0.29]*
Ziprasidone vs Olanzapine	−0.15 [−0.43 to 0.14]	−0.24 [−0.43 to −0.03]*	—	—
Ziprasidone vs Risperidone	−0.31 [−0.63 to 0.02]	−0.31 [−0.51 to −0.10]*	—	—

NOTE: CrI = credible interval; CI = confidence interval; SMD = standardized mean difference as Hedges' *g*.

All results are reported as difference in the treatment effect (SMD) of the first agent listed relative to the second.

Data for multiple-treatments meta-analyses based on the single agent trials is adapted from Yildiz, Nikodem, et al. (in press) and on the single agent and add-on trials from Cipriani et al. (2011).

* Statistically significant difference. ** Data from chemically related agents analyzed conjointly in the same node (e.g., paliperidone and risperidone or carbamazepine and oxcarbazepine).

[a] The SMD values computed for the single agent trials by the frequentist approach (CI) can be found in Yildiz et al. (2011).

carbamazepine, lithium, quetipaine, valproate, ziprasidone) and both olanzapine and risperidone against two (valproate, ziprasidone) competing interventions (Cipriani et al., 2011). Except the one on risperidone versus valproate none of these findings could be replicated in the recent MTM. Significant findings of both networks are summarized in Table 21.3. Indeed, considering that 41% of the entire evidence structure at 53 data points was different disagreements between the present and previous network were not surprising. For example, the first network allowed inclusion of add-on and combination trials while the second one allowed only monotherapy trials; a decision to be made by the meta-anlaysts according to the research question of interest, accumulated evidence, and clinical context. Within the context of acute bipolar mania, since great majority of accumulated evidence is as monotharpy and different hypotheses are being operated in the monotherapy versus add-on or combination trials, and we selected to construct a network based on monotherapy trials (Yildiz, Nikodem, et al., 2014). The initial network on the other hand, selected to include add-on or combination trials as well; yet, by treating data obtained from add-on trials in the same nodes or joints with monotherapy trials. As such, no information on the comparative efficacy of combination versus single-agent treatments could be obtained (Cipriani et al., 2011). Through that approach data coming from add-on or combination treatments pooled together with single-agent trial results as such modified computed effect-sizes of considered drug. One further difference between the two available antimanic treatment networks is the consideration of the chemically related drugs conjointly in the same joints (e.g., paliperidone and risperidone; or carbamazepine and oxcarbazepine) in the preceeding network (Cipriani et al., 2011). All these factors might have contributed to the conflicting results and different point estimates for the considered treatment alternatives (for technical details see Yildiz, Vieta, et al., 2014; and Yildiz, Nikodem, et al., 2014).

A sensitivity analysis considering drugs in groups of FGA, SGAs, and MSs tested superiority of one group to another in the context of MTM (Yildiz, Nikodem, et al., 2014). This analysis by class effect confirmed antimanic effectiveness of FGA, haloperidol with SMD values of 0.54 (95% CrI: 0.39–0.69), SGAs 0.44 (5% CrI: 0.36–0.51), and MSs 0.39 (95% CrI: 0.28–0.49) as relative to placebo, with no indication of significance among each other. Trivial effect sizes detected for SGAs versus MSs 0.05 (–0.06–0.17) or FGA versus MSs 0.16 (–0.02–0.32) did not reach significance.

TREATMENT IMPLICATIONS

Recommendations regarding initial treatment of patients with bipolar manic episodes are usually based on five considerations: the evidence base of acute treatment efficacy for a selected agent or agents; history of prior treatment response and tolerability; episode severity; relevant co-occurring psychiatric and medical illnesses and the potential for beneficial or adverse effects on these conditions; and the use of initial treatment as a potential basis for establishing a foundational regimen for long-term relapse prevention. Based on the available scientific evidence from RCTs, the efficacy of lithium, divalproex, carbamazepine, haloperidol, risperidone, paliperidone, olanzapine, quetiapine, ziprasidone, aripiprazole, asenapine, and cariprazine have demonstrated efficacy in the treatment of manic episodes as monotherapy. Greater efficacy and often more rapid improvement has been demonstrated for adjunctive therapy for risperidone, olanzapine, quetiapine, aripiprazole, and asenapine, each in combination with lithium or divalproex. Illness severity and patient safety considerations are two factors that often affect the recommendation of combination compared with monotherapy for acute manic episodes.

As treatment recommendations for acute manic episodes may also be considered in light of establishing an agent for potential long-term maintenance treatment, considerations of not just short-term but long-term tolerability and evidence maintenance efficacy become relevant. Of the agents with established efficacy in the short-term treatment of manic episodes, lithium, olanzapine, aripiprazole, quetiapine, and risperidone (long-acting, injectable) have established efficacy in maintenance treatment of patients with bipolar I disorder (Keck & McElroy, in press).

Disclosure statements: Dr. Keck is employed by the University of Cincinnati College of Medicine and University of Cincinnati Physicians. Dr. Keck is presently or has been in the past year a principal or co-investigator on research studies sponsored by Alkermes; AstraZeneca; Cephalon; GlaxoSmithKline; Eli Lilly and Company; Marriott Foundation; National Institute of Mental Health; Orexigen; Pfizer, Inc.; and Shire.

Dr. Keck has been reimbursed for consulting to, in the past year,

2012: Bristol-Myers-Squibb, Teva, Otsuka, Forest, Merck

2013: Sunovion, Alkermes, Shire, Forest, Merck

Dr. Paul E. Keck, Jr. is a co-inventor on United States Patent No. 6,387,956: Shapira, N. A., Goldsmith, T. D., & Keck, P. E. Jr. (University of Cincinnati). (2002). Methods of treating obsessive-compulsive spectrum disorder comprises the step of administering an effective amount of tramadol to an individual. Filed March 25, 1999; approved May 14, 2002. Dr. Keck has received no financial gain from this patent.

Dr. McElroy has not disclosed any conflicts of interest.

Dr. Yildiz has received research grants from or served as a consultant to, or speaker for, Abdi Ibrahim, Actavis, AliRaif, AstraZeneca, Bristol-Myers Squibb, Janssen-Cilag, Lundbeck, Pfizer, Sanofi-Aventis, and Servier.

REFERENCES

Akhondzadeh, S., Mohajari, M. R., Aminia, H., &Tehrani-Doost, M. (2006). Allopurinol as an adjunct to lithium and haloperidol for treatment of patients with acute mania: A double-blind, randomized, placebo-controlled trial. *Bipolar Disorders*, 8, 485–489.

Akhondzadeh, S., Mohajari, M. R., Reza, H. M., &Amini, H. (2003). Ritanserin as an adjunct to lithium and haloperidol for the treatment of medication-naïve patients with acute mania: A double-blind and placebo controlled trial. *BMC Psychiatry*, 3, 76–79.

American Psychiatric Association. (2013). *Diagnostic and statistical manual of mental disorders* (5th ed.). Washington, DC: Author.

Becker, B. J. (2007). Multivariate meta-analysis: Contributions of Ingram Olkin. *Statistical Science*, 22, 401–406.

Berk, M., Ichim, L., & Brook, S. (1999). Olanzapine compared to lithium in mania: double-blind randomized controlled trial. *International Journal of Clinical Psychopharmacology*, 14(6), 339–343.

Berwaerts, J., Lane, R., Nuamah, I. F., Lim, P., Remmerie, B., & Hough, D. W. (2011). Paliperidone extended-release as adjunctive therapy to lithium or valproate in the treatment of acute mania: A randomized, placebo-controlled study. *Journal of Affective Disorders*, 129, 252.

Berwaerts, J., Xu, H., Nuamah, I., Lim, P., & Hough, D. (2012). Evaluation of the efficacy and safety of paliperidone extended-release in the treatment of acute mania: randomized, double-blind, dose-response study. *Journal of Affective Disorders*, 136(1–2), 51–60.

Bose, A., Starace, A., Wang, Q., Diaz, E., Goodman, J., Ruth, A.,...Laszlovszky, I. (2012). Cariprazine in the treatment of acute mania in bipolar disorder: a double-blind, placebo-controlled, phase III trial. ClinicalTrials.gov: NCT01058096. *European Neuropsychopharmacology*, 22(Suppl 2), S285.

Bowden, C. L. (1995). Predictors of response to divalproex and lithium. *Journal of Clinical Psychiatry*, 56(Suppl.), 25–30.

Bowden, C. L., Brugger, A. M., Swann, A. C., Calabrese, J. R., Janicak, P. G., Petty, F.,...Small, J. G. (1994). Efficacy of divalproex vs lithium and placebo in the treatment of mania. *Journal of the American Medical Association*, 271(12), 918–924.

Bowden, C., Calabrese, J., Ascher, J., DeVeaugh-Geiss, J., Earl, N., Evoniuk, G.,...Paska, W. (2000). Spectrum of efficacy of Lamotrigine in bipolar disorder: Overview of double-blind, placebo-controlled studies. Study ID Number: SCAB2009. *American College of Neuropsychopharmacology 39th Annual Meeting*, San Juan, Puerto Rico.

Bowden, C. L., Grunze, H., Mullen, J., Brecher, M., Paulsson, B., Jones, M.,...Svensson, K. (2005). Randomized, double-blind, placebo-controlled efficacy and safety study of quetiapine or lithium as monotherapy for mania in bipolar disorder. *Journal of Clinical Psychiatry*, 66(1), 111–121.

Bowden, C. L., Swann, A. C., Calabrese, J. R., Rubenfaer, L. M., Wozniak, P. J., Collins, M. A.,...Depakote, E. R., Mania Study Group (2006). Randomized, placebo-controlled, multicenter study of divalproex sodium extended release in the treatment of acute mania. *Journal of Clinical Psychiatry*, 67(10), 1501–1510.

Calabrese, J. R., Keck, P. E. Jr., Starace, A., Lu, K., Ruth, A., Laszlovszky, I.,...Durgam, S. (2013). Efficacy and safety of low- and high-dose cariprazine in patients with acute mania associated with bipolar I disorder. ClinicalTrials.gov: NCT01058668. *European Neuropsychopharmacology*, 23(Suppl 2), S378–S379.

Cipriani, A., Barbui, C., Salanti, G., Rendell, J., Brown, R., Stockton, S.,...Geddes, J. R. (2011). Comparative efficacy and acceptability of antimanic drugs in acute mania: Multiple-treatments meta-analysis. *Lancet*, 378(9799), 1306–1315.

Cutler, A. J., Datto, C., Nordenhem, A., Minkwitz, M., Acevedo, L., & Darko, D. (2011). Extended-release quetiapine as monotherapy for the treatment of adults with acute mania: a randomized, double-blind, 3-week trial. *Clinical Therapeutics*, 33(11), 1643–1658.

El Mallakh, R. S., Vieta, E., Rollin, L., Marcus, R., Carson, W. H., & McQuade, R. (2010). Comparison of two fixed doses of aripiprazole with placebo in acutely relapsed, hospitalized patients with bipolar disorder I (manic or mixed) in subpopulations. Study ID Number: CN138-007. *European Neuropsychopharmacology*, 20(11), 776–783.

Freeman, T. W., Clothier, J. L., Pazzaglia, P., Lesem, M. D., & Swann, A. C. (1992). Double-blind comparison of valproate and lithium in the treatment of acute mania. *American Journal of Psychiatry*, 149(1), 108–111.

Goldberg, J. F., Garno, J. L., Leon, A. C., Kocsis, J. H., & Portera, L. (1998). Rapid titration of mood stabilizers predicts remission from mixed or pure mania in bipolar patients. *Journal of Clinical Psychiatry*, 59, 151–158.

Goldsmith, D. R., Wagstaff, A. J., Ibbotson, T., & Perry, C. M. (2003). Lamotrigine: review of its use in bipolar disorder. Study ID Number: SCAA2008. *Drugs*, 63(19), 2029–2050.

Hirschfeld, R. M. A., Bowden, C. L., Vigna, N. V., Wozniak, P., & Collins, M. (2010). A randomized, placebo-controlled, multicenter study of divalproex sodium extended-release in the acute treatment of mania. *Journal of Clinical Psychiatry*, 71(4), 426–432.

Hirschfeld, R. M., Keck, P. E., Jr, Kramer, M., Karcher, K., Canuso, C., Eerdekens, M., & Grossman, F. (2004). Rapid antimanic effect of risperidone monotherapy: 3-week multicenter, double-blind, placebo-controlled trial. *American Journal of Psychiatry*, 161(6), 1057–1065.

Hung, S. I, Chung, W. H., Jee, S. H., Chen, W. C., Chang, Y. T., Lee, W. R.,...Chen, Y. T. (2006). Genetic susceptibility to carbamazepine-induced cutaneous adverse drug reactions. *Pharmacogenetics and Genomics*, 16, 297.

Ichim, L., Berk, M., & Brook, S. (2000). Lamotrigine compared with lithium in mania: double-blind randomized controlled trial. *Annals of Clinical Psychiatry*, 12(1), 5–10.

Janicak, P. G., Sharma, R. P., Pandey, G., & Davis, J. M. (1998). Verapamil for the treatment of acute mania: double-blind, placebo-controlled trial. *American Journal of Psychiatry*, 155(7), 972–973.

Kakkar, A. K., Rehan, H. S., Unni, K. E. S., Gupta, N. K., Chopra, D., & Kataria, D. (2009). Comparative efficacy and safety of oxcarbazepine versus divalproex sodium in the treatment of acute mania: pilot study. *European Psychiatry*, 24(3), 178–182.

Katagiri, H., Takita, Y., Tohen, M., Higuchi, T., Kanba, S., & Takahashi, M. (2012). Efficacy and safety of olanzapine in the treatment of Japanese patients with bipolar I disorder in a current manic or mixed episode: randomized, double-blind, placebo- and haloperidol-controlled study. *Journal of Affective Disorders*, 136(3), 476–484.

Keck, P. E., Jr, Marcus, R., Tourkodimitris, S., Ali, M., Liebeskind, A., Saha, A., Ingenito, G., Aripiprazole Study Group (2003a).

Placebo-controlled, double-blind study of the efficacy and safety of aripiprazole in patients with acute bipolar mania. *American Journal of Psychiatry, 160*(9), 1651–1658.

Keck, P. E. Jr., & McElroy, S. L. (2009). Treatment of bipolar disorder. In A. F. & C. B. Nemeroff (Eds.), *Textbook of psychopharmacology* (pp. 1113–1133). Washington, DC: American Psychiatric Publishing.

Keck, P. E. Jr., & McElroy, S. L. (in press). Pharmacological treatments for bipolar disorder. In P. E. Nathan & J. M. Gorman (Eds.), *A guide to treatments that work* (4th ed.). New York: Oxford University Press.

Keck, P. E. Jr., McElroy, S. L., &Nemeroff, C. B. (1992). Anticonvulsants in the treatment of bipolar disorder. *Journal of Neuropsychiatry and Clinical Neuroscience, 4,* 595–605.

Keck, P. E. Jr, Orsulak, P. J., Cutler, A. J., Sanchez, R., Torbeyns, A., Marcus, R. N.,…Carson, W. H. (2009). Aripiprazole monotherapy in the treatment of acute bipolar I mania: a randomized, double-blind, placebo- and lithium-controlled study. *Journal of Affective Disorders, 112*(1–3), 36–49.

Keck, P. E., Jr, Versiani, M., Potkin, S., West, S. A., Giller, E., & Ice, K. (2003b). Ziprasidone in the treatment of acute bipolar mania: three-week, placebo-controlled, double-blind, randomized trial. *American Journal of Psychiatry, 160*(4), 741–748.

Keck, P. E. Jr., Zukin, S., Lu, K., Laszlovsky, I., Nemeth, G., & Durgam, S. (2013, May). *Cariprazine effects on YMRS items: Results of a pooled analysis of 3 randomized, double-blind, placebo-controlled trials in bipolar mania.* Paper presented at the annual meeting of the American Psychiatric Association, San Francisco, CA.

Ketter, T. A. (2008). Monotherapy versus combined treatment with second-generation antipsychotics in bipolar disorder. *Journal of Clinical Psychiatry, 73*(Suppl.), 9–15.

Khanna, S., Vieta, E., Lyons, B., Grossman, F., Eerdekens, M., & Kramer, M. (2005). Risperidone in the treatment of acute mania: double-blind, placebo-controlled study. *British Journal of Psychiatry, 187,* 229–234.

Klein, D. F. (1967). Importance of psychiatric diagnosis in prediction of clinical drug effects. *Archives of General Psychiatry, 16,* 118–126.

Knesevich, M., Papadakis, K., Bose, A., Andor, G., & Laszlovszky, I. (2009). The efficacy and tolerability of cariprazine in acute mania associated with bipolar I disorder: a phase II trial. ClinicalTrials.gov: NCT00488618. *European Neuropsychopharmacology, 19* (suppl 3), S469.

Kushner, S. F., Khan, A., Lane, R., & Olson, W. H. (2006). Topiramate monotherapy in the management of acute mania: results of four double-blind placebo-controlled trials. ClinicalTrials.gov: NCT00037674; NCT00240721; NCT00035230. *Bipolar Disorders, 8*(1), 15–27.

Leucht, S., Hierl, S., Kissling, W., Dold, M., & Davis, J. M. (2012). Putting the efficacy of psychiatric and general medicine medication into perspective: Review of meta-analyses. *The British Journal of Psychiatry, 200,* 97–106.

Li, H., Ma, C., Wang, G., Zhu, X., Peng, M., & Gu, N. (2008). Response and remission rates in Chinese patients with bipolar mania treated for 4 weeks with either quetiapine or lithium: randomized and double-blind study. ClinicalTrials.gov: NCT00448578. *Current Medical Research and Opinion, 24*(1), 1–10.

Machado-Vieria, R., Soares, J. C., Lara, D. R., Luckenbaugh, D. A., Busnello, J. V., Marca, G.,…Kapczinski, F. (2008). A double-blind, randomized, placebo-controlled 4-week study on the efficacy and safety of the purinergic agents allopurinal and dipyramidole adjunctive to lithium in acute bipolar mania. *Journal of Clinical Psychiatry, 69,* 1237–1245.

McElroy, S. L., Keck, P. E., Stanton, S. P., Tugrul, K. C., Bennett, J. A., & Strakowski, S. M. (1996). Randomized comparison of divalproex oral loading vs. haloperidol in the initial treatment of acute psychotic mania. *Journal of Clinical Psychiatry, 57*(4), 142–146.

McElroy, S. L., Martens, B., Winstanley, E. L., Creech, R., Malhotra, S., & Keck, P. E. Jr. (2010). Randomized, double-blind, placebo-controlled study of divalproex extended release loading monotherapy in ambulatory bipolar spectrum disorder with moderate-to-severe hypomania or mild mania. *Journal of Clinical Psychiatry, 71,* 557–565.

McIntyre, R. S., Brecher, M., Paulsson, B., Huizar, K., & Mullen, J. (2005). Quetiapine or haloperidol as monotherapy for bipolar mania: 12-week, double-blind, randomized, parallel-group, placebo-controlled trial. *European Neuropsychopharmacology, 15*(5), 573–585.

McIntyre, R. S., Cohen, M., Zhao, J., Alphs, L., Macek, T. A., & Panagides, J. (2010). Asenapine in the treatment of acute mania in bipolar I disorder: randomized, double-blind, placebo-controlled trial. *Journal of Affective Disorders, 122*(1–2), 27–38.

McIntyre, R. S., Cohen, M., Zhao, J., Alphs, L., Macek, T. A., & Panagides, J. (2009). Three-week, randomized, placebo-controlled trial of asenapine in the treatment of acute mania in bipolar mania and mixed states. *Bipolar Disorders, 11*(7), 673–686.

Niufan, G., Tohen, M., Qiuqing, A., Fude, Y., Pope, E., McElroy, H.,…Liang, S. (2008). Olanzapine vs. lithium in the acute treatment of bipolar mania: a double-blind, randomized, controlled trial. ClinicalTrials.gov: NCT00485680. *Journal of Affective Disorders, 105*(1–3), 101–108.

Novartis Clinical Trial Results Database (2007). Randomized, double-blind, placebo-controlled multicenter study to evaluate efficacy and tolerability of licabazepine 1000-2000 mg/d in the treatment of manic episodes of bipolar I disorder over 3 weeks. Study ID Number: CLIC477D2301. ClinicalTrials.gov: NCT00099229. (Data on file).

Perlis, R. H., Baker, R. W., Zarate, C. A., Jr, Brown, E. B., Schuh, L. M., Jamal, H. H., & Tohen, M. (2006). Olanzapine vs. risperidone in the treatment of manic or mixed States in bipolar I disorder: a randomized, double-blind trial. *Journal of Clinical Psychiatry, 67*(11), 1747–1753.

Piantadosi, S. (1997). *Clinical trials: A methodological approach.* New York: Wiley.

Pope, H. G., Jr, McElroy, S. L., Keck, P. E., Jr, & Hudson, J. I. (1991). Valproate in the treatment of acute mania: placebo-controlled study. *Achieves of General Psychiatry, 48*(1), 62–68.

Potkin, S. G., Keck, P. E., Jr, Segal, S., Ice, K., & English, P. (2005). Ziprasidone in acute bipolar mania: 21-day randomized, double-blind, placebo-controlled replication trial. *Journal of Clinical Psychopharmacology, 25*(4), 301–310.

Sachs, G. S., Chengappa, K. N. R., Suppes, T., Mullen, J. A., Brecher, M., Devine, N. A., & Sweitzer, D. E. (2004). Quetiapine with lithium or divalproex for the treatment of bipolar mania: A randomized, double-blind, placebo-controlled study. *Bipolar Disorders, 6,* 213–223.

Sachs, G. S., Grossman, F., Ghaemi, S. N., Okamoto, A., & Bowden, C. L. (2002). Combination moods stabilizer with risperidone or haloperidol for treatment of acute mania: A double- blind, placebo-controlled comparison of efficacy and safety. *The American Journal of Psychiatry, 159,* 1146–1154.

Sachs, G., Sanchez, R., Marcus, R., Stock, E., McQuade, R., Carson, W.,…Iwamoto, T., Aripiprazole Study Group (2006). Aripiprazole in the treatment of acute manic or mixed episodes in patients with bipolar I disorder: 3-week placebo-controlled study. *Journal of Psychopharmacology, 20*(4), 536–546.

Sachs, G. S., Vanderburg, D. G., Edman, S., Karayal, O. N., Kolluri, S., Bachinsky, M., & Cavus, I. (2012). Adjunctive oral ziprasidone in patients with acute mania treated with lithium or divalproex: Part 2. Influence of protocol-specific eligibility criteria on signal detection. *Journal of Clinical Psychiatry, 73,* 1420–1425.

Sachs, G. S., Vanderburg, D. G., Karayal, O. N., Kolluri, S., Bachinsky, M., &Cavus, I. (2012). Adjunctive oral ziprasidone in patients with acute mania treated with lithium or divalproex: Part 1. Results of a randomized, double-blind, placebo-controlled trial. *Journal of Clinical Psychiatry, 73,* 1412–1419.

Salanti, G., Higgins, J. P. T., Ades, A. E., & Ioannidis, J. P. A. (2008). Evaluation of networks of randomized trials. *Statistical Methods in Medical Research, 17*(3), 279–301.

Segal, J., Berk, M., & Brook, S. (1998). Risperidone compared with both lithium and haloperidol in mania: double-blind randomized controlled trial. *Clinical Neuropharmacology*, 21(3), 176–180.

Shafti, S. S. (2010). Olanzapine vs. lithium in management of acute mania. *Journal of Affective Disorders*, 122(3), 273–276.

Small, J. G., Klapper, M. H., Milstein, V., Kellams, J. J., Miller, M. J., Marhenke, J. D., & Small, I. F. (1991). Carbamazepine compared with lithium in the treatment of mania. *Achieves of General Psychiatry*, 48(10), 915–921.

Smulevich, A. B., Khanna, S., Eerdekens, M., Karcher, K., Kramer, M., & Grossman, F. (2005). Acute and continuation risperidone monotherapy in bipolar mania: 3-week placebo-controlled trial followed by 9-week double-blind trial of risperidone and haloperidol. *European Neuropsychopharmacology*, 15(1), 75–84.

Suppes, T., Dennehy, E. B., Hirschfeld, R. M. A, Altshuler, L. L., Bowden, C. L., Calabrese, J. R.,...Texas Consensus Conference of Medication Treatment of Bipolar Disorder. (2005). The Texas Implementation of Medication Algorithms: Update to the algorithms for the treatment of bipolar I disorder. *Journal of Clinical Psychiatry*, 66, 870–886.

Szegedi, A., Calabrese, J. R., Stet, L., Mackie, M., Zhao, J., Panagides, J., & Apollo Study Group. (2012). Asenapineas adjunctive treatment for bipolar mania: A placebo-controlled 12- week study and 40-week extension. *Journal of Clinical Psychopharmacology*, 32, 46–55.

Tamayo, J. M., Zarate, C. A., Vieta, E., & Vázquez, G. (2010). Level of response and safety of pharmacological monotherapy in the treatment of acute bipolar I disorder phases: A systematic review and meta-analysis. *International Journal of Neuropsychopharmacology*, 13, 813–832.

Tarr, G. P., Herbison, P., Leon de la Barra, S., & Glue, P. (2011). Study design and patient characteristics and outcome in acute mania trials. *Bipolar Disorders*, 13, 125–132.

Tohen, M., Baker, R. W., Altshuler, L. L., Zarate, C. A. Jr., Suppes, T., Ketter, T. A.,...Tollefson, G. A. (2002). Olanzapine versus divalproex in the treatment of acute mania. *The American Journal of Psychiatry*, 159(6), 1011–1017.

Tohen, M., Chengappa, K. N. R., Suppes, T., Zarate, C. A. Jr., & Calabrese, J. R. (2002). Efficacy of olanzapine in the treatment of mania in patients partially responsive to lithium or valproate. *Archives of General Psychiatry*, 59, 62–69.

Tohen, M., Jacobs, T. G., Grundy, S. L., McElroy, S. L., Banov, M. C., Janicak, P. G.,...Breier, A. (2000). Efficacy of olanzapine in acute bipolar mania: double-blind, placebo-controlled study. *Archives of General Psychiatry*, 57(9), 841–849.

Tohen, M., Goldberg, J. F., Gonzalez-Pinto Arrillaga, A. M., Azorin, J. M., Vieta, E., Hardy-Bayle, M. C.,...Breier, A. (2003). 12-week, double-blind comparison of olanzapine vs. haloperidol in the treatment of acute mania. *Archives of General Psychiatry*, 60(12), 1218–1226.

Tohen, M., Sanger, T. M., McElroy, S. L., Tollefson, G. D., Chengappa, K. N., Daniel, D. G.,...Toma, V. (1999). Olanzapine vs. placebo in the treatment of acute mania. *American Journal of Psychiatry*, 156(5), 702–709.

Tohen, M., Vieta, E., Goodwin, G., Sun, B., Amsterdam, J., Banov, M.,...Bowden, C. (2008). Olanzapine vs. divalproex vs. placebo in the treatment of mild to moderate mania: randomized, 12-week, double-blind study. *Journal of Clinical Psychiatry*, 69(11), 1776–1789.

Vasudev, K., Goswami, U., & Kohli, K. (2000). Carbamazepine and valproate monotherapy: feasibility, relative safety and efficacy, and therapeutic drug monitoring in manic disorder. *Psychopharmacology*, 150(1), 15–23.

Vieta, E., Bourin, M., Sanchez, R., Marcus, R., Stock, E., McQuade, R.,...Iwamoto, T. (2005). Effectiveness of aripiprazole vs. haloperidol in acute bipolar mania: double-blind, randomised, comparative 12-week trial. *British Journal of Psychiatry*, 187, 235–242.

Vieta, E., Nuamah, I. F., Lim, P., Yuen, E. C., Palumbo, J. M., Hough, D. W., & Berwaerts, J. (2010a). Randomized, placebo- and active-controlled study of paliperidone extended release for the treatment of acute manic and mixed episodes of bipolar I disorder.

ClinicalTrials.gov: NCT00309699. *Bipolar Disorders*, 12(3), 230–243.

Vieta, E., Ramey, T., Keller, D., English, P. A., Loebel, A. D., & Miceli, J. (2010b). Ziprasidone in the treatment of acute mania: 12-week placebo-controlled, haloperidol-referenced study. *Journal of Psychopharmacology*, 24(4), 547–558.

Vieta, E., T'joen, C., McQuade, R. D., Carson, W. H., Marcus, R. N., Sanchez, R., Owen, R., & Nameche, L. (2008). Efficacy of adjunctive aripiprazole to either valproate or lithium in bipolar mania patients partially nonresponsive to valproate/lithium monotherapy. *The American Journal of Psychiatry*, 165, 1316–1325.

Weisler, R. H., Dunn, J., & English, P. (2003, September). *Ziprasidone in adjunctive treatment of bipolar mania: A randomized, double-blind, placebo-controlled trial*. Paper presented at the 16th annual meeting of the European College of Neuropsychopharmacology, Prague, Czech Republic.

Weisler, R. H., Kalali, A. H., & Ketter, T. A. (2004). Multicenter, randomized, double-blind, placebo-controlled trial of extended-release carbamazepine capsules as monotherapy for bipolar disorder patients with manic or mixed episodes. *Journal of Clinical Psychiatry*, 65(4), 478–484.

Weisler, R. H., Keck, P. E., Jr, Swann, A. C., Cutler, A. J., Ketter, T. A., & Kalali, A. H. (2005). Extended-release carbamazepine capsules as monotherapy for acute mania in bipolar disorder: multicenter, randomized, double-blind, placebo-controlled trial. *Journal of Clinical Psychiatry*, 66(3), 323–330.

Yatham, L. N., Grossman, F., Augustyns, I., Vieta, E., & Ravindran, A. (2003). Mood stabilizers plus risperidone or placebo in the treatment of acute mania: International, double-blind, randomized, controlled trial. *The British Journal of Psychiatry*, 182, 141–147.

Yatham, L. N., Kennedy, S. H., Parikh, S. V., Schaffer, A., Beaulieu, S., Alda, M.,...Berk, M. (2013). Canadian Network for Mood and Anxiety Treatments (CANMAT) and International Society for Bipolar Disorders (ISBD) collaborative update of CANMAT guidelines for the management of patients with bipolar disorder: Update 2013. *Bipolar Disorders*, 15, 1–44.

Yatham, L. N., Paulsson, B., Mullen, J. A., &Vagaro, A. M. (2004). Quetiapine versus placebo in combination with lithium or divalproex for the treatment of bipolar mania. *Journal of Clinical Psychopharmacology*, 24, 599–606.

Yildiz, A., Guleryuz, S., Ankerst, D. P., Ongur, D., & Renshaw, P. F. (2008). Protein kinase C inhibition in the treatment of mania: A double-blind, placebo-controlled trial of tamoxifen. *Archives of General Psychiatry*, 65(3), 255–263.

Yildiz, A., Nikodem, M., Vieta, E., Correll, C. U., & Baldessarini, R. J. (2014). A network meta-analysis on comparative efficacy and all-cause discontinuation of antimanic treatments in acute bipolar mania *Psychological Medicine*, 18 July [Epub ahead of print].

Yildiz, A., Vieta, E., Correll, C. U., Nikodem, M., & Baldessarini, R. J. (2014). Critical issues on the use of network meta-analysis in psychiatry. *Harvard Review of Psychiatry*, 22(6), 367–372.

Yildiz, A., Vieta, E., Leucht, S., & Baldessarini, R. J. (2011). Efficacy of antimanic treatments: Meta- analysis of randomized controlled trials. *Neuropsychopharmacology*, 36(2), 375–389.

Young, A. H., Oren, D. A., Lowy, A., McQuade, R. D., Marcus, R. N., Carson, W. H.,...Sanchez, R. (2009). Aripiprazole monotherapy in acute mania: 12-week randomized placebo- and haloperidol-controlled study. *The British Journal of Psychiatry*, 194(1), 40–48.

Zajecka, J. M., Weisler, R., Sachs, G., Swann, A. C., Wozniak, P., & Sommerville, K. W. (2002). Comparison of the efficacy, safety, and tolerability of divalproex sodium and olanzapine in the treatment of bipolar disorder. *Journal of Clinical Psychiatry*, 63(12), 1148–1155.

Zarate, C. A. Jr., Singh, J. B., Carlson, P. J., Quiroz, J., Jolkovsky, L., Luckenbaugh, D. A., & Manji, H. K. (2007). Efficacy of a protein kinase C inhibitor (tamoxifen in the treatment of acute mania: A pilot study. *Bipolar Disorders*, 9(6), 561–570.

22.

PHARMACOLOGICAL TREATMENT
BIPOLAR DEPRESSION

Keming Gao, Renrong Wu, Heinz Grunze, and Joseph R. Calabrese

INTRODUCTION

The burden of bipolar depression is greater than that of bipolar mania, although mania may present in more dramatic ways such as impaired judgment with risky behaviors. Patients with bipolar disorder spend more time in depression than in mania/hypomania with more impairment at work, social life, and family life and an increased suicide risk during depressive phases. Significant psychosocial impairment during euthymia is more strongly predicted by the number of past depressive episodes than past manias. It is critical to treat acute depression and to prevent depressive relapse in order to reduce mortality and morbidity in patients with bipolar disorder. However, the treatment of bipolar depression has not been as widely studied as mania.

Antidepressant effects of lithium, anticonvulsants, antipsychotics, antidepressants, and some unconventional psychopharmacological agents have been studied in bipolar depression using *Diagnostic and Statistical Manual of Mental Disorders* fourth edition (*DSM-IV*) diagnostic criteria. However, only quetiapine monotherapy, olanzapine and fluoxetine combination (OFC), lurasidone monotherapy, and lurasidone adjunctive to mood stabilizer have been approved by the United States Food and Drug Administration (US FDA) for acute bipolar depression. Therefore, most treatments for acute bipolar depression are off-label and some are still controversial. To maximize benefit and minimize risk of current available agents, it is essential to understand the efficacy and safety of each medication in the treatment of bipolar depression. In this chapter, commonly used agents for bipolar depression are reviewed. Agents with large, randomized, double-blind, placebo-controlled studies are prioritized.

ATYPICAL ANTIPSYCHOTICS

OLANZAPINE AND OLANZAPINE-FLUOXETINE COMBINATION

OFC is the first agent approved by the US FDA for the acute treatment of bipolar I depression (Tohen et al., 2003). Olanzapine monotherapy or OFC exhibited significant improvement in depressive symptoms compared to placebo (see Table 22.1 and Table 22.2). OFC was significantly better than placebo and olanzapine alone. The effect size for olanzapine monotherapy was small (0.32), but the effect size of the OFC arm was moderate (0.68). The efficacy of olanzapine monotherapy was replicated in bipolar I depression with an effect size of 0.22 (Tohen et al., 2012). Limited efficacy and safety concern of olanzapine monotherapy made the US FDA approve OFC but not olanzapine monotherapy for the acute treatment of bipolar I (BPI) depression. A recent meta-analysis showed that OFCs were superior to olanzapine and placebo but not to lamotrigine (Silva, Zimmermann, Galvao, & Pereira, 2013). Adverse events were more common in patients treated with OFC than those with lamotrigine, which support the recommendation of lamotrigine over OFC as the first-line treatment for acute bipolar depression although OFC had better efficacy than lamotrigine (Suppes et al., 2005).

Both OFC and olanzapine were relatively well tolerated compared to placebo. There was a small but significantly increased risk for discontinuation due to adverse events (DAEs) with olanzapine relative to placebo with a number needed to treat to harm (NNTH) of 24 (95% confidence interval [CI]: 23–224; Gao et al., 2011). Adverse events occurred more frequently in patients treated with either olanzapine or OFC included somnolence, weight gain,

Table 22.1. SUMMARY OF RANDOMIZED, DOUBLE-BLIND, PLACEBO OR ACTIVE TREATMENT CONTROLLED STUDIES OF DRUG MONOTHERAPY OR META-ANALYSES IN THE ACUTE TREATMENT OF BIPOLAR DEPRESSION

AGENTS AND TRIALS	PATIENTS	TREATMENT ARMS	DURATION (WEEKS)	NO. OF PATIENTS	PRIMARY OUTCOME	SECONDARY OUTCOMES
Antipsychotics						
Aripiprazole Thase et al., 2008	Bipolar I depression	Aripiprazole 5–30 mg/day (15.5–17.6 mg/day) Placebo	8	337 353	Not superior to placebo in reducing MADRS	No significant difference from placebo in changes in CGI-S, remission rate, or response rate
Olanzapine Tohen et al., 2003 Tohen et al., 2012	Bipolar I depression	Olanzapine 5–20 mg/d (9.7 mg/day) Placebo	6 to 8	690 524	Superior to placebo in reducing MADRS	Significant difference from placebo in response, HAMA, CGI-S, and some items of MADRS
Quetiapine-IR Calabrese et al., 2005 Thase et al., 2006 Young et al., 2010 McElroy et al., 2010	Bipolar I or II depression BPI n =1,472 BPI n =808	Quetiapine-IR 300 mg/day Quetiapine-IR 600 mg/day Placebo	8	811 816 580	Superior to placebo in reducing MADRS	Significant difference from placebo in response, remission, HAMD, HAMA, CGI-S, and Q-LES-Q
Quetiapine-XR Suppes et al., 2008	Bipolar I or II Depression BPI n =217 BPII n =53	Quetiapine-XR 300 mg/day Placebo	8	133 137	Superior to placebo in reducing MADRS total score	Superior to placebo in response, remission, CGI-S, 8 of 10 items of MADRS
Ziprasidone Lombardo et al., 2012	Bipolar I depression	Ziprasidone 40–80 mg/day Ziprasidone 120–160 mg/day Placebo	6	288 232 364	Not superior to placebo in reducing MADRS	Not superior to placebo in any secondary outcome measure
Lurasidone Lobel et al., 2014	Bipolar I depression	Lurasidone 20–60 mg/day Lurasidone 80–120 mg/d Placebo	6	161 162 162	Superior to placebo in reducing MADRS	Superior to placebo in responder, remission, QIDS-16 HAMA, SDS, Q-LES-Q
Anticonvulsants						
Lamotrigine Geddes et al., 2009	Bipolar I or II depression BPI n = 833 BPII n = 305	Lamotrigine 100–400 mg/ day Placebo	7 to 10	541 530	Superior to placebo in response rate based on MADRS and HAMD	Superior to placebo in remission rate based on MADRS, but not based on HAMD Superior to placebo in reducing MADRS, but not HAMD
Divalproex-ER Bond et al., 2010	Bipolar I or II depression BPI n =78 BPII n =62	Divalproex Placebo	6 to 8	69 69	Superior to placebo in response rate based on ≥ 50% improvement in standard depression rating scale	Superior to placebo in remission rate based on the definition from original studies

Antidepressant		Diagnosis	Treatment		N			
Paroxetine McElroy et al., 2010		Bipolar I or II Depression BPI *n* = 150 BPII *n* = 99	Paroxetine 20 mg/day Placebo	8	121 118	Not superior to placebo in reducing MADRS	Superior to placebo in reducing HAMA, but not in other secondary outcome measures
Others							
Lithium Young et al., 2010		Bipolar I or II Depression BPI *n* = 165 BPII *n* = 100	Lithium 600–1,800 mg/day with 64.4% Li Level of 0.6–1.2 mEq/L Placebo	8	136 129	Not superior to placebo in reducing MADRS	Trended decrease in HAMD, CGI-S, SDS favoring lithium over placebo
Olanzapine+fluoxetine vs. Lamotrigine Brown et al., 2005		Bipolar I depression	Olanzapine-fluoxetine 6/25 mg/d, 6/50 mg/day, 12/25 mg or 12/50 mg/day Lamotrigine 150–200 mg/day	7	205 205	Olanzapine plus fluoxetine superior to lamotrigine in reducing CGI-S with effect size of 0.26	Olanzapine plus fluoxetine superior to lamotrigine in reducing MADRS, YMRS, CGI-I, BPRS, but not in response or remission rates based on MADRS

NOTE: BPRS = Brief Psychiatric Rating Scale; CGI-I = Clinical Global Impression—Improvement; CGI-S = Clinical Global Impression–Severity; HAMD = Hamilton Depression Rating Scale; HAMA = Hamilton Anxiety Rating Scale; MADRS = Montgomery-Åsberg Depression Rating Scale; QIDS-16 = Quick Inventory of Depressive Symptomatology–16 item; Q-LES-Q = Quality of Life, Enjoyment, and Satisfaction Questionnaire; SDS = Sheehan Disability Scale; YMRS = Young Mania Rating Scale.

Table 22.2. SUMMARY OF RANDOMIZED, DOUBLE-BLIND, PLACEBO OR ACTIVE TREATMENT CONTROLLED STUDIES OR META-ANALYSES OF DRUG ADJUNCTIVE (COMBINATION) THERAPY IN THE ACUTE TREATMENT OF BIPOLAR DEPRESSION

AGENTS AND TRIALS	PATIENTS	TREATMENT ARMS	DURATION (WEEKS)	NO. OF PATIENTS	PRIMARY OUTCOME	SECONDARY OUTCOMES
Antipsychotics						
Olanzapine-Fluoxetine Tohen et al., 2003	Bipolar I depression	Olanzapine-fluoxetine 6/25 mg/day, 6/50 mg/day, or 12/50 mg/day Placebo	8	82 355	Superior to placebo in reducing MADRS	Significant difference from placebo in response, remission, HAMA, CGI-S, and 8 of 10 items of MADRS
Ziprasidone Sachs et al., 2011	Bipolar I depression Lithium 0.6–1.2 mEq/L or valproate 50-125 µg/ml for ≥ 4 weeks	MS + ziprasidone 40–160 mg/day MS + placebo	6	145 145	Not superior to placebo in reducing MADRS	Superior to placebo in improving GAF and SDS, but not in CGI-S, HAMA, or Q-LES-Q
Lurasidone Lobel et al., 2014	Bipolar I depression Lithium or valproate in therapeutic level for 4 weeks	MS + lurasidone 20–120 mg/day MS + placebo	6	179 161	Superior to placebo in reducing MADRS	Superior to placebo in responder and remission rates and reducing QIDS-16, HAMA, SDS, Q-LES-Q, CGI-S
Antidepressant						
Antidepressant vs. Placebo Sachs et al., 2007	Bipolar I or II depression	MS + paroxetine or bupropion MS + placebo	26	179 187	Not superior to placebo in durable recovery	Not superior to placebo in transient remission, transient remission or durable recovery, treatment-effectiveness response, treatment-emergent affective switch, or discontinuation of study medication due to adverse event
Antidepressant vs. placebo[a] Gijsman et al., 2004	Bipolar I or II depression, mainly bipolar I	MS + antidepressant MS + placebo	5 to 10	213 449	Superior to placebo in response rate	Superior to placebo in remission rate No significant difference from placebo in switch rate
Antidepressant vs. placebo[b] Sidor and MacQueen, 2011	Bipolar I or II depression	MS + antidepressant MS + placebo	6 to 26	341 565	Not superior to placebo in response rate	Not significant different from placebo in remission rate
Antidepressant vs. other agents Sidor and MacQueen, 2011	Bipolar I or II depression	MS + antidepressant MS + other agents	4 to 12	235 222	Not superior to other agents in response rate	Not significant different from other agents in remission rate

Study	Population	Intervention	Duration	N	Result (response)	Result (remission)
Bupropion vs. antidepressant Sidor and MacQueen, 2011	Bipolar I or II depression	MS + bupropion MS+ antidepressant	6 to 10	119 137	Not superior to other antidepressants in response rate	Not significant different from other antidepressants in remission rate

Awake-promoting agent

Study	Population	Intervention	Duration	N	Result (response)	Result (remission)
Modafinil Frye et al., 2007	Bipolar I or II depression inadequately response to a mood stabilizer at stable doses for ≥ 2 weeks	MS + Modafinil 100–200 mg/day MS + Placebo	6	41 44	Superior to placebo in reducing IDS-C$_{30}$ total score	Superior to placebo in response and remission rate, and in improvement of 4 item of fatigue—and energy—subset of the IDS-C$_{30}$
Armodafinil Calabrese et al., 2010	Bipolar I depression nonresponse to lithium, valproic acid, or olanzapine for ≥ 8 weeks	MS + Armadofinil 150 mg/day MS + Placebo	8	124 123	Superior to placebo in Reduction of IDS-C30 with analysis of variance but no with analysis of covariance	No difference between group in response, remission, MADRS, QIDS-16, CGI-S, IDS-C30 items, MADRS items, HAMA, Q-LES-Q
Armodafinil[c] Calabrese et al., 2014	Bipolar I depression Emergence of a new depressive episode while taking a FDA-approved maintenance therapy	MS + Armadofinil 150 mg/day MS + Placebo	8	201 199	Armodafinil superior to placebo in reducing IDS-C$_{30}$ total score	Significant difference from placebo in changes in IDS-C$_{30}$ individual items of panic/phobic symptoms, increased appetite, concentration/decisions, energy/fatigability, and leaden paralysis/physical energy, and IDS-C$_{30}$ responders, but not in CGI-S responders or change in GAF

Others

Study	Population	Intervention	Duration	N	Result (response)	Result (remission)
Lamotrigine + lithium vs. Lithium alone van der Loos et al., 2009	Bipolar I or II depression BPI n =84 BPII n =40 Lithium for ≥ 2 weeks	Lithium (0.6–1.2 mEq/L) + lamotrigine 200 mg/day Lithium (0.6–1.2 mEq/L) + Placebo	8	64 60	Superior to placebo in reducing MADRS	Significant difference in MADRS responder, but not in CGI-S responder

NOTE: CGI-S = Clinical Global Impression—Severity; GAF = Global Assessment of Functioning; HAMD = Hamilton Depression Rating Scale; HAMA = Hamilton Anxiety Rating Scale; IDS-C$_{30}$ = Inventory of Depressive Symptomatology–Clinician-Rated, 30 items; MADRS = Montgomery-Asberg Depression Rating Scale; MS = mood stabilizer; QIDS-16 = Quick Inventory of Depressive Symptomatology–16 item; Q-LES-Q = Quality of Life, Enjoyment, and Satisfaction Questionnaire; SDS = Sheehan Disability Scale.

[a] In this meta-analysis, about 184 patients were not on a mood stabilizer and 54 patients did not have bipolar disorder. [b] In this meta-analysis, about 67 patients were not on a mood stabilizer but all patients had bipolar disorder. [c] In this study, a FDA-approved maintenance therapy included (a) lithium or valproate monotherapy; (b) olanzapine, aripiprazole, risperidone, or lamotrigine (either alone or in combination with lithium or valproate); or (c) ziprasidone in combination with lithium or valproate.

increased appetite, dry mouth, asthenia, and diarrhea (see Table 22.3). Treatment-emergent mania (TEM) did not differ among the olanzapine, OFC, and placebo groups. Olanzapine and OFC caused significant weight gain compared to placebo with 2.59 ± 3.24 kg, 2.79 ± 3.23 kg, and −0.47 ± 2.62 kg, respectively. The NNTH for ≥ 7% weight gain of OFC and olanzapine relative to placebo was 5 for both (Gao et al., 2011). Olanzapine and OFC also caused significantly higher cholesterol and nonfasting blood glucose levels compared to placebo.

Olanzapine has some anxiolytic effect and may be especially useful for those with depression and a high level of anxiety (Gao, Muzina, Gajwani, & Calabrese, 2006). Somnolence/sedation was the most common side effect from OFC or olanzapine and caused premature discontinuation or noncompliance (Gao et al., 2008, 2011), but the main concern is the long-term effect of olanzapine causing metabolic abnormalities. The metabolic parameters should be monitored as recommended by the Consensus Development Conference on Antipsychotic Drugs and Obesity and Diabetes (American Psychiatric Association, American Association of Clinical Endocrinologists, and North American Association for the Study of Obesity, 2004).

QUETIAPINE

Quetiapine immediate-release (quetiapine-IR) monotherapy is the second medication approved by the US FDA for acute bipolar I and II depression (see Table 22.1). Two initial studies demonstrated that quetiapine-IR 600 mg/day and 300 mg/day produced significantly greater improvement in depressive symptoms compared with placebo as early as Week 1. The effect sizes for quetiapine-IR 600 mg/day and 300 mg/day were moderate. The response and remission rates and other secondary outcome measures also showed significant superiority of quetiapine-IR over the placebo (see Table 22.1). In a subtype analysis of the first study (Calabrese et al., 2005), the effect sizes for quetiapine-IR 600 mg/day and quetiapine-IR 300 mg/day in the BPI subgroup were large but in the BPII subgroup were small. However, in the second study (Thase et al., 2006), the effect sizes for quetiapine-IR 600 mg/day and quetiapine-IR 300 mg/day were moderate in both BPI and BPII subtypes.

Quetiapine extended-release (quetiapine-XR) at 300 mg/day also exhibited superiority over placebo in reducing depressive symptoms in BPI or BPII depression with a moderate effect size (Suppes et al., 2010, see Table 22.1). In the two quetiapine-IR pivotal studies, there was minimal difference in efficacy between a fixed dose of 600 mg/

day and 300 mg/day, but there was a higher rate of DAEs in the quetiapine-IR 600 mg group (Gao et al., 2011). The NNTH for DAEs with quetiapine-IR 600 mg/day and 300 mg/day was 11 (95% CI: 8–18) and 24 (95% CI: 14–83), respectively. The most common causes for discontinuation were sedation, somnolence, and dizziness (Gao et al., 2008, 2011).

Patients treated with quetiapine-IR or -XR had significantly higher rates of dry mouth, sedation, somnolence, dizziness, and constipation than those treated with a placebo (see Table 22.3). Mean weight gain was 1.6 kg for quetiapine-IR 600 mg/day, 1.0 kg for quetiapine-IR 300 mg/day, and 0.2 kg for the placebo. The NNTH for ≥ 7% weight gain with quetiapine-IR 600 mg/day and 300 mg/day was 17 (95% CI: 12–27) and 28 (95% CI: 18–71), respectively (Gao et al., 2011). Weight gain in the quetiapine-XR was greater than in the placebo (1.3 kg vs. −0.2 kg). The NNTH for ≥ 7% weight gain was 14 (95% CI 8–39) (Gao et al., 2011). Similar to quetiapine-IR, quetiapine-XR at 300 mg/day had a significant higher rate for DAEs relative to placebo with a NNTH of 9 (95% CI: 6–20; Gao et al., 2011).

Since the most common cause for premature discontinuation from quetiapine was somnolence and sedation (Gao et al., 2008, 2011), undoubtedly it is essential to properly manage these side effects. Starting a lower dose and titrating slowly might be helpful. There has been no study on the onset and duration of somnolence sedation of antipsychotics in bipolar depression. However, a recent post hoc analysis of asenapine and olanzapine in acute mania found that the median duration of somnolence was 7 days for asenapine and 8.5 days for olanzapine (Gao, Mackle, Cazorla, Zhao, & Szegedi. 2013). Since depressed bipolar patients had lower tolerability to somnolence than those with mania or schizophrenia (Gao et al., 2008), it appears reasonable that if somnolence/sedation continues after three to four weeks, other medications should be considered.

The targeted dose of quetiapine should be 300 mg/day regardless of IR or XR formulation. For those who cannot tolerate 300 mg/day, a lower dose may be worth trying. The justification of a lower dose than 300 mg/day is based on the fact that a minimal effective dose of quetiapine has not been established. Quetiapine also has anxiolytic effects and may be especially useful for those with depression and a high level of anxiety (Gao et al., 2006).

ARIPIPRAZOLE

Aripiprazole has partial agonistic activity at D_2, D_3, and 5-HT$_{1A}$ receptors and antagonistic activity at 5-HT$_{2A}$

receptors. There were some preliminary positive results of aripiprazole in bipolar depression, but two large, randomized, placebo-controlled trials did not show superiority of aripiprazole over placebo in reducing depressive symptoms at the end of the studies. Aripiprazole did transiently reduce depressive symptoms significantly compared to placebo (Thase et al., 2008). There were also no significant differences in key secondary outcome measures between aripiprazole and placebo (see Table 22.1). Therefore, aripiprazole did not receive US FDA approval for acute bipolar depression. In contrast, aripiprazole adjunctive to antidepressant(s) was superior to placebo in patients with major depressive disorder (MDD) who failed antidepressant treatment and received US FDA approval for this indication.

The adverse events with >10% incidences in these two studies were akathisia, insomnia, nausea, fatigue, restlessness, dry mouth, and headache (see Table 22.3). Akathisia was a common, significantly higher side effect with aripiprazole relative to placebo with a NNTH of 5 (95% CI: 4–6). The NNTH for the DAEs was 14 (95% CI: 1–35; Gao et al., 2011). There was no significant difference in mean weight gain or the proportion of ≥ 7% weight gain between the two groups.

ZIPRASIDONE

Like olanzapine, ziprasidone showed efficacy in reducing depressive symptoms in patients with mixed mania as well as in bipolar depression and treatment-resistant MDD. However, ziprasidone monotherapy or adjunctive therapy to mood stabilizers in bipolar depression did not show superiority over placebo (see Table 22.1). Like aripiprazole, ziprasidone was not approved by US FDA for acute bipolar depression. Exploratory analyses of randomized, placebo-controlled studies found that 36% of patients in one study and 31% in another study did not meet moderate severity inclusion criterion at baseline as measured by the Montgomery-Åsberg Depression Rating Scale (MADRS). The inclusion of mildly depressed patients in these studies might result in the inability to detect the treatment-induced change. Serious inconsistencies in subject rating could be another potential cause for failure to detect a difference between ziprasidone and placebo (Lombardo, Sachs, Kolluri, Kremer, & Yang, 2012). Poor-quality rating at baseline by a subgroup of patients and raters were also observed in the ziprasidone adjunctive therapy study (Sachs et al., 2011; see Table 22.2).

In contrast, a six-week study in a group of patients with MDD (n = 29) and BPII depression (n = 43) who were in a mixed state showed that ziprasidone (40–160 mg/day) had superiority over the placebo at reducing depressive symptoms (Patkar et al., 2012). The benefit of patients with BPII was larger than those with MDD.

There was no significant difference in the DAEs between ziprasidone and placebo regardless of higher (120–160 mg/day) or lower (40–80 mg/day) doses. The most common side effect was somnolence (see Table 22.3), with a NNTH of 10 for the lower dose and 7 for the higher dose. At the higher dose, there was a slightly higher but statistically

Table 22.3. SUMMARY OF SIDE EFFECTS FROM MEDICATIONS STUDIED IN ACUTE BIPOLAR DEPRESSION WITH RATES OF AT LEAST ONE AND HALF TIMES HIGHER RELATIVE TO PLACEBO

MEDICATIONS	SIDE EFFECTS IN DESCENDING ORDER
Aripiprazole	Akathisia, insomnia, nausea, fatigue, restlessness, dry mouth, anxiety, increased appetite, sedation, disturbance in attention
Olanzapine	Somnolence, weight gain, increase appetite, dry month, asthenia
Olanzapine+Fluoxetine	Somnolence, weight gain, dry mouth, increase appetite, asthenia, diarrhea
Quetiapine-IR	Dry mouth, sedation, somnolence, dizziness, fatigue, constipation, dyspepsia, increased appetite, tremor
Quetiapine-XR	Dry mouth, somnolence, sedation, increased appetite, weight gain, dyspepsia, fatigue
Ziprasidone	Somnolence, sedation, dizziness, nausea, insomnia, anxiety, akathisia, restlessness
Lurasidone	Nausea, somnolence, tremor, akathisia, sedation
Lamotrigine	none
Divalproex-ER	Nausea, increased appetite, diarrhea, dry mouth, and stomach cramps
Lithium	Somnolence, dry mouth, nausea, tremor
Paroxetine	Nausea
Armodafinil	Restlessness, somnolence, dry mouth, anxiety
Lamotrigine + Lithium	Nausea, flu-like symptoms, insomnia, tremor, skin problem/mild rash

significant risk for akathisia with ziprasidone relative to placebo with a NNTH of 38 (Gao, Pappadopulos, Karayal, Kolluri, & Calabrese, 2013).

LURASIDONE

Lurasidone is a newer atypical antipsychotic approved by the US FDA for schizophrenia and bipolar depression. It has high affinity for D_2, 5-HT_{2A}, and 5HT_7 receptors (antagonist effect), moderate affinity for 5HT_{1A} (partial agonist effect) and α_{2C} receptors (antagonist effect), and no appreciable affinity for H_1 and M_1 receptors. The approval for bipolar depression was based on two studies (Loebel, Cucchiaro, Silva, Kroger, Sarma, et al., 2014; Loebel, Cucchiaro, Silva, Kroger, Hsu, et al., 2014). In a monotherapy study, lurasidone 20 to 60 mg/day and 80 to 120 mg/day monotherapy resulted in a significantly greater MADRS score reduction in BPI depression than placebo (Loebel, Cucchiaro, Silva, Kroger, Hsu, et al., 2014). The effect sizes were 0.51 for both doses of lurasidone. Both active groups separated from placebo from Week 2 onward and showed significant improvement over placebo on other secondary outcome measures (see Table 22.1). In an adjunctive therapy study (Loebel, Cucchiaro, Silva, Kroger, Sarma, et al., 2012), lurasidone 20 to 120 mg/day adjunctive to either lithium or valproate was also superior to placebo in the treatment of moderate to severe bipolar I depression (see Table 22.2).

Rates of the DAEs, as well as reported nausea and headache, were similar between lurasidone and placebo, but akathisia was higher in lurasidone than in the placebo (see Table 22.3). There were minimal changes in weight, lipids, and measures of glycemic control.

Lurasidone is the third antipsychotic showing efficacy in acute bipolar depression and approved by US FDA for this indication. Although its effect size of 0.51 is smaller than that of quetiapine or OFC, its favorable safety and tolerability profile suggests that it may be used even before trying quetiapine or OFC. Since lurasidone was also efficacious for anxiety symptoms, it may be considered as a first-line medication over lamotrigine for patients with bipolar depression and anxiety symptoms.

ANTICONVULSANTS

LAMOTRIGINE

Lamotrigine monotherapy

The first randomized, double-blind, placebo-controlled study of lamotrigine monotherapy in the acute bipolar depression was published in 1999 (Calabrese et al., 1999). Afterward, none of four similar studies showed a separation between lamotrigine and placebo in reducing depressive symptoms (Calabrese et al., 2008). Therefore lamotrigine was not approved for acute bipolar depression. In the first study, lamotrigine 200 mg/day demonstrated significant efficacy not on the primary but on several secondary outcome measures compared to placebo, but lamotrigine 50 mg/day was superior only to the placebo in a few outcome measures. In a combined analysis of a single patient dataset from these five studies with a total of 1,072 participants, more patients treated with lamotrigine than a placebo responded to treatment as measured with either the Hamilton Depression Rating Scale (HAMD) or the MADRS (Geddes, Calabrese, & Goodwin, 2009). The number needed to treat to benefit (NNTB) for response based on MADRS and HAMD was 13 and 11, respectively. Remission rate of lamotrigine based on MADRS but not based on HAMD was significantly higher than that of placebo (see Table 22.1). In a group of patients with a baseline HAMD total score of > 24, the efficacy of lamotrigine was superior to placebo. However, in a group of patients with a baseline HAMD total score of ≤ 24, the efficacy of lamotrigine was not superior to placebo.

During these studies, patients treated with lamotrigine had a significantly higher rate of headache compared with those treated with placebo (32% vs. 17%) in the first study but no difference in the other four studies (Calabrese et al., 2002, 2008). The incidence of rash did not differ between placebo and treatment arms. However, rash is generally recognized as a side effect likely to complicate the drug's clinical use. In early epilepsy trials, rash lead to hospitalization and treatment discontinuation or Stevens-Johnson syndrome in 0.3% of adults treated with lamotrigine. According to GlaxoSmithKline, manufacturer of lamotrigine, the incidence of serious rashes, including Stevens-Johnson syndrome, is approximately 0.8% (8 per 1,000) in pediatric patients (2 to 16 years of age) receiving lamotrigine as adjunctive therapy for epilepsy and 0.3% (3 per 1,000) in adults on adjunctive therapy for epilepsy (per package insert). In clinical trials of bipolar and other mood disorders, the rate of serious rash was 0.08% (0.8 per 1,000) in adult patients receiving lamotrigine monotherapy and 0.13% (1.3 per 1,000) in adult patients receiving lamotrigine as adjunctive therapy. Severe rashes are more likely to occur in child and adolescents, especially in those younger than 12 years old, forced titration, or co-administration with valproate. Therefore, standard titration schedules should be followed. In addition, during the postmarketing era, rare cases of aseptic meningitis were reported (Simms, Kortepeter, & Avigan, 2012).

Lamotrigine versus OCF

OFC was the first medication approved by the US FDA for acute bipolar depression, but lamotrigine was commonly recommended as the first-line medication for this condition instead. A head-to-head seven-week comparison study of OFC and lamotrigine in the acute treatment of bipolar depression found OFC to be significantly superior to lamotrigine in the primary outcome, the CGI-S (Clinical Global Impression-Severity) score, but did not find significant difference between the two treatments in response and remission rates (Brown et al., 2005; see Table 22.1). Adverse event rates of suicidal and self-injurious behavior were significantly more common among patients treated with lamotrigine (3.4%) as compared with OFC (0.5%). However, significant differences favored treatment with lamotrigine on measures such as hemoglobin A1c, prolactin, and lipids. More important, the rate of ≥ 7% body weight gain in OFC was significantly higher than in lamotrigine (23.4% versus 0%).

Lamotrigine versus lithium

Lithium is the most accepted standard treatment for bipolar disorder. However, its efficacy in acute bipolar depression was never established in rigorous randomized controlled trials. Maintenance studies showed that lithium was more effective in preventing prevent manic relapses, but lamotrigine was more effective in preventing depressive relapses. A 16-week single-blind comparison of lamotrigine ($n = 41$) with lithium ($n = 49$) monotherapy in BPII depression found that both lamotrigine 200 mg/day and lithium ≥ 900 mg/day (0.6–1.2 mEq/L) significantly reduced depressive symptoms from baseline to endpoint with no significant difference between the two groups (Suppes et al., 2008).

Lamotrigine adjunctive therapy to lithium

Maintenance data suggests that the combination of these two agents may have more benefit than either alone. In a randomized, placebo-controlled trial, lamotrigine adjunctive therapy to lithium versus placebo adjunctive to lithium supported the superiority of the combination of these two agents over lithium alone in BPI and BPII depression (van der Loos et al., 2009; see Table 22.2). The rates of DAEs

were 6.3% in lamotrigine and 3.3% in placebo. There were no significant differences between lamotrigine and placebo in common side effects (see Table 22.3). These data support the use of lithium and lamotrigine together in acute bipolar depression, especially in those who do not respond to either medication alone.

Valproate/divalproex

Valproate is one of most studied anticonvulsants in bipolar disorder and is approved for acute mania. However, its efficacy in acute bipolar depression has never been studied in large, randomized, placebo-controlled trials. In the largest study of divalproex-ER in the acute treatment of patients with BPI ($n = 20$) or BPII ($n = 34$) depression who were naïve to mood stabilizer, divalproex-ER (1,000–2,000 mg/day) treatment produced statistically significant improvement in MADRS total scores compared with placebo from Week 3 onward (Muzina et al., 2011). Subgroup analysis revealed significant difference between divalproex-ER and placebo in patients with BPI depression but not in those with BPII depression.

A meta-analysis of four trials with 142 patients found that response (39.3% vs.17.5%) and remission (40.6% vs. 24.3%) rates were significantly greater for divalproex than placebo (Bond, Lam, & Yatham, 2010; see Table 22.1). Subjects receiving divalproex-ER compared to placebo reported increased nausea, increased appetite, diarrhea, dry mouth, and stomach cramps (see Table 22.3). There were no clinically relevant differences between groups in vital signs, electrocardiograms, hematology, or clinical chemistry parameters, but patients receiving divalproex gained more weight than those with placebo (4.9 lbs vs. –0.5 lbs).

Topiramate and levetiracetam

There is no double-blinded, placebo-controlled study of topiramate in acute bipolar depression. A small, randomized, placebo-controlled study did not find levetiracetam adjunctive therapy or monotherapy ($n =17$) superior to placebo ($n = 15$) in reducing depressive symptoms in patients with bipolar depression who failed previous treatments (Saricicek et al., 2011). A single-blind study ($n = 36$) comparing topiramate (50–300 mg/day) with bupropion-SR (100-400 mg/day) adjunctive to a mood stabilizer(s) in BPI or BPII depression found that there was no significant difference between two drugs in reducing depressive symptoms, although addition of both drugs produced a significant decrease in depression from baseline to endpoint (McIntyre et al., 2002). Rates of the majority side effects were comparable, but the bupropion group had a significantly higher rate of sleeping difficulty (28% vs. 16%). The topiramate group had more weight loss than the bupropion group (5.8 kg vs. 1.2 kg).

LITHIUM

The efficacy of lithium in the treatment of bipolar mania and maintenance treatment of bipolar disorder has been long established. However, its efficacy in acute bipolar depression was unsettled because there had never been a large study of lithium monotherapy in acute bipolar depression. A recent study of quetiapine-IR in acute bipolar depression has included lithium (Young et al., 2010). Lithium had numerically greater but not statistically significant improvement in MADRS total score compared with placebo (see Table 22.1). Post hoc analyses according to lithium concentration of ≥ 0.8 mEq/L or < 0.8 mEq/L revealed no significant difference from placebo in the improvement of MADRS total score. Quetiapine 600 mg/day and 300 mg/day were superior to placebo in reducing MADRS total scores. Both doses of quetiapine-IR were associated with significant improvements over placebo in MADRS total score in patients with BPI depression, but patients treated with lithium did not show a significant improvement over the placebo in patient with either BPI or BPII depression.

Significantly increased adverse events of quetiapine-IR over placebo were somnolence, dry mouth, sedation, and/or constipation. Significantly increased adverse events of lithium over placebo were dry mouth, nausea, and tremor (see Table 22.3). There were small but significant differences in weight gain and body mass index increases between placebo and the three active treatment arms. However, rates of ≥ 7% weight gain were 8.8% for quetiapine-IR 600 mg/day, 4.6% for quetiapine-IR 300 mg/day, 2.4% for lithium, and 3.3% for the placebo. Triglycerides increased with quetiapine-IR but decreased with lithium and placebo. The other changes, including HbA1c, glucose, insulin, total cholesterol, high-density lipoprotein cholesterol, low-density lipoprotein cholesterol, and prolactin, were generally similar across the treatment arms.

ANTIDEPRESSANTS

Monotherapy

The controversy on the efficacy and safety of antidepressants, especially antidepressant monotherapy, in acute bipolar depression remains unsettled. Evidence suggests that monotherapy with certain antidepressants for bipolar depression may increase the risk for manic/hypomanic switch (Chen, Fang, Kemp, Calabrese, & Gao, 2010; see Chapter 30). The possibility of such risk has made regulatory agencies and professional organizations advise clinicians not to use antidepressant monotherapy for bipolar depression. The best data for the efficacy so far are from a double-blind, placebo-controlled study of quetiapine-IR and paroxetine in bipolar depression (McElroy et al., 2010). Similar to previous studies of quetiapine-IR in BPI or BPII depression, quetiapine-IR 600 mg/day and 300 mg/day were significantly more effective than placebo in reducing depressive symptoms, but paroxetine did not result in a statistically significant improvement in depression compared with placebo at any time point during the study period (see Table 22.1). Bipolar subtype analysis did not find superiority of paroxetine over placebo in BPI or BPII depression. The study has been criticized for the apparent low dosing of paroxetine (20mg/day), which might have compromised the results.

The rates of the DAEs were similar from 8.1% with placebo to 13.2% with paroxetine. The rates of dry mouth, somnolence, and sedation were higher in quetiapine groups than that in the placebo or paroxetine group. The rate for nausea was higher in the paroxetine group than in other groups (see Table 22.3). The rates of TEM were not significantly different, from 2.1% with quetiapine-IR 300 to 10.8% with paroxetine.

The finding that paroxetine was not more effective than placebo in reducing depressive symptoms in BPI or BPII depression confirmed previous speculations that antidepressants at best have only limited efficacy in bipolar depression. However, antidepressants are a diverse group. The efficacy of other antidepressant monotherapy in bipolar depression needs to be studied separately. A similar risk for TEM of paroxetine as placebo should not be considered as the evidence of the safety for using antidepressant monotherapy in bipolar depression. Again, the relative low dose of paroxetine might explain the apparent low switch risk. Also patients with more frequent cycling courses and recent substance use disorder were excluded from the study. These groups of patients are more likely to have TEM (Chen et al., 2010; see Chapter 30).

In a small, randomized, double-blind, placebo-controlled study including 32 patients with BPI depression and 2 with BPII depression, fluoxetine monotherapy 10 to 30 mg/day, olanzapine monotherapy 5 to 20 mg/day, and fluoxetine 10 to 40 mg/day plus olanzapine 3 to 15 mg/day, and placebo for up to eight weeks were all effective in reducing depressive symptoms without significant differences among the groups (Amsterdam & Shults, 2005). No patients met the criteria for a manic episode. In contrast, there was a significant reduction in manic symptoms in patients treated with fluoxetine monotherapy. Randomized studies also found that fluoxetine and venlafaxine were as effective and safe as lithium in BPII depression (Amsterdam & Shults, 2005, 2008, 2010).

Adjunctive therapy to mood stabilizer

Antidepressant adjunctive therapy to mood stabilizer(s) has been recommended as an option for the acute treatment of bipolar depression, but good data supporting this practice are lacking. With the exception of OFC, there is no large, randomized, placebo-controlled study demonstrating that an antidepressant is effective in acute bipolar depression. A recent meta-analysis of 15 randomized, double-blind, placebo or active drug-controlled antidepressant adjunctive to mood stabilizer clinical trials ($n = 2,373$) found that antidepressants were not superior to placebo or other active treatments for bipolar depression (Sidor & MacQueen, 2011; see Table 22.2). In five placebo-controlled studies including the OFC study (Tohen et al., 2003) and a Systematic Treatment Enhancement Program for Bipolar Disorder (STEP-BD) study (Sachs et al., 2007), the relative risk for clinical response and remission with antidepressant relative to placebo was 1.18 (95% CI: 0.99–1.40) and 1.20 (95% CI: 0.98–1.47), respectively. In four studies with antidepressants versus other agents, the relative risk for clinical response and remission was 1.12 (95% CI: 0.98–1.28) and 1.17 (95% CI: 0.97–1.41), respectively, favoring antidepressants over other drugs. In bupropion versus antidepressant studies, bupropion did not show any advantage over other antidepressants (see Table 22.2).

In an earlier meta-analysis of antidepressants for acute bipolar depression, the analysis of five trials with placebo as comparison, including the OCF study, showed that antidepressants were superior to placebo in short-term treatment of bipolar depression (Gijsman, Geddes, Rendell., Nolen, & Goodwin, 2004). This analysis included patients without bipolar disorder and some patients who were not on a mood stabilizer (see Table 22.2). The positive results from this analysis were believed due to the inclusion of the OCF study, in which a large number of patients on placebo were included and the OCF had a relatively large effect size compared to the placebo. The diverging outcomes of these two large meta-analyses suggest that results of meta-analyses in bipolar depression critically depend on study selection. Therefore caution should be used when interpreting findings from different meta-analyses.

There was no increased risk for manic/hypomanic switch or any individual adverse event with antidepressant relative to placebo (Sidor & MacQueen, 2011), but different risks for TEM from different antidepressants were reported. Tricyclic antidepressants had higher TEM than other antidepressants combined (10% vs. 3.2%; Gijsman et al., 2004). Venlafaxine adjunctive to mood stabilizer also had a higher risk for TEM than sertraline or bupropion adjunctive to mood stabilizer in bipolar depression (Chen et al., 2010).

Monotherapy or adjunctive therapy from nonrandomized and/or non-double-blind studies

Clinical trials with randomization and double-blind design can minimize variances in treatment arms, reduce bias from researchers and participants, and provide relatively fair comparisons between treatment arms. However, bias from randomized, double-blind, head-to-head comparison trials was observed in pharmaceutical company-sponsored studies (Heres et al., 2006). Potential sources of bias were identified in areas of doses and dosage escalation, study inclusion criteria and study populations, statistics and methods, reporting of results, and wording of findings. In addition, patients in company-sponsored pivotal studies were highly selected with strict inclusion criteria (Grunze et al., 2009). Therefore the results from such studies may not generalizable to routine clinical practice. In contrast, nonrandomized, non-double-blind studies commonly include patients with complicate presentations but may cause additional biases due to lack of randomization and blinded assessment. With this in mind, we should be more cautious when interpreting findings from nonrandomized and non-double-blind studies.

An early study from the Stanley Foundation Bipolar Network (SFBN) showed that about 15% of patients (84 of 549) who received at least one antidepressant treatment with a mood stabilizer(s) might benefit from antidepressant treatment (Altshuler et al., 2003). However, among those who completed at least a 60-day antidepressant treatment, the remission rate was 44% (84 of 189). High response rates (> 60%) were reported in open-label studies and other naturalistic studies of antidepressants in bipolar depression.

Results from some studies even suggested that patients with bipolar depression, especially with BPII depression, had higher response rates than those with MDD. In a study of 1,036 patients with BPI, BPII, or MDD, 59% of patients with BPI, 80% with BPII, and 91% with MDD received antidepressant treatments for 12 weeks (Tondo,

Baldessarini, Vázquez, Lepri, & Visioli, 2013), response rate without manic/hypomanic switching was 77% for BPII, 72% for BPI, and 62% for MDD, respectively. An earlier study with 2,032 inpatients also found that patients with BPI depression and those with MDD had similar response to antidepressant treatments (Möller, Bottlender, Grunze, Strauss, & Wittmann, 2001). This is in line with most open studies showing that adjunctive different antidepressants to mood stabilizer had equal or similar efficacy in reducing depressive symptoms in bipolar disorder.

One of the main reasons for the discontinuation of antidepressants after acute treatments is fear of manic switching. A majority of studies have shown that antidepressant adjunctive therapy to mood stabilizers did not have an increased risk for TEM. However, the data from the SFBN showed that acute or continuation treatment with venlafaxine plus mood stabilizers had a higher risk for TEM compared to sertraline or bupropion plus mood stabilizers (Chen et al., 2010, see Chapter 30). It remains unclear if venlafaxine has a higher risk for TEM than placebo. In addition, there are also inconsistent data on the benefit from continuation of antidepressant treatments. The SFBN studies showed that the continuation of antidepressants is beneficial in those who responded initially (Altshuler et al., 2003; 2009). A more recent study of the STEP-BD found that antidepressant continuation trended toward less severe depressive symptoms based on *DSM-IV* depression diagnostic criteria and mildly delayed depressive episode relapse without increased manic symptoms based on *DSM-IV* mania diagnostic criteria. There were no benefits in prevalence or severity of new depressive or manic episodes or overall time in remission. BPII did not predict enhanced antidepressant response, but rapid-cycling course predicted three times more depressive episodes with antidepressant continuation (Ghaemi et al., 2010).

A consensus on the role of antidepressants in bipolar disorders has recently been developed by the International Society for Bipolar Disorder Task-Force, which consisted of 65 international experts in bipolar disorders (Pacchiarotti et al., 2013). The Task-Force found that there was striking disparity between the wide use and the weak evidence base for the efficacy and safety of antidepressants in bipolar disorders. Integrating the evidence and clinical experience of the Task-Force members, a consensus was reached on 12 statements on the use of antidepressants in bipolar disorders. For acute treatment of bipolar depression, the Task-Force recommended that adjunctive antidepressant to mood stabilizer(s) may be used for BP I or BPII acute depressive episode when there is a history of positive response to antidepressant(s), but adjunctive antidepressant(s) should be avoided for an acute BPI or BPII depressive episode with two or more concomitant core manic symptoms in the presence of psychomotor retardation or rapid cycling. The Task-Force also recommended antidepressant monotherapy be avoided in BPI or BPII depression with two or more concomitant core manic symptoms. Regarding the long-term use of antidepressant, the Task-Force recommended maintenance treatment with adjunctive antidepressant(s) be considered if a patient has had a relapse into a depressive episode after stopping antidepressant therapy in the past.

WAKEFULNESS-PROMOTING AGENT

Modafinil

Modafinil, a wakefulness-promoting agent, has been approved by the US FDA for improving wakefulness in patients with excessive sleepiness associated with narcolepsy, obstructive sleep apnea, and shift-work sleep disorder. The first study of its efficacy and safety in acute bipolar depression was carried out in 85 patients with BPI or BPII depression who were inadequately responsive to a standard treatment, which could include mood stabilizer, antidepressants, and/or antipsychotics (Frye et al., 2007). The endpoint scores on the Inventory of Depression Symptomatology-Clinician Rated Scale–30 items (IDS-C$_{30}$), four-item Fatigue and Energy subscale, and the CGI-S were significantly improved in the modafinil group ($n = 41$) compared with the placebo group ($n = 44$; see Table 22.2). The effect sizes were from small to moderate with 0.47 for the IDS-C$_{30}$, 0.56 for the four items, and 0.63 for the CGI-S.

Armodafinil

Armodafinil, a longer-lasting isomer of modafinil, has also been approved in the United States for the same indication as modafinil. The first study of armodafinil adjunctive to lithium, olanzapine, and/or valproic acid found that the difference in the changes in IDS-C$_{30}$ between armodafinil and a placebo was significant with analysis of variance but was not significant when analyzed with analysis of covariance (with baseline score as a covariate, $p = 0.0742$; Calabrese et al., 2010). Differences between the two arms in secondary outcome measures were not significant (see Table 22.2).

A more recent study showed that adjunctive armodafinil to a mood stabilizer(s) was superior to placebo in reducing depressive symptoms in patients with BPI treatment-refractory depression (Calabrese Frye, Yang, & Ketter, 2014). There were also significant greater decrease at the item level of IDS-C$_{30}$, including panic/phobic symptoms, increased appetite, concentration/decisions, energy/fatigability, and leaden paralysis/physical energy (see Table 22.2). The significant difference between armodafinil and placebo started at Week 7. The responder rate was significantly greater in the armodafinil 150 mg group versus the placebo at Week 8 (55% vs. 39%). The NNTB for IDS-C$_{30}$ responder of armodafinil 150 mg relative to the placebo was 9. The most common adverse events in both arms were headache, insomnia, and diarrhea (see Table 22.3). There were no significant differences between armodafinil and placebo in the DAEs, TEM, and changes in clinical laboratory values, electrocardiogram, body weight, body mass index, glucose level, and cholesterol level.

DOPAMINE 2/3 RECEPTOR AGONIST

Pramipexole

Pramipexole, a synthetic aminothiazole derivative, is a dopamine 2/3 receptor agonist that is approved for the treatment of Parkinson's disease. The first study in bipolar depression was carried out in 21 patients with BPII depression who were treated with lithium or valproate prior to randomization (Zarate et al., 2004). Addition of pramipexole 1.7 ± 0.9 mg/day (n = 10) to the mood stabilizer for six weeks decreased MADRS and 24-item HAMD scores significantly more than the placebo (n = 10). The second study enrolled 22 patients who had treatment-resistant bipolar depression (BPI n = 15, BPII n = 7). Adjunctive pramipexole (1.7 ± 1.3 mg/day) to a mood stabilizer(s) for six weeks was superior to placebo in reducing depressive symptoms (Goldberg, Burdick, & Endick, 2004). Insomnia, nausea/vomiting, agitation/anxiety, somnolence, gastrointestinal complaints, weight loss, headache, lassitude, and hypomanic/manic exacerbation were commonly reported (>10%) in both groups of pramipexole and placebo, but the differences between two groups were not significant. Tremor appeared to be more common in the pramipexole group (50% vs. 18%).

POLYUNSATURATED FATTY ACIDS

Omega-3 fatty acids

Common omega-3 fatty acids in the body are (alpha) linolenic acid, eicosapentaenoic acid (EPA), and docosahexaenoic acid (DHA). DHA is found in high levels in neurons of the central nervous system as a form of scaffolding for structural support. When omega-3 intake is inadequate, neuron becomes stiff as cholesterol and omega-6 fatty acids are substituted for omega-3. When a neuron becomes rigid, proper neurotransmission from cell to cell and within cells is compromised. While DHA provides structure and helps to ensure normal neurotransmission, EPA may be more important in the signaling within neurons. Normalizing communications within neurons has been suggested as an important factor in alleviating depressive symptoms.

A number of studies have examined national and international fish consumption data and compared them to rates of depression. Higher fish consumption was correlated with lower risk of depression, postpartum depression, seasonal affective disorder, and bipolar disorder. However, the results of omega-3 fatty acids in the treatment of bipolar disorder have been inconsistent. A recent meta-analysis of six randomized controlled studies of omega-3 for bipolar disorder with a total of 291 patients revealed a significant effect on reducing depressive symptoms favoring omega-3 over placebo with a small effect size of 0.34 (Sarris, Mischoulon, & Schweitzer, 2012), but the effect on manic symptoms was not significantly different between omega-3 and placebo.

The most common adverse effect in both the omega-3 and control groups was mild gastrointestinal tract distress, generally characterized by loose stools. Omega-3 fatty acids might have a mood-stabilizing effect, but good-quality data are lacking. At the current stage, it is reasonable to use omega-3 as a supplement but not as a major mood-stabilizing agent. Omega-3 fatty acids have different components, and it remains unclear what the best combination of these components should be for commercially available products. A meta-analysis of the effects of EPA in 15 randomized, double-blind, placebo-controlled clinical trials with 916 participants with MDD or bipolar disorder showed that supplements with EPA ≥ 60% were effective in reducing depressive symptom with an effect size of 0.53 (Sublette et al., 2011). However, the supplements with < 60% of EPA were ineffective. A similar meta-analysis of 28 randomized, placebo-controlled trials found a similar result; that is, EPA but not DHA were responsible for reducing depressive symptoms in patients with bipolar or unipolar depression. Therefore supplements containing ≥ 60% of total EPA+DHA in a dose range of 200 to 2,200 mg/day of EPA in excess of DHA were effective against primary depression (Sublette et al., 2011).

THYROID HORMONES

Thyroid function has been associated with response to treatment in patients with bipolar depression. Both lower values of free thyroxin index and higher values of thyroid-stimulating hormone were significantly associated with longer time to remission during the treatment with mood stabilizer. Supraphysiological doses (250–500 mcg/day) of thyroxine (T_4) were effective in the acute and maintenance treatment of bipolar or unipolar patients with treatment-refractory depression. Augmentation with triiodothyronine (T_3) (13–188 mcg/day) was also effective in reducing depressive symptoms in patients with bipolar disorder. A neuroimaging study in women showed that supraphysiological doses of T4 improved mood and decreased relative activity in brain regions related to mood regulation (Bauer et al., 2005).

ANTICHOLINERGICS

Scopolamine

Scopolamine is a muscarinic receptor antagonist and commonly used for nausea and motion sickness. Intravenous infusions of scopolamine hydrobromide (4 µg/kg) in a mixed group of patients with MDD ($n = 15$) or bipolar disorder ($n = 12$) were significantly superior to placebo infusions in reducing depressive symptoms with an effect size of 2.7. The significant difference was observed within three days of first infusion. Placebo-adjusted remission rates were 56% and 45% for the initial and a replication study, respectively (Drevets, Zarate, & Furey, 2013). However, oral scopolamine augmentation to citalopram in the treatment of moderate to severe MDD did not produce robust results. The effect size of scopolamine relative to placebo was 0.9, which was much smaller than that of intravenous infusions (Khajavi et al., 2012).

Mecamylamine

Mecamylamine is a nonselective and noncompetitive nicotinic receptor antagonist and has been used for autonomic dysreflexia and hypertension. Its mood stabilizing effect in two patients with bipolar disorder was observed in a study of mecamylamine (up to 7.5 mg/day) treatment for Tourette's syndrome (Shytle, Silver, & Sanberg, 2000).

GLUTAMATERGIC MODULATING AGENTS

Riluzole

Riluzole is an FDA-approved medication for the treatment of amyotrophic lateral sclerosis and can rapidly inhibit presynaptic release of glutamate. In a small open study, riluzole 5 to 20 mg/day adjunctive to lithium significantly reduced depressive symptoms in bipolar depression (Zarate et al., 2005).

Ketamine

Ketamine is a noncompetitive N-methyl-D-aspartate (NMDA) antagonist and has been used as an anesthetic. Intravenous infusion of a subanesthetic dose of ketamine for 40 minutes produced significantly more improvement in depressive symptoms than a placebo in bipolar patients (BPI $n = 8$, BPII $n = 10$) who did not respond to the treatment with lithium or valproate (Zarate et al., 2012). The significant improvement lasted through Day 3 although the largest difference between the two groups was at Day 2 with an effect size of 0.8.

Memantine

Memantine is a low-affinity NMDA receptor antagonist and is approved for the treatment of Alzheimer's disease. Addition of memantine to lamotrigine ($n = 14$) was not superior to a placebo ($n = 15$) in reducing depressive symptoms in bipolar patients who had inadequate response to lamotrigine (Anand et al., 2012).

Glutamate receptor antagonists may represent a third-generation of antidepressants with fast onset and large effect size. A recent review of ketamine found that all controlled trials used a within-subject, cross-over design with an inactive placebo as the control. Ketamine administration was not recommended outside of the hospital setting (Aan Het Rot, Zarate, Charney, & Mathew, 2012).

CONCLUSION

Only quetiapine-IR and –XR monotherapy, OFC, and lurasidone monotherapy and lurasidone adjunctive to mood stabilizer have been approved by the US FDA for the acute treatment of bipolar depression. Lurasidone has a more favorable safety and tolerability profile than quetiapine and OFC and may be used as a first-line agent. Combination of lithium and lamotrigine may be considered since it is more effective than lithium alone.

The role of antidepressants as a heterogeneous group for the treatment of bipolar depression remains under debate. More controlled studies for individual antidepressants are needed on efficacy and risk of TEM. In addition, we need to learn more about characteristics of potential responders to antidepressants and who will be on the risk of harm.

Armodafinil and, to a lesser extent, pramipexole, may be used for treatment-resistant bipolar depression, especially for those who have symptoms of low energy, poor concentration, and/or lack of motivation. Agents targeting anticholinergic and glutamatergic symptoms may represent new classes of antidepressants with fast onset of action in bipolar depression.

Somnolence and sedation are common side effects for all atypical antipsychotics, but akathisia from aripiprazole is the highest among atypicals. Weight gain and metabolic side effects, especially from olanzapine and quetiapine, are a major concern. Metabolic parameters should be monitored closely when an antipsychotic is prescribed. In contrast, attention should be paid to TEM when antidepressant and/or a wake-promoting agent is indicated. More important, a majority of these studies were carried out in the United States and European countries and in relatively "pure" populations of patients with bipolar depression. The results from these studies may not be generalizable to routine clinical practice.

Disclosure statement: Dr. Calabrese has not disclose any conflict of interest. Dr. Gao is on a speaker's bureau of Sunovion. He receives research grant support from the Brain & Behavior Research Foundation and Cleveland Foundation. To his knowledge, all of Dr. Heize Grunze's possible conflicts of interest, financial or otherwise, including direct or indirect financial or personal relationships, interests, and affiliations, whether or not directly related to the subject of the chapter, are as follows: Grant support: National Institute for Health Research United Kingdom, Medical Research Council United Kingdom, Northumberland, Tyne & Wear National Health Service Foundation Trust, Otsuka Pharmaceuticals. Receipt of honoraria or consultation fees: Gedeon-Richter, Desitin, Lundbeck, Hofmann-LaRoche. Participation in a company sponsored speaker's bureau: Astra Zeneca, Bristol-Myers Squibb, Otsuka, Lundbeck, Servier.

Dr. Wu receives grant support from the National Natural Science Foundation of China (Grant No. 81371481). She has no conflicts to disclose.

REFERENCES

Aan Het Rot, M., Zarate, C. A. Jr., Charney, D. S., & Mathew, S. J. (2012). Ketamine for depression: Where do we go from here? *Biological Psychiatry, 72*(7), 537–547.

Altshuler, L., Suppes, T., Black, D., Nolen, W. A., Keck, P. E. Jr., Frye, M. A.,…Post R. (2003). Impact of antidepressant discontinuation after acute bipolar depression remission on rates of depressive relapse at 1-year follow-up. *The American Journal of Psychiatry, 160*(7), 1252–1262.

Altshuler, L. L., Post, R. M., Hellemann, G., Leverich, G. S., Nolen, W. A., Frye, M. A.,…Suppes, T. (2009). Impact of antidepressant continuation after acute positive or partial treatment response for bipolar depression: A blinded, randomized study. *Journal of Clinical Psychiatry, 70*(4), 450–457.

American Diabetes Association, American Psychiatric Association, American Association of Clinical Endocrinologists, and North American Association for the Study of Obesity. (2004). Consensus development conference on antipsychotic drugs and obesity and diabetes. *Diabetes Care, 27*(2), 596–601.

Amsterdam, J. D., & Shults, J. (2005). Comparison of fluoxetine, olanzapine, and combined fluoxetine plus olanzapine initial therapy of bipolar type I and type II major depression—Lack of manic induction. *Journal of Affective Disorders, 87*(1), 121–130.

Amsterdam, J. D., & Shults, J. (2008). Comparison of short-term venlafaxine versus lithium monotherapy for bipolar II major depressive episode: A randomized open-label study. *Journal of Clinical Psychopharmacology, 28*(2), 171–181.

Amsterdam, J. D., & Shults, J. (2010). Efficacy and safety of long-term fluoxetine versus lithium monotherapy of bipolar II disorder: A randomized, double-blind, placebo-substitution study. *The American Journal of Psychiatry, 167*(7), 792–800.

Anand, A., Gunn, A. D., Barkay, G., Karne, H. S., Nurnberger, J. I., Mathew, S. J., & Ghosh, S. (2012). Early antidepressant effect of memantine during augmentation of lamotrigine inadequate response in bipolar depression: A double-blind, randomized, placebo-controlled trial. *Bipolar Disorders, 14*(1), 64–70.

Bauer, M., London, E. D., Rasgon, N., Berman, S. M., Frye, M. A., Altshuler, L. L.,…Whybrow, P. C. (2005). Supraphysiological doses of levothyroxine alter regional cerebral metabolism and improve mood in bipolar depression. *Molecular Psychiatry, 10*(5), 456–469.

Bond, D. J., Lam, R. W., & Yatham, L. N. (2010). Divalproex sodium versus placebo in the treatment of acute bipolar depression: A systematic review and meta-analysis. *Journal of Affective Disorders, 124*(3), 228–234.

Brown, E. B., McElroy, S. L., Keck, P. E. Jr., Deldar, A., Adams, D. H., Tohen, M., & Williamson, D. J. (2005). A 7-week, randomized, double-blind trial of olanzapine/fluoxetine combination versus lamotrigine in the treatment of bipolar I depression. *Journal of Clincial Psychiatry, 67*(7), 1025–1133.

Calabrese, J. R., Bowden, C. L., Sachs, G. S., Ascher, J. A., Monaghan, E., & Rudd, G. D. (1999). A double blind placebo-controlled study of lamotrigine monotherapy in outpatients with bipolar I depression. Lamictal 602 Study Group. *Journal of Clincial Psychiatry, 60*, 79–88.

Calabrese, J. R., Huffman, R. F., White, R. L., Edwards, S., Thompson, T. R., Ascher, J. A.,...Leadbetter, R. A. (2008). Lamotrigine in the acute treatment of bipolar depression: Results of five double-blind, placebo-controlled clinical trials. *Bipolar Disorders, 10*(2), 323–233.

Calabrese, J. R., Keck, P. E. Jr., Macfadden, W., Minkwitz, M., Ketter, T. A., Weisler, R. H.,...Mullen, J. (2005). A randomized, double-blind, placebo-controlled trial of quetiapine in the treatment of bipolar I or II depression. *The American Journal of Psychiatry, 162*, 1351–1360.

Calabrese, J. R., Ketter, T. A., Youakim, J. M., Tiller, J. M., Yang, R., & Frye, M. A. (2010). Adjunctive armodafinil for major depressive episodes associated with bipolar I disorder: A randomized, multicenter, double-blind, placebo-controlled, proof-of-concept study. *Journal of Clinical Psychiatry, 71*(10), 1363–1370.

Calabrese, J. R., Frye, M. A., Yang, R., Ketter, T. A., Armodafinil Treatment Trial Study Network. (2014). Efficacy and safety of adjunctive armodafinil in adults with major depressive episodes associated with bipolar I disorder: a randomized, double-blind, placebo-controlled, multicenter trial. *Journal of Clinical Psychiatry, 75*(10), 1054–1061.

Calabrese, J. R., Sullivan, J. R., Bowden, C. L., Suppes, T., Goldberg, J. F., Sachs, G. S.,...Kusumakar, V. (2002). Rash in multicenter trials of lamotrigine in mood disorders: Clinical relevance and management. *Journal of Clinical Psychiatry, 63*(11), 1012–1019.

Chen, J., Fang, Y., Kemp, D. E., Calabrese, J. R., & Gao, K. (2010). Switching to hypomania and mania: Differential neurochemical, neuropsychological, and pharmacologic triggers and their mechanisms. *Current Psychiatry Reports, 12*(6), 512–521.

Drevets, W. C., Zarate, C. A. Jr., & Furey, M. L. (2013). Antidepressant effects of the muscarinic cholinergic receptor antagonist scopolamine: A review. *Biological Psychiatry, 73*(12), 1156–1163.

Frye, M. A., Grunze, H., Suppes, T., McElroy, S. L., Keck, P. E. Jr., Walden, J.,...Post, R. M. (2007). A placebo-controlled evaluation of adjunctive modafinil in the treatment of bipolar depression. *The American Journal of Psychiatry, 164*(8), 1242–1249.

Gao, K., Ganocy, S. J., Gajwani, P., Muzina, D. J., Kemp, D. E., & Calabrese, J. R. (2008). A review of sensitivity and tolerability of antipsychotics in patients with bipolar disorder or schizophrenia: Focus on somnolence. *Journal of Clinical Psychiatry, 69*(2), 302–309.

Gao, K., Kemp, D. E., Fein, E., Wang, Z., Fang, Y., Ganocy, S. J., & Calabrese, J. R. (2011). Number needed to treat to harm for discontinuation due to adverse events in the treatment of bipolar depression, major depressive disorder, and generalized anxiety disorder with atypical antipsychotics. *Journal of Clinical Psychiatry, 72*(8), 1063–1071.

Gao, K., Mackle, M., Cazorla, P., Zhao, J., & Szegedi, A. (2013). Comparison of somnolence associated with asenapine, olanzapine, risperidone, and haloperidol relative to placebo in patients with schizophrenia or bipolar disorder. *Neuropsychiatric Disease Treatment, 9*, 1145–157.

Gao, K., Muzina, D., Gajwani, P., & Calabrese, J. R. (2006). Efficacy of typical and atypical antipsychotics for primary and comorbid anxiety symptoms or disorders: a review. *Journal of Clinical Psychiatry, 67*(9), 1327–1340.

Gao, K., Pappadopulos, K., Karayal, O. N., Kolluri, S., & Calabrese, J. R. (2013). Risk for discontinuation due to adverse events with ziprasidone monotherapy versus placebo during acute treatment for bipolar depression, bipolar mania, and schizophrenia. *Journal of Clinical Psychopharmacology, 33*, 425–431.

Geddes, J. R., Calabrese, J. R., & Goodwin, G. M. (2009). Lamotrigine for treatment of bipolar depression: Independent meta-analysis and meta-regression of individual patient data from five randomized trials. *The British Journal of Psychiatry, 194*(1), 4–9.

Ghaemi, S. N., Ostacher, M. M., El-Mallakh, R. S., Borrelli, D., Baldassano, C. F., Kelley, M. E.,...Baldessarini, R. J. (2010). Antidepressant discontinuation in bipolar depression: A Systematic Treatment Enhancement Program for Bipolar Disorder (STEP-BD)

randomized clinical trial of long-term effectiveness and safety. *Journal of Clinical Psychiatry, 71*(4), 372–380.

Gijsman, H. J., Geddes, J. R., Rendell, J. M., Nolen, W. A., & Goodwin, G. M. (2004). Antidepressants for bipolar depression: A systematic review of randomized, controlled trials. *The American Journal of Psychiatry, 161*(9), 1537–1547.

Goldberg, J. F., Burdick, K. E., & Endick, C. J. (2004). Preliminary randomized, double-blind, placebo-controlled trial of pramipexole added to mood stabilizers for treatment-resistant bipolar depression. *The American Journal of Psychiatry, 61*, 564–566.

Grunze, H., Vieta, E., Goodwin, G. M., Bowden, C., Licht, R. W., Moller, H. J., & Kasper, S. (2009). The World Federation of Societies of Biological Psychiatry (WFSBP) guidelines for the biological treatment of bipolar disorders: Update 2009 on the treatment of acute mania. *World Journal of Biological Psychiatry, 10*(2), 85–116.

Heres, S., Davis, J., Maino, K., Jetzinger, E., Kissling, W., & Leucht, S. (2006). Why olanzapine beats risperidone, risperidone beats quetiapine, and quetiapine beats olanzapine: An exploratory analysis of head-to-head comparison studies of second-generation antipsychotics. *The American Journal of Psychiatry, 163*(2), 185–194.

Khajavi, D., Farokhnia, M., Modabbernia, A., Ashrafi, M., Abbasi, S. H., Tabrizi, M., & Akhondzadeh, S. (2012). Oral scopolamine augmentation in moderate to severe major depressive disorder: A randomized, double-blind, placebo-controlled study. *Journal of Clinical Psychiatry, 73*(11), 1428–1433.

Loebel, A., Cucchiaro, J., Silva, R., Kroger, H., Hsu, J., Sarma, K., & Sachs, G. (2014). Lurasidone monotherapy in the treatment of bipolar I depression: a randomized, double-blind, placebo-controlled study. *The American Journal of Psychiatry, 171*(2), 160–168.

Loebel, A., Cucchiaro, J., Silva, R., Kroger, H., Sarma, K., Xu, J., & Calabrese, J. R. (2014). Lurasidone as adjunctive therapy with lithium or valproate for the treatment of bipolar I depression: a randomized, double-blind, placebo-controlled study. *The American Journal of Psychiatry, 171*(2), 169–177.

Lombardo, I., Sachs, G., Kolluri, S., Kremer, C., & Yang, R. (2012). Two 6-week, randomized, double-blind, placebo-controlled studies of ziprasidone in outpatients with bipolar I depression: Did baseline characteristics impact trial outcome? *Journal of Clinical Psychopharmacology, 32*(4), 470–478.

McElroy, S. L., Weisler, R. H., Chang, W., Olausson, B., Paulsson, B., Brecher, M.,...EMBOLDEN II (Trial D1447C00134) Investigators. (2010). A double-blind, placebo-controlled study of quetiapine and paroxetine as monotherapy in adults with bipolar depression (EMBOLDEN II). *Journal of Clinical Psychiatry, 71*(2), 163–174.

McIntyre, R. S., Mancini, D. A., McCann, S., Srinivasan, J., Sagman, D., & Kennedy, S. H. (2002). Topiramate versus bupropion SR when added to mood stabilizer therapy for the depressive phase of bipolar disorder: A preliminary single-blind study. *Bipolar Disorders, 4*, 207–213.

Möller, H. J., Bottlender, R., Grunze, H., Strauss, A., & Wittmann, J. (2001). Are antidepressants less effective in the acute treatment of bipolar I compared to unipolar depression? *Journal of Affective Disorders, 67*(1–3), 141–146.

Muzina, D. J., Gao, K., Kemp, D. E., Khalife, S., Ganocy, S. J., Chan, P. K.,...Calabrese, J. R. (2011). Acute efficacy of divalproex sodium versus placebo in mood stabilizer-naive bipolar I or II depression: A double-blind, randomized, placebo-controlled trial. *Journal of Clinical Psychiatry, 72*(6), 813–819.

Pacchiarotti, I., Bond, D. J., Baldessarini, R. J., Nolen, W. A., Grunze, H., Licht, R. W.,...Vieta, E. (2013). The International Society for Bipolar disorder (ISBD) Task-Force report on antidepressant use in bipolar disorder. *The American Journal of Psychiatry, 170*(11), 1249–1262.

Patkar, A., Gilmer, W., Pae, C. U., Vöhringer, P. A., Ziffra, M., Pirok, E.,...Ghaemi, S. N. (2012). A 6 week randomized double-blind placebo-controlled trial of ziprasidone for the acute depressive mixed state. *PLoS One, 7*(4), e34757.

Sachs, G. S., Ice, K. S., Chappell, P. B., Schwartz, J. H., Gurtovaya, O., Vanderburg, D. G., & Kasuba, B. (2011). Efficacy and safety of adjunctive oral ziprasidone for acute treatment of depression in patients with bipolar I disorder: A randomized, double-blind, placebo-controlled trial. *Journal of Clinical Psychiatry, 72*(10), 1413–1422.

Sachs, G. S., Nierenberg, A. A., Calabrese, J. R., Marangell, L. B., Wisniewski, S. R., Gyulai, L.,...Thase, M. E. (2007). Effectiveness of adjunctive antidepressant treatment for bipolar depression. *New England Journal of Medicine, 356*(17), 1711–1722.

Saricicek, A., Maloney, K., Muralidharan, A., Ruf, B., Blumberg, H. P., Sanacora, G.,...Bhagwagar, Z. (2011). Levetiracetam in the management of bipolar depression: A randomized, double-blind, placebo-controlled trial. *Journal of Clinical Psychiatry, 72*(6), 744–750.

Sarris, J., Mischoulon, D., & Schweitzer, I. (2012). Omega-3 for bipolar disorder: Meta-analyses of use in mania and bipolar depression. *Journal of Clinical Psychiatry, 73*(1), 81–86.

Shytle, R. D., Silver, A. A., & Sanberg, P. R. (2000). Comorbid bipolar disorder in Tourette's syndrome responds to the nicotinic receptor antagonist mecamylamine (Inversine). *Biological Psychiatry, 48*(10), 1028–1031.

Sidor, M. M., & Macqueen, G. M. (2011). Antidepressants for the acute treatment of bipolar depression: A systematic review and meta-analysis. *Journal of Clinical Psychiatry, 72*(2), 156–167.

Silva, M. T., Zimmermann, I. R., Galvao, T. F., & Pereira, M. G. (2013). Olanzapine plus fluoxetine for bipolar disorder: A systematic review and meta-analysis. *Journal of Affective Disorders, 146*(3), 310–148.

Simms, K. M., Kortepeter, C., & Avigan, M. (2012). Lamotrigine and aseptic meningitis. *Neurology, 78*(12), 921–927.

Sublette, M. E., Ellis, S. P., Geant, A. L., & Mann, J. J. (2011). Meta-analysis of the effects of eicosapentaenoic acid (EPA) in clinical trials in depression. *Journal of Clinical Psychiatry, 72*(12), 1577–1584.

Suppes, T., Datto, C., Minkwitz, M., Nordenhem, A., Walker, C., & Darko, D. (2010). Effectiveness of the extended release formulation of quetiapine as monotherapy for the treatment of acute bipolar depression. *Journal of Affective Disorders, 121*(1–2), 106–115.

Suppes, T., Dennehy, E. B., Hirschfeld, R. M., Altshuler, L. L., Bowden, C. L., Calabrese, J. R.,...Texas Consensus Conference Panel on Medication Treatment of Bipolar Disorder. (2005). The Texas implementation of medication algorithms: Update to the algorithms for treatment of bipolar I disorder. *Journal of Clinical Psychiatry, 66*(7), 870–886.

Suppes, T., Marangell, L. B., Bernstein, I. H., Kelly, D. I., Fischer, E. G., Zboyan, H. A.,...Gonzalez, R. (2008). A single blind comparison of lithium and lamotrigine for the treatment of bipolar II depression. *Journal of Affective Disorders, 111*(2–3), 334–343.

Thase, M. E., Jonas, A., Khan, A., Bowden, C. L., Wu, X., McQuade, R. D.,...Owen, R. (2008). Aripiprazole monotherapy in nonpsychotic bipolar I depression: results of 2 randomized, placebo-controlled studies. *Journal of Clinical Psychopharmacology, 28*(1), 13–20.

Thase, M. E., Macfadden, W., Weisler, R. H., Chang, W., Paulsson, B., Khan, A.,...BOLDER II Study Group. (2006). Efficacy of quetiapine monotherapy in bipolar I and II depression: A double-blind, placebo-controlled study (the BOLDER II study). *Journal of Clinical Psychopharmacology, 26*(6), 600–609.

Tohen, M., McDonnell, D. P., Case, M., Kanba, S., Ha, K., Fang, Y. R.,...Gomez, J. C. (2012). Randomized, double-blind, placebo-controlled study of olanzapine in patients with bipolar I depression. *The British Journal of Psychiatry, 201*(5), 376–382.

Tohen, M., Vieta, E., Calabrese, J., Ketter, T. A., Sachs, G., Bowden, C.,...Breier, A. (2003). Efficacy of olanzapine and olanzapine-fluoxetine combination in the treatment of bipolar depression. *Archives of General Psychiatry, 60*, 1079–1088.

Tondo, L., Baldessarini, R. J., Vázquez, G., Lepri, B., & Visioli, C. (2013). Clinical responses to antidepressants among 1036 acutely depressed patients with bipolar or unipolar major affective disorders. *Acta Psychiatrica Scandinavica, 127*(5), 355–364.

van der Loos, M. L., Mulder, P. G., Hartong, E. G., Blom, M. B., Vergouwen, A. C., de Keyzer, H. J.,...LamLit Study Group. (2009). Efficacy and safety of lamotrigine as add-on treatment to lithium in bipolar depression: A multicenter, double-blind, placebo-controlled trial. *Journal of Clinical Psychiatry, 70*(2), 223–231.

Young, A. H., McElroy, S. L., Bauer, M., Philips, N., Chang, W., Olausson, B... EMBOLDEN I (Trial 001) Investigators. (2010). A double-blind, placebo-controlled study of quetiapine and lithium monotherapy in adults in the acute phase of bipolar depression (EMBOLDEN I). *Journal of Clinical Psychiatry, 71*(2), 150–162.

Zarate, C. A. Jr., Brutsche, N. E., Ibrahim, L., Franco-Chaves, J., Diazgranados, N., Cravchik, A.,...Luckenbaugh, D. A. (2012). Replication of ketamine's antidepressant efficacy in bipolar depression: A randomized controlled add-on trial. *Biological Psychiatry, 71*(11), 939–946.

Zarate, C. A. Jr., Payne, J. L., Singh, J., Quiroz, J. A., Luckenbaugh, D. A., Denicoff, K. D.,...Manji, H. K. (2004). Pramipexole for bipolar II depression: A placebo-controlled proof of concept study. *Biological Psychiatry, 56*(1), 54–60.

Zarate, C. A. Jr., Quiroz, J. A., Singh, J. B., Denicoff, K. D., De Jesus, G., Luckenbaugh, D. A.,...Manji, H. K. (2005). An open-label trial of the glutamate-modulating agent riluzole in combination with lithium for the treatment of bipolar depression. *Biological Psychiatry, 57*(4), 430–432.

23.

MAINTENANCE TREATMENTS IN BIPOLAR DISORDER

Paul A. Kudlow, Danielle S. Cha, Roger S. McIntyre, and Trisha Suppes

INTRODUCTION

Following remission of a bipolar mood episode, patients require maintenance treatments to delay or prevent further mood episodes. Preventing further mood episodes is among the most challenging aspects of treating bipolar disorder (BD) and is important for preventing adverse clinical outcomes and progression. Evidence indicates that up to 60% to 80% will experience recurrence of mood symptoms after discontinuation of lithium or antipsychotic therapy, and 20% to 50% during ongoing therapy have been reported for BD (Calabrese et al., 2003; Tohen et al., 2005; Yatham et al., 2005; Yazici, Kora, Polat, & Saylan, 2004). Multiyear (i.e., five years) studies suggest that recurrence rates in BD are up to 85% (Keller, Lavori, Coryell, Endicott, & Mueller, 1993). Although many of these patients will experience recurrence only a few times in their lifetime, up to 10% to 15% will suffer more than 10 episodes (Pfennig et al., 2010). Furthermore, a substantial proportion of patients with BD, even those patients who undergo intensive ongoing therapy, will experience considerable illness-related morbidity. Treatment guidelines suggest that maintenance therapy consists of pharmacotherapy plus adjunctive psychotherapy, and where psychotherapy is not available, pharmacotherapy alone is reasonable (Yatham et al., 2013). Details of psychotherapy are beyond the scope of this chapter but are reviewed at greater length elsewhere (Beynon, Soares-Weiser, Woolacott, Duffy, & Geddes, 2008; Miklowitz, 2008). The overarching aim of treatment in BD should not be limited to achieving and sustaining euthymia but also preventing, limiting, and eliminating undesirable treatment-related side effects that impact global functioning. Typical side effects that lead to treatment discontinuation include sedation, cognitive impairment, tremor, weight gain, and rash. The goals of maintenance therapy should be to reduce residual symptoms, delay and prevent recurrence of new mood episodes, reduce the risk of suicide, and enhance psychosocial functioning. We begin this chapter with a review of factors that affect relapse in BD. This is followed by a review of the evidence supporting maintenance pharmacological treatments of bipolar I and II disorder as well as mixed episodes.

ADHERENCE

In the outpatient setting, it has been reported that more than 50% of individuals with BD are classified as being nonadherent to treatment (Bates, Whitehead, Bolge, & Kim, 2010; Yatham et al., 2013). An important cause of recurrence in BD depends on adherence to treatment regimens and is associated with higher rates of both hospitalization and suicide (Yatham et al., 2005). Recognizing factors that negatively impact adherence (Table 23.1) may improve treatment selection and discontinuation by identifying individuals at greater risk of nonadherence. Several lines of evidence indicate that adherence depends on a myriad of factors. For example, adherence is positively associated with higher satisfaction with medication, treatment with monotherapy medication, a college degree, and fear of relapse (Devulapalli et al., 2010; Gonzalez-Pinto, Reed, Novick, Bertsch, & Haro, 2010; Sajatovic et al., 2009). In addition, adherence has been found to be increased by other factors associated with medication use, such as route of administration (e.g., long-acting injectable versus oral administration; Quiroz et al., 2010); adjunctive psychosocial intervention–customized adherence enhancement (i.e., needs-based, manualized approach intended to improve medication adherence in individuals with BD; Sajatovic et al., 2012); and the use of text-messaging and other mobile technology-based interventions (Depp et al., 2010). Medication adherence has been found to be negatively associated with illness factors (e.g., substance use, previous hospitalizations, psychotic symptoms, reduced

Table 23.1. LEVELS OF EVIDENCE CRITERION

1. Meta-analysis or replicated double-blind, randomized controlled trial that includes a placebo condition
2. At least one double-blind, randomized controlled trial with placebo or active comparison condition
3. Prospective uncontrolled trial with at least ten or more subjects
4. Anecdotal reports or expert opinion

NOTE: Adapted from Yatham et al. (2013).

insight into illness), medication factors (e.g., side effects, no perceived daily benefit, difficulties with medication routines), and patient attitudes (e.g., belief that medications are unnecessary, negative attitudes toward medications, etc.; Bates et al., 2010; Gianfrancesco, Sajatovic, Tafesse, & Wang, 2009; Hou, Cleak, & Peveler, 2010; Lang et al., 2011). Suboptimal utilization of pharmacotherapy may in some situations contribute to nonadherence. In a retrospective cohort study ($N = 27,751$), controlling for confounding variables, patients receiving lower doses of ziprasidone had significantly higher discontinuation rates than those receiving medium or high doses (Citrome et al., 2009). Taken together, evidence suggests that nonadherence is a multifactorial phenomenon; strategies to prevent nonadherence include, but are not limited to, enhanced therapeutic alliance, early intervention, group setting, and psychoeducation. By assessing adherence risk factors and tolerability, physicians can increase adherence and improve clinical outcomes of patients with BD.

Nonadherence in BD represents a barrier to effective treatment and commonly results in adverse clinical outcomes. Several lines of evidence indicate that nonadherence is associated with a high frequency of mood episodes (particularly depressive episodes); a higher risk of suicide, hospitalization, and emergency room visits; and higher employee costs of absenteeism, short-term disability, and workers' compensation (Bagalman et al., 2010; Gutierrez-Rojas, Jurado, Martinez-Ortega, & Gurpegui, 2010; Hassan & Lage, 2009; Lage & Hassan, 2009; Lang et al., 2011). Evidence also suggests that nonadherence to treatment in BD is associated with greater economic costs. In an analysis of data from the United Kingdom ($N = 792$), investigators reported that direct costs of care were two to three times higher in patients with BD following an acute manic or mixed episode compared to those who did not experience a recurrent mood episode over the 6- to 12-month follow-up period (Hong et al., 2010). Increased costs related to nonadherence and relapse of mood episodes have been amply documented (Yatham et al., 2013).

PREDICTORS OF RECURRENCE

While adherence to treatment in patients with BD is an important component in reducing risk of recurrence, several other factors have been identified. Evidence indicates that up to 50% of individuals with BD will experience recurrence of mood symptoms after initial treatment at two-year follow-up (Perlis et al., 2006). Recurrence in BD represents a significant clinical concern as it increases the risk of suicide attempts and is associated with poorer social and occupational functioning (Yatham et al., 2013). In observational studies, predictors of symptomatic remission and recovery using baseline indices during one to two years of follow-up in patients with manic episodes included being Caucasian, maintained social functioning (i.e., limited work or social impairment, not living independently or without a spouse/partner), outpatient treatment, and being neither satisfied nor dissatisfied with life (Dikeos et al., 2010; Haro et al., 2011; Yatham et al., 2013). Notwithstanding the results from the foregoing observational studies, future controlled studies are needed to discern predictors of symptomatic remission and recovery.

Following treatment, replicated studies indicate that the presence of residual symptoms after resolution of a major mood episode is indicative of a significant risk for a rapid relapse and/or recurrence (Judd et al., 2008; Perlis et al., 2006). Some investigators have posited that this may be due to a progression of pathology through a "kindling" phenomenon (Bender & Alloy, 2011; Post, 1992)—a process first discovered in 1967 in epilepsy wherein neurons become sensitized. The kindling hypothesis has yet to be elucidated; however, it is posited that if mood episodes in BD continue to recur unmonitored, the brain becomes kindled or sensitized. This kindling or sensitization of various pathways inside the central nervous system may be reinforced over time, leading to a greater frequency of future episodes of depression, hypomania, or mania. Indeed, robust data indicate that more previous mood episodes are associated with future episodes, significant neurocognitive dysfunction (Kessler et al., 2013), decreased quality of life and psychosocial functioning, poorer response to treatment, and longer hospitalizations (Yatham et al., 2005). A study completed by Berk et al. (2011) suggested that BD may be more effectively treated if the bipolar illness was staged based on the number of mood recurrences. Results of the study indicated that response rates for mania ranged from 52% to 69% and maintenance studies ranged from 10% to 50% for individuals with one to five previous episodes, whereas individuals with fewer than five previous episodes had response rates for mania ranging from 29% to

59% versus 11% to 40% across maintenance studies (Berk et al., 2011). These data indicate that the number of episodes prior to treatment initiation influences recurrence vulnerability or at least the response to treatment during maintenance therapy in BD. The potential consequences of multiple episodes underlie the recommendation that initiating therapy early, even after the first manic episode, is justified.

The use and timing of certain medications may also be predictors of recurrence. For example, evidence indicates that prescription of typical antipsychotics and prescription of antidepressants at the first visit of the long-term treatment phase may be an independent predictor of lower remission and recovery rates (Haro et al., 2011). There is also some evidence that switching medication after an acute response may predict poorer outcomes during maintenance therapy (McElroy et al., 2008). However, there is not a "one-size-fits-all" strategy for maintenance therapy to reduce recurrence. Intuitively, one might assume that acute efficacy of a medication is synonymous with recurrence prevention efficacy. That turns out not to be the case for many agents. For example, divalproex, which is unequivocally antimanic, has not consistently demonstrated recurrence prevention over and above placebo in bipolar I disorder (Bowden et al., 2000). Conversely, lamotrigine, which has demonstrated recurrence prevention efficacy in bipolar depression (and to a lesser extent bipolar mania), has also been reported to be inefficacious for acute mania and acute depression (Cipriani et al., 2011); however, the latter results remain controversial (Geddes, Calabrese, & Goodwin, 2009)

The symptoms experienced and the subtype of BD (e.g., manic episodes vs. rapid cycling; Yatham et al., 2013) are also predictors of recurrence. As compared to other subtypes of BD, those patients who experience rapid cycling episodes exhibit increased rates of recurrence and decreased rates of remission and recovery (Gao et al., 2010). In those patients with rapid cycling treated with lithium or divalproex, increased risk for recurrence was associated with a history of recent substance use disorder, early-life verbal abuse, female gender, and late onset of first depressive episode (Gao et al., 2010; Pfennig et al., 2010). In addition, quality of long-term efficacy of lithium therapy is influenced by a number of illness factors. For example, the risk of recurrence has been shown to be higher in those with atypical features (i.e., mood-incongruent psychotic symptoms), interepisodic residual symptoms, and rapid cycling (Pfennig et al., 2010).

Recurrence is a clinically significant concern in BD; however, evidence suggests that the risk can be reduced by a number of different strategies, including improving adherence to medications/treatment, adjunctive psychotherapy, and medication choice. Treatment guidelines suggest that targeting residual symptoms during maintenance therapy may reduce risk of recurrence and progression of BD.

PHARMACOLOGICAL TREATMENTS FOR MAINTENANCE THERAPY—BIPOLAR I DISORDER

In general, maintenance pharmacotherapy consists of the same regimen that successfully treated the acute bipolar episode. This observation has been confirmed in two studies. In a randomized controlled trial (RCT) of 148 acutely manic patients who initially remitted with open-label divalproex and were then assigned to maintenance treatment with divalproex, lithium, or placebo, time to recurrence was significantly longer with divalproex compared with lithium or placebo (McElroy et al., 2008). This result was replicated in an RCT ($N = 1,172$) that investigated the efficacy and safety of quetiapine monotherapy as maintenance treatment in bipolar I disorder compared to switching to placebo or lithium. It was found that for those patients with a manic, depressive, or mixed episode who were initially stabilized with open-label quetiapine and then assigned to maintenance quetiapine, lithium, or placebo, time to recurrence was significantly longer with quetiapine compared to lithium or placebo (Weisler et al., 2011). In addition, in patients stabilized during acute quetiapine treatment, continuation of quetiapine significantly increased time to recurrence of any mood, manic, or depressive event compared with switching to placebo.

Often clinicians are faced with the question of whether they should combine medications. While some patients require medication combinations for maintenance therapy, it is recommended that clinicians initially attempt to manage patients with monotherapy in order to maximize chances of adherence and minimize side effects and costs. See the section "To Combine or Not to Combine?", as well as Table 23.4, for a review of the evidence in support of combination maintenance pharmacotherapy.

There are, however, methodological issues that affect the interpretation of data on maintenance treatments in BD. For example, the majority of long-term studies have used "enriched" designs wherein the patient's acute symptoms had to respond to a given medication during open-label treatment to the point of syndromal remission before randomization. This results in sample "enrichment" for acute responders. While an enriched design may address the pragmatic clinical question of whether the drug that was used for an acute episode should be maintained beyond the achievement of remission, it also introduces a number of limitations to the data. More specifically, an enriched design (a) limits the generalizability of study results to patients treated under similar conditions, (b) favors the test drug with respect to an active comparator if introduced at randomization, and (c) may lead to a higher frequency of early relapses in the placebo and/or comparator arms of a study versus the open phase due to possible discontinuation effects of the drug under investigation.

FIRST-LINE OPTIONS

The evidence for effective maintenance therapy of BD is the most comprehensive for lithium, divalproex, olanzapine, and quetiapine (for both bipolar depression and mania), as well as lamotrigine (primarily for preventing bipolar depression), risperidone long-acting injection (LAI), and ziprasidone (primarily for preventing mania). These medication choices should be considered first-line monotherapy options for maintenance treatment of BD (Table 23.1). Quetiapine, risperidone LAI, aripiprazole, and ziprasidone are also recommended as adjunctive therapy with lithium or divalproex (Table 23.1) (Yatham et al., 2013).

A systematic review and meta-analysis of pharmacological treatment options for the prevention of relapse in BD included 34 RCTs and open-label trials and concluded that, in comparison to placebo, lithium, olanzapine, and aripiprazole had significant clinical effects in the prevention of manic relapses (Beynon, Soares-Weiser, Woolacott, Duffy, & Geddes, 2009). The study also found that divalproex, lamotrigine, and imipramine had robust effectiveness in the prevention of depressive symptoms. These pooled data were replicated in a meta-analysis of 20 RCTs ($N = 5,364$) that sought to examine the effectiveness of maintenance therapies in BD. The study confirmed the efficacy of lithium, divalproex, lamotrigine, and a number of atypical antipsychotic agents (most robust evidence for quetiapine) in preventing relapse to any episode versus placebo (Vieta et al., 2011). While methodological quality was noted to vary between studies and the strength of evidence was not equal for all treatments and for all comparisons, these data support the maintenance treatment recommendations outlined in Table 23.2.

An important methodological issue to remember is that almost all studies have enrolled individuals who have recently recovered from mania. This implies that this enriched enrolled population has a greater proclivity toward manic recurrence than depressive recurrence. Only

Table 23.2. TREATMENT RECOMMENDATIONS

First line	Level 1 or Level 2 evidence plus clinical support for efficacy and safety
Second line	Level 3 evidence or higher plus clinical support for efficacy and safety
Third line	Level 4 evidence or higher plus clinical support for efficacy and safety
Not recommended	Level 1 or Level 2 evidence for lack of efficacy

NOTE: Adapted from Yatham et al. (2013).

lamotrigine and quetiapine have been studied for individuals recovering from a depressive episode (in the case of quetiapine it was from depressive or manic episode). As a result, much of the evidence to date supports prevention of manic episodes in bipolar I disorder.

The following sections discuss the relevant evidence for all of the first-line maintenance treatment options in bipolar I disorder.

Lithium

Lithium has long been considered the gold standard for long-term maintenance therapy in BD. There is comprehensive evidence to support lithium from meta-analyses (Burgess et al., 2001; Geddes, Burgess, Hawton, Jamison, & Goodwin, 2004) and RCTs (Bowden et al., 2003; Calabrese et al., 2006; Yazici et al., 2004; Tables 23.2 and 23.3:

Table 23.3. FACTORS NEGATIVELY INFLUENCING TREATMENT ADHERENCE

Patient Factors

> Younger age
> Single status
> Male gender
> Low education level
> Lack of psychosocial support

Illness Factors

> Hypomanic denial
> Psychosis
> Comorbid personality disorders
> Comorbid substance abuse
> Poor insight

Treatment Factors

> Side effects of medications
> Unfavorable personal attitudes toward treatment

NOTE: Adapted from Sajatovic et al. (2004).

Level 1). Lithium has been more widely studied than any other maintenance treatment for BD. A meta-analysis of five RCTs (753 patients with BD) found relapses occurred in significantly fewer patients who received lithium compared with placebo (41% vs. 61%, respectively; Smith, Cornelius, Warnock, Bell, & Young, 2007). Several lines of evidence suggest that the benefit with lithium is greater for the prevention of manic episodes than it is for preventing depressive symptomatology (Bowden et al., 2003; Calabrese et al., 2003). These data provide support for the use of lithium monotherapy maintenance treatment in bipolar I disorder.

The use of lithium in the treatment of bipolar I disorder also reduces the risk of suicide. A meta-analysis of 33 RCTs and observational studies (1970–2000) yielded 13-fold lower rates of suicide (and reported attempts) during long-term lithium treatment when compared to no lithium treatment or after its discontinuation (Baldessarini, Tondo, & Hennen, 2001). However, as with all observational studies, there are some limitations that affect the interpretation of these data. For example, there were highly variable sample sizes and inconsistent reporting on risks with and without lithium; in addition, most of the studies included were not aimed specifically at assessing suicidal risk. Notwithstanding these limitations, this result has been replicated in many other trials, as well as observational studies of health plans and a nationwide medical registry monitoring studies confirming the association of lithium use in treatment of BD and decreased suicide risk.

The initial dose of lithium is 300 mg once a day. It is then titrated to achieve a target 12-hour serum trough level of 0.8 to 1.2 mEq/L, and taken once per day. The serum level can be reduced to 0.6 mEq/L (or lower if necessary) for patients unable to tolerate higher levels. There is also emerging evidence to suggest that the often-cited target of 0.8 mEq/L might not be necessary. A reanalysis of lithium data during maintenance treatment suggested that whatever the plasma level is that "gets you better" during acute treatment is the level that "keeps you better" (Perlis et al., 2002). Therefore, while physicians are encouraged to check plasma lithium levels, it is equally if not more important to titrate lithium levels to clinical effect. Common side effects include weight gain, tremor, gastrointestinal distress, impaired ability to concentrate, urine, polyuria, and hypothyroidism (Frye et al., 2009).

Rapid discontinuation with lithium can pose a problem for recurrence in BD even after good response and a lengthy illness-free period. If lithium needs to be discontinued, it should be done gradually, as abrupt discontinuation is associated with a higher rate of recurrence (Suppes, Baldessarini, Faedda, & Tohen, 1991). A two-year naturalistic follow-up study compared illness recurrence among patients who continued ($n = 159$) or discontinued ($n = 54$) lithium after an extended period of clinical stability on monotherapy (Biel, Peselow, Mulcare, Case, & Fieve, 2007). Patients who continued on lithium had a five-fold lower risk of recurrence; the authors therefore concluded that discontinuation of lithium is not recommended. Evidence suggests that discontinuation of lithium is motivated by similar features to that of adherence in general, such as patients' knowledge regarding lithium treatment, general opposition to prophylaxis, fear of side effects, denial of therapeutic effectiveness, and illness severity; these factors were directly correlated to treatment adherence (Rosa et al., 2007). Addressing these factors may improve patients' adherence to lithium maintenance pharmacotherapy.

Divalproex

There is reasonable evidence to support the use of divalproex for maintenance therapy in BD. Several lines of evidence indicate that divalproex is more effective in preventing depressive episodes in BD rather than mania (Beynon et al., 2009). Although one RCT failed to demonstrate that divalproex was superior to placebo in preventing recurrence of bipolar episodes (Bowden et al., 2000), multiple RCTs have demonstrated that divalproex is as effective as lithium or olanzapine in the prevention of recurrence, especially for prevention of depressive episodes (Lambert & Venaud, 1987; Tohen et al., 2003). There is also some hypothesis-generating evidence to suggest that divalproex may be superior to other agents for severely ill bipolar patients—however, this evidence arises from nonblinded open studies (Bowden et al., 2000). Several lines of evidence also indicate that if patients respond to acute treatment with divalproex, maintenance treatment with divalproex is superior compared with lithium or placebo (McElroy et al., 2008). However, as mentioned, these data are derived from enriched study designs that tend to favor the test drug over comparators. Notwithstanding enriched study designs, the fact that multiple double-blind RCTs have shown at least equivalency of divalproex and active comparators, together with extensive clinical experience and good tolerability of the medication, divalproex is recommended as a first-line monotherapy treatment option in bipolar I disorder (Table 23.2; Beynon et al., 2009).

Divalproex is prescribed at a dose of 500 mg once per day initially and titrated to achieve a target 12-hour serum trough level of 50 to 125 mcg/mL. Long-acting preparations are available that can be prescribed once per day as well. When converting stable patients with

BD from twice-daily divalproex delayed release to once daily extended release (ER), the total daily dose should be increased by 250 to 500 mg to ensure maintenance of therapeutic levels of valproic acid. Common side effects from divalproex include somnolence, weight gain, gastrointestinal distress, elevated transaminases, tremor, decreased platelet counts, and alopecia. Divalproex should also be avoided during pregnancy due to the risk of teratogenicity. In addition, divalproex has been associated with increased risk of polycystic ovarian syndrome. Polycystic ovarian syndrome has been reported to occur in approximately 10% of women during maintenance; in addition, 50% of women reported menstrual problems (McIntyre et al., 2005; Morrell et al., 2008; Thase, 2007).

Lamotrigine

Multiple RCTs have demonstrated the effectiveness of lamotrigine in the prevention of relapse of mood episodes in BD (Bowden et al., 2003; Calabrese et al., 2000; van der Loos et al., 2011; Table 23.2: Level 1). Data from meta-analyses suggest that lamotrigine reduces the risk of relapse by 16% to 20% compared with placebo (Vieta et al., 2011). However, some evidence suggests that lamotrigine, while effective in prolonging time to intervention for depressive episodes, did not demonstrate efficacy for prevention of manic episodes (Calabrese et al., 2003). Treatment guidelines therefore do not recommend lamotrigine be used as monotherapy for bipolar patients if the primary objective of maintenance is the prevention of manic episodes. If prevention of manic episodes were a treatment priority, the recommendation would be to either combine lamotrigine with an antimanic agent such as lithium or try monotherapy with lithium or divalproex.

Treatment guidelines recommend that lamotrigine be started at a dose of 25 mg per day for the first two weeks, though titration may be slower or faster depending on concomitant medications. For Weeks 3 and 4, the dose is increased to 50 mg per day, taken into two divided doses. Following this, the dose can then be titrated up by 25 to 50 mg per day, one week at a time for each increase. This slow titration is important to markedly decrease the risk of serious and life-threatening skin rash (0.1% risk of Stevens-Johnson syndrome [toxic epidermal necrolysis]). The target dose generally ranges from 50 to 200 mg per day, taken in two divided doses; however, doses up to 400 mg per day may be required. An ER formulation is also available for once-a-day dosing. Common side effects include nausea, dyspepsia, pain, insomnia, and benign cutaneous reactions.

Olanzapine

Randomized-controlled trial (Vieta et al., 2012) and meta-analytic (Cipriani, Rendell, & Geddes, 2010) data suggest that olanzapine is an effective maintenance treatment for preventing relapses in BD, particularly that of manic episodes, and is recommended as a first-line treatment option. A 48-week RCT reported that time to symptomatic relapse into any mood episode (median 174 days vs. 22 days) and relapse rate (46.7% vs. 80.1%) was significantly superior with olanzapine compared to placebo (Tohen et al., 2003). Furthermore, a meta-analysis of five RCTs (Cipriani et al., 2010) found that olanzapine as a monotherapy or an adjunct to lithium or divalproex was more effective than adjunct placebo in preventing manic but not composite outcomes of all mood episodes. The analysis concluded that olanzapine may prevent further manic episodes only in patients who have responded to olanzapine in an acute manic or mixed episode and who have not previously had a satisfactory response to lithium or valproate (Cipriani et al., 2010). In addition, a large, observational cohort study (EMBLEM) included 1,076 patients in a comparison of olanzapine monotherapy or as an adjunct and found no significant difference in rates of improvement, remission, or recovery but significantly lower relapse rates with olanzapine alone compared to adjunctive olanzapine over the two-year follow-up. Given these data, treatment guidelines recommend olanzapine as a possible first-line maintenance treatment in BD.

Emerging evidence suggests that in comparison to other second-generation antipsychotics, olanzapine may be more effective in preventing relapse in BD. In two RCTs olanzapine was included as an active control arm, and in both studies patients receiving olanzapine had a significantly longer time to recurrence of a mood episode than either risperidone LAI (Vieta et al., 2012) or paliperidone ER (Berwaerts, Melkote, Nuamah, & Lim, 2012).

Notwithstanding proven efficacy of olanzapine for the maintenance treatment of BD, olanzapine has a number of potentially serious metabolic side effects. For example, olanzapine leads to weight gain and increases the risk of developing type II diabetes mellitus. Other side effects include increased cholesterol and triglycerides, dyspepsia, constipation, dry mouth, somnolence, fatigue, insomnia, extrapyramidal symptoms, and hyperprolactinemia. The dose of olanzapine is typically 5 to 20 mg/day at bedtime. Given the side effect profile, some treatment guidelines recommend the use of olanzapine as second-line therapy, whereas others recommend it as first line. The decision of whether to start a patient on olanzapine should be assessed on an individual basis.

Quetiapine

Multiple RCTs have demonstrated the efficacy of quetiapine alone or in combination with lithium/divalproex for maintenance therapy in BD (Suppes et al., 2009; Weisler et al., 2011). In all these studies, patients in remission, after acute treatment, were randomized to quetiapine or placebo maintenance therapy with the primary outcome being the recurrence of any mood event. For example, two double-blind RCTs, EMBOLDEN I and II, assessed quetiapine monotherapy in patients in remission at eight weeks. Data from these studies demonstrated that the acute efficacy of quetiapine in bipolar depression was maintained in continuation treatment for 26 to 52 weeks compared with placebo (McElroy et al., 2010; Young et al., 2010). In a pooled analysis, recurrence of a mood event was reported in 24.5% (71/290) of patients in the quetiapine group and 40.5% (119/294) of patients in the placebo group. The risk of recurrence of any mood event or a depression event was reported to be significantly lower with quetiapine than placebo. Interpretation of these data may be limited by the use of enriched samples, wherein patients randomized to comparators may have an exaggerated relapse rate due to discontinuation of an effective treatment regimen. In another example, a 104-week RCT compared the efficacy of quetiapine, lithium, or placebo monotherapy in patients who were stable for at least four weeks following up to 24 weeks of quetiapine therapy. At 56 weeks, an interim analysis found that quetiapine was significantly more effective than placebo in reducing the risk of any mood event, including both manic and depressive episodes, or any episode (Weisler et al., 2011). Lithium was also more effective than placebo on all three measures. Quetiapine was also more effective than lithium for prevention of any event or depressive events, but the two therapies were similar for prevention of manic events.

In addition to the recommendation as a first-line monotherapy agent, quetiapine is also recommended as a first-line adjunctive agent to maintenance therapy. This recommendation is supported by two RCTs that have assessed the efficacy of adjunctive quetiapine maintenance therapy. In these studies, patients were randomized to lithium or divalproex plus quetiapine or placebo after achieving at least 12 weeks remission with open-label lithium or divalproex plus quetiapine (Suppes et al., 2009; Vieta, Suppes, et al., 2008). Pooled and individually, these studies demonstrated that quetiapine in combination with lithium or divalproex was significantly more effective than lithium or divalproex alone in the prevention of mood episodes during continuation treatment for up to 104 weeks.

Generally, in the maintenance phase, patients continue to receive the same dosage of quetiapine on which they were initially stabilized. Typically the dosage falls into the range of 400 to 800 mg/day. Similar to other second-generation antipsychotics such as olanzapine, quetiapine can cause clinically meaningful increases in insulin resistance, which, although controversial, may lead to new or exacerbated cases of type II diabetes mellitus (Newcomer, 2007). Other common (>10%) side effects include dizziness, dry mouth, headache, and somnolence. Further study is necessary to accurately estimate incidence and risk of these side effects since RCTs to date have not been designed to assess these side effects.

Risperidone intramuscular injection

Risperidone LAI is currently recommended as first-line maintenance monotherapy as well as an adjunctive medication. The treatment guidelines recommendation is based on results of two RCTs ($N = 799$ total), finding that time to recurrence of any mood episode was significantly longer with risperidone LAI compared to placebo (Level 1; Berwaerts et al., 2012; Quiroz et al., 2010; Yatham et al., 2013). Similar to olanzapine, risperidone LAI was more efficacious in preventing mania relapses than depression; however, it was found to be less effective in preventing overall relapse compared to olanzapine (Berwaerts et al., 2012). There are no large trials to date that have evaluated the use of oral risperidone for maintenance treatment in BD. However, since risperidone is the active component in the risperidone LAI, some treatment guidelines recommend both risperidone oral and risperidone LAI as first-line treatment options for maintenance treatments in BD.

Patient preference toward long-acting injectable as a route of administration is mixed. Observational data indicate that the use of risperidone LAI independently improves treatment adherence, reductions in any relapse rate, and reductions in rehospitalization rates with adjunctive risperidone LAI. At study endpoint 14 patients (48%) were very much improved according to the Clinical Global Impressions scale (Malempati et al., 2011; Vieta, Nieto, et al., 2008). Evidence also suggests that risperidone LAI may be particularly effective in treating patients with psychotic BD (Malempati et al., 2011). While no trials have been completed on patients poorly adherent to treatment, given that administration of risperidone LAI independently improves adherence, outcomes may be superior in this group in comparison to oral medications.

The usual starting dose of long-acting injectable risperidone is 25 mg every two weeks, but patients with a lower body mass index or with an increased sensitivity to side effects may benefit from an initial dose of 12.5 mg. After the first injection, oral risperidone is continued for three weeks (then discontinued) to maintain adequate therapeutic plasma concentrations prior to the main release phase of risperidone from the injection site. The dose of long-acting injectable risperidone can be increased to 37.5 or 50 mg every two weeks in patients with a larger body mass index or persistent or recurrent symptoms; a minimum of four weeks should elapse between dose adjustments. In addition, patients may benefit from intermittent use of oral risperidone to treat subsyndromal symptoms that occur during maintenance treatment with risperidone LAI—however, this has yet to be evaluated in RCTs.

Aripiprazole

Two of three RCTs have found both aripiprazole adjunctive and monotherapy efficacious for maintenance treatments of patients with bipolar I disorder. Similar to other atypical antipsychotics, evidence to date suggests that aripiprazole is more effective in preventing manic relapse but not depressive relapse (Yatham et al., 2009). For example a 100-week RCT ($N = 161$) reported that aripiprazole monotherapy was superior to placebo in delaying manic relapse but not depressive relapse (Keck et al., 2007). Results have been similar in RCTs involving aripiprazole as an adjuvant therapy. This was demonstrated in a 52-week, relapse-prevention RCT ($N = 337$) that examined the efficacy of aripiprazole as an adjunct to lithium or divalproex in patients with manic/mixed episodes displaying inadequate response to lithium or divalproex (Marcus et al., 2011). Results of the study indicated that patients in remission for 12 weeks who were randomized to continue adjunctive aripiprazole had a lower rate of relapse to manic but not depressive episodes. Since adjunctive aripiprazole demonstrated efficacy for the prevention of any mood episode or manic episodes but not depressive episodes, treatment guidelines recommended aripiprazole as both first-line adjunct and monotherapy maintenance for the prevention of manic episodes in BD.

Aripiprazole is initially started at a dose of 10 or 15 mg once per day and can be increased to 15 or 30 mg once per day. Common side effects are similar to other second-generation antipsychotics, including weight gain, headache, agitation, anxiety, nausea, dry mouth, tremor, akathisia, and other extrapyramidal symptoms. It should also be noted that the incidence of extrapyramidal symptoms might be higher in individuals taking aripiprazole in comparison to other antipsychotics such as quetiapine or olanzapine. Starting with a lower dose of 2 or 5 mg per day may help prevent side effects.

Ziprasidone

Several lines of evidence derived from RCTs suggest that adjunctive ziprasidone is efficacious for maintenance treatment of BD. This was demonstrated in a six-month RCT in 239 patients with bipolar I disorder who were stabilized for at least eight weeks on open-label therapy (Level 2; Bowden et al., 2010; Yatham et al., 2009). The time to intervention for a mood episode was significantly longer with ziprasidone. In the study, 19.7% of patients in the ziprasidone group versus 32.4% of patients receiving placebo required intervention for a mood episode. In addition, evidence indicates that ziprasidone's efficacy is most consistent for the prevention of manic but not depressive episodes. No studies to date have examined whether ziprasidone is an effective monotherapy maintenance treatment in BD.

For maintenance treatment, ziprasidone is recommended as an adjunct to lithium or divalproex therapy starting at 40 mg twice per day but can be increased to 160 mg/day according to tolerance and efficacy. As with other maintenance medications, it is advised the same dose be continued at which the patient was initially stabilized. Common side effects (>10%) include somnolence and headache. Less common side effects include extrapyramidal symptoms. However, the hazard for tardive dyskinesia does not appear to be worse in treated versus placebo-treated subjects (Bowden et al., 2010).

SECOND-LINE OPTIONS

Carbamazepine

While several lines of evidence suggest that carbamazepine has good efficacy in preventing relapses in BD, its effectiveness in clinical practice is not as robust as other first-line treatment options such as lithium. There is also evidence to suggest that carbamazepine recurrence-prevention effects may be greater in those with bipolar II disorder as compared to those with bipolar I disorder; however, these data are derived from post hoc analyses and are limited by small sample size (Greil, Kleindienst Nikolaus, Erazo Natalia, & Müller-Oerlinghausen, 1998). A meta-analysis of four RCTs, including 464 patients, supports the conclusion that maintenance treatment with carbamazepine has similar efficacy to lithium for rates of relapses, with the main caveat that there were fewer withdrawals reported due to adverse events with lithium (Ceron-Litvoc, Soares, Geddes, Litvoc, & de Lima, 2009). These data suggest that carbamazepine is not as well tolerated as first-line treatment options such as lithium. Given the significant tolerability issues with carbamazepine and the difficulty with combining this agent with other psychotropic medications (carbamazepine is an inducer of cytochrome P450 enzymes), treatment guidelines recommend carbamazepine as a second-line maintenance treatment option for BD.

Carbamazepine is initially prescribed at a dose of 200 mg twice per day and can be increased in increments of 200 mg per day. The maximum daily dose is 800 mg, twice per day. A long-acting preparation can be given as a single daily dose. Many clinicians attempt to achieve a target 12-hour serum trough level of 4 to 8 mcg/mL, but there are no studies that have documented a relationship between this blood-level range and efficacy for maintenance treatment of BD. Common side effects include dizziness, somnolence, ataxia, gastrointestinal distress, and elevated transaminases; a slow dose titration to below an individual's side effect threshold may decrease the occurrence of these side effects. Serious side effects include blood dyscrasias and life-threatening rashes.

Olanzapine/fluoxetine combination

While the evidence is mixed, several lines of evidence suggest that the combination of olanzapine and fluoxetine (OFC) may be an effective maintenance treatment for BD. A six-month RCT comparing OFC and lamotrigine monotherapy found that those patients on OFC had a significant improvement in depressive and manic symptoms. However, there were no differences in relapse rates among responders to acute treatment of OFC or lamotrigine monotherapy (Brown et al., 2009). These data are buttressed by results from observational studies showing that adjunctive olanzapine is less effective than olanzapine monotherapy in preventing any relapse (Gonzalez-Pinto et al., 2011). In contrast, an open-label continuation study ($N = 114$) reported that patients with BD who initially responded to OFC and subsequently maintained on OFC maintained their response and had less relapse compared to those patients on olanzapine monotherapy (Tamayo et al., 2009). However, these results may be limited by the effects of an enriched study design wherein patients randomized to comparators may have an exaggerated relapse rate due to discontinuation of an effective treatment regimen. Given the mixed evidence for efficacy of OFC in prophylaxis of BD, this treatment option is treated as second-line.

Daily starting of OFC is 25 mg/6 mg per day (fluoxetine/olanzapine), which may be titrated up to 75 mg/18 mg per day, depending on efficacy and tolerability. Serious metabolic side effects are possible from olanzapine, including obesity, increased insulin resistance, and type II diabetes mellitus. Metabolic indices should be frequently monitored in patients starting this combination of medication.

Paliperidone ER

Evidence derived from one well-designed RCT indicates that paliperidone may be an efficacious maintenance treatment for BD. A two-year RCT compared paliperidone ER with placebo in 290 patients with BD who initially remitted from acute manic or mixed episodes with paliperidone. The median time to recurrence was longer in patients who received paliperidone than placebo (558 vs. 283 days). The study also included 82 patients who remitted with olanzapine and were maintained on it. In this nonrandomized arm, olanzapine was found to be more effective in preventing relapse than in either the randomized paliperidone or placebo arms (Level 2; Berwaerts et al., 2012). While more RCTs are needed to determine if olanzapine is superior to paliperidone ER and if this agent should be recommended as first-line treatment, these data provide sufficient evidence to justify the use of paliperidone ER as a second-line maintenance treatment option for BD.

Paliperidone can be started at 6 mg per day, and the dose can be titrated up by 3 mg every two to three days within a range of 3 to 12 mg per day. Common side effects include headache, somnolence, dizziness, nausea, and akathisia.

THIRD-LINE OPTIONS

Asenapine

Asenapine is an atypical antipsychotic that has been shown to provide some efficacy for maintenance treatment in BD. A 49-week extension study from two pooled, three-week RCTs compared asenapine with olanzapine for treatment of acute manic or mixed episodes. At one year, a worsening of mania was reported in 2.6% of asenapine patients and 1.9% of olanzapine patients, while a switch to a depressive episode occurred in 0% of asenapine and 3.0% of olanzapine patients. Time to response was significantly longer with asenapine compared to olanzapine. In addition, 40-week extension phase results indicated that of the original 318 patients, improvements in mania and depression were comparable for asenapine and the olanzapine treatment groups with 71 patients having completed the 40-week extension. Taken together, these data suggest the efficacy of asenapine maintenance treatment to be potentially comparable to olanzapine. However, in the absence of relapse-prevention data and clinical experience, asenapine should be recommended as a third-line option for maintenance therapy for BD (McIntyre et al., 2010).

Asenapine is typically prescribed at a dose of 5 to 10 mg twice per day. Common side effects include weight gain, sedation, dizziness, insomnia, and extrapyramidal symptoms.

Oxcarbazepine

There is limited evidence to support the use of oxcarbazepine in the maintenance treatment of BD. A 52-week RCT in 55 patients with bipolar I and II disorder found a lower risk of recurrence with oxcarbazepine as adjuncts to lithium (38%) compared to placebo (59%), but this difference was not statistically significant (Level 2, negative; Vieta, Cruz, et al., 2008). However, investigators postulated that the lack of significant difference could be attributed to a lack of power due to smaller sample size in the study, as the differences in relapse were substantial between the two groups. Buttressing the results of the aforementioned data, a systematic review found insufficient evidence to recommend oxcarbazepine for maintenance treatment of BD.

Notwithstanding the foregoing results, oxcarbazepine is a possible alternative to carbamazepine, based on limited evidence of effectiveness in treating acute mood episodes and its structural similarity to carbamazepine. Data has shown that there is also a trend toward fewer depressive episodes and improved psychosocial function in those patients treated with adjunct oxcarbazepine (Vieta, Cruz, et al., 2008). In addition, oxcarbazepine is generally better tolerated and is easier to prescribe because it does not induce its own metabolism, as carbamazepine does. Therefore, oxcarbazepine remains a third-line adjuvant option. However, there is insufficient data to support the use of oxcarbazepine monotherapy in the maintenance treatment of bipolar I disorder.

The initial dose of oxcarbazepine is 300 mg taken twice daily, which is titrated by 600 mg/day at weekly intervals to a target dose of 1,200 to 2,400 mg/day, taken twice daily. Common side effects include dizziness, ocular disturbances, gastrointestinal distress, and somnolence. Clinicians should monitor serum sodium because oxcarbazepine can cause hyponatremia, especially early in treatment.

Clozapine

Given the risks of potentially lethal agranulocytosis, few studies have investigated the use of clozapine in the maintenance treatment of bipolar I disorder. Data from small, open-label prospective and retrospective studies suggest that clozapine added to any combination of lithium, anticonvulsants, antidepressants, or anxiolytics may effectively delay or prevent relapse of bipolar mood episodes. For example, adjunctive treatment with clozapine was significantly better than treatment as usual in a small RCT ($N = 38$) of 12 months duration (Suppes et al., 1999). In addition, clozapine may be useful as a treatment for refractory bipolar I disorder as an effective medication to simplify polypharmacy regimens. Evidence also indicates that clozapine may have antisuicidal properties, which suggests a role for this agent in some patients with bipolar I disorder (Meltzer et al., 2003). These data provide some support for the use of adjuvant clozapine in the treatment of bipolar I disorder, particularly in cases with limited response to other agents.

Given the risks of agranulocytosis, clozapine requires regular monitoring of white blood cell counts every one or two weeks. In addition, clozapine should not be combined with carbamazepine because they both adversely affect hematopoiesis.

Electroconvulsive therapy

There is evidence from case series that suggests that maintenance electroconvulsive therapy (ECT), usually adjunctive to medication, is effective in reducing hospitalizations in bipolar I disorder (Level 3; Vaidya, Mahableshwarkar, & Shahid, 2003). However, a nonsystematic review suggested that while ECT may have an acute beneficial effect, it is unlikely to have long-term stabilizing prosperities as a maintenance treatment in BD (Sharma, 2001). Randomized controlled trials are needed to discern to what extent, if any, ECT can be used as an effective maintenance treatment in bipolar I disorder.

Omega-3 fatty acids

While there is limited high-quality RCT data available, there is some evidence to suggest adjunctive omega-3 fatty acids may provide some benefit to maintenance treatments of BD. A meta-analysis of five RCTs of variable methodological quality found that adjunctive treatment with omega-3 fatty acids showed positive effects for depressive, but not manic, relapses in BD (Montgomery & Richardson, 2008). These findings were buttressed by a separate meta-analysis of five pooled datasets ($N = 291$), which provided strong evidence that bipolar depressive symptoms may be improved by adjunctive use of omega-3 fatty acids (Sarris, Mischoulon, & Schweitzer, 2012). However, these results are limited in part by the methodological quality of the studies included for analysis. Further study is needed before firm conclusions can be drawn. However, given the relatively benign nature and possible benefits of daily omega-3 fatty acid use, adjunctive omega-3 fatty acids are a reasonable third-line maintenance treatment option for BD.

NOT RECOMMENDED

Benzodiazepines

Benzodiazepines are not recommended for maintenance treatment in BD. An observational study from the Systematic Treatment Enhancement Program for Bipolar Disorder (STEP-BD) examined 1,365 bipolar I and II patients who recovered from a mood episode and found that the use of a benzodiazepine on a standing or as-needed basis following recovery was associated with an increased risk of recurrence (Perlis et al., 2010). However, as these are observational data, they are subject to effects of residual confounders (e.g., individuals receiving benzodiazepines are also more likely to be severely ill). In addition to likely increasing risk of recurrence, the use of benzodiazepines is associated with issues of dependence, rebound anxiety, memory impairment, and discontinuation syndrome. For all these reasons, treatment guidelines recommend the gradual titration of these agents to either discontinuation or to the lowest effective dose for essential symptomatic management (Yatham et al., 2005).

Antidepressant adjunctive and monotherapy

While antidepressants may have some efficacy in acute depressive episodes, antidepressant monotherapy is not recommended as a maintenance treatment in BD; adjunctive antidepressant therapy should be used with caution. Despite these recommendations, studies from the United States and Europe indicate that antidepressants are prescribed to 50% to 80% of patients with BD (Yatham et al., 2013). Antidepressant monotherapy for BD is not recommended because use of these agents is associated with concerns that they are not effective and that may harm patients by causing switches from depression to mania, as well as rapid cycling. Several studies support these concerns (Fountoulakis, Grunze, Panagiotidis, & Kaprinis, 2008). In a seminal maintenance study, manic episodes occurred in 12% of patients on lithium, 33% of patients on placebo, and 66% of patients on imipramine monotherapy (Prien, Klett, & Caffey, 1973). These data were buttressed by a meta-analysis of seven RCTs (predominantly tricyclic antidepressants [TCAs]) examining monotherapy or adjunctive antidepressant treatment and concluded that they were ineffective in preventing relapse (Ghaemi, Lenox, & Baldessarini, 2001). In another study of one-year duration, 50% of patients randomized to desipramine as add-on to mood-stabilizers experienced a manic switch compared with only 11% of patients randomized to bupropion add-on treatment (Sachs et al., 1994). These results clearly suggest that TCAs destabilize the course of BD whether used in monotherapy or in combination with lithium or divalproex. In contrast to these data, a study by Amsterdam & Shults (2010) has suggested that long-term fluoxetine monotherapy may provide superior relapse-prevention benefit relative to lithium monotherapy after recovery from a bipolar II major depressive episode without an increase in hypomanic mood conversion episodes; however, these results should be interpreted with caution as they have yet to be replicated.

There is some evidence to suggest that adjunctive antidepressant therapy may be beneficial for individuals who initially stabilize on antidepressants during an acute episode—particularly for those that experience a depressive episode. Altshuler et al. (2009) completed a study ($N = 83$) in which subjects with bipolar depression were treated with a mood stabilizer plus one of three randomly assigned blinded antidepressants administered during an acute depressive episode. At the study endpoint of 10 weeks, 42 (69%) of the 61 acute positive responders maintained positive response and 32 (53%) achieved remission. Patients who achieved a positive acute antidepressant response to 10 weeks of antidepressant treatment, adjunctive to a mood stabilizer, were more likely to maintain response with the same continued treatment. The switch rate into mania for patients being treated with an antidepressant adjunctive to a mood stabilizer was not found to be higher than the reported rate for patients on mood stabilizer monotherapy. Nevertheless, RCTs replicating these results are needed before firm clinical recommendations can be made pertaining to the benefits of adjunctive antidepressant therapy for maintenance treatment of BD.

It has yet to be established whether the risk of switching into mania/hypomania is class specific among antidepressants, because most drugs have not been compared in head-to-head trials. In general, the evidence suggests that switching polarity during treatment of bipolar depression appears to occur more often with venlafaxine or tricyclics compared with bupropion, selective-serotonin reuptake inhibitors, and placebo. This generalization is supported by several other studies. Two RCTs found that 15% of patients ($N = 95$) who received adjunct venlafaxine plus mood stabilizers experienced a switch to hypo/mania (Post et al., 2006; Vieta et al., 2002). A meta-analysis of six RCTs ($N = 370$) found that switching occurred in more patients who received TCAs (clomipramine, desipramine, imipramine) than other antidepressants (bupropion, fluoxetine, fluvoxamine, moclobemide, paroxetine, or tranylcypromine; 10% vs. 3%; Gijsman, Geddes, Rendell, Nolen, & Goodwin, 2004). In a separate meta-analysis of two RCTs ($N = 240$), switching occurred in fewer patients who received bupropion than other antidepressants (paroxetine, sertraline, or venlafaxine; 5% vs. 13%); Sidor & Macqueen, 2011).

Although a few RCTs have suggested that antidepressant monotherapy may be effective and safe for some patients with BD, most were small and lacked a placebo control group. Given the evidence of lack of prophylaxis efficacy and the risks of switching, antidepressant monotherapy is not recommended for maintenance treatment of BD. While the concomitant use of mood stabilizers lowers the risk of switching, adjunctive antidepressant therapy has not been found to reduce the risk of relapses and should be prescribed with caution.

Other treatments

There are several other agents that are not recommended for maintenance treatment in BD (Table 23.2). The typical antipsychotic, flupenthixol has been relatively well studied and does not appear to have prophylactic efficacy in patients with BD (Level 2, negative) (Yatham et al., 2005). Another typical antipsychotic, perphenazine, in combination with a mood stabilizer was not superior to mood stabilizer alone and in fact was found to increase the incidence of depressive episodes in BD. In addition, agents such as gabapentin, topiramate, and calcium channel blockers have been investigated for use in BD, but insufficient data exist to recommend their use as monotherapy maintenance treatments in BD.

TO COMBINE OR NOT TO COMBINE?

Despite treatment with monotherapy, relapses frequently occur in BD. There is still debate whether first-line agents should be combined or if monotherapy is most effective for maintenance therapy and prevention of relapse episodes. The Bipolar Affective Disorder Lithium/Anti-Convulsant Evaluation (BALANCE) study randomized 330 patients with BD to open-label lithium monotherapy, divalproex

monotherapy, or the combination after an active run-in period of four to eight weeks on the combination. Both the combination and lithium monotherapy were significantly more effective than divalproex monotherapy in preventing relapse during the two-year follow-up period. Combination therapy was not found to be significantly more effective than lithium alone. While this study was randomized, it had a number of important methodological limitations, including a nonblinded and open design; these findings need to be confirmed with double-blind trials before firm clinical conclusions can be drawn. Buttressing these results, the LITMUS study, an effectiveness trial designed to determine if low-dosage lithium added to an optimized personalized treatment regimen improves clinical outcome for bipolar I and bipolar II patients, found that low-dosage lithium did not provide any additional benefit beyond guideline-concordant care (Nierenberg et al., 2013).

In contrast to these data, several lines of evidence support the use of combination therapy for maintenance treatment of BD. The majority of evidence gathered has tested medication combinations in patients who were initially treated with a medication combination for the acute episode. Following remission, patients are randomly assigned to maintenance treatment with the combination or monotherapy (by substituting placebo for one of the medications in the combination). Evidence suggests that combination therapy should be maintained for maintenance therapy as the benefits of the combination therapy often outweigh the increased side effects and costs (Grunze et al., 2009). Furthermore, for those patients who have a partial but inadequate response to monotherapy, and it is tolerated, should be put on a combination therapy as opposed to augmenting the initial monotherapy treatment (according to several guidelines; Grunze et al., 2009; Yatham et al., 2005). In terms of which combinations to use, several guidelines recommend lithium or divalproex plus an atypical antipsychotic. Several new trials have shown atypical antipsychotics to be more effective than lithium or divalproex monotherapy. In situations where a second-generation antipsychotic is not tolerated or desirable, lithium with the addition of divalproex, carbamazepine, or lamotrigine are the suggested alternatives.

Should a clinician decide to put a patient on a combination therapy, there are several principles to keep in mind (Preskorn & Lacey, 2007). Some of the recommendations are to (a) minimize combination therapy when possible; (b) try to limit the number of medications to two, although three may be necessary; (c) keep in mind the combination should not pose significant safety or tolerability risks; and (d) keep in mind the combination of medications should

Table 23.4. RECOMMENDATIONS FOR
MAINTENANCE PHARMACOTHERAPY OF
BIPOLAR DISORDER

First line	Monotherapy: lithium, lamotrigine (limited efficacy in preventing mania), divalproex, olanzapine,[a] quetiapine, risperidone LAI,[b] aripiprazole[b]
	Adjunctive therapy with lithium or divalproex: quetiapine, risperidone LAI,[b] aripiprazole,[b] ziprasidone[b]
Second line	*Monotherapy:* carbamazepine, palideridone ER[c]
	Combination therapy: lithium + divalproex, lithium + carbamazepine, lithium or divalproex + olanzapine, lithium + risperidone, lithium + lamotrigine, olanzapine + fluoxetine
Third line	*Monotherapy:* asenapine[c]
	Adjunctive therapy: phenytoin, clozapine, ECT, topiramate, omega-3-fatty acids, oxcarbazepine, gabapentin, asenapine[c]
Not recommended	*Monotherapy:* gabapentin, topiramate, or antidepressants
	Adjunctive therapy: flupenthixol

NOTE: LAI = long-acting injection; ER = extended release; ECT = electroconvulsive therapy. Adapted from Yatham et al. (2013).

[a] Given the metabolic side effects, use should be carefully monitored.

[b] Mainly for the prevention of mania.

[c] New or change to recommendation.

not have the same or opposing mechanism of action. In addition, physicians should be well advised of potential metabolic/pharmacokinetic implications of combination therapy. For example, carbamazepine is an inducer of hepatic P450 enzymes and therefore will decrease drug levels of medications metabolized by that system; in contrast, divalproex is an inhibitor of that same enzyme system and therefore will cause medication levels to rise. In the following section we discuss the evidence for specific combination therapies. Table 23.4 provides the ratings of evidence for the different combinations of therapy.

Lithium or divalproex plus an atypical antipsychotic

Multiple RCTs have found that lithium or divalproex in combination with an atypical antipsychotic leads to significantly less relapse compared to lithium or divalproex monotherapy for maintenance treatment. These data underpin the recommendations set out by treatment guidelines recommending, in order of preference, adjunctive quetiapine, risperidone LAI, ziprasidone, or olanzapine (Table 23.2; Yatham et al., 2013). The evidence for quetiapine is the strongest. In two RCTs (N = 1334), patients were treated with either lithium or divalproex; relapse occurred in significantly fewer individuals on adjunctive quetiapine when compared with placebo (19 and 20 vs. 49% and 52%, respectively; Suppes et al., 2009; Vieta, Suppes, et al., 2008). Similar findings have been found for adjunctive risperidone LAI, ziprasidone, or olanzapine (Yatham et al., 2013). In addition, there are some prospective open-label and retrospective data that supports the use of clozapine added to lithium and/or divalproex monotherapy. However, clozapine should be used with caution, needs to be monitored for potentially fatal agranulocytosis, and therefore requires monitoring of white blood cells every one to two weeks.

Lithium plus an anticonvulsant

While there have been few well-designed RCTs completed to date, data indicates that lithium combined with an anticonvulsant such as divalproex or carbamazepine may be more effective in preventing relapse in BD (Pies, 2002). However, most of the data is derived from RCTs with few participants, open-label studies, as well as expert clinical consensus. Therefore this treatment combination is recommend as a second-line option (Table 23.2; Yatham et al., 2013).

DISCONTINUATION

Most patients with bipolar I disorder require maintenance treatment for many years and, for some, their entire lives (data is not as strong for bipolar II disorder). Often there is motivation to discontinue maintenance treatment because of side effects, inadequate response, medical illness, pregnancy, attitudes toward the use of medication, lack of insight, or a wish to be medication-free after a prolonged period of euthymia (Yatham et al., 2013). However, several lines of evidence indicate that discontinuation of maintenance treatment often leads to relapse and recurrence of mood episodes. In a meta-analysis completed on 14 studies involving bipolar I patients (N= 257) stable on medications for an average of 30 months, greater than 50% of new mood episodes occurred within 10 weeks of stopping and about 90% relapsed within the first year off treatment (Suppes et al., 1991). Evidence indicates that even with a prolonged maintenance therapy of five years, the risk of relapse is as high as 50% to 60% within one year of stopping treatment (Baldessarini et al., 1996).

Besides the risk of recurrence of mood episodes, cessation of treatment increases the risks of increased hospitalization and utilization, persistent subsyndromal symptoms (e.g., cognitive dysfunction), family and economic losses, as well as morbidity and mortality associated with suicide. Psychoeducation that teaches patients and family members about BD, including its etiology, clinical features, diagnosis, treatment, and prognosis, can help to discourage discontinuation and increase adherence. Despite these efforts, should a patient still choose to discontinue maintenance treatment, it is advised that the medications be tapered slowly over the course of weeks to months as opposed to abrupt cessation. Clinicians are advised to monitor for prodromal features of recurrence (e.g., sleep disturbances, irritability) and intervene as necessary. Evidence indicates that even with slow taper strategies, the majority of patients (> 95% of bipolar disorder I) still experience a relapse. Treatment guidelines recommend that patients, particularly patients with bipolar I disorder, be encouraged to stay on maintenance therapy.

PHARMACOLOGICAL TREATMENTS FOR MAINTENANCE THERAPY—BIPOLAR II DISORDER

Evidence indicates that patients being treated for bipolar II disorder spend 37 times more days experiencing depressive symptoms than hypomanic symptoms (Judd et al., 2003). In comparison to bipolar I disorder, patients with bipolar II disorder are at less risk of rapid cycling—although this finding remains controversial(Kupka et al., 2005). A few pharmacological maintenance treatments for bipolar I disorder are also indicated for bipolar II disorder; often trials are done with both bipolar I and II patients together. However, the focus of long-term therapy for patients with bipolar II disorder should be primarily on prevention of depressive episodes (Ketter & Calabrese, 2002). In most situations, clinicians will often continue patients on the acute treatment regimen, and some will require additional pharmacotherapy. Lithium, lamotrigine, and quetiapine are recommended as first-line agents for maintenance treatment of bipolar II disorder (Table 23.5). In the following section we outline the evidence that supports the first-line maintenance treatment options in bipolar II disorder. We also provide second- and third-line treatment options based on available evidence and clinical guideline consensus (Tables 23.5 and 23.6). In comparison to bipolar I disorder, the

Table 23.5. STRENGTH OF EVIDENCE FOR EFFICACY OF MAINTENANCE MONOTHERAPY FOR BIPOLAR I DISORDER

AGENT	LEVEL OF EVIDENCE
Lithium	1
Anticonvulsants	
Divalproex	2
Lamotrigine	Depression: 1
	Mania: 2
Carbamazepine	2
Gabapentin	4
Topiramate	4
Oxcarbazepine	4
Atypical Antipsychotic	
Olanzapine	2
Anpiprazole	Mania: 2
Risperidone	3
Quetiapine	3
Clozapine	4
Other Treatments	
ECT	4
Tricyclic antidepressants	2 (−ye)

NOTE. ECT = electroconvulsive therapy. Adapted from Yatham et al. (2005).

evidentiary base of maintenance treatments for bipolar II disorder is limited. It is therefore necessary to combine the evidence from expert clinical opinions to formulate treatment guidelines for bipolar II disorder.

FIRST-LINE OPTIONS

Lithium

While the prophylactic clinical benefits of lithium in patients with bipolar II disorder have been replicated in a limited number of RCTs, there have been some inconsistencies in the data (Suppes & Dennehy, 2002). For example, in one trial the prophylactic benefit of lithium was less clear in bipolar II patients than in bipolar I patients (Fieve, Kumbaraci, & Dunner, 1976). In a separate study, only the reduction in depressive episodes was statistically significant (Dunner, Stallone, & Fieve, 1976). Notwithstanding

Table 23.6. STRENGTH OF EVIDENCE FOR EFFICACY OF MAINTENANCE COMBINATION THERAPY FOR BIPOLAR I DISORDER

AGENT	LEVEL OF EVIDENCE
Lithium + Divalproex	2
Lithium + Carbarmazepine	2
Lithium or Divalproex + Olanzapine	2
Lithium or Divalproex + Risperidone	3
Lithium or Divalproex + Quetiapine	3
Lithium or Divalproex + Clozapine	3
Lithium + TCA	2 (−vet)
Lithium + SSRI	3
Lithium or Divalproex + Oxcarbazepine	3
Lithium or Divalproex + Omega-3-Fatty Acids	2
Adjunctive Phenytoin	3
Adjunctive Gabapentin	3
Adjunctive Topiramate	3
Lithium or Divalproex + ECT	3
Lithium + Flupenthixol	2 (−ye)

NOTE. ECT = electroconvulsive therapy; SSRI = selective-serotonin reuptake inhibitor; TCA = tricyclic antidepressant. Adapted from Yatham et al. (2005).

these inconsistencies, long-term observational data suggest that lithium maintenance therapy has clinical benefits in bipolar II patients. Bipolar II patients on maintenance lithium experience significantly fewer episodes per year, and significantly less time ill, compared to the time prior to initiation of lithium therapy (Tondo, Baldessarini, & Floris, 2001).

Lamotrigine

Lamotrigine is currently recommended as first-line monotherapy for maintenance treatment of bipolar II disorder. Several studies support this recommendation. In a large, six-month RCT ($N = 324$), significantly more patients treated with lamotrigine compared to placebo were stable without recurrence at six months among patients with bipolar II disorder (46% vs. 18%; Calabrese et al., 2000). Open-label and naturalistic data also support the monotherapy use of lamotrigine in bipolar II patients for the prevention of depressive symptoms (Calabrese et al., 1999).

Quetiapine

Several lines of evidence suggest that quetiapine is an effective maintenance treatment for bipolar II disorder. A pooled analysis of data from placebo-controlled RCTs found that among patients with bipolar II disorder ($N = 231$), those who achieved remission during acute-phase treatment with quetiapine monotherapy were significantly less likely to experience a relapse into any mood episode. The risk of a mood episode was also found to be dependent on the dose of quetiapine given to patients. Patients on 600 mg of quetiapine had greater than a 60% decrease in risk of a mood relapse in comparison to the lower dose of 300 mg (Suppes, Hirschfeld, Vieta, Raines, & Paulsson, 2008). These data support the first-line recommendation of quetiapine for maintenance treatment of bipolar II disorder.

SECOND- AND THIRD-LINE OPTIONS

There are a number of second- and third-line treatment options for bipolar II disorder. These are outlined in Table 23.5; the evidence in support of these recommendations is ranked in Table 23.6. The evidence base for effective treatments for bipolar II disorder is nascent; more studies are needed to determine optimal maintenance treatments.

PHARMACOLOGICAL TREATMENTS FOR MAINTENANCE THERAPY—MIXED EPISODES

While the risk of recurrence and treatment challenges are often greatest in individuals with mixed episodes, there have been relatively few high-quality studies to determine the optimal medications (Table 23.7). Several open-label and post hoc analyses suggest a role for atypical antipsychotic agents in the management of patients with mixed episodes or psychotic symptoms. In a post hoc analysis of patients with mixed episodes enrolled in a continuation study ($N = 121$), where responders to olanzapine were randomized to continue or switch to placebo, there were significant reductions in relapse rates with olanzapine compared to placebo (59.2% vs. 91.1%; Tohen, Sutton, Calabrese, Sachs, & Bowden, 2009). In another open-label extension study ($N = 65$), 52 weeks of flexible dosed ziprasidone (40–160 mg/day), showed comparable improvements in symptoms for patients initially treated for bipolar mania, regardless of whether the baseline episode was manic or

Table 23.7. RECOMMENDATIONS FOR MAINTENANCE TREATMENT OF BIPOLAR II DISORDER

First line	Lithium, lamotrigine, quetiapine[a]
Second line	Divalproex; lithium or divalproex or atypical antipsychotic + antidepressant; adjunctive quetiapine[a] adjunctive lamotrigine[a]; combination of two of: lithium, divaiproex, or atypical antipsychotic
Third line	Carbarmazepine, oxcarbazepine, atypical antipsychotic agent, ECT, fluoxetine[a]
Not recommended	Gabapentin

NOTE: ECT = electroconvulsive therapy. Adapted from Yatham et al. (2013).
[a] New or change to recommendation.

mixed or involved psychotic symptoms (Keck, Versiani, Warrington, Loebel, & Horne, 2009). Furthermore, evidence of efficacy for adjunctive risperidone was observed in a 24-week, open-label trial in 114 patients with mixed or manic episodes, finding a significant reduction from

Table 23.8. STRENGTH OF EVIDENCE FOR MAINTENANCE TREATMENTS OF BIPOLAR II DISORDER

LEVEL OF AGENT	EVIDENCE
Lithium	2
Anticonvulsants	
Divalproax	3
Lamotrigine	2
Carbamazepine	3
Gabapentin	4
Atypical antipsychotics	
Adjunctive Risperidone	3
Antidepressants	
Fluexetine	3
Imiprarnine	2 (–ve)
Combination therapy	
Lithium + Imipramine	2 (–ve)
Lithium + SSRI, Venlafaxine or Bupropion	4
Electroconvulsive therapy	4

NOTE: SSRI = selective serotonin reuptake inhibitor.

baseline in manic, depressive, and overall symptom scores with combination therapy in both the manic and mixed groups (Woo et al., 2010). However, all of these studies are limited by an enriched sample design, which may lead to a higher frequency of early relapse in the placebo and comparator arms of a study due to possible discontinuation effect of the drug under investigation. Future studies utilizing alternative study designs (e.g., nonenriched samples, length of stabilization before randomization, length of experimental phase, and recurrence outcome criteria; Gitlin, Abulseoud, & Frye, 2010) are needed to determine optimal medications for the maintenance treatment of mixed episodes (Table 23.8).

CONCLUSION

Bipolar disorder is a chronic, highly recurrent, and, in some cases, progressive illness. There are a myriad of evidence-based pharmacological maintenance treatment options to choose from for BD. Clinicians are advised to recognize factors that negatively influence medication adherence (e.g., side effects, patient factors, illness factors) as these may improve treatment selection and discontinuation by identifying individuals at greater risk of nonadherence. Bipolar disorder often show pluri-potential courses that are not deterministic but modifiable, some of which are open to intervention and others that are not. It should also be noted that multiepisode recurrences in BD foster incident comorbidity (e.g., neurocognitive impairment), which only synergizes the underlying pathological processes. Thus the goals for maintenance therapy should include delaying or preventing recurrence of new mood episodes, reducing subsyndromal symptoms and the risk of suicide, and promoting psychosocial functioning. It is important to educate patients about the chronic nature of BD and the need for ongoing pharmacological maintenance therapy to optimize clinical outcomes.

Disclosure statement: Ms. Danielle S. Cha has no conflicts of interest. Dr. Paul Kudlow has received no financial support for the production of this book chapter. Dr. Paul Kudlow declares no conflicts of interest. Dr. Roger McIntyre has no conflicts of interest. Dr. Trisha Suppes has no conflicts of interest.

REFERENCES

Altshuler, L. L., Post, R. M., Hellemann, G., Leverich, G. S., Nolen, W. A., Frye, M. A.,…Suppes, T. (2009). Impact of antidepressant continuation after acute positive or partial treatment response for bipolar depression: a blinded, randomized study. *Journal of Clinical Psychiatry, 70*(4), 450–457.

Amsterdam, J. D., & Shults, J. (2010). Efficacy and safety of long-term fluoxetine versus lithium monotherapy of bipolar II disorder: A randomized, double-blind, placebo-substitution study. *The American Journal of Psychiatry, 167*(7), 792–800. doi:10.1176/appi.ajp.2009.09020284

Bagalman, E., Yu-Isenberg, K. S., Durden, E., Crivera, C., Dirani, R., & Bunn, W. B., 3rd. (2010). Indirect costs associated with nonadherence to treatment for bipolar disorder. *Journal of Occupational and Environmental Medicine, 52*(5), 478–485. doi:10.1097/JOM.0b013e3181db811d

Baldessarini, R. J., Tondo, L., Faedda, G. L., Suppes, T. R., Floris, G., & Rudas, N. (1996). Effects of the rate of discontinuing lithium maintenance treatment in bipolar disorders. *Journal of Clinical Psychiatry, 57*(10), 441–448.

Baldessarini, R. J., Tondo, L., & Hennen, J. (2001). Treating the suicidal patient with bipolar disorder: Reducing suicide risk with lithium. *Annals of the New York Academy of Science, 932*, 24–38; discussion 39–43.

Bates, J. A., Whitehead, R., Bolge, S. C., & Kim, E. (2010). Correlates of medication adherence among patients with bipolar disorder: Results of the bipolar evaluation of satisfaction and tolerability (BEST) study: A nationwide cross-sectional survey. *Prim Care Companion to Journal of Clinical Psychiatry, 12*(5). doi:10.4088/PCC.09m00883yel

Bender, R. E., & Alloy, L. B. (2011). Life stress and kindling in bipolar disorder: Review of the evidence and integration with emerging biopsychosocial theories. *Clinical Psychological Review, 31*(3), 383–398. doi:10.1016/j.cpr.2011.01.004

Berk, M., Brnabic, A., Dodd, S., Kelin, K., Tohen, M., Malhi, G. S.,...McGorry, P. D. (2011). Does stage of illness impact treatment response in bipolar disorder? Empirical treatment data and their implication for the staging model and early intervention. *Bipolar Disorders, 13*(1), 87–98. doi:10.1111/j.1399-5618.2011.00889.x

Berwaerts, J., Melkote, R., Nuamah, I., & Lim, P. (2012). A randomized, placebo- and active-controlled study of paliperidone extended-release as maintenance treatment in patients with bipolar I disorder after an acute manic or mixed episode. *Journal of Affective Disorders, 138*(3), 247–258. doi:10.1016/j.jad.2012.01.047

Beynon, S., Soares-Weiser, K., Woolacott, N., Duffy, S., & Geddes, J. R. (2008). Psychosocial interventions for the prevention of relapse in bipolar disorder: systematic review of controlled trials. *The British Journal of Psychiatry, 192*(1), 5–11. doi:10.1192/bjp.bp.107.037887

Beynon, S., Soares-Weiser, K., Woolacott, N., Duffy, S., & Geddes, J. R. (2009). Pharmacological interventions for the prevention of relapse in bipolar disorder: a systematic review of controlled trials. *Journal of Psychopharmacology, 23*(5), 574–591. doi:10.1177/0269881108093885

Biel, M. G., Peselow, E., Mulcare, L., Case, B. G., & Fieve, R. (2007). Continuation versus discontinuation of lithium in recurrent bipolar illness: A naturalistic study. *Bipolar Disorders, 9*(5), 435–442. doi:10.1111/j.1399-5618.2007.00389.x

Bowden, C. L., Calabrese, J. R., McElroy, S. L., Gyulai, L., Wassef, A., Petty, F.,...Wozniak, P. J. (2000). A randomized, placebo-controlled 12-month trial of divalproex and lithium in treatment of outpatients with bipolar I disorder. Divalproex Maintenance Study Group. *Archives of General Psychiatry, 57*(5), 481–489.

Bowden, C. L., Calabrese, J. R., Sachs, G., Yatham, L. N., Asghar, S. A., Hompland, M.,...Lamictal 606 Study, Group. (2003). A placebo-controlled 18-month trial of lamotrigine and lithium maintenance treatment in recently manic or hypomanic patients with bipolar I disorder. *Archives of General Psychiatry, 60*(4), 392–400. doi:10.1001/archpsyc.60.4.392

Bowden, C. L., Vieta, E., Ice, K. S., Schwartz, J. H., Wang, P. P., & Versavel, M. (2010). Ziprasidone plus a mood stabilizer in subjects with bipolar I disorder: A 6-month, randomized, placebo-controlled, double-blind trial. *Journal of Clinical Psychiatry, 71*(2), 130–137. doi:10.4088/JCP.09m05482yel

Brown, E., Dunner, D. L., McElroy, S. L., Keck, P. E., Adams, D. H., Degenhardt, E.,...Houston, J. P. (2009). Olanzapine/fluoxetine combination vs. lamotrigine in the 6-month treatment of bipolar I depression. *International Journal of Neuropsychopharmacology, 12*(6), 773–782. doi:10.1017/S1461145708009735

Burgess, S., Geddes, J., Hawton, K., Townsend, E., Jamison, K., & Goodwin, G. (2001). Lithium for maintenance treatment of mood disorders. *Cochrane Database System Review, 3*, CD003013. doi:10.1002/14651858.CD003013

Calabrese, J. R., Bowden, C. L., McElroy, S. L., Cookson, J., Andersen, J., Keck, P. E., Jr.,...Ascher, J. A. (1999). Spectrum of activity of lamotrigine in treatment-refractory bipolar disorder. *The American Journal of Psychiatry, 156*(7), 1019–1023.

Calabrese, J. R., Bowden, C. L., Sachs, G., Yatham, L. N., Behnke, K., Mehtonen, O. P.,...Lamictal 605 Study, Group. (2003). A placebo-controlled 18-month trial of lamotrigine and lithium maintenance treatment in recently depressed patients with bipolar I disorder. *Journal of Clinical Psychiatry, 64*(9), 1013–1024.

Calabrese, J. R., Goldberg, J. F., Ketter, T. A., Suppes, T., Frye, M., White, R.,...Thompson, T. R. (2006). Recurrence in bipolar I disorder: A post hoc analysis excluding relapses in two double-blind maintenance studies. *Biological Psychiatry, 59*(11), 1061–1064. doi:10.1016/j.biopsych.2006.02.034

Calabrese, J. R., Suppes, T., Bowden, C. L., Sachs, G. S., Swann, A. C., McElroy, S. L.,...Monaghan, E. T. (2000). A double-blind, placebo-controlled, prophylaxis study of lamotrigine in rapid-cycling bipolar disorder. Lamictal 614 Study Group. *Journal of Clinical Psychiatry, 61*(11), 841–850.

Ceron-Litvoc, D., Soares, B. G., Geddes, J., Litvoc, J., & de Lima, M. S. (2009). Comparison of carbamazepine and lithium in treatment of bipolar disorder: A systematic review of randomized controlled trials. *Human Psychopharmacology, 24*(1), 19–28. doi:10.1002/hup.990

Cipriani, A., Barbui, C., Salanti, G., Rendell, J., Brown, R., Stockton, S.,...Geddes, J. R. (2011). Comparative efficacy and acceptability of antimanic drugs in acute mania: a multiple-treatments meta-analysis. *Lancet, 378*(9799), 1306–1315. doi:10.1016/S0140-6736(11)60873-8

Cipriani, A., Rendell, J., & Geddes, J. R. (2010). Olanzapine in the long-term treatment of bipolar disorder: a systematic review and meta-analysis. *Journal of Psychopharmacology, 24*(12), 1729–1738. doi:10.1177/0269881109106900

Citrome, L., Reist, C., Palmer, L., Montejano, L. B., Lenhart, G., Cuffel, B.,...Sanders, K. N. (2009). Impact of real-world ziprasidone dosing on treatment discontinuation rates in patients with schizophrenia or bipolar disorder. *Schizophrenia Research, 115*(2–3), 115–120. doi:10.1016/j.schres.2009.09.023

Depp, C. A., Mausbach, B., Granholm, E., Cardenas, V., Ben-Zeev, D., Patterson, T. L.,...Jeste, D. V. (2010). Mobile interventions for severe mental illness: design and preliminary data from three approaches. *Journal of Nervous Mental Disorders, 198*(10), 715–721. doi:10.1097/NMD.0b013e3181f49ea3

Devulapalli, K. K., Ignacio, R. V., Weiden, P., Cassidy, K. A., Williams, T. D., Safavi, R.,...Sajatovic, M. (2010). Why do persons with bipolar disorder stop their medication? *Psychopharmacological Bulletin, 43*(3), 5–14.

Dikeos, D., Badr, M. G., Yang, F., Pesek, M. B., Fabian, Z., Tapia-Paniagua, G.,...Treuer, T. (2010). Twelve-month prospective, multinational, observational study of factors associated with recovery from mania in bipolar disorder in patients treated with atypical antipsychotics. *World Journal of Biological Psychiatry, 11*(4), 667–676. doi:10.3109/15622970903544638

Dunner, D. L., Stallone, F., & Fieve, R. R. (1976). Lithium carbonate and affective disorders: V. A double-blind study of prophylaxis of depression in bipolar illness. *Archives of General Psychiatry, 33*(1), 117–120.

Fieve, R. R., Kumbaraci, T., & Dunner, D. L. (1976). Lithium prophylaxis of depression in bipolar I, bipolar II, and unipolar patients. *The American Journal of Psychiatry, 133*(8), 925–929.

Fountoulakis, K. N., Grunze, H., Panagiotidis, P., & Kaprinis, G. (2008). Treatment of bipolar depression: An update. *Journal of Affective Disorders, 109*(1–2), 21–34. doi:10.1016/j.jad.2007.10.016

Frye, M. A., Yatham, L., Ketter, T. A., Goldberg, J., Suppes, T., Calabrese, J. R.,…Adams, B. (2009). Depressive relapse during lithium treatment associated with increased serum thyroid-stimulating hormone: Results from two placebo-controlled bipolar I maintenance studies. *Acta Psychiatrica Scandinavica, 120*(1), 10–13. doi:10.1111/j.1600-0447.2008.01343.x

Gao, K., Kemp, D. E., Wang, Z., Ganocy, S. J., Conroy, C., Serrano, M. B.,…Calabrese, J. R. (2010). Predictors of non-stabilization during the combination therapy of lithium and divalproex in rapid cycling bipolar disorder: A post-hoc analysis of two studies. *Psychopharmacological Bulletin, 43*(1), 23–38.

Geddes, J. R., Burgess, S., Hawton, K., Jamison, K., & Goodwin, G. M. (2004). Long-term lithium therapy for bipolar disorder: Systematic review and meta-analysis of randomized controlled trials. *The American Journal of Psychiatry, 161*(2), 217–222.

Geddes, J. R., Calabrese, J. R., & Goodwin, G. M. (2009). Lamotrigine for treatment of bipolar depression: Independent meta-analysis and meta-regression of individual patient data from five randomised trials. *The British Journal of Psychiatry, 194*(1), 4–9. doi:10.1192/bjp.bp.107.048504

Ghaemi, S. N., Lenox, M. S., & Baldessarini, R. J. (2001). Effectiveness and safety of long-term antidepressant treatment in bipolar disorder. *Journal of Clinical Psychiatry, 62*(7), 565–569.

Gianfrancesco, F. D., Sajatovic, M., Tafesse, E., & Wang, R. H. (2009). Association between antipsychotic combination therapy and treatment adherence among individuals with bipolar disorder. *Annals of Clinical Psychiatry, 21*(1), 3–16.

Gijsman, H. J., Geddes, J. R., Rendell, J. M., Nolen, W. A., & Goodwin, G. M. (2004). Antidepressants for bipolar depression: A systematic review of randomized, controlled trials. *The American Journal of Psychiatry, 161*(9), 1537–1547. doi:10.1176/appi.ajp.161.9.1537

Gitlin, M. J., Abulseoud, O., & Frye, M. A. (2010). Improving the design of maintenance studies for bipolar disorder. *Current Medical Research Opinion, 26*(8), 1835–1842. doi:10.1185/03007995.2010.489830

Gonzalez-Pinto, A., Reed, C., Novick, D., Bertsch, J., & Haro, J. M. (2010). Assessment of medication adherence in a cohort of patients with bipolar disorder. *Pharmacopsychiatry, 43*(7), 263–270. doi:10.1055/s-0030-1263169

Gonzalez-Pinto, A., Vieta, E., Reed, C., Novick, D., Barraco, A., Aguado, J., & Haro, J. M. (2011). Effectiveness of olanzapine monotherapy and olanzapine combination treatment in the long term following acute mania—Results of a two year observational study in bipolar disorder (EMBLEM). *Journal of Affective Disorders, 131*(1–3), 320–329. doi:10.1016/j.jad.2010.11.037

Greil, W., Kleindienst, N., Dipl-Stat, Erazo, N., & Müller-Oerlinghausen, B. (1998). Differential response to lithium and carbamazepine in the prophylaxis of bipolar disorder. *Journal of Clinical Psychopharmacology, 18*(6), 455–460.

Grunze, H., Vieta, E., Goodwin, G. M., Bowden, C., Licht, R. W., Moller, H. J., & Kasper, S. (2009). The World Federation of Societies of Biological Psychiatry (WFSBP) guidelines for the biological treatment of bipolar disorders: Update 2009 on the treatment of acute mania. *World Journal of Biological Psychiatry, 10*(2), 85–116. doi:10.1080/15622970902823202

Gutierrez-Rojas, L., Jurado, D., Martinez-Ortega, J. M., & Gurpegui, M. (2010). Poor adherence to treatment associated with a high recurrence in a bipolar disorder outpatient sample. *Journal of Affective Disorders, 127*(1–3), 77–83. doi:10.1016/j.jad.2010.05.021

Haro, J. M., Reed, C., Gonzalez-Pinto, A., Novick, D., Bertsch, J., Vieta, E., & Board, Emblem Advisory. (2011). 2-year course of bipolar disorder type I patients in outpatient care: Factors associated with remission and functional recovery. *European Neuropsychopharmacology, 21*(4), 287–293. doi:10.1016/j.euroneuro.2010.08.001

Hassan, M., & Lage, M. J. (2009). Risk of rehospitalization among bipolar disorder patients who are nonadherent to antipsychotic therapy after hospital discharge. *American Journal of Health-System Pharmacy, 66*(4), 358–365. doi:10.2146/ajhp080374

Hong, J., Reed, C., Novick, D., Haro, J. M., Windmeijer, F., & Knapp, M. (2010). The cost of relapse for patients with a manic/mixed episode of bipolar disorder in the EMBLEM study. *Pharmacoeconomics, 28*(7), 555–566. doi:10.2165/11535200-000000000-00000

Hou, R., Cleak, V., & Peveler, R. (2010). Do treatment and illness beliefs influence adherence to medication in patients with bipolar affective disorder? A preliminary cross-sectional study. *European Psychiatry, 25*(4), 216–219. doi:10.1016/j.eurpsy.2009.09.003

Judd, L. L., Akiskal, H. S., Schettler, P. J., Coryell, W., Endicott, J., Maser, J. D.,…Keller, M. B. (2003). A prospective investigation of the natural history of the long-term weekly symptomatic status of bipolar II disorder. *Archives of General Psychiatry, 60*(3), 261–269.

Judd, L. L., Schettler, P. J., Akiskal, H. S., Coryell, W., Leon, A. C., Maser, J. D., & Solomon, D. A. (2008). Residual symptom recovery from major affective episodes in bipolar disorders and rapid episode relapse/recurrence. *Archives of General Psychiatry, 65*(4), 386–394. doi:10.1001/archpsyc.65.4.386

Keck, P. E. Jr., Calabrese, J. R., McIntyre, R. S., McQuade, R. D., Carson, W. H., Eudicone, J. M.,…Aripiprazole Study Group. (2007). Aripiprazole monotherapy for maintenance therapy in bipolar I disorder: A 100-week, double-blind study versus placebo. *Journal of Clinical Psychiatry, 68*(10), 1480–1491.

Keck, P. E. Jr., Versiani, M., Warrington, L., Loebel, A. D., & Horne, R. L. (2009). Long-term safety and efficacy of ziprasidone in subpopulations of patients with bipolar mania. *Journal of Clinical Psychiatry, 70*(6), 844–851.

Keller, M. B., Lavori, P. W., Coryell, W., Endicott, J., & Mueller, T. I. (1993). Bipolar I: A five-year prospective follow-up. *Journal of Nervous Mental Disorders, 181*(4), 238–245.

Kessler, U., Schoeyen, H. K., Andreassen, O. A., Eide, G. E., Hammar, A., Malt, U. F.,…Vaaler, A. E. (2013). Neurocognitive profiles in treatment-resistant bipolar I and bipolar II disorder depression. *BMC Psychiatry, 13*, 105. doi:10.1186/1471-244X-13-105

Ketter, T. A., & Calabrese, J. R. (2002). Stabilization of mood from below versus above baseline in bipolar disorder: a new nomenclature. *Journal of Clinical Psychiatry, 63*(2), 146–151.

Kupka, R. W., Luckenbaugh, D. A., Post, R. M., Suppes, T., Altshuler, L. L., Keck, P. E. Jr.,…Nolen, W. A. (2005). Comparison of rapid-cycling and non-rapid-cycling bipolar disorder based on prospective mood ratings in 539 outpatients. *The American Journal of Psychiatry, 162*(7), 1273–1280. doi:10.1176/appi.ajp.162.7.1273

Lage, M. J., & Hassan, M. K. (2009). The relationship between antipsychotic medication adherence and patient outcomes among individuals diagnosed with bipolar disorder: A retrospective study. *Annals of General Psychiatry, 8*, 7. doi:10.1186/1744-859X-8-7

Lambert, P. A., & Venaud, G. (1987). Use of valpromide in psychiatric therapeutics. *Encephale, 13*(6), 367–373.

Lang, K., Korn, J., Muser, E., Choi, J. C., Abouzaid, S., & Menzin, J. (2011). Predictors of medication nonadherence and hospitalization in Medicaid patients with bipolar I disorder given long-acting or oral antipsychotics. *Journal of Medical Economics, 14*(2), 217–226. doi:10.3111/13696998.2011.562265

Malempati, R. N., Bond, D. J., Kunz, M., Malemati, C., Cheng, A., & Yatham, L. N. (2011). Long-term efficacy of risperidone long-acting injectable in bipolar disorder with psychotic features: A prospective study of 3-year outcomes. *International Journal of Clinical Psychopharmacology, 26*(3), 146–150. doi:10.1097/YIC.0b013e328343ba60

Marcus, R., Khan, A., Rollin, L., Morris, B., Timko, K., Carson, W., & Sanchez, R. (2011). Efficacy of aripiprazole adjunctive to lithium or valproate in the long-term treatment of patients with bipolar I disorder with an inadequate response to lithium or valproate monotherapy: A multicenter, double-blind, randomized study. *Bipolar Disorders*, 13(2), 133–144. doi:10.1111/j.1399-5618.2011.00898.x

McElroy, S. L., Bowden, C. L., Collins, M. A., Wozniak, P. J., Keck, P. E. Jr., & Calabrese, J. R. (2008). Relationship of open acute mania treatment to blinded maintenance outcome in bipolar I disorder. *Journal of Affective Disorders*, 107(1–3), 127–133. doi:10.1016/j.jad.2007.08.014

McElroy, S. L., Weisler, R. H., Chang, W., Olausson, B., Paulsson, B., Brecher, M., . . . Investigators, Embolden Ii. (2010). A double-blind, placebo-controlled study of quetiapine and paroxetine as monotherapy in adults with bipolar depression (EMBOLDEN II). *Journal of Clinical Psychiatry*, 71(2), 163–174. doi:10.4088/JCP.08m04942gre

McIntyre, R. S., Cohen, M., Zhao, J., Alphs, L., Macek, T. A., & Panagides, J. (2010). Asenapine for long-term treatment of bipolar disorder: A double-blind 40-week extension study. *Journal of Affective Disorders*, 126(3), 358–365. doi:10.1016/j.jad.2010.04.005

McIntyre, R. S., Mancini, D. A., Pearce, M. M., Silverstone, P., Chue, P., Misener, V. L., & Konarski, J. Z. (2005). Mood and psychotic disorders and type 2 diabetes: A metabolic triad. *Canadian Journal of Diabetes*, 29(2), 122–132.

Meltzer, H. Y., Alphs, L., Green, A. I., Altamura, A. C., Anand, R., Bertoldi, A., . . . International Suicide Prevention Trial Study Group. (2003). Clozapine treatment for suicidality in schizophrenia: International Suicide Prevention Trial (InterSePT). *Archives of General Psychiatry*, 60(1), 82–91.

Miklowitz, D. J. (2008). Adjunctive psychotherapy for bipolar disorder: State of the evidence. *The American Journal of Psychiatry*, 165(11), 1408–1419. doi:10.1176/appi.ajp.2008.08040488

Montgomery, P., & Richardson, A. J. (2008). Omega-3 fatty acids for bipolar disorder. *Cochrane Database System Reviews*, 2, CD005169. doi:10.1002/14651858.CD005169.pub2

Morrell, M. J., Hayes, F. J., Sluss, P. M., Adams, J. M., Bhatt, M., Ozkara, C., . . . Isojarvi, J. (2008). Hyperandrogenism, ovulatory dysfunction, and polycystic ovary syndrome with valproate versus lamotrigine. *Annals of Neurology*, 64(2), 200–211. doi:10.1002/ana.21411

Newcomer, J. W. (2007). Metabolic considerations in the use of antipsychotic medications: A review of recent evidence. *Journal of Clinical Psychiatry*, 68(Suppl. 1), 20–27.

Nierenberg, A. A., Friedman, E. S., Bowden, C. L., Sylvia, L. G., Thase, M. E., Ketter, T., . . . Calabrese, J. R. (2013). Lithium treatment moderate-dose use study (LiTMUS) for bipolar disorder: A randomized comparative effectiveness trial of optimized personalized treatment with and without lithium. *The American Journal of Psychiatry*, 170(1), 102–110. doi:10.1176/appi.ajp.2012.12060751

Perlis, R. H., Ostacher, M. J., Miklowitz, D. J., Smoller, J. W., Dennehy, E. B., Cowperthwait, C., . . . Sachs, G. S. (2010). Benzodiazepine use and risk of recurrence in bipolar disorder: A STEP-BD report. *Journal of Clinical Psychiatry*, 71(2), 194–200. doi:10.4088/JCP.09m05019yel

Perlis, R. H., Ostacher, M. J., Patel, J. K., Marangell, L. B., Zhang, H., Wisniewski, S. R., . . . Thase, M. E. (2006). Predictors of recurrence in bipolar disorder: primary outcomes from the Systematic Treatment Enhancement Program for Bipolar Disorder (STEP-BD). *The American Journal of Psychiatry*, 163(2), 217–224. doi:10.1176/appi.ajp.163.2.217

Perlis, R. H., Sachs, G. S., Lafer, B., Otto, M. W., Faraone, S. V., Kane, J. M., & Rosenbaum, J. F. (2002). Effect of abrupt change from standard to low serum levels of lithium: A reanalysis of double-blind lithium maintenance data. *The American Journal of Psychiatry*, 159(7), 1155–1159.

Pfennig, A., Schlattmann, P., Alda, M., Grof, P., Glenn, T., Müller-Oerlinghausen, B., . . . Berghofer, A. (2010). Influence of

atypical features on the quality of prophylactic effectiveness of long-term lithium treatment in bipolar disorders. *Bipolar Disorders*, 12(4), 390–396. doi:10.1111/j.1399-5618.2010.00826.x

Pies, R. (2002). Combining lithium and anticonvulsants in bipolar disorder: A review. *Annals of Clinical Psychiatry*, 14(4), 223–232.

Post, R. M. (1992). Transduction of psychosocial stress into the neurobiology of recurrent affective disorder. *The American Journal of Psychiatry*, 149(8), 999–1010.

Post, R. M., Altshuler, L. L., Leverich, G. S., Frye, M. A., Nolen, W. A., Kupka, R. W., . . . Mintz, J. (2006). Mood switch in bipolar depression: Comparison of adjunctive venlafaxine, bupropion and sertraline. *The British Journal of Psychiatry*, 189, 124–131. doi:10.1192/bjp.bp.105.013045

Preskorn, S. H., & Lacey, R. L. (2007). Polypharmacy: When is it rational? *Journal of Psychiatric Practice*, 13(2), 97–105. doi:10.1097/01.pra.0000265766.25495.3b

Prien, R. F., Klett, C. J., & Caffey, E. M., Jr. (1973). Lithium carbonate and imipramine in prevention of affective episodes: A comparison in recurrent affective illness. *Archives of General Psychiatry*, 29(3), 420–425.

Quiroz, J. A., Yatham, L. N., Palumbo, J. M., Karcher, K., Kushner, S., & Kusumakar, V. (2010). Risperidone long-acting injectable monotherapy in the maintenance treatment of bipolar I disorder. *Biological Psychiatry*, 68(2), 156–162. doi:10.1016/j.biopsych.2010.01.015

Rosa, A. R., Marco, M., Fachel, J. M., Kapczinski, F., Stein, A. T., & Barros, H. M. (2007). Correlation between drug treatment adherence and lithium treatment attitudes and knowledge by bipolar patients. *Progress in Neuro-Psychopharmacology & Biological Psychiatry*, 31(1), 217–224. doi:10.1016/j.pnpbp.2006.08.007

Sachs, G. S., Lafer, B., Stoll, A. L., Banov, M., Thibault, A. B., Tohen, M., & Rosenbaum, J. F. (1994). A double-blind trial of bupropion versus desipramine for bipolar depression. *Journal of Clinical Psychiatry*, 55(9), 391–393.

Sajatovic, M., Davies, M., & Hrouda, D. R. (2004). Enhancement of treatment adherence among patients with bipolar disorder. *Psychiatric Services*, 55(3), 264–269.

Sajatovic, M., Ignacio, R. V., West, J. A., Cassidy, K. A., Safavi, R., Kilbourne, A. M., & Blow, F. C. (2009). Predictors of nonadherence among individuals with bipolar disorder receiving treatment in a community mental health clinic. *Comprehensive Psychiatry*, 50(2), 100–107. doi:10.1016/j.comppsych.2008.06.008

Sajatovic, M., Levin, J., Tatsuoka, C., Micula-Gondek, W., Williams, T. D., Bialko, C. S., & Cassidy, K. A. (2012). Customized adherence enhancement for individuals with bipolar disorder receiving antipsychotic therapy. *Psychiatric Services*, 63(2), 176–178. doi:10.1176/appi.ps.201100133

Sarris, J., Mischoulon, D., & Schweitzer, I. (2012). Omega-3 for bipolar disorder: Meta-analyses of use in mania and bipolar depression. *Journal of Clinical Psychiatry*, 73(1), 81–86. doi:10.4088/JCP.10r06710

Sharma, V. (2001). The effect of electroconvulsive therapy on suicide risk in patients with mood disorders. *Canadian Journal of Psychiatry*, 46(8), 704–709.

Sidor, M. M., & Macqueen, G. M. (2011). Antidepressants for the acute treatment of bipolar depression: A systematic review and meta-analysis. *Journal of Clinical Psychiatry*, 72(2), 156–167. doi:10.4088/JCP.09r05385gre

Smith, L. A., Cornelius, V., Warnock, A., Bell, A., & Young, A. H. (2007). Effectiveness of mood stabilizers and antipsychotics in the maintenance phase of bipolar disorder: A systematic review of randomized controlled trials. *Bipolar Disorders*, 9(4), 394–412. doi:10.1111/j.1399-5618.2007.00490.x

Suppes, T., Baldessarini, R. J., Faedda, G. L., & Tohen, M. (1991). Risk of recurrence following discontinuation of lithium treatment in bipolar disorder. *Archives of General Psychiatry*, 48(12), 1082–1088.

Suppes, T., & Dennehy, E. B. (2002). Evidence-based long-term treatment of bipolar II disorder. *Journal of Clinical Psychiatry, 63*(Suppl. 10), 29–33.

Suppes, T., Hirschfeld, R. M., Vieta, E., Raines, S., & Paulsson, B. (2008). Quetiapine for the treatment of bipolar II depression: Analysis of data from two randomized, double-blind, placebo-controlled studies. *World Journal of Biological Psychiatry, 9*(3), 198–211. doi:10.1080/15622970701317265

Suppes, T., Vieta, E., Liu, S., Brecher, M., Paulsson, B., & Trial Investigators. (2009). Maintenance treatment for patients with bipolar I disorder: Results from a north american study of quetiapine in combination with lithium or divalproex (trial 127). *The American Journal of Psychiatry, 166*(4), 476–488. doi:10.1176/appi.ajp.2008.08020189

Suppes, T., Webb, A., Paul, B., Carmody, T., Kraemer, H., & Rush, A. J. (1999). Clinical outcome in a randomized 1-year trial of clozapine versus treatment as usual for patients with treatment-resistant illness and a history of mania. *The American Journal of Psychiatry, 156*(8), 1164–1169.

Tamayo, J. M., Sutton, V. K., Mattei, M. A., Diaz, B., Jamal, H. H., Vieta, E.,…Tohen, M. (2009). Effectiveness and safety of the combination of fluoxetine and olanzapine in outpatients with bipolar depression: An open-label, randomized, flexible-dose study in Puerto Rico. *Journal of Clinical Psychopharmacol, 29*(4), 358–361. doi:10.1097/JCP.0b013e3181ad223f

Thase, M. E. (2007). STEP-BD and bipolar depression: What have we learned? *Current Psychiatry Reports, 9*(6), 497–503.

Tohen, M., Greil, W., Calabrese, J. R., Sachs, G. S., Yatham, L. N., Oerlinghausen, B. M.,…Bowden, C. L. (2005). Olanzapine versus lithium in the maintenance treatment of bipolar disorder: A 12-month, randomized, double-blind, controlled clinical trial. *The American Journal of Psychiatry, 162*(7), 1281–1290. doi:10.1176/appi.ajp.162.7.1281

Tohen, M., Ketter, T. A., Zarate, C. A., Suppes, T., Frye, M., Altshuler, L.,…Baker, R. W. (2003). Olanzapine versus divalproex sodium for the treatment of acute mania and maintenance of remission: A 47-week study. *The American Journal of Psychiatry, 160*(7), 1263–1271.

Tohen, M., Sutton, V. K., Calabrese, J. R., Sachs, G. S., & Bowden, C. L. (2009). Maintenance of response following stabilization of mixed index episodes with olanzapine monotherapy in a randomized, double-blind, placebo-controlled study of bipolar 1 disorder. *Journal of Affective Disorders, 116*(1–2), 43–50. doi:10.1016/j.jad.2008.11.003

Tondo, L., Baldessarini, R. J., & Floris, G. (2001). Long-term clinical effectiveness of lithium maintenance treatment in types I and II bipolar disorders. *The British Journal of Psychiatry, 178*(Suppl. 41), S184–190.

Vaidya, N. A., Mahableshwarkar, A. R., & Shahid, R. (2003). Continuation and maintenance ECT in treatment-resistant bipolar disorder. *The Journal of ECT, 19*(1), 10–16.

van der Loos, M. L., Mulder, P., Hartong, E. G., Blom, M. B., Vergouwen, A. C., van Noorden, M. S.,…LamLit Study Group. (2011). Long-term outcome of bipolar depressed patients receiving lamotrigine as add-on to lithium with the possibility of the addition of paroxetine in nonresponders: A randomized, placebo-controlled trial with a novel design. *Bipolar Disorders, 13*(1), 111–117. doi:10.1111/j.1399-5618.2011.00887.x

Vieta, E., Cruz, N., Garcia-Campayo, J., de Arce, R., Manuel Crespo, J., Valles, V.,…Comes, M. (2008). A double-blind, randomized, placebo-controlled prophylaxis trial of oxcarbazepine as adjunctive treatment to lithium in the long-term treatment of bipolar I and II disorder. *International Journal of Neuropsychopharmacol, 11*(4), 445–452. doi:10.1017/S1461145708008596

Vieta, E., Gunther, O., Locklear, J., Ekman, M., Miltenburger, C., Chatterton, M. L.,…Paulsson, B. (2011). Effectiveness of psychotropic medications in the maintenance phase of bipolar disorder: A meta-analysis of randomized controlled trials. *International Journal of Neuropsychopharmacology, 14*(8), 1029–1049. doi:10.1017/S1461145711000885

Vieta, E., Martinez-Aran, A., Goikolea, J. M., Torrent, C., Colom, F., Benabarre, A., & Reinares, M. (2002). A randomized trial comparing paroxetine and venlafaxine in the treatment of bipolar depressed patients taking mood stabilizers. *Journal of Clinical Psychiatry, 63*(6), 508–512.

Vieta, E., Montgomery, S., Sulaiman, A. H., Cordoba, R., Huberlant, B., Martinez, L., & Schreiner, A. (2012). A randomized, double-blind, placebo-controlled trial to assess prevention of mood episodes with risperidone long-acting injectable in patients with bipolar I disorder. *European Neuropsychopharmacology, 22*(11), 825–835. doi:10.1016/j.euroneuro.2012.03.004

Vieta, E., Nieto, E., Autet, A., Rosa, A. R., Goikolea, J. M., Cruz, N., & Bonet, P. (2008). A long-term prospective study on the outcome of bipolar patients treated with long-acting injectable risperidone. *World Journal of Biological Psychiatry, 9*(3), 219–224. doi:10.1080/15622970701530917

Vieta, E., Suppes, T., Eggens, I., Persson, I., Paulsson, B., & Brecher, M. (2008). Efficacy and safety of quetiapine in combination with lithium or divalproex for maintenance of patients with bipolar I disorder (international trial 126). *Journal of Affective Disorders, 109*(3), 251–263. doi:10.1016/j.jad.2008.06.001

Weisler, R. H., Nolen, W. A., Neijber, A., Hellqvist, A., Paulsson, B., & Trial 144 Study Investigators. (2011). Continuation of quetiapine versus switching to placebo or lithium for maintenance treatment of bipolar I disorder (Trial 144: a randomized controlled study). *Journal of Clinical Psychiatry, 72*(11), 1452–1464. doi:10.4088/JCP.11m06878

Woo, Y. S., Bahk, W. M., Jon, D. I., Chung, S. K., Lee, S. Y., Ahn, Y. M.,…Yoon, B. H. (2010). Risperidone in the treatment of mixed state bipolar patients: Results from a 24-week, multicenter, open-label study in Korea. *Psychiatry Clin Neurosci, 64*(1), 28–37. doi:10.1111/j.1440-1819.2009.02026.x

Yatham, L. N., Kennedy, S. H., O'Donovan, C., Parikh, S., MacQueen, G., McIntyre, R.,…Canadian Network for Mood and Treatments. (2005). Canadian Network for Mood and Anxiety Treatments (CANMAT) guidelines for the management of patients with bipolar disorder: Consensus and controversies. *Bipolar Disorders, 7*(Suppl. 3), 5–69. doi:10.1111/j.1399-5618.2005.00219.x

Yatham, L. N., Kennedy, S. H., Parikh, S. V., Schaffer, A., Beaulieu, S., Alda, M.,…Berk, M. (2013). Canadian Network for Mood and Anxiety Treatments (CANMAT) and International Society for Bipolar Disorders (ISBD) collaborative update of CANMAT guidelines for the management of patients with bipolar disorder: update 2013. *Bipolar Disorders, 15*(1), 1–44. doi:10.1111/bdi.12025

Yatham, L. N., Kennedy, S. H., Schaffer, A., Parikh, S. V., Beaulieu, S., O'Donovan, C.,…Kapczinski, F. (2009). Canadian Network for Mood and Anxiety Treatments (CANMAT) and International Society for Bipolar Disorders (ISBD) collaborative update of CANMAT guidelines for the management of patients with bipolar disorder: Update 2009. *Bipolar Disorders, 11*(3), 225–255. doi:10.1111/j.1399-5618.2009.00672.x

Yazici, O., Kora, K., Polat, A., & Saylan, M. (2004). Controlled lithium discontinuation in bipolar patients with good response to long-term lithium prophylaxis. *Journal of Affective Disorders, 80*(2–3), 269–271. doi:10.1016/S0165-0327(03)00133-2

Young, A. H., McElroy, S. L., Bauer, M., Philips, N., Chang, W., Olausson, B.,…Investigators Embolden I. (2010). A double-blind, placebo-controlled study of quetiapine and lithium monotherapy in adults in the acute phase of bipolar depression (EMBOLDEN I). *Journal of Clinical Psychiatry, 71*(2), 150–162. doi:10.4088/JCP.08m04995gre

24.

IMPROVING EARLY DIAGNOSIS

AN UNMET NEED FOR EARLY INTERVENTION IN BIPOLAR DISORDERS

Gabriele Sani and Giacomo Salvadore

INTRODUCTION

Bipolar disorder (BD) is a severe, lifelong illness characterized by recurrent episodes of mania or hypomania and depression, with variable interpolations of relatively asymptomatic periods, called euthymic, during which, however, some psychopathological symptoms may persist (Judd et al., 2002; Judd et al., 2003; Merikangas et al., 2011). Epidemiological studies estimate a lifetime prevalence of 0.6% to 1% for bipolar type I disorder (BD-I), 0.4% to 1.1% for bipolar type II disorder (BD-II), and 2.4% to 5.1% for subthreshold BD (Judd & Akiskal, 2003, Merikangas et al., 2007).

Although classic descriptions of patients affected by manic-depressive illness reported generally positive outcomes (Kraepelin, 1896), highlighting the absence of progression into "dementia," evidence from the past few decades has provided a dramatically different clinical picture. Bipolar disorder is a condition with high rates of non-recovery, recurrence, and chronicity and is one of the leading causes of disability worldwide due to psychosocial consequences, long-term unemployment, medical comorbidity, and suicide (Fagiolini, Frank, Scott, Turkin, & Kupfer, 2005; Sani et al., 2011). Furthermore, BD is a progressive and accelerating condition, associated with neurostructural changes and cognitive deterioration (Martinez-Aran et al., 2004).

Different levels of evidence suggest that it is important to identify individuals at risk for developing BD before full-blown illness is manifest. There is typically a several-year lag between the appearance of the first clinical symptoms and the correct diagnosis of BD (Ghaemi, Boiman, & Goodwin, 2000). Patients with BD are often misdiagnosed early in course of illness as suffering from schizophrenia, borderline personality disorder, or major depression and prescribed suboptimal treatments such as antidepressants. Pharmacological treatments, mainly antidepressants, might be associated with iatrogenic complications that worsen the course of the illness, such as triggering switch to the opposite polarity phase (Valentí et al., 2012), causing rapid cyclicity (Koukopoulos et al., 2003), and mixed states (Koukopoulos, Albert, Sani, Koukopoulos, & Girardi, 2005).

There is also substantial evidence that the number of previous affective episodes is a risk factor for episode recurrence, chronicity, and suicide. Appropriate treatment early on would likely decrease the risk for these negative outcomes (Kessing & Andersen, 2005). Independent studies have shown that both in major depression and BD, the risk of episode recurrence increases as the number of previous and new illness episodes increase (Kessing, 1998; Kessing & Andersen, 1999; Kessing, Hansen, Andersen, & Angst, 2004) and that the treatment response rate decreases as the number of previous disease episodes increases (Berk et al., 2011).

Finally, evidence from neuropsychological studies suggests that degree of cognitive impairment, an aspect likely to affect functioning, is significantly correlated with duration of illness and the number of previous episodes (Kessing, 1998; Martinez-Aran et al., 2004). Thus one way that early intervention in subjects vulnerable to BD might improve long-term outcome is by diminishing the number of affective recurrences. It is therefore necessary to recognize persons at risk of developing BD as early as possible in order to avoid misdiagnosis/mistreatments and possibly intercept disease course and prevent negative long-term outcome. Unfortunately, this effort is made difficult by the nature of the disorder itself. It is now well established that BD evolves in evident clinical stages from nonspecific disorders (such as anxiety or sleep disorders), to subthreshold mood instability, and then to a major disorder, typically depression, in adolescence (Duffy, Alda, Hajek, & Grof, 2009). Moreover, some disorders, like attention deficit hyperactivity disorder (ADHD), share several clinical signs and symptoms with BDs and are sometimes difficult to distinguish (Skirrow, Hosang, Farmer, & Asherson, 2012). The complex pathologic process called "bipolar disorder" is constituted by heterogeneous phases. It is possible to state that BD includes not only the classical three phases of depression, (hypo)mania, and symptom-free interval (or euthymia) but also different phenomenological presentations during the lifespan. In other words, we can state that different phenotypes stem into the same genotype. This modern knowledge incredibly resembles Aretaeus' observation made almost 2,000 years ago: "The modes and species of Mania are myriad, but the genus only one." (Aretaeus, I sec DC). In this essence, we fully share Jamison's (1995) view: "the word 'bipolar' seems to me to obscure and minimize the illness it is supposed to represent."

The debate over whether to intervene early in patients who display subsyndromal symptoms or who appear to be at high risk for psychotic disorders has raised obvious ethical and methodological issues. Although there is now a general consensus that targeted early intervention is helpful, the question remains of how early is too early and, in addition, what constitutes the most appropriate treatment (Scott & Meyer, 2007). These are extremely challenging questions, also in light of the fact that prodromal symptoms have in general low specificity and that only a small proportion of young individuals who display mood lability, sleep disturbances, or other attenuated clinical features end up developing BD (Parker, 2010).

EARLY STAGE BIPOLAR DISORDER CLINICAL RESEARCH

PRODROME CLINICAL STUDIES

Clinically detecting the prodromal phase of BD in the general population is a very challenging paradigm; naturalistic studies showed that full-blown bipolar symptoms that require medical care are usually preceded by subtle, attenuated symptoms up to 10 years before the acute onset of the illness, even though some studies have described a much shorter prodromal period (reviewed in Skjelstad et al., 2010).

Recently, Faedda and collaborators (Faedda et al., 2014) reviewed prospective studies to characterize affective

clinical predictors of BD and to evaluate their predictive value. These authors found that precursors of BD, mainly manic or depressive symptoms, emotional instability, over-arousal, dysregulation of sleep and activity, and dysthymic and cyclothymic traits, typically arise years prior to syndromal onset, often with clinically significant morbidity and disability. Interestingly, prospective findings regarding precursors of BD were found generally consistent with retrospective and family-risk studies.

As shown by a recent retrospective study, subthreshold symptoms usually represent attenuated forms of full-blown manic and depressive episodes (Correll et al., 2007). These include mood lability, increased energy with lack of impulse control, hyperactivity, racing thoughts, and disinhibition (Correll et al., 2007; Egeland, Hostetter, Pauls, & Sussex, 2000; Thompson et al., 2003; Yung & McGorry, 1996). Other studies have suggested that, when patients present with a first episode of major depression, a personal history of labile mood, fluctuating symptoms, sleep inefficiency, and family history of BD may help distinguish BD patients from those with major depression. Other symptoms that might suggest the presence of an underlying bipolar diathesis are early age of onset, psychomotor retardation, and atypical symptoms (Goodwin & Jamison, 2007). A recent large prospective study in 3,024 subjects ages 14 to 24 years showed that the presence of individual bipolar symptoms as well as their persistence across time was associated with increased likelihood of a full-blown bipolar episodes at the 10-year follow-up and higher mental health-care resources utilization (Tijssen et al., 2010); however, the risk of developing a (hypo)manic episode at follow-up was overall small (i.e., 1.6%–2.3% for subjects with increasing loading of bipolar symptoms and 2.4% in the case of persistence of symptoms across two visits).

It remains unclear at this time whether exposing subjects with these attenuated and nonspecific symptoms to pharmacological and nonpharmacological interventions would lead to benefits that outweigh the potential risks associated with drug treatment, especially in light of the low predictive power and specificity of prodromal symptoms (Parker, 2010). More studies are needed to address this later point.

HIGH-RISK STUDIES

An intriguing approach to better understand early phases of BD is studying populations at risk of developing BD, such as the offspring of families in which one or both parents have BD (Chang, Steiner, Dienes, Adleman, & Ketter, 2003). Twins and family studies, in fact, report that the disorder has a 59% to 87% heritability, and first-degree relatives of probands with BD are at very high risk for BD themselves (Smoller & Finn, 2003). Concordance rates among monozygotic twins average 57% and among dizygotic twins 14% (Alda, 1997). Twins and adoption studies empirically support the notion that genetic factors are the vulnerability factors with the largest effect size (Barnett & Smoller, 2009).

These studies suggest that offspring of parents with BD have a four-fold increased risk of developing any mood disorder compared with the general population, as well as increased risk for other psychiatric disorders such as ADHD, anxiety disorders, or disruptive disorders (Lapalme, Hodgins, & LaRoche, 1997). The range of estimates for the risk of BD in high-risk populations is wide (3%–50%) but is consistently much higher than in the general population (1.6%–2.1%) (Kessler et al., 2005; Merikangas et al., 2007) and varies depending on the length of observation and the operational criteria applied (e.g., whether or not to consider bipolar spectrum diagnoses). In addition, the morbidity risk of major affective disorder of first-degree relatives of a bipolar patient is about 23% (about 9% bipolar and 14% major depressive disorder; Smoller & Finn, 2003), and the estimated risk for illness is 10-fold the risk of individuals in control families (McGuffin et al., 2003).

In addition, there is now accumulating published evidence that high-risk subjects have impaired neuropsychological function compared to healthy controls (HCs) in some specific cognitive domain (e.g., executive function, memory), which are usually also impaired—albeit by greater extent—in subjects with full-blown BD (Arts, Jabben, Krabbendam, & van Os, 2008).

Unfortunately, most studies of high-risk populations for BD have several limitations: small sample sizes, retrospective and descriptive designs, and lack of data about which symptoms are the most informative predictors for developing BD in the follow-up period. Additionally, most relatives of individuals with BD do not develop BD (Smoller & Finn, 2003).

In addition to genetic vulnerability and cognitive functioning, other biological markers have been studied to strengthen the predictability of the development of BD. Neuroimaging studies indicate functional and structural impairment in BD patients (Pan, Keener, Hassel, & Phillips, 2009). However, it is still unclear whether these abnormalities precede the onset of the BD or are due to the chronicity of the disease or to the medical treatment. For these reasons, these findings are not helpful in improving the predictability of the illness.

In the following we review findings from neuropsychological studies and studies with different imaging modalities that have been performed in subjects at risk for BD (AR-BD; i.e., twins or offspring of subjects with a BD diagnosis). We do not discuss findings in patients who have already experienced a first episode of mania; these are reviewed comprehensively in other publications (Salvadore, Drevets, Henter, Zarate, & Manji, 2008a, 2008b).

NEUROPSYCHOLOGICAL STUDIES IN THE OFFSPRING AND UNAFFECTED TWINS OF PROBANDS WITH BIPOLAR DISORDER

Neuropsychological impairment is one of the most salient aspects of BD and is also present during periods of prolonged euthymia (Martinez-Aran et al., 2004). Almost a decade ago, neuropsychological impairment was proposed as a potential endophenotype of BD because it met the key prerequisite associated with endophenotype definition (i.e., heritability, association with the illness, independence from clinical state, cosegregation with the illness within a family with some degree of impairment present in first-degree relatives; Glahn, Bearden, Niendam, & Escamilla, 2004). At that time, there were only a handful of published studies about neuropsychological functioning in subjects at risk for BD, which were indicative of a possible impairment in the domains of verbal memory and executive function in high-risk subjects.

A meta-analysis of neuropsychological studies in first-degree relatives of probands with BD that summarized findings from 14 studies across several cognitive domains showed a significant impairment in executive function and verbal memory (immediate recall), albeit with a small effect size (Arts et al., 2008), confirming previous observations. Subjects with BD showed deficits across several domains, including working memory, sustained attention, concept shifting, and mental speed. Interestingly, the domains that were impaired in high-risk subjects (i.e, executive function, verbal memory) showed a large effect size in subjects with full-blown disorder, further supporting their validity as candidate endophenotypes.

A subsequent meta-analysis, which included a slightly higher number of studies, showed neuropsychological deficits in high-risk subjects in executive function and verbal memory, as well as sustained attention, response inhibition, and set shifting (Bora, Yucel, & Pantelis, 2009). The effect sizes reported were all small, with the exception of a moderate effect size in the Stroop task ($d = 0.51$). Deficits in processing speed, visual memory, and verbal fluency were found only in BD subjects; a secondary analysis that took into account the medication status at the time of testing showed a potential confounding effect of current medications on processing speed. Another more recent study with a relatively large sample size in patients with familial, psychotic BD, their non-BD, nonpsychotic relatives, and controls failed to detect significant impairment in sustained attention in at-risk relatives (Walshe et al., 2012).

A large-scale study in 45 families with at least two siblings with BD investigated neuropsychological functioning with a comprehensive computerized cognitive battery in 230 subjects with a broad bipolar phenotype (i.e., BD-I, BD-II, BD—not otherwise specified, schizoaffective bipolar), 243 unaffected first-degree, 86 unaffected second-degree, and 42 unaffected third-degree relatives of BD subjects (Glahn et al., 2010). All but 2 of the 22 neuropsychological measures assessed in that study were found to be heritable; non-BD first-degree relatives showed impairment in processing speed, working memory, and facial memory with a moderate to large effect size ($d = 0.50-0.86$). Those domains overall were shown to be heritable, impaired in individuals with the illness and their nonbipolar relatives, and genetically correlated with affection status and thus promising candidate endophenotypes.

However, whether first-degree relatives of subjects with BD show cognitive impairment compared to healthy subjects is still a controversial topic, as conflicting results also exist in the literature. For example Jabben and colleagues (2012) investigated attention and memory in probands with schizophrenia spectrum disorder (SSD) or BD and their first-degree relatives and found no evidence of impairment in relatives of BD subjects compared to HCs, while relatives of subjects with SSD performed worse than controls in measures of verbal memory and sustained attention (Jabben et al., 2012).

A recent report from the Bipolar and Schizophrenia Network on Intermediate Phenotypes (B-SNIP) Study, which is a large-scale consortium to investigate diagnostic boundaries and candidate intermediate phenotypes in probands with SSD or BD with psychosis and their relatives, found that first-degree relatives of BD subjects ($n = 259$) were no different from controls ($n = 295$) on the neuropsychological measures captured by the Brief Assessment of Cognition in Schizophrenia battery (Hill et al., 2013). However, while relatives of probands with SSD showed neuropsychological impairment regardless of the presence of elevated cluster A or B personality traits, first-degree relatives of BD subjects with higher cluster A or B personality traits had worse cognitive performance than HCs. This suggests that the mechanism underlying familiar transmission of cognitive impairment might be different across SSD and BD.

A few twin studies have investigated cognitive function in nonaffected twins of probands with BD. In one of the first twin cognitive studies in BD, Gourovitch and colleagues (1999) found that the unaffected twins performed significantly worse than HCs on measures of verbal learning and memory. Similar impairment in verbal learning and memory has also been reported in nonaffected female twins by an independent study (Kieseppä et al., 2005); studies that have investigated other cognitive domains in twins discordant for BD report negative or conflicting results: for example, no deficits in spatial working memory was detected in a study 22 bipolar patients, 16 of unaffected co-twins, and 100 controls (Pirkola et al., 2005). Impairment in response inhibition using the Stroop test has been described by Juselius, Kieseppä, Kaprio, Lönnqvist, and Tuulio-Henriksson (2009), but it was not replicated in an independent study (Kravariti et al., 2009).

In summary, several independent reports have described mild deficits in memory and executive function in AR-BD subjects. These deficits are likely to be influenced by the presence of psychosis in the family, as well as the degree of subthreshold symptoms and the sensitivity of the neuropsychological test battery utilized. The few reports that have included first-degree relatives of SSD subjects in the same study consistently indicate that, even when present, the cognitive impairment in AR-BD subjects is of a smaller magnitude than the one detected in first-degree relatives of SSD subjects. In future studies it will be important to investigate the temporal profile of cognitive performance in AR-BD subjects through longitudinal studies, as well as the relationship with the development of clinically relevant symptoms.

BRAIN IMAGING STUDIES IN THE OFFSPRING AND UNAFFECTED TWINS OF PROBANDS WITH BIPOLAR DISORDER

STRUCTURAL IMAGING

Volumetric studies

Most of the studies in the literature are cross-sectional in design and involve mono- or dizygotic twins or first- or second-degree relatives of BD patients (AR-BD group). Table 24.1 presents the main findings from the reviewed articles.

Gray matter studies

In a twin study, Noga, Vladar, and Torrey (2001) found a bilateral increase in volume of the caudate nucleus in BD twins and in their well co-twins compared to HCs, while right hippocampal volume was smaller in the sick versus well bipolar twins. However, reduced hippocampal volume was not detected by the majority of investigators who performed volumetric studies in individuals at risk for BD (Connor et al., 2004, Hajek et al., 2009, Karchemskiy et al., 2011; Kempton et al, 2009, McDonald et al. 2006; McIntosh et al., 2004).

McDonald et al. (2004) used voxel-based morphometry (VBM) to investigate volumetric differences between BD patients, their first-degree relatives, and HCs. Their findings suggest that a genetic risk for BD is associated with a decrease of gray matter (GM) in the right anterior cingulate gyrus and the ventral striatum and decrease of white matter (WM) volume in bilateral frontal, left temporoparietal, and right parietal regions, and in the anterior corpus callosum. In a follow-up study, the same authors also found a trend toward larger cerebral volume in AR-BD compared to HCs (McDonald et al., 2006). Forcada and colleagues (2011) employed the same technique without finding any significant morphometric difference between the groups, while Hajek and colleagues (2012) found a significant and common GM volume increase in right inferior frontal gyrus both in AR-BD and BD groups compared to healthy subjects.

McIntosh et al. (2004, 2005, 2006) conducted several VBM studies and reported that the only brain abnormality present both in AR-BD and BD group was a reduction of GM density in the left anterior thalamus, as compared to HCs. Other abnormalities were present only in BD (anterior limb of internal capsule reduction), or in the AR-BD group (GM density reduction in the caudate), compared to HCs.

In a recent VBM study that used a preprocessing algorithm that provides more accurate segmentation (i.e., Diffeomorphic Anatomical Registration Through Exponentiated Lie algebra, or DARTEL), Matsuo and colleagues (2012) found reduced left anterior insular GM volume in BD and AR-BD subjects. This finding conflicts with previous evidence of increased left insular GM volume in AR-BD subjects described by Kempton et al. (2009) using VBM. Ladouceur and colleagues (2008) used VBM to compare GM volume in bipolar offspring and HC subjects and found increased GM volume in the left parahippocampal/hippocampal gyrus in the AR-BD group while no differences were apparent in a priori regions of interest, such as the amygdala and the orbitomedial prefrontal cortex.

Hajek and colleagues (2009) found increased caudate volume in the AR-BD subjects compared to controls, failing to find any other differences in subgenual cingulate (Hajek et al., 2008a, 2010), pituitary (Hajek et al., 2008b), putamen (Hajek et al., 2009), and amygdala (Hajek et al., 2009). Other independent studies confirmed that pituitary alterations do not reflect genetic predisposition to BD but rather may be associated with disease expression for BD (Mondelli et al., 2008; Takahashi et al., 2010). Finally, no significant differences were found in the studies that investigated structural abnormalities in the prefrontal cortex, thalamus, striatum, and amygdala (Karchemskiy et al., 2011; Kempton et al., 2009; Singh, Delbello, Adler, Stanford, & Strakowski, 2008).

White matter volumetric studies

A few studies have investigated WM volumetric abnormalities in AR-BD subjects using VBM or other semiautomated morphometric techniques. Kieseppä et al. (2003) found decreased left hemispheric WM volume both in AR-BD and BD twins, suggesting that this alteration may reflect genetic factors predisposing to the disorder. In two subsequent studies, van der Schot and colleagues (2009, 2010) found decreased WM density in the superior longitudinal fasciculus bilaterally, as well as GM density in the right medial frontal gyrus, precentral gyrus, and insula. In addition,

Decreased WM volume in the medial prefrontal cortex in AR-BD but not in BD subjects has been reported recently by Matsuo and colleagues (Matsuo et al., 2012). Also, no evidence of size or shape alterations of the corpus callosum in AR-BD subjects has been found in a study that compared callosal morphometry in 70 BD, 45 AR-BD, and 75 HC subjects (Walterfang et al., 2009).

Finally, three studies have qualitatively studied the presence of brain alterations in patients and their relatives. Ahearn and colleagues (1998), studying a family with a substantial history of BDs, first observed that all bipolar patients and 60% of their healthy relatives had either WM or subcortical gray nuclei lesions. Gulseren, Gurcan, Gulseren, Gelal, and Erol (2006) noticed a higher presence of subcortical, but not deep or periventricular, WM hyperintensities in bipolar patients (67%), compared to their unaffected siblings (17%) or HCs (33%). In a more

Table 24.1. VOLUMETRIC IMAGING STUDIES IN POPULATIONS AT RISK FOR BIPOLAR DISORDER

STUDY/TYPE OF DESIGN	AR-BD	COMPARISON GROUP	TECHNIQUE	BRAIN AREAS ANALYZED	MAJOR FINDINGS
Ahearn et al., 1998	10 unaffected family members of BD pts F: not reported Mean age: 38.5 (range 12–66) Other Axis I diagnoses: none	9 family members with BD F: not reported Mean age: 47 (range 20–65) Other Axis I diagnoses: none 2 family members with MDD (F: not reported) Mean age: 27 (range 20–54) Other Axis I diagnoses: none	1.5 T Qualitative	Whole brain	6 AR-BD (60%) had lesions in the subcortical gray nuclei, 1 had a WM lesion. All 9 BD (100%) had MRI findings: 4 had deep WM changes and 8 had lesions of the subcortical gray nuclei. Neither of the 2 (0%) family members with MDD had MRI findings.
Noga et al., 2001	6 unaffected MZ twins of BD pts F: 83% Mean age: 34.5 (SD: 10.5) Other Axis I diagnoses: none	6 MZ twins with BD F: 83% Mean age: 34.5 (SD: 10.5) Other Axis I diagnoses: none 22 (11 pairs) healthy MZ twins HC F: 83% Mean age: 29.9 (SD: 10.3) Other Axis I diagnoses: none	1.5 T ROI	Basal ganglia: striatum (bilateral caudate nuclei and putamen/globus pallidus); bilateral amygdala-hippocampus; cerebral hemispheric volumes	AR-BD vs HC: ↑ bilateral caudate nuclei, no differences in hemispheric volume; AR-BD vs BD: ↓ right caudate nuclei, ↑ right hippocampus, > rightward asymmetry in the hippocampus, no differences in hemispheric volume; BD vs HC: ↑ bilateral caudate nuclei, < rightward asymmetry in the hippocampus, no differences in hemispheric volume.
Kieseppä et al., 2003	15 unaffected twins of BD pts F: 60% Mean age: 44.5 (range 40.9–48.2) Other Axis I diagnoses: 13.3% lifetime alcohol dependence, 13.3% lifetime anxiety disorder.	24 twins with BD I F: 45.8% Mean age: 44.4 (range 41.2–47.6) Other Axis I diagnoses: 29.2% lifetime alcohol dependence, 4.2% current alcohol dependence, 29.2% lifetime anxiety disorder 27 healthy twins HC F: 48.1% Mean age: 46.7 (range 44–49.6) Other Axis I diagnoses: 11.1% lifetime alcohol dependence, 3.7% current alcohol dependence, 3.7% lifetime anxiety disorder	1 T ROI	Bilateral ventricles, frontal and temporal lobes	AR-BD vs HC: ↓ left hemispheric WM, no changes in GM or ventricular volume; AR-BD vs BD: no WM or GM differences; BD vs HC: ↓ bilateral hemispheric WM, no changes in GM or ventricular volume.
Connor et al., 2004	54 FDR of BD pts F: 52% Mean age: 44 (SD: 16) Other Axis I diagnoses: none	39 BD F: 61% Mean age: 41 (SD: 12) 219 HC F: 47% Mean age: 34 (SD: 12) Other Axis I diagnoses: none	1.5 T ROI	Hippocampus	AR-BD vs BD vs HC: no significant differences.
McDonald et al., 2004	50 FDR of BD pts F: 52% Mean age: 44.1 (SD: 15.7) Other Axis I diagnoses: 18% (mostly MDD)	37 BD F: 59.5% Mean age: 40.7 (SD: 11.6) Other Axis I diagnoses: none	1.5 T VBM	Whole brain	Genetic risk for bipolar disorder is associated with: ↓ GM in the right anterior cingulate gyrus and ventral striatum, and ↓ WM in the bilateral frontal, left temporoparietal, and right parietal regions, and in the anterior corpus callosum.

Study	Sample 1	Sample 2	Technique	Region	Results
McIntosh et al., 2004	22 FDR or SDR of BD pts F: 59% Mean age: 34.7 (*SD*: 12.6) Other Axis I diagnoses: none	26 BD F: 46% Mean age: 40.5 (*SD*: 12.1) Other Axis I diagnoses: none 49 HC F: 53% Mean age: 35.3 (*SD*: 11.1) Left-handed: 6% Other Axis I diagnoses: none	1.5 T VBM	Whole brain (SVC: amygdala, hippocampus, thalamus)	AR-BD vs HC: ↓ in left anterior thalamic and caudate GM density; AR-BD vs BD: No significant differences; BD vs HC: ↓ in bilateral anterior thalamic GM density.
McIntosh et al., 2005	22 FDR or SDR of BD pts F: 59% Mean age: 34.7 (*SD*: 12.6) Other Axis I diagnoses: none	26 BD F: 46% Mean age: 40.5 (*SD*: 12.1) Other Axis I diagnoses: none 49 HC F: 53% Mean age: 35.3 (sd:11.1) Other Axis I diagnoses: none	1.5 T VBM	Whole brain (SVC: frontal subgyral WM, ALIC)	AR-BD vs HC: No significant differences; AR-BD vs BD: Not tested; BD vs HC: ↓ in left ALIC
Gulseren et al., 2006	12 FDR of BD pts F: 50% Mean age: 29.5 (*SD*: 5.8) Other Axis I diagnoses: none	12 BD F: 33.3% Mean age: 30.9 (*SD*: 3.6) Other Axis I diagnoses: none 12 HC F: 33% Mean age: 30.4 (*SD*: 3.6) Left-handed: not reported Other Axis I diagnoses: none	0.5 T Qualitative	Frontal, parietal, temporal, occipital lobe, internal capsule	AR-BD vs HC: ↑ presence of deep WM hyperintensities in the right cerebral hemisphere; BD vs AR-BD: ↑ presence of subcortical WM hyperintensities in the right cerebral hemisphere; BD vs HC: ↑ presence of deep WM hyperintensities in the right cerebral hemisphere, ↑ presence of subcortical WM hyperintensities in the right cerebral hemisphere.
McDonald et al., 2006	52 FDR of BD pts F: 52% Mean age: 44 (*SD*: 15.4) Other Axis I diagnoses: 19.3% lifetime alcohol or substance abuse or dependence, 3.8% lifetime alcohol or substance abuse or dependence, 1.9% PAD without agoraphobia	38 BD F: 60.5% Mean age: 41 (*SD*: 11.7) Other Axis I diagnoses: 21.1% lifetime alcohol or substance abuse or dependence 54 healthy subjects HC F: 64% Mean age: 40.2 (*SD*: 15.3) Other Axis I diagnoses: 21.1% lifetime alcohol or substance abuse or dependence, 9.2% MDD	1.5 T ROI	Cerebral volume, bilateral ventricular volume, third ventricular volume, bilateral hippocampus	AR-BD vs HC: no significant differences in ventricular or hippocampal volume; trend toward larger cerebral volume in AR-BD; AR-BD vs BD: no significant differences; BD vs HC: no significant differences.
McIntosh et al., 2006	22 FDR or SDR of BD pts F: 59% Mean age: 34.7 (*SD*: 12.6) Other Axis I diagnoses: none	26 BD F: 46% Mean age: 40.5 (*SD*: 12.1) Other Axis I diagnoses: none	1.5 T VBM	Whole brain (SVC: prefrontal cortex, temporal lobe, amygdala-hippocampal complex, thalamus)	AR-BD vs BD: no structural deficits related with an increased liability to BD were found.

(continued)

Table 24.1. CONTINUED

STUDY/TYPE OF DESIGN	AR-BD	COMPARISON GROUP	TECHNIQUE	BRAIN AREAS ANALYZED	MAJOR FINDINGS
Hajek et al., 2008	24 unaffected FDR or SDR of BD pts F: 62.5% Mean age: 19.8 (*SD*: 3.2) Other Axis I diagnoses: none	19 affected FDR or SDR of BD pts F: 73.7% Mean age: 21.3 (*SD*: 3.5) Axis I diagnoses: 52.6% MDD, 15.7% BD-I, 15.7% BD-II, 5.2% BD-NOS, 5.2% dysthymia, 5.2% psychosis NOS. 31 HC F: 64.5% Mean age: 20.6 (*SD*: 3.3) Left-handed: 10% Other Axis I diagnoses: none	1.5 T ROI	Subgenual cingulate	AR-BD vs affected subjects vs HC: no significant differences.
Hajek et al., 2008	24 unaffected FDR or SDR of BD pts F: 62.5% Mean age: 19.8 (*SD*: 3.2) Other Axis I diagnoses: none	19 affected FDR or SDR of BD pts F: 73.7% Mean age: 21.3 (*SD*: 3.5) Axis I diagnoses: 52.6% MDD, 15.7% BD-I, 15.7% BD-II, 5.2% BD-NOS, 5.2% dysthymia, 5.2% psychosis NOS. 31 HC F: 64.5% Mean age: 20.6 (*SD*: 3.3) Other Axis I diagnoses: none	1.5 T ROI	Pituitary	AR-BD vs affected subjects vs HC: no significant differences.
Ladouceur et., 2008	20 FDR of BD pts F: 55% Mean age: 13 (*SD*: 2.7) Other Axis I diagnoses: 10% anxiety disorder	22 HC F: 68% Mean age: 14 (*SD*: 2.6) Other Axis I diagnoses: none	3 T VBM	Whole brain (SVC: amygdala, OMPFC)	AR-BD vs HC: ↑ GM volume in left parahippocampal gyrus, extending into left hippocampus.
Mondelli et., 2008	24 FDR of BD pts F: 50% Mean age: 42.2 (*SD*: 2.6) Other Axis I diagnoses: 21.1% regular cannabis use	29 BD patients F: 62% Mean age: 40.5 (*SD*: 3.5) Other axis I diagnoses: 21.1% regular cannabis use. 46 HC F: 52% Mean age: 39.7 (*SD*: 2.2) Other Axis I diagnoses: 28.3% regular cannabis use.	1.5 T ROI	Pituitary	AR-BD vs BD vs HC: no significant differences.
Singh et al., 2008	21 FDR of BD pts F: 43% Mean age: 9.7 (*SD*: 1.5)	24 HC F: 54% Mean age: 10.1 (*SD*: 1.5) Other Axis I diagnoses: none	1.5 T ROI	PFC, thalamus, striatum, amygdala	AR-BD vs HC: no significant differences.

Study	FDR/SDR sample	BD patients / HC sample	Method	Brain region	Results
	Other Axis I diagnoses: 24% anxiety disorder, 19% MDD, 19% ADHD, 14% dysthymia, 9.5% ODD, 9.5% cyclothymia				
Kempton et al., 2009	50 FDR of BD pts F: 52% Mean age: 33.8 (*SD*: 12.7) Other Axis I diagnoses: MDD	30 BD patients F: 50% Mean age: 39.4 (*SD*: 9.8) Other Axis I diagnoses: none 52 HC F: 48% Mean age: 35.2 (*SD*: 13.0) Other Axis I diagnoses: none.	1.5 T VBM + ROI	Whole brain (ROI: amygdala, anterior and posterior cingulate, subgenual PFC, hippocampus)	**AR-BD vs HC:** ↑ volume of left insula. **AR-BD vs BD:** ↓volume of substantia nigra; **BD vs HC:** ↑ volume of left insula, ↑ volume of substantia nigra. **AR-BD without MDD vs BD and HC:** ↑ volume of left cerebellum. **AR-BD with MDD vs BD and HC:** no significant difference in left cerebellum volume.
Hajek et al., 2009	26 FDR or SDR of BD pts F: 65.4% Mean age: 19.6 (*SD*: 3.1) Other Axis I diagnoses: none	20 affected FDR or SDR of BD pts F: 75% Mean age: 21.0 (*SD*: 3.7) Axis I diagnoses: 55% MDD, 15% BD-I, 15% BD-II, 5% BD-NOS, 5% dysthymia, 5% psychosis NOS 31 HC F: 64.5% Mean age: 20.6 (sd:3.3) Other Axis I diagnoses: none	1.5 T ROI	Caudate, putamen	**AR-BD vs HC:** ↑ caudate volume; **AR-BD vs affected subjects:** no significant differences; Affected subjects vs HC: no significant differences.
Hajek et al., 2009	26 FDR or SDR of BD pts F: 65.4% Mean age: 19.6 (*SD*: 3.1) Other Axis I diagnoses: none	20 affected FDR or SDR of BD pts F: 75% Mean age: 21.0 (sd:3.7) Axis I diagnoses: 55% MDD, 15% BD-I, 15% BD-II, 5%, BD-NOS, 5% dysthymia, 5% psychosis NOS 31 HC F: 64.5% Mean age: 20.6 (*SD*: 3.3) Other Axis I diagnoses: none	1.5 T ROI	Hippocampus, amygdala	**AR-BD vs affected subjects vs HC:** no significant differences.
Walterfang et al., 2009	45 FDR of BD pts F: 51.1% Mean age: 34.8 (*SD*: 12.5) Other Axis I diagnoses: none	70 BD patients F: 52.8% Mean age: 43.6 (*SD*: 11.8) Other axis I diagnoses: none 75 HC F: 48% Mean age: 36.1 (*SD*: 13.5) Other Axis I diagnoses: none	1.5 T ROI	Corpus callosum	**AR-BD vs HC:** no significant differences; **BD vs AR-BD:** ↓ CC area and thickness; **BD vs HC:** ↓ CC area and thickness.

(*continued*)

Table 24.1. CONTINUED

STUDY/TYPE OF DESIGN	AR-BD	COMPARISON GROUP	TECHNIQUE	BRAIN AREAS ANALYZED	MAJOR FINDINGS
van der Schot et al., 2009	37 MZ or DZ twins of BD pts F: not reported Mean age: 40.2 (*SD*: not reported) Other Axis I diagnoses: alcohol use disorder, borderline personality disorder, depressive disorder NOS, dissociative disorder NOS, MDD, mood disorder due to hyperthyroidism, OCD, PAD without agoraphobia, personality disorder NOS, schizophrenia (paranoid type)	63 MZ or DZ twins with BD pts F: not reported Mean age: 40.6 (*SD*: not reported) Other Axis I diagnoses: alcohol use disorder, borderline personality disorder, depressive disorder NOS, dissociative disorder NOS, MDD, mood disorder due to hyperthyroidism, OCD, PAD without agoraphobia, personality disorder NOS, schizophrenia (paranoid type) 134 unaffected twins HC F: 57.4% Mean age: 39.0 (*SD*: not reported) Left-handed: 14.1% Other Axis I diagnoses: none	1.5 T ROI	GM and WM of cerebrum, lateral and third ventricular volume, cerebellum	Decrease in WM volume is related to the genetic risk of developing bipolar disorder.
Hajek et al., 2010	20 FDR of BD pts F: 55% Mean age: 20.2 (*SD*: 4.2) Other Axis I diagnoses: none	15 affected offspring of BD pts F: 73.3% Mean age: 22.1 (*SD*: 4.8) Axis I diagnoses: 40% MDD, 33.3% BD-I, 26.6% BD-II 18 unaffected offspring of healthy subjects HC F: 61.1% Mean age: 23.0 (*SD*: 3.5) Other Axis I diagnoses: none	1.5 T ROI	Subgenual cingulate	AR-BD vs affected subjects vs HC: no significant differences.
van der Schot et al., 2010	36 MZ or DZ twins of BD pts F: not reported Mean age: 40.3 (*SD*: not reported) Other Axis I diagnoses: alcohol use disorder, borderline personality disorder, depressive disorder NOS, dissociative disorder NOS, MDD, mood disorder due to hyperthyroidism, OCD, PAD without agoraphobia, personality disorder NOS, schizophrenia (paranoid type)	62 MZ or DZ twins with BD pts F: not reported Mean age: 40.3 (*SD*: not reported) Other Axis I diagnoses: alcohol use disorder, borderline personality disorder, depressive disorder NOS, dissociative disorder NOS, MDD, mood disorder due to hyperthyroidism, OCD, PAD without agoraphobia, personality disorder NOS, schizophrenia (paranoid type). 134 unaffected twins HC F: 57.4% Mean age: 39.0 (*SD*: not reported) Other Axis I diagnoses: none	1.5 T VBM	Whole brain	The genetic risk to develop bipolar disorder was related to decreased GM density in the right medial frontal gyrus, precentral gyrus and insula, and with decreased WM density in the SLF bilaterally.

Takahashi et al., 2010	49 FDR of BD pts F: 53% Mean age: 33.9 (*SD*: 12.7) Other Axis I diagnoses: 30.6% MDD	29 BD patients F: 48.2% Mean age: 39.6 (*SD*: 9.9) Other axis I diagnoses: none 52 HC F: 46.1% Mean age: 35.8 (*SD*: 13.6) Other Axis I diagnoses: none	1.5 T ROI	Pituitary	AR-BD vs HC: no significant differences; BD vs AR-BD: ↑ pituitary volume; BD vs HC: ↑ pituitary volume.
Gunde et al., 2011	44 FDR or SDR of BD pts F: 62.9% Mean age: 19.8 (*SD*: 3.6) Other Axis I diagnoses: none	35 affected FDR or SDR of BD pts F: 74.1% Mean age: 21.3 (*SD*: 3.5) Axis I diagnoses: none 49 HC F: 62.8% Mean age: 21.5 (*SD*: 3.5) Other Axis I diagnoses: none	1.5 T Qualitative	PVWMHs, DWMHs, SCWMHs	AR-BD vs affected subjects vs HC: no significant differences.
Forcada et al., 2011	27 FDR of BD pts F: 52%[a] Mean age: 33.7 (*SD*: 12.7)[a] Other Axis I diagnoses: none	41 BD patients F: 51.2% Mean age: 44.3 (*SD*: 11.8) Other axis I diagnoses: none 23 affected FDR of BD pts F: 52%[a] Mean age: 33.7 (*SD*: 12.7)[a] Axis I diagnoses: 65.2% MDD, 26% past SUD, 8.7% anxiety disorders	1.5 T VBM	Whole brain	AR-BD vs affected subjects vs BD: no significant differences in GM and WM volumes. WM volume was associated with functional outcome in BD patients, but not in their relatives.
Karchemskiy et al., 2011	22 bipolar offspring F: 51.1% Mean age: 31.8 (*SD*: not reported) Other Axis I diagnoses: 100% ADHD, 40.9% MDD, 40.9% ODD, 36.4% anxiety disorders	22 HC F: 51.1% Mean age: 31.8 (*SD*: not reported) Other axis I diagnoses: none	3 T ROI	Amygdala, hippocampus, thalamus.	AR-BD vs HC: no significant differences.

(continued)

Table 24.1. CONTINUED

STUDY/TYPE OF DESIGN	AR-BD	COMPARISON GROUP	TECHNIQUE	BRAIN AREAS ANALYZED	MAJOR FINDINGS
Hajek et al., 2012	50 FDR of BD pts F: 62% Mean age: 19.8 (range 15–30) Other Axis I diagnoses: none	36 affected offspring of BD pts F: 72.2% Mean age: 21.5 (range 15–30) Axis I diagnoses: 52.7% MDD, 22.2% BD-I, 19.4% BD-II, 11.1% anxiety disorders, 8.3% SUD, 2.7% ADHD, 2.7% bulimia 49 HC F: 63.2% Mean age: 21.8 (range 15–30) Other Axis I diagnoses: none 19 BD pts F: 63.2% Mean age: 26.5 (range 17–30) Axis I diagnoses: 84.2% BD-I, 15.8% BD-II, 15.7% anxiety disorders, 5.3% SUD	1.5 T VBM	GM in the cortical regions	AR-BD + Affected subjects vs HC: ↑ GM volume in rIFG. BD vs HC: ↑ GM volume in rIFG.
Matsuo et al., 2012	20 FDR of BD pts F: 75% Mean age: 46.2 (SD: 10.7) Other Axis I diagnoses: none	35 BD-I pts F: 77.1% Mean age: 40.8 (SD: 9.2) Axis I diagnoses: 17.1% anxiety disorders 40 HC F: 60% Mean age: 41.6 (SD: 9.1)	3 T VBM with DARTEL ROI	Ventromedial and dorsolateral prefrontal cortex, anterior cingulate, striatum, hippocampus and amygdala	AR-BD vs HC: ↓ GM volume in the left insula; ↓ WM volume in the right medial frontal white matter BD vs HC:↓ GM volume in the left insula; ↓ GM volume in the right medial frontal gyrus

NOTE: ADHD = attention deficit hyperactivity disorder; ALIC = anterior limb of internal capsule; AR-BD = at risk for bipolar disorder; BD = bipolar disorder; CC = corpus callosum; DARTEL = diffeomorphic anatomical registration through exponentiated lie algebra; DW MHs = deep white matter hyperintensities; F = female; FDR = first-degree relatives; GM = gray matter; HC= healthy controls; MDD = major depressive disorder; MZ = monozygotic; DZ = dizygotic; NOS = not otherwise specified; OCD = obsessive-compulsive disorder; ODD = oppositional defiant disorder; OMPFC = orbital medial prefrontal cortex; PAD = panic attack disorder; PFC = prefrontal cortex; PV WMHs = periventricular white matter hyperintensities; rIFG = right inferior frontal gyrus; ROI = regions of interest; SCWMHs = subcortical white matter hyperintensities; SDR = second-degree relatives; SLF = superior longitudinal fasciculus; SUD = substance use disorders; SVC = small volume correction; VBM = voxel-based morphometry; WM = white matter.

a Affected plus unaffected relatives.

recent study, however, Gunde and colleagues (2011) found a proportion of periventricular-, deep-, or subcortical WM hyperintensities not significantly different between the unaffected high-risk, affected familial and control groups.

DIFFUSION TENSION IMAGING

Diffusion tensor imaging (DTI) is a quantitative, noninvasive neuroimaging technique for assessing the integrity of WM fiber tracts indirectly via measurement of the directionality of water diffusion (fractional anisotropy [FA]; Pierpaoli & Basser, 1996). FA reflects axonal diameter, axonal density, and fiber tract complexity (Beaulieu, 2002). More specifically, reduced FA can be attributed to degradation of both myelin sheaths and axonal membranes (Pierpaoli et al., 2001), abnormalities of myelin, or reduced density of axonal fibers (Song et al., 2005). Mean diffusivity is another parameter that indicates the overall mean-squared movement of water molecules (Neil, Miller, Mukherjee, & Hüppi, 2002) and reflects cellular density and extracellular volume (Sotak, 2004). Thus low FA and high mean diffusivity is associated with less organized myelin and/or axonal structure (Pfefferbaum & Sullivan, 2005).

Table 24.2 presents the main DTI findings from the studies in AR-BD subjects.

DTI imaging studies recruited first-degree relatives (; Chaddock et al., 2009; Frazier et al, 2007; Versace et al., 2010) and first- or second-degree relatives (in this case the subjects must have at least two second-degree relatives affected) of patients with BD (Sprooten et al., 2011) as AR-BD. With the exception of one study (Frazier et al., 2007), where the subjects were psychiatric patients with a nonbipolar *Diagnostic and Statistical Manual of Mental Disorder* (fourth edition [*DSM-IV*]) Axis I diagnosis, all subjects had no psychiatric diagnosis. Most of the studies found consistent differences between AR-BD and their respective groups in WM integrity.

Frazier and colleagues (2007) confirmed their a priori hypothesis, according to which AR-BD have findings similar to patients with BD but attenuated in magnitude. Comparing BD to HCs, in fact, they found FA reduction in the superior frontal tracts of the bilateral superior longitudinal fasciculus and cingulate-paracingulate in the left orbital frontal cortex and the right corpus callosum body. Comparing BD to AR-BD, they found FA reduction in the right and left cingulate-paracingulate and a trend toward reduced FA in the left orbital frontal cortex and the right corpus callosum body in subjects with BD. Finally, comparing AR-BD and HCs, they found that FA was reduced bilaterally in the bilateral superior longitudinal fasciculus,

but the magnitude of this reduction was less than that seen between BD and HCs.

The study by Chaddock and colleagues (2009) showed data derived from 21 first-degree relative of patients with BP-I (AR-BD), 19 patients with BD-I, and 18 HCs. Comparing BD-I patients and HCs, the authors found a significant reduction of FA in a bilateral frontal cluster, extending from deep frontal WM to include the genu of corpus callosum and a left lateralized portion of internal capsule, in a right temporal cluster, which extended superiorly toward the parietal lobe, as well as in a superior frontal cluster. Between AR-BD and HCs, no significant difference was detected; however, a linear trend was confirmed within all clusters, indicating that the mean FA value of AR-BD is intermediate between to the BD patients and the HCs. Furthermore, independently of the clinical diagnosis, the authors correlated the Genetic Liability Scale scores and FA. Chaddock and colleagues found a negative association between Genetic Liability Scale score and FA in cerebellum and the brainstem, the temporal lobe bilaterally (corresponding to the inferior and superior longitudinal fascicule and uncinate), bilateral deep frontal WM (extending to the genu of corpus callosum corresponding to the anterior regions of the fronto-occipital fasciculus), posterior brain regions (corresponding to bilateral portions of the inferior fronto-occipital and inferior longitudinal fasciculi), splenium of corpus callosum, and corona radiata, and a positive association (in 11 clusters, with one cluster having a spatial threshold greater than 50 voxels) in left parietal WM, posterior to the splenium of corpus callosum.

Linke and colleagues (2013) provided further evidence of WM abnormalities as putative endophenotypes of BD, as reduced FA in the right anterior limb of the internal capsule and right uncinate fasciculus was detected in both BD-I patients and their healthy first-degree relatives. Furthermore, WM abnormalities were associated with impairment in executive function tasks (Linke et al., 2013).

However, a recent large-scale DTI study conducted as part of the B-SNIP consortium in 82 BD psychotic subjects and 83 first-degree relatives found only minor WM tracts abnormalities in AR-BD subjects (i.e., lower FA than the HCs in the left posterior corona radiate), while BD subjects had widespread abnormalities that were distributed in a similar pattern as schizophrenia patients (Skudlarski et al., 2013).

Versace and colleagues (2010) used probabilistic tractography to investigate WM abnormalities in AR-BD compared to HCs. AR-BD subjects showed a linear decrease in FA and an increase in radial diffusivity with age in the left corpus callosum and right inferior longitudinal fasciculus.

Table 24.2. DIFFUSION IMAGING STUDIES IN POPULATION AT RISK FOR BIPOLAR DISORDER

STUDY/TYPE OF DESIGN	AR-BD	COMPARISON GROUP	DTI ACQUISITION	WHITE MATTER TRACTS	MAJOR FINDINGS
Frazier et al., 2007	7 FDR of BD pts F: 43% Mean age: 8.9 (SD:3.0) Other Axis I diagnoses: Anxiety disorder 71.4%, ADHD 57.1%, C/ODD 42.9%, PTSD 14.3%, Asperger's disorder 14.3%. One AR-BD on medication (stimulant).	10 BD F: 60% Mean age: 9.2 (SD:3.0) Other Axis I diagnoses: ADHD 80%, C/ODD 80%, MD 70%, Anxiety disorder 60%, Psychosis 40% TD 20%. All BD children on medications [antypsychotics (n:8); anticonvulsants (n:5); antidepressants (n:3); alpha agonist (n:2); benzodiazepines (n:1); atomoxetine (N:3)] 8 HC F:37.5% Mean age 9.2 (SD:2.4)	1.5T 6 non-collinear directions b=1125.28 s/mm² ROI-based analysis Non parametric statistics FA measured	ROIs of any significant clusters within SLF I and CG-PAC established on *a priori* knowledge of topographic human neuro-anatomy. SLF I contains WM of superior parietal lobule, precuneus, postcentral gyrus, and posterior part of the superior frontal gyrus as well as the supplementary motor area. CG-PAC$_{wm}$ defined as tracts to/ from the anterior and posterior cingulated and paracingulate gyri.	BD vs HC: ↓FA superior frontal tracts in bilateral SLF I and CG-PAC$_{wm}$, left OFC$_{wm}$ and the right CC3. AR-BD vs HC: ↓ FA in bilateral SLF I BD vs AR-BD: ↓FA in the right and left CG-PAC$_{wm}$; trend to↓ FA in left OFC$_{wm}$, right CC3,
Chaddock et al., 2009	21 FDR of BD-I pts F:43% Mean age: 42.5 (SD: 13.6)	19 BD-I F:52.6% Mean age: 43.3 (SD: 10.2) 15 BD-I pts on medications [antypsychotics (n:8); anticonvulsants (n:5); antidepressants (n:3); alpha agonist (n:2); benzodiazepines (n:1); atomoxetine (N:3)] 18 HC F:44.4% Mean age: 41.7 (SD: 12.2)	1.5T 64 optimized directions uniformly distributed in space, b=1300 s/mm² Voxel-by-voxel analysis Non-parametric statistics Mean T$_2$-weighted and FA measured	Bilateral deep frontal white matter and genu of corpus callosum: corresponding to anterior portions of the fronto-occipital fasciculus and superior longitudinal fasciculus. Superior frontal white matter: corresponding to the superior longitudinal fasciculus and corona radiata. Parietotemporal junction: incorporating temporal white matter and extending to parieto/occipital regions: corresponding to the inferior longitudinal fasciculus and posterior portions of the inferior fronto-occipital fasciculus	BD I vs HC: ↓↓ FA bilateral frontal cluster extending from deep frontal WM to include the genu of corpus callosum; a left lateralized portion of internal capsule; a right temporal cluster which extended superiorly towards the parietal lobe; and a superior frontal cluster. AR-BD vs HC: no significant difference in FA was detected; however, a linear trend was confirmed within all clusters, indicating that the mean FA value of AR-BD is intermediary to the BD 1 and HC. ↑ GLS associated to ↓ FA in cerebellum and brainstem, bilateral temporal lobe, bilateral deep frontal WM, posterior brain regions, splenium of corpus callosum and corona radiata. ↑ GLS associated to ↑ FA in left parietal WM.
Versace et al., 2010	20 FDR of BD pts F:55% Mean age:13.2 (SD:2.5)	25 HC F:72% Mean age:13.9 (SD:2.6) FDR of HC with no Axis I disorder.	3T 6 non-coplanar directions b=850 s/mm² TBSS analysis Non-parametric statistics FA, RD and LD measured.	Corpus callosum. Inferior longitudinal fasciculus.	Left CC: positive relation between FA and age in HC, and negative relation in HBO; negative relation between age and RD in HC and positive relation in HBO. ILF in the temporal lobe: positive relation between age and FA in the right ILF in HC, no relation in HBO; negative relation between age and RD in HC, no relation in HBO.

Study	Sample	Methods	Region	Results
Sprooten et al., 2011	117 FDR of BD-I pts F:53% Mean age: 21.03 (SD:2.75) No difference in history of SUD compared to HC group.	79 HC F:53.2% Mean age:20.78 (SD:2.27) No difference in history of SUD compared to AR-BD group	1.5T 64 non-collinear directions b=1000 s/mm² TBSS analysis Non parametric/parametric statistics FA values with DTIFIT	Whole skeleton	AR-BD vs HC: ↓ FA in one large diffuse cluster extending over most of the WM skeleton, including the corpus callosum, internal and external capsules (including anterior thalamic radiations), inferior and superior longitudinal fasciculi, inferior fronto-occipital fasciculi, uncinate fasciculi, parts of the corticospinal tract, and subcortical WM around the central sulci. CT and FA: negative association in the internal capsules bilaterally connected via deep subthalamic white matter and in the left hemisphere contained several fronto-temporal and fronto-thalamic connections, including the external capsule, inferior longitudinal fasciculus, anterior parts of the left arcuate fasciculus, dorsal left uncinate fasciculus, as well as left occipital white matter.
Linke et al., 2013	22 FDR of BD-I pts F: 50% Mean age: 28 (SD: 11)	22 HC F: 50% Mean age: 28 (SD:10)	3.0 T 40 noncollinear directions b=1000 sec/mm² TBSS analysis ROI-based analysis Permutation statistics FA, LD, RD, and the mode of anisotropy also analyzed	Anterior limb of internal capsule Uncinate fasciculus Corpus callosum	AR-BD vs HC: ↓ FA and ↑ RD in the right ALIC; ↓ FA in the right UF
Skudlarski et al., 2013	83 FDR of psychotic BD-I F: 66.3% Mean age: 40.6 (SD:2.5)	104 HC F: 58.7% Mean age: 38.9 (SD:1.3)	Two different scanners Both 3.0 T Scanner 1: 32 directions b=1000 sec/mm² Scanner 2: 30 directions b=1000 sec/mm² ROI-based analysis whole skeleton analysis Permutation statistics	29 pre-specified regions	AR-BD vs HC: ↓ FA in the left posterior corona radiata

Positive relation between age and LD in HC, negative relation in HBO in the visual cortex. HBO vs HC: ↑ FA and ↓ RD in CC; ↓ RD in right ILF; ↑ LD in the visual cortex.

NOTE: ADHD = attention deficit hyperactivity disorder; ALIC = anterior limb of internal capsule; AR-BD = at risk for bipolar disorder; BD = bipolar disorder; CC = corpus callosum; CC3 = corpus callosum body; CG-PAC = cingulate-paracingulate; C/ODD = conduct/oppositional defiant disorder; CT = cyclothymic temperament; FA = fractional anisotropy; FLIRT = FMRIB's Linear Image Registration Tool; FDR = first-degree relatives; FSL = FMRIB Software Library; GLS = genetic liability scale; HC = healthy controls; ILF = inferior longitudinal fasciculus; LD = longitudinal diffusivity; MD = major depression; OFC = orbital frontal cortex; PTSD =posttraumatic stress disorder; RD = radial diffusivity; ROIs = regions of interest; SLF I = superior longitudinal fasciculus; TBSS = Tract-Based Spatial Statistics; TD = tic disorder; WM = white matter.

Table 24.3. FUNCTIONAL MAGNETIC RESONANCE IMAGING STUDIES IN POPULATION AT RISK FOR BIPOLAR DISORDER

STUDY/TYPE OF DESIGN	AR-BD	COMPARISON GROUP	TASK/CONDITION	FIELD STRENGTH	AREAS ANALYZED	MAJOR FINDINGS
Drapier et al., 2008	20 FDR of BD pts F: 40% Mean age: 43 (SD:13.8) Other axis I diagnoses: 15% MDD, 5% substance-induced mood disorder.	20 BD pts F: 55% Mean age: 42.7 (SD:10.4) Other axis I diagnoses: 5% alcohol dependence syndrome, 5% PAD. 20 HC F: 50% Mean age: 41.9 (SD:11.6) Other Axis I diagnoses: 10% past MDD, 5% alcohol abuse.	N-back working memory	1.5 T	Whole brain	**AR-BD vs HC:** ↑ activation in the left frontal pole in 1-back and 2-back conditions; **BD vs HC:** trend ↑ activation in the left frontal pole in 1-back condition.
Costafreda et al., 2009	7 MZ twins of BD pts F: 85.7% Mean age: 39.4 (SD:15.8) Other axis I diagnoses: none.	28 MZ twins with BD pts F:57.1% Mean age: 40.0 (SD:12.4) Other Axis I diagnoses: none. 48 HC F:47.9% Mean age: 37.4 (SD: 9.8%) Other Axis I diagnoses: none.	Verbal fluency	1.5 T	Bilateral inferior frontal cortex	**AR-BD vs affected subjects vs HC:** no significant differences in activation of the analyzed area.
Thermenos et al., 2010	18 FDR of BD pts F: 55.6% Mean age: 36.3 (SD:2) Other axis I diagnoses: alcohol or drug abuse or dependence.	19 BD pts F: 42.2% Mean age: 41.1 (SD:3.1) Other axis I diagnoses: alcohol or drug abuse or dependence. 19 HC F: 52.6% Mean age: 39.2 (SD:2.7) Other Axis I diagnoses: none.	N-back working memory	1.5 T	Whole brain + ROIs	**AR-BD vs HC:** ↑ activation in left anterior insula (BA 13), ↑ activation in the left frontopolar cortex (BA 10), ↑ activation in the left OFC (BA 47) and superior parietal cortex; **BD vs AR-BD:** ↓ activation in the left frontopolar cortex (BA 10); **BD vs HC:** ↑ activation in left anterior insula (BA 13), ↓ activation in the left frontopolar cortex (BA 10).
Allin et al., 2010	19 FDR of BD pts F: 57.8% Mean age: 42.1 (SD:13.9) Other axis I diagnoses: 15.8% MDD, 5% substance-induced mood disorder.	18 BD pts F: 61.1% Mean age: 39.2 (SD:11.5) Other axis I diagnoses: none. 19 HC F: 47.3% Mean age: 39.9 (SD:11.0) Other Axis I diagnoses: 10.5% MDD, 5% pts alcohol abuse.	Verbal fluency	1.5 T	Whole brain	**AR-BD vs HC:** in the easy condition ↑ activation in the retrosplenial/posterior cingulate cortex and the precuneus, ↓ activation in the left frontotemporal areas; in the hard condition ↑ activation in the retrosplenial/posterior cingulate cortex, ↓ activation in the medial frontal cortex. **BD vs AR-BD:** in the easy condition ↑ activation in the ventrolateral prefrontal cortex; in the hard condition ↓ activation in the retrosplenial/posterior cingulate cortex, ↑ activation in the medial frontal cortex. **BD vs HC:** in the easy condition ↑ activation in the retrosplenial/posterior cingulate cortex, ↓ activation in the left frontal cortex; in the hard condition ↑ activation in the retrosplenial/posterior cingulate cortex.

Study	Sample (FDR)	Sample (BD/HC)	Task	Field	Analysis	Results
Surguladze et al., 2010	20 FDR of BD pts F: 55% Mean age: 43 (*SD*:13.8) Axis I diagnoses: 15% MDD, 5% substance-induced mood disorder.	20 BD pts F: 40% Mean age: 42.7 (*SD*:10.4) Other axis I diagnoses: 5% alcohol dependence syndrome, 5% PAD. 20 HC F: 50% Mean age: 41.9 (*SD*:11.6) Other Axis I diagnoses: 10% past MDD, 5% alcohol abuse.	Emotional faces	1.5 T	Whole brain + ROIs	AR-BD vs HC: ↑ activation in medial PFC, left putamen and amygdala; BD vs HC: ↑ activation in medial PFC, left putamen and amygdala;
Whalley et al., 2011	93 FDR or SDR of BD pts F: 51.6% Mean age: 21.0 (*SD*:2.83) Other Axis I diagnoses: lifetime substance misuse.	70 HC F: 54.2% Mean age: 20.9 (*SD*:2.3) Other Axis I diagnoses: lifetime substance misuse.	Hayling sentence completion test	1.5 T	Whole brain	AR-BD vs HC: ↑ activation in left amygdala.
Pompei et al., 2011a,b	25 FDR of BD pts without MDD F: 48% Mean age: 35 (*SD*:13.7) 14 FDR of BD pts with MDD F: 48% Mean age: 31.2 (*SD*:10.3)	39 BD pts F: 51.2% Mean age: 39.4 (*SD*:11.5) Other axis I diagnoses: none. 48 HC F: 47.9% Mean age: 36.3 (*SD*:12.8) Other Axis I diagnoses: none.	Stroop test	1.5 T	Whole brain	ARBD vs HC: ↓ activity in the superior and inferior parietal lobuli AR-BD without MDD vs HC: ↓ FC between VLPFC and ventral ACC and INS. AR-BD with MDD vs HC: ↓ FC between VLPFC and ventral ACC, CN, GP and INS. BD vs HC: ↓ activity in the left caudate and the right IFG; ↓ FC between VLPFC and ventral ACC, CN, and GP.
Thermenos et al., 2011	10 FDR of BD pts F: 50% Mean age: 18.4 (*SD*:4.2) Other Axis I diagnoses: none.	10 HC F: 54.2% Mean age: 20.9 (*SD*:2.3) Other Axis I diagnoses: none.	N-back working memory	1.5 T	Whole brain + ROIs	AR-BD vs HC: ↓ modulation (activation from 0-back to 2-back condition) in the CV, insula and amygdala/parahippocampal region, ↑ modulation in the frontopolar cortex and brainstem.
Kim et al., 2012	13 FDR of BD pts F: 54% Mean age: 13.9 (*SD*:2.01) Other axis I diagnoses: none.	28 BD pts F: 57% Mean age: 14.3 (*SD*:2.6) Other axis I diagnoses: 64% ADHD, 36% anxiety disorders, 32% ODD/CC. 21 HC (F: 38%) Mean age: 13.7 (*SD*:1.96) Axis I diagnoses: none.	Change task	3 T	Whole brain	AR-BD vs HC: ↑ activity in right VLPFC (BA44/45/47), ↑ activity in right IPL during successful response switching; ↑ activity in right caudate during failed response switching. AR-BD vs BD: ↑ activity in right VLPFC (BA44/45/47) during successful response switching; ↓ activity in right sgACC during failed response switching. BD vs HC: ↑ activity in right VLPFC (BA45), ↑ activity in right IPL during successful response switching; ↑ activity in right caudate, ↑ activity in the right subgenual ACC during failed response switching.

(continued)

Table 24.3. CONTINUED

STUDY/TYPE OF DESIGN	AR-BD	COMPARISON GROUP	TASK/ CONDITION	FIELD STRENGTH	AREAS ANALYZED	MAJOR FINDINGS
Mourão-Miranda et al., 2012	13 FDR of BD pts F: 46% Mean age: 14.0 (SD:2.4) Other axis I diagnoses: none.	16 healthy bipolar offspring F: 56.2% Mean age: 15.3 (SD:1.2) Other Axis I diagnoses: none. 16 HC F: 56.2% Mean age: 14.8 (SD:1.8) Axis I diagnoses: none.	Emotional faces gender-labeling (machine learning analysis)	3 T	Whole brain	Activity to neutral faces presented during the happy experiment significantly differentiated AR-BD from HC with 75% accuracy (sensitivity 75%, specificity 75%). The spatial pattern that best discriminated the groups included VMPFC and STS. GPC predictive probabilities were significantly higher for the 6 AR-BD who subsequently met DSM-IV criteria for MDE (n=3) or anxiety disorders (n=3) than for AR-BD who remained well at follow-up.
Olsavsky et al., 2012	13 FDR of BD pts F: 65.3% Mean age: 40.6 (SD:13.0) Other axis I diagnoses: none.	32 BD pts F: 46% Mean age: 14.0 (SD:2.4) Other axis I diagnoses: 47% anxiety disorders, 41% ADHD, 22% ODD. 21 HC F: 54% Mean age: 14.0 (SD:2.6) Axis I diagnoses: none.	Emotional faces	3 T	Amygdala	AR-BD vs HC: ↑ activation in right amygdala to fearful faces. AR-BD vs BD: no significant differences. BD vs HC: ↑ activation in right amygdala to fearful faces.
Meda et al., 2012	13 FDR of BD pts F: 65.3% Mean age: 40.6 (SD:13.0) Other axis I diagnoses: none.	64 BD pts F: 45.3% Mean age: 14.0 (SD:2.4) Other axis I diagnoses: none. 118 HC F: 53.4% Mean age: 36.4 (SD:10.8) Axis I diagnoses: none.	Resting state	3 T	Whole brain	Three network pairs containing five different RSNs identified in the study: (A) fronto/occipital, (B) a DMN/prefrontal, (C) meso/paralimbic, (D) fronto-temporal/paralimbic, (E) sensory-motor). AR-BD vs HC: ↓ FC between networks A-B and between networks C-E. BD vs HC: ↓ FC between networks A-B, ↑ FC between networks CD,
Linke et al.,2012	22 FDR of BD pts F: 50% Mean age: 28 (SD:11)	22 HC F: 50% Mean age: 28 (SD:10)	Probabilistic reversal learning task	3 T	Five bilateral regions of interest: the medial and lateral orbitofrontal cortex, the amygdala, the anterior cingulate cortex, and the striatum	↑ activation in response to reward and reward reversal contingencies in the right medial orbitofrontal cortex in AR-BD group vs HC ↑ activation of the amygdala in response to reward and reward reversal in AR-BD groups vs HC

Study	FDR/SDR group	BD/HC group	Task		Analysis	Results
Sepede et al., 2012	22 FDR of BD-I pts F: 68.2% Mean age: 31.5 (SD: 7.3)	24 BD-I pts F: 58.3% Mean age: 34.8 (SD: 8.0) 24 HC F: 66.7% Mean age: 32.5 (SD: 6.2)	Continuous Performance Test	1.5 T	Whole brain	AR-BD vs HC: ↑ deactivation in the PCC during correct target condition; ↑activation in the bilateral IPL and left insula during the degraded condition; ↑activation in the MCC and bilateral insula during incorrect target condition BD vs AR-BD: ↓ activation in the right insula during correct target condition BD vs HC: ↓ activation in the right insula during correct target condition; ↑activation in the MCC and bilateral insula during incorrect target condition
Whalley et al., 2013	20 FDR or SDR of BD pts who developed MDD at follow-up F: 60% Mean age: 20.6 (SD: 2.9) 78 FDR or SDR of BD pts who did not develop MDD at follow-up F: 46.2% Mean age: 21.1 (SD: 3.7)	58 HC F: 56.9% Mean age: 31.5 (SD: 7.3)	Hayling sentence completion test	1.5 T	Whole brain	No group differences in baseline comparisons, all the significant differences were found from linear "parametric" contrast of brain activation with increasing task difficulty. AR-BD who developed MDD vs HC and AR-BD who remained well: ↑ bilateral insula activation with increasing task difficulty (i.e., lack of disengagement with increasing difficulty)
Roberts et al., 2013	47 FDR of BD pts F: 53.2% Mean age: 24.6 (SD: 3.8)	49 HC F: 65.3% Mean age: 23.2 (SD: 3.4)	Facial-emotion go/no-go task	3 T	Whole brain	Reduced activation of the left IFG when inhibiting responses to fearful faces in the AR-BD group
Khadka et al., 2013	52 FDR of psychotic BD pts F: 65.3% Mean age: 40.6 (SD: 13)	118 HC F: 53.3% Mean age: 36.4 (SD:10.8)	Resting state	3 T	Analysis across the 16 networks identified through the Independent Component Analysis (ICA)	AR-BD group showed abnormalities in the fronto-occipital (↓FC in the cuneus), frontal/thalamic/basal ganglia (↓FC in the right thalamus and right putamen), sensorimotor networks (↑FC in the superior and medial frontal gyrus) vs. healthy controls

NOTE: ADHD = attention deficit hyperactivity disorder; aDMN = anterior default-mode network; ACC = anterior cingulate cortex; AR-BD = at risk for bipolar disorder; BA = Brodmann area; BD = bipolar disorder; CC = conduct disorder; CN = caudate nucleus; CV =cerebellar vermis; DGKH = diacylglycerol kinase eta; DLPFC = dorsolateral prefrontal cortex; FC = functional connectivity; FDR = first-degree relatives; fMRI = functional magnetic resonance imaging; GP = globus pallidus; GPC = Gaussian Process Classifier (a machine learning approach); HC = healthy controls; IFG = inferior frontal gyrus; INS = insula; IPL = inferior parietal lobe; MCC = midcingulate cortex; MDD= major depressive disorder; OFC = orbitofrontal cortex; ODD = oppositional defiant disorder; PCC = posterior cingulate cortex; PFC = prefrontal cortex; PET = positron emission tomography; PNOS = psychosis not otherwise specified; PPI = psychophysiological interaction; RISK+= homozygotes for the risk haplotype; RISK– = not carriers or heterozygotes for the risk haplotype; ROI = region of interest; RSN = resting states network; SDR = second-degree relatives; STS = superior temporal sulcus; VLPFC = ventrolateral prefrontal cortex; VMPFC = ventromedial prefrontal cortex.

Sprooten and colleagues (2010) reported data concerning 117 AR-BD subjects and 79 HCs without family history for psychiatric disorders. In the AR-BD compared to the HC subjects they observed a FA reduction in one large diffuse cluster extending over most of the WM skeleton, including the corpus callosum, the internal and external capsules (including anterior thalamic radiations), the inferior and superior longitudinal fasciculi, the inferior fronto-occipital fasciculi, the uncinate fasciculi, parts of the corticospinal tract, and the subcortical WM around the central sulci. Finally, cyclothymic temperament scores, measured by the short version of the Temperament Evaluation of Memphis, Pisa, Paris and San Diego-autoquestionnaire (Akiskal et al., 2005), were significantly higher in the unaffected relatives compared to the control subjects. Interestingly, a negative association of FA with cyclothymic temperament was found in the internal capsules bilaterally connected via deep subthalamic WM and in the left hemisphere contained several fronto-temporal and fronto-thalamic connections, including the external capsule, inferior longitudinal fasciculus, anterior parts of the left arcuate fasciculus, dorsal left uncinate fasciculus, as well as left occipital WM.

FUNCTIONAL IMAGING STUDIES

The main findings from the functional imaging studies in AR-BD subjects are summarized in Table 24.3.

Functional magnetic resonance imaging

Drapier and colleagues (2008) used the N-back working memory task in AR-BD subjects and observed greater activation in left frontal polar cortex in AR-BD subjects and in BD patients compared to control groups. The authors suggested that this finding is associated with genetic liability for BD and represents a potential neurobiological endophenotype for the illness. A more recent study (Thermenos et al., 2010, 2011) confirmed this preliminary finding. Compared to HCs, the AR-BD group failed to deactivate left frontopolar cortex, together with left anterior insula and superior parietal cortex, during a working memory task.

Abnormal insular activity has also been described during a sustained attention task in at AR-BD subjects, as well as increased activity in the bilateral inferior parietal lobule bilaterally and an augmented deactivation of the posterior cingulate/retrosplenial cortex (Sepede et al., 2012); interestingly insular hyperactivity at baseline during an executive function task was found to differentiate between the AR-BD subjects who later developed major depressive disorder and subjects who remained well (Whalley et al.,

2013). Using a verbal fluency task, Costafreda and colleagues (2009) did not notice different activation between unaffected twins, their bipolar co-twins, and HCs in the inferior frontal cortex. In contrast, Allin and colleagues (2010), using the same task, found increased activation (namely, reduced deactivation) in the retrosplenial cortex and decreased activation in the left frontal cortex, both in AR-BD and BD groups compared to HCs. These data suggest that abnormality of the neural network incorporating the left prefrontal cortex and bilateral retrosplenial cortex might be a potential genetic predisposition to BD. Parietal and prefrontal abnormalities have also been described by two studies that investigated response inhibition in AR-BD subjects compared to HCs (Pompei et al., 2011b; Roberts et al., 2013).

Surguladze and colleagues (2010), using an emotional faces task, found that bipolar patients and AR-BD subjects shared the same abnormal pattern of activation in the medial prefrontal cortex, the left putamen, and the left amygdala in response to fearful (putamen, medial prefrontal cortex) and happy faces (amygdala, medial prefrontal cortex) compared to healthy subjects. Abnormal activation in right amygdala (Olsavsky et al., 2012) in the AR-BD group in response to fearful but not to happy faces has been also reported in the literature. Hyperactivity of the amygdala in AR-BD subjects has also been described during nonemotional tasks, such as a sentence-completion task and a probabilistic reversal learning reward task (Linke et al., 2012; Whalley et al., 2011). Taking together, these data suggest that amygdala hyperactivation may be a candidate endophenotype in BD. However, evidence of amygdala hyperactivity to negative stimuli has also been associated with unipolar depression (Arnone et al., 2012) and anxiety disorders (Killgore et al., 2014), possibly challenging the specificity of this finding to a pure BD diathesis. Results from a study performed by Kim and colleagues (2012) suggest that abnormal activity in ventrolateral prefrontal cortex, inferior parietal cortex, and striatum during a cognitive flexibility task may be also considered as potential endophenotypes for BD.

A few studies have investigated functional connectivity in AR-BD subjects during task-based or resting-state functional magnetic resonance imaging (fMRI). Pompei, Dima, Rubia, Kumari, and Frangou (2011a) investigated functional connectivity of the ventrolateral prefrontal cortex during a Stroop Color and Word Test using psychophysiological interaction analysis. The authors found decreased connectivity between ventrolateral prefrontal cortex and ventral anterior cingulate cortex in both AR-BD and BD groups compared to HCs, demonstrating that dysregulation in the coupling of prefrontal with limbic/paralimbic regions is a correlate of predisposition to BD. Additional dysfunction in the coupling of prefrontal with basal ganglia regions was seen both in BD patients and their relatives with major depressive disorder.

Another recent study investigated how different resting-state networks interact in BD patients and in their relatives (Meda et al., 2012). AR-BD and BD subjects were found to share the same abnormal low-frequency resting-state networks interaction, namely a reduced connectivity between network A (fronto/occipital) and network B (anterior default-mode network/prefrontal). Abnormal functional connectivity has also been suggested as a potential endophenotype of BD by a recent study that used independent component analysis applied to resting state fMRI data in 64 psychotic BD probands and 52 first-degree relatives. Both patients and at-risk subjects showed abnormalities in the fronto-occipital, frontal/thalamic/basal ganglia, and sensorimotor networks compared to HC subjects (Khadka et al., 2013).

Finally, Mourão-Miranda and colleagues (2012) recently applied machine learning to fMRI data during an emotional faces gender-labeling task; they used Gaussian Process Classifiers, a machine learning approach that assigns to an individual a predictive probability to be part of a group based on the confidence of a classifiers computed preprocessed fMRI scans. Activity to happy faces accurately and significantly differentiated AR-BD from HCs with 75% accuracy (sensitivity 75%, specificity 75%). The spatial pattern that best discriminated the groups included ventromedial prefrontal cortex and superior temporal sulcus activity. Moreover, using Gaussian Process Classifiers, predictive probabilities were significantly higher for the six AR-BD who subsequently met *DSM-IV* criteria for a major depressive episode ($n = 3$) or anxiety disorders ($n = 3$) than for AR-BD who remained well at follow-up.

Positron emission tomography

One study measured regional cerebral blood flow (rCBF) using positron emission tomography (Krüger et al., 2006) in AR-BD subjects. The authors enrolled euthymic bipolar lithium responders and their healthy siblings. A sadness induction protocol was used in the study by asking the subjects to draft a short autobiographical script describing a sad life event. The scan was done one minute after the subjects reached the peak negative emotion. Siblings shared with lithium-treated patients the same pattern of rCBF changes, namely increased rCBF in the premotor cortex, dorsal and rostral anterior cingulate, anterior insula, and cerebellum and decreased rCBF in the orbitofrontal cortex and inferior

temporal cortex. Discordant patterns in the two groups were detected in the medial frontal cortex: metabolic increase and decrease was found in the AR-BD and the BD group, respectively.

Magnetic resonance spectroscopy

Magnetic resonance spectroscopy is an MRI-based procedure that enables the quantification of the concentrations of different neurochemicals in vivo, such as N-acetylaspartate (NAA), choline (Cho), myoinositol (mI), creatine/phospocreatine (CR), and glutamate (Glu).

Cecil, DelBello, Sellars, and Strakowski (2003) found significantly different NAA/Cho concentrations in cerebellar vermis of bipolar offspring with mood disorders compared to HC. Furthermore, they noticed a trend of increase mI levels in the medial frontal cortex in the AR-BD group. In one study, bipolar offspring with subsyndromal mood symptoms (i.e., AR-BD) were compared to bipolar offspring with previous episodes of mania and HCs (Singh et al., 2010). Decreased absolute Glu and Glu/Cr concentrations were found in the bipolar offspring with previous episodes of mania group compared to HCs in the anterior cingulate cortex. No significant differences were apparent in nonsymptomatic AR-BD subjects compared to HC subjects. In a follow-up study, Singh and colleagues (2011) investigated cerebellar neurochemical abnormalities in AR-BD subjects with subsyndromal mood symptoms and found decreased mI, Cho, and Cho/Cr and a trend to a decreased mI/Cr concentration in the AR-BD group compared to the HC group, possibly indicating decreased cellular metabolism as an early marker of susceptibility to BD. Two other studies in AR-BD subjects (Gallelli et al., 2005; Hajek et al., 2008c) failed to find significant differences in the concentrations of NAA and other metabolites in the prefrontal cortex when comparing them with BD patients or HC subjects.

SUMMARY

Recently, several studies with different imaging techniques have been performed in AR-BD subjects to investigate potential endophenotypes of BD that are evident before the occurrence of frank (hypo)manic episodes. While findings from GM structural VBM studies are encouraging, there still are several inconsistencies. Evidence for WM pathology as a putative endophenotype of BD is accumulating, especially generated from studies that used DTI. Unlike T_1-weighted MRI, DTI seems to be less susceptible to the signal generated by non-neuronal tissue components (Hui,

Cheung, Chan, & Wu, 2010). Evidence from studies of primary demyelinating conditions suggests that it is both a valid and a more sensitive technique than conventional MRI (Guo, MacFall, & Provenzale, 2002). This technique may play an important role in early identification of people either at risk for BD or at an initial phase of illness.

Results in AR-BD subjects confirm that WM alterations are a common marker not only in patients with BD but also in people at risk for BD. It is also noteworthy that DTI has also been proven effective to detect "soft bipolarity," such as cyclothymic temperament (Sprooten et al., 2011), strengthening the idea that cyclothymia is per se part of the bipolar spectrum (Akiskal, Djenderedjian, Rosenthal, & Khani, 1997).

CONCLUSION AND FUTURE DIRECTIONS

Early recognition of people likely to develop BD is an urgent need in psychiatry. Despite actual improvements in clinical and research psychiatry, a long delay is still observed between the onset of the disorder and its treatment (Ghaemi et al., 2000). The delay can lead to misdiagnosis, mistreatment, and worsening of clinical picture and course of the disorder.

Lack of research in prevention strategies for BD can be in part responsible for this void. In fact, in recent years, although considerable clinical and research interest has been directed at the early and prepsychotic phases of psychotic disorders, research on early phase of affective disorders has been a relatively neglected area (Conus & McGorry, 2002). However, this is not the only problem. Compared to psychotic disorders, BD's complexity makes early detection harder. BD is a recurrent polyphasic disorder. Its first clinical manifestation is often different from a mood episode and its course hardly predictable; BD can assume different forms and can be dramatically influenced by treatments or substance abuse. Moreover, although the peak age of onset is between 15 and 24 years, almost 20% of patients with BD have the first clinically evident episodes of mania or hypomania later in life. Finally, the limit between premorbid characteristics (i.e., "normal" adolescent turmoil) or personality and temperamental traits and the onset of the disorder is not clearly identified.

Clinical studies are, for the most part, retrospective and are somehow consistent in finding premorbid and early signs of bipolarity in patients who later develop full-blown BD (for a review, see Skjelstad, Malt, & Holte, 2010). Key issues are how to clearly define the concept of prodrome of BD and how to identify which symptoms or signs have the highest specificity for BD.

Combining clinical and biological data is probably a more promising strategy to improve our knowledge of BD and enhance possibility for early detection. Recently, Brietzke and colleagues (2012) proposed an interesting multivariate prediction algorithm for BD integrating both phenomenological and biological markers. The authors proposed the "three pillars" to prediction BD: genetic high risk, environmental high risk, and biomarkers profile.

In this context, neuroimaging studies play a fundamental role. In particular, relatively novel techniques such as DTI and fMRI used in populations at high risk for BD have already showed interesting pilot results.

Further studies are needed to fully understand the role of these neuroimaging techniques in the prevention strategy of BD. Specifically, it is necessary to verify if combining neuroimaging with neurobiological (e.g., genetic), neuropsychological, and clinical findings will help us learn more about the pathophysiology of this disease to identify "prodromal" BD and at-risk subjects who might benefit from early pharmacological or nonpharmacological interventions.

Given the varied nature of presentation and variability in course of BD, separating and appropriately treating at-risk individuals constitutes a serious challenge. Careful selection of the subjects who might benefit from an early intervention and appropriate prospective study designs to correctly evaluate outcome are still needed.

Disclosure statement: Dr. Salvadore is a full-time employee and shareholder of Janssen Pharmaceuticals INC. Dr. Gabriele Sani has no conflicts of interest.

REFERENCES

Ahearn, E. P., Steffens, D. C., Cassidy, F., Van Meter, S. A., Provenzale, J. M., Seldin, M. F.,…Krishnan, K. R. (1998). Familial leukoencephalopathy in bipolar disorder. *The American Journal of Psychiatry, 155,* 1605–1607.

Akiskal, H. S., Djenderedjian, A. M., Rosenthal, R. H., & Khani, M. K. (1997). Cyclothymic disorder: Validating criteria for inclusion in the bipolar affective group. *The American Journal of Psychiatry, 134,* 1227–1233.

Akiskal, H. S., Mendlowicz, M. V., Jean-Louis, G., Rapaport, M. H., Kelsoe, J. R., Gillin, J. C., & Smith, T. L. (2005). TEMPS-A: Validation of a short version of a self-rated instrument designed to measure variations in temperament. *Journal of Affective Disorders, 85,* 45–52.

Alda, M. (1997). Bipolar disorder: From families to genes. *Canadian Journal of Psychiatry, 42,* 378–387.

Allin, M. P., Marshall, N., Schulze, K., Walshe, M., Hall, M. H., Picchioni, M.,…McDonald, C. (2010). A functional MRI study of verbal fluency in adults with bipolar disorder and their unaffected relatives. *Psychological Medicine, 40,* 2025–2035.

Arnone, D., McKie, S., Elliott, R., Thomas, E. J., Downey, D., Juhasz, G., ... Anderson, I. M. (2012). Increased amygdala responses to sad but not fearful faces in major depression: Relation to mood state and pharmacological treatment. *The American Journal of Psychiatry, 169*, 841–850.

Arts, B., Jabben, N., Krabbendam, L., & van Os, J. (2008). Meta-analyses of cognitive functioning in euthymic bipolar patients and their first-degree relatives. *Psychological Medicine, 38*, 771–785.

Barnett, J. H., & Smoller, J. W. (2009). The genetics of bipolar disorder. *Neuroscience, 164*, 331–343.

Beaulieu, C. (2002). The basis of anisotropic water diffusion in the nervous system—a technical review. *NMR in Biomedicine, 15*, 435–455.

Beaulieu, C., Plewes, C., Paulson, L. A., Roy, D., Snook, L., Concha, L., ... Phillips, L. (2005). Imaging brain connectivity in children with diverse reading ability. *Neuroimage, 25*, 1266–1271.

Berk, M., Brnabic, A., Dodd, S., Kelin, K., Tohen, M., Malhi, G. S., et al. (2011). Does stage of illness impact treatment response in bipolar disorder? Empirical treatment data and their implication for the staging model and early intervention. *Bipolar Disorders, 13*, 87–98.

Bora, E., Yucel, M., & Pantelis, C. (2009). Cognitive endophenotypes of bipolar disorder: A meta-analysis of neuropsychological deficits in euthymic patients and their first-degree relatives. *Journal of Affective Disorders, 113*, 1–20.

Brietzke, E., Mansur, R. B., Soczynska, J. K., Kapczinski, F., Bressan, R. A., & McIntyre, R. S. (2012). Towards a multifactorial approach for prediction of bipolar disorder in at risk populations. *Journal of Affective Disorders, 140*, 82–91.

Cecil, K. M., DelBello, M. P., Sellars, M. C., & Strakowski, S. M. (2003). Proton magnetic resonance spectroscopy of the frontal lobe and cerebellar vermis in children with a mood disorder and a familial risk for bipolar disorders. *Journal of Child and Adolescent Psychopharmacology, 13*, 545–555.

Chaddock, C. A., Barker, G. J., Marshall, N., Schulze, K., Hall, M. H., Fern, A., ... McDonald, C. (2009). White matter microstructural impairments and genetic liability to familial bipolar I disorder. *The British Journal of Psychiatry, 194*, 527–534.

Chang, K., Steiner, H., Dienes, K., Adleman, N., & Ketter, T. (2003). Bipolar offspring: A window into bipolar disorder evolution. *Biological Psychiatry, 53*, 945–951.

Connor, S. E., Ng, V., McDonald, C., Schulze, K., Morgan, K., Dazzan, P., & Murray, R. M. (2004). A study of hippocampal shape anomaly in schizophrenia and in families multiply affected by schizophrenia or bipolar disorder. *Neuroradiology, 46*, 523–534.

Conus, P. O., & McGorry, P. (2002). First-episode mania: A neglected priority for early intervention. *Australia and New Zealand Journal of Psychiatry, 36*, 158–172.

Correll, C. U., Penzer, J. B., Frederickson, A. M., Richter, J. J., Auther, A. M., Smith, C. W., ... Cornblatt, B. A. (2007). Differentiation in the preonset phases of schizophrenia and mood disorders: Evidence in support of a bipolar mania prodrome. *Schizophrenia Bulletin, 33*, 703–714.

Costafreda, S. G., Fu, C. H., Picchioni, M., Kane, F., McDonald, C., Prata, D. P., ... McGuire, P. K. (2009). Increased inferior frontal activation during word generation: A marker of genetic risk for schizophrenia but not bipolar disorder? *Human Brain Mapping, 30*, 3287–3298.

Drapier, D., Surguladze, S., Marshall, N., Schulze, K., Fern, A., Hall, M. H., ... McDonald, C. (2008). Genetic liability for bipolar disorder is characterized by excess frontal activation in response to a working memory task. *Biological Psychiatry, 64*, 513–520.

Duffy, A., Alda, M., Hajek, T., & Grof, P. (2009). Early course of bipolar disorder in high-risk offspring: Prospective study. *The British Journal of Psychiatry, 195*, 457–458.

Egeland, J. A., Hostetter, A. M., Pauls, D. L., & Sussex, J. N. (2000). Prodromal symptoms before onset of manic-depressive disorder suggested by first hospital admission histories. *Journal of the American Academy of Child & Adolescent Psychiatry, 39*, 1245–1252.

Faedda, G., Serra, G., Marangoni, C., Salvatore, P., Sani, G., Vazquez, G., ... Koukopoulos, A. (2014). Clinical risk factors for bipolar disorders: a systematic review of prospective studies. *Journal of Affective Disorders, 168*, 314–321.

Fagiolini, A., Frank, E., Scott, J. A., Turkin, S., & Kupfer, D. J. (2005). Metabolic syndrome in bipolar disorder: Findings from the Bipolar Disorder Center for Pennsylvanians. *Bipolar Disorders, 7*, 424–430.

Forcada, I., Papachristou, E., Mur, M., Christodoulou, T., Jogia, J., Reichenberg, A., ... Frangou, S. (2011). The impact of general intellectual ability and white matter volume on the functional outcome of patients with Bipolar Disorder and their relatives. *Journal of Affective Disorders, 130*, 413–420.

Frazier, J. A., Breeze, J. L., Papadimitriou, G., Kennedy, D. N., Hodge, S. M., Moore, C. M., ... Makris, N. (2007). White matter abnormalities in children with and at risk for bipolar disorder. *Bipolar Disorders, 9*, 799–809.

Gallelli, K. A., Wagner, C. M., Karchemskiy, A., Howe, M., Spielman, D., Reiss, A., & Chang, K. D. (2005). N-acetylaspartate levels in bipolar offspring with and at high-risk for bipolar disorder. *Bipolar Disorders, 7*, 589–597.

Ghaemi, S. N., Boiman, E. E., & Goodwin, F. K. (2000). Diagnosing bipolar disorder and the effect of antidepressants: A naturalistic study. *Journal of Clinical Psychiatry, 61*, 804–808.

Glahn, D. C., Almasy, L., Barguil, M., Hare, E., Peralta, J. M., Kent, J. W. Jr., ... Escamilla, M. A. (2010). Neurocognitive endophenotypes for bipolar disorder identified in multiplex multigenerational families. *Archives of General Psychiatry, 67*, 168–177.

Glahn, D. C., Bearden, C. E., Niendam, T. A., & Escamilla, M. A. (2004). The feasibility of neuropsychological endophenotypes in the search for genes associated with bipolar affective disorder. *Bipolar Disorders, 6*, 171–182.

Goodwin, F. K., & Jamison, K. R. (2007). *Manic-depressive illness: Bipolar disorders and recurrent depression*. New York: Oxford University Press.

Gourovitch, M. L., Torrey, E. F., Gold, J. M., Randolph, C., Weinberger, D. R., & Goldberg, T. E. (1999). Neuropsychological performance of monozygotic twins discordant for bipolar disorder. *Biological Psychiatry, 45*, 639–646.

Gulseren, S., Gurcan, M., Gulseren, L., Gelal, F., & Erol, A. (2006). T2 hyperintensities in bipolar patients and their healthy siblings. *Archives of Medica Research, 37*, 79–85.

Gunde, E., Novak, T., Kopecek, M., Schmidt, M., Propper, L., Stopkova, P., ... Hajek, T. (2011). White matter hyperintensities in affected and unaffected late teenage and early adulthood offspring of bipolar parents: A two-center high-risk study. *Journal of Psychiatric Research, 45*, 76–82.

Guo, A. C., MacFall, J. R., & Provenzale, J. M. (2002). Multiple sclerosis: Diffusion tensor MR imaging for evaluation of normal-appearing white matter. *Radiology, 222*, 729–736.

Hajek, T., Gunde, E., Bernier, D., Slaney, C., Propper, L., Grof, P., ... Alda, M. (2008a). Subgenual cingulate volumes in affected and unaffected offspring of bipolar parents. *Journal of Affective Disorders, 108*, 263–269.

Hajek, T., Gunde, E., Bernier, D., Slaney, C., Propper, L., Macqueen, G., ... Alda, M. (2008b). Pituitary volumes in relatives of bipolar patients: High-risk study. *European Archives of Psychiatry and Clinical Neuroscience, 258*, 357–362.

Hajek, T., Bernier, D., Slaney, C., Propper, L., Schmidt, M., Carrey, N., ... Alda, M. (2008c). A comparison of affected and unaffected relatives of patients with bipolar disorder using proton magnetic resonance spectroscopy. *J Psychiatry Neurosci, 33*, 531–540.

Hajek, T., Cullis, J., Novak, T., Kopecek, M., Blagdon, R., Propper, L., ... Alda, M. (2012). Brain structural signature of familial predisposition for bipolar disorder: Replicable evidence for involvement of the right inferior frontal gyrus. *Biological Psychiatry, 73*, 144–152.

Hajek, T., Gunde, E., Slaney, C., Propper, L., MacQueen, G., Duffy, A., & Alda, M. (2009). Striatal volumes in affected and unaffected relatives of bipolar patients—High-risk study. *Journal of Psychiatric Research, 43,* 724–729.

Hajek, T., Gunde, E., Slaney, C., Propper, L., MacQueen, G., Duffy, A., & Alda, M. (2009). Amygdala and hippocampal volumes in relatives of patients with bipolar disorder: A high-risk study. *Canadian Journal of Psychiatry, 54,* 726–733.

Hajek, T., Novak, T., Kopecek, M., Gunde, E., Alda, M., & Höschl, C. (2010). Subgenual cingulate volumes in offspring of bipolar parents and in sporadic bipolar patients. *European Archives of Psychiatry and Clinical Neuroscience, 260,* 297–304.

Hill, S. K., Reilly, J. L., Keefe, R. S., Gold, J. M., Bishop, J. R., Gershon, E. S., . . . Sweeney, J. A. (2013). Neuropsychological impairments in schizophrenia and psychotic bipolar disorder: Findings from the Bipolar and Schizophrenia Network on Intermediate Phenotypes (B-SNIP) Study. *The American Journal of Psychiatry, 170,* 1275–1284.

Hui, E. S., Cheung, M. M., Chan, K. C., & Wu, E. X. (2010). B-value dependence of DTI quantitation and sensitivity in detecting neural tissue changes. *Neuroimage, 49,* 2366–2374.

Jabben, N., Arts, B., Jongen, E. M., Smulders, F. T., van Os, J., & Krabbendam, L. (2012). Cognitive processes and attitudes in bipolar disorder: A study into personality, dysfunctional attitudes and attention bias in patients with bipolar disorder and their relatives. *Journal of Affective Disorders, 143,* 265–268.

Jamison, K. R. (1995). *An unquiet mind*: A memoir of moods and madness. New York: A. A. Knopf, 181–182.

Judd, L. L., & Akiskal, H. S. (2003). The prevalence and disability of bipolar spectrum disorders in the US population: Re-analysis of the ECA database taking into account subthreshold cases. *Journal of Affective Disorders, 73,* 123–131.

Judd, L. L., Akiskal, H. S., Schettler, P. J., Coryell, W., Endicott, J., Maser, J., . . . Keller, M. B. (2003). A prospective investigation of the natural history of the long-term weekly symptomatic status of bipolar II patients. *Archives of General Psychiatry, 60,* 261–269.

Judd, L. L., Akiskal, H. S., Schettler, P. J., Endicott, J., Maser, J., Solomon, D. A., . . . Keller, M. B. (2002). The long-term natural history of the weekly symptomatic status of bipolar I disorder. *Archives of General Psychiatry, 59,* 530–537.

Juselius, S., Kieseppä, T., Kaprio, J., Lönnqvist, J., & Tuulio-Henriksson, A. (2009). Executive functioning in twins with bipolar I disorder and healthy co-twins. *Archives of Clinical Neuropsychology, 24,* 599–606.

Karchemskiy, A., Garrett, A., Howe, M., Adleman, N., Simeonova, D. I., Alegria, D., . . . Chang, K. (2011). Amygdalar, hippocampal, and thalamic volumes in youth at high risk for development of bipolar disorder. *Psychiatry Research: Neuroimaging, 194,* 319–325.

Kempton, M. J., Haldane, M., Jogia, J., Grasby, P. M., Collier, D., & Frangou, S. (2009). Dissociable brain structural changes associated with predisposition, resilience, and disease expression in bipolar disorder. *Journal of Neuroscience, 2(29),* 10863–10868.

Kessing, L. V. (1998). Cognitive impairment in the euthymic phase of affective disorder. *Psychological Medicine, 28,* 1027–1038.

Kessing, L. V., & Andersen, P. K. (1999). The effect of episodes on recurrence in affective disorder: A case register study. *Journal of Affective Disorders, 53,* 225–231.

Kessing, L. V., Hansen, M. G., Andersen, P. K., & Angst, J. (2004). The predictive effect of episodes on the risk of recurrence in depressive and bipolar disorders—A life-long perspective. *Acta Psychiatrica Scandinavica, 109,* 339–344.

Kessing, L. V., & Andersen, P. K. (2005). Predictive effects of previous episodes on the risk of recurrence in depressive and bipolar disorders. *Current Psychiatry Reports, 7,* 413–420.

Kessler, R. C., Berglund, P., Demler, O., Jin, R., Merikangas, K. R., & Walters, E. E. (2005). Lifetime prevalence and age-of-onset distributions of DSM-IV disorders in the National Comorbidity Survey Replication. *Archives of General Psychiatry, 62,* 593–602.

Khadka, S., Meda, S. A., Stevens, M. C., Glahn, D. C., Calhoun, V. D., Sweeney, J. A., . . . Pearlson, G. D. (2013). Is aberrant functional connectivity a psychosis endophenotype? A resting state functional magnetic resonance imaging study. *Biological Psychiatry,* in press.

Kieseppä, T, van Erp, T. G., Haukka, J., Partonen, T., Cannon, T. D., Poutanen, V. P., . . . Lönnqvist, J. (2003). Reduced left hemispheric white matter volume in twins with bipolar I disorder. *Biological Psychiatry, 54,* 896–905.

Kieseppä, T., Tuulio-Henriksson, A., Haukka, J., Van Erp, T., Glahn, D., Cannon, T. D., . . . Lönnqvist, J. (2005). Memory and verbal learning functions in twins with bipolar-I disorder, and the role of information-processing speed. *Psychological Medicine, 35,* 205–215.

Killgore, W. D., Britton, J. C., Schwab, Z. J., Price, L. M., Weiner, M. R., Gold, A. L., . . . Rauch, S. L. (2014). Cortico-limbic responses to masked affective faces across PTSD, panic disorder and specific phobia. *Depression and Anxiety, 31,* 150–159.

Kim, P., Jenkins, S. E., Connolly, M. E., Deveney, C. M., Fromm, S. J., Brotman, M. A., . . . Leibenluft, E. (2012). Neural correlates of cognitive flexibility in children at risk for bipolar disorder. *Journal of Psychiatric Research, 46,* 22–30.

Koukopoulos, A., Sani, G., Koukopoulos, A. E., Minnai, G. P., Girardi, P., Pani, L., . . . Reginaldi, D. (2003). Duration and stability of the rapid-cycling course: A long-term personal follow-up of 109 patients. *Journal of Affective Disorders, 73,* 75–85.

Koukopoulos, A., Albert, M. J., Sani, G., Koukopoulos, A. E., & Girardi, P. (2005). Mixed depressive states: Nosologic and therapeutic issues. *International Review of Psychiatry, 17,* 21–37.

Koukopoulos, A., Sani, G., Koukopoulos, A. E., Albert, M. J., Girardi, P., & Tatarelli, R. (2006). Endogenous and exogenous cyclicity and temperament in bipolar disorder: Review, new data and hypotheses. *Journal of Affective Disorders, 96,* 165–175.

Kraepelin, E. (1896). *Psychiatric: Ein lehrbuch für studierende und arzte* (5th ed.). Leipzig: Barth.

Kravariti, E., Schulze, K., Kane, F., Kalidindi, S., Bramon, E., Walshe, M., . . . Murray, R. M. (2009). Stroop-test interference in bipolar disorder. *The British Journal of Psychiatry, 194,* 285–286.

Krüger, S., Alda, M., Young, L. T., Goldapple, K., Parikh, S., & Mayberg, H. S. (2006). Risk and resilience markers in bipolar disorder: Brain responses to emotional challenge in bipolar patients and their healthy siblings. *The American Journal of Psychiatry, 163,* 257–264.

Ladouceur, C. D., Almeida, J. R., Birmaher, B., Axelson, D. A., Nau, S., Kalas, C., . . . Phillips, M. L. (2008). Subcortical gray matter volume abnormalities in healthy bipolar offspring: potential neuroanatomical risk marker for bipolar disorder? *Journal of the American Academy of Child & Adolescent Psychiatry, 47,* 532–539.

Lapalme, M., Hodgins, S., & LaRoche, C. (1997). Children of parents with bipolar disorder: A meta-analysis of risk for mental disorders. *Canadian Journal of Psychiatry, 42,* 623–631.

Linke, J., Witt, S. H., King, A. V., Nieratschker, V., Poupon, C., Gass, A., . . . Wessa, M. (2012). Genome-wide supported risk variant for bipolar disorder alters anatomical connectivity in the human brain. *Neuroimage, 15(59),* 3288–3296.

Linke, J., King, A. V., Poupon, C., Hennerici, M. G., Gass, A., & Wessa, M. (2013). Impaired anatomical connectivity and related executive functions: Differentiating vulnerability and disease marker in bipolar disorder. *Biological Psychiatry, 74,* 908–916.

Martinez-Aran, A., Vieta, E., Reinares, M., Colom, F., Torrent, C., Sanchez-Moreno, J., . . . Salamero, M. (2004). Cognitive function across manic or hypomanic, depressed, and euthymic states in bipolar disorder. *The American Journal of Psychiatry, 161,* 262–270.

Matsuo, K., Kopecek, M., Nicoletti, M. A., Hatch, J. P., Watanabe, Y., Nery, F. G., . . . Soares, J. C. (2012). New structural brain imaging endophenotype in bipolar disorder. *Molecular Psychiatry, 17,* 412–420.

McDonald, C., Bullmore, E. T., Sham, P. C., Chitnis, X., Wickham, H., Bramon, E., Murray, R. M. (2004). Association of genetic risks for schizophrenia and bipolar disorder with specific and generic brain structural endophenotypes. *Archives of General Psychiatry*, 61, 974–984.

McDonald, C., Marshall, N., Sham, P. C., Bullmore, E. T., Schulze, K., Chapple, B.,...Murray, R. M. (2006). Regional brain morphometry in patients with schizophrenia or bipolar disorder and their unaffected relatives. *The American Journal of Psychiatry*, 163, 478–487.

McGuffin, P., Rijsdijk, F., Andrew, M., Sham, P., Katz, R., & Cardno, A. (2003). The heritability of bipolar affective disorder and the genetic relationship to unipolar depression. *Archives of General Psychiatry*, 60, 497–502.

McIntosh, A. M., Job, D. E., Moorhead, T. W., Harrison, L. K., Forrester, K., Lawrie, S. M., & Johnstone, E. C. (2004). Voxel-based morphometry of patients with schizophrenia or bipolar disorder and their unaffected relatives. *Biological Psychiatry*, 15(56), 544–552.

McIntosh, A. M., Job, D. E., Moorhead, T. W., Harrison, L. K., Lawrie, S. M., & Johnstone, E. C. (2005). White matter density in patients with schizophrenia, bipolar disorder and their unaffected relatives. *Biological Psychiatry*, 1(58), 254–257.

McIntosh, A. M., Job, D. E., Moorhead, W. J., Harrison, L. K., Whalley, H. C., Johnstone, E. C., & Lawrie, S. M. (2006). Genetic liability to schizophrenia or bipolar disorder and its relationship to brain structure. *American Journal of Medical Genetics Part B: Neuropsychiatric Genetics*, 5(141B), 76–83.

Meda, S. A., Gill, A., Stevens, M. C., Lorenzoni, R. P., Glahn, D. C., Calhoun, V. D.,...Pearlson, G. D. (2012). Differences in resting-state functional magnetic resonance imaging functional network connectivity between schizophrenia and psychotic bipolar probands and their unaffected first-degree relatives. *Biological Psychiatry*, 71, 881–889.

Merikangas, K. R., Akiskal, H. S., Angst, J., Greenberg, P. E., Hirschfeld, R. M., Petukhova, M., & Kessler, R. C. (2007). Lifetime and 12-month prevalence of bipolar spectrum disorder in the National Comorbidity Survey replication. *Archives of General Psychiatry*, 64, 543–552.

Merikangas, K. R., Jin, R., He, J. P., Kessler, R. C., Lee, S., Sampson, N. A.,...Zarkov, Z. (2011). Prevalence and correlates of bipolar spectrum disorder in the world mental health survey initiative. *Archives of General Psychiatry*, 68, 241–251.

Mondelli, V., Dazzan, P., Gabilondo, A., Tournikioti, K., Walshe, M., Marshall, N.,...Pariante, C. M. (2008). Pituitary volume in unaffected relatives of patients with schizophrenia and bipolar disorder. *Psychoneuroendocrinology*, 33, 1004–1012.

Mourão-Miranda, J., Oliveira, L., Ladouceur, C. D., Marquand, A., Brammer, M., Birmaher, B.,...Phillips, M. L. (2012). Pattern recognition and functional neuroimaging help to discriminate healthy adolescents at risk for mood disorders from low risk adolescents. *PLoS One*, 7(2), e29482.

Neil, J., Miller, J., Mukherjee, P., & Hüppi, P. S. (2002). Diffusion tensor imaging of normal and injured developing human brain—A technical review. *NMR in Biomedicine*, 15, 543–552.

Noga, J. T., Vladar, K., & Torrey, E. F. (2001). A volumetric magnetic resonance imaging study of monozygotic twins discordant for bipolar disorder. *Psychiatry Research*, 106, 25–34.

Olsavsky, A. K., Brotman, M. A., Rutenberg, J. G., Muhrer, E. J., Deveney, C. M., Fromm, S. J.,...Leibenluft, E. (2012). Amygdala hyperactivation during face emotion processing in unaffected youth at risk for bipolar disorder. *Journal of the American Academy of Child & Adolescent Psychiatry*, 51, 294–303.

Pan, L., Keener, M. T., Hassel, S., & Phillips, M. L. (2009). Functional neuroimaging studies of bipolar disorder: Examining the wide clinical spectrum in the search for disease endophenotypes. *International Review of Psychiatry*, 21, 368–379.

Parker, G. (2010). Predicting onset of bipolar disorder from subsyndromal symptoms: A signal question? *The British Journal of Psychiatry*, 196, 87–88.

Pfefferbaum, A., & Sullivan, E. V. (2005). Disruption of brain white matter microstructure by excessive intracellular and extracellular fluid in alcoholism: Evidence from diffusion tensor imaging. *Neuropsychopharmacology*, 30, 423–432.

Pierpaoli, C., & Basser, P. J. (1996). Toward a quantitative assessment of diffusion anisotropy. *Magnetic Resonance in Medicine*, 36, 893–906.

Pierpaoli, C., Barnett, A., Pajevic, S., Chen, R., Penix, L. R., Virta, A., & Basser, P. (2001). Water diffusion changes in Wallerian degeneration and their dependence on white matter architecture. *Neuroimage*, 13, 1174–1185.

Pirkola, T., Tuulio-Henriksson, A., Glahn, D., Kieseppä, T., Haukka, J., Kaprio, J.,...Cannon, T. D. (2005). Spatial working memory function in twins with schizophrenia and bipolar disorder. *Biological Psychiatry*, 58, 930–936.

Pompei, F., Dima, D., Rubia, K., Kumari, V., & Frangou, S. (2011a). Dissociable functional connectivity changes during the Stroop task relating to risk, resilience and disease expression in bipolar disorder. *Neuroimage*, 57, 576–582.

Pompei, F., Jogia, J., Tatarelli, R., Girardi, P., Rubia, K., Kumari, V., Frangou, S. (2011b). Familial and disease specific abnormalities in the neural correlates of the Stroop Task in Bipolar Disorder. *Neuroimage*, 56, 1677–1684.

Roberts, G., Green, M. J., Breakspear, M., McCormack, C., Frankland, A., Wright, A.,...Mitchell, P. B. (2013). Reduced inferior frontal gyrus activation during response inhibition to emotional stimuli in youth at high risk of bipolar disorder. *Biological Psychiatry*, 74, 55–61.

Salvadore, G., Drevets, W. C., Henter, I. D., Zarate, C. A., & Manji, H. K. (2008a). Early intervention in bipolar disorder, part I: Clinical and imaging findings. *Early Intervention in Psychiatry*, 2, 122–135.

Salvadore, G., Drevets, W. C., Henter, I. D., Zarate, C. A., & Manji, H. K. (2008b). Early intervention in bipolar disorder, part II: Therapeutics. *Early Intervention in Psychiatry*, 2, 136–146.

Sani, G., Tondo, L., Koukopoulos, A., Reginaldi, D., Kotzalidis, G. D., Koukopoulos, A. E.,...Tatarelli, R. (2011). Suicide in a large population of former psychiatric inpatients. *Psychiatry and Clinical Neurosciences*, 65, 286–295.

Scott, J., & Meyer, T. D. (2007). Editorial: Prospects for early intervention in bipolar disorders. *Early Intervention in Psychiatry*, 1, 111–113.

Sepede, G., De Berardis, D., Campanella, D., Perrucci, M. G., Ferretti, A., Serroni, N.,...Gambi, F. (2012). Impaired sustained attention in euthymic bipolar disorder patients and non-affected relatives: An fMRI study. *Bipolar Disorders*, 14, 764–779.

Singh, M. K., Delbello, M. P., Adler, C. M., Stanford, K. E., & Strakowski, S. M. (2008). Neuroanatomical characterization of child offspring of bipolar parents. *Journal of the American Academy of Child & Adolescent Psychiatry*, 47, 526–531.

Singh, M., Spielman, D., Adleman, N., Alegria, D., Howe, M., Reiss, A., Chang, K. (2010). Brain glutamatergic characteristics of pediatric offspring of parents with bipolar disorder. *Psychiatry Research*, 182, 165–171.

Singh, M. K., Spielman, D., Libby, A., Adams, E., Acquaye, T., Howe, M.,...Chang, K. D. (2011). Neurochemical deficits in the cerebellar vermis in child offspring of parents with bipolar disorder. *Bipolar Disorders*, 13, 189–197.

Skirrow, C., Hosang, G. M., Farmer, A. E., & Asherson, P. (2012). An update on the debated association between ADHD and bipolar disorder across the lifespan. *Journal of Affective Disorders*, 141, 143–159.

Skjelstad, D. V., Malt, U. F., & Holte, A. (2010). Symptoms and signs of the initial prodrome of bipolar disorder: A systematic review. *Journal of Affective Disorders*, 126, 1–13.

Skudlarski, P., Schretlen, D. J., Thaker, G. K., Stevens, M. C., Keshavan, M. S., Sweeney, J. A.,...Pearlson, G. D. (2013). Diffusion tensor imaging white matter endophenotypes in patients with schizophrenia or psychotic bipolar disorder and their relatives. *The American Journal of Psychiatry, 170,* 886–898.

Smoller, J. W., & Finn, C. T. (2003). Family, twin, and adoption studies of bipolar disorder. *The American Journal of Medical Genetics Part C: Seminars in Medical Genetics, 123,* 48–58.

Song, S. K., Yoshino, J., Le, T. Q., Lin, S. J., Sun, S. W., Cross, A. H., & Armstrong, R. C. (2005). Demyelination increases radial diffusivity in corpus callosum of mouse brain. *Neuroimage, 26,* 132–140.

Sotak, C. H. (2004). Nuclear magnetic resonance (NMR) measurement of the apparent diffusion coefficient (ADC) of tissue water and its relationship to cell volume changes in pathological states. *Neurochemistry International, 45,* 569–582.

Sprooten, E., Sussmann, J. E., Clugston, A., Peel, A., McKirdy, J., Moorhead, T. W.,...McIntosh, A. M. (2011). White matter integrity in individuals at high genetic risk of bipolar disorder. *Biological Psychiatry, 70,* 350–356.

Surguladze, S. A., Marshall, N., Schulze, K., Hall, M. H., Walshe, M., Bramon, E.,...McDonald, C. (2010). Exaggerated neural response to emotional faces in patients with bipolar disorder and their first-degree relatives. *Neuroimage, 53,* 58–64.

Takahashi, T., Walterfang, M., Wood, S. J., Kempton, M. J., Jogia, J., Lorenzetti, V.,...Frangou, S. (2010). Pituitary volume in patients with bipolar disorder and their first-degree relatives. *Journal of Affective Disorders, 124,* 256–261.

Thermenos, H. W., Goldstein, J. M., Milanovic, S. M., Whitfield-Gabrieli, S., Makris, N., Laviolette, P.,...Seidman, L. J. (2010). An fMRI study of working memory in persons with bipolar disorder or at genetic risk for bipolar disorder. *American Journal of Medical Genetics Part B: Neuropsychiatric Genetics, 153,* 120–131.

Thermenos, H. W., Makris, N., Whitfield-Gabrieli, S., Brown, A. B., Giuliano, A. J., Lee, E. H.,...Seidman, L. J. (2011). A functional MRI study of working memory in adolescents and young adults at genetic risk for bipolar disorder: Preliminary findings. *Bipolar Disorders, 13,* 272–286.

Thompson, K. N., Conus, P. O., Ward, J. L., Phillips, L., Koutsogiannis, J., Leicester, S., McGorry, P. D. (2003). The initial prodrome to bipolar affective disorder: Prospective case studies. *Journal of Affective Disorders, 77,* 79–85.

Tijssen, M. J., van Os, J., Wittchen, H. U., Lieb, R., Beesdo, K., Mengelers, R., & Wichers, M. (2010). Prediction of transition from common adolescent bipolar experiences to bipolar disorder: 10-year study. *The British Journal of Psychiatry, 196,* 102–108.

Valentí, M., Pacchiarotti, I., Bonnín, C. M., Rosa, A. R., Popovic, D., Nivoli, A. M.,...Vieta, E. (2012). Risk factors for antidepressant-related switch to mania. *Journal of Clinical Psychiatry, 73,* e271–276.

van der Schot, A. C., Vonk, R., Brans, R. G., van Haren, N. E., Koolschijn, P. C., Nuboer, V., et al. (2009). Influence of genes and environment on brain volumes in twin pairs concordant and discordant for bipolar disorder. *Archives of General Psychiatry, 66,* 142–151.

van der Schot, A. C., Vonk, R., Brouwer, R. M., van Baal, G. C., Brans, R. G., van Haren, N. E.,...Khan, R. S. (2010). Genetic and environmental influences on focal brain density in bipolar disorder. *Brain, 133,* 3080–3092.

Versace, A., Ladouceur, C. D., Romero, S., Birmaher, B., Axelson, D. A., Kupfer, D. J., & Phillips, M. L. (2010). Altered development of white matter in youth at high familial risk for bipolar disorder: A diffusion tensor imaging study. *Journal of the American Academy of Child & Adolescent Psychiatry, 49,* 1249–1259.

Walshe, M., Schulze, K. K., Stahl, D., Hall, M. H., Chaddock, C., Morris, R.,...Kravariti, E. (2012). Sustained attention in bipolar I disorder patients with familial psychosis and their first-degree relatives. *Psychiatry Research, 199,* 70–73.

Walterfang, M., Wood, A. G., Barton, S., Velakoulis, D., Chen, J., Reutens, D. C.,...Frangou, S. (2009). Corpus callosum size and shape alterations in individuals with bipolar disorder and their first-degree relatives. *Progress in Neuro-Psychopharmacology & Biological Psychiatry, 33,* 1050–1057.

Whalley, H. C., Sussmann, J. E., Chakirova, G., Mukerjee, P., Peel, A., McKirdy, J.,...McIntosh, A. M. (2011). The neural basis of familial risk and temperamental variation in individuals at high risk of bipolar disorder. *Biological Psychiatry, 70,* 343–349.

Whalley, H. C., Sussmann, J. E., Romaniuk, L., Stewart, T., Papmeyer, M., Sprooten, E.,...McIntosh, A. M. (2013). Prediction of depression in individuals at high familial risk of mood disorders using functional magnetic resonance imaging. *PLoS One, 8,* e57357.

Yung, A., & McGorry, P. (1996). The initial prodrome in psychosis: Descriptive and qualitative aspects. *Australia and New Zealand Journal of Psychiatry, 30,* 587–599.

25.

ALTERNATIVE AND COMPLEMENTARY TREATMENTS FOR BIPOLAR DISORDER

Janet Wozniak

INTRODUCTION

Like any organ, the brain is affected by nutritional intake. There is no debate that the brain's functions, including thinking, feeling, and behavior can be affected by or corrected by dietary measures. But many questions remain, such as: Which interventions improve which functions? At what age can these interventions exert effects (infancy versus old age)? To what extent and to what degree can positive effects occur? (Bourre, 2006). And, perhaps most important, what are the potential downsides of averting treatment with known efficacious pharmacological agents?

Bipolar disorder (BPD) is associated with high levels of morbidity and documented disability, and unfortunately none of the current conventional treatments can claim a high level of efficacy combined with a low level of adverse events for all individuals. Adverse effects and noncompliance are significant problems in the management of BPD throughout the life cycle (Sajatovic et al., 2008). In particular, the side effects of weight gain, tremors, dyskinesias, acne, gastrointestinal distress, and need for frequent blood test monitoring can minimize adherence to treatment. Individuals, including school-aged children and adolescents but those in the workforce as well, are concerned about cognitive impairments and interference with learning. Increasingly, clinicians, researchers, and patients and their families are turning to an array of natural products and interventions considered complementary and alternative treatments. While these agents have little evidence of efficacy, the fact that they appear to be safe and even healthful make them attractive options to try as monotherapy, especially those with only mild to moderate distress, or as supplements to conventional treatment in many more cases. (Sarris, Lake, & Hoenders, 2011; Sarris, Mischoulon, & Schweitzer, 2012) While studies of these agents generally report disappointing efficacy rates, the fact that

complementary treatments are usually part of a normal diet and likely to have no or minimal side effects leaves many individuals and clinicians seeing little downside in trying them, especially as augmentors. Furthermore, as BPD is often a lifelong condition and is diagnosed at younger and younger ages, the urgent need for early and aggressive treatment needs to be balanced against the side effects of early and lengthy exposure to agents with serious side effects (Jerrell & Prewette, 2008). Alternative treatments offer a healthy option for treating developing youth with psychiatric disturbance. As BPD is severely impairing, lack of intervention is usually not an option. Alternative treatments may be acceptable to a subset of individuals throughout the lifecycle who refuse treatment with conventional agents.

In this chapter, we review some of the agents noted to have mood stabilizing or antidepressant action and that have some evidence base for use in the treatment of BPD, although this is by no means an exhaustive list nor is it an endorsement of the agents described. The use of an alternative treatment must always be weighed against the risk of not using an agent with known antimanic effect on a case-by-case basis. Even positive studies of natural treatments have effect sizes lower than those seen in conventional treatments. Negative studies in adults need not rule out the possibility that used in developing brains, and proximal to the onset of illness, alternative and complementary treatments could play a more robust therapeutic role in pediatric populations.

OMEGA-3 FATTY ACIDS

The notion that inflammatory processes are etiologic in a variety of psychiatric conditions, including BPD, has led to an interest in agents that have anti-inflammatory action, notably omega-3 fatty acids. Fatty acids fall into the family called lipids, and lipids make up over half the mass of the brain, especially important in the structure and function of cell membranes. Cell membrane functioning is critical for cell-to-cell communication as receptor proteins and ion channels sit in the cell membrane. Eicosapentaeonic acid (EPA; 20:5n-3) is an essential fatty acid and metabolite of alpha-linolenic acid (found in flaxseed oil). EPA in turn is metabolized to form docosahexanoic acid (DHA; 22:6n-3). Essential fatty acids, in large part EPA and DHA, make up 20% of the brain's dry weight and are important components of cell membranes and important for cell-to-cell communication.

A fatty acid is "highly unsaturated" if it contains more than four double bonds in its long chain. Double bonds result in greater flexibility of the fatty acid, leading to greater cell membrane fluidity. The term *omega-3* is a chemistry term that refers to the position of the first of these bonds. That is, for omega-3s, the first double bond is located three carbons from the end (or "omega") carbon atom of the molecule. Certain nutrients are considered "essential" and must be ingested, as our body cannot construct them from other molecules. Essential nutrients include the essential amino acids (8 of the 20), vitamins (organic molecules), minerals (inorganic molecules), and essential fatty acids. EPA is an essential fatty acid that can be metabolized to DHA. EPA is a component of the human diet if fish, especially salmon, cod, and tuna, is consumed. Our bodies do have a process for manufacturing EPA via another essential fatty acid, alpha linoleic acid (ALA). ALA is fairly common in our diet, found in vegetable sources such as flaxseed, walnuts and canola oil. ALA can be converted to DHA and EPA. However, this process is not very efficient, so less than 10% of the ALA consumed is converted to EPA and DHA.

Omega-6 fatty acids are fairly common in our diet, primarily from vegetable oils and in particular from corn, safflower, and soybean. The role of the ratio of omega-6 fatty acids to omega-3 acids has been implicated in increasing rates of depression. Arachadonic acid is a common omega-6 fatty acid. In the absence of omega-3 fatty acids, our bodies will use omega-6 fatty acids in our cell membranes. These omega-6 fatty acids, due to the configuration of the double bonds, are less flexible than the omega-3 fatty acids and speculatively result in less efficient cell membrane performance. Arachidonic acid plays a central role in the production of inflammatory eicosanoids, and increase in inflammation from the products of the arachidonic acid pathway has been implicated in cardiovascular disease, joint disease, and mental illness. In contrast, the omega-3 fatty acids are anti-inflammatory. Omega-3 fatty acids and other polyunsaturated fatty acids act as precursors for prostaglandins and second messengers in normal cell physiology.

Omega-3s are known for their healthy effect on the cardiovascular system (Stoll et al., 1999) and their anti-inflammatory properties (versus the unhealthy saturated fats that contribute to coronary artery disease and the omega-6s, which have a proinflammatory effect). Omega-3 fatty acids are known to lower serum lipids, decrease platelet aggregation, maintain arterial elasticity, and play a role in the prevention of diabetes (Terano et al., 1983). Decrease in platelet aggregation, while beneficial in the prevention of atherosclerotic plaques, can lead to increase in bleeding time, but no study has suggested that this is a clinically significant adverse effect. Studies supplementing infant formula with omega-3 fatty acids find positive effects on development and cognition (Willatts, 2002). Indeed, it is now routine to find infant formula supplemented with omega-3 fatty acids.

Clinical evidence suggests that the omega-3 fatty acids EPA and/or DHA may play a therapeutic role in the management of mood disorders. In his letter to the editor in *Lancet*, Hibbeln (1998) linked fish consumption (rich in omega-3 fatty acids) to worldwide rates of depression, initiating a careful look at the role of diet and omega-3 fatty acids in the prevention and treatment of mood disorders. Noaghiul and Hibbeln, (2003) have also noted an association with fish consumption and BPD. Both EPA and DHA are found in large quantities in the brain, particularly in cell membranes. Abnormalities in fatty acid composition of phospholipids in cell membranes have been described in psychiatric disorders in general and in BPD in particular (Horrobin & Bennett, 1999; Horrobin, Glen, & Vaddadi, 1994; Peet, Murphy, Shay, & Horrobin, 1998; Stoll et al., 1999). Patients with depression have increased plasma and red blood cell (RBC) membrane arachidonic acid (omega-6) to EPA (omega-3) ratios (Adams, Lawson, Sanigorski, & Sinclair, 1996). A significant depletion of RBC fatty acids, particularly DHA, was noted in depressed subjects relative to healthy control subjects. Greater severity of depression has been associated with lower RBC membrane levels and low dietary intake of omega-3 fatty acids.

The use of omega-3 fatty acids for the treatment of BPD has been addressed in scientific studies (Horrobin & Bennett, 1999; Post et al., 2003; Stoll et al., 1999). The first study of omega-3 fatty acids for BPD was a four-month, double-blind, placebo-controlled study in which the authors added EPA+DHA, a total of 9.6g (6.2g and 3.4 g, respectively) to ongoing treatment in 30 adults with BPD (Stoll et al., 1999). The authors reported a significantly longer period of remission for those supplemented with omega-3s. Furthermore, these omega-3 supplemented subjects performed better on the Clinical Global Improvement scale (CGI), Global Assessment Scale (GAS), and the Hamilton Depression Rating Scale (HAM-D) than the placebo group (there was no difference in the Young Mania Rating Scale (YMRS)). On the other hand, a discouraging outcome was reported by authors associated with the Stanley Foundation Bipolar Network, which conducted a four-month, double-blind, randomized-controlled study of EPA monotherapy (unlike the previous study in which EPA was added to existing therapy) in 116 bipolar adults. This long-term large-scale study failed to show efficacy. Six grams of EPA daily used as monotherapy was compared with placebo for four months in the treatment of either acute depression or rapid cycling illness (Post et al., 2003). The authors note that this dose may not have been ideal for demonstrating efficacy. Dose-ranging studies in depression and schizophrenia found efficacy at lower dose levels (1–3 g) but not for higher doses. For example, Frangou, Lewis, and McCrone (2006) studied 1 g versus 2 g in a 12-week, double-blind, placebo-controlled trial of bipolar I and II depression. These authors reported improved clinical outcomes compared with placebo on the Hamilton Depression Rating Scale and the CGI but not on the YMRS, with no difference between the treatment groups. Peet & Horrobin (2002) studied 1 g, 2 g, and 4 g in a randomized, double-blind, placebo-controlled trial of depression and found that the 1 g (but not the 2 g or 4 g) per day group performed better than placebo on all three depression rating scales used. A dose-ranging study of DHA suggests that lower doses are more effective (Mischoulon et al., 2008). Pediatric studies in particular could benefit from a study on dosing of omega-3 fatty acids for mood disorders. In one study, effectiveness was noted in those individuals receiving 2 g or greater, but doses beyond 2 g were not associated with greater improvement (Wozniak et al., 2007).

A meta-analysis of five pooled data sets from studies of omega-3 fatty acids for augmentation in BPD ($N = 291$) addressed the relative use of omega-3 fatty acids for mania and bipolar depression. The authors reported statistically significant results in the treatment of bipolar depression with an effect size of 0.34 and a trend toward improvement but nonsignificant findings in the treatment of mania with an effect size of 0.20. They concluded that strong evidence supports the use of omega-3s as an adjunctive treatment for bipolar depression but that the evidence does not support a role in treating mania (Sarris, Mischoulon, & Schweitzer).

Because of the documented efficacy of omega-3 fatty acids in the treatment of adult depression (Nemets, Stahl, & Belmaker, 2002; Peet & Horrobin, 2002), and since depression is a prominent feature of the mixed presentation of pediatric BPD, more work is needed to explore the effectiveness of these compounds in the treatment of pediatric BPD. Negative studies in adults need not rule out the possibility that, used in developing brains proximal to the onset of illness, omega-3 fatty acids could play a therapeutic role. In an eight-week open-label trial in a pediatric population, Wozniak et al. (2007) found that monotherapy with EPA plus DHA was associated with modest improvements in manic symptoms. A 16-week trial of flax oil (ALA) in youth with BPD did not demonstrate efficacy versus placebo (Gracious et al., 2010).

The phospholipid hypothesis of mental illness proposes that neurotransmitter receptor functioning is affected by the fatty acid composition of the phospholipids of the cell membrane (Horrobin & Bennett, 1999). With reduced omega-3 fatty acids, the fatty acid composition of the cell membrane phospholipids would be altered, possibly leading to altered neurotransmitter binding and psychopathology. Several studies have shown reduced levels of omega-3 fatty acids in the RBC membranes, fibroblasts, and even in the postmortem brain tissue of schizophrenic patients (Yao, Leonard, & Reddy, 2000). Other studies demonstrate increased uptake of omega-3 fatty acids into the RBC membrane of treated subjects, raising the question as to whether subjects have a dietary deficiency in omega-3 fatty acids that can be corrected by supplementation. No clear guidelines exist on normal blood levels of omega-3 fatty acids, but the increase in blood levels with supplementation may be an indicator of a relatively depleted state.

As omega-3 fatty acids have also been shown to be protective against coronary heart disease, a relative deficiency of omega-3 fatty acids may help explain the observed link between heart disease, cardiac mortality, and depression. (Stoll et al., 1999) Converging evidence thus suggests that omega-3 fatty acids may be protective for both heart disease and mood disorder, which has important clinical implications, especially given the increased risk for diabetes associated with the atypical antipsychotics commonly used in the treatment of BPD.

Omega-3 fatty acids are part of normal metabolism, thus the likelihood of unwanted side effects is low. The only adverse effects reported with omega-3 fatty acids are the mild gastrointestinal disturbance (loose stool), minimized by taking them with food. A "fishy" taste or fishy burps decrease compliance, but this can be mitigated by taking with food or switching brands. A recent study linked omega-3 fatty acids to cancer, but whether this will change recommendations for use is unclear (DiNicolantonio, 2013).

INOSITOL

Inositol is a precursor for, as well as a product of the phosphatidylinositol (PI) cycle and therefore common and widely found, located primarily within cell membranes (Baraban, 1989). The PI cycle is the second messenger system for numerous neurotransmitter receptors, including cholinergic muscarinic, alpha 1 noradrenergic, serotonin (5-HT$_{2A}$ and 5-HT$_{2C}$), and dopaminergic D$_1$ receptors. Inositol has been referred to as vitamin B8 and is a structural isomer of glucose. Myoinositol comprises 95% of total free inositol in the human body (Clements, 1980; Moore et al., 1999). Inositol is present in numerous different foods in low amounts; it is present in higher amounts in beans, grains, nuts, and many fruits (Clements, 1980). The average adult human consumes about 1 g of inositol in the daily diet (Baraban, 1989).

Lithium may, among other actions, exert clinical effects due to its actions on the phosphoinositol second messenger system (PI cycle). This, coupled with the finding that inositol was shown to be decreased in the cerebrospinal fluid (CSF) of depressed patients with depression, has formed a rationale for its use in mood disorders. However, Levine et al., 1993 studied CSF inositol in patients treated with inositol for depression and found that baseline CSF inositol did not predict response to inositol treatment.

Increased levels of the monophosphatase enzyme that breaks down inositol have been reported in patients with depression and schizophrenia. Inositol is also decreased in the frontal cortex of postmortem brains of patients with BPD and in those who completed suicide compared with normal controls (Shimon, Agam, Belmaker, Hyde, & Kleinman, 1997). Silverstone showed that chronic treatment with either lithium or sodium valproate in bipolar patients may normalize PI-cycle functioning. Berridge, Downes, and Hanley (1989) et al suggested that lithium may treat BPD by inhibiting the enzyme inositol-1-monophosphatase and causing a relative inositol deficiency, leading to the speculation that mania is a disorder of excess inositol and depression results from its deficit. In addition, in animal models of depression, inositol has been shown to reduce depressive behaviors. Positive studies of inositol in humans have been reported in the treatment of depression, panic disorder, obsessive-compulsive disorder, and bulimia (Levine, 1997; Mukai, Kishi, Matsuda, & Iwata, 2014). In Europe, over-the-counter inositol has long been used as a folk remedy for depression (Belmaker et al., 1996).

The mechanism of action of inositol remains unclear. From the available evidence, we indirectly presume that subjects with mood disorders experience a decrease in brain myo-inositol, which adversely affects the functioning of the PI second messenger system, which in turns results in mood changes. Dietary supplement with inositol, therefore, could improve the functioning of the PI system and treat the depressive symptoms. Lithium may operate conversely by lowering or blocking myo-inositol, the so-called inositol depletion hypothesis: that is, lithium produces a lowering of myo-inositol in the brain, via inositol monophosphatase, bringing about a mood-stabilizing effect (Atack et al., 1998; Silverstone et al., 2005).

Mood stabilizer medications may be better thought of as producing an action that stabilizes inositol and its actions. Lithium, valproate, and carbamazepine act in human astrocyte cells to decrease inositol uptake at high inositol concentrations and increase inositol uptake at low inositol concentrations, suggesting a much more complicated mode of action (Kaya, Ozerdem, Guner, & Tunca, 2004; Wolfson, Bersudsky, Hertz, et al., 2000; Wolfson, Bersudsky, Zinger, et al., 2000; Wolfson, Einat, et al., 2000). Kaya et al. found that erythrocyte IMPase activity was higher in lithium treated euthymic patients than nonlithium-treated patients; increased IMPase activity by chronic lithium use suggests paradoxically, over time, an upregulation of the enzyme activity (Kaya, 2004).

In response to the seemingly contradictory findings, Belmaker (1997) evolved the inositol polyphosphate signal suppression hypothesis and hypothesized that inositol's effect in the brain was much more complex than simply being a matter of too much or too little (Belmaker, 1997; Belmaker et al., 1996). He suggests a complex regulation with a "pendulum" effect where a push from either direction, high or low concentration, causes an identical effect. When inositol supplements lithium treatment, it reverses the effects of lithium on protein kinase C levels, but inositol monotherapy has effects similar to those of lithium. Further, because the PI cycle serves as a second messenger for several balancing and mutually interactive neurotransmitters, Belmaker hypothesizes that exogenous inositol could hypothetically alleviate inositol deficiency in one system without increasing inositol above normal levels in another (Belmaker, 1997; Belmaker et al., 1996).

Trials with inositol in pediatric BPD are limited to measuring levels in neurochemical spectroscopic studies; despite its safety and ease of administration, there are no clinical trials examining the efficacy of inositol in the treatment of pediatric BPD. Davanzo et al. (2001) measured changes in myo-inositol levels in the anterior cingulate cortex of 11 children (mean age 11.4 years) diagnosed with BPD, currently manic, hypomanic, or mixed before and after lithium therapy (mean serum level of 0.64 mEq/L) and in 11 case-matched controls at baseline and at Day 7 using proton magnetic resonance spectroscopy (^{1}H MRS). There was a significant decrease in anterior cingulate myo-inositol/Cr ratio following seven days of lithium therapy in children and adolescents with BPD. When responders and nonresponders were compared at Week 1, myo-inositol/Cr was decreased at one week versus baseline in the lithium-responder group, but not in the lithium nonresponder group consistent with report by Moore et al., 1999, but contrasting with report by Silverstone et al., 2005. These same authors compared myo-inositol levels in the anterior cingulate of 10 youth on various medications with bipolar I disorder (most recent episode manic or mixed), 10 youth with intermittent explosive disorder, and 13 normal comparison youth using ^{1}H MRS (Davanzo et al., 2003). The patients with BPD had significantly higher mean anterior cingulate myo-inositol and myo-inositol/creatinine-phosphocreatine measures than the patients with intermittent explosive disorder and the normal comparison subjects. There were no significant differences in levels between the youth with intermittent explosive disorder and the normal comparison subjects. There was no significant difference in levels between groups in the occipital cortex.

Patel et al. (2006) reported on an open-label study of 28 inpatient adolescents (12 to 18 years old; mean age 15.5 years) who met *Diagnostic and Statistical Manual of Mental Disorders* (fourth edition [*DSM-IV*]; American Psychiatric Association, 1994) criteria for diagnosis of bipolar I disorder, currently depressed, given lithium doses adjusted to serum levels of 1.0 to 1.2 mEq/L. Myo-inositol concentrations in the medial as well as the left and right lateral prefrontal cortices were measured using ^{1}H MRS scan at baseline, Day 7, and Day 42 of treatment. Lithium administration did not result in significant changes from baseline in myo-inositol concentrations in the medial as well as the left and right lateral prefrontal cortices. Consistent with previous studies (Moore et al., 1999), these authors suggested that the insositol-depletion hypothesis may not be the mechanism of action of lithium in patients with bipolar depression.

Magnetic resonance spectroscopic studies have also been completed on adult subjects. Frey et al. (1998) studied 22 unmedicated depressed bipolar and unipolar patients and found reduced myo-inositol concentrations in the frontal lobes compared with 22 healthy controls, although this finding was significant only when the groups were paired by age (<40 years old). Moore et al. (1999) found an initial significant increase of myo-inositol/Cr levels in the occipital cortex gray matter and parietal white matter of 17 healthy subjects taking a dietary supplement of 12g/day inositol, but this level returned to baseline by Day 8. Moore et al. also investigated lithium's effects on in vivo brain myo-inositol levels in 12 adults (mean age 36.6 years) diagnosed with *DSM-IV* diagnosis of BPD, most recently depressed. Patients underwent a drug washout period of at least 14 days, then underwent a baseline MRS scan prior to initiation of treatment with lithium. Brain myo-inositol levels were measured by ^{1}H MRS after acute (five to seven days) and chronic (three to four weeks) lithium treatment. In the right frontal lobe, the myo-inositol concentrations during both acute and chronic treatment were significantly lower than at baseline before correction for multiple comparisons but not after correction. Lowering of myo-inositol levels per se did not appear to be associated with therapeutic efficacy. The authors hypothesized that the initial reduction of myo-inositol initiates a cascade of secondary changes in the protein kinase C signaling pathway and gene expression in the central nervous system, effects that may ultimately be responsible for lithium's therapeutic efficacy. No significant differences were found in the temporal, occipital, and parietal lobes.

Taken together, these neuroimaging studies suggest that inositol is implicated in the pathophysiology of BPD and that treatment with exogenous inositol or with medications that affect brain inositol levels (lithium) results in brain chemistry changes associated with clinical improvement. The conflicting results lend credence to Belmaker's statements highlighting the complex, pendulum like, role of inositol.

Double-blind, controlled trials of inositol treatment of depression in adults offer conflicting evidence regarding the use of inositol in clinical practice. A recent meta-analysis of seven RCTs concluded that inositol may be beneficial for depression, especially for premenstrual dysphoric disorder, but that there are too few studies to draw firm conclusions (Mukai et al., 2014). Levine et al. conducted a four-week study of 27 adults with *Diagnostic and Statistical Manual of Mental Disorders* (third edition, revised [*DSM-III-R*]; American Psychiatric Association, 1980) diagnosis for major depression or BPD, depressed, who had failed antidepressant treatment or dropped out due to side effects. Subjects were given either inositol 12 g/day or a placebo. Treatment with inositol resulted in significantly greater improvement in Hamilton Depression Rating Scale score than for placebo in females (but not in males) with unipolar depression at four weeks (there was no difference at two weeks). In a follow-up study, half of the patients who had responded well to inositol relapsed rapidly after inositol discontinuation, whereas none of those who responded to placebo relapsed rapidly after placebo cessation.

Several studies in adults have addressed the utility of inositol as an adjunctive treatment to selective serotonin reuptake inhibitors (SSRIs) or other treatment for depression. Adding inositol to SSRI treatment under double-blind conditions in 27 adults with *DSM-IV* diagnosis of major depression resulted in no improvement of effect and no side effects (Levine et al., 1999). Forty-two depressed adults who were failing a three to four-week trial of SSRI were randomized to receive as an adjunct either inositol 12g/day or a placebo. Inositol was found to have no effect for augmenting the response to SSRI therapy in depression (Nemets et al., 1999).

Three studies of inositol as an adjunctive treatment in bipolar adults have suggested at best a modest clinical effect of inositol. Twenty-two adults diagnosed with *DSM-IV* bipolar depression were given either inositol 12 g/day or placebo as add-on treatment to current medication. There was a nonsignificant but encouraging difference between the two groups, with 50% of inositol subjects improving versus 30% of placebo subjects (Chengappa et al., 2000). The authors concluded that a controlled study with an adequate sample size may demonstrate efficacy for inositol in bipolar depression.

Sixty-six bipolar adults, currently depressed, were randomized to receive lamotrigine, risperidone, or inositol (target dose 10–25 mg) added on to regular treatment for eight weeks (Nierenberg et al., 2006). There were no significant between-group differences; however, post hoc analysis suggested that lamotrigine may be superior to inositol and risperidone in improving treatment-resistant bipolar depression. Recovery rate with lamotrigine was 23.8%, with risperidone 4.6%, and with inositol 17.4%. A similar study by Evins et al. (2006) randomized 17 depressed bipolar adults on therapeutic levels of lithium or valproate to receive either inositol 5 to 20 g/day or a placebo as adjunct treatment. While 44% on inositol versus 0% on the placebo met response criteria for symptoms of depression, this finding was not statistically significant.

A study of inositol for attention deficit hyperactivity disorder in 11 children failed to demonstrate efficacy, but this study demonstrated that treatment was well tolerated in children in doses of 200 mg per kg body weight (Levine, 1997). A review of controlled trials of inositol in psychiatry reported no changes found in hematology, kidney, or liver function tests (Levine, 1997). There is no established recommended daily allowance for inositol. Studies of adults have used dosages ranging from 6 to 25 g/day of inositol or myo-inositol given in divided doses. One study suggested that 12 g/day of inositol has been shown to raise CSF inositol levels by 70% (Levine et al., 1993). Studies

for inositol in pediatric mood disorders are lacking, but the two studies of inositol in psychiatry for children used a dose of 200 mg per kg and offers initial evidence of the safety and tolerability of this dose (Levine, 1997).

Regarding safety, like many nutraceutical agents, inositol has been found to be generally well tolerated in adult and pediatric trials. Side effects reported in available studies include mild increases in glucose, flatus, nausea, sleepiness and insomnia, dizziness, and headache. Inositol has been studied as an adjunctive agent, and no drug interactions have been reported to date. There have been case reports of inositol-induced mania, suggesting caution in those with BPD.

N-ACETYLCYSTEINE

N-acetylcysteine, also known as acetylcysteine or N-acetyl-L-cysteine (NAC), has generated excitement as a natural treatment/dietary supplement that may be useful in psychiatry due both to its known physiological targets as well as emerging clinical trials. N-acetylcysteine is an acetylated amino acid and a precursor of glutathione that acts as an antioxidant in the brain to reduce oxidative stress, which has been implicated in BPD and major depression (Magalhaes et al., 2011). Further, NAC may modulate glutamatergic pathways and play a role in modulating inflammation. Because NAC breaks disulfide bonds in mucous, making it less viscous, it has also been commonly used in cough medications or as a mucolytic in patients with pulmonary mucous. When ingested, NAC provides increased cysteine levels leading to the synthesis of more glutathione in the brain. NAC is perhaps best known to physicians as an antidote to acetaminophen/paracetamol (Tylenol) overdose. Acetaminophen overdose results in life-threatening liver damage, which occurs via an acetaminophen metabolite that is normally cleared via conjugation with the body's supply of glutathione. In case of overdose, this normal pathway becomes overwhelmed, glutathione is depleted, and the reactive metabolite builds up, which is directly toxic to the hepatocyte cell membranes, resulting in liver necrosis. NAC is a precursor for glutathione; NAC increases the liver's supply of glutathione and thus assists in the clearance of the toxic metabolite. Ingesting glutathione itself is not helpful due to poor absorption and rapid metabolism, and therefore it never reaches the brain. NAC, however, crosses the blood-brain barrier with ease (Dean, Giorlando, & Berk, 2011; Witschi, Reddy, Stofer, & Lauterburg, 1992).

Oxidation biology, or the study of oxidative stress with subsequent cellular damage, has been considered a possible mechanism contributing to brain cell malfunction and consequent psychiatric symptoms. The main interest in psychiatry involves NAC as a precursor to glutathione, which acts as a potent antioxidant diminishing free radicals that can lead to cell damage and death. Glutathione is the major endogenous antioxidant in the brain. Glutathione is a molecule comprising three peptides: glutamate, cysteine, and glycine. The addition of the cysteine is the rating limiting step, and NAC provides this key substrate for the creation of glutathione. Glutathione neutralizes potentially damaging oxidative free radicals in a cascade of biochemical reactions in the mitochondria. Mitochondrial structure and activity have been implicated in psychiatric conditions, especially schizophrenia. Mitochondria are the source of damaging free radicals, a by-product of energy production. Low glutathione levels have long been noted psychiatric illness. Omega-3 fatty acids, useful in BPD, also increase brain glutathione.

The cystine portion of NAC is a key player in the transport of glutamate out of the cell. Through a feedback mechanism with astrocytes, this can result in diminished release of glutamate into the extracellular space. Thus this additional role, regulating glutamate levels, may additionally play a therapeutic role, as malfunctions in the glutamate system result in consequent excito-toxic damage from activation of the N-methyl-D-aspartate glutamate receptor. NAC in a similar way regulates the release of dopamine from presynaptic terminals. NAC is also an anti-inflammatory.

Coupled with the purported mechanism of action, a large, lengthy clinical trial with placebo control has provided compelling interest in NAC as an evidence-based treatment for BPD. In this double-blind, randomized, placebo-controlled trial of 1,000 mg twice a day (BID) NAC (or placebo) added to treatment as usual, 75 bipolar subjects were assessed over six months. Large decreases in the Montgomery-Asberg Depression Rating Scale and the Bipolar Depression Rating Scale scores were seen in the treated versus the placebo group. In addition, global improvement was noted. In those with bipolar II disorder, six of the seven treated with NAC attained remission of both depression and mania, versus only two of seven in the placebo group. These positive effects were lost after treatment discontinuation (Berk et al., 2008; Berk et al., 2011; Magalhaes et al., 2011).

This treatment's utility in moderate depression in BPD was investigated in an open-label eight-week trial of NAC 1000 mg BID with 149 subjects. One hundred thirty-two completed the trial. There was a statistically significant decrease in depression rating scale scores as well as improvements in functioning and quality of life with open-label NAC added to treatment as usual (Berk et al., 2008; Berk et al., 2011). This trial was part of a double-blind, randomized, placebo-controlled trial. After the eight-week open-label trial, participants were randomized to placebo or continued NAC for 24 more weeks. Of the 132 subjects in the open-label trial, 121 were randomized with at least one follow-up visit. Because of the very low level of symptoms in this double-blind phase, between-group differences could not be discerned and so the trial was considered failed rather than negative (Berk et al., 2012).

NAC has been shown to be helpful in a multitude of disorders, including the treatment of marijuana, nicotine and cocaine addictions, gambling, obsessive-compulsive disorder, skin picking, nail biting, trichotillomania, schizophrenia, and BPD, suggesting that it may address the end of the line pathway targets common to multiple disturbances. Which disorders are more robustly treated is unclear, as is the best dose. Generally well tolerated, concern about asthma results from idiosyncratic adverse events, and animal (but not human) subjects have developed pulmonary hypertension with high doses. Seizures have been reported with high doses (Berk, Malhi, Gray, & Dean, 2013).

S-ADENOSYL-L-METHIONINE

S-adenosyl-L-methionine (SAMe) has been routinely prescribed in Europe as treatment for depression since the 1970s and has gained popularity in the United States since its release as an over-the-counter dietary supplement in 1999. It is one of the better-studied natural agents used to treat depression. SAMe is produced in mammals from the essential amino acid L-methionine and adenosine triphosphate. Adequate concentrations of folate and vitamin B_{12} are required for the production of SAMe. SAMe is found throughout the human body, although particularly high concentrations have been measured in the liver, adrenal glands, and pineal gland (Mischoulon & Fava, 2002). Concentrations are highest in childhood and decrease with age.

SAMe serves as a crucial intermediate of three major pathways in all biological systems: methylation, transulfuration, and aminopropylation. These pathways are known to be involved in the synthesis of nucleic acids, proteins, phospholipids, hormones, neurotransmitters, antioxidants, polyamines, catecholamines, and other biogenic amines; it is required for the synthesis of norepinephrine, dopamine, and serotonin (Mischoulon & Fava, 2002).

Bottiglieri et al. (1990) demonstrated that CSF SAMe was significantly lower in severely depressed patients compared to neurological control groups and significantly increased following intravenous SAMe 200 mg/day or oral SAMe 1,200 mg/day. Bell et al. (1994) conducted a double-blind, randomized study comparing oral SAMe 1,600 mg/day with oral desipramine 250 mg/day in 26 depressed adults for four weeks. Sixty-two percent of the patients treated with SAMe and 50% of the patients treated with desipramine significantly improved. Responders (50% decrease in their HAM-D score), regardless of type of treatment, showed a significant increase in plasma SAMe concentration with treatment.

Because SAMe takes part in many metabolic pathways, defining the mechanisms of action of SAMe's antidepressant effect is difficult. Possible direct or indirect metabolic or receptor effects on monoamine neurotransmission (e.g., norepinephrine, dopamine, and serotonin) or on neuronal membrane structure and function in the brain has been theorized to play a role in SAMe's antidepressant effects. In addition, Williams (2005) discussed the potential role SAMe plays in reversing regional brain volume loss in depressive rat models.

A number of adult studies have evaluated SAMe's antidepressant effectiveness. In 2002 the Agency for Healthcare Research and Quality published a meta-analysis of placebo-controlled SAMe trials for the treatment of depression, osteoarthritis, and liver disease (Hardy et al., 2003). This meta-analysis noted that the majority of the 28 depression studies they evaluated enrolled small numbers of patients and varied greatly in their quality. The authors determined that, compared to placebo, treatment with SAMe was associated with an improvement of approximately 6 points in the score of the Hamilton Rating Scale for Depression measured at three weeks. This was a statistically as well as clinically significant, albeit partial, response. When compared to treatment with tricyclic antidepressants, treatment with SAMe was not associated with a statistically significant difference in outcomes (though not all of these trials were adequately powered to discern a difference between SAMe and the tricyclics; some used only low to moderate doses of tricyclics; and a majority involved parenteral formulations of SAMe). Some studies have suggested a faster onset of action for SAMe than for conventional antidepressants and report that it may even accelerate the effect of conventional antidepressants (Mischoulon & Fava, 2002). Alpert et al. (2004) conducted a six-week open trial of 30 adults (23 completed the trial) with major depression to evaluate the safety, tolerability, and efficacy of oral SAMe when used as an adjunct among partial or nonresponders to SSRI antidepressants or venlafaxine. Subjects started with SAMe 400 mg BID to augment current treatment,

then increased to 800 mg BID after 2 weeks. There was a significant decrease in depression severity from baseline to endpoint. No patient experienced serious adverse events, including serotonin syndrome. There was a significant but modest (4.9%) decrease in pretreatment to posttreatment homocysteine levels.

Very limited data exist on the use of SAMe for treatment of pediatric depression. Schaller, Thomas, and Bazzan (2004) described three case reports of the use of SAMe for pediatric major depression. In Case 1, an 11-year-old girl (34 kg) diagnosed with *Diagnostic and Statistical Manual of Mental Disorders* (fourth edition, text revision [*DSM-IV-TR*]; American Psychiatric Association, 2000) major depression was placed on 200 mg SAMe enteric-coated tabled each morning for one week, then increased to 400 mg every morning. Improvement began four days after increasing the dose, with modest improvement over three weeks. At three weeks, the dose was increased to 600 mg every morning, which resulted in complete resolution of depressive symptoms two days after the dose increase. She had no signs of mania or anxiety. Her Children's Depression Inventory (CDI) fell from 34 to 4. She had been on this dose for six months at the time of the report without complications and with continued efficacy.

In Case 2, an eight-year-old girl (24 kg) with *DSM-IV TR* major depression and a CDI score of 29 was treated with 200 mg of SAMe. She started showing improvement by Day 2 and was at baseline by Day 11. She had increased sadness at three months and was increased to 200 mg BID, with a resultant decrease of CDI score to 6. She had been on this dose for six months at the time of the report without complications and with continued efficacy.

In Case 3, a 16-year-old male diagnosed with *DSM-IV TR* major depression and oppositional defiant disorder who refused traditional antidepressants but agreed to a trial of SAMe was started on 200 mg with an increase in dose to 1,800 mg/day over 10 days. He experienced slight tremor and anxiety on 1,800 mg/day, but after decrease to 1,400 mg/day the side effects abated. His mood and function improved to baseline over one to two weeks, although he continued to have residual oppositional behavior. After two to three months he stopped taking SAMe, which resulted in relapse over the next three weeks. Restarting 800 mg every morning and 400 mg every afternoon restored him to baseline in five to eight days.

The recommended adult dose of SAMe ranges from 400 to 1,600 mg/day, although some individuals may require doses of 3,000 mg/day or more to alleviate depression (Mischoulon & Fava, 2002); there is no established dose range for children and adolescents. It is available in capsule and powder form.

Enteric-coated formulation have helped address the chemical instability of older formulations (Alpert et al., 2004).

Although short-term trials have suggested that SAMe is safe, no long-term data exist. Potential adverse effects include gastrointestinal side effects (primarily flatulence and diarrhea), headache, dizziness, dry mouth, nausea, and cold or flu-like symptoms. In addition, mild nausea, restlessness, and moderate increase in anxiety have been observed in some patients (Bell et al., 1994).

Several reports of mania while on SAMe exist in the literature. In patients with personal or family history of BPD SAMe should likely be avoided unless patients are also taking a mood stabilizer. Iruela et al. (1993) published a case report describing altered mentations, fever, hyperreflexia, and elevated creatinine phosphokinase when SAMe (100 mg intramuscular) was combined with clomipramine 75 mg in a 71-year-old woman. Similar symptoms suggesting serotonin syndrome have not been described in controlled studies evaluating the efficacy and safety of SAMe administered in conjugation with older antidepressants (Alpert et al., 2004). Since SAMe is ultimately metabolized to homocysteine, it is theoretically possible that SAMe administration could lead to increased homocysteine levels. In contrast, due to SAMe-associated elevations in 5-methyltetrahydrofolate, a cofactor of homocysteine metabolism, SAMe has been postulated to be effective in treating elevated homocysteine. Thomas et al. (1987) performed a double-blind, placebo-controlled trial in which 20 subjects with depression were given SAMe; they found a highly significant fall in prolactin concentrations in the SAM-treated group after 14 days of treatment. Fava et al. (1990) investigated the effects of treatment with SAMe on TSH and prolactin response to thyrotropin-releasing-hormone (TRH) stimulation in 7 depressed outpatient women (without childbearing potential) and 10 depressed outpatient men in a six-week open study of oral SAMe (maximum dose of 1,600 mg/day) in the treatment of major depression. There was a significant reduction after treatment with SAMe in the response of both prolactin and TSH to TRH stimulation in the group of depressed men but not in the women. Interactions with other drugs are not well known. Theoretically, SAMe may potentiate the activity and/or toxicities of MAO inhibitors, tricyclic antidepressants, or SSRIs, though this has not been documented.

ST. JOHN'S WORT

St. John's wort (*Hypericum perforatum*), a five-petal perennial flowering plant that grows in many areas of the world, is one of the most extensively studied of the medicinal plants (Butterweck, 2003; Findling et al., 2003). Studied in psychiatric disorders, including depression, seasonal affective disorder, anxiety, obsessive-compulsive disorder, and social phobia, it has been used for depression in Europe for centuries and is approved for treatment of depression in Germany. In fact, St. John's wort products and tricyclic antidepressants account for more that 80% of antidepressant use in Germany's children and adolescents. While a number of biologically active constituents of St. John's wort have been identified, hypericin and hyperforin have been most often related to St. John's wort's antidepressant effects.

The exact antidepressant mechanism of action of St. John's wort is not fully understood. It has been reported to modulate neurotransmitter levels and receptors including serotonin and norepinephrine, as well as γ-aminobutyric acid and glutamate amino acid. While there have been reports that St. John's wort inhibits monoamine oxidase (MAO), subsequent investigations have reported only a weak potency as a MAO inhibitor that is not strong enough to have relevance in the antidepressant effect of St. John's wort (Butterweck, 2003). Additional proposed mechanisms of action include modification of inflammatory cytokines, inhibition of cortisol production, modulation of neuronal ionic conductance, elevation of intracellular sodium concentration, and induction of neurogenesis and neuroprotection (Nierenberg, Lund, & Mischoulon, 2008).

While many studies (mostly conducted in Europe) have supported the antidepressant effects of St. John's wort, several key adult studies in the United States have been negative. Linde & Knuppel (2005) conducted a meta-analysis of randomized controlled trials in which they investigated 23 trials involving placebo-controlled groups and 13 trials comparing hypericum extracts with standard antidepressants. They reported that, in adults with mild to moderate depression, *Hypericum perforatum* extracts improved symptoms more than placebo and similarly to standard antidepressants. They reported, however, that pooled analysis of six large, more recent, and more precise trials restricted to patients with major depression showed only minimal benefits of *Hypericum* extract compared with placebo. This meta-analysis found that *Hypericum* extracts caused fewer adverse effects than older antidepressants and might have caused slightly fewer adverse effects than SSRIs. Since the 2005 meta-analysis, there have been at least six positive studies and at least two large negative studies regarding the antidepressant effect of St. John's wort (Fava et al., 2005).

St. John's wort has been studied for treatment of pediatric depression. In 2005, Simeon et al. (2005) published an eight-week, open-label pilot study of 26 adolescents (12 to 17 years old) diagnosed with major depressive disorder (MDD) who were given St. John's wort (300 mg three times daily). Nine patients out of the 11 who completed the study (82%) showed significant clinical improvement at Week 8. Statistically significant clinical improvements appeared during the first week and continued to be noted until Week 8. Mild and transient side effects were noted and included restlessness, dry mouth, nightmares, confusion, loss of attentiveness, nausea, and fatigue. There were no significant changes in blood tests, urinalysis, weight, blood pressure, and electrocardiogram. Of note, 15 patients withdrew from the study due to persisting or worsening depression or noncompliance. In 2003, Findling and colleagues (2003) published results of an eight-week, open-label pilot study of 30 youth (6 to 16 years old) diagnosed with MDD of at least moderate severity. They were given 150 to 300 mg of St. John's wort three times daily. Twenty-four percent met response criteria at the end of Week 4 (83% at the end of the study). Ninety-three percent of the patients who completed eight weeks chose to continue their treatment with St. John's wort after their participation in the study ended. The most common side effects were generally mild and transient and included dizziness, increased appetite, and loose stools. No clinically significant changes in weight, vitals, laboratory parameters, or electrocardiogram were noted. In addition, to investigate its pharmacodynamics in vivo, fasting predose morning 5-HT levels were obtained at baseline, at Week 4, and at the end of the study. End of Week 4 or 8 5-HT levels did not significantly differ from baseline (Findling 2003). Finally, in 2001 Hubner et al. reported on a multicenter postmarketing surveillance study (Hubner, 2001). One hundred one children under 12 years with symptoms of depression and psychovegetative disturbances were treated for four to six weeks with St. John's wort 300 to 900 mg/ day (one coated tablet containing 300 mg *Hypericum perforatum* extract was standardized to contain 900µg hypericin). Compliance, tolerability, and efficacy were assessed every two weeks by physicians and parents. Physicians rating of effectiveness as "good" or "excellent" was 72% after two weeks, 97% after four weeks, and 100% after six weeks, though the amount of missing data also increased with time, with results based on 94% of the initial sample at two weeks, 89% at four weeks, and 76% at the final assessment. No adverse events were reported. Dropouts were due to achievement of therapeutic goal, inadequate therapeutic effect, difficulty swallowing tablets, and going on holiday.

Doses of 300 to -900 mg/day have been studied in children and 900 to 1,800 mg/day in adults. Capsules generally are standardized to contain 0.3% to 0.5% hypericin and/or 3% to 5% hyperforin per dose. Given that hyperforin and hypericin content can vary between commercially available St. John's wort products, users are encouraged to use the same brand on a regular basis to help ensure consistency in response (Wurglics et al., 2001).

The most commonly reported side effects of St. John's wort include dry mouth, gastrointestinal symptoms (such as constipation), dizziness/confusion, tiredness/sedation, urinary frequency, anorgasmia, and swelling (Knuppel & Linde, 2004). In addition, St. John's wort can cause photosensitivity. A review of data from 35 double-blind randomized trials showed that dropout and adverse effects rates in patients receiving hypericum extracts were similar to placebo, lower than with older antidepressants, and slightly lower than with SSRI (Knuppel & Linde, 2004).

Caution should be used in patients with personal or family history of BPD, as St. John's wort has been reported to induce mania and worsen anxiety (Nierenberg et al. 1999). Also, St. John's wort has been theorized to cause an increase in thyroid-stimulating hormone, though a clear link has not been established. Finally, in 2008, Karalapillai and Bellomo (2007) reported a case of a 16-year-old-girl who presented with a seizure due to an overdose of St. John's wort. She reportedly took up to fifteen 300µg tablets a day in the two weeks leading to her seizure, plus an additional 50 tabs just before presentation.

St. John's wort has been shown to significantly induce the activity of the cytochrome P-450 system, mostly CYP 3A4 (but also CYP2C9 and CYP1A2) and the drug transporter P-glycoprotein, which may result in diminished clinical effectiveness or increased dosage requirements for substrates. In addition, combination with SSRIs, MAOIs, and other antidepressants may result in serotonin syndrome (Whitten, 2006).

LECITHIN

Lecithin has been examined for its possible role in the treatment of many neurological disorders, including mania, memory impairment, tardive dyskinesia, Gilles de la Tourette's disease, Friedreich's ataxia, levodopa-induced dyskinesia, Huntington's, Alzheimer's, spastic spinocerebellar degeneration, myasthenic syndromes, and tardive dyskinesia (Wood & Allison, 1982). Discovered by French scientist Maurice Gobley in 1805, lecithin is a naturally occurring phospholipid that acts as an emulsifier; it is found in several foods, including egg yolks, soybeans, nuts, and whole grains, as well as in organ meats. It often is used as an emulsification agent in processed foods. Dietary lecithin intake varies, but generally ranges from 1 to 5 grams per day. It has been theorized that low-fat and low-cholesterol diets may lower the amount of lecithin consumed, thus creating a deficit (Wood & Allison, 1982). Commercially available lecithin is a complex mixture of phosphatidyl esters, mainly phosphatidylcholine, phosphatidylethanolamine, phosphatidylserine, and PI. Phosphatidyl choline is an important structural component of cellular membranes. Choline is the precursor of the neurotransmitter acetylcholine. Underactivity of central cholinergic mechanisms has been hypothesized as an underlying feature in a number of neuropsychiatric disorders, including mania (Rosenberg & Davis, 1982). Neuroimaging studies have demonstrated altered membrane phospholipid metabolism in the frontal lobes and basal ganglia of patients with BPD; Cecil, DelBello, Morey, and Strakowski (2002) have reported lowered choline levels within the orbital frontal gray matter in adolescents and young adults with bipolar disorder, manic phase, found on MR spectroscopy. The effect of lecithin taken orally has been noted to be considerably greater and more prolonged than ingestion of an equivalent amount of choline chloride (Wurtman, 1977). In addition to its role in increasing acetylcholine, lecithin has been noted to cause changes in neurotransmitter receptor availability in cell membranes (Cohen et al., 1980, 1982).

In 1979 Cohen et al. reported on an open trial they had conducted at a private psychiatric hospital in which eight newly admitted patients with manic-depressive illness, manic phase, were treated with lithium and/or neuroleptics + either Lethicon (51%–55% pure lecithin) or Phospholipon 100 (>90% pure lecithin). Subjects received a dose of 15 g/day of lecithin in the first week and 30 g/day of lecithin in the second week. Manic subjects were found to be intolerant of 15 g/day of lecithin in the 50% pure form but were reported to be tolerant of as much as 30 g/day in the 90% pure form. All subjects who received Phospholipon 100 improved rapidly, and three of four showed some worsening following its withdrawal. Three years later, Cohen and colleagues (1982) reported on augmentation with lecithin in a double-blind, placebo-controlled trial of six adult psychiatric inpatients with *DSM-III* diagnosis of BPD, manic phase (except one patient with schizoaffective disorder). All patients had been on a stable medication regimen for one month prior to the study and remained on that regimen throughout the course of the study. Patients were given either 10 mg three times daily of >90% pure lecithin or a placebo. Lecithin resulted in significant improvement compared to the placebo and was noted to have a clear therapeutic effect in five of six patients studied. Lecithin did not lead to the appearance of depressive symptoms in any of the patients studied.

While there have been no similar trials in children and adolescents, in 1981 Schreier reported a case of a 13-year-old manic girl who did not respond to neuroleptics or lithium but appeared to respond to 15 to 23 g/day of 90% pure lecithin monotherapy with a remission lasting at least 13 months (Schreier, 1981).

Because lecithin is not considered an essential nutrient, no recommended daily allowance has been set. Doses of 1 to 45 g/day have been used for various conditions (Wood, & Allison, 1982). As it is a dietary supplement, lecithin has not undergone the rigorous safety testing required for prescription drugs, though generally it has been regarded as safe for most adults, except in those highly allergic to soy. High intakes of lecithin (>25g per day) or choline have been reported to cause acute gastrointestinal distress, sweating, salivation, and anorexia (Wood & Allison, 1982).

Caution must be used with lecithin, as it is possible that some patients may become depressed with increased cholinergic activity. Wood and Allison (1982) also discussed concerns regarding the development of supersensitivity of dopamine receptors and disturbance of the cholinergic-dopaminergic-serotonergic balance with prolonged, repeated intakes of large amounts of lecithin (Rosenberg & Davis, 1982; Wood & Allison, 1982). Drug interactions have not been well documented with lecithin.

MELATONIN

Melatonin (N-acetyl-5-methoxytryptamine or 5-methoxy, N-acetyltryptamine), a hormone secreted from the pineal gland, is the principal hormone of the circadian system (Zhdanova & Friedman, 2008). The amino acid L-trypotphan is converted to serotonin (5HT), then eventually to melatonin. Melatonin secretion starts between the third to sixth months of life. It then increases rapidly, with a peak in nocturnal melatonin concentrations between ages three to seven years (Waldhauser, 1984). In addition to effects on sleep and circadian body rhythm, melatonin has been proposed to affect mood (it has been studied in BPD, depression, and seasonal affective disorder), regulate the secretion of growth hormone and gonadotropic hormones, and have antioxidant activity. Food does not supply meaningful amounts of melatonin.

Rapid-cycling BPD has been proposed to be associated with unstable circadian rhythms (Leibenluft, 1997). Patients with BPD have been reported to have lower baseline levels of melatonin and increased sensitivity to dim light (with dim light causing increased melatonin suppression in bipolar patients compared to healthy controls;

Nathan, 1999), though other reports do not support these data (Whalley, Perini, Shering, & Bennie, 1991).

There is conflicting evidence regarding the efficacy of melatonin in the treatment of BPD. In 2000 Bersani and Garavini published an open-label trial in which 11 outpatient ages 22 to 43 years who met *DSM-IV* criteria for bipolar disorder, manic type, and experienced insomnia not responding to usual hypnotic therapies were given melatonin 3 mg nightly at 10:30 PM for 30 days. They found that, by the end of the treatment, all patients showed a longer sleep duration compared to baseline (mean hours of sleep increased from 2.43 ± 0.76 to 5.24 ± 1.51 per night) and a significant decrease in severity of mania Brief Psychiatric Rating Scale (BPRS total scores decreased from 22.72 ± 4.45 to 14.09 ± 4.43; Bersani, 2000). In 1997 Leibenluft and colleagues reported a double-blind, placebo-controlled evaluation of five outpatients diagnosed with rapid-cycling *DSM-III-R* BPD treated with melatonin 10 mg daily at 10:00 PM for 12 weeks (added on to a stable medication regimen) and found that the administration of melatonin had no significant effects on mood or sleep. They noted that the administration of exogenous melatonin may have caused partial suppression of endogenous melatonin secretion in two of the patients and melatonin withdrawal led to marked instability in the sleep–wake cycle of one of the patients. They hypothesized that bipolar patients may be more sensitive than controls to suppressive effects of exogenous melatonin on endogenous melatonin secretion. One patient was withdrawn from the study after 35 days on melatonin due to acute worsening of mood and overdose on clonazepam and wine (Leibenluft, 1997)

While there are no studies available evaluating the use of melatonin for treatment of pediatric BPD, Robertson and Tanguay (1997) described the clinical course of a 10-year-old boy diagnosed with BPD nonresponsive to combinations of lithium (levels up to 1.5mEq/L), thioridazine up to 80 mg/day, and valproic acid to 750 mg/day. While this child did respond to a combination of lithium and carbamazepine, he developed adverse reaction that required discontinuation of carbmazepine. He required numerous inpatient psychiatric hospitalizations due to manic symptoms and aggression. His insomnia and manic episode responded rapidly to a trial of melatonin 3 mg nightly, with recurrence of symptoms when efforts to stop the melatonin were made one month after starting it. Subsequent recurrence of symptoms responded to dose increase to 9 mg/day, then to 12 mg/day augmented by alprazolam 0.375 mg/day. At the time of the publication, the boy had been stable for 15 months without recurrence of full-blown manic episode on melatonin 12 mg/day + alprazolam 0.375 mg/day (Robertson, 1997).

Melatonin has been investigated as an adjunct to buspirone, and a double-blind, placebo-controlled trial comparing placebo to buspirone monotherapy to buspirone (15 mg) plus melatonin (3 mg) for the treatment of MDD (6 weeks, $N = 134$ adults) demonstrated superior response in symptoms of depression to the combination therapy: 58.2% of the MDD subjects treated with the combination were responders using the CGI scale compared to only 36.4% of the placebo subjects and 38.2% of the buspirone along subjects. The combination was well tolerated (Fava et al., 2012).

There is no established dose range for melatonin in the use of BPD. Usual doses of melatonin range from 0.1 to 5 mg/day, though staying in the range of 0.1 to 0.3 mg/day has been recommended. Dose ranges are separated by "physiologic" and "pharmacologic" doses, and dose timing is determined by whether melatonin is used for circadian regulation or for acute sleep-promoting effects. Typical physiologic nocturnal peak serum concentrations of melatonin are around 60 to 200 pg/mL, while daytime levels are as low as 3 to 10 pg/mL. Taking 0.1 to 0.3 mg of oral melatonin typically induces physiologic serum melatonin levels. Ingestion of 10 mg of melatonin can result in a 1,000-fold increase in plasma melatonin when compared to peak melatonin levels normally occurring at night in a young healthy adult. Physiologic doses of melatonin have been reported not to cause substantial changes in sleep architecture, though this is not the case with doses greater than 5 mg per day (Zhdanova & Friedman, 2008).

The circadian effect largely depends on the time of melatonin administration and can produce opposite effects: morning administration may delay the onset of evening sleepiness by delaying the phase of the circadian rhythms, while evening ingestion can advance the circadian rhythms and sleep onset. Of note, rather than produce a rapid increase in subjective sleepiness or drowsiness, at physiologic doses melatonin has been reported to induce a behavioral state that resembles quiet wakefulness, which usually enables sleep initiation. It leads to minimal alterations in performance ability. Therefore, sleep results if the environmental conditions are appropriate for sleep and an individual can override the melatonin's effects with stimuli such as turning lights on or sitting (Zhdanova & Friedman, 2008).

Melatonin is generally well tolerated. The most common side effects that have been noted include drowsiness, headache, dizziness, and nausea. (Buscemi et al., 2005) Additional reported side effects include transient depressive symptoms, mild tremor, mild anxiety, abdominal cramps, irritability, reduced alertness, confusion, vomiting, and hypotension.

Long-term clinical and experimental studies are needed to address questions regarding adverse effects of melatonin. Concerns have been raised that taking pharmacologic doses of melatonin could induce a circadian rhythm disorder by disrupting the body's natural circadian body rhythms (Leibenluft, 1997). There is some evidence to suggest that altered melatonin levels may lead to increased levels of prolactin and to disorders of the hypothalamic-pituitary-gonadal axis (delayed puberty, precocious puberty, hypothalamic amenorrhea; Cavallo, 2007). In light of this possibility, melatonin should be used with caution in developing children. In addition, exacerbation of seizure disorder in three neurologically disabled patients during melatonin treatment has been reported (Sheldon, 1998).

Melatonin inactivation occurs in the liver by the P450-dependent microsomal mixed-function oxidase enzyme system. Thus medication affecting this pathway could influence the metabolism of melatonin. In addition, data exists that melatonin may inhibit the CYP1A2 and CYP2C9 isoenzymes, theoretically affecting medications metabolized through these pathways (including theophylline, caffeine, clozapine, haloperidol, tacrine and NSAIDs, phenytoin, warfarin, and zafirlukast). Since production of melatonin depends on increased noradrenergic innervation of the pineal gland at nighttime and serotonin as a precursor for melatonin synthesis, psychotropic medications that affect norepinephrine or serotonin levels may affect the production of melatonin.

MAGNESIUM

Scientific speculation has addressed the role of magnesium in depression and mania, as it is involved in numerous metabolic processes, activating enzymes and affecting the metabolism and release of myriad neurotransmitters. Magnesium is a calcium channel blocker and noncompetitive antagonist of the N-methyl-D-aspartate channel. As magnesium inhibits calcium activity and promotes membrane stabilization, it is thought to mimic some of the actions of lithium and carbamazepine.

As with many natural treatments, the evidence supporting magnesium supplementation is spare and indirect. One study found that patients who responded to antidepressant treatment had higher baseline magnesium levels ($N = 123$) compared with nonresponders, although all the patients had magnesium levels in the normal range (Camardese et al., 2012). Another study found hypermagnesaemia

in drug-naive first-episode MDD patients (Cubala, Landowski, Szyszko, & Czarnowski, 2013). Regarding other disorders in psychiatry, a relatively large number (six) studies address the use of magnesium for attention deficit hyperactivity disorder, but none are randomized, double-blind, placebo-controlled or monotherapy studies (Ghanizadeh, 2013). A study of suicidal schizophrenic subjects found higher concentrations of platelet magnesium and lower concentrations of serum calcium in patients with attempted suicide versus those without suicidal behavior (Ruljancic, Mihanovic, Cepelak, & Bakliza, 2013). A large sample ($N = 5,708$) of adults in a Norwegian health study found an association between magnesium intake and depression (Jacka et al., 2009). A study of postpartum depression suggests that trace elements including magnesium could play a role in the pathophysiology of postpartum depression and calls for studies of these supplements in this population (Etebary, Nikseresht, Sadeghipour, & Zarrindast, 2010). A case series reported that IV magnesium was a useful adjunctive treatment to lithium, haloperidol, and clonazepam for treatment-resistant, severely impairing mania with agitation in 10 patients. This intervention resulted in a decrease in mania severity and improvements in global functioning. Seven patients showed marked improvement. In addition, the adjunctive magnesium permitted a tapering of the dose of concomitant medications. Although bradycardia was noted as a side effect, the treatment was well tolerated (Heiden et al., 1999).

Magnesium in the form of 375 mg magnesium oxide was tested in randomized clinical trial versus placebo over 16 weeks ($N = 20$) as an adjunct to treatment with verapamil in bipolar subjects. The authors reported a statistically significant reduction in BPRS scores in the treated group. Magnesium was chosen as an apt adjunct to verapamil due to some shared properties, including inhibiting calcium activity and enhancing membrane stabilization. Based on these findings, the authors concluded that magnesium could augment the antimanic effects of verapamil during maintenance therapy in BPD. Nine patients with rapid cycling BPD were treated with a magnesium preparation in open label study for 32 weeks. The authors report that 50% of these patients had a clinical result similar to that of lithium (Chouinard, Beauclair, Geiser, & Etienne, 1990).

Although bradycardia was noted as a side effect in one study, the treatment was overall well tolerated (Heiden et al., 1999). As a caveat with magnesium, whether increasing levels of magnesium in the serum alters brain levels has been questioned with animal research results (Kim et al., 1996).

MICRONUTRIENT COMBINATION

A micronutrient supplement that appears to have potential benefit in a variety of mental disorders, BPD in particular, is a propriety trademarked product called EMPowerplus, accessed via a website called Truehope. The 36-ingredient supplement consists of 16 minerals, 14 vitamins, 3 amino acids, and 3 antioxidants. Due to many testimonials and case reports indicating remission of symptoms, this product has gained popularity among patients and parents of patients. Like many natural treatments, most of the evidence for efficacy is limited to compelling case series and case reports, although this product also has two open-label trials, one in adults and one in children. The lack of evidence from a double-blind, placebo-controlled trial is notable.

The earliest report of success with this produce came from Popper in 2001, who published the success of this product via naturalistic clinical practice follow-up. He described the case of a 10-year-old boy with early onset BPD characterized by severe daily temper outbursts lasting for hours. After two days of EMP+, the behavior was much improved, and, after five days, all the irritability and outbursts had stopped. When the nutritional supplement was discontinued, the outbursts returned. Treatment with a different supplement did not bring about improvement. When the EMP+ was restarted, the symptoms again remitted. In addition, this same author followed 22 child, adolescent, and adult patients with BPD in clinical practice and reported on remarkably positive outcomes: 86% had a positive response to this supplement and 11 of 15 patients who had been taking conventional treatments were able to stop these treatments with good result with nutritional product monotherapy (Popper, 2001).

Published in tandem was an open-label trial of 11 adult patients ages 19 to 46 with BPD who were treated with this broad-based nutritional supplement and assessed at six months. Symptom reduction ranged from 55% to 66% on HAM-D, BPRS, and YMRS scales. The number of psychotropic medications decreased from mean of 2.7 to mean of 1.0. Some patients stopped conventional treatment. Ten children with pediatric BPD were treated in open-label trial with this supplement. The authors reported a 37% decrease in depression scores and 45% decrease in mania scores over eight weeks in open-label trial (Frazier, Fristad, & Arnold, 2012).

A letter to the editor outlined experience with this supplement in a private clinical practice and described that 12 of 19 adults with bipolar spectrum disorder improved markedly and 13 subjects completely stopped their original psychiatric medication with stability over an average of 13 months follow-up (Frazier et al., 2012).

Kaplan et al reported on-and-off use in two boys with mood lability, describing marked improvements in mood. Mood lability and explosive outbursts dissipated with treatment, returned when not taking the supplement, and remitted when the nutritional supplement was reintroduced. The two patients were followed with good result for two years. This same author reported a case series of 11 children ages 8 to 15 years with mood/behavioral problems, 3 with BPD. For the nine who completed the trial, significant improvements were noted on the YMRS (Frazier et al., 2012).

One author reported on a 12-year-old with treatment-resistant bipolar I disorder beginning at age six who was moved to monotherapy with this nutritional treatment and followed for 14 months with remission of all symptoms. In this case report, the boy was noted to have severely impairing psychotic features with severe impairment. The authors describe aggressive conventional pharmacotherapy from age 6 to 12 years, which did not bring consistent improvement. Over the course of 19 days, he was cross-tapered off pharmacotherapy and onto the nutritional supplement EMP+. Notable improvements in global functioning occurred immediately. After one month of treatment, all diagnoses had remitted (Frazier et al., 2012).

ACUPUNCTURE

Acupuncture, one of the oldest medical procedures in the world, has long been used for disorders including depression, anxiety, stress, and insomnia in China, Japan, and Korea (Wang et al., 2008). Acupuncture describes a family of procedures involving the stimulation of anatomical points on the body through a variety of styles and techniques. Common styles include traditional Chinese, Japanese, Korean, Vietnamese, and French acupuncture, as well as specialized forms such as hand, auricular, and scalp acupuncture. Common techniques include the insertion of ultra fine needles to stimulate acupoints, as well as the use of manual pressure, electrical stimulation, magnets, low-power lasers, heat, and ultrasound. There are many schools of acupuncture (e.g., Chinese, Japanese, Korean, Indian), each with its own approach to diagnosis and allocation of acupoints. (Samuels, Gropp, Singer, & Oberbaum, 2008).

One of the central treatments of traditional Chinese medicine, acupuncture gained popularity in the United States in 1971, when *New York Times* reporter James Reston wrote about his experience with acupuncture to ease his postsurgical pain. Acupuncture is now one of the most popular complementary therapies in the West (Wang et al., 2008).

Acupuncture is based on the traditional Chinese medicine concept that disease results from the disruption in the flow of energy, *Qi* (pronounced *chee*), along a series of points that connect bodily organs, *meridians*. Disease is thought to result when there is disharmony or imbalance in the body's energy system. By using acupuncture at certain points on the body that connect with meridians, *Qi* can be unblocked, thus restoring flow and balance. There are at least 2,000 acupuncture points on the body (Samuels et al., 2008; Wang et al., 2008). The exact mechanism of action of acupuncture is unknown, though its effect has been reported to be due to the stimulation of afferent Group III nerve fibers that transmit impulses to various parts of the central nervous system and induce release of serotonin, norepinephrine, substance P, dopamine, b-endorphin, enkephalin, and dynorphins. (Samuels et al., 2008; Wang et al., 2008).

Three adult reports address the use of acupuncture to treat BPD, though two are case reports that are published in Chinese-language journals and are not available in English. The third study evaluated traditional Chinese medicine acupuncture with manual stimulation against an active, nonspecific acupuncture control and against medication alone in 26 bipolar patients with depression refractory to treatment. Augmentation of medication with acupuncture yielded significant improvement over medication alone in the primary outcome measures, including the Inventory of Depressive Symptomatology and the Global Assessment of Functioning, but there were no significant differences between groups (Suppes et al., 2007).

Though more studies address the role of acupuncture in the treatment of depression, the research is still limited. Because of the heterogeneity of acupuncture treatments, conducting randomized trials is difficult. Wang et al. (2008) conducted a meta-analysis of eight randomized clinical trials that compared acupuncture with sham acupuncture in depression patients. While this meta-analysis concluded that results supported acupuncture as an effective treatment that could significantly reduce the severity of major depression and depressive neurosis, these results should be read with caution due to high heterogeneity of the studies and many limitations. Samuels et al. (2008) published a review that summarized clinical trials addressing acupuncture treatment of depression, anxiety, schizophrenia, and substance abuse. They noted that, due to poor design and limited number of studies, there is insufficient evidence that acupuncture is effective for treatment of depression. This agreed with a previous report by Leo & & Ligot (2007) in which they reviewed available RCTs looking at acupuncture in treating depression and determined that results were inconclusive and limited by varied methodology and study design. Further evaluation of the role of acupuncture in treating depression is warranted.

There are no child and adolescent studies addressing the use of acupuncture for the treatment of BPD or depression. In 2000 Kemper and colleagues published a retrospective study in which they spoke with 47 children and adolescents (or their parents) who received acupuncture after referral from the Pain Treatment Service to assess their qualitative experiences. Most families found acupuncture to be a positive, pleasant, and relaxing experience (67% compared with 13% who found it negative/unpleasant/scary and 20% who found it other/neutral/strange); although some patients began with anxiety about the needles, many developed more positive perceptions over the course of treatment.

Acupuncture appears to be safe when provided by qualified acupuncturists. In 2001 Ernst and Adrian published a systematic review of nine studies that evaluated the safety of nearly a quarter of a million acupuncture treatments (Ernst & White, 2001). They found that the most common adverse events were needle pain (range from 0.2% to 59% across studies), tiredness (2.3% to 41%), bleeding (0.03% to 38%), feeling faint (0.02% to 7%), and nausea (0.01% to 0.2%). Serious side effects were rare but included two cases of pneumothorax and two cases of needle fracture requiring surgical removal of the fragment (0.001% for both). Few studies commented on long-term follow-up; thus long-term complications, such as nerve injury, may have been underestimated. In a subsequent prospective investigation of adverse effects of acupuncture in 97,733 patients (over 760,000 acupuncture sessions) administered by 7,050 German physicians with at least 140 hours of formal acupuncture, a total of five potentially serious adverse effect were noted in six patients: pneumothorax in two patients (both recovered), exacerbation of depression, acute hypertensive crisis, vasovagal reaction, and acute asthma attack with angina and hypertension (Melchart, 2004). Complications can arise from inadequate sterilization of needles and improper delivery of treatments (Wang et al., 2008). In the United States, acupuncturists should be certified by the National Certification Commission for Acupuncture and Oriental Medicine or the American Board of Medical Acupuncture. The US Food and Drug Administration regulates acupuncture needles for use by licensed practitioners. Local contraindications to acupuncture include active infection or malignancy at insertion sites. No drug interactions have been reported. Some insurance carriers will cover acupuncture.

ADDITIONAL INTERVENTIONS

As there is growing evidence for the link between the mind and body, attention to diet and exercise play a role in promoting healthy mood. Bipolar patients have been reported being more likely to engage in poor exercise habits and suboptimal eating behaviors compared with individuals without serious mental illness (Kilbourne et al., 2007). Improvements in cardiorespiratory fitness have been reported to have positive effects on depression, anxiety, mood status, and self-esteem in children and adolescents (Ortega, Ruiz, Castillo, & Sjostrom, 2008). While exercise has not been extensively studied in BPD, there is data supporting exercise as an effective intervention (Sylvia, Ametrano, & Nierenberg, 2010), though other reports are less conclusive, largely due to the limitations of the available studies (Lawlor & Hopker, 2001). In 2005 Dunn and colleagues published data of their DOSE trial in which 80 adults diagnosed with mild to moderate depression were randomized into one of five groups: total weekly energy expenditure of 7 kcal/kg/week (low dose) for three days or five days a week, total weekly energy expenditure of 17.5 kcal/kg/week (consensus public health recommended dose) for three days or five days a week, or placebo (three days/week of stretching flexibility exercise for 15 to 20 minutes per session) to determine not only whether or not exercise was effective for treatment of depression but also whether energy expenditure or frequency of exercise had an impact on the efficacy. They found that exercise at the public health dose (17.5kcal/kg/week) was significantly more effective than low dose and placebo, which both showed nonsignificant improvements in symptoms. There was no difference between exercising three days per week versus five days per week in improvement of depressive symptoms, suggesting that energy expenditure is the determining factor in the reduction of depressive symptoms (Dunn, Trivedi, Kampert, Clark, & Chambliss, 2005).

While there is some data supporting the possible use of relaxation and massage to benefit depression and anxiety symptoms in children and adolescents (von Knorring, Soderberg, Austin, & Uvnas-Moberg, 2008), two recent reviews of available randomized control trials did not support a significantly positive effect of massage therapy on pediatric depression (Beider & Moyer, 2007).

The role of vitamins and minerals in healthy mood has been hypothesized and evaluated, though available data is limited, especially in the pediatric population in which such interventions might be surmised to have the biggest impact due to ongoing development (Sylvia, Peters, Deckersbach, & Nierenberg, 2013). Data supporting the use of nutrients is both correlational (e.g., deficiency of a specific nutrient has been found in patients with depression) and investigational (e.g., taking a specific nutritional supplement has been shown to improve depressive symptoms). Vitamin C has been linked to mood disorders (Naylor, 1981). B vitamins of particular interest included vitamins B9 (folate), B6 (pyridoxine), and B1 (thiamine) for the treatment of depression, as well as B12 (cobalamin) repletion to address vitamin deficiency-induced depressive and manic symptoms. Behzadi, Omrani, Chalian, Asadi, and Ghadiri (2009) added folic acid to sodium valproate for three weeks in patients with mania and found that those patients who received the folic acid had improvement in symptoms of mania. In addition, in light of the idea that mood disorders usually are not due to a single deficiency but rather an imbalance of an array of micronutrients, emerging data supports mutlivitamin supplements. While most of the available data are from adults, some pediatric studies have shown promising preliminary results. Even with evidence of usefulness of attention to proper nutrition, difficulty arises in identifying and treating deficiencies, as individuals differ in optimal requirements for vitamins and minerals. (Kaplan, Crawford, Field, & Simpson, 2007). Deficiencies of various minerals have also been evaluated for their potential roles in affective symptoms: calcium in depression (Kaplan, Crawford, Field, & Simpson, 2007), chromium to treat rapid cycling BPD (depressive episode), and zinc to address depressive symptoms (Lakhan & Vieira, 2008). In addition, the amino acids tryptophan (precursor of serotonin; Chouinard, 1983), tyrosine (converted to dopamine and norepinephrine), phenylalanine (precursor of tyrosine; Sabelli et al., 1986), and methoinine (combined with adenosine triphosphate to produce SAMe) have been reported to be helpful in treating mood disorders (Lakhan, 2008).

CONCLUSION

The severe impairment caused by BPD throughout the life cycle often leads to the need for aggressive interventions, requiring clinicians, patients, and parents of patients to weigh risks versus benefits when deciding on specific treatment regimens. In light of high rates of relapse, moderate efficacy, difficult side-effect profiles, and poor adherence associated with conventional mood-stabilizing medications, there has been growing interest in complementary and alternative treatments. Although intriguing due to purported mechanisms of action and "good for overall health" qualities, data supporting natural interventions in lieu of conventional treatment is lacking. In particular, caution must be exerted when enthusiasm for a natural intervention crowds out the use of a known pharmacological agent with strong medical evidence base for efficacy, especially for a condition as seriously impairing as BPD.

This chapter covered select complementary and alternative treatments that have some data, in BPD, both mania and depression. While some studies document that treatments are safe and well tolerated in short-term treatment, longer term data are lacking. Most of the treatments do not have clear recommended doses, especially in the pediatric patient population. Mechanisms of antidepressant or antimanic action, similar to conventional treatments, have been theorized but remain to be fully elucidated. Given that drug interactions and long-term effects are not completely known for many of the treatments, use with conventional medications should be monitored closely.

Disclosure statement: In 2013–2014, Janet Wozniak received research support from Merck/Schering-Plough and income from MGH Psychiatry Academy. In the past she has received research support, consultation fees, or speaker's fees from: Eli Lilly, Janssen, Johnson and Johnson, McNeil, Pfizer, and Shire. She is the author of the book *Is Your Child Bipolar* (Bantam Books, 2008).

In 2013–2014, her spouse received income from Associated Professional Sleep Societies, Cambridge University Press, Gerson Lerman Group, MGH Psychiatry Academy, Summer Street Partners, UCB, and Cantor Colburn. In the past, he has received research support, consultation fees, royalties, or speaker's fees from Axon Labs, Boehringer-Ingelheim, Cambridge University Press, Covance, Cephalon, Eli Lilly, GlaxoSmithKline, Impax, Jazz Pharmaceuticals, King, Luitpold, Novartis, Neurogen, Novadel Pharma, Pfizer, Sanofi-Aventis, Sepracor, Takeda, UCB (Schwarz) Pharma, UptoDate, Wyeth, Xenoport, and Zeo.

REFERENCES

Adams, P. B., Lawson, S., Sanigorski, A., & Sinclair, A. J. (1996). Arachidonic acid to eicosapentaenoic acid ratio in blood correlates positively with clinical symptoms of depression. *Lipids, 31*(Suppl.), S157–S161.

Alpert, J. E., Papakostas, G., Mischoulon, D., Worthington, J. J., Petersen, T., Mahal, Y.,...Fava, M. (2004). S-Adenosyl-L-Methionine (SAMe) as an adjunct for resistant major depressive disorder. *Journal of Clinical Psychopharmacology, 24*(6), 661–664.

American Psychiatric Association. (1980). *Diagnostic and statistical manual of mental disorders* (3rd ed., rev.). Washington, DC: Author.

American Psychiatric Association. (1994). *Diagnostic and statistical manual of mental disorders* (4th ed.). Washington, DC: Author.

American Psychiatric Association. (2000). *Diagnostic and statistical manual of mental disorders* (4th ed., text rev.). Washington, DC: Author.

Baraban, J. M., Worley, P. F., & Snyder, S. H. (1989). Second messenger systems and psychoactive drug action: Focus on the phosphoinositide system and lithium. *The American Journal of Psychiatry, 146*(10), 1251–1260.

Behzadi, A. H., Omrani, Z., Chalian, M., Asadi, S., & Ghadiri, M. (2009). Folic acid efficacy as an alternative drug added to sodium valproate in the treatment of acute phase of mania in bipolar disorder: A double-blind randomized controlled trial. *Acta Psychiatrica Scandanavia, 120*(6), 441–445. doi:10.1111/j.1600-0447.2009.01368.x

Bell, K. M., Potkin, S. G., Carreon, D., & Pion, L. (1994). S-adenosylmethionine blood levels in major depression: changes with drug treatment. *Acta Neurologica Scandinavica, 154*, 15–18.

Belmaker, R. H. (1997). The inositol depletion hypothesis: Promise and problems. *Biological Psychiatry, 42*, 1S–297S.

Belmaker, R. H., Bersudsky, Y., Agam, G., Levine, J., & Kofman, O. (1996). How does lithium work on manic depression? Clinical and psychological correlates of the inositol theory. *Annual Review of Medicine, 47*, 47–56.

Berk, M., Copolov, D. L., Dean, O., Lu, K., Jeavons, S., Schapkaitz, I.,...Bush, A. I. (2008). N-acetyl cysteine for depressive symptoms in bipolar disorder—A double-blind randomized placebo-controlled trial. *Biological Psychiatry, 64*(6), 468–475. doi:10.1016/j.biopsych.2008.04.022

Berk, M., Dean, O., Cotton, S. M., Gama, C. S., Kapczinski, F., Fernandes, B. S.,...Malhi, G. S. (2011). The efficacy of N-acetylcysteine as an adjunctive treatment in bipolar depression: An open label trial. *Journal of Affective Disorders, 135*(1–3), 389–394. doi:10.1016/j.jad.2011.06.005

Berk, M., Dean, O. M., Cotton, S. M., Gama, C. S., Kapczinski, F., Fernandes, B.,...Malhi, G. S. (2012). Maintenance N-acetyl cysteine treatment for bipolar disorder: a double-blind randomized placebo controlled trial. *BMC Medicine, 10*, 91. doi:10.1186/1741-7015-10-91

Berk, M., Malhi, G. S., Gray, L. J., & Dean, O. M. (2013). The promise of N-acetylcysteine in neuropsychiatry. *Trends in Pharmacological Science, 34*(3), 167–177. doi:10.1016/j.tips.2013.01.001

Berridge, M. J., Downes, C. P., & Hanley, M. R. (1989). Neural and developmental actions of lithium: A unifying hypothesis. *Cell, 59*, 411–419.

Bersani, G., & Garavini, A. (2000). Melatonin add-on in manic patients with treatment resistant insomnia. *Progress in Neuropsychopharmacology & Biological Psychiatry, 24*, 185–191.

Beider, S., & Moyer, C. A. (2007). Randomized control trials of pediatric massage: a review. *eCAM, 4*, 23–34.

Bottiglieri, T., Godfrey, P., Flynn, T., Carney, M. W. P., Toone, B. K., & Reynolds, E. H. (1990). Cerebrospinal fluid S-adenosylmethionine in depression and dementia: effects of treatment with parental and oral S-adenosylmethionine. *Journal of Neurology, Neurosurgery, and Psychiatry, 53*, 1096–1098.

Bourre, J. M. (2006). Effects of nutrients (in food) on the structure and function of the nervous system: Update on dietary requirements for brain: Part 1. Micronutrients. *The Journal of Nutrition, Health & Aging, 10*(5), 377–385.

Buscemi, N., Vandermeer, B., Hooton, N., Pandya, R., Tjosvold, L., Hartling, L.,...Vohra, S. (2005). The efficacy and safety of exogenous melatonin for primary sleep disorders. A meta-analysis. *Journal of General Internal Medicine, 20*(12), 1151–1158. doi:JGI243

Butterweck, V. (2003). Mechanism of action of St. John's wort in depression. *CNS Drugs, 17*(8), 539–562.

Camardese, G., De Risio, L., Pizi, G., Mattioli, B., Buccelletti, F., Serrani, R.,...Janiri, L. (2012). Plasma magnesium levels and treatment outcome in depressed patients. *Nutrition Neuroscience, 15*(2), 78–84. doi:10.1179/1476830512Y.0000000002

Cavallo, A. (2007). Melatonin and human puberty: Current perspectives. *Journal of Pineal Research, 15*(3), 15–121.

Cecil, K. M., DelBello, M. P., Morey, R., & Strakowski, S. M. (2002). Frontal lobe differences in bipolar disorder as determined by proton MR spectroscopy. *Bipolar Disorders, 4,* 357–365.

Chengappa, K. N., Levine, J., Gershon, S., Mallinger, A. G., Hardan, A., Vagnucci, A.,…Kupfer, D. J. (2000). Inositol as an add-on treatment for bipolar depression. *Bipolar Disorders, 2*(1), 47–55.

Chouinard, G., Beauclair, L., Geiser, R., & Etienne, P. (1990). A pilot study of magnesium aspartate hydrochloride (Magnesiocard) as a mood stabilizer for rapid cycling bipolar affective disorder patients. *Progress in Neuro-Psychopharmacology & Biological Psychiatry, 14*(2), 171–180.

Chouinard, G. (1983). Tryptophan in the treatment of depression and mania. *Advances in Biological Psychiatry, 10,* 46–66.

Clements, R. S., & Darnell, B. (1980). Myo-inositol content of common foods: Development of a high-myo-inositol diet. *The American Journal of Clinical Nutrition, 33,* 1954–1967.

Cohen, B. M., Lipinski, J. F., & Altesman, R. I. (1982). Lecithin in the treatment of mania: Double-blind, placebo-controlled trials. *The American Journal of Psychiatry, 139*(9), 1162–1164.

Cubala, W. J., Landowski, J., Szyszko, M., & Czarnowski, W. (2013). Magnesium in drug-naive patients with a short-duration, first episode of major depressive disorder: Impact on psychopathological features. *Magnesium Research, 26*(4), 192–198. doi:10.1684/mrh.2014.0355

Davanzo, P., Thomas, M. A., Yue, K., Oshiro, T., Belin, T., Strober, M., & McCracken, J. (2001). Decreased anterior cingulate myo-inositol/creatine spectroscopy resonance with lithium treatment in children with bipolar disorder. *Neuropsychopharmacology, 24*(4), 359–369.

Davanzo, P., Yue, K., Thomas, M. A., Belin, T., Mintz, J., Venkatraman, T. N.,…McCracken, J. (2003). Proton magnetic resonance spectroscopy of bipolar disorder versus intermittent explosive disorder in children and adolescents. *The American Journal of Psychiatry, 160*(8), 1442–1452.

Dean, O., Giorlando, F., & Berk, M. (2011). N-acetylcysteine in psychiatry: Current therapeutic evidence and potential mechanisms of action. *Journal of Psychiatry Neuroscience, 36*(2), 78–86.

DiNicolantonio, J. J., McCarty, M. F., Lavie, C. J., & O'Keefe, J. H. (2013). Do omega-3 fatty acids cause prostate cancer? *Molecular Medicine, 110*(4), 293–295.

Dunn, A. L., Trivedi, M. H., Kampert, J. B., Clark, C. G., & Chambliss, H. O. (2005). Exercise treatment for depression: Efficacy and dose response. *American Journal of Preventative Medicine, 28*(1), 1–8. doi:S0749-3797(04)00241-7 [pii]

Ernst, E. White A. R. (2001). Prospective studies of the safety of acupuncture: A systematic review. *The American Journal of Medicine, 110,* 481–485.

Etebary, S., Nikseresht, S., Sadeghipour, H. R., & Zarrindast, M. R. (2010). Postpartum depression and role of serum trace elements. *Iran Journal of Psychiatry, 5*(2), 40–46.

Evins, E. A. D., Demopulos, C., Yovel, I., Culhane, M., Ogutha, J., Grandin, L. D.,…Gary S. (2006). Inositol augmentation of lithium or valproate for bipolar depression. *Bipolar Disorders, 8,* 168–174.

Fava, M., Targum, S. D., Nierenberg, A. A., Bleicher, L. S., Carter, T. A., Wedel, P. C.,…Barlow, C. (2012). An exploratory study of combination buspirone and melatonin SR in major depressive disorder (MDD): A possible role for neurogenesis in drug discovery. *Journal of Psychiatric Research, 46*(12), 1553–1563. doi:10.1016/j.jpsychires.2012.08.013

Fava, M., Alpert, J., Nierenberg, A. A., Mischoulon, D., Otto, M. W., Zajecka, J.,…Rosenbaum, J. (2005). A double-blind, randomized trial of St. John's wort, fluoxetine, and placebo in major depressive disorder. *Journal of Clinical Psychopharmacology, 25*(5), 441–447.

Fava, M., Rosenbaum, J. F., MacLaughlin, R., Falk, W. E., Pollack, M. H., Cohen, L. S.,…Pill, L. (1990). Neuroendocrine effects of s-adenosyl-l-methionine, A novel putative antidepressant. *Journal of Psychiatric Research, 24*(2), 177–184.

Findling, R. L., McNamara, N. K., O'Riordan, M. A., Reed, M. D., Demeter, C. A., Branicky, L. A., & Blumer, J. L. (2003). An open-label pilot study of St. John's Wort in juvenile depression. *Journal of the American Academy of Child & Adolescent Psychiatry, 42*(8), 908–914.

Frangou, S., Lewis, M., & McCrone, P. (2006). Efficacy of ethyl-eicosapentaenoic acid in bipolar depression: Randomised double-blind placebo-controlled study. *The British Journal of Psychiatry, 188,* 46–50.

Frazier, E. A., Fristad, M. A., & Arnold, L. E. (2012). Feasibility of a nutritional supplement as treatment for pediatric bipolar spectrum disorders. *Journal of Alternative and Complementary Medicine, 18*(7), 678–685. doi:10.1089/acm.2011.0270

Frey, R., Metzler, D., Fischer, P., Heiden, A., Moser, E., & Kasper, S. (1998). Myo-inositol in depressive and healthy subjects by means of frontal H-magnetic resonance spectroscopy. *Biological Psychiatry, 42,* 1S–297S.

Ghanizadeh, A. (2013). A systematic review of magnesium therapy for treating attention deficit hyperactivity disorder. *Archives of Iranian Medicine, 16*(7), 412–417. doi:013167/AIM.0010

Gracious, B. L., Chirieac, M. C., Costescu, S., Finucane, T. L., Youngstrom, E. A., & Hibbeln, J. R. (2010). Randomized, placebo-controlled trial of flax oil in pediatric bipolar disorder. *Bipolar Disorders, 12*(2), 142–154. doi:10.1111/j.1399-5618.2010.00799.x

Hardy, M., Coulter, I., Morton, S. C., Favreau, J., Venuturupalli, S., Chiappelli, F.,…Shekelle, P. (2003). S-adenosyl-L-methionine for treatment of depression, osteoarthritis, and liver disease. *Evidence Report/Technology Assessment (Summary), 64,* 1–3.

Heiden, A., Frey, R., Presslich, O., Blasbichler, T., Smetana, R., & Kasper, S. (1999). Treatment of severe mania with intravenous magnesium sulphate as a supplementary therapy. *Psychiatry Research, 89*(3), 239–246.

Hibbeln, J. R. (1998). Fish consumption and major depression. *Lancet, 351*(9110), 1213. doi:S0140-6736(05)79168-6

Horrobin, D. F., & Bennett, C. N. (1999). Depression and bipolar disorder: Relationships to impaired fatty acid and phospholipid metabolism and to diabetes, cardiovascular disease, immunological abnormalities, cancer, ageing and osteoporosis. Possible candidate genes. *Prostaglandins Leukotrienes and Essential Fatty Acids, 60*(4), 217–234.

Horrobin, D. F., Glen, A. I., & Vaddadi, K. (1994). The membrane hypothesis of schizophrenia. *Schizophrenia Research, 13*(3), 195–207.

Hubner, W. D., Kirste, T. (2001). Experience with St. John's wort (hypericum perforatum) in children under 12 years with symptoms of depression and psychovegetative disturbances. *Phytotherapy Research, 15,* 367–370.

Iruela, L. M., Minguez, L., Merino, J., & Monedero, G. (1993). Toxic interaction of S-adenosylmethionine and clomipramine. *American Journal of Psychiatry, 150*(3), 522.

Jacka, F. N., Overland, S., Stewart, R., Tell, G. S., Bjelland, I., & Mykletun, A. (2009). Association between magnesium intake and depression and anxiety in community-dwelling adults: The Hordaland Health Study. *Australian and New Zealand Journal of Psychiatry, 43*(1), 45–52. doi:10.1080/00048670802534408

Jerrell, J. M., & Prewette, E. D. II. (2008). Outcomes for youths with early- and very-early-onset bipolar I disorder. *Journal of Behavioral Health Services Research, 35*(1), 52–59. doi:10.1007/s11414-007-9081-3

Karalapillai, D. C., & Bellomo, R. (2007). Convulsions associated with an overdose of St John's wort. *Medical Journal of Australia, 186*(4), 213–214. doi:letters_190207_fm-2

Kaya, N., Resmi, H., Ozerdem, A., Guner, G., & Tunca, Z. (2004). Increased inositol-monophosphatase activity by lithium treatment in bipolar patients. *Progress in Neuropsychopharmacology & Biological Psychiatry, 28*(3), 521–527.

Kilbourne, A. M., Rofey, D. L., McCarthy, J. F., Post, E. P., Welsh, D., & Blow, F. C. (2007). Nutrition and exercise behavior among patients with bipolar disorder. *Bipolar Disorders, 9*(5), 443–452

Kim, Y. J., McFarlane, C., Warner, D. S., Baker, M. T., Choi, W. W., & Dexter, F. (1996). The effects of plasma and brain magnesium concentrations on lidocaine-induced seizures in the rat. *Anesthesia & Analgesia, 83*(6), 1223–1228.

Knuppel, L., & Linde, K. (2004). Adverse effects of St. John's wort: A systematic review. *Journal of Clinical Psychiatry, 65*(11), 1470–1479.

Lakhan, S. E., & Vieira, K. F. (2008). Nutritional therapies for mental disorders. *Nutrition Journal, 21;7:2.*

Lawlor, D. A., & Hopker, S. W. (2001). The effectiveness of exercise as an intervention in the management of depression: Systematic review and meta-regression analysis of randomised controlled trials. *British Medical Journal, 322*(7289), 763–767.

Leibenluft, E., Feldman-Naim, S., Turner, E. H., Wehr, T. A., & Rosenthal, N. E. (1997). Effects of exogenous melatonin administration and withdrawal in five patients with rapid-cycling bipolar disorder. *Journal of Clinical Psychiatry, 58,* 383–388.

Leo, R. J., & Ligot, J. S. (2007). A systematic review of randomized controlled trials of acupuncture in the treatment of depression. *Journal of Affective Disorders, 97,* 13–22.

Levine, J. (1997). Controlled trials of inositol in psychiatry. *European Neuropsychopharmacology, 7*(2), 147–155. doi:S0924-977X(97)00409-4 [pii]

Levine, J., Mishori, A., Susnosky, M., Martin, M., & Belmaker, R. H. (1999). Combination of inositol and serotonin reuptake inhibitors in the treatment of depression. *Biological Psychiatry, 45,* 270–273.

Levine, J, Rapaport, A., Lev, L., Bersudsky, Y., Kofman, O., Belmaker, R. H., Shapiro, J., & Agam, G. (1993). Inositol treatment raises CSF inositol levels. *Brain Research, 627,* 168–170.

Linde, K., & Knüppel L. (2005). Large-scale observational studies of hypericum extracts in patients with depressive disorders—A systematic review. *Phytomedicine, 12*(1–2), 148–157.

Magalhaes, P. V., Dean, O. M., Bush, A. I., Copolov, D. L., Malhi, G. S., Kohlmann, K.,…Berk, M. (2011). N-acetylcysteine for major depressive episodes in bipolar disorder. *Rev Bras Psiquiatr, 33*(4), 374–378.

Melchart, D., Weidenhammer, W., Streng, A., Reitmayr, S., Hoppe, A., Ernst, E., & Linde, K. (2004). Prospective investigation of adverse effects of acupuncture in 97,733 patients. *Archives of Internal Medicine, 164,* 104–105.

Mischoulon, D., Best-Popescu, C., Laposata, M., Merens, W., Murakami, J. L., Wu, S. L.,…Fava, M. (2008). A double-blind dose-finding pilot study of docosahexaenoic acid (DHA) for major depressive disorder. *European Neuropsychopharmacology, 18*(9), 639–645.

Mischoulon, D., & Fava, M. (2002). Role of S-adenosyl-L-methionine in the treatment of depression: A review of the evidence. *The American Journal of Clinical Nutrition, 76,* 1158S–1161S.

Moore, C. M., Breeze, J. L., Kukes, T. J., Rose, S. L., Dager, S. R., Cohen, B. M., & Renshaw, P. F. (1999). Effects of myo-inositol ingestion on human brain myo-inositol levels: A proton magnetic resonance spectroscopic imaging study. *Biological Psychiatry, 45,* 1197–1202.

Mukai, T., Kishi, T., Matsuda, Y., & Iwata, N. (2014). A meta-analysis of inositol for depression and anxiety disorders. *Human Psychopharmacology, 29*(1), 55–63. doi:10.1002/hup.2369

Nathan, P. J., Burrows, G. D., Norman, T. R. (1999). Melatonin sensitivity to dim white light in affective disorders. *Neuropsychopharmacology, 21,* 408–413.

Naylor, G. J., & Smith, A. H. (1981). Vanadium: A possible aetiological factor in manic-depressive illness. *Psychological Medicine, 11* (2), 249–256.

Nemets, B., Stahl, Z., & Belmaker, R. H. (2002). Addition of omega-3 fatty acid to maintenance medication treatment for recurrent unipolar depressive disorder. *The American Journal of Psychiatry, 159*(3), 477–479.

Nemets, B., Mishory, A., Levine, J., & Belmaker, R. H. (1999). Inositol addition does not improve depression in SSRI treatment failures. *Journal of Neural Transmission, 106,* 795–798.

Nierenberg, A. A., Lund, H. G., & Mischoulon, D. (2008). St. John's wort: A critical evaluation of the evidence for antidepressant effects. In D. Mischoulon & J. F. Rosenbaum (Eds.), *Natural medications for psychiatry: Considering the alternatives* (2nd ed., pp. 27–29). Philadelphia: Lippincott Williams & Wilkins.

Nierenberg, A. A., Ostacher, M. J., Calabrese, J. R., Ketter, T. A., Marangell, L. B., Miklowitz, D. J.,…Sachs, G. S. (2006). Treatment-resistant bipolar depression: A STEP-BD equipoise randomized effectiveness trial of antidepressant augmentation with lamotrigine, inositol, or risperidone. *The American Journal of Psychiatry, 163*(2), 210–216. doi:163/2/210 [pii] 10.1176/appi.ajp.163.2.210

Nierenberg, A. A., Burt, T., Matthews, J., & Weiss, A. P. (1999). Mania associated with St. John's wort. *Biological Psychiatry, 46,* 1707–1708.

Noaghiul, S., & Hibbeln, J. R. (2003). Cross-national comparisons of seafood consumption and rates of bipolar disorders. *The American Journal of Psychiatry, 160*(12), 2222–2227.

Ortega, F. B., Ruiz, J. R., Castillo, M. J., & Sjostrom, M. (2008). Physical fitness in childhood and adolescence: A powerful marker of health. *International Journal of Obesity, 32*(1), 1–11. doi:0803774 [pii] 10.1038/sj.ijo.0803774

Patel, N. C., DelBello, M. P., Cecil, K. M., Adler, C. M., Bryan, H. S., Stanford, K. E., & Strakowski, S. M. (2006). Lithium treatment effects on myo-inositol in adolescents with bipolar depression. *Biological Psychiatry, 60,* 998–1004.

Peet, M., & Horrobin, D. F. (2002). A dose-ranging study of the effects of ethyl-eicosapentaenoate in patients with ongoing depression despite apparently adequate treatment with standard drugs. *Archives of General Psychiatry, 59*(10), 913–919.

Peet, M., Murphy, B., Shay, J., & Horrobin, D. (1998). Depletion of omega-3 fatty acid levels in red blood cell membranes of depressive patients. *Biological Psychiatry, 43*(5), 315–319.

Popper, C. W. (2001). Do vitamins or minerals (apart from lithium) have mood-stabilizing effects? *Journal of Clinical Psychiatry, 62*(12), 933–935.

Post, R., Leverich, G., Nolen, W., Kupka, R., Altshuler, L., Frye, M.,…Walden, J. (2003). A re-evaluation of the role of antidepressants in the treatment of bipolar depression: Data from the Stanley Foundation Bipolar Network. *Bipolar Disorders, 5*(6), 396–406.

Robertson, J. M., & Tanguay, P. E. (1997). Case study: The use of melatonin in a boy with refractory bipolar disorder. *Journal of the American Academy of Child & Adolescent Psychiatry, 36*(6), 822–825.

Rosenberg, G. S, & Davis, K. L. (1982). The use of cholinergic precursors in neuropsychiatric diseases. *The American Journal of Clinical Nutrition, 36,* 709–720.

Ruljancic, N., Mihanovic, M., Cepelak, I., & Bakliza, A. (2013). Platelet and serum calcium and magnesium concentration in suicidal and non-suicidal schizophrenic patients. *Psychiatry Clinical Neuroscience, 67*(3), 154–159. doi:10.1111/pcn.12038

Ruljancic, N., Mihanovic, M., Cepelak, I., Bakliza, A., & Curkovic, K. D. (2013). Platelet serotonin and magnesium concentrations in suicidal and non-suicidal depressed patients. *Magnesium Research, 26*(1), 9–17. doi:10.1684/mrh.2013.0332

Sabelli, H. C., Fawcett, J., Gusovsky, F., Javaid, J. I., Wynn, P., Edwards, J., & Jeffriess, H., Kravitz, H. (1986). Clinical studies on the phenylethylamine hypothesis of affective disorder: Urine and blood phenylacetic acid and phenylalanine dietary supplements. *Journal of Clinical Psychiatry, 47*(2), 66–70.

Sajatovic, M., Biswas, K., Kilbourne, A. K., Fenn, H., Williford, W., & Bauer, M. S. (2008). Factors associated with prospective long-term treatment adherence among individuals with bipolar disorder. *Psychiatric Services, 59*(7), 753–759. doi:10.1176/appi.ps.59.7.753

Samuels, N., Gropp, C., Singer, S. R., & Oberbaum, M. (2008). Acupuncture for psychiatric illness: A literature review. *Behavioral Medicine, 34*(2), 55–64. doi:10.3200/BMED.34.2.55–64

Sarris, J., Lake, J., & Hoenders, R. (2011). Bipolar disorder and complementary medicine: Current evidence, safety issues, and clinical considerations. *Journal of Alternative and Complementary Medicine, 17*(10), 881–890. doi:10.1089/acm.2010.0481

Sarris, J., Mischoulon, D., & Schweitzer, I. (2012). Omega-3 for bipolar disorder: Meta-analyses of use in mania and bipolar depression. *Journal of Clinical Psychiatry, 73*(1), 81–86. doi:10.4088/JCP.10r06710

Schaller, J. T., Thomas, J., & Bazzan, A. J. (2004). SAMe use in children and adolescents. *European Child and Adolescent Psychiatry, 13*, 332–334.

Schreier, H. A. (1981). Mania responsive to lecithin in a 13-year-old girl. *The American Journal of Psychiatry, 139*(1), 108–110.

Sheldon, S. H. (1998). Pro-convulsant effects of oral melatonin in neurologically disabled children. *Lancet, 351*, 1254.

Shimon, H., Agam, G., Belmaker, R. H., Hyde, T. M., & Kleinman, J. E. (1997). Reduced frontal cortex inositol levels in postmortem brain of suicide victims and patients with bipolar disorder. *The American Journal of Psychiatry, 154*(8), 1148–1150.

Silverstone, P. H., McGrath, B. M., Brent, M., & Kim, H. (2005). Bipolar disorder and myo-inositol: A review of the magnetic resonance spectroscopy findings. *Bipolar Disorders, 7*, 1–10.

Simeon, J., Nixon, M. K., Milin, R., Jovanovic, R., & Walker, S. (2005). Open-label pilot study of St. John's wort in adolescent depression. *Journal of Child Adolescent Psychopharmacology, 15*(2), 293–301.

Stoll, A., Severus, E., Freeman, M., Rueter, S., Zhoyan, H., Diamond, E., ...Marangell, L. (1999). Omega 3 fatty acids in bipolar disorder. *Archives of General Psychiatry, 56*, 407–412.

Suppes, T., Bersntein, I., Dennehy, E. et al. (2009). The safety, acceptability, and effectiveness of acupuncture as adjunctive treatment for bipolar disorder. *Journal of Clinical Psychiatry, 70*(6), 897–905.

Sylvia, L. G., Ametrano, R. M., & Nierenberg, A. A. (2010). Exercise treatment for bipolar disorder: Potential mechanisms of action mediated through increased neurogenesis and decreased allostatic load. *Psychotherapy and Psychosomatics, 79*(2), 87–96. doi:10.1159/000270916

Sylvia, L. G., Peters, A. T., Deckersbach, T., & Nierenberg, A. A. (2013). Nutrient-based therapies for bipolar disorder: a systematic review. *Psychotherapy and Psychosomatics, 82*(1), 10–19. doi:10.1159/000341309

Terano, T., Hirai, A., Hamazaki, T., Kobayashi, S., Fujita, T., Tamura, Y., & Kumagai, A. (1983). Effect of oral administration of highly purified eicosapentaenoic acid on platelet function, blood viscosity and red cell deformability in healthy human subjects. *Atherosclerosis, 46*(3), 321–331.

Thomas, C. S., Bottiglieri, T., Edeh, J., Carney, M. W., Reynolds, E. H., & Toone, B. K. (1987). The influence of S-adenosylmethionine (SAM) on prolactin in depressed patients. *International Clinical Psychopharmacology, 2*(2), 97–102.

von Knorring, A. L., Soderberg, A., Austin, L., & Uvnas-Moberg, K. (2008). Massage decreases aggression in preschool children: A long-term study. *Acta Paediatrica, 97*(9), 1265–1269.

Waldhauser, F., Weiszenbacher, G., Frisch, H., Zeitlhuber, U., Waldhauser, M., & Wurtman, R. J. (1984). Fall in nocturnal serum melatonin during prepuberty and pubescence. *Lancet, 1*(8373), 362–365.

Wang, H., Qi, H., Wang, B-S., Cui, Y.-Y., Zhu, L. Rong, Z-X., Chen, H-Z. (2008). Is acupuncture beneficial in depression: A meta-analysis of 8 randomized controlled trials? *Journal of Affective Disorders, 1*–10.

Whalley, L. J., Perini, T., Shering, A., & Bennie, J. (1991). Melatonin response to bright light in recovered, drug-free, bipolar patients. *Psychiatry Research, 38*, 13–19.

Willatts, P. (2002). Long chain polyunsaturated fatty acids improve cognitive development. *Journal of Family Health Care, 12*(Suppl. 6), 5.

Williams, A., Girard, C., Jui, D., Sabina, A., & Katz, D. L. (2005). S-Adenosylmethionine (SAMe) as Treatment for Depression: A Systematic Review. *Clinical and Investigative Medicine, 28*(3), 132–139.

Wolfson, M., Bersudsky, Y., Zinger, E., Simkin, M., Belmaker, R. H., & Hertz, L. (2000). Chronic treatment of human astrocytoma cells with lithium, carbamazepine or valproic acid decreases inositol uptake at high inositol concentrations but increases it at low inositol concentrations. *Brain Research, 855*(1), 158–161. doi:S0006-8993(99)02371-9 [pii]

Wood, J. L., & Allison, R. G. (1982). Effects of consumption of choline and lecithin on neurobiological and cardiovascular systems. *Federation Proceedings, 41*(14), 3015–3021.

Wood, J. L, & Allison, R. G. (1982). Effects of consumption of choline and lecithin on neurological and cardiovascular systems. *Federation Proceedings, 41*(14), 3015–3021.

Wozniak, J., Biederman, J., Mick, E., Waxmonsky, J., Hantsoo, L., Best, C., ...Laposata, M. (2007). Omega-3 fatty acid monotherapy for pediatric bipolar disorder: A prospective open-label trial. *European Neuropsychopharmacology, 17*(6–7), 440–447. doi:S0924-977X(06)00256-2 [pii]

Zhdanova, I. V., & Friedman, L. (2008). Therapeutic potential of melatonin in sleep and circadian disorders. In D. Mischoulon & J. F. Rosenbaum (Eds.), *Natural medications for psychiatry: Considering the alternatives* (2nd ed., pp. 140–162). Philadelphia: Lippincott Williams & Wilkins.

PART II

SOMATIC NONPHARMACOLOGICAL TREATMENTS

26.

ELECTROCONVULSIVE THERAPY AND BIPOLAR DISORDER

Lauren S. Liebman, Gabriella M. Ahle, Mimi C. Briggs, and Charles H. Kellner

INTRODUCTION

Electroconvulsive therapy (ECT) is an important treatment for patients with severe bipolar disorder. It is an effective treatment for all three phases of the illness. While ECT is most commonly used for the treatment of bipolar depression, it is also used for refractory mania and mixed states. Despite widespread clinical use, review articles on the treatment of bipolar disorder often only mention it cursorily (Geddes & Miklowitz, 2013; Kellner, Goldberg, Briggs, Liebman, & Ahle, 2013). Yet there is a large body of evidence-based literature supporting its use for bipolar disorder. Searching PubMed for "bipolar disorder electroconvulsive therapy" returns over 1,000 citations; over 500 citations for the search terms "bipolar depression ECT;" and over 600 for the search terms "mania ECT." Despite its proven efficacy and safety in bipolar disorder, stigma remains the largest obstacle to the more widespread use of ECT (Fink, 1997; Wilkinson & Daoud, 1998). In this chapter, we review the literature on ECT for bipolar depression, mania, and mixed states and provide recommendations for the selection of patients and technique.

PATIENT REFERRAL FOR ECT

In contemporary psychiatric medical practice, ECT is almost always reserved for patients who have failed multiple trials of psychotropic medications (Kellner et al., 2012). The rare exception is the patient who is so urgently ill (because of suicidality, agitation from psychosis, or medical comorbidity) that he or she needs to be treated urgently. In such situations, ECT may become the treatment of choice because of its rapid speed of response (Husain et al., 2004). Typical patients will often have been allowed to remain severely ill, undergoing multiple medication trials, before ECT is considered. Referral for ECT is typically made by the treating psychiatrist to an ECT expert practitioner consultant (Kellner, 2012).

The ECT consultation should include careful review of the patient's current, past, and family psychiatric history; medical history; and discussion of informed consent (Kellner, 2012). Evaluation of a patient's psychiatric history allows the practitioner to assess severity, episodicity, and heritability of the illness (Kellner, Popeo, Pasculli, Briggs, & Gamss, 2012). Symptoms in the current episode that compel serious consideration of ECT include suicidal acts and thoughts, catatonia, severe functional disability and poor self-care, and inanition due to weight loss or dehydration. A comprehensive medical history is critical for identifying any comorbidities that may need to be managed by the ECT team during the procedure (Tess & Smetana, 2009). Of particular concern is the status of patient's cardiac and pulmonary functions. The most common serious medical comorbidity that needs careful management is coronary artery disease. Modern anesthetic techniques allow control of heart rate and blood pressure within safe ranges. Prior to starting ECT patients are required to have a medical evaluation that typically consists of a complete history and physical, electrocardiogram, basic metabolic panel, complete blood count, and, in some cases, a chest x-ray or other additional, specific diagnostic testing (Kellner, 2012). An anesthesiology consultation is also performed prior to the procedure; close collaboration with the anesthesiologist in the development of the ECT treatment plan is essential to optimum ECT practice (Kellner & Bryson, 2012).

As with any other medical procedure, informed consent is a crucial part of ECT. The vast majority of patients, despite being seriously psychiatrically ill, are able to provide fully informed consent. The informed consent process for ECT is more comprehensive than that for most medical procedures because of the intense scrutiny to which ECT has been subjected. For the small minority of patients who are too ill to have decisional capacity for their medical treatments, a substituted consent procedure is instituted. Specific regulations about substituted consent vary by jurisdiction (Kellner et al., 2012).

Although ECT is appropriate only for a small percentage of the most seriously ill psychiatric patients, because psychiatric illness is so prevalent, this remains an absolutely large number. ECT should be available widely and in fact continues to be offered at most major medical centers on an inpatient and/or outpatient basis (Case et al., 2013). The clinical and scientific evidence base for ECT is large, spanning several decades; more recently developed, experimental somatic and pharmacologic treatments for mood disorders have yet to establish themselves as clinically viable alternatives for seriously ill patients (Fink, 2014).

OVERVIEW OF ECT TECHNIQUE

ECT technique for the treatment of bipolar depression does not differ from that for unipolar depression (ECT technique in mania is discussed later). Clinical decisions about electrode placement, stimulus dose, and treatment schedule are based on the same clinical factors as for other psychiatric indications. Severity of illness is the most important determinant of electrode placement; bilateral electrode placement is preferred in the most severely ill patients (Kellner et al., 2010; Kellner, Tobias, & Wiegand, 2010). Right unilateral (RUL) electrode placement, in which the stimulus is applied across the nondominant hemisphere for language (the right hemisphere in over 90% of the population), may be preferred for the nonurgently ill patient with the intent of minimizing adverse cognitive effects (American Psychiatric Association, 2001). Patient preference may play a role in this decision; many patients with cognitively demanding occupations may opt to try RUL before considering bilateral placement.

Stimulus dosing in ECT continues to evolve. Recent advances in technique include the use of a dose titration method to empirically determine an individual's seizure threshold at the first treatment. Additionally, an accumulating body of evidence suggests that stimulus pulse widths of less than 0.5 msec (referred to as ultrabrief pulse stimuli) may result in less cognitive impairment (Sienaert, Vansteelandt, Demyttenaere, & Peuskens, 2010).

Strategies for electrical stimulus dosing aim to maximize antidepressant/mood stabilizing/antipsychotic efficacy and speed of response while minimizing adverse cognitive effects (Prudic, 2008). Current guidelines suggest conservative stimulus dosing with bilateral electrode placement (1.5–2x seizure threshold, or the half-age method) (Petrides et al., 2009) whereas with RUL placement, stimulus dosing is more liberal (at least 5 times the seizure threshold; American Psychiatric Association, 2001; Sackeim et al., 2000).

It should be remembered that modern ECT technique always involves full general anesthesia, muscle relaxation, and hyperventilation with 100% oxygen. Standard anesthesia induction agents are methohexital, thiopental, and propofol; alternative agents include etomidate and ketamine. The muscle relaxant of choice for ECT is succinylcholine. This is administered at a dose of approximately 1.0 mg/kg once the patient is rendered unconscious by the induction anesthetic agent. A blood pressure cuff is inflated to above systolic pressure on the patient's ankle for the purpose of excluding the succinylcholine from that foot, in order to observe the motor manifestations of the seizure. Modern ECT standard of care also involves recording of the electroencephalograph (EEG) for the purposes of confirming that the seizure has been initiated and, equally important, for confirming that the seizure has ended. Modern ECT devices allow for measurement of at least two EEG channels, typically recorded from each hemisphere using right and left frontal and mastoid leads (Kellner, 2012; Weiner, Coffey, & Krystal, 1991).

When given for the remediation of symptoms for an acute episode of mood disorder, the treatment series is referred to as "an acute course of ECT" or "an index course of ECT." The treatment schedule for bipolar depressed patients is the same as for unipolar depressed patients: typically three times per week but sometimes twice per week to allow cognitive recovery between treatments. Treatments in the acute course are typically continued until the patient has reached remission of the current episode. However, post–ECT relapse is an important problem. By convention, continuation ECT refers to those treatments delivered in the six-month period following remission, while maintenance refers to the treatments provided after six months. Current practice is often to taper the acute course, with increasing intervals between treatments with the goal of reducing relapse (Rabheru, 2012). When maintenance treatment is provided, the interval between treatments is gradually increased and many patients are treated approximately once every three to five weeks on an outpatient basis. No specific fixed schedule has been agreed on in the field, and it is typical for maintenance schedules to be adjusted based on patient illness characteristics. True maintenance ECT is provided to patients who are well at the time, with the goal of preventing the onset of a subsequent mood episode.

ECT AND BIPOLAR DEPRESSION

The treatment of bipolar depression is by far the most common and important use of ECT in bipolar disorder. Similar to its use in unipolar depression, ECT is typically reserved for the most severely ill patients who have failed to respond to multiple pharmacological interventions. Such patients may be urgently ill on the basis of suicidal thoughts and behavior, psychosis, and medical risk from poor self-care.

There is a large evidence base in the literature suggesting that ECT is an equally effective treatment for unipolar and bipolar depression. In a cohort of 220 patients, Bailine et al. (2010) compared the efficacy of ECT for the treatment of unipolar ($n = 170$) and bipolar ($n = 50$) depression. Remission was defined as 24-item Hamilton Rating Scale for Depression ($HRSD_{24}$) scores of less than or equal to 10 and at least a 60% reduction in $HRSD_{24}$ score from baseline. Patients were treated with either bifrontal, bitemporal, or RUL electrode placements. Overall, 61.8% of patients remitted, and there was no significant difference in remission rates between unipolar (61.2%) and bipolar (64%) patients. Additionally, there was no significant interaction between electrode placement, remission, and diagnosis (Bailine et al., 2010).

A meta-analysis by Dierckx, Heijnen, van den Broek, & Birkenhager (2012) reviewed six of the largest studies that compare ECT response and remission outcome in bipolar ($n = 790$) and unipolar ($n = 316$) depressed patients, including the Bailine et al. (2010) study previously mentioned. In general, response criteria were defined as a decrease of greater than or equal to 50% from the baseline HRSD (17-item [$HRSD_{17}$] or 24-item) score. Remission criteria were mostly defined as a $HRSD_{24}$ less than or equal to 10 or a $HRSD_{17}$ less than or equal to 7. Dierckx et al. found no significant difference in rates of remission between unipolar (50.9%) and bipolar (53.2%) patients.

While response and remission rates were similar among bipolar and unipolar depressed patients, some studies found that bipolar patients required fewer treatments to achieve response and remission. Using "moderate" ($HRSD_{17} \leq 10$, "remitter 10") or "strict" ($HRSD_{17} \leq 7$, "remitter 7") remission criteria, Sienaert et al. (2009) found that bipolar depressed patients ($n = 13$) required approximately seven treatments to achieve response and eight treatments to achieve remitter-10

status. On the other hand, unipolar patients ($n = 51$) required an average of 9 treatments to achieve response and 11 treatments to achieve remitter-10 status. Despite the fact that bipolar patients initially required fewer treatments to achieve a $HRSD_{17}$ score of 10, there was no significant difference in additional treatments needed to get to a $HRSD_{17}$ of 7 between the two groups. Both bipolar and unipolar patients were treated with either RUL ultrabrief pulse or bifrontal ultrabrief pulse ECT (Sienaert, Vansteelandt, Demyttenaere, & Peuskens, 2009). Similarly, Daly et al. (2001) in a reanalysis of data from three prior studies found that by the sixth ECT, bipolar patients ($n = 66$) showed a 54.9% ($SD = 31.9$%) reduction in $HRSD_{24}$ score compared with a 43.9% ($SD = 29.8$%) reduction among unipolar patients ($n = 162$). These patients were treated with either RUL (at four different stimulus intensities) or bilateral (at two different stimulus intensities) ECT; while high stimulus dose and bilateral placement were associated with greater efficacy, bipolar patients responded more quickly than unipolar patients overall. (Daly et al., 2001). Sackeim and Prudic (2005) in a naturalistic sample of patients treated at seven community hospitals also found that bipolar patients ($n = 54$) showed a more rapid response to ECT compared to unipolar patients ($n = 279$) when treated with either RUL or bilateral ECT (Sackeim & Prudic, 2005). While other studies suggest that speed of response to ECT is similar between bipolar and unipolar patients (Abrams & Taylor, 1974; Bailine, et al., 2010; Black, Winokur, & Nasrallah, 1986), these results provide evidence that bipolar patients may, in fact, require fewer treatments.

SAFETY AND TOLERABILITY

Safety and tolerability data for ECT are derived largely from studies in which diagnosis was of secondary importance. As such, most of these data are from patients with unipolar depression. However, there is no reason to believe that different diagnoses have an impact on the safety and tolerability of ECT. Therefore, in this section we review overall data about the safety and tolerability of ECT.

The mortality of ECT is generally reported to be 1 per 10,000 patients (American Psychiatric Association, 2001). This is likely to be derived from a largely healthy population. However, since many ECT patients are elderly and have multiple systemic medical illnesses, the true rate may be somewhat higher. A recent survey of adverse events (between 1999 and 2010) related to ECT in the Veterans Affairs National Center for Patient Safety database found that the mortality rate of ECT was less than 1 death per 73,440 treatments, suggesting that ECT is even safer than previously reported (Watts, Groft, Bagian, & Mills, 2011). Additionally, a 2013 case report found no significant morphological brain changes postmortem in an 84-year-old man who had received 422 ECT treatments (with bilateral electrode placement and maximum stimulus dosing; Anderson, Wollmann, & Dinwiddie, 2013).

Medical risks

The most significant morbidity of ECT involves cardiovascular events. These are rare enough that a true base rate is very difficult to ascertain. The greatest risk in ECT is in patients with coronary artery disease; this puts them at risk for myocardial ischemia during a period of increased oxygen demand induced by the ECT seizure (Zielinski, Roose, Devanand, Woodring, & Sackeim, 1993). Of theoretical but much less practical importance because of its rarity, the risk of ECT in patients with neurological illnesses associated with increased intracranial pressure is substantial. It has been stated that the only true medical contraindication to ECT is the presence of an intracranial tumor associated with increased intracranial pressure (Kellner, 1996).

Cognitive risks

Historically, the side effect that has most limited the use of ECT is that of memory loss. Modern ECT techniques result in markedly diminished memory impairment compared to ECT techniques of the past, and concern about cognitive outcome should no longer be considered a major impediment to prescribing the treatment for appropriately selected patients (Kellner, 2013). In other words, concerns about cognitive risk should not be the overriding consideration for seriously ill bipolar depressed patients who have failed to respond to pharmacotherapy. The adverse cognitive effects can be divided into three types: (a) an acute confusional state, (b) anterograde amnesia, and (c) retrograde amnesia. The acute confusional state and anterograde amnesia are of relatively little concern because they are almost always time limited. Retrograde amnesia, the erasing of some recent memories, has been the effect of most concern. The extent of retrograde amnesia is commensurate with the type and intensity of ECT that a patient receives: patients who remit with short courses of RUL ECT may have very minor retrograde amnesia, compared with more significant effects in patients who require longer courses with bilateral electrode placement

(Lisanby, 2007). Interestingly, and often overlooked, is the fact that many of the cognitive impairments related to depression will be reversed by ECT and a patient's overall cognition will be improved following a course of ECT (Stoudemire, Hill, Morris, & Dalton, 1995).

CONCOMITANT MEDICATIONS

The concomitant use of medications with ECT for patients with bipolar depression is little different from that of other ECT patients. The controversial nature of treating bipolar depression with antidepressants notwithstanding, many bipolar depressed patients coming to ECT will be on antidepressant medications. In recent years, there has been a tendency to liberalize concomitant use of antidepressants and ECT. In fact, new evidence suggests that some antidepressants will add to the antidepressant effect of ECT (Sackeim et al., 2009). Even monoamine oxidase inhibitors, once believed to present unacceptable risks during ECT, are now considered relatively safe (Dolenc, Habl, Barnes, & Rasmussen, 2004). In general, it is believed that most antidepressants, used at conventional doses, are quite safe in conjunction with ECT (Yildiz et al., 2010). However, use of antidepressants in bipolar disorder necessitates caution, and their prudent administration should follow the most recent statements provided in the International Society for Bipolar Disorders Task Force Report on Antidepressant Use in Bipolar Disorders (Pacchiarotti et al., 2013).

KETAMINE ANESTHESIA AS A POTENTIAL ANTIDEPRESSANT ADJUNCT

Recent demonstration of the intrinsic antidepressant effect of ketamine has rekindled interest in ketamine as an anesthetic for ECT (Murrough et al., 2013). Ketamine has been used as an alternative anesthetic in ECT for the past several decades. However, its use has been limited by the adverse side-effect profile, including dissociative symptoms and hypertension (Rasmussen, Jarvis, & Zorumski, 1996). There is no reason to believe that bipolar depressed patients will respond to ketamine differently than ECT patients with other diagnoses. A fairly extensive literature documenting ketamine's use in ECT demonstrates only modest increased antidepressant efficacy (Kranaster, Kammerer-Ciernioch, Hoyer, & Sartorius, 2011). The hope that there would be dramatic synergistic effects between ketamine and ECT has not been realized. Ketamine remains a useful alternative anesthetic for any ECT patient in whom seizure elicitation has become difficult, because of its mildly proconvulsant properties (Krystal et al., 2003).

ECT AND MANIA

In addition to its well-known use as an antidepressant, ECT is among the treatment options for the manic phase of bipolar disorder. In fact, mania is one of the six "cleared indications" listed for ECT devices by the United States Food and Drug Administration (FDA Executive Summary, 2011). Additionally, all major international guidelines for the use of ECT list mania as an indication (American Psychiatric Association, 2001; National Institute for Clinical Excellence, 2003). Despite this ubiquitous recognition for the use of ECT to treat mania, it is used far less for this indication than for depression. ECT is often recommended as a second-line treatment option for medication-refractory mania, which is a relatively uncommon condition. Most manic patients will respond to medications if given high enough doses (of single or multiple agents) for an adequate time.

In a review published in *The American Journal of Psychiatry* in 1994, Mukherjee et al. reviewed 50 years' experience of using ECT to treat mania. They concluded that ECT resulted in "marked clinical improvement or clinical remission…in 80% of 589 manic patients" (p. 171). Many of these patients had been unresponsive to pharmacotherapy. They reviewed the earlier study of Black et al. (1986) that reported approximately 60% remission rates in manic patients with poor response to lithium or neuroleptics. They also reviewed technical aspects of ECT and mania (see section on "ECT Technique in Mania") as well as concomitant use of lithium and neuroleptics (discussed later). More recently, Loo, Katalinic, Mitchell, & Greenberg (2011) again reviewed the literature on the use of ECT to treat acute mania. Little had changed since the findings of Mukherjee et al. (1994) 15 years earlier; Loo et al. added reviews of two studies comparing bifrontal and bitemporal electrode placement for mania. Both studies found good efficacy for both techniques and slightly discrepant results regarding differential cognitive outcomes (see section on "ECT Technique in Mania"; Barekatain, Jahangard, Haghighi, & Ranjkesh, 2008; Hiremani, Thirthalli, Tharayil, & Gangadhar, 2008.

DELIRIOUS MANIA

Delirious mania, also known as excited catatonia and malignant catatonia, is a rare syndrome characterized by sudden onset delirium, mania, and psychosis that has recently gained attention as a unique diagnostic entity (Maldeniya & Vasudev, 2013). As defined by Fink (1999), delirious mania "is a syndrome of the acute onset of the excitement, grandiosity, emotional lability, delusions, and insomnia characteristic of mania and the disorientation and altered consciousness characteristic of delirium" (p. 59). It is often accompanied by fever, dehydration, and autonomic instability, making it a medical emergency. Initial treatment is supportive, and definitive treatment is often with ECT, sometimes on a schedule of daily treatments until response is achieved (Kellner, 2012).

ECT TECHNIQUE IN MANIA

Given that most patients with refractory mania who are treated with ECT are urgently ill, it seems reasonable that the most potent and effective form of ECT should be used. In fact, it has been the standard of the field to recommend bilateral ECT at moderately high stimulus doses, sometimes on a daily schedule, for such urgently ill patients (Mukherjee, Sackeim, & Schnur, 1994). However, there is also considerable clinical trial and case report data to suggest that RUL ECT is effective in some manic patients (Mukherjee, Sackeim, & Lee, 1988; Robinson, Penzner, Arkow, Kahn, & Berman, 2011). Despite these reports, prudent clinical practice would suggest continuing the use of the most potent forms of ECT in patients with urgent clinical indications (Milstein et al., 1987).

In their review of the literature to date, Mukherjee et al. (1994) concluded that the speed of response to ECT in mania did not differ from the speed of response in major depression. Thirthalli, Kumar, Bangalore, & Gangadhar (2009), in a retrospective chart review, noted that manic patients showed clinical improvement with significantly fewer treatments with treatment at higher, compared to lower, stimulus doses.

CONCOMITANT MEDICATIONS IN MANIA AND ECT

Lithium

Because of its common usage in the treatment of bipolar disorder, lithium is a medication that ECT practitioners will encounter frequently in their practice. There is an extensive literature on the concurrent administration of lithium and ECT, which concludes that, in general, the practice is relatively safe (Dolenc & Rasmussen, 2005). Many patients have been treated safely while continuing to take lithium. However, it is clear that in certain situations lithium may increase the risk of a prolonged seizure or increased cognitive impairment/delirium with ECT (Weiner, Whanger, Erwin, & Wilson, 1980). These factors mandate the prudent coadministration of lithium and ECT and result in the common recommendation that lithium levels be decreased to the low therapeutic range when ECT is given. In practice, lithium doses are commonly held for 24 to 48 hours prior to each ECT procedure (Kellner, 2012). Given the pharmacokinetics of lithium, this typically results in a reduction of serum lithium levels by approximately 50%. This liberal attitude toward the concurrent administration of lithium and ECT allows patients to benefit from the mood-stabilizing effects of lithium and ECT simultaneously.

Anticonvulsants

Anticonvulsants, including valproate, carbamazepine, and lamotrigine, are frequently administered as mood stabilizers in all phases of bipolar disorder and present specific challenges with concomitant ECT use. Obviously, since the therapeutic goal of ECT is to induce a seizure, anticonvulsant medications may interfere either with the induction of a seizure or the therapeutic potency of an induced seizure. In general, it is recommended that anticonvulsants given for psychiatric indications either be tapered or discontinued prior to ECT (American Psychiatric Association, 2001). An accumulating evidence base suggests that many patients can be treated successfully while on concomitant anticonvulsants, but it may be prudent to at least withhold doses prior to treatment such that blood levels are lower (Rubner, Koppi, & Conca, 2009; Sienaert & Peuskens, 2007; Virupaksha, Shashidhara, Thirthalli, Kumar, & Gangadhar, 2010).

Antipsychotics

Both first- and second-generation antipsychotic medications have been used safely and effectively in conjunction with ECT. There is an extensive literature, going back decades, suggesting that concomitant use of first-generation antipsychotics with ECT in patients with psychotic depression, psychotic symptoms in mania, and schizophrenia is a helpful strategy for early remediation of symptoms (Haskett & Loo, 2010). Because of the potential for cardiovascular adverse effects with low potency first-generation antipsychotics, these drugs should be used cautiously in conjunction with ECT (Grinspoon & Greenblatt, 1963). There is an accumulating literature about the safety of concomitant use of second-generation (atypical) antipsychotics and ECT. Because these medications are increasingly prescribed for their antidepressant and mood-stabilizing effects, they are likely to be used more frequently with ECT in the future.

ECT INDUCING MANIC SWITCHES

All effective antidepressants are capable of switching depressed bipolar patients into hypomania or mania, and ECT is no exception. However, fears of this complication have been greatly exaggerated, and the extant literature suggests that this is a relatively uncommon phenomenon. When it does occur, it most commonly results in a brief period of hypomania and, only very rarely, frank mania. In a cohort of 220 depressed patients, (170 unipolar, 50 bipolar), Bailine et al. (2010) reported that approximately 9% (21/220) of patients received scores in the mild to moderate range on the Clinician-Administered Rating Scale for Mania Outcome at some point during the ECT course. Of these 21 patients, only one patient received a score in the moderate range after the course of ECT (Bailine et al., 2010). Management of such a switch can be temporary cessation of ECT with continued medication management or continuation of the ECT treatment course with the expectation that the ECT itself will treat the induced hypomania. It should be remembered that a hypomanic patient is almost always less seriously ill than a profoundly depressed one; therefore, such switches into hypomania, unless they evolve to full-blown mania or cycle acceleration, may often be regarded as relative therapeutic successes.

ECT AND BIPOLAR MIXED STATES

The literature in ECT and mixed states is necessarily small because this diagnostic entity is much less commonly identified. Since ECT works at both poles of bipolar illness (depression and mania), there is no intuitive reason to suspect that it would not also work equally well for mixed states. The literature on mixed states includes a review by Valenti et al. (2008) in which the only three papers on the subject are discussed in detail. Given the evidence that suicide risk may be particularly high in mixed states (because of the coexistence of depressed mood and increased energy), the well-known rapid antisuicide effect of ECT should be kept in mind (Kellner et al., 2005).

Devanand et al. (2000) conducted a chart review comparing treatment response and clinical course in 38 bipolar depressed, 5 bipolar manic, and 10 bipolar mixed patients. The three patient groups exhibited robust response to ECT, but the mixed group had longer hospital stays and there was a trend for them to require a greater number of ECT treatments. Gruber, Dilsaver, Shoaib, and Swann (2000) reported on seven patients in mixed states who were pharmacotherapy-resistant and referred for ECT; all seven patients remitted. Ciapparelli et al. (2001) reported on 41 patients with mixed states and compared them to 23 patients with bipolar depression. The mixed-mania patients showed a significantly greater decrease in depression rating scores than bipolar depressed patients, a greater reduction in suicidality, and a more rapid response. Despite minor differences in the findings of the above studies, it is clear that mixed affective states respond robustly to ECT.

CONSENT FOR ECT

The consent process for ECT, while always more comprehensive than that for most other medical procedures, is particularly difficult in the case of a bipolar patient experiencing a severe and/or psychotic mood episode. In both depressive and manic or mixed phases of bipolar disorder, patients may be agitated and psychotic with delusional thinking and very limited attention span. Such patients often lack capacity for informed medical decision making and will need to have substituted consent. The specific procedure for obtaining such substituted consent will vary by jurisdiction and may be constrained by the country or the US state laws that are considered by some to be overly restrictive and prejudicial to certain patient populations (Kellner et al., 2012; Wachtel et al., 2013). In certain states this will be a relatively simple matter of invoking emergency procedures, while in others it will involve an ECT-specific court-mandated process. Once a bipolar patient has begun to improve after one or several ECT, it may then be possible to obtain informed consent from the patient him or herself. In rare instances, patients and providers have collaborated to create advanced directives such that euthymic bipolar patients may be able to express their preference for future treatments, including ECT, should they have another severe episode.

CONCLUSION

The existing literature makes it clear that ECT is an important and efficacious treatment for severe bipolar disorder in all phases of the illness. Efficacy is almost uniformly reported as high, as are safety and tolerability. In bipolar disorder, as in all other major psychiatric illnesses for which ECT is indicated, ECT use continues to be limited because of stigma and lack of familiarity with, or availability of, the treatment. Consent issues, always a focus of treatment with contemporary ECT, are no different for bipolar depressed patients than for unipolar depressed patients;

however, patients with psychotic features or in manic phase of the illness present particular challenges to obtaining fully informed consent, such that substituted consent with recourse to mandated judicial requirements may be necessary for some severely ill patients.

Disclosure statement: Dr. Charles H. Kellner has received grant support from the National Institute of Mental Health, royalties from Cambridge University Press, and honoraria from UpToDate, Psychiatric Times, and North Shore-LIJ Health System.

Lauren S. Liebman has no conflicts of interest. Gabriella M. Ahle has no conflicts of interest. Mimi C. Briggs has no conflicts of interest.

REFERENCES

Abrams, R., & Taylor, M. A. (1974). Unipolar and bipolar depressive illness. Phenomenology and response to electroconvulsive therapy. *Archives of General Psychiatry, 30*(3), 320–321.

American Psychiatric Association. (2001). *The practice of ECT: Recommendations for treatment, training, and privileging* (2nd ed.). Washington DC: American Psychiatric Press.

Anderson, D., Wollmann, R., & Dinwiddie, S. H. (2014). Neuropathological evaluation of an 84-year-old man after 422 ECT treatments. *The Journal of ECT, 30*(3), 248–250.

Bailine, S., Fink, M., Knapp, R., Petrides, G., Husain, M. M., Rasmussen, K.,…Kellner, C. H. (2010). Electroconvulsive therapy is equally effective in unipolar and bipolar depression. *Acta Psychiatrica Scandinavica, 121*(6), 431–436.

Barekatain, M., Jahangard, L., Haghighi, M., & Ranjkesh, F. (2008). Bifrontal versus bitemporal electroconvulsive therapy in severe manic patients. *The Journal of ECT, 24*(3), 199–202.

Black, D. W., Winokur, G., & Nasrallah, A. (1986). ECT in unipolar and bipolar disorders: A naturalistic evaluation of 460 patients. *Convulsive Therapy, 2*(4), 231–237.

Case, B. G., Bertollo, D. N., Laska, E. M., Price, L. H., Siegel, C. E., Olfson, M., & Marcus, S. C. (2013). Declining use of electroconvulsive therapy in U.S. general hospitals is not restricted to unipolar depression. *Biological Psychiatry, 74*(10), e19–e20.

Ciapparelli, A., Dell'Osso, L., Tundo, A., Pini, S., Chiavacci, M. C., Di Sacco, I., & Cassano, G. B. (2001). Electroconvulsive therapy in medication-nonresponsive patients with mixed mania and bipolar depression. *Journal of Clinical Psychiatry, 62*(7), 552–555.

Daly, J. J., Prudic, J., Devanand, D. P., Nobler, M. S., Lisanby, S. H., Peyser, S.,…Sackeim, H. A. (2001). ECT in bipolar and unipolar depression: Differences in speed of response. *Bipolar Disorders, 3*(2), 95–104.

Devanand, D. P., Polanco, P., Cruz, R., Shah, S., Paykina, N., Singh, K., & Majors, L. (2000). The efficacy of ECT in mixed affective states. *The Journal of ECT, 16*(1), 32–37.

Dierckx, B., Heijnen, W. T., van den Broek, W. W., & Birkenhager, T. K. (2012). Efficacy of electroconvulsive therapy in bipolar versus unipolar major depression: A meta-analysis. *Bipolar Disorders, 14*(2), 146–150.

Dolenc, T. J., Habl, S. S., Barnes, R. D., & Rasmussen, K. G. (2004). Electroconvulsive therapy in patients taking monoamine oxidase inhibitors. *The Journal of ECT, 20*(4), 258–261.

Dolenc, T. J., & Rasmussen, K. G. (2005). The safety of electroconvulsive therapy and lithium in combination: A case series and review of the literature. *The Journal of ECT, 21*(3), 165–170.

FDA Executive Summary. (2011). Washington, DC: US Food and Drug Administration. http://www.fda.gov/downloads/Advisory Committees/CommitteesMeetingMaterials/MedicalDevices/ MedicalDevicesAdvisoryCommittee/NeurologicalDevices Panel/ UCM240933.pdf

Fink, M. (1997). Prejudice against ECT: Competition with psychological philosophies as a contribution to its stigma. *Convulsive Therapy, 13*(4), 253–265; discussion 266–258.

Fink, M. (1999). Delirious mania. *Bipolar Disorders, 1*(1), 54–60.

Fink, M. (2014). What was learned: Studies by the consortium for research in ECT (CORE) 1997–2011. *Acta Psychiatrica Scandinavica, 129*(6), 417–426.

Geddes, J. R., & Miklowitz, D. J. (2013). Treatment of bipolar disorder. *Lancet, 381*(9878), 1672–1682.

Grinspoon, L., & M. Greenblatt (1963). pharmacotherapy combined with other treatment methods. *Comprehensive Psychiatry, 4,* 256–262.

Gruber, N. P., Dilsaver, S. C., Shoaib, A. M., & Swann, A. C. (2000). ECT in mixed affective states: A case series. *The Journal of ECT, 16*(2), 183–188.

Haskett, R. F., & Loo, C. (2010). Adjunctive psychotropic medications during electroconvulsive therapy in the treatment of depression, mania, and schizophrenia. *The Journal of ECT, 26*(3), 196–201.

Hiremani, R. M., Thirthalli, J., Tharayil, B. S., & Gangadhar, B. N. (2008). Double-blind randomized controlled study comparing short-term efficacy of bifrontal and bitemporal electroconvulsive therapy in acute mania. *Bipolar Disorders, 10*(6), 701–707.

Husain, M. M., Rush, A. J., Fink, M., Knapp, R., Petrides, G., Rummans, T.,...Kellner, C. H. (2004). Speed of response and remission in major depressive disorder with acute electroconvulsive therapy (ECT): A Consortium for Research in ECT (CORE) report. *Journal of Clinical Psychiatry, 65*(4), 485–491.

Kellner, C. H. (1996). The CT scan (or MRI) before ECT: A wonderful test has been overused. *Convulsive Therapy, 12*(2), 79–80.

Kellner, C. H. (2012). *Brain stimulation in psychiatry: ECT, DBS, TMS, and other modalities.* Cambridge, UK: Cambridge University Press.

Kellner, C. H. (2013). The cognitive effects of ECT: tolerability versus safety. *Psychiatric Times, 30*(3).

Kellner, C. H., & Bryson, E. O. (2012). Anesthesia advances add to safety of ECT. *Psychiatric Times, 29*(1), 12–15.

Kellner, C. H., Fink, M., Knapp, R., Petrides, G., Husain, M., Rummans, T.,...Malur, C. (2005). Relief of expressed suicidal intent by ECT: A consortium for research in ECT study. *The American Journal of Psychiatry, 162*(5), 977–982.

Kellner, C. H., Goldberg, J. F., Briggs, M. C., Liebman, L. S., & Ahle, G. M. (2013). Somatic treatments for severe bipolar disorder. *Lancet, 382*(9891), 505–506.

Kellner, C. H., Greenberg, R. M., Murrough, J. W., Bryson, E. O., Briggs, M. C., & Pasculli, R. M. (2012). ECT in treatment-resistant depression. *The American Journal of Psychiatry, 169*(12), 1238–1244.

Kellner, C. H., Knapp, R., Husain, M. M., Rasmussen, K., Sampson, S., Cullum, M.,...Petrides, G. (2010). Bifrontal, bitemporal and right unilateral electrode placement in ECT: randomised trial. *The British Journal of Psychiatry, 196*(3), 226–234.

Kellner, C. H., Popeo, D. M., Pasculli, R. M., Briggs, M. C., & Gamss, S. (2012). Appropriateness for electroconvulsive therapy (ECT) can be assessed on a three-item scale. *Medical Hypotheses, 79*(2), 204–206.

Kellner, C. H., Tobias, K. G., & Wiegand, J. (2010). Electrode placement in electroconvulsive therapy (ECT): A review of the literature. *The Journal of ECT, 26*(3), 175–180.

Kranaster, L., Kammerer-Ciernioch, J., Hoyer, C., & Sartorius, A. (2011). Clinically favourable effects of ketamine as an anaesthetic for electroconvulsive therapy: A retrospective study. *European Archives of Psychiatry in Clinical Neuroscience, 261*(8), 575–582.

Krystal, A. D., Weiner, R. D., Dean, M. D., Lindahl, V. H., Tramontozzi, L. A. III, Falcone, G., & Coffey, C. E. (2003). Comparison of seizure duration, ictal EEG, and cognitive effects of ketamine and methohexital anesthesia with ECT. *The Journal of Neuropsychiatry & Clinical Neurosciences, 15*(1), 27–34.

Lisanby, S. H. (2007). Electroconvulsive therapy for depression. *New England Journal of Medicine, 357*(19), 1939–1945.

Loo, C., Katalinic, N., Mitchell, P. B., & Greenberg, B. (2011). Physical treatments for bipolar disorder: A review of electroconvulsive therapy, stereotactic surgery and other brain stimulation techniques. *Journal of Affective Disorders, 132*(1–2), 1–13.

Maldeniya, P. M., & Vasudev, A. (2013). Is the concept of delirious mania valid in the elderly? A case report and a review of the literature. *Case Reports in Psychiatry, 2013,* 432568.

Milstein, V., Small, J. G., Klapper, M. H., Small, I. F., Miller, M. J., & Kellams, J. J. (1987). Uni- versus bilateral ect in the treatment of mania. *Convulsive Therapy, 3*(1), 1–9.

Mukherjee, S., Sackeim, H. A., & Lee, C. (1988). Unilateral ECT in the treatment of manic episodes. *Convulsive Therapy, 4*(1), 74–80.

Mukherjee, S., Sackeim, H. A., & Schnur, D. B. (1994). Electroconvulsive therapy of acute manic episodes: A review of 50 years' experience. *The American Journal of Psychiatry, 151*(2), 169–176.

Murrough, J. W., Iosifescu, D. V., Chang, L. C., Al Jurdi, R. K., Green, C. E., Perez, A. M.,...Mathew, S. J. (2013). Antidepressant efficacy of ketamine in treatment-resistant major depression: A two-site randomized controlled trial. *The American Journal of Psychiatry, 170*(10), 1134–1142.

National Institute for Clinical Excellence. (2003). *Guidance on the use of electroconvulsive therapy.* London: National Institute for Clinical Excellence.

Pacchiarotti, I., Bond, D. J., Baldessarini, R. J., Nolen, W. A., Grunze, H., Licht, R. W.,...Vieta, E. (2013). The International Society for Bipolar Disorders (ISBD) Task Force report on antidepressant use in bipolar disorders. *The American Journal of Psychiatry, 170,* 1249–1269. doi:10.1176/appi.ajp.2013.13020185. [Epub ahead of print]

Petrides, G., Braga, R. J., Fink, M., Mueller, M., Knapp, R., Husain, M.,...Kellner, C. (2009). Seizure threshold in a large sample: implications for stimulus dosing strategies in bilateral electroconvulsive therapy: A report from CORE. *The Journal of ECT, 25*(4), 232–237.

Prudic, J. (2008). Strategies to minimize cognitive side effects with ECT: Aspects of ECT technique. *The Journal of ECT, 24*(1), 46–51.

Rabheru, K. (2012). Maintenance electroconvulsive therapy (M-ECT) after acute response: Examining the evidence for who, what, when, and how? *The Journal of ECT, 28*(1), 39–47.

Rasmussen, K. G., Jarvis, M. R., & Zorumski, C. F. (1996). Ketamine anesthesia in electroconvulsive therapy. *Convulsive Therapy, 12*(4), 217–223.

Robinson, L. A., Penzner, J. B., Arkow, S., Kahn, D. A., & Berman, J. A. (2011). Electroconvulsive therapy for the treatment of refractory mania. *Journal of Psychiatric Practice, 17*(1), 61–66.

Rubner, P., Koppi, S., & Conca, A. (2009). Frequency of and rationales for the combined use of electroconvulsive therapy and antiepileptic drugs in Austria and the literature. *World Journal of Biological Psychiatry, 10*(4 Pt. 3), 836–845.

Sackeim, H. A., Dillingham, E. M., Prudic, J., Cooper, T., McCall, W. V., Rosenquist, P.,...Haskett, R. F. (2009). Effect of concomitant pharmacotherapy on electroconvulsive therapy outcomes: Short-term efficacy and adverse effects. *Archives of General Psychiatry, 66*(7), 729–737.

Sackeim, H. A., & Prudic, J. (2005). Length of the ECT course in bipolar and unipolar depression. *The Journal of ECT, 21*(3), 195–197.

Sackeim, H. A., Prudic, J., Devanand, D. P., Nobler, M. S., Lisanby, S. H., Peyser, S.,...Clark, J. (2000). A prospective, randomized, double-blind comparison of bilateral and right unilateral electroconvulsive therapy at different stimulus intensities. *Archives of General Psychiatry, 57*(5), 425–434.

Sienaert, P., & Peuskens, J. (2007). Anticonvulsants during electroconvulsive therapy: Review and recommendations. *The Journal of ECT*, *23*(2), 120–123.

Sienaert, P., Vansteelandt, K., Demyttenaere, K., & Peuskens, J. (2009). Ultra-brief pulse ECT in bipolar and unipolar depressive disorder: Differences in speed of response. *Bipolar Disorders*, *11*(4), 418–424.

Sienaert, P., Vansteelandt, K., Demyttenaere, K., & Peuskens, J. (2010). Randomized comparison of ultra-brief bifrontal and unilateral electroconvulsive therapy for major depression: Cognitive side-effects. *Journal of Affective Disorders*, *122*(1–2), 60–67.

Stoudemire, A., Hill, C. D., Morris, R., & Dalton, S. T. (1995). Improvement in depression-related cognitive dysfunction following ECT. *The Journal of Neuropsychiatry & Clinical Neurosciences*, *7*(1), 31–34.

Tess, A. V., & Smetana, G. W. (2009). Medical evaluation of patients undergoing electroconvulsive therapy. *New England Journal of Medicine*, *360*(14), 1437–1444.

Thirthalli, J., Kumar, C. N., Bangalore, R. P., & Gangadhar, B. N. (2009). Speed of response to threshold and suprathreshold bilateral ECT in depression, mania and schizophrenia. *Journal of Affective Disorders*, *117*(1–2), 104–107.

Valenti, M., Benabarre, A., Garcia-Amador, M., Molina, O., Bernardo, M., & Vieta, E. (2008). Electroconvulsive therapy in the treatment of mixed states in bipolar disorder. *European Psychiatry*, *23*(1), 53–56.

Virupaksha, H. S., Shashidhara, B., Thirthalli, J., Kumar, C. N., & Gangadhar, B. N. (2010). Comparison of electroconvulsive therapy (ECT) with or without anti-epileptic drugs in bipolar disorder. *Journal of Affective Disorders*, *127*(1–3), 66–70.

Wachtel, L. E., Dhossche, D. M., Fink, M., Jaffe, R., Kellner, C. H., Weeks, H., & Shorter, E. (2013). ECT for developmental disability and severe mental illness. *The American Journal of Psychiatry*, *170*(12), 1498–1499.

Watts, B. V., Groft, A., Bagian, J. P., & Mills, P. D. (2011). An examination of mortality and other adverse events related to electroconvulsive therapy using a national adverse event report system. *The Journal of ECT*, *27*(2), 105–108.

Weiner, R. D., Coffey, C. E., & Krystal, A. D. (1991). The monitoring and management of electrically induced seizures. *The Psychiatric Clinics of North America*, *14*(4), 845–869.

Weiner, R. D., Whanger, A. D., Erwin, C. W., & Wilson, W. P. (1980). Prolonged confusional state and EEG seizure activity following concurrent ECT and lithium use. *The American Journal of Psychiatry*, *137*(11), 1452–1453.

Wilkinson, D., & Daoud, J. (1998). The stigma and the enigma of ECT. *International Journal of Geriatrics Psychiatry*, *13*(12), 833–835.

Yildiz, A., Mantar, A., Simsek, S., Onur, E., Gokmen, N., & Fidaner, H. (2010). Combination of pharmacotherapy with electroconvulsive therapy in prevention of depressive relapse: A pilot controlled trial. *The Journal of ECT*, *26*(2), 104–110.

Zielinski, R. J., Roose, S. P., Devanand, D. P., Woodring, S., & Sackeim, H. A. (1993). Cardiovascular complications of ECT in depressed patients with cardiac disease. *The American Journal of Psychiatry*, *150*(6), 904–909.

27.

NEUROMODULATIVE TREATMENTS FOR BIPOLAR DISORDER

REPETITIVE TRANSCRANIAL MAGNETIC STIMULATION, VAGUS NERVE STIMULATION, AND DEEP BRAIN STIMULATION

Christina Switala, Sabrina Maria Gippert, Sarah Kayser,

Bettina Heike Bewernick, and Thomas Eduard Schlaepfer

INTRODUCTION

In psychiatric disorders, targets have been chosen using knowledge derived from lesion and imaging studies as well as from current understanding of the pathophysiology of the disorder. In the contrary to neurological diseases, there is not a single pathological structure in psychiatric illness. Several brain structures presumably play different roles in the development, as well as in the maintenance of symptoms. Some targets are in close anatomical or functional relationship (neural networks) and an overlap of effect is plausible. It has been shown that several targets can lead to remission. Thus different targets manipulate the pathological network at different nodes.

So far, the management of treatment-resistant unipolar or bipolar depression is a therapeutic challenge, as many such patients continue to lack adequate treatment options. Current data point to the fact that the neurobiology of bipolar depression is very similar to unipolar major depression. Especially in severe, therapy-resistant forms, a differentiation between unipolar and bipolar depression has become unnecessary.

Hence, for these patients alternative treatment methods are urgently needed. This chapter introduces the methods of repetitive transcranial magnetic stimulation (rTMS), vagus nerve stimulation (VNS), and deep brain stimulation (DBS) as possible treatment options for bipolar disorder (BD).

REPETITIVE TRANSCRANIAL MAGNETIC STIMULATION AND DEEP REPETITIVE TRANSCRANIAL MAGNETIC STIMULATION

REPETITIVE TRANSCRANIAL MAGNETIC STIMULATION

Repetitive transcranial magnetic stimulation (rTMS) refers to the administration of series of pulsed magnetic stimuli to the brain for the purpose of altering brain function (Figure 27.1). This treatment method was originally invented by Barker, Jalinous, and Freeston (1985) and delivers magnetic pulses to the cortex using a stimulating coil, which is applied directly to the head. The equipment necessary to deliver rTMS consists of two parts: a stimulator, which generates brief pulses of strong electrical currents whose frequency and intensity can be varied, and a stimulation coil connected to the stimulator. The magnetic field generated at the coil passes unimpeded through scalp and skull and induces an electrical current in the underlying tissue, which in turn depolarizes neurons (George et al., 2003; Schlaepfer & Kosel., 2004a). The main advantage of this method is its noninvasiveness and the possibility to stimulate relatively small brain volumes. With recent technology, single, paired, or repetitive magnetic pulses can be generated and delivered (Schlaepfer, George, & Mayberg, 2010). A repetitively application of TMS pulses can modulate cortical excitability (i.e., increasing or decreasing it), depending

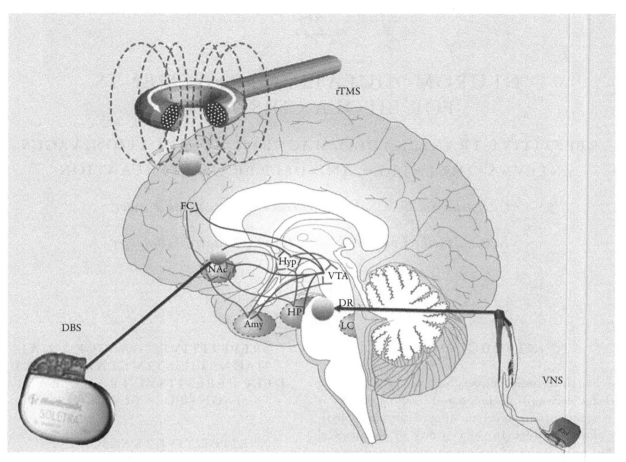

Figure 27.1 Repetitive transcranial magnetic stimulation (rTMS), vagus nerve stimulation (VNS) and deep brain stimulation (DBS) (exemplary Nucleus Accumbens) as neuromodulative treatments. (See color insert)

on the parameters of stimulation (Fitzgerald, Fountain, & Daskalakis, 2006). Because rTMS can reversibly alter cortical function, it is being actively researched in many disorders such as depression, negative symptoms in schizophrenia, hallucinations, anxiety, posttraumatic stress disorder, obsessive-compulsive disorder, tinnitus, and migraine (Schlaepfer, et al., 2010).

DEEP REPETITIVE TRANSCRANIAL MAGNETIC STIMULATION

Deep rTMS, as a modification of rTMS, is mainly used for the treatment of drug-resistant Major depressive disorder (MDD), but there are also ongoing studies investigating its use for the treatment of other psychiatric, neurological and medical diseases like BD, posttraumatic stress disorder, autism, Asperger's syndrome, addictions, alcoholism, Alzheimer's disease, Parkinson's disease, schizophrenia, tinnitus, migraine, cognitive deficits, multiple sclerosis, and neuropathic pain (Bersani, Minichino, et al., 2013). Whereas rTMS is mostly applied with a figure-of-eight coil

(8-coil), deep rTMS can be applied with different types of coils: the H-coil (Roth, Zangen, & Hallett, 2002), the C-core coil (Davey & Riehl, 2006), and the circular crown coil (Deng, Peterchev, & Lisanby, 2008). The H-coil, however, is the only coil whose safety and effectiveness has been tested.

Even though both rTMS and deep rTMS can modulate cortical excitability positively or negatively by inducing changes in those neural circuits that are supposed to be dysfunctional, the H-coil is able to modulate cortical excitability up to a maximum depth of 6 cm (Roth, Amir, Levkovitz, & Zangen, 2007). The 8-coil, on the other hand, has biological effects on the nerve cells within 1.5 to 2.5 cm from the scalp. Therefore, the induced electromagnetic field considerably decreases in intensity when approaching deeper brain regions. This exponential decay of the electromagnetic signal can be regarded as a function of the distance from the coil, due to the characteristics of the cerebral tissue acting as a conductor. Thus the H-coil modulates the activity not only of the cerebral cortex but also of deeper neural circuits (Bersani, Minichino, et al., 2013).

TREATMENT ADMINISTRATION

Before the onset of treatment, the motor threshold (MT) must be identified—a global measure of corticospinal excitability that represents the lowest stimulation intensity required to evoke a motor potential of at least 50 μV or the contraction of abductor brevis pollicis muscle in 5 out of 10 stimulations. As MT is affected by such factors as medications, abuse of substances, electroconvulsive therapy, and pathological events, it should be measured daily during therapy with TMS. After the identification of the MT, the coil is moved from the motor cortex to the specific target cortical region. In the treatment of MDD and bipolar depression, the target area is the left dorsolateral prefrontal cortex (Harel et al., 2011; Levkovitz et al., 2009). Further, the frequency (the effect of the stimulation on the cortical excitability) and the intensity (the depth of the stimulation) of the electromagnetic stimulation are considered. In detail, frequencies equal or less than 1 Hz produce an inhibitory effect and frequencies more than 1 Hz an excitatory effect. The intensity is measured from 1 to 100. This number represents a percentage value with regard to the maximum intensity of the neurostimulator. The correct intensity is measured in relation to the MT, for example 100% of MT, 110% of MT, and so on (Bersani, Minichino, et al., 2013).

CONTRAINDICATIONS AND SIDE EFFECTS

Repetitive transcranial magnetic stimulation

In general, rTMS is regarded as safe and without enduring side effects. There have been no reported lasting neurological, cognitive, or cardiovascular sequelae as a result of rTMS (Schlaepfer, et al., 2010). Inducing a seizure is the primary safety concern with rTMS. A summary document from an international safety meeting on rTMS reported 12 cases of seizures induced with rTMS (Wassermann, 1997). The authors estimated these 12 cases occurred with a sample size of several thousand. This puts the risk at less than 0.5 percent. Most of these patients were healthy volunteers without a history of epilepsy. Fortunately, there are no reports that the individuals affected experienced recurrence. Also, all of the seizures occurred during rTMS administration when the patient was sitting down and near an investigator, and all of the seizures were self-limited without needing medications or other interventions. Of the reported cases, the majority were receiving rTMS to the motor cortex—the most epileptogenic region of the cortex. Additionally, most (but not all) were receiving trains of stimulation outside of suggested limits. These cases suggest that rTMS-induced seizures will remain a small but significant adverse event even in patients without a history of seizures and even when rTMS is used within suggested guidelines. One patient reported a temporary hearing loss after rTMS. In light of this, an extensive study of auditory threshold was conducted before and after four weeks of rTMS in over 300 patients. No changes were found. However, patients and TMS operators should wear earplugs when receiving TMS. Headaches are the most common complaint after rTMS, typically relieved by non-narcotic analgesics such as aspirin. The incidence of headache did not differ between active and sham in the largest clinical trials to date (Janicak et al., 2008). Repeated analysis of cognitive functioning of rTMS patients has not found any enduring negative effects from the procedure (Janicak, et al., 2008; Little et al., 2000; Schulze-Rauschenbach et al., 2005). After a session, patients are able to drive home and return to work. When conducting rTMS, safety criteria on the basis of two consensus conferences (Rossi, Hallett, Rossini, & Pascual-Leone, 2009; Wassermann, 1998) must be considered. Based on the results of a study by O'Reardon and colleagues (2007), rTMS was approved by the US Food and Drug Administration (FDA) in 2008 for the treatment of modest treatment-resistant depression (TRD). Furthermore, there is evidence for rTMS either as a mono- or add-on therapy for the treatment of modest TRD (evidence-based medicine, Level 1).

Deep repetitive transcranial magnetic stimulation

Patients showing the following physiological or pathological conditions are discouraged from undergoing deep rTMS treatment for safety reasons: a history of seizures or epilepsy in first-degree relatives and the presence of any known factor that can lower the seizure threshold (sleep deprivation, caffeine, abuse substance, etc.); previous head injury and the presence of metallic implants in the cephalic region (e.g., aneurysm clips, shunts, stimulators, cochlear implants, electrodes) with the exception of dental fillings and the presence of cardiac pacemakers, neurostimulators, surgical clips, or other electronic equipment; the presence of an acute or chronic cardiac disease; deafness or hearing loss; metabolic or systemic diseases; and comorbidity with several neurological disorders (e.g., increased intracranial pressure, space-occupying lesion, history of stroke or transient ischemic attack, brain aneurysm). Overall, deep rTMS can be considered a safe and tolerable treatment. Nevertheless, side effects like scalp discomfort, transient headache, and dizziness, as well as dizziness associated with nausea, insomnia, sensation of foul smell, bad taste and repulsive smell, numbness in the right temporal and right cervical zone, and generalized seizures have been reported

(Bersani, Minichino, et al., 2013). On the one hand, high stimulation intensities used in deep rTMS can overstimulate cortical regions and facial nerves, which in turn can lead to epileptic seizures or other undesirable side effects (Marcolin & Padberg, 2007). On the other hand, patients who are additionally in treatment with high doses of antidepressant drugs are more likely to experience seizures (Pisani, Spina, & Oteri, 1999).

REPETITIVE TRANSCRANIAL MAGNETIC STIMULATION AS A TREATMENT FOR UNIPOLAR DEPRESSION

Repetitive transcranial magnetic stimulation

Largely because of its noninvasiveness, rTMS has been investigated in several neuropsychiatric disorders. Depression has been the most widely studied disorder using TMS (George et al., 2003; Kosel & Schlaepfer, 2005; Schlaepfer & Kosel, 2004a, 2005). To investigate response, remission and drop-out rates following high-frequency rTMS (HF-rTMS; frequencies ≥ 5 Hz) for MDD, a meta-analysis including data from 29 randomized, double-blind, and sham-controlled trials (N = 1371 subjects with MDD) was conducted (Berlim, van den Eynde, Tovar-Perdomo, & Daskalakis, 2013). Response was defined as a ≥ 50% reduction in posttreatment scores on the Hamilton Depression Rating Scale (HADRS) or on the Montgomery–Åsberg Depression Rating Scale (MADRS) at the end of the blinded treatment. Remission was based on the primary efficacy measure (e.g., 17- or 21-item HADRS scores ≤ 7 or ≤ 8, respectively, or MADRS scores ≤ 6 at the end of the blinded treatment). Briefly, the results showed that this neuromodulation technique is significantly more effective than sham rTMS in terms of both response (29.3% vs. 10.4% in sham rTMS) and remission rates (18.6% vs. 5% in sham rTMS). Furthermore, HF-rTMS seems to be equally effective as an augmentation strategy or monotherapy for MDD when it is used in patients with defined TRD or in patients with less resistant depressive disorder and in samples with unipolar MDD or in mixed samples with unipolar and bipolar depression. Moreover, alternative stimulation parameters were not associated with differential efficacy estimates. Finally, HF- and sham rTMS groups did not differ in terms of baseline depressive symptomatology and drop-out rates. Therefore, the authors concluded that HF-rTMS seems to be a suitable treatment for depression that is associated with clinically relevant antidepressant effects and a benign tolerability profile.

Deep repetitive transcranial magnetic stimulation

So far, deep rTMS has achieved the greatest therapeutic effects in the treatment of depression, and it is regarded as a valid method to become a new treatment for drug-resistant depressed patients or those who cannot be treated with medications (Bersani, Minichino, et al., 2013).

The prefrontal cortex is the brain region that is mostly involved in the modulation of mood and emotional behavior. In this respect, the greatest efficacy was obtained by excitatory stimulation applied to the left dorsolateral prefrontal cortex using standard rTMS (Broadbent et al., 2011). The left dorsolateral prefrontal cortex, in turn, is a region that is hypoactive (reduced metabolism and blood flow) during episodes of declined mood (Drevets, 2000). Alternatively, the reward circuit is a system that has gained increasing focus in the study of MDD. The main component of this circuit is the mesolimbic dopaminergic pathway consisting of the nucleus accumbens and the ventral tegmentum area, which are both interconnected with the dorsal and ventral lateral prefrontal cortices. It is assumed that the nucleus accumbens and the ventral tegmentum area contribute substantially to the pathophysiology and symptomatology of depression (Nestler & Carlezon, 2006).

Therefore, even though rTMS has proved to be moderately effective in treating drug-resistant depression and has been shown to be effective in stimulating the prefrontal cortex, it is conceivable that deep rTMS stimulation, which reaches a much greater depth, might show greater effects as the magnetic field generated by rTMS is not sufficient to reach deeper cortical, subcortical, and limbic areas (Bersani, Minichino, et al., 2013). To date, seven studies have been published investigating the efficacy of deep rTMS in patients suffering from drug-resistant depression (Harel et al., 2012; Isserles et al., 2011; Levkovitz, et al., 2009; Levkovitz et al., 2011; Rosenberg et al., 2011; Rosenberg, Shoenfeld, Zangen, Kotler, & Dannon, 2010; Rosenberg, Zangen, Stryjer, Kotler, & Dannon, 2010). Overall, the results indicate that deep rTMS is an effective, safe, and well-tolerated method of treatment for patients suffering from drug-resistant unipolar depression both as a monotherapy and as an add-on treatment.

REPETITIVE TRANSCRANIAL MAGNETIC STIMULATION AS A TREATMENT FOR BIPOLAR DEPRESSION

Repetitive transcranial magnetic stimulation

Studies investigating the efficacy of rTMS in bipolar depression are mixed with some studies showing rather positive results (Erfurth, Michael, Mostert, & Arolt, 2000; George, Speer, Molloy, et al., 1998; Tamas, Menkes, & El-Mallakh, 2007) and some negative trials (Nahas, Kozel, Li, Anderson, & George, 2003; Tharayil, Gangadhar, Thirthalli, & Anand, 2005). It must be pointed out that as the baseline mood changes more quickly because patients cycle into and out of a depression naturally, in general it takes larger samples to show effects in bipolar patients (George et al., 2009).

Deep repetitive transcranial magnetic stimulation

There is only one clinical trial present in the scientific literature so far where deep rTMS was used to treat patients suffering from bipolar depression (Harel et al., 2011). Nineteen patients under psychopharmacological treatment were enrolled and received prefrontal deep rTMS with H-coil every weekday for four consecutive weeks. All pulses were delivered in trains of 20 Hz at 120% of MT. Each session consisted of 42 trains with a 2- second duration for each and a 20-second intertrain interval (a total of 1,680 magnetic pulses delivered per session). Response was defined as a 50% reduction on the HDRS one week after the last treatment session; remission was defined as an HDRS score less than 10. Concerning these criterions, 12 of 19 patients (63.2%) were classified as responders; 10 of 19 patients (52.6%) achieved remission. Despite the limitations of a small sample taking concomitant medications and the lack of placebo stimulation in this study, the results nevertheless suggest a higher efficacy of deep rTMS than rTMS. In this respect, a response rate of 54% and a remission rate of 36.3% in a study using rTMS were observed (Dell'Osso et al., 2009). In this study, 11 subjects with bipolar I or bipolar II disorder and MDD who did not respond to previous pharmacological treatment were treated with three weeks of open-label rTMS at 1 Hz, 110% of MT, 300 stimuli/day. In 2013, a case report assessing efficacy and safety of add-on deep rTMS in drug-resistant bipolar depression, as well as its ability to protect from subsequent episodes of any polarity, was published (Bersani, Girardi, et al., 2013). It is the first published report to show efficacy of deep rTMS in treatment-resistant bipolar depression so far. The authors presented the achieved data from one patient suffering from BD that has been treated with 20 daily consecutive deep rTMS sessions and with one deep rTMS session every two weeks for the following three months with the same parameters used in the acute phase: 18 Hz for 2 seconds for 55 trains at 120% of the MT. Depressive symptoms improved rapidly. Thus the patient started improving by the first week of deep rTMS and

clinical remission was achieved after 2 weeks of treatment (10 sessions). Furthermore, the safety of deep rTMS in this case, also in terms of cognitive improvements, could be confirmed. Moreover, the patient reported only mild and transient side effects such as nausea, diaphoresis, mild headaches, and scalp discomfort. During continuation sessions the patient was in stable remission. He showed no depressive relapses and no manic switches. The authors concluded that deep rTMS can be useful in treatment-resistant bipolar depression and in preventing bipolar episodes of any polarity, even though this case report presents a relatively short follow-up and the improvements cannot solely be attributed to the deep rTMS treatment as it was an add-on study on medications. Further, there is a lack of double-blind, placebo-controlled studies investigating the efficacy and safety of deep rTMS, as well as clinical trials comparing deep rTMS with other brain stimulation techniques, and more factors associated with successful treatment should be identified (Bersani, Minichino, et al., 2013).

VAGUS NERVE STIMULATION

BACKGROUND

Vagus nerve stimulation (VNS) therapy is an invasive brain stimulation method whereby a small electrical pulse is administered through an implanted neurostimulator to a bipolar lead fixed to the left vagus nerve (George et al., 2000; Schlaepfer & Kosel, 2004a) (Figure 27.1). Ben-Menachem et al. (1995) studied this procedure in patients with treatment-resistant epilepsy, and subsequently the VNS device was approved by the FDA for epilepsy in 1997. Interestingly, significant and clinically meaningful antidepressant effects of VNS therapy in epilepsy patients have been described independently of reduction of seizure frequency (Elger, Hoppe, Falkai, Rush, & Elger, 2000). Thus in 2005 the FDA approved VNS therapy for the adjunctive long-term treatment of chronic or recurrent depression (unipolar or bipolar) for patients over the age of 18 who are undergoing a major depressive episode and have not had an adequate response to two or more antidepressant treatments.

MECHANISM OF ACTION

Both vagus nerves carry signals from the brain to the heart, lungs, and intestines and to areas of the brain that control mood, sleep, and other functions. So far, no precise mechanism of action has been reported for antiseizure effects of

VNS therapy or for the antidepressant efficacy. It was demonstrated in brain imaging studies that VNS affects the metabolism of limbic structures and of the prefrontal cortex, which are both relevant to mood regulation (Drevets, Bogers, & Raichle, 2002; Henry et al., 1999). Another putative mechanism of action, supported by animal and human studies, might be the influence of VNS on monoaminergic neurotransmission (Dorr & Debonnel, 2006; Roosevelt, Smith, Clough, Jensen, & Browning, 2006), for example, serotonin, norepinephrine, gamma-aminobutyric acid, and glutamate (George et al., 2000). Serotonergic and noradrenergic systems are especially involved in both the pathophysiology of depression and the mechanisms of action of antidepressants. Different from other antidepressants (e.g., electroconvulsive therapy, antidepressant drugs), VNS therapy does not seem to be associated with an initial reduction in the firing rates of serotonergic neurons, which could be an explanation for the slow and progressive increase of antidepressant response in clinical VNS studies (Dorr & Debonnel, 2006). However, these findings are not consistent with those in functional neuroimaging studies (e.g., PET, SPECT, fMRI; Chae et al., 2003).

VAGUS NERVE STIMULATION PROCEDURE AND STIMULATION PARAMETERS

The VNS therapy system consists of the implantable pulse generator, the lead, and the external programming system used to change stimulation parameters. The generator is surgically implanted under the skin of the left chest. An electrical lead is connected from the generator to an electrode partially wrapped around the left midcervical region of the vagus nerve. Intermittent electrical signals are sent via the wire from the generator to the vagus nerve and via nucleus tractus solitarius to various regions of the brain (Schachter & Schmidt, 2001). The handheld device allows noninvasive programming, device diagnostics, and data check back. Usually, electrical pulses that last about 30 seconds are forwarded about every five minutes from the generator to the vagus nerve; other parameters consist of a current intensity of 0.20 to 2.50 mA, a pulse width of 500 ms and a pulse frequency of 20 Hz.

ANTIDEPRESSANT EFFICACY RESULTS

A number of clinical studies assessing antidepressant properties of VNS therapy in patients suffering from TRD have been conducted yet (see Table 27.1). Researchers have suggested acute and longer-term antidepressants effects, but different response rates were demonstrated. The one- and two-year results were significantly superior by outcomes in comparison of patients receiving treatment as usual (TAU). Additionally, many of the patients who had a significant response within the first year of treatment continued to have a similar degree of response through two years. However, VNS therapy is most effective in patients with moderate but not extreme levels of resistance to conventional antidepressant treatments. The averaged response rates of VNS therapy plus TAU measured by the MADRS was 12% after 12 weeks (TAU only 4%), 18% after 24 weeks (TAU only 7%), 28% after 48 weeks (TAU only 12%), and 32% after 96 weeks (TAU only 14%). Finally, despite FDA approval, VNS therapy continues to be a controversial treatment for depression because antidepressant results of studies have been inconsistent. Altogether, the incidence of manic reaction or manic depressive reaction was 44% in D01, 12% in D02, 11% in D03, as described in detail in the following, and for all bipolar patients combined 22%. In published clinical studies, no difference in response rates between MDD and BD were described.

The first open-label, unblinded, four-center pilot study (D01) in patients suffering from TRD, evaluating VNS

Table 27.1. OVERVIEW OF CLINICAL STUDIES ASSESSING ANTIDEPRESSANT PROPERTIES OF VNS THERAPY IN PATIENTS SUFFERING FROM TRD

VARIABLE	VNS THERAPY + TAU (N = 1,035)					TAU ONLY (N = 425)	
	D01	D02	D03	D21	D23	D04	D23
Number of patients	60	235	74	331	335	124	301
MDD (%)	73.3	89.4	73	77.9	71	87.9	76.4
BP I and II (%)	26.7	10.6	27	22.1	29	12.1	23.6
MADRS baseline Mean (SD)	33.4 (5.1)	31.7 (6.2)	32.9 (6.4)	33.7 (4.8)	33.1 (7.9)	29.4 (6.9)	33.4 (5.1)

NOTE: MDD = major depressive disorder; BP = bipolar disorder; MADRS = Montgomery–Åsberg Depression Rating Scale; TAU = treatment as usual.

therapy plus TAU over 24 months, was conducted in 1998 (Nahas et al., 2005; Rush et al., 2000; Sackeim et al., 2001). Patients suffering from bipolar depressive disorder (26.7% of the whole sample) were required to demonstrate a resistance to lithium treatment, have a medical contraindication to lithium, or be intolerant to lithium. The results demonstrated a 31% response rate during the acute study (after three months) and one-year response rates of 45% (Rush et al., 2000). These results led to a subsequent randomized, double-blind, multisite, sham-controlled pivotal clinical study (D02,) which was initiated in 2000 to evaluate safety and effectiveness of VNS therapy following a 12-week acute phase and during a 12-month follow-up evaluation period. Patients were treated with VNS therapy plus TAU or TAU only. Twenty-five patients had a baseline diagnosis of BD. The response rates of 15.2% in the active VNS therapy group and of 10% in the sham control group measured after three months were alike (Rush, Marangell, et al., 2005; Rush, Sackeim, et al., 2005). Concerning side effects, a total of six patients experienced a manic/hypomanic reaction during the study. However, there was a significant improvement in 30% of the patients over 12 months of VNS therapy. These results were superior to outcome rates of 12.5% after 12 months in a cluster-matched sample of patients receiving only TAU (George et al., 2005). In both samples, medications, psychotherapy, and other nonpharmacological treatments (electroconvulsive therapy, TMS) could be used, which could have led to the different one-year outcome results. The two-year outcome demonstrated response rates of 42% in a total sample of 52 patients. Thus TRD patients showed long-term benefits of the treatment with VNS therapy (Nahas et al., 2005). The postapproval study D21 evaluated three different doses of VNS therapy in 331 patients (Aaronson et al., 2013). During the acute phase of 22 weeks, patients received low dose (0.25 mA, 130 μsec), medium dose (0.5–1.0 mA, 250 μsec), or high dose (1.25–1.5 mA, 250 μsec) of VNS therapy. The D23 study is a long-term (60 months), open-label, observational registry of patients receiving VNS plus TAU (335 patients) or TAU only (301 patients). The observational study D04 was initiated to collect long-term clinical data for 124 patients. The purpose of this study was to compare clinical outcomes in similar depressed patients, who received VNS therapy and TAU (D02 study) and TAU only (Dunner et al., 2006; George et al., 2005). 15 patients (*SD* 12) with BD were enrolled in this study. Patients with a history of rapid cycling were excluded. Four percent of the patients improved after 12 months, in comparison to 12% in the D02 study.

The VNS therapy was approved for commercial distribution in the European Union countries in 2001. This study (D03) continued as a Phase IV European postmarketing study and includes an acute treatment phase, as well as a long-term follow-up phase (24 months). Antidepressant properties of VNS therapy (plus TAU) in extremely treatment-resistant patients were demonstrated, even if due to the protocol limitation that the putative contribution of the placebo effect cannot be assessed (Schlaepfer et al., 2008). The VNS therapy D05 study was a videotape assessment of the D02 study to examine interrater reliability for the depression assessments. Finally, the D06 VNS therapy pilot study included patients with rapid cycling BD.

SIDE EFFECTS

Patients receiving VNS therapy may experience various side effects, including infection from the implant surgery, hoarse voice, cough, and shortness of breath; difficulty in swallowing; and neck pain, some of which may persist as long as the device is active. Long-term side effects are unknown. The VNS therapy cannot be used in patients who have had their vagus nerve cut or who will be exposed to diathermy.

DEEP BRAIN STIMULATION

DEEP BRAIN STIMULATION AS A PUTATIVE TREATMENT METHOD IN SEVERE PSYCHIATRIC DISORDERS

Electric stimulation of the brain began in 1879, when limb movement were elicited by stimulating the motor cortex in dogs; human studies followed in 1884 (Gildenberg, 2005). Insights from lesioning studies, imaging studies, and animal models have contributed to the development of DBS. DBS is the stereotaxic placement of unilateral or bilateral electrodes connected to a permanently implanted, battery-powered neurostimulator, usually placed subcutaneously in the chest area (Figure 27.1). Although the exact neurobiological mechanisms by which DBS exerts effects on brain tissue are not yet fully understood (Hardesty & Sackeim, 2007), the hypothesis is that chronic HF (130–185 Hz) stimulation reduces neural transmission through inactivation of voltage-dependent ion channels (Breit, Schulz, & Benabid, 2004). Chronic DBS was invented in the 1980s by Benabid, Pollak, Louveau, Henry, and de Rougemont (1987) for the treatment of movement disorders, especially Parkinson's disease. In the mid-20th century, the first chronic brain stimulation was performed, when the Nucleus Caudatus was stimulated for eight weeks in a case of a severe depressed patient (Fins, 2003). Today this method is clinically used for the treatment of tremor associated with Parkinson's disease, chronic pain, and dystonia. The observation of induced psychiatric side effects (e.g., changes in mood, hypomania, reduction of anxiety) initiated the attempt to try DBS for psychiatric disorders (Mallet et al., 2002). Another reason was the fact that the effective but irreversible ablative neurosurgical interventions could now be emulated using DBS with a focused, fully reversible, and titratable technique.

DBS can be seen as an improved alternative to ablative neurosurgical procedures, which are used for well-defined groups of patients with extremely severe treatment-refractory mental disorders, such as anterior cingulotomy (for obsessive-compulsive disorder, MDD, and pain; Greenberg et al., 2003), subcaudate tractotomy (for obsessive-compulsive disorder and MDD), limbic leucotomy (for obsessive-compulsive disorder, MDD, and self-mutilation; Price et al., 2001) and anterior capsulotomy (for obsessive-compulsive disorder).

On the neuronal level, excitatory and inhibitory processes might play a role (McIntyre, Savasta, Kerkerian-Le Goff, & Vitek, 2004). Most probably DBS leads to a functional lesion of the surrounding tissue. Further mechanisms are depolarization blockade of current dependent ion channels (Beurrier, Bioulac, Audin, & Hammond, 2001), exhaustion of the neurotransmitter pool (Zucker & Regehr, 2002), or synaptic inhibition (Dostrovsky et al., 2000). Today it is unknown which part of the neuron (e.g., cell body, axon) is primarily modulated by DBS. Certainly the stimulation volume is not a fixed area around the electrode and the effect on neuronal tissue is variable. The effect of DBS on neurons depends on different factors: the physiological properties of the surrounding brain tissue, the geometric configuration of the electrode, as well as the distance and orientation of the neuronal elements toward the electrode (Kringelbach, Jenkinson, Owen, & Aziz, 2007). Stimulation parameters (frequency, amplitude, pulse width, duration) also clearly have an impact on the effect (Ranck, 1975). With commonly used parameters, a relatively large volume of neural tissue is influenced (Kringelbach, et al., 2007).

Neurophysiologic recordings during stimulation have demonstrated that the oscillatory activity between brain structures is modulated by DBS in patients with movement disorders (Kringelbach, et al., 2007). Also, changes in neurotransmitter release (glutamate, dopamine) have been reported (Hilker et al., 2002; Stefani et al., 2006). Functional neuroimaging data have demonstrated that DBS changes the activity of brain areas far beyond the targeted region. Thus complex neural networks are modulated (Kringelbach, et al., 2007; Mayberg et al., 2005; Schnitzler & Gross, 2005; Stefurak et al., 2003). These results are in line with the long-term changes described in psychiatric patients.

In summary, short time processes might well explain acute effects in movement disorder. Especially in psychiatric disorders, long-term changes in symptoms have been described. This can only result from long-lasting, complex modulation of neural networks (McIntyre et al., 2004).

BIPOLAR DISORDER AND MAJOR DEPRESSION

Bipolar disorder is often misdiagnosed as MDD because of the high frequency of depressive symptomatology in many patients with BD. Depressive episodes that are resistant to treatment may also be associated with a worse course of illness in BD, but we do not yet understand all the factors in the connection between BD and depression.

Symptoms of depression in the context of BD are generally not the same as in unipolar major depression (Belmaker, 2004). Bipolar depression tends to be atypical with prominent fatigue, hypersomnia, and reverse diurnal mood variability (Berns & Nemeroff, 2003). Nonetheless, current data point to the fact that the neurobiology of bipolar depression is very similar to unipolar major depression, especially regarding striatal dysfunction (Kupferschmidt & Zakzanis, 2011; Marchand & Yurgelun-Todd, 2010). In addition, anhedonia and lack of motivation are also prominent in bipolar patients suffering from treatment-resistant depression.

Similar to major depression, the pharmacological treatment and psychotherapy of chronic BD does not seem to be effective enough despite the availability of many pharmacological substances (Gijsman, Geddes, Rendell, Nolen, & Goodwin, 2004; Papadimitriou, Dikeos, Soldatos, & Calabrese, 2007), and there have been few prospective, randomized studies on the subject (Bowden, 2005). In face of the remarkable increase in medications in BD, treatment is still plagued by inadequate response to acute manic or depressive episodes or long-term preventive maintenance treatment (Gitlin, 2006).

Current data point to the fact that the neurobiology of bipolar depression is very similar to unipolar major depression. For instance, the subsyndrome of anhedonia is the same. Most of the approaches for treatment-resistant bipolar depression are relatively similar to those used in unipolar depression, with the possible exception of a more prominent place for atypical neuroleptics (with an often underestimated side effect burden), prescribed either alone or in combination with antidepressants (Gitlin, 2006; Nemeroff, 2005). Therefore, bipolar patients suffering from depression, especially anhedonia, could possibly profit from DBS.

DEEP BRAIN STIMULATION IN BIPOLAR DEPRESSION

Actual studies in TRD are targeting the nucleus accumbens (NAcc) (Bewernick et al., 2010; Schlaepfer et al., 2007), the medial forebrain bundle (Coenen, Schlaepfer, Maedler, & Panksepp, 2010), the anterior cingulate cortex (Lozano et al., 2008; Mayberg et al., 2005; Puigdemont et al., 2011), and the anterior limb of the capsula interna (Malone et al., 2009). These targets are in close anatomical or functional relationship (neural networks) and an overlap of effect is probable (Figure 27.2).

Encouraging antidepressant results in patients suffering from TRD led to a study by Holtzheimer and colleagues (2012) who included seven bipolar II patients together with 10 MDD patients stimulating subcallosal cingulate white matter. It has been shown that DBS can possibly induce manic or hypomanic states (Bewernick, et al., 2010; Haq et al., 2010); therefore, bipolar patients were assessed carefully for hypomanic symptoms. No hypomanic effects occurred in bipolar patients in this study. The authors stated that antidepressant effects in bipolar patients were similar to unipolar depressed patients. A single blind discontinuation (sham stimulation) phase was introduced in the protocol after 24 months of open stimulation; during the course of the study, this phase was eliminated due to symptom worsening and distress of the first three patients (Holtzheimer et al., 2012). Only three of the seven bipolar patients finished the second year, thus larger samples are needed to evaluate efficacy and safety of DBS in BD.

Another DBS study, which was conducted in Bonn by Schlaepfer, Bewernick, Kayser, Mädler, and Coenen (2013), included one bipolar II patient stimulating the medial forebrain bundle. This patient showed similar and stable antidepressant effects like the patients diagnosed with TRD; no manic or hypomanic states occurred.

A second study is currently being carried out that explores antidepressant effects and the risk of hypomania in bipolar patients stimulated at NAcc (registered at clinicaltrials.gov identifier NCT01372722). A single case study, carried out by Schlaepfer and colleagues (2013) with a bipolar II patient stimulated at the NAcc showed comparable results.

SIDE EFFECTS AND RISKS

The adverse reactions caused by DBS can be differentiated in those who are connected to the surgical implantation itself and those who are linked to the stimulation. The main risk caused by the implantation is associated with the fact that a very small amount of brain tissue will be suppressed. This suppression might cause an injury of vessels. Seizures, bleeding, and infection are also possible but are very rare consequences of the implantation. Former studies using DBS to improve neurological symptoms report the frequency of seizure with 1% to 3%, 1% to 5% for bleeding, and 2% to 25% for infection. Most of these infections are superficial and related to the tissue directly connected with the sensor and its connecting wires. An infection of the brain or even an abscess of the brain is very rare.

In contrast, the side effects of the stimulation might occur more frequently, but these are reversible since

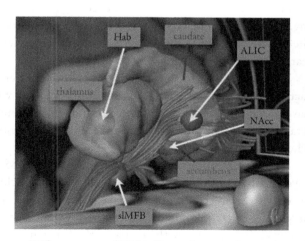 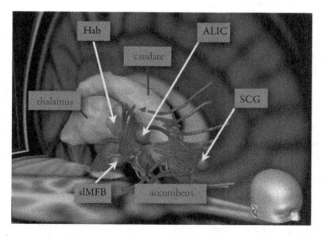

Figure 27.2 Different targets of DBS in Depression in nucleus caudatus, thalamus and nucleus accumbens (Hab = habenula, ALIC = anterior limb of the capsula interna, NAcc = nucleus accumbens, sIMFB = superolateral branch of the medial forebrain bundle). (See color insert)

adjustments of the stimulation parameters are always possible. These side effects involve paresthesia, muscle contraction, dysarthria, and diplopia.

ETHICAL CONSIDERATIONS

Advantages of DBS are its reversibility; the ability to continuously adjust stimulation variables for each patient individually, thereby maximizing effects and minimising side effects; and the possibility of assessing efficacy in controlled protocols (separate investigation of on-and-off cycles; Bewernick, Kayser, Sturm, & Schlaepfer, 2012; Greenberg & Rezai, 2003).

Because former well-established conservative treatment options failed to achieve an adequate response, the benefit for such patients will be the opportunity to experience a new promising treatment. This is even more important when taking into account that these patients suffer from severe depressive symptoms, including suicidal ideations.

Bipolar depression is a mental disease with a high mortality rate (15% to 20 %), which leads to an immense restriction of quality of life. Because many patients do not profit from any conventional treatment, it is essential to do research about new treatment options. It is expected that DBS improves depression in BD, decreases suicidality, and improves quality of life; thus the possible stated risks are ethically justifiable.

Since DBS is already a conventional treatment method for treatment-resistant movement disorders (e.g., Parkinson's disease, tremor), the outcome of this method is well established. Serious side effects are possible, but one should consider that improvements and/or the minimization of symptoms within the particular neurologic disease are possible. Thus DBS has become a very attractive therapeutic option for patients suffering from serious and massive functional limitation caused by their neurologic disease.

Nonetheless, there are some differences as compared to the mentioned neurological diseases. The main difference is based on the historical way of doing research in psychiatry. Because in the past neurosurgical methods were applied without any research-based method, this early destructive neurosurgical method still has a bad reputation—especially if recalling the frontal lobotomy, which was practiced in the middle of the 20th century. Many patients were treated with this method before any secure, long-term data were confirmed. Based on this, a multidisciplinary research group was founded that examines the efficiency and safety of DBS for neurological diseases. This research group has already published some ethical guidelines for DBS for treatment-resistant obsessive-compulsive disorder, a neuropsychiatric disease.

Due to notable risks of surgery (e.g., intracerebral bleeding and wound infection) and lacking broad efficacy, DBS research needs to adhere to highest ethical standards. Obligatory rules for patient inclusion and target selection are needed. Inclusion criteria based on severity, chronicity, disability, and treatment refractoriness (Nuttin et al., 2002) need to be internationally standardized and defined for each psychiatric disease.

Especially in depression with an elevated risk for suicide associated with the disease, careful patient monitoring is necessary. Before surgery, patients need to be seen at regular intervals over at least several months to control for changes in severity and assure inclusion criteria. It is extremely important to clarify the patient's expectations before surgery and to closely follow the patients after the operation to avoid stress, catastrophic thinking, hypomania, or suicidal ideation, especially in the event of suboptimal acute therapy effect. After surgery, visits should take place weekly and, after amelioration of symptoms and parameter adjustment, at monthly intervals for one year at least in order to evaluate long-term effects. In case of nonresponse or acute aggravation of symptoms, hospitalization or other treatment options (psychotherapy, change in medication, or electroconvulsive therapy) should be offered.

In psychiatric disorders the process of diagnosis is less verifiable and observable than in neurology lacking neurobiological markers. Thus it is essential to corroborate the patient's life history, course of illness, and psychopathology. Each case must be documented according to high scientific and administrative expectations (standardized diagnostic with clinical scales, evaluation of cognitive parameters with psychological tests, quality of life, report of parameter changes, other therapies, etc.). In addition to the evaluation of the clinical effects, basic neuroscience (e.g., brain imaging, intracranial EEG, genetics, and anatomic estimation of the individual electrical field) should be applied in order to learn most about each patient.

This requires a team of surgeons (experienced in stereotactic surgery), psychiatrists, and neuropsychologists who have developed proficiency. These standards are most straightforwardly fulfilled in tertiary-care academic centers where such resources are available.

In addition, minimal requirements for using DBS in psychiatric conditions (Nuttin et al., 2002) should include an ethics committee to consider the study protocol and ongoing projects. Despite any committee review, clinical responsibility remains with the patient's clinicians and is

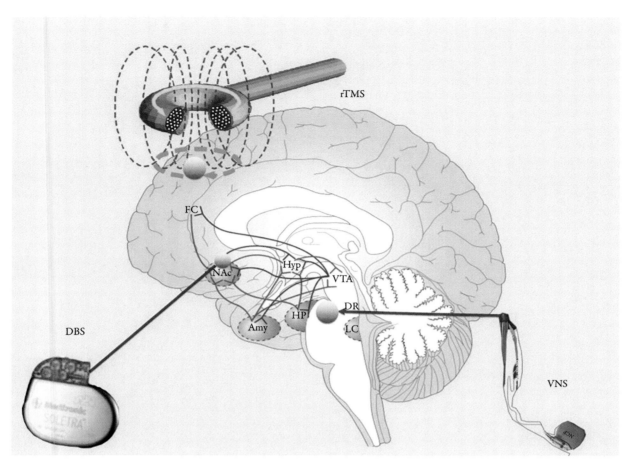

Figure 27.1 Repetitive transcranial magnetic stimulation (rTMS), vagus nerve stimulation (VNS) and deep brain stimulation (DBS) (exemplary Nucleus Accumbens) as neuromodulative treatments.

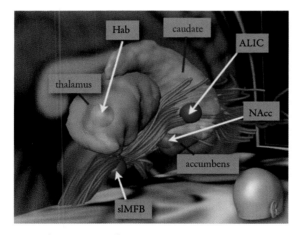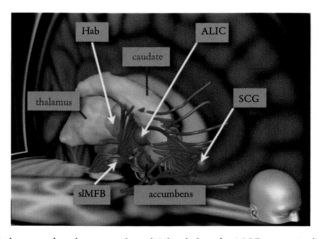

Figure 27.2 Different targets of DBS in Depression in nucleus caudatus, thalamus and nucleus accumbens (Hab = habenula, ALIC = anterior limb of the capsual interna, NAcc = nucleus accumbens, sIMFB = superolateral branch of the medial forebrain bundle).

not shared by review committees. Scientific quality standards for target selection need to be established with clear anatomical and functional hypotheses.

Disclosure statement: The authors have no conflicts of interest to disclose.

REFERENCES

Aaronson, S. T., Carpenter, L. L., Conway, C. R., Reimherr, F. W., Lisanby, S. H., Schwartz, T. L., Bunker, M. (2013). Vagus nerve stimulation therapy randomized to different amounts of electrical charge for treatment-resistant depression: Acute and chronic effects. *Brain Stimulation, 6*(4), 631–640. doi:10.1016/j.brs.2012.09.013S1935-861X(12)00188-X

Barker, A. T., Jalinous, R., & Freeston, I. L. (1985). Non-invasive magnetic stimulation of human motor cortex. *Lancet, 1*(8437), 1106–1107. doi:S0140-6736(85)92413-4 [pii]

Belmaker, R. H. (2004). Bipolar disorder. *New England Journal of Medicine, 351*(5), 476–486. doi:10.1056/NEJMra035354351/5/476 [pii]

Ben-Menachem, E., Hamberger, A., Hedner, T., Hammond, E. J., Uthman, B. M., Slater, J., … Wilder, B. J. (1995). Effects of vagus nerve stimulation on amino acids and other metabolites in the CSF of patients with partial seizures. *Epilepsy Research, 20*(3), 221–227. doi:0920121194000839 [pii]

Benabid, A. L., Pollak, P., Louveau, A., Henry, S., & de Rougemont, J. (1987). Combined (thalamotomy and stimulation) stereotactic surgery of the VIM thalamic nucleus for bilateral Parkinson disease. *Applied Neurophysiology, 50*(1–6), 344–346.

Berlim, M. T., van den Eynde, F., Tovar-Perdomo, S., & Daskalakis, Z. J. (2013). Response, remission and drop-out rates following high-frequency repetitive transcranial magnetic stimulation (rTMS) for treating major depression: A systematic review and meta-analysis of randomized, double-blind and sham-controlled trials. *Psychological Medicine, 44*(2), 225–239., 1–15. doi:S0033291713000512 [pii]10.1017/S0033291713000512

Berns, G. S., & Nemeroff, C. B. (2003). The neurobiology of bipolar disorder. *American Journal of Medical Genetics: Part C, Seminars in Medical Genetics, 123*(1), 76–84.

Bersani, F. S., Girardi, N., Sanna, L., Mazzarini, L., Santucci, C., Kotzalidis, G. D., Girardi, P. (2013). Deep transcranial magnetic stimulation for treatment-resistant bipolar depression: A case report of acute and maintenance efficacy. *Neurocase, 19*(5), 451–457. doi:10.1080/13554794.2012.690429

Bersani, F. S., Minichino, A., Enticott, P. G., Mazzarini, L., Khan, N., & Antonacci, G., Biondi, M. (2013). Deep transcranial magnetic stimulation as a treatment for psychiatric disorders: A comprehensive review. *European Psychiatry, 28*(1), 30–39. doi:10.1016/j.eurpsy.2012.02.006S0924-9338(12)00022-3 [pii]

Beurrier, C., Bioulac, B., Audin, J., & Hammond, C. (2001). High-frequency stimulation produces a transient blockade of voltage-gated currents in subthalamic neurons. *Journal of Neurophysiology, 85*(4), 1351–1356.

Bewernick, B., Hurlemann, R., Matusch, A., Kayser, S., Grubert, C., Hadrysiewicz, B., & Schlaepfer, T. E. (2010). Nucleus accumbens deep brain stimulation decreases ratings of depression and anxiety in treatment-resistant depression. *Biological Psychiatry, 67*(2), 110–116. doi:S0006-3223(09)01094-4 [pii]10.1016/j.biopsych.2009.09.013

Bewernick, B., Kayser, S., Sturm, V., & Schlaepfer, T. E. (2012). Long-term effects of deep brain stimulation for treatment-restistant depression—Evidence for sustained efficacy. *Neuropsychopharmacology, 37*(9), 1975–1985.

Bowden, C. L. (2005). Treatment options for bipolar depression. *Journal of Clinical Psychiatry, 66*(Suppl. 1), 3–6.

Breit, S., Schulz, J. B., & Benabid, A. L. (2004). Deep brain stimulation. *Cell Tissue Research, 318*(1), 275–288.

Broadbent, H. J., van den Eynde, F., Guillaume, S., Hanif, E. L., Stahl, D., David, A. S., Schmidt, U. (2011). Blinding success of rTMS applied to the dorsolateral prefrontal cortex in randomised sham-controlled trials: A systematic review. *World Journal of Biological Psychiatry, 12*(4), 240–248. doi:10.3109/15622975.2010.541281

Chae, J. H., Nahas, Z., Lomarev, M., Denslow, S., Lorberbaum, J. P., Bohning, D. E., & George, M. S. (2003). A review of functional neuroimaging studies of vagus nerve stimulation (VNS). *Journal of Psychiatric Research, 37*(6), 443–455.

Coenen, V. A., Schlaepfer, T. E., Maedler, B., & Panksepp, J. (2010). Cross-species affective functions of the medial forebrain bundle: Implications for the treatment of affective pain and depression in humans. *Neuroscience & Biobehavioral Reviews, 35*, 1971–1981. doi:S0149-7634(10)00210-1 [pii]10.1016/j.neubiorev.2010.12.009

Davey, K. R., & Riehl, M. (2006). Suppressing the surface field during transcranial magnetic stimulation. *IEEE Transactions in Biomedical Engineering, 53*(2), 190–194. doi:10.1109/TBME.2005.862545

Dell'Osso, B., Mundo, E., D'Urso, N., Pozzoli, S., Buoli, M., Ciabatti, M., Altamura, A. C. (2009). Augmentative repetitive navigated transcranial magnetic stimulation (rTMS) in drug-resistant bipolar depression. *Bipolar Disorders, 11*(1), 76–81. doi:10.1111/j.1399-5618.2008.00651.xBDI651 [pii]

Deng, Z. D., Peterchev, A. V., & Lisanby, S. H. (2008). Coil design considerations for deep-brain transcranial magnetic stimulation (dTMS). *Conference Proceedings of IEEE Engineering in Medicine and Biology Society*, 5675–5679. doi:10.1109/IEMBS.2008.4650502

Dorr, A. E., & Debonnel, G. (2006). Effect of vagus nerve stimulation on serotonergic and noradrenergic transmission. *Journal of Pharmacology and Experimental Therapy, 318*(2), 890–898.

Dostrovsky, J. O., Levy, R., Wu, J. P., Hutchison, W. D., Tasker, R. R., & Lozano, A. M. (2000). Microstimulation-induced inhibition of neuronal firing in human globus pallidus. *Journal of Neurophysiology, 84*(1), 570–574.

Drevets, W. C. (2000). Neuroimaging studies of mood disorders. *Biological Psychiatry, 48*(8), 813–829. doi:S0006-3223(00)01020-9 [pii]

Drevets, W. C., Bogers, W., & Raichle, M. E. (2002). Functional anatomical correlates of antidepressant drug treatment assessed using PET measures of regional glucose metabolism. *European Neuropsychopharmacology, 12*(6), 527–544. doi:S0924977X02001025 [pii]

Dunner, D. L., Rush, A. J., Russell, J. M., Burke, M., Woodard, S., Wingard, P., & Allen, J. (2006). Prospective, long-term, multicenter study of the naturalistic outcomes of patients with treatment-resistant depression. *Journal of Clinical Psychiatry, 67*(5), 688–695.

Elger, G., Hoppe, C., Falkai, P., Rush, A. J., & Elger, C. E. (2000). Vagus nerve stimulation is associated with mood improvements in epilepsy patients. *Epilepsy Research, 42*(2–3), 203–210. doi:S0920-1211(00)00181-9 [pii]

Erfurth, A., Michael, N., Mostert, C., & Arolt, V. (2000). Euphoric mania and rapid transcranial magnetic stimulation. *The American Journal of Psychiatry, 157*(5), 835–836.

Fins, J. J. (2003). From psychosurgery to neuromodulation and palliation: History's lessons for the ethical conduct and regulation of neuropsychiatric research. *Neurosurgery Clinics of North America, 14*(2), 303–319.

Fitzgerald, P. B., Fountain, S., & Daskalakis, Z. J. (2006). A comprehensive review of the effects of rTMS on motor cortical excitability and inhibition. *Clinical Neurophysiology, 117*(12), 2584–2596. doi:S1388-2457(06)00976-X [pii]10.1016/j.clinph.2006.06.712

George, M. S., Nahas, Z., Lisanby, S. H., Schlaepfer, T., Kozel, F. A., & Greenberg, B. D. (2003). Transcranial magnetic stimulation. *Neurosurgery Clinics of North America, 14*(2), 283–301.

George, M. S., Padberg, F., Schlaepfer, T. E., O'Reardon, J. P., Fitzgerald, P. B., Nahas, Z. H., & Marcolin, M. A. (2009). Controversy: Repetitive transcranial magnetic stimulation or transcranial direct current stimulation shows efficacy in treating psychiatric diseases (depression, mania, schizophrenia, obsessive-complusive disorder, panic, posttraumatic stress disorder). *Brain Stimulation*, 2(1), 14–21. doi:10.1016/j.brs.2008.06.001S1935-861X(08)00037-5 [pii]

George, M. S., Rush, A. J., Marangell, L. B., Sackeim, H. A., Brannan, S. K., Davis, S. M., Goodnick, P. (2005). A one-year comparison of vagus nerve stimulation with treatment as usual for treatment-resistant depression. *Biological Psychiatry*, 58(5), 364–373.

George, M. S., Sackeim, H. A., Rush, A. J., Marangell, L. B., Nahas, Z., Husain, M. M., Ballenger, J. C. (2000). Vagus nerve stimulation: a new tool for brain research and therapy. *Biological Psychiatry*, 47(4), 287–295.

George, M. S., Speer, A. M., Molloy, M., Nahas, Z., Teneback, C. C., Craig Risch, S., ... Post, R. M. (1998). Low frequency daily left prefrontal rTMS improves mood in bipolar depression-a placebo-controlled case report. *Human Psychopharmacology*, 13(4), 271–275.

Gijsman, H. J., Geddes, J. R., Rendell, J. M., Nolen, W. A., & Goodwin, G. M. (2004). Antidepressants for bipolar depression: a systematic review of randomized, controlled trials. *The American Journal of Psychiatry*, 161(9), 1537–1547. doi:10.1176/appi.ajp.161.9.1537161/9/1537

Gildenberg, P. L. (2005). Evolution of neuromodulation. *Stereotactic and Functional Neurosurgery*, 83(2–3), 71–79.

Gitlin, M. (2006). Treatment-resistant bipolar disorder. *Molecular Psychiatry*, 11(3), 227–240. doi:4001793 [pii]10.1038/sj.mp.4001793

Greenberg, B. D., Price, L. H., Rauch, S. L., Friehs, G., Noren, G., Malone, D., & Rasmussen, S. A. (2003). Neurosurgery for intractable obsessive-compulsive disorder and depression: critical issues. *Neurosurgery Clinics of North America*, 14(2), 199–212.

Greenberg, B. D., & Rezai, A. R. (2003). Mechanisms and the current state of deep brain stimulation in neuropsychiatry. *CNS Spectrum*, 8(7), 522–526.

Haq, I. U., Foote, K. D., Goodman, W. K., Ricciuti, N., Ward, H., & Sudhyadhom, A., Okun, M. S. (2010). A case of mania following deep brain stimulation for obsessive compulsive disorder. *Stereotactic and Functional Neurosurgery*, 88(5), 322–328. doi:000319960 [pii]10.1159/000319960

Hardesty, D. E., & Sackeim, H. A. (2007). Deep brain stimulation in movement and psychiatric disorders. *Biological Psychiatry*, 61(7), 831–835. doi:10.1016/j.biopsych.2006.08.028

Harel, E. V., Rabany, L., Deutsch, L., Bloch, Y., Zangen, A., & Levkovitz, Y. (2012). H-coil repetitive transcranial magnetic stimulation for treatment resistant major depressive disorder: An 18-week continuation safety and feasibility study. *World Journal of Biological Psychiatry*, 15(4), 298–306. doi:10.3109/15622975.2011.639802

Harel, E. V., Zangen, A., Roth, Y., Reti, I., Braw, Y., & Levkovitz, Y. (2011). H-coil repetitive transcranial magnetic stimulation for the treatment of bipolar depression: an add-on, safety and feasibility study. *World Journal of Biological Psychiatry*, 12(2), 119–126. doi: 10.3109/15622975.2010.510893

Henry, T. R., Votaw, J. R., Pennell, P. B., Epstein, C. M., Bakay, R. A., & Faber, T. L., Hoffman, J. M. (1999). Acute blood flow changes and efficacy of vagus nerve stimulation in partial epilepsy. *Neurology*, 52(6), 1166–1173.

Hilker, R., Voges, J., Thiel, A., Ghaemi, M., Herholz, K., Sturm, V., & Heiss, W. D. (2002). Deep brain stimulation of the subthalamic nucleus versus levodopa challenge in Parkinson's disease: Measuring the on- and off-conditions with FDG-PET. *Journal of Neural Transmission*, 109(10), 1257–1264.

Holtzheimer, P. E., Kelley, M. E., Gross, R. E., Filkowski, M. M., Garlow, S. J., Barrocas, A., & Mayberg, H. S. (2012). Subcallosal cingulate deep brain stimulation for treatment-resistant unipolar and bipolar depression. *Archives of General Psychiatry*, 69(2), 150–158. doi:10.1001/archgenpsychiatry.2011.1456archgenpsychiatry.2011.1456

Isserles, M., Rosenberg, O., Dannon, P., Levkovitz, Y., Kotler, M., Deutsch, F., Zangen, A. (2011). Cognitive-emotional reactivation during deep transcranial magnetic stimulation over the prefrontal cortex of depressive patients affects antidepressant outcome. *Journal of Affective Disorders*, 128(3), 235–242. doi:10.1016/j.jad.2010.06.038S0165-0327(10)00466-0

Janicak, P. G., O'Reardon, J. P., Sampson, S. M., Husain, M. M., Lisanby, S. H., Rado, J. T., & Demitrack, M. A. (2008). Transcranial magnetic stimulation in the treatment of major depressive disorder: A comprehensive summary of safety experience from acute exposure, extended exposure, and during reintroduction treatment. *Journal of Clinical Psychiatry*, 69(2), 222–232. doi:ej07m03619

Kosel, M., Schlaepfer, T. E. (2005). *Brain stimulation*. New York: Marce Dekker.

Kringelbach, M. L., Jenkinson, N., Owen, S. L., & Aziz, T. Z. (2007). Translational principles of deep brain stimulation. *Nature Reviews Neuroscience*, 8(8), 623–635.

Kupferschmidt, D. A., & Zakzanis, K. K. (2011). Toward a functional neuroanatomical signature of bipolar disorder: Quantitative evidence from the neuroimaging literature. *Psychiatry Research*, 193(2), 71–79. doi:10.1016/j.pscychresns.2011.02.011

Levkovitz, Y., Harel, E. V., Roth, Y., Braw, Y., Most, D., Katz, L. N., & Zangen, A. (2009). Deep transcranial magnetic stimulation over the prefrontal cortex: evaluation of antidepressant and cognitive effects in depressive patients. *Brain Stimulation*, 2(4), 188–200. doi:10.1016/j.brs.2009.08.002S1935-861X(09)00082-5 [pii]

Levkovitz, Y., Sheer, A., Harel, E. V., Katz, L. N., Most, D., Zangen, A., & Isserles, M. (2011). Differential effects of deep TMS of the prefrontal cortex on apathy and depression. *Brain Stimulation*, 4(4), 266–274. doi:10.1016/j.brs.2010.12.004S1935-861X(10)00206-8

Little, J. T., Kimbrell, T. A., Wassermann, E. M., Grafman, J., Figueras, S., Dunn, R. T., Post, R. M. (2000). Cognitive effects of 1- and 20-hertz repetitive transcranial magnetic stimulation in depression: Preliminary report. *Neuropsychiatry, Neuropsychology, and Behavorial Neurology*, 13(2), 119–124.

Lozano, A. M., Mayberg, H. S., Giacobbe, P., Hamani, C., Craddock, R. C., & Kennedy, S. H. (2008). Subcallosal cingulate gyrus deep brain stimulation for treatment-resistant depression. *Biological Psychiatry*, 64(6), 461–467. doi:10.1016/j.biopsych.2008.05.034

Mallet, L., Mesnage, V., Houeto, J. L., Pelissolo, A., Yelnik, J., Behar, C., & Agid, Y. (2002). Compulsions, Parkinson's disease, and stimulation. *Lancet*, 360(9342), 1302–1304.

Malone, D. A. Jr., Dougherty, D. D., Rezai, A. R., Carpenter, L. L., Friehs, G. M., Eskandar, E. N., & Greenberg, B. D. (2009). Deep brain stimulation of the ventral capsule/ventral striatum for treatment-resistant depression. *Biological Psychiatry*, 65(4), 267–275. doi:10.1016/j.biopsych.2008.08.029

Marchand, W. R., & Yurgelun-Todd, D. (2010). Striatal structure and function in mood disorders: A comprehensive review. *Bipolar Disorders*, 12(8), 764–785. doi:10.1111/j.1399-5618.2010.00874.x

Marcolin, M. A., & Padberg, F. (2007). Transcranial brain stimulation for treatment in mental disorders. *Advances in Biological Psychiatry*, 23, 204–225.

Mayberg, H., Lozano, A., Voon, V., McNeely, H., Seminowicz, D., Hamani, C., & Kennedy, S. (2005). Deep brain stimulation for treatment-resistant depression. *Neuron*, 45(5), 651–660.

Mayberg, H. S., Lozano, A. M., Voon, V., McNeely, H. E., Seminowicz, D., Hamani, C., & Kennedy, S. H. (2005). Deep brain stimulation for treatment-resistant depression. *Neuron*, 45, 651–660.

McIntyre, C. C., Savasta, M., Kerkerian-Le Goff, L., & Vitek, J. L. (2004). Uncovering the mechanism(s) of action of deep brain stimulation: Activation, inhibition, or both. *Clinical Neurophysiology, 115*(6), 1239–1248.

Nahas, Z., Kozel, F. A., Li, X., Anderson, B., & George, M. S. (2003). Left prefrontal transcranial magnetic stimulation (TMS) treatment of depression in bipolar affective disorder: A pilot study of acute safety and efficacy. *Bipolar Disorders, 5*(1), 40–47.

Nahas, Z., Marangell, L. B., Husain, M. M., Rush, A. J., Sackeim, H. A., Lisanby, S. H., & George, M. S. (2005). Two-year outcome of vagus nerve stimulation (VNS) for treatment of major depressive episodes. *Journal of Clinical Psychiatry, 66*(9), 1097–1104.

Nemeroff, C. B. (2005). Use of atypical antipsychotics in refractory depression and anxiety. *Journal of Clinical Psychiatry, 66*(Suppl. 8), 13–21.

Nestler, E. J., & Carlezon, W. A. Jr. (2006). The mesolimbic dopamine reward circuit in depression. *Biological Psychiatry, 59*(12), 1151–1159. doi:10.1016/j.biopsych.2005.09.018

Nuttin, B., Gybels, J., Cosyns, P., Gabriels, L., Meyerson, B., Andreewitch, S., & Fins, J. J. (2002). Deep brain stimulation for psychiatric disorders. *Neurosurgery, 51*(2), 519.

O'Reardon, J. P., Solvason, H. B., Janicak, P. G., Sampson, S., Isenberg, K. E., Nahas, Z., & Sackeim, H. A. (2007). Efficacy and safety of transcranial magnetic stimulation in the acute treatment of major depression: A multisite randomized controlled trial. *Biological Psychiatry, 62*(11), 1208–1216. doi:10.1016/j.biopsych.2007.01.018

Papadimitriou, G. N., Dikeos, D. G., Soldatos, C. R., & Calabrese, J. R. (2007). Non-pharmacological treatments in the management of rapid cycling bipolar disorder. *Journal of Affective Disorders, 98*(1–2), 1–10. doi:10.1016/j.jad.2006.05.036

Pisani, F., Spina, E., & Oteri, G. (1999). Antidepressant drugs and seizure susceptibility: from in vitro data to clinical practice. *Epilepsia, 40*(Suppl. 10), S48–S56.

Price, B. H., Baral, I., Cosgrove, G. R., Rauch, S. L., Nierenberg, A. A., Jenike, M. A., & Cassem, E. H. (2001). Improvement in severe self-mutilation following limbic leucotomy: A series of 5 consecutive cases. *Journal of Clinical Psychiatry, 62*(12), 925–932.

Puigdemont, D., Perez-Egea, R., Portella, M. J., Molet, J., de Diego-Adelino, J., Gironell, A., & Perez, V. (2011). Deep brain stimulation of the subcallosal cingulate gyrus: Further evidence in treatment-resistant major depression. *International Journal of Neuropsychopharmacology, 15*(1), 121–133. doi:10.1017/S1461145711001088

Ranck, J. B., Jr. (1975). Which elements are excited in electrical stimulation of mammalian central nervous system? A review. *Brain Research, 98*(3), 417–440.

Roosevelt, R. W., Smith, D. C., Clough, R. W., Jensen, R. A., & Browning, R. A. (2006). Increased extracellular concentrations of norepinephrine in cortex and hippocampus following vagus nerve stimulation in the rat. *Brain Research, 1119*(1), 124–132. doi:10.1016/j.brainres.2006.08.048

Rosenberg, O., Isserles, M., Levkovitz, Y., Kotler, M., Zangen, A., & Dannon, P. N. (2011). Effectiveness of a second deep TMS in depression: A brief report. *Progress in Neuro-Psychopharmacology & Biological Psychiatry, 35*(4), 1041–1044. doi:10.1016/j.pnpbp.2011.02.015S0278-5846(11)00071-6 [pii]

Rosenberg, O., Shoenfeld, N., Zangen, A., Kotler, M., & Dannon, P. N. (2010). Deep TMS in a resistant major depressive disorder: A brief report. *Depression and Anxiety, 27*(5), 465–469. doi:10.1002/da.20689

Rosenberg, O., Zangen, A., Stryjer, R., Kotler, M., & Dannon, P. N. (2010). Response to deep TMS in depressive patients with previous electroconvulsive treatment. *Brain Stimulation, 3*(4), 211–217. doi:10.1016/j.brs.2009.12.001S1935-861X(09)00110-7

Rossi, S., Hallett, M., Rossini, P. M., & Pascual-Leone, A. (2009). Safety, ethical considerations, and application guidelines for the use of transcranial magnetic stimulation in clinical practice and research. *Clinical Neurophysiology, 120*(12), 2008–2039. doi:10.1016/j.clinph.2009.08.016S1388-2457(09)00519-7

Roth, Y., Amir, A., Levkovitz, Y., & Zangen, A. (2007). Three-dimensional distribution of the electric field induced in the brain by transcranial magnetic stimulation using figure-8 and deep H-coils. *Journal of Clinical Neurophysiology, 24*(1), 31–38. doi:10.1097/WNP.0b013e31802fa39300004691-200702000-00006

Roth, Y., Zangen, A., & Hallett, M. (2002). A coil design for transcranial magnetic stimulation of deep brain regions. *Journal of Clinical Neurophysiology, 19*(4), 361–370.

Rush, A. J., George, M. S., Sackeim, H. A., Marangell, L. B., Husain, M. M., Giller, C., & Goodmann, R. (2000). Vagus nerve stimulation (VNS) for treatment-resistant depression: A multicenter study. *Biological Psychiatry, 47*, 276–286.

Rush, A. J., Marangell, L. B., Sackeim, H. A., George, M. S., Brannan, S. K., Davis, S. M., & Cooke, R. G. (2005). Vagus nerve stimulation for treatment-resistant depression: A randomized, controlled acute phase trial. *Biological Psychiatry, 58*(5), 347–354.

Rush, A. J., Sackeim, H. A., Marangell, L. B., George, M. S., Brannan, S. K., Davis, S. M., & Barry, J. J. (2005). Effects of 12 months of vagus nerve stimulation in treatment-resistant depression: A naturalistic study. *Biological Psychiatry, 58*(5), 355–363.

Sackeim, H. A., Rush, A. J., George, M. S., Marangell, L. B., Husain, M. M., & Nahas, Z., Goodman, R. R. (2001). Vagus nerve stimulation (VNS) for treatment-resistant depression: Efficacy, side effects, and predictors of outcome. *Neuropsychopharmacology, 25*(5), 713–728. doi:10.1016/S0893-133X(01)00271-8

Schachter, S. C., & Schmidt, D. (Eds.). (2001). *Vagus nerve stimulation*. London: CRC Press.

Schlaepfer, T. E., Bewernick, B., Kayser, S., Mädler, B., & Coenen, V. (2013). Rapid effects of deep brain stimulation for treatment resistant major depression. *Biological Psychiatry, 73*(12), 1204–1212.

Schlaepfer, T. E., Cohen, M. X., Frick, C., Kosel, M., Brodesser, D., Axmacher, N., & Sturm, V. (2007). Deep brain stimulation to reward circuitry alleviates anhedonia in refractory major depression. *Neuropsychopharmacology, 33*, 368–377.

Schlaepfer, T. E., Frick, C., Zobel, A., Maier, W., Heuse, I, Bajbouj, M., & Hasdemir, M. (2008). Vagus nerve stimulation for depression: Efficacy and safety in a european study. *Psychological Medicine, 38*(5), 651–662.

Schlaepfer, T. E., George, M. S., & Mayberg, H. (2010). WFSBP guidelines on brain stimulation treatments in psychiatry. *World Journal of Biological Psychiatry, 11*(1), 2–18. doi:10.3109/15622970903170835

Schlaepfer, T. E., & Kosel, M. (2004a). Novel physical treatments for major depression: Vagus nerve stimulation, transcranial magnetic stimulation and magnetic seizure therapy. *Current Opinion in Psychiatry, 17*, 15–20.

Schlaepfer, T. E., & Kosel M. (2004b). *Transcranial magnetic stimulation in depression*. Washington, DC: American Psychiatric Press.

Schlaepfer, T. E., & Kosel M. (2005). *Brain stimulation in depression*. London: John Wiley.

Schnitzler, A., & Gross, J. (2005). Normal and pathological oscillatory communication in the brain. *Nature Reviews Neuroscience, 6*(4), 285–296.

Schulze-Rauschenbach, S. C., Harms, U., Schlaepfer, T. E., Maier, W., Falkai, P., & Wagner, M. (2005). Distinctive neurocognitive effects of repetitive transcranial magnetic stimulation and electroconvulsive therapy in major depression. *The British Journal of Psychiatry, 186*, 410–416.

Stefani, A., Fedele, E., Galati, S., Raiteri, M., Pepicelli, O., Brusa, L., & Mazzone, P. (2006). Deep brain stimulation in Parkinson's disease patients: Biochemical evidence. *Journal of Neural Transmission, 70*(Suppl.), 401–408.

Stefurak, T., Mikulis, D., Mayberg, H., Lang, A. E., Hevenor, S., Pahapill, P., & Lozano, A. (2003). Deep brain stimulation for Parkinson's disease dissociates mood and motor circuits: A functional MRI case study. *Movement Disorders, 18*(12), 1508–1516.

Tamas, R. L., Menkes, D., & El-Mallakh, R. S. (2007). Stimulating research: A prospective, randomized, double-blind, sham-controlled study of slow transcranial magnetic stimulation in depressed bipolar patients. *The Journal of Neuropsychiatry & Clinical Neurosciences, 19*(2), 198–199. doi:10.1176/appi.neuropsych.19.2.198

Tharayil, B. S., Gangadhar, B. N., Thirthalli, J., & Anand, L. (2005). Seizure with single-pulse transcranial magnetic stimulation in a 35-year-old otherwise-healthy patient with bipolar disorder. *The Journal of ECT, 21*(3), 188–189. doi:00124509-200509000-000 14 [pii]

Wassermann, E. M. (1998). Risk and safety of repetitive transcranial magnetic stimulation: report and suggested guidelines from the International Workshop on the Safety of Repetitive Transcranial Magnetic Stimulation, June 5–7, 1996. *Electroencephalography and clinical Neurophysiology, 108*(1), 1–16.

Zucker, R. S., & Regehr, W. G. (2002). Short-term synaptic plasticity. *Annual Reviews in Physiology, 64*, 355–405.

PART III

ADVERSE TREATMENT EFFECTS

28.

MANAGEMENT OF METABOLIC AND ENDOCRINE EFFECTS OF MEDICATIONS USED TO TREAT BIPOLAR DISORDERS

Richard Balon

INTRODUCTION

The management of metabolic and endocrine effects of medications used to treat bipolar disorders is a complicated matter. The complexity is due to the fact that these medications can induce metabolic and endocrine abnormalities, but also the disorder itself seems to be associated with metabolic and endocrine abnormalities. The area of managing metabolic and endocrine abnormalities in bipolar disorder patients has been gradually gaining importance and prominence over the past two decades, partially due to the introduction of new medications and partially due to new research focusing on metabolic, endocrine, immunological, and cardiovascular risk factors associated with bipolar disorders. Two or three decades ago, the majority of these abnormalities were not fully appreciated or considered in treatment planning—the classic text, *Manic-Depressive Illness*, by Goodwin and Jamison (1990) mentions only thyroid abnormalities associated with lithium administration and does not discuss any metabolic abnormalities.

This chapter focuses on the management of endocrine and metabolic effects of medications used for the treatment of acute mania and mood stabilization—carbamazepine, lamotrigine, lithium, oxcarbazepine, topiramate, valproic acid, and other mood stabilizers, and antipsychotic drugs used in these indications.

ENDOCRINE AND METABOLIC CHANGES ASSOCIATED WITH BIPOLAR DISORDER

The prevalence of comorbid physical health conditions in patients with bipolar disorder is twice that of the general population (Young & Grunze, 2013). Bipolar disorder patients are prone to developing type 2 diabetes mellitus, dyslipidemia, hyperglycemia, and obesity (Young & Grunze, 2013). In bipolar disorder patients, general medical illness comorbidity seems to occur at an earlier age than in the general population (Kilbourne et al., 2004).

About 30 years ago, Liliker (1980) reported that the prevalence of diabetes mellitus in one state facility in the preceding 10 years was 10%. Her study had numerous limitations, for example, retrospective chart review and no data on medications used (e.g., antipsychotics). Nevertheless, her finding probably could not be explained by treatment with antipsychotic drugs or medications for physical illness, as the prevalence of diabetes in bipolar patients was much higher than in patients with other diagnoses, such as schizophrenia (presumably receiving antipsychotics too). Interestingly, Cassidy, Ahearn, and Carroll (1999) reported a similar prevalence of diabetes mellitus (9.9%) in their sample of 345 bipolar patients. The bipolar patients with comorbid diabetes in their study had significantly more lifetime psychiatric hospitalizations than nondiabetic patients, which suggests a more severe course of illness. This study did not control for the use of medications either. Nevertheless, as the prevalence of diabetes was higher than expected from national norms (3.4%), this finding suggests that patients suffering from bipolar disorder are at greater risk of diabetes mellitus. More recent findings further confirm this association. Crump, Sunquist, Winkleby, and Sundquist (2013) reported that in a Swedish national cohort study, patients with bipolar disorder had increased mortality from diabetes. The association between mortality from chronic diseases, including diabetes, and bipolar disorder was weaker among those with a prior diagnosis of these conditions than among those without a prior diagnosis of these conditions.

Finally, adolescents with schizophrenia or bipolar disorder had a significantly increased risk of developing diabetes and dyslipidemia than adolescents without these disorders (the adjusted hazard ration for bipolar disorder was 1.66; 95% confidence interval [CI]: 1.22–2.28) (Enger, Jones, Kryzhanovskaya, Doherty, & McAfee, 2013).

During the past decade, more studies have reported the association of bipolar disorder and metabolic syndrome (Newcomer, 2007b). For instance, in a small study by Fiedorowicz, Palagummi, Forman-Hoffman, Miller, and Haynes (2008), most patients with bipolar disorder were overweight or obese and nearly half were obese. Among those with all requisite data ($n = 60$), over 50% met criteria for metabolic syndrome (double the expected prevalence) and there was a trend toward greater prevalence of metabolic syndrome among patients on second-generation antipsychotics. In a recent systematic review and meta-analysis Vancampfort and colleagues (2013) reported that patients with bipolar disorder had higher metabolic syndrome rates than the general population (odds ratio [OR] = 1.98; 95% CI = 1.74–2.25). Metabolic syndrome was also significantly more prevalent among patients currently treated with antipsychotics than in those who were antipsychotics free (45.3% vs. 32.4%).

The association between diabetes mellitus and bipolar disorder and between metabolic syndrome and bipolar disorder seem to be clear. However, the underlying mechanism(s) of these associations is not. As Taylor and MacQueen (2006) and Vancampfort and colleagues (2013) pointed out, various factors such as unhealthy lifestyle (lack of exercise due to fatigue in depression, substance abuse, smoking), poor access to health care, and adverse effects of pharmacological agents used for the treatment of bipolar disorder can increase the risk of diabetes mellitus and metabolic syndrome in bipolar disorder. Nevertheless, there may be other factors involved, such as genetic ones; the impact of chronic stress (which leads to chronically elevated glucocorticoids, which in turn impact the ability of insulin to promote glucose uptake—Taylor and MacQueen, 2006); or impairment of immune function (chronic inflammation may contribute to the development of depression and endocrine disease).

The association of thyroid disease and bipolar disorder, though studied over decades, remains unclear. Various reports suggested the role of hypothyroidism in the development of rapid cycling bipolar depression. Some studies reported antithyroid antibodies in up to 20% of depressed patients (Nemeroff, Simon, Haggerty, & Evans, 1985). Several studies reported blunted thyroid stimulating hormone (TSH) response to thyrotropin-releasing hormone (TRH) in depressed and manic patients. Most of the reports on thyroid function abnormalities in bipolar disorder patients are complicated by the fact that those patients were receiving lithium (which has antithyroid properties—reviewed later in this chapter) and were females. The changes in thyroid function in bipolar patients are usually subtle, and their significance remains to be elucidated.

Various other endocrine abnormalities (e.g., changes of growth hormone, melatonin, plasma cortisol and prolactin levels, variable dexamethasone suppression test responses) have been observed in bipolar patients. These abnormalities do not seem to have clinical significance (at least judged by our present level of knowledge).

ENDOCRINE AND METABOLIC ABNORMALITIES ASSOCIATED WITH MEDICATIONS USED TO TREAT BIPOLAR DISORDER

ANTIPSYCHOTICS

Antipsychotics are frequently associated with both serious endocrine and metabolic adverse effects. The most important "pure" endocrine effect is hyperprolactinemia caused by the blockade of D2 dopamine receptors in the pituitary gland (prolactin secretion is regulated by tonic inhibition by dopamine and thus when dopamine is blocked by antipsychotics, prolactin is increasingly released from the pituitary gland). The typical or older antipsychotics are associated with hyperprolactinemia more frequently than the newer ones. Correll and Carlson (2006) estimated that the relative potency of antipsychotic drugs in inducing hyperprolactinemia is, roughly: risperidone > haloperidol > olanzapine > ziprasidone > quetiapine > clozapine > aripiprazole. The rates of hyperprolactinemia with newer antipsychotics such as asenapine and lurasidone are probably fairly low, and intermediate with drugs such as iloperidone and paliperidone. The symptoms of hyperprolactinemia include amenorrhea, oligomenorrhea, galactorrhea, gynecomastia (in men and women), sexual dysfunction (erectile dysfunction in men—prolonged erections, priapism; decreased libido in both genders), decreased bone density and osteoporosis, and possibly hirsutism in women (Maguire, 2002).

Metabolic effects of antipsychotic medications include weight gain (particularly troubling in children and adolescents), lipid abnormalities (increased cholesterol and low-density lipoprotein-cholesterol levels, decreased high-density lipoprotein-cholesterol levels, elevated triglyceride levels), diabetes mellitus, and metabolic syndrome (constellation of physical features and laboratory findings predisposing to cardiovascular disease, diabetes, stroke—see Table 28.1; Grundy, Brewer, Cleeman, Smith, & Lenfant, 2004; Grundy et al., 2005). The metabolic syndrome is a predisposing factor for the development of type 2 diabetes mellitus and atherosclerotic cardiovascular disease (Grundy et al., 2005). The underlying risk factors for metabolic syndrome are abdominal obesity and insulin resistance; other associated risk conditions can include physical inactivity, aging, and hormonal imbalance (for a review see Grundy et al., 2005).

The risk of metabolic syndrome and diabetes mellitus associated with antipsychotics has been clearly established in numerous studies, the review of which is beyond the scope of this chapter (for a review see, e.g., Buse, 2002; Malhotra & McElroy, 2002; Newcomer, 2007a; De Hert, Detraux, van Winkel, Yu, & Correll, 2012). Most literature focuses on metabolic syndrome and related side effects of antipsychotics in schizophrenia, but it has become more obvious that these serious adverse effects occur during treatment of bipolar disorder too. Quetiapine decreased thyroxine levels in some studies (Correll & Carlson, 2006).

CARBAMAZEPINE, LAMOTRIGINE, OXCARBAZEPINE, TOPIRAMATE, VALPROIC ACID

Carbamazepine may alter the hypothalamic-pituitary-adrenal axis function. It is less likely to cause weigh gain compared to lithium, valproic acid, and antipsychotics. Carbamazepine and oxcarbazepine may be associated with usually asymptomatic hyponatremia. The mechanism of hyponatremia associated with these drugs is not known, but it is possible that these drugs influence the secretion of antidiuretic hormone (Correll & Carlson, 2006). The side effects of oxcarbazepine are usually milder/less frequent than those of carbamazepine. Lamotrigine is considered to be weight-neutral and is not associated with clinically significant endocrine effects, while topiramate has been known to be associated with decreased appetite and weight loss and has been actually used in antipsychotic-associated weight gain.

Valproic acid may negatively impact thyroid functioning and cause mild increase of TSH in some patients. Valproic acid seems to be also occasionally associated with polycystic ovarian syndrome, menstrual abnormalities, and increased levels of androgens (e.g., Joffe et al., 2006). Interestingly, while valproic acid may decrease lipid levels, it is associated with weight gain in up to 20% of patients (3–24 lbs over 3–12 months; Bowden, 2003). Valproic acid weight gain is associated with metabolic disturbances such as hyperinsulinemia and insulin resistance, hyperleptinemia, and leptin resistance (Belcastro, D'Egidio, Striano, & Verrotti, 2013). Patients treated with valproic acid (and other valproate preparations) may develop metabolic syndrome.

LITHIUM

The adverse endocrine effects of lithium include inhibition of various aspects of thyroid functioning (e.g., release of thyroid hormone from the thyroid gland) and hypothyroidism. Lithium-associated hypothyroidism may be accompanied by goiter. Some patients maybe more susceptible to the adverse effects of lithium on the thyroid gland, for example, those with autoimmune Hashimoto's thyroiditis, those with a family history of thyroid disease, females, tobacco smokers, those with a thyroid gland damaged by radiation, and those taking valproic acid (Correll & Carlson, 2006). The estimates of frequency of lithium-associated hypothyroidism vary from study to study with a frequency of around 10% to 20% of patients treated with lithium.

Less well known is the adverse effect of lithium on the parathyroid gland resulting in increased levels of parathyroid hormone and usually mild hypercalcemia. The hypercalcemia is usually benign and nonprogressive in adults (Correll & Carlson, 2006) and usually reversible when lithium is stopped (Mallette & Eichorn, 1986). Lithium has also been known to increase weight—in a review of 14 randomized clinical trials clinically significant weight gain (>7%) was more frequent in patients receiving lithium than those receiving placebo but lower than those receiving olanzapine (McKnight et al., 2012).

MANAGEMENT OF METABOLIC AND ENDOCRINE ADVERSE EFFECTS ASSOCIATED WITH MEDICATIONS USED FOR TREATMENT OF BIPOLAR DISORDER

Management of adverse effects should start at the primary and/or secondary prevention level. Primary prevention focuses on avoiding the occurrence of disease or, in this case, side effects, and secondary prevention focuses on diagnosing and treating disease or side effects in early stages before significant consequences or morbidity occur. Regular screening and monitoring for side effects should be implemented as part of primary and secondary prevention. Developed side effects should be treated accordingly and regularly monitored for.

Table 28.1. CRITERIA FOR CLINICAL DIAGNOSIS OF METABOLIC SYNDROME

ANY 3 OF 5 CONSTITUTE DIAGNOSIS OF METABOLIC SYNDROME

RISK FACTOR/MEASURE	DEFINING LEVEL/CATEGORICAL CUTPOINT
Abdominal obesity, given as waist circumference [a, b] Men Women	> 102 cm (>40 in) > 88 cm (> 35 in)
Triglycerides	≥ 150 mg/dL or on drug treatment for elevated triglycerides
HDL cholesterol Men Women	< 40 mg/dL < 50 mg/dL or on drug treatment for reduced HDL-C
Blood pressure	≥130/≥85 mm Hg or on antihypertensive drug therapy in a patient with a history of hypertension
Fasting glucose	≥100 mg/dL [c] (previously > 110 mg/dL) or on drug treatment for elevated glucose

NOTE: Body mass index is calculated as weigh in kg/(height in meters)^2 or (weight in pounds) × 703/(height in inches)^2.

[a] Overweight and obesity are associated with insulin resistance and the metabolic syndrome. However, the presence of abdominal obesity is more highly correlated with the metabolic risk factors than is an elevated body mass index. Therefore a simple measure of waist circumference is recommended to identify the body weight component of the metabolic syndrome.

[b] Some male patients can develop multiple metabolic risk factors when the waist circumference is only marginally increased (e.g., 94 to 102 cm [37–39 in]). Such patients may have a strong genetic contribution to insulin resistance. They should benefit from changes in life habits, similarly to men with categorical increases in waist circumference.

[c] The American Diabetes Association has recently established a cutpoint of > 100 mg/dL, above which persons have pre-diabetes (impaired fasting glucose) or diabetes. This new cutpoint should be applicable for identifying the lower boundary to define an elevated glucose as one criterion for the metabolic syndrome.

Further risks of metabolic syndrome include family history of type 2 diabetes mellitus; hypertension; cardiovascular disease; polycystic ovary syndrome; advanced age; sedentary lifestyle; ethnic groups having high risk for type 2 diabetes.

Adapted from Grundy et al. (2004) and Grundy et al. (2005).

METABOLIC SYNDROME, WEIGHT GAIN, DIABETES MELLITUS

The first step in the management of weight gain, metabolic syndrome, and diabetes mellitus should be preventive measures, such as promotion of a healthy lifestyle in bipolar patients in general, screening for diabetes and metabolic syndrome, and using medications that are associated with less weight gain and less chance of developing diabetes mellitus (examples include aripiprazole or ziprasidone).

BASELINE

The promotion of a healthy lifestyle should include recommendations of regular exercise, healthy diet (e.g., Mediterranean diet), avoiding smoking, smoking cessation in smokers, and avoiding alcohol and drugs of abuse. A healthy lifestyle could be promoted as a part of patient psychoeducation (Stafford & Colom, 2013), cognitive-behavioral therapy, or interpersonal and social rhythm therapy (Frank, Swartz, & Kupfer, 2000). Psychoeducation should include the discussion of possible severe consequences of weight gain, obesity, metabolic syndrome (such as diabetes), cardiovascular disease, and non-alcoholic steatohepatitis (which may progress to cirrhosis and liver failure). As Grundy et al. (2005) pointed out, if lifestyle change is not sufficient, then drug therapies for abnormalities in the individual risk factors may be indicated. They also stated that there was an insufficient evidence for primary use of drugs that target the underlying cause of metabolic syndrome. On the other hand, Andrade (2013) recently suggested that statins should be considered for the primary prevention of cardiovascular and cerebrovascular events in psychiatric patients, especially for those with a high risk of developing these events and/or metabolic syndrome.

Screening prior to starting treatment with antipsychotics and mood stabilizers should include personal and family medical history, dietary habits, appetite level, height, weight, blood pressure, heart rate, fasting glucose level, and lipid profile. Patients who are overweight (body mass index [BMI] > 25 kg/m²) or obese (BMI ≥30 kg/m²; for calculation of BMI see legend to Table 28.1) at baseline should be guided to start exercise and diet or offered weight management sessions or tailored exercise. Table 28.2 outlines some healthy dietary behaviors. A behavioral weight-loss intervention significantly reduced weight over a period of 18 months in overweight and obese adults with severe mental illness (schizophrenia, schizoaffective disorder, bipolar disorder, major depression) in a study by Daumit and colleagues (2013). Severely obese patients could be offered medications for obesity, though none of the available agents has been found consistently useful and effective (see later). Some overweight or obese patients with already developed significant comorbidity (e.g., type 2 diabetes mellitus) may be offered referral to a bariatric specialist or an endocrinologist and may even opt for bariatric surgery.

Even patients who are not overweight and are started on a mood stabilizer or other medication should be counseled about the possible development of weight gain and metabolic syndrome and recommended dietary and health lifestyle habits as outlined in Table 28.2.

As noted, patients may be started on medications with lesser propensity for weight gain. These include aripiprazole and ziprasidone among antipsychotics. The mood-stabilizing agent lamotrigine was associated with stable body weight during one year of treatment and was comparable to placebo in mean weight change in a report by Sachs and colleagues (2006), and obese patients with bipolar I disorder lost weight while taking lamotrigine in another study (Bowden et al., 2006). Antidepressants are used in bipolar disorder also (mostly in combination with mood stabilizers), and thus one should remember that some of them (e.g., amitriptyline, clomipramine, mirtazapapine, and paroxetine) may be associated with weight gain; the only one not associated with weight gain seems to be bupropion. Lithium and other mood stabilizers (e.g., valproic acid) may also be associated with weight gain, and thus some of the management strategies for weight gain (monitoring, diet, exercise) described here may apply to patients treated with these medications as well.

MONITORING

Monitoring patients who are on medications that potentially cause weight gain and metabolic syndrome should include body weight, height, and calculation of BMI at every visit or measuring waist circumference every three months (Correll & Carlson, 2006). Fasting serum lipids should be obtained possibly 3 months after starting the medication and every 6 to 12 months thereafter if BMI is

Table 28.2. HEALTHY DIETARY AND LIFESTYLE HABITS/BEHAVIORS

1. Replace all sugar-containing drinks (soda, juices, punch) or whole milk with at least 2 L of water and moderate amounts of unsweetened tea or low-fat milk. Recommend no cream, milk, or sugar in coffee. Drinks that contain artificial sweeteners should be avoided too, as they may increase food intake.

2. Eat three meals a day; avoid snacks whenever possible. Do not snack when full. If snacking, use fruits, vegetables, or small amount of nuts. Nuts are healthy.

3. Eat small portions at meals.

4. Eat breakfast every morning.

5. Eat slowly, drink an ample amount of water between bites, and avoid second helpings or take one only after a delay.

6. Do not eat fast food if possible, or maximally once per week.

7. Replace refined white flour and processed sugar products with whole grain and other foods that have a low glycemic index (i.e., ≤ 55; http://www.glycemicindex.com)

8. Limit saturated fat intake but avoid extensive consumption of processed fat-free food items.

9. Eat at least 25–30 g/day of soluble fiber from fruits, vegetables, and/or whole nuts.

10. If not eating it regularly, introduce fish into your regular diet, eat least once or twice a week.

11. Perform moderate to vigorous physical activity for at least 30–60 min/day.

12. Walk and climb stairs whenever suitable/possible.

NOTE: Adapted from Correll and Carlson (2006).

stable and results of the lipid test are normal at baseline and first follow-up (Correll & Carlson, 2006). Measuring blood pressure and heart rate regularly is also recommended. Monitoring for diabetes mellitus should include a fasting blood glucose test three months after starting the medication and then every six months or quarterly in patients with a high risk for developing diabetes (Correll & Carlson, 2006). Patients should be also asked about symptoms of hyperglycemia (polyuria, polydipsia). Ng and colleagues (2009) recommend HbA1C (glycosylated hemoglobin) be reserved as a monitoring aid for patients with diabetes mellitus rather than as a screening parameter. They suggested another set of monitoring recommendations: monthly weight measurements for the first three months, followed by measures every three months for the duration of treatment; blood pressure and fasting glucose at three-month intervals for the first year then annually; and a fasting lipid profile at three months after initiation of atypical antipsychotic therapy, to be repeated at annual intervals thereafter.

Patients with significant weight gain after the first three months (5% of weight) or thereafter should be encouraged to exercise and diet and may be considered for either a medication switch or treatment with adjunctive medication (discussed later). Grundy and colleagues (2005) recommended that in patients with metabolic syndrome the physician should

> consistently encourage weight maintenance/reduction through appropriate balance of physical activity, caloric intake, and formal behavior-modification programs when indicated to maintain/achieve waist circumference of < 40 inches in men and < 35 inches in women. Aim initially at slow reduction of about 7% to 10% from baseline weight. Even small amounts of weight loss are associated with significant health benefits. (p. 2741)

TREATMENT

Psychiatrists are usually hesitant and resistant to treat physical illness or physical, metabolic, and endocrine adverse effects of medications. Thus for those who are not comfortable initiating treatment after measures such as diet, exercise, and switching to another medication(s) with lower metabolic risk profile (Grande, Bernardo, Bones, Sainz-Ruiz, & Alamo, 2014) fail, referral to the patient's primary care physician, internist, or endocrinologist may be the next step.

Grundy and colleagues (2005) review the treatment of metabolic syndrome in general, whereas McIntyre et al. (2012) summarize the recommendation of the Canadian Network for Mood and Anxiety Treatments Task Force for patients with mood disorders and comorbid metabolic disorders:

1. In regard to medication management of weight gain in this population, the authors suggest that, according to World Health Organization recommendations, individuals with a BMI of ≥27 and weight-related morbidity (e.g., diabetes mellitus) or BMI > 30 without weight related morbidity may be considered for "bariatric" medicines. These may include phentermine (probably not recommended in bipolar disorder as it may induce hypomania/mania); orlistat (poorly tolerated by patients because of loose stools, abdominal pain, flatulence); naltrexone-bupropion; modafinil; and a host of other medications such as topiramate (which may be useful in bipolar disorder as it is also used as a mood stabilizer), metformin, reboxetine (not available in the United States), zonisamide, nizatidine, and amantadine. They suggested that in bipolar disorder, behavioral/diet modification/cognitive intervention should be the first-line approach; metformin, topiramate, modafinil, and orlistat the second-line approach; and other drugs the third-line approach. They did not recommend using phentermine and pointed out that the naltrexone-bupropion combination has not been properly studied in this population. It is worth noting that metformin was recently found modestly effective in reducing weight and other risk factors for cardiovascular disease in clinically stable, overweight outpatients with chronic schizophrenia or schizoaffective disorder over 16 weeks in a double-blind, placebo-controlled study by Jarskog and colleagues (2013). Such a study is not available in bipolar patients at the present time, but results suggest the usefulness in reducing weight in this population too.

2. For treatment of dyslipidemia, McIntyre and colleagues (2012) recommend behavioral and dietary strategies. They point out that no studies have evaluated the effects of antilipidemic therapy in mood disorder population so far.

3. Finally, for dysglycemic patients and patients with diabetes mellitus, the authors suggest treatment behavioral/diet modification/cognitive intervention as

the first-line approach for dysglycemia and commonly used antidiabetic agents, including insulin, metformin, and possibly pioglitazone (although this medication has been withdrawn from the market in some countries because of association with bladder cancer, it is still available in the United States though with appropriate warning).

Most of these medications should be used in coordination with the primary care physician, internist, or endocrinologist, or patients should be referred to these physicians.

ENDOCRINE ADVERSE EFFECTS

THYROID FUNCTION

As noted, lithium therapy is associated with thyroid dysfunction, namely hypothyroidism. Thus the treating physician should obtain baseline thyroid function tests (TSH) and free thyroxine (T_4) and possibly triiodothyronine (T_3) (most of the time TSH is sufficient) in every patient considered for treatment with lithium. These tests should be rechecked 1 to 2 months after the initiation of lithium therapy and repeated every 6 to 12 months. Some suggest repeating these tests only yearly in patients stable on lithium. In addition, patients should be routinely questioned for symptoms of hypothyroidism, such as fatigue, weight gain, and newly developed cold intolerance. If hypothyroidism is detected, patients should be started on thyroid hormone replacement (various preparations, preferably thyroxine). The treatment should be guided by laboratory indices, and the goal should be a normal level of TSH (depending on one's local laboratory). One should start with a minimal dose of thyroxine (e.g., 25 mcg/day) and titrate upward guided by TSH levels repeated every approximately six to eight weeks. Some specialists may start treating patients with TSH within the upper limits of normal levels. Patients treated with thyroxine whose TSH levels are stabilized within the normal limits should still be regularly monitored and their TSH levels should be repeated every 6 to 12 months (in some patients TSH may normalize after a year or two, thus a decrease of thyroxine supplementation with subsequent checking of TSH may be indicated). Thyroid augmentation is also used in mood disorders and could be occasionally used in lithium-treated patients. Finally, hypothyroidism is not a contraindication for treatment with lithium. It may just require more careful monitoring and thyroxine-dose adjustment during lithium treatment.

Valproate may alter thyroid function and quetiapine may decrease T_4. Thus some suggest monitoring thyroid function in bipolar patients treated with these medications. However, this has not been a routine practice. Nevertheless, yearly monitoring of TSH in patients on valproate may be prudent.

PARATHYROID FUNCTION

Lithium may have an adverse effect on calcium homeostasis; chronic lithium exposure has been linked to hyperparathyroidism, hypercalcemia (usually mild, 10.5–11.5 mg/dL), and hyperparathormonemia (Saunders, Saunders, & Gauger, 2009). Correll and Carlson (2006) recommend obtaining a baseline calcium level prior to starting lithium and monitoring it 1, 6, and 12 months after staring lithium and yearly thereafter (Mallette & Eichorn, 1986). However, this has not been a common practice. Calcium levels may normalize when lithium is discontinued (this, according to Correll and Carlson [2006], does not need to be done unless serum calcium is >11.5 mg/dL). There may be a role for calcimimetic drug therapy or even surgery in case of severe hyperparathyroidism (Saunders et al., 2009).

PROLACTIN LEVELS AND HYPERPROLACTINEMIA

The development of hyperprolactinemia associated with antipsychotic medications is unpredictable and, at times, inconsequential. At times, increased prolactin levels may be noted when one obtains comprehensive laboratory assessment without signs of hyperprolactinemia. In cases of increased prolactin level, one may ask about symptoms of hyperprolactinemia more carefully (nipple discharge, amenorrhea, changes in sexual functioning) and in women about the possibility of pregnancy and use of hormonal contraceptives (both may increase prolactin; Correll & Carlson, 2006). Thyroid function, blood urea nitrogen, and creatinine could be also checked as hypothyroidism and renal failure may increase prolactin levels. However, if there are no symptoms of hyperprolactinemia and other causes of hyperprolactinemia are ruled out, treatment may not be necessary (one should not treat abnormal laboratory levels without the clinical context).

If symptoms of hypeprolactinemia occur, the patient's prolactin level should be checked, and if levels are less than 200 ng/mL, the antipsychotic dose should be reduced, or the antipsychotic medication should be switched either to an antipsychotic with lesser impact on prolactin (e.g., aripiprazole, quetiapine) or to another mood stabilizer if using antipsychotics for mood stabilization. An MRI scan of the sella turcica to look for pituitary adenoma should be obtained if levels of prolactin remain increased after medication is changed or if prolactin level is more than 200 ng/dL (Correll & Carlson, 2006). Hyperprolactinemia has been treated with dopamine agonists such as amantadine, bromocriptine, and cabergoline in the past. However, these medications may be associated with worsening of psychosis and thus should be avoided. After dopamine agonists fail, pituitary adenoma is usually treated surgically.

OTHER ENDOCRINE EFFECTS

Female patients treated with valproate may develop polycystic ovary syndrome. If symptoms of this syndrome occur, the most prudent management approach would be substitution with another mood stabilizer and referral to an endocrinologist to address oligomenorrhea and other complications. Sexual side effects may occur during the treatment with various medications used for treatment of bipolar disorder, including antipsychotics and lithium. The sexual side effects associated with antipsychotics are frequently explained by hyperprolactinemia but may be also due to dopamine blockade (low libido) and other effects of antipsychotics. The rare sexual effects associated with lithium are poorly understood. Possible sexual side effects of valproate may be explained by its effects on various hormones. The management of sexual side effects of drugs used for bipolar disorder may employ various strategies such as decreasing the dose, changing to a different medication or use of some "antidotes" (e.g., phosphodiesterase-5 inhibitors such as avanafil, sildenafil, tadalafil, and vardenafil in case of erectile dysfunction). Some of these strategies (switching the mood stabilizer, decreasing the dose) may not always be suitable in an unstable bipolar patient and need to be considered in the clinical context of the illness.

CONCLUSION

Endocrine- and metabolic-adverse effects of drugs used in the management of bipolar disorder may pose a serious obstacle in the management of the disorder, as they are associated with serious health consequences. Addressing these adverse effects must be proactive and of a preventive nature, as fully developed adverse effects, especially metabolic ones, are usually very difficult to reverse. There are not enough controlled studies on the management of metabolic-adverse effects in the area of bipolar disorder, but the management

strategies used in other disorders (e.g., schizophrenia) can be helpful. Management of these adverse effects may frequently require collaboration with a primary care physician or endocrinology specialist. Collaboration with these physicians within the framework of comprehensive patient management is strongly advised.

Disclosure statement: The author has no conflict of interest related to the material in this chapter. He has authored/edited books for various publishing houses, but that does not present any conflict of interest.

REFERENCES

Andrade, C. (2013). Primary prevention of cardiovascular events in patients with major mental illness: A possible role for statins. *Bipolar Disorders*, *15*(8), 813–823.

Bowden, C. L. (2003). Valproate. *Bipolar Disorders*, 5, 189–202.

Bowden, C. L., Calabrese, J. R., Ketter, T. A., Sachs, G. S., White, R. L., & Thompson, T. R. (2006). Impact of lamotrigine and lithium on weight in obese and nonobese patients with bipolar I disorder. *American Journal of Psychiatry*, *163*, 1199–1201.

Belcastro, V., D'Edigio, C., Striano, P., & Verrotti, A. (2013). Metabolic and endocrine effects of valproic acid chronic treatment. *Epilepsy Research*, *107*, 1–8.

Buse, J. B. (2002). Metabolic side effects of antipsychotics: Focus on hyperglycemia and diabetes. *Journal of Clinical Psychiatry*, *63*(Suppl. 4), 37–41.

Cassidy, F., Ahearn, E., & Carroll, B. J. (1999). Elevated frequency of diabetes mellitus in hospitalized manic-depressive patients. *American Journal of Psychiatry*, *156*, 1417–1420.

Correll, C. U., & Carlson, H. E. (2006). Endocrine and metabolic adverse effects of psychotropic medications in children and adolescents. *Journal of the American Academy of Child & Adolescent Psychiatry*, *45*, 771–791.

Crump, C., Sunquist, K., Winkleby, M. A., & Sundquist, J. (2013). Comorbidities and mortality in bipolar disorder: A Swedish national cohort study. *JAMA Psychiatry*, *70*, 931–939.

Daumit, G. L., Dickerson, F. B., Wang, N-Y., Dalcin, A., Jerome, G. J., Anderson, C. A. M.,…Appel, L. J. (2013). A behavioral weight-loss intervention in persons with serious mental illness. *New England Journal of Medicine*, *368*, 1594–1602.

De Hert, M., Detraux, J, van Winkel, R., & Correll, C. U. (2012). Metabolic and cardiovascular adverse effects associated with antipsychotic drugs. *Nature Reviews Endocrinology*, *8*, 114–126.

Enger, C., Jones, C. M., Kryzhanovskaya, L., Doherty, M., & McAfee, A. T. (2013). Risk of developing diabetes and dyslipidemia among adolescents with bipolar disorder or schizophrenia. *International Journal of Adolescent Medicine and Health*, *25*, 3–11.

Fiedorowicz, J. G., Palagummi, N. M., Forman-Hoffman, V. L., Miller, D. D., & Haynes, W. G. (2008). Elevated prevalence of obesity, metabolic syndrome, and cardiovascular risk factors in bipolar disorder. *Annals of Clinical Psychiatry*, *20*, 131–137.

Frank, E., Swartz, H. A., & Kupfer, D. J. (2000). Interpersonal and social rhythm therapy: Managing the chaos of bipolar disorder. *Biological Psychiatry*, *48*, 593–604.

Goodwin, F. K., & Jamison, K. R. (1990). *Manic-depressive illness*. New York: Oxford University Press.

Grande, I., Bernardo, M., Bobes, J., Saiz-Ruiz, J., Alamo, C., & Vieta, E. (2014). Antipsychotic switching in bipolar disorders: A systematic review. *International Journal of Neuropsychopharmacology*, *17*(3), 497–507.

Grundy, S. M., Brewer, H. B., Cleeman, J. I., Smith, S. C. Jr., & Lenfant, C. (2004). Definition of metabolic syndrome: Report of the National Heart, Lung and Blood Institute/American Heart Association Conference on scientific issues related to definition. *Circulation, 109*, 433–438.

Grundy, S. M., Cleeman, J. I., Daniels, S. R., Donato, K. A., Eckel, R. H., Franklin, B. A.,...Costa, F. (2005). Diagnosis and management of the metabolic syndrome. An American Heart Association/National Heart, Lung, and Blood Institute Scientific Statement. *Circulation, 112*, 2735–2752.

Joffe, H., Cohen, L. S., Suppes, T., McLaughlin, W. L., Lavori, P., Adams, J. M.,...Sachs, G. S. (2006). Valproate is associated with new-onset oligoamenorrhea with hyperandrosteronism in women with bipolar disorder. *Biological Psychiatry, 59*, 1078–1086.

Jarskog, L. F., Hamer, R. M., Catellier, D. J., Stewart, D. D., LaVange, L., Ray, N.,...Stroup, T. S. (2013). Metformin for weight loss and metabolic control in overweight outpatients with schizophrenia and schizoaffective disorder. *American Journal of Psychiatry, 170*, 1032–1040.

Kilbourne, A. M., Cornelius, J. R., Han, X., Pincus, H. A., Shad, M., Salloum, I.,...Haas, G. L. (2004). Burden of general medical conditions among individuals with bipolar disorder. *Bipolar Disorders, 6*, 368–373.

Liliker, S. L. (1980). Prevalence of diabetes in a manic-depressive population. *Comprehensive Psychiatry, 21*, 271–275.

Maguire, G. A. (2002). Prolactin elevation with antipsychotic medications: Mechanism of action and clinical consequences. *Journal of Clinical Psychiatry, 63*(Suppl. 4), 56–62.

Malhotra, S., & McElroy, S. L. (2002). Medical management of obesity associated with mental disorders. *Journal of Clinical Psychiatry, 63*(Suppl. 4), 24–32.

Mallette, L. E., & Eichorn, E. (1986). Effects of lithium carbonate on human calcium metabolism. *Archives of Internal Medicine, 146*, 770–776.

McIntyre, R. S., Alsuwaidan, M., Goldstein, B. I., Taylor, V. H., Schaffer, A., Beaulieu, S.,...Canadian Network for Mood and Anxiety Treatments (CANMAT) Task Force. (2012). The Canadian Network for Mood and Anxiety Disorders Treatments (CANMAT) Task Force recommendation for the management of patients with mood disorders and comorbid metabolic disorders. *Annals of Clinical Psychiatry, 24*, 69–81.

McKnight, R. F., Adida, M., Budge, K., Stockton, S., Goodwin, G. M., & Geddes, J. R. (2012). Lithium toxicity profile: A systemic review and meta-analysis. *Lancet, 379*, 721–728.

Nemeroff, C. B., Simon, J. S., Haggerty, J. J. Jr., & Evans, D. L. (1985). Antithyroid antibodies in depressed patients. *American Journal of Psychiatry, 142*, 840–843.

Newcomer, J. W. (2007a). Antipsychotic medications: Metabolic and cardiovascular risk. *Journal of Clinical Psychiatry, 68*(Suppl. 4), 8–13.

Newcomer, J. W. (2007b). Metabolic syndrome and mental illness. *American Journal of Managed Care, 13*(Suppl. 7), S170–S177.

Ng, F., Mammen, O. K., Wilting, I., Sachs, G. S., Ferrier, I. N., Cassidy, F....Berk, M. (2009). The International; Society for Bipolar Disorders (ISBD) consensus guidelines for the safety monitoring of bipolar disorder treatments. *Bipolar Disorders, 11*, 559–595.

Sachs, G., Bowden, C., Calabrese, J. R., Ketter, T., Thompson, T., White, R., & Bentley, B. (2006). Effects of lamotrigine and lithium on body weight during maintenance treatment of bipolar disorder. *Bipolar Disorders, 8*, 175–181.

Saunders, B. D., Saunders, E. F., & Gauger, P. G. (2009). Lithium therapy and hyperparathyroidism: An evidence-based assessment. *World Journal of Surgery, 33*, 2314–2324.

Stafford, N., & Colom, F. (2013). Purpose and effectiveness of psychoeducation in patients with bipolar disorder in a bipolar disorder clinic setting. *Acta Psychiatrica Scandinavica, 127*(Suppl. 442), 11–18.

Taylor, V., & MacQueen, G. (2006). Association between bipolar disorder and metabolic syndrome: A review. *Journal of Clinical Psychiatry, 67*, 1034–1041.

Vancampfort, D., Vansteelandt, K., Correll, C. U., Mitchell, A. J., De Hert, A., Sienaert, P.,...De Hert, M. (2013). Metabolic syndrome and metabolic abnormalities in bipolar disorder. *American Journal of Psychiatry, 170*, 265–274.

Young, A. H., & Grunze, H. (2013). Physical health of patients with bipolar disorder. *Acta Psychiatrica Scandinavica, 127*(Suppl. 442), 3–10.

29.

NEUROLOGICAL, COGNITIVE, AND NEUROPROTECTIVE EFFECTS OF TREATMENTS USED IN BIPOLAR DISORDER

Janusz K. Rybakowski

NEUROBIOLOGY OF BIPOLAR DISORDER: INTRODUCTION

In the fifth edition of the *Diagnostic and Statistical Manual of Mental Disorder* (American Psychiatric Association, 2013), bipolar disorders (BPDs) have been classified as a separate category of mental disorders. BPD is a recurrent and sometimes chronic mental disorder that is characterized by episodes of mania, hypomania, depression, and mixed states. BPD has a worldwide prevalence of 2% to 5% of the population (Merinkangas & Tohen, 2011); the prevalence of BPD with mania (bipolar I) is about 1%, while the remaining types amount to about 3% to 4%. Genetic predisposition is one of the highest among psychiatric disorders, and the heritability index is estimated to be 0.85 (McGuffin et al., 2003). BPD is a serious mental illness, the cause of significant suffering for patients and burden for their families, and approximately 10% to 20% of patients commit suicide over the course of their illness (Rihmer & Kiss, 2002). The prognosis of BPD is encumbered with high rates of relapse, lingering residual symptoms, cognitive impairments, and diminished well-being. However, adequate treatment may allow for long-term remission and good functioning in a proportion of patients.

Since the 1960s, the brain systems receiving the greatest attention in the neurobiology of BPD have been the monoaminergic neurotransmitter systems (i.e., serotonergic, noradrenergic, and dopaminergic). The therapeutic mechanisms of some medications used for the treatment of BPD (i.e., antipsychotic and antidepressant drugs) have been mostly explained on the basis of involving these systems. In the past two decades, several new pathogenic pathways of BPD have been identified such as hypothalamic-pituitary-adrenal axis pathology, inflammatory and oxidative stress disturbances, as well as impairment of neuroplasticity and neuroresilience in the central nervous system. Furthermore, such changes have been considered in the context of the process of allostasis, as well as of staging and neuroprogression in BPD (Gama, Kunz, Magalhaes, & Kapczinski, 2013).

The impairment of neurotrophic processes and neuroplasticity has been now regarded as an important pathogenic mechanism in BPD (Soeiro-de-Souza et al., 2012). Impairment of synaptic strength and cellular plasticity in this illness has been shown to involve changes in pathways regulating neurotrophic factors and neuroprotective protein levels and expression. Among neurotrophins, the most important seems to be the brain-derived neurotrophic factor (BDNF). Other neurotrophins include nerve growth factor, neurotrophin(NT)-3, NT-4, NT-5, and NT-6. BDNF and other neurotrophins are necessary for the survival and function of neurons. BDNF modulates the activity of such neurotransmitters as glutamate, gamma-aminobutyric acid, dopamine, and serotonin. A transcription of the *BDNF* gene is activated by the cyclic adenosine monophosphate (c-AMP) response element binding (CREB). Other important factors connected with neuroplasticity include glycogen synthase kinase-3 (GSK-3), the phosphatidylinositide (PI) pathway, protein kinase C (PKC) and B-cell lymphoma 2 (Bcl-2). GSK-3 is a serine/threonine kinase that regulates diverse cellular processes and specifically cell apoptosis. Therefore GSK-3 inhibition directly influences gene transcription leading to antiapoptotic effects and improved cell structural stability. The PI pathway plays a key role in signal transduction pathways, which are connected to receptors of various neurotransmitters. PKC is an enzyme closely connected with the PI pathway that regulates both pre- and postsynaptic aspects of neurotransmission and several cellular processes. Bcl-2 is an important protein for cellular resilience and plasticity, exerting mostly antiapoptotic effects. Other neurobiological changes related to impaired neuroplasticity

Table 29.1. NEUROLOGICAL SIDE EFFECTS OF TREATMENTS USED IN BIPOLAR DISORDERS

TREATMENT	NEUROLOGICAL SIDE EFFECTS
Lithium	Tremor—most frequent (20% of patients) Rare: extrapyramidal and oculomotor symptoms Culmination of neurological symptoms with lithium intoxication (cerebellar and extrapyramidal symptoms) The syndrome of irreversible lithium-effectuated neurotoxicity (SILENT)
Anticonvulsants	High doses (levels): tremor, nystagmus, ataxia Valproate—hyperammonemic encephalopathy
Antipsychotics	Extrapyramidal (parkinsoninsm, dystonia, akathisia, tardive dyskinesia): the risk differs between antipsychotic drugs (lowest: quetiapine, clozapine) Neuroleptic malignant syndrome Seizures Increased risk of cardiovascular events in elderly
Antidepressants	Serotonin syndrome Seizures Rare: extrapyramidal symptoms
Electroconvulsive therapy	Rare: subdural hematoma

include calcium dysregulation and mitochondrial/endoplasmic reticulum dysfunction (Soeiro-de-Souza et al., 2012).

On neuroimaging levels, disturbances in neurotrophic processes and neuroplasticity in BPD are reflected in reductions in volume, density, number, and size of neurons and glial cells in such brain structures as the dorsal anterolateral and subgenual prefrontal cortex, orbital cortex, hippocampus, amygdala, basal ganglia, and dorsal raphe nuclei. They may be also connected to the presence of white matter abnormalities that are repeatedly reported in patients with BPD (Hajek, Carrey, & Alda, 2005; Lenox, Gould, & Manji, 2002; Rajkowska, Halaris, & Selemon, 2001).

Disturbances of neurotrophic processes and neuroplasticity can now be regarded as a molecular target of treatment procedures in this illness. On the one hand, it has been demonstrated that the effect on them may be associated with therapeutic efficacy of mood-stabilizing drugs, especially of lithium. On the other hand, any new procedures that may prevent, treat, or reverse such changes may constitute promising strategies for developing improved treatment of BPD.

BIOLOGICAL TREATMENTS OF BIPOLAR DISORDER

Drugs, collectively known as mood stabilizers, have been most widely used for the treatment of BPD. A mood stabilizer can be defined as a drug that, if used as monotherapy, it (a) acts therapeutically in mania or/and in depression; (b) acts prophylactically against manic or/and depressive episodes, as demonstrated in a trial of at least one year's duration; and (b) does not worsen any therapeutic or prophylactic aspect of the illness outlined previously. A classification of mood stabilizers based on the chronology of their introduction for the treatment of bipolar mood disorder has been proposed (Rybakowski, 2007).

In 2013 we observed the 50th anniversary of the first publication on long-term mood-stabilizing properties of lithium in mood disorders (Hartigan, 1963), initiating the first generation of mood-stabilizing drugs. In the 1960s and 1970s, publications appeared pointing to a possible mood-stabilizing effect (*thymoregulatrice*—in French) exerted by valproates (Lambert, Carraz, Borselli, & Carbel, 1966; Lambert, Borselli, Marcou, Bouchardy, & Cabrol, 1971). In the early 1970s, Japanese researchers obtained evidence for a mood-stabilizing effect of carbamazepine (Takezaki & Hanaoka, 1971; Okuma, Kishimoto, & Inue, 1973). Since these drugs preceded introduction of new mood-stabilizing substances by more than two decades, it has therefore been proposed to name lithium, carbamazepine, and valproate first-generation mood stabilizers (Rybakowski, 2007).

The first suggestion that the atypical antipsychotic drug clozapine had a mood-stabilizing action was advanced in the mid-1990s (Zarate, Tohen, Banov, Weiss, & Cole, 1995). In the following years, mood-stabilizing properties, as defined previously, have been confirmed for such atypical antipsychotic drugs as olanzapine, quetiapine, aripiprazole, and risperidone (Quiroz et al., 2010a; Rybakowski, 2007, 2008a). A suggestion for lamotrigine being a mood-stabilizing drug was made in the early

Table 29.2. COGNITIVE SIDE EFFECTS OF TREATMENT USED IN BIPOLAR DISORDERS

TREATMENT	COGNITIVE SIDE EFFECTS
Lithium	Slight impairment of cognitive functions, probably dose-related Possibility of preserving cognitive functions with long-term treatment Excellent lithium responders: cognitive functions comparable to healthy people
Anticonvulsants	Carbamazepine and valproate: moderate impairment of cognitive functions, dose-related, increased with combination treatment Lamotrigine: favorable effect on cognitive functions both in pediatric and in adult bipolar patients
Antipsychotics	Better effect on cognitive functions of atypical than typical antipsychotics Quetiapine may be less impairing than olanzapine and risperidone
Antidepressants	Cognitive performance improves with amelioration of depressive symptoms with antidepressants Tricyclic antidepressants may be more impairing than SSRI
Electroconvulsive therapy	Cognitive abnormalities occur mostly in the first three days posttreatment Memory disturbances in some patients may persist for several weeks

2000s (Ketter & Calabrese, 2002). Therefore, atypical antipsychotics fulfilling the aforementioned criteria and lamotrigine could be considered second-generation mood stabilizers (Rybakowski, 2007).

Historically, typical antipsychotics were, besides lithium, the oldest drugs in the treatment of mania, and they remain still of value in this condition. Haloperidol has been the most frequently used, and its antimanic properties score very favorably compared with other mood-stabilizing drugs (Cipriani et al., 2011; Yildiz, Nikodem, Vieta, Correll, & Baldessarini, in press).

Antidepressant drugs have been widely used in the treatment of BPD, although their adequate application, especially as monotherapy, in the treatment of bipolar depression is a subject of debate. As there is a general consensus that in bipolar I depression they should be accompanied by mood-stabilizing drug(s), some researchers try to advise on antidepressant monotherapy, even for several months' duration, in bipolar II depression (Amsterdam, Luo, & Shults, 2013). The International Society for Bipolar Disorders' report on using antidepressant drugs in BDP appeared recently in *The American Journal of Psychiatry* (Pacchiarotti et al., 2013).

Finally, electroconvulsive therapy (ECT) has been recommended for treatment-refractory depression, both unipolar and bipolar. Recent meta-analysis showed that the efficacy of ECT in bipolar depression is at least equal to that of unipolar depression (Dierckx, Heijnen, van den Broek, & Birkenhager, 2012). In some therapeutic standards, ECT has been also recommended for treatment-resistant mania (Yatham et al., 2013).

In this chapter the effects of all of these treatments used in BPD are reviewed in terms of their neurotoxic and neuroprotective effects. First, neurotoxic effects, reflected as clinical neurological symptoms, are discussed, along with the possibility of their management. Second, the effect of these treatments on cognitive functions in bipolar patients is presented. In this context, it should be kept in mind that neurocognitive functions may already be compromised in BPD by the disease process itself. Recent meta-analysis involving 31 primary data sets as a single large sample of 2,876 patients showed that at least three neuropsychological measures, such as the Verbal Learning Task, Digit Span, and Trail Making Test, were impaired in euthymic bipolar patients (Bourne et al., 2013).

The treatments used in BPD can also either favorably or adversely influence neurotrophic processes and cellular plasticity. This chapter reviews such effects demonstrated both in experimental studies, as well as in clinical settings, including patients with BPD. The most extensive data in this respect exist on neuroprotective properties of lithium.

LITHIUM

Lithium, the oldest mood-stabilizing drug, is still considered the gold standard for treatment of BPD, especially for a long-term prevention of recurrences. Neurological effects of lithium are mostly connected with its higher serum level and culminate during lithium intoxication. Cognitive effects may be also dependent on serum level and can be associated with a degree of therapeutic response. Furthermore, neuroprotective effects of lithium in BPD have been demonstrated to a greater extent than for any other mood-stabilizing drug.

Table 29.3. NEUROPROTECTIVE EFFECTS OF TREATMENT USED IN BIPOLAR DISORDERS

TREATMENT	NEUROPROTECTIVE EFFECTS
Lithium	Stimulation of BDNF Inhibition of GSK-3 activity Inhibition of PI pathway Inhibiton of PKC Increasing expression of bcl-2 Increase of cerebral grey matter volume
Anticonvulsants	Inhibition of PI pathway (carbamazepine, valproate) Inhibition of PKC (valproate) Stimulation of BDNF system (valproate, lamotrigine) Preventing glutamate-induced neurotoxicity (lamotrigine)
Antipsychotics	Typical antipsychotics: devoid of neuroprotective effects Atypical antipsychotics (clozapine, olanzapine, quetiapine, aripiprazole, risperidone) stimulate BDNF system and exert anti-apoptotic action
Antidepressants	Stimulation of BDNF Reversing neurotoxicity of hypercortisolemia Stimulation of neurogenesis and synaptogenesis
Electroconvulsive therapy	Effect on BDNF system Stimulation of neurogenesis in experimental studies

NOTE: BDNF = brain-derived neurotrophic factor, GSK-3 = glucogen synthase kinase-3, PI = phosphatidyl inositol, PKC = protein kinase C.

Neurological effects

The most frequent neurological adverse effect of lithium is a fine tremor of the upper limbs occurring as postural tremor or during any type of active movements (action tremor). This tremor looks like an exaggeration of physiologic tremor with a similar frequency range between 8 and 13 Hz, differing from resting Parkinsonian tremor, which has a frequency of 4 to 6 Hz. The incidence rate of tremor, which may occur as early as several weeks after beginning treatment, is about 20% of lithium-treated patients. Predisposing factors include high lithium level; older age; and concomitant treatment with antidepressant, anticonvulsant, or antipsychotic drugs. Lithium-induced tremor is usually mild and often disappears after dose reduction. However, if a reduction of lithium dosage is not possible and if the tremor is considered clinically relevant (i.e., interfering with the patients' daily activities), administration of low-dose beta blockers, usually propranolol at 30 to 80 mg/day, can be used with good results.

Infrequent neurological adverse effects of lithium involving central nervous system include extrapyramidal and oculomotor symptoms. Sometimes they may occur even with lithium concentration within therapeutic dose. Similarly as in tremor, predisposing factors include high lithium levels; older age; and concomitant treatment with antidepressant, anticonvulsant, or antipsychotics drugs. Any preexisting cerebral abnormalities may also constitute a risk factor. Extrapyramidal symptoms may include Parkinsonism, akathisia, or tardive dyskinesia and occur mostly in patients who receive co-treatment with antipsychotic drugs. These symptoms do not favorably respond to anti-Parkinsonian medications. Lithium-induced nystagmus is usually reversible under reduction of lithium dose or lithium discontinuation. Neurological adverse effects of lithium involving the peripheral nervous system include complaints of muscle weakness with subtle decrease of motor nerve conduction. Although of doubtful clinical significance, attention should be given in the case of giving lithium to patients with muscular disorders or peripheral neuropathies (Fountoulakis, Vieta, Bouras, Notaridis, Giannakopoulos, Kaprinis & Akiskal, 2007; Pogarell, Folkerts, & Hegerl, 2006).

All neurological side effects of lithium markedly increase during lithium intoxication, leading to a loss of consciousness, occasionally with the occurrence of convulsions. In most lithium-intoxicated patients, a range of neurological symptoms can be observed, especially cerebellar signs such as tremor, nystagmus, dysarthria, vertigo, ataxia or extrapyramidal Parkinsonian, or choreoathetotic motor symptoms. Treatment of lithium intoxication includes supportive care and enhancement of lithium elimination with intravenous saline. Hemodialysis is the method of choice for treating patients with severe intoxication and high lithium levels (> 2 mmol/l). In some patients, persisting neurological and cognitive deficits following lithium intoxication such as short-term memory disturbances and cerebellar dysfunctions (especially ataxia) can ensue. They are named the syndrome of irreversible lithium-effectuated neurotoxicity (SILENT) (Aditanjee, Munshi, & Thampy, 2005).

Cognitive effects

Early clinical observations in bipolar patients receiving lithium on a long-term basis suggested either no effect or a slight impairment of cognitive function. In one recent clinical study, impaired verbal memory and otherwise spared cognition in remitted bipolar patients on monotherapy with lithium was found, while in others, a lower performance on episodic verbal and visual verbal memory tests of bipolar patients compared to the healthy subjects was observed. However, no difference between lithium-treated bipolar patients and those receiving no medication was found (Dias, Balanza-Martinez, Soeiro-de-Souza, Moreno, Figueira, Machado-Vieira, & Vieta, 2012).

On the other hand, the results of recent animal research point unanimously to lithium having a favorable effect on cognitive function, as demonstrated on various models. Lithium treatment protects irradiated hippocampal neurons from apoptosis and improves cognitive performance in irradiated mice. Such procognitive effect of lithium was attributed to the inhibition of GSK-3ß and to an increase in Bcl-2 protein expression (Yazlovitskaya et al., 2006). In another study, using three different positive reinforcement spatial cognitive tasks in rats, it was demonstrated that lithium magnifies learning in all three tasks, which may be associated with enhancing hippocampal synaptic plasticity (Nocjar, Hammonds, & Shim, 2007).

In our own studies, we have attempted to correlate cognitive functions in lithium-treated patients with a quality of lithium prophylactic effect. We found that non-responders to lithium had significantly worse performance on many domains of the Wisconsin Card Sorting Test compared to excellent and partial responders (Rybakowski, Permoda-Osip, & Borkowska, 2009). In a recent study, using neuropsychological tests from a Cambridge Neuropsychological Test Automated Battery that measured spatial working memory and sustained attention, we demonstrated that bipolar patients who are excellent lithium responders have cognitive functions comparable to those of matched control subjects, thereby probably constituting a specific subgroup of bipolar patients in which long-term lithium administration can produce complete normality in this respect. As a decreased BDNF serum level was proposed as a marker of later stage of bipolar mood disorder, it should be noted that the excellent lithium responders in our study, receiving lithium for a mean 15 years,

concomitantly with their normal cognitive functions, also had normal serum BDNF levels (Rybakowski & Suwalska, 2010).

Several mechanisms may be responsible for a favorable effect of lithium on cognitive functions in excellent lithium responders. Probably the most important is a total prevention of affective episodes, which themselves cause a deterioration of cognitive functions. Neuroprotective effect of lithium can obviously play a significant role. A possible mechanism could also be connected with antiviral properties of lithium. Dickerson, Boronow, Stallings, Origoni, Cole, Krivogorsky, & Yolken (2004) demonstrated that infection with herpes simplex virus was associated with cognitive deficits in BPD whereas, in our study, long-term lithium administration was connected with attenuation, or remission, of herpes infection (Rybakowski & Amsterdam, 1991).

Related to the lithium effect on cognitive functions, there is a possibility that this ion exerts a preventive effect against dementia in patients with BD. Nunes, Forlenza, and Gattaz (2007) found in their group of 114 bipolar patients that those receiving long-term lithium therapy had a decreased prevalence of Alzheimer's disease compared with patients not receiving recent lithium therapy. In the Danish epidemiological study of Kessing, Forman, & Andersen (2010), a total of 4,856 patients with a diagnosis of a manic or mixed episode BPD at their first psychiatric contact were investigated over the study period of 1995 to 2005. Among these patients, 50.4% were exposed to lithium, 36.7% to anticonvulsants, 88.1% to antidepressants, and 80.3% to antipsychotics. A total of 216 patients received a diagnosis of dementia during follow-up (103.6/10,000 person-years). Analysis revealed that continued treatment with lithium was associated with a reduced rate of dementia in patients with BPD in contrast to continued treatment with anticonvulsants, antidepressants, or antipsychotics.

Neuroprotective effects

Lithium is the main mood-stabilizing drug for which the evidence for neurotrophic and neuroprotective effects has increasingly accumulated over the past two decades. The neurotrophic and neuroprotective effects of this ion are now regarded as important therapeutics mechanisms in mood disorders (Gray & McEwen, 2013). They may be also responsible for the favorable influence of lithium on cognitive functions and for an increase in cerebral grey matter volume in lithium-treated patients with BPD. The evidence for a neuroprotective effect of lithium also makes this ion a possible candidate for use as a therapeutic drug in neurology, especially in neurodegenerative disorders (Rybakowski, 2011).

Several biochemical targets have been involved in the neurotrophic and neuroprotective effect of lithium. They include increased expression of neurotrophins (mainly BDNF), the inhibition of GSK-3, modulation of c-AMP–mediated signal transduction, with a special role of CREB and PI cascade, PKC inhibition, and increased Bcl-2 expression. As a result of such action, lithium increases cell survival by promoting neurogenesis in the adult brain and by inhibiting cell death (apoptosis) cascades. In experimental studies it was demonstrated that lithium activates CREB and increases BDNF expression. In clinical studies lithium treatment results in an increase of blood level of BDNF. We found that the Val66Met *BDNF* gene polymorphism is associated with the degree of prophylactic response to lithium (Rybakowski, 2008b). Since 1996, the evidence has been accumulating using various experimental models showing that lithium inhibits GSK-3 activity and that this enzyme can be regarded as one of the therapeutic targets of lithium. Clinical studies demonstrated that GSK-3 activity is altered in mania and regulated after treatment with mood stabilizers, including lithium (Quiroz et al., 2010).

The effect of lithium on the PI pathway has long been considered one of the main therapeutic mechanisms of this ion in mood disorders and led to a formulation of the inositol-depletion hypothesis of lithium action. Lithium exerts effect on many steps of PI pathways, the most important being inhibition of inositol monophosphatase. In one of the genome-wide association studies in bipolar illness, the strongest association was related to a genetic variation in the diacylglycerol kinase *(DGKH)* gene, which encodes a key protein in the lithium-sensitive phosphatidyl inositol pathway (Baum et al., 2008). An inhibition of the collapse of sensory neuron growth and an increase of growth cone area, the processes dependent on PI pathway have been proposed as a common mechanism of therapeutic action of three mood-stabilizing drugs of the first generation (i.e. lithium, carbamazepine, and valproates; Williams, Cheng, Mudge, & Harwood, 2002). Recently it has been found that lithium inhibits sodium myo-inositol transporter 1; similar action was also attributed to carbamazepine and valproates (Quiroz et al., 2010).

Lithium inhibits the activity of PKC and decreases the levels of phosphorylation of myristoylated alanine-rich C-kinase substrate, a major PKC substrate that has been implicated in signaling and neuroplastic events associated with cytoskeletal architecture. Lithium treatment also results in an increase of Bcl-2 in the brain of experimental animals. Lithium increases the expression of Bcl-2

associated athanogene, which is known to attenuate glucocorticoid receptor nuclear translocation, thus potentiating the antiapoptotic effect. In patients with BPD, polymorphism of the *bcl-2* gene is associated with an abnormality of the PI system (Quiroz et al., 2010).

Neuroimaging evidence for lithium neuroprotective action started with a provocative research letter in 2000 to the *Lancet* submitted by Moore, Bebchuk, Wilds, Chen & Manji (2000), postulating a lithium-induced increase in human brain grey matter. The results of several studies on this issue have been reported mainly over the past five years. The target brain structures that could presumably be influenced by either short-term or long-term lithium treatment were the hippocampus and prefrontal cortex (including the anterior cingulated region). Moore, Shepherd, Eccleston, Macmillan, Goswami, McAllister, & Ferrier (2001) extended their results published nine years earlier as they found that an increase in total grey matter volume in the prefrontal cortex of bipolar depressed subjects after four weeks of lithium administration was significant only in lithium responders. American researchers focusing on prefrontal grey matter showed greater cortical gray matter density in lithium-treated patients with BPD, especially in the right anterior cingulate region. In the second study, they gave lithium in therapeutic doses to healthy individuals for four weeks. By conducting vaxel-based morphometry analysis they showed that lithium caused a significant increase in grey matter in the left and right dorsolateral prefrontal cortices and the left anterior cingulated region (Monkul et al., 2007). Canadian investigators demonstrated a bilateral increase in hippocampal volume after both short-term (up to eight weeks), as well as long-term (two to four years) lithium administration in patients with BPD (Yucel et al., 2008). A similar study was that of Bearden et al. (2008) who, using three-dimensional mapping of hippocampal anatomy, demonstrated that total hippocampal volume in lithium-treated bipolar patients was significantly larger compared to that of both unmedicated bipolar patients and healthy control subjects. The localized difference applied to the right hippocampus in regions corresponding primarily to cornu Ammonis subfields. A recent study by the International Group of Lithium-Treated Patients comparing bipolar patients receiving or not receiving lithium showed that the lithium group had significantly greater hippocampal volume, independent of long-term response (Hajek et al., 2014).

In 2010 the reports of two neuroimaging studies appeared that compared the effects of lithium with those of anticonvulsants and antipsychotics possessing mood-stabilizing properties. In Lyoo, Dager, Kim, Yoon,

Friedman, Dunner, & Renshaw (2010) paper, the course and magnitude of cerebral gray matter volume changes in 22 bipolar patients treated with either lithium or valproate was studied. The authors found that lithium caused an increase in grey matter volume, peaking at Week 10 to 12 and maintained through 16 weeks of treatment and that this increase was associated with a positive clinical response. By contrast, valproate-treated patients did not show grey matter volume changes over time. Germana et al. (2010) performed a cross-sectional structural brain magnetic resonance imaging study of 74 remitted bipolar patients receiving long-term prophylactic treatment with lithium, valproate, carbamazepine, or antipsychotics. They found that volume of grey matter in the subgenual anterior cingulate gyrus on the right and in the postcentral gyrus, the hippocampus/amygdala complex, and the insula on the left was greater in patients on lithium treatment compared to all other treatments.

In summary, there is considerable evidence for lithium causing an increase in cerebral grey matter volume in patients with BPD, which may reflect a neuroprotective effect of lithium at a clinical level. Such an effect has not been demonstrated for any other mood-stabilizing drug.

ANTICONVULSANTS WITH MOOD-STABILIZING PROPERTIES

In this chapter, we review the neurotoxic and neuroprotective effects only of anticonvulsants for which mood-stabilizing properties have been amply demonstrated (i.e., carbamazepine and valproate as the representatives of first-generation mood stabilizers and lamotrigine as the second-generation mood-stabilizer).

NEUROLOGICAL EFFECTS

Neurological effects of anticonvulsants are usually associated with their higher serum level and co-administration of other drugs. They include drowsiness, slurred speech, blurred vision, ataxia, and tremor. Tremor is especially prominent during combination of mood-stabilizing drugs of the first generation (carbamazepine, valproate, lithium). In a recent review of side effects associated with psychotropic medication, based on the analysis of patients from the Systematic Treatment Enhancement Program for Bipolar Disorder and from the Clinical Outcome and Psycho-Education for Bipolar Disorder, Serretti et al. (2013) found that the use of the first-generation mood stabilizers was specifically associated with neurological side

effects, mainly tremor. Symptoms of neurotoxicity were also described when valproate was added to lamotrigine. The management of these side effects include a decrease of anticonvulsant dose or discontinuation of one of the drugs.

A specific neurotoxic effect of valproate is hyperammonemic encephalopathy, due to valproate-induced elevated plasma ammonia. This may occur in people with normal liver function and therapeutic serum levels of valproate. The cases of such complication were also described in bipolar patients, sometimes even after a long period of valproate administration. Hyperammonemic encephalopathy may necessitate withdrawal of valproate, although improvement was also reported with L-carnitine treatment (Amanat et al., 2013).

COGNITIVE EFFECTS

Similar to neurotoxic effects, cognitive effects of anticonvulsants are usually dose-related and more likely to occur if these drugs are taken in combination. Studies on anticonvulsants' effect on neurocognition in patients with BPD are not numerous; most data were obtained from studies conducted on healthy volunteers and patients with epilepsy (Goldberg & Burdick, 2001). Of three anticonvulsants discussed here, monotherapy with lamotrigine appears to have better neurocognitive profile than carbamazepine and valproate. This was confirmed in a study by Gualtieri and Johnson (2006) including 159 patients with BPD ages 18 to 70 years, of whom 16 were treated with carbamazepine, 38 with lamotrigine, 19 with oxcarbazepine, 19 with topiramate, 27 with valproate, and 30 with lithium. Significant group differences were detected in tests of memory, psychomotor speed, processing speed, reaction time, cognitive flexibility, and attention. Rank order analysis showed superiority for lamotrigine (1.8), followed by oxcarbazepine (2.1), lithium (3.3), topiramate (4.3), valproate (4.5), and carbamazepine (5.0).

In healthy subjects and epileptic patients, valproate may exert some subtle negative effect on such cognitive functions as attention and concentration, memory attention, and motor speed. Dosage reductions of valproate by half did not alleviate these deficits, but drug discontinuation led to progressive improvement over one year. Similar effect were found with carbamazepine except for a negative influence on motor speed but prolonged visual stimulus evaluation time. However, data from epilepsy trials suggest that both drugs cause little cognitive impairment when used as monotherapy and their blood levels are maintained within the therapeutic range (Goldberg & Burdick, 2001). In patients with BPD, both drugs caused more cognitive impairment than lithium in one study (Gualtieri & Johnson, 2006), but in one earlier study carbamazepine was not different than lithium (Joffe, MacDonald, & Kutcher, 1988).

Lamotrigine stands out positively from both anticonvulsants mentioned here. An acute administration of lamotrigine in healthy subjects has not been associated with cognitive deficit and may even improve some cognitive functions such as concentration, sustained attention, and verbal fluency. This was also reflected during treatment of patients with BPD where favorable effects of lamotrigine on cognitive functions both in pediatric and adult patients were reported. Lamotrigine improved cognitive functions in bipolar I patients independent of concomitant treatment with valproate, antidepressants, or antipsychotics (Dias, Balanza-Martinez, Soeiro-de-Souza, Moreno, Figueira, Machado-Vieira, & Vieta, 2012).

NEUROPROTECTIVE EFFECTS

The basis for possible neuroprotective effects of carbamazepine and valproate is derived from studies in which these two drugs were used as comparators to lithium. The effect on the PI pathway (inhibition of the collapse of sensory neuron growth and an increase growth cone area) have been proposed as a common mechanism of therapeutic action of lithium, carbamazepine, and valproates (Williams et al., 2002). Recently it has been found that, besides lithium, carbamazepine and valproate inhibit sodium myo-inositol transporter 1. Similar to lithium, valproate inhibits the activity of PKC and exerts a stimulating effect on the BDNF system (Quiroz et al., 2010).

Neuroprotective effects of lamotrigine can be attributed to an increase of activity in the BDNF system and to preventing glutamate-induced neurotoxicity to hippocampus and other brain structures (Dias, Balanza-Martinez, Soeiro-de-Souza, Moreno, Figueira, Machado-Vieira, & Vieta, 2012; Li, He, Zhang, Qi, Li, Zhu, & He, 2011).

ANTIPSYCHOTICS

In recent years there has been an increasing tendency to use atypical antipsychotics in the treatment of BPD. Some of these drugs have already fulfilled the aforementioned criteria for mood-stabilizing drugs (clozapine, olanzapine, quetiapine, aripiprazole, risperidone). In addition, some new atypical antipsychotics have gained recommendation for treatment of some aspects of BPD (i.e., ziprasidone and asenapine for mania, lurasidone for bipolar depression;

Yatham et al., 2013). However, some typical antipsychotics for the treatment of manic states are still used, with haloperidol being the most important in this respect. In Europe, zuclopenthixol decanoate injection is fairly popular in the treatment of acute manic states.

NEUROLOGICAL EFFECTS

Extrapyramidal syndromes are the most frequent neurological complications of antipsychotic drugs. These include Parkinsonism, dystonia, akathisia, and tardive dyskinesia. Parkinsoninsm consists of a triad of bradykinesia, tremor, and rigidity. Acute dystonia denotes the contraction of a voluntary muscle to its maximal degree, which leads to a postural distortion. Akathisia consists of a subjective and objective element; the first includes unease, distress, dysphoria, and inner restlessness. Objectively, repetitive movements of the legs and feet occur with pacing and walking on the spot and inability to sit steadily. Tardive dyskinesia starting after months or years of treatment with antipsychotic drugs typically manifests with involuntary movements of the tongue, lips, mouth, or face (Haddad & Dursun, 2008). A susceptibility to extrapyramidal syndromes may slightly differ between patients with BPD and schizophrenia. For example, the former appear to have a higher risk of developing tardive dyskinesia than the latter (Kane, 1999).

The risk of extrapyramidal symptoms differs between antipsychotic drugs. Such disorders may be significantly less frequent in patients treated with second- than with first-generation antipsychotic drugs (Barnes & McPhillips, 1998). However, second-generation antipsychotic drugs, including those with evidenced mood-stabilizing properties, also show differences in this regard. Among them, risperidone is associated with more use of anti-Parkinson medication than clozapine, olanzapine, and quetiapine (Rummel-Kluge et al., 2012). On the other hand, aripirazole seems to have the highest propensity for developing akathisia (Kane et al., 2010).

Acute dystonia and Parkinsonism can be treated with anticholinergic drugs. The evidence for treating akathisia is strongest for beta-blockers and benzodiazepines. However, the occurrence of all three syndromes is less likely if antipsychotic dosages are kept low. In the case of tardive dyskinesia, when further antipsychotic treatment is necessary, one should consider switching to an antipsychotic with a low propensity to cause the disorder—either quetiapine or clozapine. Other pharmacological interventions have also been suggested (e.g., tetrabenazine, benzodiazepines, vitamin E, or donepezil).

Neuroleptic malignant syndrome (NMS) is the most severe complication of treatment with antipsychotic drugs, although it may rarely appear with other kinds of medications. The incidence of NMS in patients treated with antipsychotic drugs amounts to 0.2%, and it has been reported with all the atypical antipsychotics, including clozapine and quetiapine in monotherapy (Ananth, Parameswaran, Gunatilake, Burgoyne, & Sidhom, 2004). Although specific research has not been performed, it is probable that the frequency of NMS may be similar in neuroleptic-treated bipolar patients and those with schizophrenia (Chen, Guo, Steinbuch, Buckley, & Patel, 2009). The main symptoms of NMS include muscular rigidity, pyrexia, change in consciousness level (from mild confusion to coma), and autonomic disturbances (diaphoresis, tachycardia, hypersalivation, and blood pressure changes; Haddad & Dursun, 2008). If NMS is suspected, all antipsychotic medications should be stopped. Regular physical observations and daily serum creatinine phosphate kinase levels should be monitored. Dopamine agonists (bromocriptine, amantadine) and muscle relaxants (dantrolene, benzodiazepines) are used. In severe cases, ECT may be performed.

Other neurological effects of antipsychotic drugs include seizures; among atypical antipsychotics, the risk is highest with clozapine, amounting to 1%, with doses of clozapine below 300 mg/day and several times higher with higher doses. In such cases, anticonvulsants (e.g., valproate) can be added. In recent years, concern has focused on an increased risk of cerebrovascular events and mortality when atypical antipsychotics are used in elderly populations (Schneider, Dagerman, & Insel, 2006).

COGNITIVE EFFECTS

The majority of data concerning neurocognitive effects of antipsychotic drugs in clinical settings have been obtained from schizophrenic patients. First experiences with second-generation antipsychotic drugs were promising as they found them superior in this respect to first-generation antipsychotics. Although preclinical data suggested that second-generation antipsychotics can potentially reduce cognitive impairments, subsequent large clinical trials indicated only modest, if any, cognitive benefits relative to first-generation antipsychotics in schizophrenic patients (Galderisi et al., 2009; Hill, Bishop, Palumbo, & Sweeney, 2010).

As in schizophrenia, cognitive deficits are an important feature of BPD, although their severity may be lower than in schizophrenia. Cognitive impairments in BPD show a tendency to increase during acute episode of the illness (especially depression), although they are discernible also

in the euthymic state (Bourne et al., 2013). Therefore the question arises regarding how antipsychotic drugs used in the treatment of BPD may influence such deficits. Torrent et al. (2011) found that nonmedicated bipolar patients showed better cognitive performance than those receiving antipsychotic drugs with mood-stabilizing properties such as olanzapine, quetiapine, and risperidone. Among drug-treated patients, those on quetiapine showed less impairment in measures of verbal memory than those on the other drugs. This may correspond to data in adolescent BPD patients receiving quetiapine whereby cognitive function was found similar to that of healthy control subjects. There are also data showing some improvement of cognitive performance by risperidone and olanzapine in BPD patients (Dias, Balanza-Martinez, Soeiro-de-Souza, Moreno, Figueira, Machado-Vieira, & Vieta, 2012). Clozapine has been found superior to haloperidol for improving cognitive performance in patients with schizophrenia (Potkin, Fleming, Jin, & Gulasekaram, 2001); however, such studies with bipolar patients have been not performed. Clearly more studies are needed to find any cognitive benefits from second-generation antipsychotics in BPD.

NEUROPROTECTIVE EFFECTS

Experimental and clinical studies in the past decade have shown that the area of neuroprotection is one that allows differentiation of typical and atypical antipsychotic drugs. The two groups exert opposing effect on these processes (Nandra & Agius, 2012). Haloperidol, the main representative of typical antipsychotic drugs, exerts a negative effect on neuroprotection by promoting apoptosis and lowering BDNF levels. In contrast, favorable effect on BDNF expression in experimental studies and/or increase of BDNF levels in a clinical setting was found for clozapine, olanzapine, quetiapine, aripipazole, and risperidone (Gonzáles-Pinto et al. 2010; Nandra & Agius, 2012; Park, Lee, Kim, Yoon, & Kim, 2006). Furthermore, in experimental studies, olanzapine has been shown, similar to lithium, to upregulate Bcl-2, a CREB (Hammonds & Shim, 2009). These findings may show that atypical antipsychotics can favorably influence some mechanisms connected with neuroprotection.

ANTIDEPRESSANTS

The use of antidepressants in BPD is widespread, although restrictions for such a practice have been voiced in therapeutic guidelines, pointing to a propensity of antidepressants for increased risk of switching into (hypo)manic or mixed episode or producing a rapid cycling course. It has been also suggested that the use of antidepressants should be confined to acute episodes, since there is no evidence of any benefit from their long-term administration in BPD.

NEUROLOGICAL EFFECTS

Main neurological complications of antidepressant drugs include serotonin syndrome, seizures, and extrapyramidal effects. Serotonin toxicity is connected with drugs increasing serotonergic neurotransmission used in high doses, most frequently with co-prescription of two drugs increasing such transmission by different pathways (i.e., selective serotonin reuptake inhibitors [SSRIs], clomipramine, lithium, or monoamine oxidase inhibitor). The main symptoms of serotonin syndrome include altered mental state (agitation, excitement, confusion), neuromuscular hyeractivity (tremor, clonus, myoclonus), and autonomic disturbances (diaphoresis, pyrexia, mydriasis, tachycardia, and tachypnoea; Haddad & Dursun, 2008). If the syndrome is suspected, all serotonergic medications should be stopped. Depending on severity, patients may require respiratory and cardiovascular monitoring, reduction of pyrexia, and prevention of renal failure. Sometimes the treatment should take place in an intensive care unit.

Most antidepressant drugs lower the seizure threshold, and, in this respect, tricyclic antidepressants and bupropion are regarded as more epileptogenic than the SSRIs. This should be taken into account when using antidepressant in patients with a history of seizures. Extrapyramidal symptoms associated with antidepressant are rare phenomenon; most reported cases were connected with duloxetine and SSRIs (Madhusoodanan, Alexeenko, Sanders, & Brenner, 2010).

COGNITIVE EFFECTS

Antidepressant effect on cognition are disease specific and directly influenced by mood symptoms. Depression in both unipolar and bipolar mood disorder is associated with cognitive impairment, although some studies point out greater impairment in bipolar depression (Borkowska & Rybakowski, 2001). Significant correlations between depression severity and numerous domains of cognitive functions were found. Generally, antidepressants do not induce major cognitive side effects; however, tricyclic antidepressants are more likely than SSRIs to cause such effects, mostly because of their anticholinergic activity. In depressed patients receiving antidepressants, cognitive performance improves with amelioration of depressive symptoms; therefore, a specific effect of these drugs on cognition is difficult to delineate. To date, no study has specifically examined the cognitive effects of antidepressants in BPD (Dias et al., 2012).

NEUROPROTECTIVE EFFECTS

Neuroprotective effects of antidepressants have been suggested in the context of possible stimulation of neurogenesis processes in the adult brain exerted by these drugs. Antidepressants are postulated to facilitate neuroprotection by reversing neurotoxic effect of hypercortisolemia and suppressed synthesis of BDNF occurring during depressive episodes. Santarelli et al (2003) hypothesized that stimulation of hippocampal neurogenesis may be essential for a therapeutic effects of antidepressant drugs. However, Tang, Helmeste, and Leonard (2012) indicate that neurogenesis is not specific to depression or to antidepressant drugs' action and that neuroprotective effects of antidepressant drugs are mostly related to increased synaptogenesis.

ELECTROCONVULSIVE THERAPY

The use of ECT in BPD has been mainly applied for treatment-refractory bipolar depression, although some guidelines have proposed it as a second-line indication for treatment-resistant mania (Yatham et al., 2013). Adverse cognitive effects of this procedure, mainly memory impairment, have long been reported. In recent years, a possibility of some neurotrophic effect of ECT has also been suggested.

NEUROLOGICAL EFFECTS

Somatic complication of ECT constitute less than 1% of treated patients, the majority being cardiac complications, mostly arrhythmias (Nuttall et al., 2004). Neurological complications are extremely rare when neurological contra-indications for ECT are taken into account. In the literature, sporadic cases of subdural hematoma after ECT have been reported (Kulkarni & Melkundi, 2012).

COGNITIVE EFFECTS

Cognitive side effects of ECT have long been observed, witih memory impairment the most prominent symptom.

Recently Semkovska and McLoughlin (2010) conducted a meta-analysis of cognitive symptoms after ECT based on 84 studies including nearly 3,000 participants. The authors concluded that cognitive abnormalities associated with ECT are mainly limited to the first three days after completing the procedure. Pretreatment functioning levels are subsequently recovered. After two weeks posttreatment, processing speed, working memory, anterograde memory, and some aspects of executive function improve beyond beaseline levels. Despite this optimistic report, there is still a possibility that, in some individual patients, some memory impairment may persist for a longer period of time (even months). In such cases, additional administration of procognitive drugs (piracetam, memantine) may be helpful.

NEUROPROTECTIVE EFFECTS

In view of the evidence of disturbances in neurotrophic processes and cellular plasticity in BPD and marked therapeutic efficacy of ECT, it is conceivable that this procedure may exert some neurotrophic action. A number of experimental and clinical studies indicate that ECT influences the BDNF system both in the brain and in periphery. However, whether this is directly connected with therapeutic effect is a controversial issue (Taylor, 2008). Another aspect of ECT could be a stimulation of neurogenesis. In one recent experimental study it was found that ECT causes stimulation of neurogenesis not only in the hippocampus but also in the frontal region (Inta et al., 2013). (See Tables 29.1, 29.2, and 29.3)

CONCLUSION

In this chapter the management of various neurological side effects of treatment used in BPD was described, as these effects are drug-specific. No specific management for cognitive impairment due to individual drug is feasible, besides lowering the dose of the drug used. Also, a majority of patients receive a combination of two or more drugs. Therefore, a more global approach is needed, such as cognitive-enhancing techniques ("cognitive remediation"). This refers to an empirically validated intervention that is designed to remediate neurocognitive deficits and improve functioning. In recent years, the trials of cognitive remediation, which had previously started in schizophrenia, have been extended to mood disorders, including BPD (Bowie, Gupta, & Holshausen, 2013). A novel approach described by Spanish researchers (Martínez-Aran, Torrent, Sole, Bonnin, Rosa, Sanchez-Moreno, & Vieta, 2011) called "functional remediation" goes beyond the scope of cognitive enhancement and includes communication, interpersonal relationship, and stress management strategies.

Certainly one of the most important issues connected with BPD today is that of neuroprotection, in terms of the role of its impairment in the pathogenesis of BPD and its augmentation used for treatment of this illness. The research on this topic has greatly accelerated, and it is hoped that it will bring some promising results.

Disclosure statement: During the past three years, Janusz K. Rybakowski has acted as a consultant or a speaker for the following companies: AstraZeneca, Bristol-Myers-Squibb, Eli Lilly, Janssen-Cilag, Lundbeck, Sanofi-Aventis, and Servier

REFERENCES

Aditanjee, Munshi, K., & Thampy, A. (2005). The syndrome of irreversible lithium-effectuated neurotoxicity. *Clinical Neuropharmacology, 28*, 38–49.

Amanat, S., Shahbaz, N., & Hassan, Y. (2013). Valproic acid induced hyperammonaemic encephalopathy. *Journal of Pakistanian Medical Association, 63*, 72–75.

American Psychiatric Association. (2013). *Diagnostic and statistical manual of mental disorder* (5th ed.). Washington, DC: Author.

Amsterdam, J. D., Luo, L., & Shults, J. (2013). Effectiveness and mood conversion rate during long-term fluoxetine monotherapy in rapid and nonrapid cycling bipolar II disorder. *British Journal of Psychiatry, 202*, 301–306.

Ananth, J., Parameswaran, S., Gunatilake, S., Burgoyne, K., & Sidhom, T. (2004). Neuroleptic malignant syndrome and atypical antipsychotic drugs. *Journal of Clinical Psychiatry, 65*, 464–470.

Barnes, T. R., & McPhillips, M. A. (1998). Novel antipsychotics, extrapyramidal side effects and tardive dyskinesia. *International Clinical Psychopharmacology, 13*(Suppl. 3), S49–S57.

Baum, A. E., Akula, N., Habanero, M., Cardona, I., Corona, W., Klemens, B., & Schulze, T. G. (2008). A genome-wide association study implicates diacylglycerol kinase eta (DGKH) and several other genes in the etiology of bipolar disorder. *Molecular Psychiatry, 13*, 197–207.

Bearden, C. E., Thompson, P. M., Dutton, R. A., Frey, B. N., Peluso, M. A., Nicoletti, M., & Dierschke, N. (2008). Three-dimensional mapping of hippocampal anatomy in unmedicated and lithium-treated patients with bipolar disorder. *Neuropsychopharmacology, 33*, 1229–1238.

Borkowska, A., & Rybakowski, J. K. (2001). Neuropsychological frontal lobe tests indicate that bipolar depressed patients are more impaired than unipolar. *Bipolar Disorders, 3*, 88–94.

Bourne, C., Aydemir, O., Balanzá-Martínez, V., Bora, E., Brissos, S., Cavanagh, J. T., & Clark, J. (2013). Neuropsychological testing of cognitive impairment in euthymic bipolar disorder: An individual patient data meta-analysis. *Acta Psychiatrica Scandinavica, 128*, 149–162.

Bowie, C. R., Gupta, M., & Holshausen, K. (2013). Cognitive remediation therapy for mood disorders: Rationale, early evidence, and future directions. *Canadian Journal of Psychiatry, 58*, 19–25.

Chen, Y., Guo, J. J., Steinbuch, M., Buckley, P. F., & Patel, N. C. (2009). Risk of neuroleptic malignant syndrome in patients with bipolar disorder: A retrospective, population-based case-control study. *Indian Journal of Psychiatry and Medicine, 39*, 439–450.

Cipriani, A., Barbui, C., Salanti, G., Rendell, J., Brown, R., Stockton, S., & Purgato, M. (2011). Comparative efficacy and acceptability of antimanic drugs in acute mania: A multiple-treatments meta-analysis. *Lancet, 278*, 1306–1315.

Dias, V. V., Balanzá-Martinez, V., Soeiro-de-Souza, M. G., Moreno, R. A., Figueira, M. L., Machado-Vieira & Vieta, E. (2012). Pharmacological approaches in bipolar disorders and the impact on cognition: A critical overview. *Acta Psychiatrica Scandinavica, 126*, 315–331.

Dickerson, F. B., Boronow, J. J., Stallings, C., Origoni, A. E., Cole, S., Krivogorsky, B., & Yolken, R. H. (2004). Infection with herpes simplex virus type 1 is associated with cognitive deficits in bipolar disorder. *Biological Psychiatry, 55*, 588–593.

Dierckx, B., Heijnen, W. T., van den Broek, W. W., & Birkenhager, T. K. (2012). Efficacy of electroconvulsive therapy in bipolar versus unipolar major depression: A meta-analysis. *Bipolar Disorders, 14*, 146–150.

Fountoulakis, K. N., Vieta, E., Bouras, C., Notaridis, G., Giannakopoulos, P., Kaprinis, G., & Akiskal, H. (2007). A systematic review of existing data on long-term lithium therapy: Neuroprotective or neurotoxic? *International Journal of Neuropsychopharmacology, 11*, 269–287.

Galderisi, S., Davidson, M., Kahn, R. S., Mucci, A., Boter, H., Gheorghe, M. D., & Rybakowski, J. K. (2009). Correlates of cognitive impairment in first episode schizophrenia: The EUFEST study. *Schizophrenia Research, 115*, 104–114.

Gama, C. S., Kunz, M., Magalhaes, P. V. S., & Kapczinski, F. (2013). Staging and neuroprogression in bipolar disorder: A systematic review of the literature. *Revista Brasileira de Psiquiatria, 35*, 070–074.

Germana, C., Kempton, M. J., Sarnicola, A., Christodoulou, T., Haldane, M., Hadjulis, M., & Girardi, P. (2010). The effects of lithium and anticonvulsants on brain structure in bipolar disorder. *Acta Psychiatrica Scandinavica, 122*, 481–487.

Goldberg, J. F., & Burdick, K. E. (2001). Cognitive side effects of anticonvulsants. *Journal of Clinical Psychiatry, 62*(Suppl. 14), 27–33.

González-Pinto, A., Mosquera, F., Palomino, A., Alberich, S., Gutiérrez, A., Haidar, K., & Vega, P. (2010). Increase in brain-derived neurotrophic factor in first episode psychotic patients after treatment with atypical antipsychotics. *International Clinical Psychopharmacology, 25*, 241–245.

Gray, J. D., & McEwen, B. S. (2013). Lithium's role in neural plasticity and its implications for mood disorders. *Acta Psychiatrica Scandinavica, 128*(5), 347–361.

Gualtieri, C. T., & Johnson, L. G. (2006). Comparative neurocognitive effects of 5 psychotropic anticonvulsants and lithium. *Medscape General Medicine, 23*, 46.

Haddad, P. M., & Dursun, M. D. (2008). Neurological complications of psychiatric drugs: clinical features and management. *Human Psychopharmacology, 23*, 15–26.

Hajek, T., Bauer, M., Simhandl, C., Rybakowski, J., O'Donovan, C., Pfennig, A., & König, B. (2014). Neuroprotective effect of lithium on hippocampal volumes in bipolar disorder independent of long-term treatment response. *Psychological Medicine, 44*(3), 507–517.

Hajek, T., Carrey, N., & Alda, M. (2005). Neuroanatomical abnormalities as risk factors for bipolar disorder. *Bipolar Disorders, 7*, 741–752.

Hammonds, M. D., & Shim, S. S. (2009). Effects of 4-week treatment with lithium and olanzapine on levels of brain-derived neurotrophic factor, B-cell CLL/lymphoma 2 and phosphorylated cyclic adenosine monophosphate response element-binding protein in the sub-regions of the hippocampus. *Basic and Clinical Pharmacology and Toxicology, 105*, 113–119.

Hartigan, G. P. (1963). The use of lithiu salts in affective disorders. *British Journal of Psychiatry, 109*, 810–814.

Hill, S. K., Bishop, J. R., Palumbo, D., & Sweeney, J. A. (2010). Effect of second-generation antipsychotics on cognition: Current issues and future challenges. *Expert Review of Neurotherapy, 10*, 43–57.

Inta, D., Lima-Ojeda, J. M., Lau, T., Tang, W., Dormann, C., Sprengel, R., & Schloss, P. (2013). Electroconvulsive therapy induces neurogenesis in frontal rat brain areas. *PLoS One, 8*, e69869.

Joffe, R. T., MacDonald, C., & Kutcher, S. P. (1988). Lack of differential cognitive effects of lithium and carbamazepine in bipolar affective disorder. *Journal of Clinical Psychopharmacology, 8*, 425–428.

Kane, J. M. (1999). Tardive dyskinesia in affective disorders. *Journal of Clinical Psychiatry, 60*(Suppl. 5), 43–47.

Kane, J. M., Barnes, T. R., Correll, C. U., Sachs, G., Buckley, P., Eudicone, J., & McQuade, R. (2010). Evaluation of akathisia in patients with schizophrenia, schizoaffective disorder, or bipolar I disorder: A post hoc analysis of pooled data from short- and long-term aripiprazole trials. *Journal of Psychopharmacology, 24*, 1019–1029.

Kessing, L. V., Forman, J. L., & Andersen, P. K. (2010). Does lithium protect against dementia? *Bipolar Disorders, 12*, 97–94.

Ketter, T., & Calabrese, J. R. (2002). Stabilization of mood from below versus above baseline in bipolar disorder: A new nomenclature. *Journal of Clinical Psychiatry, 63*, 146–151.

Kulkarni, R. R., & Melkundi, S. (2012). Subdural hematoma: an adverse event of electrconvulsive therapy—case report and iterature review. *Case Reports in Psychiatry, 2012*, 585303.

Lambert, P. A., Carraz, G., Borselli, S., & Carbel, S. (1966). Action neuropsychotrope d'un nouvel anti-epileptique: Le depamide. *Annales Médico-Psychologiques, 1*, 707–710.

Lambert, P. A., Borselli, S., Marcou, G., Bouchardy, M., & Cabrol, G. (1971). Action thymoregulatrice a long terme de Depamide dans la psychose maniaco-depressive. *Annales Médico-Psychologiques, 2*, 442–447.

Lenox, R. H., Gould, T. D., & Manji, H. K. (2002). Endophenotypes in bipolar disorder. *American Journal of Medical Genetics, 111*, 391–406.

Li, N., He, X., Zhang, Y., Qi, X., Li, H., Zhu, X., & He, S (2011). Brain-derived neurotrophic factor signaling mediates antidepressant effects of lamotrigine. *International Journal of Neuropsychopharmacology, 14*, 1091–1098.

Lyoo, K., Dager, S. R., Kim, J. E., Yoon, S. J., Friedman, S. D., Dunner, D. L., & Renshaw, P. E. (2010). Lithium-induced grey matter volume increase as a neural correlate of treatment response in bipolar disorder: A longitudinal brain imaging study. *Neuropsychopharmacology, 35*, 1743–1750.

Madhusoodanan, S., Alexeenko, L., Sanders, R., & Brenner, R. (2010). Extrapyramidal symptoms associated with antidepressants: A review of the literature and an analysis of spontaneous reports. *Annals of Clinical Psychiatry, 22*, 148–156.

Martínez-Arán, A., Torrent, C., Solé, B., Bonnín, C. M., Rosa, A. R., Sánchez-Moreno, J., & Vieta (2011). Functional remediation for bipolar disorder. *Clinical Practice and Epidemiology in Mental Health, 7*, 112–116.

McGuffin, P., Rijsdijk, F., Andrew, M., et al. (2003). The heritability of bipolar affective disorder and the genetic relationship to bipolar depression. *Archives of General Psychiatry, 60*, 497–502.

Merinkangas, K. R., & Tohen, M. (2011). Epidemiology of bipolar disorder in adults and children. In M. T. Tsuang, M. T. Tohen, & P. B. Jones PB (Eds.), *Textbook in psychiatric epidemiology* (pp. 329–342). Chichester, UK: John Wiley.

Monkul, E. S., Matsuo, K., Nicoletti, M. A., Dierschke, N., Hatch, J. P., Dalwani, M., & Brambilla, P. (2007). Prefrontal gray matter increases in healthy individuals after lithium treatment: A voxel-based morphometry study. *Neuroscience Letters, 429*, 7–11.

Moore, G. J., Bebchuk, J. M., Wilds, I. B., Chen, G., & Manji, H. K. (2000). Lithium-induced increase in human brain grey matter. *Lancet, 356*, 1241–1242.

Moore, P. B., Shepherd, D. J., Eccleston, D., Macmillan, I. C., Goswami, U., McAllister, V. L., & Ferrier, I. N. (2001). Cerebral white matter lesions in bipolar affective disorder: Relationship to outcome. *The British Journal of Psychiatry, 178*, 172–176.

Nandra, K. S., & Agius, M. (2012). The differences between typical and atypical antipsychotics: The effects on neurogenesis. *Psychiatria Danubina*, 24(Suppl. 1), 95–99.

Nocjar, C., Hammonds, M. D., & Shim, S. S. (2007). Chronic lithium treatment magnifies learning in rats. *Neuroscience, 150*, 774–788.

Nunes, P. V., Forlenza, O. V., & Gattaz, W. F. (2007). Lithium and risk for Alzheimer's disease in elderly patients with bipolar disorder. *The British Journal of Psychiatry, 190*, 359–360.

Nuttall, G. A., Bowersox, M. R., Douglass, S. B., McDonald, J., Rasmussen, L. J., Decker, P. A., & Oliver, W. C. Jr. (2004). Morbidity and mortality in the use of electroconvulsive therapy. *The Journal of ECT, 20*, 237–241.

Okuma, T., Kishimoto, A., & Inue, K. (1973). Anti-manic and prophylactic effect of carbamazepine (Tegretol) on manic depressive psychosis. *Folia Psychiatrica et Neurologica Japonica, 27*, 283–297.

Pacchiarotti, I., Bond, D. J., Baldessarini, R. J., Nolen, W. A., Grunze, H., Licht, R. W., & Post, R. M. (2013). The International Society for Bipolar Disorders (ISBD) Task Force report on antidepressant use in bipolar disorders. *The American Journal of Psychiatry 170*(11), 1249–1262.

Park, S. W., Lee, S. K., Kim, J. M., Yoon, J. S., & Kim, Y. H. (2006). Effects of quetiapine on the brain-derived neurotrophic factor expression in the hippocampus and neocortex of rats. *Neuroscience Letters, 402*, 25–29.

Pogarell, O., Folkerts, M., & Hegerl, U. (2006). Adverse neurological and neurotoxic effects of lithium therapy. In M. Bauer, P. Grof, & B. Müller-Oerlinghausen (Eds.), *Lithium in neuropsychiatry: The comprehensive guide* (pp. 271–282). London: Informa.

Potkin, S. G., Fleming, K., Jin, Y., & Gulasekaram, B. (2001). Clozapine enhances neurocognition and clinical symptomatology more than standard neuroleptics. *Journal of Clinical Psychopharmacology, 21*, 479–483.

Quiroz, J. A., Yatham, L. N., Palumbo, J. M., Karcher, K., Kushner, S., & Kusumakar, V. (2010). Risperidone long-acting injectable monotherapy in the maintenance treatment of bipolar I disorder. *Biological Psychiatry, 68*, 156–162.

Quiroz, J. A., Machado-Vieira, R., Zarate, C. A. Jr., & Manji, H. K. (2010). Novel insights into lithium's mechanism of action: neurotrophic and neuroprotective effects. *Neuropsychobiology, 62*, 50–60.

Rajkowska, G., Halaris, A., & Selemon, L. D. (2001). Reductions in neuronal and glial density characterize the dorsolateral prefrontal cortex in bipolar disorder. *Biological Psychiatry, 49*, 741–752.

Rihmer, Z., & Kiss, K (2002). Bipolar disorders and suicidal behavior. *Bipolar Disorders, 4*(Suppl. 1), 21–25.

Rummel-Kluge, C., Komossa, K., Schwarz, S., Hunger, H., Schmid, F., Kissling, W., & Davis, J. M. (2012). Second-generation antipsychotic drugs and extrapyramidal side effects: A systematic review and meta-analysis of head-to-head comparisons. *Schizophrenia Bulletin, 38*, 167–177.

Rybakowski, J. K. (2007). Two generations of mood stabilizers. *International Journal of Neuropsychopharmacology, 10*, 709–711.

Rybakowski, J. K. (2008a). Aripiprazole joins the family of second-generation mood stabilizers. *Journal of Clinical Psychiatry, 69*, 862–863.

Rybakowski, J. K. (2008b). BDNF gene: Functional Val66Met polymorphism in mood disorders and schizophrenia. *Pharmacogenomics, 9*, 1589–1593.

Rybakowski, J. K. (2011). Lithium in neuropsychiatry: A 2010 update. *World Journal of Biological Psychiatry, 12*, 340–348.

Rybakowski, J. K., & Amsterdam, J. D. (1991). Lithium prophylaxis and recurrent labial herpes infections. *Lithium, 2*, 43–47.

Rybakowski, J. K., Permoda-Osip, A., & Borkowska, A. (2009). Response to prophylactic lithium in bipolar disorder may be associated with a preservation of executive cognitive functions. *European Neuropsychopharmacology, 19*, 791–795.

Rybakowski, J. K., & Suwalska, A. (2010). Excellent lithium responders have normal cognitive functions and plasma BDNF levels. *International Journal of Neuropsychopharmacology, 13*, 617–622.

Santarelli, L., Saxe, M., Gross, C., Surget, A., Battaglia, F., Dulawa, S., Weisstaub, N. et al (2003). Requirement of hippocampal neurogenesis for the behavioral effects of antidepressants. *Science, 301*, 805–809.

Schneider, L. S., Dagerman, K., & Insel, P. S. (2006). Efficacy and adverse effects of atypical antipsychotics for dementia: Meta-analysis of randomized, placebo-controlled trials. *American Journal of Geriatric Psychiatry, 14*, 191–210.

Semkovska, M., & McLoughlin, D. M. (2010). Objective cognitive performance associated with electroconvulsive therapy for depression: A systematic review and meta-analysis. *Biological Psychiatry, 68*, 568–577.

Serretti, A., Chiesa, A., Calati, R., Fabbri, C., Sentissi, O., De Ronchi, D., Mendlewicz, J. et al (2013). Side effects associated with psychotropic medications in patients with bipolar disorder: Evidence from two independent samples. *Journal of Psychopharmacology, 27*, 616–628.

Soeiro-de-Souza, M. G., Dias, V. V., Figueira, M. L., Forlenza, O. V., Gattaz, W. F., Zarate C. A. Jr., & Machado-Vieira, R. (2012). Translating neurotrophic and cellular plasticity: From pathophysiology to improved therapeutics for bipolar disorder. *Acta Psychiatrica Scandinavica, 126*, 332–341.

Takezaki, H., & Hanaoka, M. (1971). The use of carbamazepine in the control of manic-depressive psychosis and other manic-depressive states. *Clinical Psychiatry, 13*, 173–183.

Tang, S. W., Helmeste, D., & Leonard, B. (2012). Is neurogenesis relevant in depression and in the mechanism of antidepressant drug action? A critical review. *World Journal of Biological Psychiatry, 13*, 402–412.

Taylor, S. M. (2008). Electroconvulsive therapy, brain-derived neurotrophic factor, and possible neurorestorative benefit of the clinical application of electroconvulsive therapy. *The Journal of ECT, 24*, 160–165.

Torrent, C., Martinez-Arán, A., Daban, C., Amann, B., Balanzá-Martínez, V., del Mar Bonnín, C., & Cruz, N. (2011). Effects of atypical antipsychotics on neurocognition in euthymic bipolar patients. *Comprehensive Psychiatry, 52*, 613–622.

Williams, R. S., Cheng, L., Mudge, A. W., & Harwood, A. J. (2002). A common mechanism of action for three mood-stabilizing drugs. *Nature, 417*, 292–295.

Yatham, L. N., Kennedy, S. H., Parikh, S. V., Schaffer, A., Beaulieu, S., Alda, M., O'Donovan, C. et al (2013). Canadian Network for Mood and Anxiety Treatments (CANMAT) and International Society for Bipolar Disorders (ISBD) collaborative update of CANMAT guidelines for the management of patients with bipolar disorder: update 2013. *Bipolar Disorders, 15*, 1–44.

Yazlovitskaya, E. M., Edwards, E., Thotala, D., Fu, A., Osusky, K. L., Whetsell, W. O., Boone, B. et al. 2006. Lithium treatment prevents neurocognitive deficit resulting from cranial irradiation. *Cancer Research, 66*, 11179–11186.

Yildiz, A., Nikodem, M., Vieta, E., Correll, C. U., & Baldessarini, R. J. (in press). A network meta-analysis on comparative efficacy and acceptability of antimanic treatments in acute bipolar mania. *Psychological Medicine*.

Yucel, K., Taylor, V. H., McKinnon, M. C., Macdonald, K., Alda, M., & Young, L. T. (2008). Bilateral hippocampal volume increase in patients with bipolar disorder and short-term lithium treatment. *Neuropsychopharmacology, 13*, 361–367.

Zarate, C. A, Jr, Tohen, M., Banov, M. D., Weiss, M. K., & Cole J. O. (1995). Is clozapine a mood stabilizer? *Journal of Clinical Psychiatry, 56*, 108–112.

30.

TREATMENT-INDUCED MOOD INSTABILITY

TREATMENT-EMERGENT AFFECTIVE SWITCHES
AND CYCLE ACCELERATION

Renrong Wu, Keming Gao, Joseph R. Calabrese, and Heinz Grunze

INTRODUCTION

The circular nature of bipolar disorder (BPD) has been described since the 1850s (Angst & Sellaro, 2000). Circular madness, *folie circulaire*, was defined as manic and melancholic episodes separated by symptom-free intervals. The term *folie á double forme* was used to describe cyclic (manic-melancholic) episodes without symptom-free intervals. In categorical but comprehensive *Diagnostic and Statistical Manual of Mental Disorders* (fifth edition) and *International Classification of Disease* (10th edition) terms, BPD is characterized just by episodic manic/hypomanic symptoms; thus, mania/hypomania is considered as the hallmark of BPD, not the cyclicity of mood swings, as the traditional term *manic-depressive* illness still comprises. In the context of this chapter, readers should always be aware that an episode can not only be triggered by psychological and pharmacologic factors but also occur spontaneously as a genuine part of the disorder (Angst & Sellaro, 2000; Perlis et al., 2010). Both kinds of episodes are difficult to predict when they will occur. To separate spontaneous from triggered mood changes is even more difficult.

Treatment-emergent mania/hypomania (TEM) following major depressive episodes (MDE) in BPD was observed from the very beginning of the introduction of somatic treatments including antidepressants (Wehr & Goodwin, 1987). However, the controversy on the causal relationship between antidepressant use and TEM and cycle acceleration has never been settled. Some early observational studies and placebo-controlled studies supported that antidepressants could precipitate mania in patients with BPD and induce mania in patients with major depressive disorder (MDD; Koukopoulos et al., 1980; Peet, 1994; Wehr & Goodwin,

1987). However, retrospective data of hospitalized patients between 1920 and 1981 from a Zurich sample did not support the emergence of a substantial drug-induced manic switch rate after antidepressants were introduced (Angst & Sellaro, 2000).

The inconsistency of previous studies on TEM could be at least in part due to the heterogeneity of BPD. There is convincing evidence supporting that BPD constitutes a very heterogeneous group (Angst et al., 2004; Gao et al., 2013; Merikangas et al., 2007). Overall, current available data suggest that a small number of patients are vulnerable for TEM, but reliable predictors for such a group are still lacking. Until very large double-blind, placebo-controlled, longitudinal studies include diverse groups of patients with BPD, a causal relationship between treatment, a manic/hypomanic switch, and patient characteristics will be difficult to establish. Accordingly, clinicians will continue to face the lack of a predictive reliability in knowing who will have TEM. Therefore, it is important that clinicians remain aware of reported causes for TEM in order to prevent or minimize the effect of affective switches. The aim of this chapter is to systematically review potential mechanisms, pharmacological and nonpharmacological treatments, and risk factors of affective mood switches.

RELEVANT BIOLOGY OF MOOD SWITCHING

The monoamine, cholinergic, glutamatergic, melatonergic, endogenous opioid and cannabinoid systems, as well as the hypothalamus-pituitary-adrenal (HPA) gland axis and hypothalamus-pituitary-thyroid (HPT) gland axis are involved in the regulation of mood. Any change caused by any pharmacological or nonpharmacological factor in these systems can potentially induce affective switches.

MONOAMINE SYSTEM

Norepinephrine

As early as in 1965, norepinephrine was believed to be a main culprit in both depression and mania; that is, depression resulted from a relatively low level of norepinephrine, and mania resulted from a relatively higher level of norepinephrine (Salvadore et al., 2010; Schildkraut, 1965). Increased norepinephrine activity was observed in manic episodes, but higher levels of urinary dopamine, not urinary norepinephrine, accompanied manic episodes in patients with rapid cycling BPD. Recent data support synergistic effects between norepinephrine and dopamine in prefrontal cortical networks. The right ventral prefrontal cortex in humans is a key structure for behavioral inhibition (Arnsten, 2007). Suppression of the ventral and orbital prefrontal cortex function is believed to be the cause of some manic symptoms during a manic episode. An increase in the release of norepinephrine and dopamine in the prefrontal cortex caused by uncontrollable stress has been speculated to trigger intracellular cascades reducing the prefrontal cortex function leading to subsequent manic symptoms (Arnsten, 2007).

Dopamine

Higher levels of norepinephrine and dopamine metabolites in the cerebral spinal fluid (CSF) have been associated with mania and lower levels have been associated with depression (Gerner et al., 1984; Roy et al., 1985; Swann et al., 1983). An increase in norepinephrine and dopamine during mania is indirectly supported by the efficacy of treatment with lithium, antipsychotics, and other antimanic agents, which can extracellularly and/or intracellularly block the signal transmission of these two neurotransmitters. Increased dopamine transmission in mania leads to secondary downregulation of dopamine receptor sensitivity and decreased dopaminergic transmission, which might correspond to the depressive phase of BPD (Berk et al., 2007).

Serotonin

Although the involvement of serotonin in MDD is well established, its role in BPD remains to be determined. Some early studies found that decreased central serotonergic function might be involved in both depression and mania, but other studies support the hypothesis that a serotonin deficit is mainly involved in mania, and the enhancement of serotonin neurotransmission exerts a mood-stabilizing effect (Shiah & Yatham, 2000). However, this is inconsistent with the observation that rapid tryptophan depletion reduces manic symptoms, suggesting that an increased serotonin activity might also be involved in mania (Applebaum, Bersudsky, & Klein, 2007). In summary, the role of serotonin in BPD remains ambiguous.

CHOLINERGIC SYSTEM

The role of the cholinergic system in BPD was hypothesized as an imbalance between the cholinergic and adrenergic systems; that is, depression would be a clinical presentation of a state of cholinergic dominance, whereas mania would correspond to the dominance of the adrenergic system. An early study showed that physostigmine, a reversible cholinesterase inhibitor, produced a state of psychomotor retardation and increased the severity of depression in a variety of psychiatric patients with depressive symptoms; however, donepezil, an acetylcholine esterase inhibitor, adjunctive to mood stabilizer was not effective in reducing manic symptoms (Chen, Fang, Kemp, Calabrese, & Gao, 2010). Both muscarinic and nicotinic acetylcholine receptors seem to be involved in the acetylcholine "depressogenic" action, but the results for anticholinergic agents as treatment of depression have been inconsistent. Best positive evidence exists for the anticholinergic drug scopolamine (4 mcg/kg), which, intravenously infused in patients with MDD or BPD, significantly reduced depressive symptoms within three days with a large effect size (see Chapter 22).

GABAERGIC/GLUTAMATERGIC SYSTEM

A role of γ-aminobutyric acid (GABA) dysfunction in mood disorders was proposed more than three decades ago and reviewed more recently (Brambilla, Perez, Barale, Schettini, & Soares, 2003). Some early studies showed that the concentration of GABA in CSF and/or blood serum was lower in patients with bipolar depression or mania than healthy controls. Increased glutamatergic activity in the anterior cingulated cortex and the parieto-occipital cortex was observed in patients with mania. A number of studies have shown that chronic treatment with lithium or valproate can increase the blood level of GABA and decrease the level of glutamate, suggesting that the balance of these two systems may play a role in mood regulation. Evidence supporting GABA and glutamate dysfunction in BPD also stems from treatment trials. Clonazepam was efficient and safe in the treatment of acute mania (Curtin

& Schulz, 2004). Intravenous infusion of ketamine, a non-competitive N-methyl-D-aspartate antagonist, produced a rapid decrease in depressive symptoms in patients with treatment-resistant bipolar depression (see Chapter 22). More recently, ketamine-induced mania in a nonbipolar patient has been reported (Ricke, Snook, & Anand, 2011).

NEUROENDOCRINE SYSTEMS

HPA axis

Dysfunction of the HPA axis in BPD has been observed, but the exact role of corticosteroids in each phase of BPD remains unclear (Chen et al., 2010).). Enduring dysfunction of the HPA axis in euthymic bipolar patients has also been reported (Watson, Gallagher, Ritchie, Ferrier, & Young, 2004). In a longitudinal study of 15 patients with BPD, the mean basal and postdexamethasone cortisol levels were increased during the phase of depression, but not during mania or euthymia (Maj, Ariano, Arena, & Kemali, 1984). In contrast, patients with mixed or pure mania were reported to have elevated levels of cortisol in CSF and urine compared to healthy controls, but no difference was observed when compared to patients in depression (Swann et al., 1992). The corticosteroid receptor antagonist mifepristone (RU-486) was superior to placebo in reducing depressive symptoms in BPD (Young et al., 2004). Moreover, two variants of the polymorphism of glucocorticoid receptor gene were reported to be associated with mania and hypomania (Spijker et al., 2009), suggesting the HPA axis has the potential of being involved in TEM.

HPT axis

It is known that low thyroid function is related to the depressive phase of BPD and that thyroid hormone has antidepressant effects in women with bipolar depression (Bauer et al., 2005; see Chapter 22). However, the results of a thyrotropin-releasing hormone (TRH) challenge test measuring the corresponding release of thyroid-stimulating hormone (TSH) were inconsistent in patients with BPD. A decreased response to TRH was reported during both manic and depressive phases. Clearly, the relationship of the HPT axis and thyroid hormones to different phases of BPD also needs further clarification. Interestingly, patients admitted due to bipolar depression and with lower levels of basal TSH had a significantly higher rate of switching to mania compared to those with higher levels of basal TSH (Bottlender, Rudolf, Strauss, & Möller, 2000).

MELATONERGIC SYSTEM

The cyclic nature of BPD, diurnal variations in its symptomatology, and a frequently disturbed sleep–wake cycle suggest that a dysfunction involving *zeitgebers* may be involved in the pathophysiology in BPD (Chen et al., 2010). Studies have shown that not only the levels but also the timing of melatonin secretion is altered in patients with BPD. Low nocturnal output of melatonin was found in MDD and BPD and was normalized after treatment with antidepressants. Bright light therapy, a melatonin suppressor and circadian phase shifter, is used for the treatment of depression with seasonal pattern, but no firm data for bipolar depression have been reported so far.

PURINERGIC SYSTEM

Purines (adenosine triphosphate and adenosine) are essential for energy metabolism and neurotransmission. Allopurinol, a purine analog, showed antimanic efficacy in patients with BPD. Adenosine is a widespread neuromodulator in the central nervous system. The antimanic action of carbamazepine may be, in part, related to its agonistic effect on adenosine receptors (Biber, Fiebich, Gebicke-Härter, & van Calker, 1999). Caffeine is an adenosine antagonist. Caffeine-induced mania and affective relapse have been reported. These data suggest that using adenosine antagonists in patients with BPD may cause TEM (Zarate & Manji, 2008).

ENDOGENOUS OPIOID SYSTEM

The endogenous opioid system is involved in the mediation, modulation, and regulation of stress responses. The widespread distribution of enkephalin and endorphins throughout the limbic system is consistent with a direct role in the modulation of mood and stress responses. Blockade of kappa opiate receptors have been shown to result in antidepressant-like properties in animals. A nonselective kappa agonist (pentazocine) showed antimanic effect in humans (Zarate & Manji, 2008). In line with this, naltrexone, an opioid receptor antagonist, produced manic-like symptoms in a patient with BPD (Losekam, Kluge, Nittel, Kircher, & Konrad, 2013).

ARACHIDONIC ACID SYSTEM

Arachidonic acid is a polyunsaturated fatty acid and is involved in second messenger systems and the inflammatory process that is believed to be a part of the pathophysiology of mood disorders. Chronic treatment with lithium and valproate in rats could selectively reduce the turnover rate of the arachidonic acid system in the brain, which is believed to be hyperactive in mania. Administration of nonselective cyclooxygenase inhibitors, indomethacin and piroxicam, could prevent amphetamine-stimulated locomotors activity and blocked cocaine sensitization in animals. Adjunctive cyclooxygenase 2 inhibitor, celecoxib (400 mg/day), to a mood stabilizer in bipolar I or II depression was superior to placebo for transient reduction in depressive symptoms (Zarate & Manji, 2008). TEM with nonsteroid, anti-inflammatory drugs have been reported (Austin & Tan, 2012; Bishop, Bisset, & Benson, 1987).

ENDOGENOUS CANNABINOID SYSTEM

Changes in the endogenous cannabinoid system in patients with neurological and psychiatric illnesses have been reported. Patients with BPD who carry cannabinoid 1 receptor gene (CNR1) variants may be more susceptible to BPD (Monteleone et al., 2010). A growing body of evidence supports that the endocannabinoid system plays a very importance role in mood disorders (Micale, Di Marzo, Sulcova, Wotjak, & Drago, 2013).

PHARMACOLOGICAL TREATMENT-EMERGENT MANIA/HYPOMANIA

Many pharmacological and nonpharmacological treatments have been reported to induce TEM in patients with or without BPD (see Table 30.1). With the exception of antidepressants and stimulants, TEM following other psychotropic medication is based on case reports. Even with antidepressants and stimulants, data are usually post hoc and ambiguous. So far there has been no study specifically designed to examine the risk for TEM in BPD.

ANTIDEPRESSANTS

Antidepressant monotherapy or adjunctive therapy with randomized, placebo-controlled trial designs

There is only a limited number of studies of antidepressant monotherapy or adjunctive therapy in the acute treatment of bipolar I and II depression (Chen et al., 2010; see Chapter 22). Overall, there were no significant differences in switching rates between active treatment arms and placebo. However, it is impossible to compare the switch rates in different studies because diverse study designs, inclusion and exclusion criteria, study duration, and definition of manic/hypomanic switching were used. For example, in a

long-term study of fluoxetine ($n = 28$), lithium ($n = 26$), and placebo ($n = 27$) in bipolar II depression (Amsterdam & Shults, 2010), the rates of switching differed based on definitions applied. If using *Dignostic and Statistical Manual of Mental Disorders* (fourth edition) criteria for a hypomanic episode, 10 patients (3 on fluoxetine, 2 on lithium, and 5 on placebo) switched to a hypomanic episode. If using subsyndromal hypomania criteria defined as an episode lasting ≤ 3 days with ≥ 4 symptoms or lasting ≥ 4 days with ≤ 3 symptoms, 21 patients (10 on fluoxetine, 7 on lithium, and 4 on placebo) had TEM. If using a Young Mania Rating Scale (YMRS) score ≥ 8 to define hypomania, rates of a switch were 21.4% in the fluoxetine group, 7.7% in the lithium group, and 11.1% in the placebo group, respectively. If using a YMRS score ≥ 12 to define a hypomanic switch, the rates of a switch were 10.7% in the fluoxetine group, 7.7% in the lithium group, and 7.2% in the placebo group, respectively. This illustrates the virtual impossibility to establish uniform switch rates and compare them across studies.

Antidepressant monotherapy or adjunctive therapy with randomized, open or double-blind, non-placebo-controlled trials

The majority of non-placebo-controlled studies are small (Chen et al., 2010). In the largest randomized study comparing bupropion, sertraline, and venlafaxine (Post et al., 2006), patients treated with venlafaxine had a significantly higher rate of TEM, especially those with rapid cycling. Duration of treatment appeared to affect the rate of TEM. During a 10-week acute phase of bupropion, sertraline, or venlafaxine treatment, switch rates were similar in the three treatment arms. However, during a one-year continuation phase, venlafaxine-treated patients had the significantly highest rate of switches among the three groups, with venlafaxine 48%, sertraline 31%, and bupropion 29% (Leverich et al., 2006). In another study, venlafaxine adjunctive to a mood stabilizer(s) also had a significantly higher rate of TEM compared to those with paroxetine plus a mood stabilizer(s) (Vieta et al., 2002).

Nonrandomized prospective or retrospective studies

Data from nonrandomized prospective or retrospective studies on the risk of TEM are inconsistent (Goldberg & Truman, 2003). In an overview of TEM in BPD, Goldberg and Truman concluded that about one-quarter to one-third of bipolar patients may be inherently susceptible to antidepressant-induced manias. Even in patients with rapid

Table 30.1. PHARMACOLOGICAL AND NONPHAR-
MACOLOGICAL FACTORS REPORTED WITH
INCREASED RISK FOR TREATMENT-EMERGENT
MANIA/HYPOMANIA IN PATIENTS WITH OR
WITHOUT BIPOLAR DISORDER

PHARMACOLOGICAL FACTORS	EVIDENCE
Antidepressants	
Tricyclics	Randomized, double-blind, placebo-controlled trials
Selective serotonin reuptake inhibitors	Randomized, double-blind, placebo-controlled trials
Bupropion	Randomized, open-label trial, and case reports
Serotonin norepinephrine reuptake inhibitors	Randomized, open-label trial, and case reports
Monoamine oxidase inhibitors	Randomized, open-label trial, and case reports
Mirtazepine	Case reports
Nefazodone	Case reports, open-label study
Stimulants and ADHD-related medication	
Amphetamine	Case reports
Methylphenidate	Case reports
Atomoxetine	Case series and case reports
Wake promoting agents	
Modafinil	Case reports
Armodaninil	Case reports
Cholinergic related agents	
Anticholinergics	Case series
Varenicline	Case reports
Acetylcholine esterase inhibitors	Case reports
Glutamate related agents	
Ketamine	Case report
Non-steroid anti-inflammatory drugs	Case reports
Opioid receptor antagonist Naltrexone	Case report
Hormones	
Steroids	Case reports
Thyroid hormone or analogs	Case reports
Male sex hormone	Case reports
Nonpharmacological factors	
Electroconvulsive therapy	Case reports
Vagal nerve stimulation	Case reports
Repetitive transcranial magnetic stimulation	Case reports
Sleep deprivation	Case reports
Light therapy	Case series

NOTE: ADHD, attention deficit hyperactivity disorder

cycling BPD who were treated with antidepressant monotherapy, only about 49.3% patients reported having at least one
TEM, and 29.1% of treatment trials were associated with TEM
(Gao et al., 2008). More important, some patients appeared to
be more vulnerable to developing TEM than others, such as
having TEM on every antidepressant trial, whereas some never
had TEM with multiple antidepressant trials.

Possible causes for inconsistent findings

The inconsistent findings could be due to, but not limited to, the following factors. First, study designs differ
(monotherapy vs. adjunctive therapy and double-blind vs.
open-label), as do study duration, definition of switching, and dosing of antidepressants. Second, the inclusion
and exclusion criteria differ. Patients with BPD are a very
heterogeneous group. Almost all industry-sponsored randomized controlled studies excluded patients with current
substance use disorder (SUD). Large pivotal studies also
excluded patients with rapid cycling BPD, especially those
with more than eight episodes in a 12-month period. Third,
baseline manic severity appears to be a risk factor for TEM,
but again, most studies excluded patients with high baseline
manic symptoms in bipolar depression studies. It is reasonable to believe that there is a group of patients with a higher
risk for TEM who were included in naturalistic studies
but not in "enriched" studies. Fourth, antidepressants are
a diverse group, and some antidepressants appeared more
likely to cause switch than others. Until all these factors are
more closely examined and standardized in future trials, the
debate on antidepressant TEM will continue. Meanwhile,
the use of antidepressant for BPD will be inevitable due to
the shortage of approved alternatives for bipolar depression
(Möller & Grunze, 2000; Pacchiarotti et al., 2013).

Risk factors for antidepressant-induced mania/hypomania

There is no good evidence supporting the use of antidepressant monotherapy in bipolar depression, although a small
group of patients may benefit from the combination of
an antidepressant and a mood stabilizer (see Chapter 22).
Antidepressant monotherapy increases the risk for manic
switching compared to a combination therapy with a mood
stabilizer(s) (Pacchiarotti et al., 2011). Clinicians should
avoid antidepressant monotherapy and take some risk factors into consideration when using antidepressant for bipolar depression (see Table 30.2; Pacchiarotti et al., 2013).

Although some studies suggested that patients
with bipolar II disorder were more susceptible for

antidepressant TEM, a meta-analysis found that patients with bipolar I disorder had higher rates of TEM than those with bipolar II disorder in both acute and maintenance trials: 14.3% versus 7.1% and 23.4% versus 13.9%, respectively (Bond, Noronha, Kauer-Sant'Anna, Lam, & Yatham, 2008). The relative risk of TEM in bipolar I versus bipolar II was 1.78 (95% confidence interval [CI]: 1.24–2.58). Tricyclic antidepressants have been consistently reported to have a higher risk for mood switching compared to second-generation antidepressants (Goldberg & Truman, 2003). Among the second-generation antidepressants, venlafaxine was reported to have a higher risk for manic switching than other antidepressants (Chen et al., 2010). In a report from the Systematic Treatment Enhancement Program for Bipolar Disorder (STEP-BD), a history of SUD and previous antidepressant TEM, the number of previous depressive episodes, lifetime and recent rapid cycling, and previous suicide attempt were associated with a greater transition rate from depression to mania (Perlis et al., 2010). A lower rate of response to antidepressant treatment and an earlier age of onset bipolar illness are also significant risk factors for TEM (Valentí et al., 2012).

In bipolar depressed patients, the number of manic symptoms (mixed depression) at admission such as flight of idea, racing thoughts, aggression, increased drive, and irritability was associated with an increased risk for manic switching (Bottlender et al., 2004). Higher baseline YMRS total scores and some item scores of the YMRS were also associated with an increased risk for TEM (Frye et al., 2009; see Table 30.2). These findings were consistent with the results of a STEP-BD study, in which residual manic symptoms at recovery or proportion of days with elevated mood in the preceding year were significantly associated with a shorter time to the recurrence of manic, hypomanic, or mixed episodes (Perlis et al., 2006). A more recent analysis of the STEP-BD data showed that greater manic symptom severity at baseline was associated with an increased risk for manic transition among both antidepressant-treated and antidepressant-untreated patients (Perlis et al., 2010). Similarly, a post hoc analysis of the study of olanzapine monotherapy, the combination of olanzapine and fluoxetine, and placebo in the acute treatment of bipolar I depression found that patients with an elevated baseline YMRS score of ≥ 12 were at a greater risk (4.5 times) for developing TEM compared to those with a baseline YMRS < 12, independent of treatments.

Besides those clinically observable risk factors, first results are now available pointing toward a genetic risk for TEM. A meta-analysis of all six published

Table 30.2. SUMMARY OF RISK FACTORS ASSOCIATED WITH ANTIDEPRESSANT TREATMENT-EMERGENT MANIA/HYPOMANIA IN BIPOLAR DISORDER

VARIABLE	RISK
Disorder subtypes	
Bipolar I versus Bipolar II	Bipolar I > Bipolar II
Bipolar disorder versus MDD	Bipolar > MDD
Rapid cycling versus nonrapid cycling	RC > non-RC
Antidepressants	
Tricyclics versus SSRIs	Tricyclics > SSRIs
Bupropion versus SSRIs	Bupropion ≈ SSRIs
SNRIs versus SSRIs	SNRIs > SSRIs
Tricyclics versus MAOIs	Tricyclics > MAOIs
Baseline manic severity	
Young Mania Rating Scale	Higher > lower
Manic item of increased motor activity	Higher > lower
Manic item of increased speech	Higher > lower
Manic item of increased distractibility	Higher > lower
Manic item of racing thoughts	Higher > lower
Residual manic symptoms	More > less
Historical variables	
History of current substance use disorder	Present > absent
History of lifetime substance use disorder	Present > absent
History of substance-induced manic switch	Present > absent
History of lifetime rapid cycling	Present > absent
History of current rapid cycling	Present > absent
History of previous suicide attempt	Present > absent
Number for previous depressive episodes	More > less
Age of onset	Early > late
Response to antidepressant treatment	Non-response > response
Pharmacogenetics	
5HTTLPR polymorphism	"S" allele carriers > "L/L" allele carriers

NOTE: 5HTTLPR = serotonin transporter-linked polymorphic region; MAOIs = monoamine oxidase inhibitors; MDD = major depressive disorder; SNRIs = serotonin norepinephrine reuptake inhibitors; SSRIs = selective serotonin reuptake inhibitors; RC = rapid cycling, "S" =, short; "L" = long.

studies including one in a pediatric population found that the 5HTTLPR polymorphism appeared to have a moderate effect size (35% increased risk) for an association between S-allele carriers and TEM in BPD (Daray, Thommi, & Ghaemi, 2010). However, another meta-analysis, in which the pediatric study was not included, concluded that there were insufficient data to confirm an association between the 5HTTLPR polymorphism and TEM (Biernacka et al., 2012). Other potential genetic markers including variants within the brain-derived neurotrophic factor gene, 5-HT2A receptor gene, polymorphism in the multi-drug-resistant 1 P-glycoprotein gene, polymorphisms of tryptophan hydroxylase, G-protein beta 3 unit, monoamine oxidase A, catechol-O-methyltransferase, serotonin receptor 2A, dopamine receptor D2, and dopamine receptor have also been studied, but none of these genetic markers was significantly associated with TEM.

STIMULANTS AND DOPAMINE-RELATED AGENTS

Stimulants

Stimulants and other dopamine-related agents may be used for treatment-resistant depression, for residual symptoms of depression such as lack of energy or motivation, to counteract side effects from other medications like fatigue or sedation, or to treat patients with comorbid attention deficit hyperactivity disorder (ADHD). Since dopamine may play a very important role in the pathogenesis of mania, stimulant-induced mania has attracted attention from the very beginning of the introduction of stimulants. A systematic review of the occurrence of hallucinations or mania associated with the use of ADHD drugs in children including 49 randomized, controlled trials found that the rate of psychosis or mania per 100 person-years for the pooled active drug group was 1.48 but was zero in patients who received a placebo (Mosholder et al., 2009). Among the more than 800 spontaneous postmarketing reports of psychosis or mania, about 90% of these cases never had a history of a similar condition.

Some clinical studies in patients with ADHD and some manic symptoms showed that psychostimulants did not worsen manic symptoms or transform ADHD to BPD while ADHD symptoms showed significant improvement (Goldsmith, Singh, & Chang, 2011). Two randomized, placebo-controlled, cross-over studies of children and adolescents with BPD and ADHD found that stimulants did not bear an increased risk for TEM (Findling et al., 2007; Scheffer, Kowatch, Carmody, & Rush, 2005). However, the dosage of stimulants in these two studies was low, with a maximal dose of amphetamine salts of 10 mg/day (Scheffer et al., 2005) and methylphenidate of 30 mg/day (Findling et al., 2007). In contrast, several studies

in children and adolescents with BPD and ADHD have shown that co-administration of a psychostimulant to a mood stabilizer(s) caused adverse mood or behavioral changes including mania, hypomania, and suicidality in up to 10% of patients (Goldsmith et al., 2011). More important, among those who had destabilized moods with a stimulant, the mood instability resolved quickly after the causative agent was discontinued.

Wakefulness-promoting agents

Modafinil and armodafinil are wakefulness-promoting agents and have been approved by the US Food and Drug Admnistration for improving wakefulness in patients with excessive sleepiness associated with narcolepsy, obstructive sleep apnea, and shift-work sleep disorder. In two separate studies, armodafinil adjunctive therapy to a mood stabilizer in the treatment of bipolar I or II depression did not have an increased risk for TEM relative to placebo (Calabrese, Frye, Yang, & Ketter, 2014; Calabrese et al., 2010). However, there are case reports of modafinil-induced mania in patients with bipolar I disorder (Fountoulakis et al., 2008; Wolf, Fiedler, Anghelescu, & Schwertfeger, 2006).

Dopamine 2/3 receptor agonist

Pramipexole is a dopamine D2/D3 receptor agonist that is approved for the treatment of Parkinson's disease. Randomized, double-blind, placebo-controlled studies did not find pramipexole to have an increased risk for TEM or increasing manic severity relative to placebo (Zarate et al., 2004). However, pramipexole-induced mania/hypomania was observed in case reports of patients with or without a history of BPD (see Table 30.1).

CHOLINERGIC AND ANTICHOLINERGIC DRUGS

Psychotropic medications targeting the cholinergic system include varenicline for nicotine dependence, cholinesterase inhibitors (tacrine, donepezil, rivastigmine, galantamine) for dementia, and anticholinergics (atropine, scopolamine) for preoperation preparation, postoperative nausea and vomiting, and motion sickness. Varenicline may be indicated in patients with BPD and nicotine dependence. Cognitive deficits are also common in patients with BPD (see Chapter 16). Therefore, cholinesterase inhibitors may be used to improve cognition in patients with BPD. More important, scopolamine has shown a large antidepressant effect size with a fast onset in bipolar and unipolar depression (see Chapter 22). With the increase in use of these agents, TEM in patients with or without history of BPD have been reported (see Table 30.1).

ROLE OF COMORBID SUBSTANCE USE DISORDER IN TREATMENT-EMERGENT MOOD SWITCH

The effect of SUD on treatment-emergent mood switching may be through direct or indirect ways. The direct way is by a specific action on neurons and neuronal circuits. The indirect way is through nonadherence to pharmacological treatments or changes in metabolism of psychotropic drugs, which lead to a reduction in efficacy of pharmacological treatments.

Alcohol

Rates of alcohol abuse and/or dependence are higher than any other SUD in BPD (Gao et al., 2013; Merikangas et al, 2007). A longitudinal study after the first hospitalization for mania found that patients with alcohol use disorder following the onset of BPD had a significant greater percentage of full affective episodes (manic or mixed) during follow-up periods than those with no alcohol use disorder or those with an onset of alcohol use disorder prior to BPD (Strakowski et al., 2005).

Cannabis

Cannabis is the second most abused substance in BPD. Cannabis-induced mania and psychotic symptoms have been reported for more than four decades. The Netherlands Mental Health Survey and Incidence Study found that any use of cannabis at baseline predicted a very strong increase in the risk for a first BPD episode with an odds ratio (OR) of 4.98 (95% CI: 1.80–13.81) during a three-year follow-up period (van Laar, van Dorsselaer, Monshouwer, & de Graaf, 2007). Among the 4,815 patients who were followed for three years, the use of cannabis at baseline increased the risk of manic symptoms with an OR of 2.7 (95% CI: 1.54–4.75). The association between cannabis use and mania were independent of the prevalence and the incidence of psychotic symptoms. A longitudinal study after the first hospitalization for mania showed that patients with an onset of BPD prior to cannabis use disorder had a significantly higher percentage of manic or mixed episodes during follow-up periods than those without cannabis use disorder or those with an onset of cannabis use disorder prior to BPD (Strakowski et al., 2007).

Cocaine

It is well known that cocaine can produce manic/hypomanic–like behaviors in animals. Cocaine-induced mania in patients with or without BPD has been reported.

These data suggest that patients with BPD and co-occurring SUD, especially those with an onset of BPD first, may have an increased risk of mood instability compared to those without a history of SUD. The mood instability in this group could be a manifestation of inherent risk factors that differentiate patients with SUD from those without SUD. An analysis from the STEP-BD examined 2,154 patients who had a new-onset MDE and were followed prospectively for up to two years (Ostacher et al., 2010). During the follow-up period, 457 of them switched to a manic, hypomanic, or mixed episode prior to recovery. Past or current SUD did not predict time to recovery from a MDE relative to no SUD comorbidity. However, those with current or past SUD were more likely to have switched from depression directly to a manic, hypomanic, or mixed episode. More important, the switch rates were similar between patients with past SUD and those with current SUD, suggesting that factors inherent in patients with BPD at risk for SUD may also confer a greater likelihood of manic/hypomanic switching.

PLACEBO TREATMENT-EMERGENT MANIA/HYPOMANIA

Placebo TEM has been reported in the majority of acute bipolar depression studies (Calabrese et al., 2005, 2008; Lobel et al., 2014; McElory et a., 2010; Suppes et al., 2010; Thase et al., 2006, 2008; Tohen et al., 2003; Young et al., 2010), but the rates of placebo TEM varied in different studies, even with the same design, inclusion and exclusion criteria, and study durations (see Table 30.3). The rates of placebo TEM in these relatively "pure" populations of patients with BPD were lower than the rates of antidepressant TEM of some open-label studies in patients with more complex presentations (Chen et al., 2010; Post et al., 2006). The lower rates of placebo TEM in those pivotal studies could be a selection bias because patients with risk factors for TEM including a recent history of SUDs are commonly excluded from pivotal studies (see Table 30.3). In contrast, the higher rates of antidepressant TEM in those open-label studies could be the effect of antidepressant or the natural mood changes in patients with more complex presentations. Since a

Table 30.3. SUMMARY OF RATES OF MANIC/HYPOMANIC SWITCHING WITH PLACEBO IN RANDOMIZED, DOUBLE-BLIND, PLACEBO-CONTROLLED, MONOTHERAPY CLINICAL TRIALS IN BIPOLAR DEPRESSION

STUDY	INCLUSION CRITERIA	EXCLUSION CRITERIA	RC (%)	NO. OF PATIENTS	SR (%)	DURATION (WEEKS)	SWITCH DEFINITION
Calabrese et al., 2008	Bipolar I or II HAMD-17≥ 18 YMRS < 10	Rapid cycling Panic disorder, OCD, social phobia, bulimia nervosa in past 12 months	0	530	3.3	7–10	YMRS≥16 on 2 consecutive visits or at final assessment or reported as an adverse events
Tohen et al., 2003	BPI depression MADRS ≥ 20 RC	Substance dependence within 3 months	35.0	377	6.7	8	YMRS<15 at baseline and ≥15 at any subsequent visit
Calabrese et al. 2005	BPI and BPII HAMD-17≥ 20 YMRS ≤12	Axis I disorder—primary focus within 6 months SUDs within 12 months	20.7	169	3.9	8	YMRS≥16 on 2 consecutive visits or at final assessment or reported as an adverse events
Thase et al., 2006	BPI and BPII HAMD-17≥ 20 YMRS ≤12	Axis I disorder—primary focus within 6 months SUDs within 12 months	32.9	167	6.6	8	YMRS≥16 on 2 consecutive visits or at final assessment or reported as an adverse events
McElroy et al., 2010	BPI and BPII RC, but ≤ 8 episodes per year HAMD-17≥ 20 YMRS ≤12	Axis I disorder—primary focus within 6 months SUDs within 12 months	19.8	124	8.9	8	YMRS≥16 on 2 consecutive visits or at final assessment or reported as an adverse events
Young et al., 2010	BPI and BPII RC, but ≤ 8 episodes per year HAMD-17≥ 20 YMRS ≤12	Axis I disorder—primary focus within 6 months SUDs within 12 months	3.9	133	0.8	8	YMRS≥16 on 2 consecutive visits or at final assessment or reported as an adverse events
Suppes et al., 2010	BPI and BPII RC, but ≤ 8 episodes per year HAMD-17≥ 20 YMRS ≤12	Axis I disorder—primary focus within 6 months SUDs within 12 months	27.7	140	6.4	8	YMRS≥16 on 2 consecutive visits or at final assessment or reported as an adverse events
Thase et al., 2008	Bipolar I HAMD-17≥18 YMRS<12 RC, but < 6 episodes per year	Primary other Axis disorder with depression, late-set depression Substance abuse 3 months Dependence 6 months; OCD, bulimia nervosa, or ADHD	n/a	367	1.6	8	Unknown
Lobel et al., 2014	Bipolar I depression MADRS≥20 YMRS≤12	n/a	n/a	168	1	6	n/a

NOTE: ADHD = attention deficit hyperactivity disorder; BPI = bipolar I disorder; BPII = bipolar II disorder; HAMD-17 = Hamilton Depression Rating Scale–17 Item; MADRS = Montgomery-Åsberg Depression Ratings Scale; n/a, = not available; OCD = obsessive compulsive disorder; RC = rapid cycling; SR = switching rate; SUDs = substance use disorders; YMRS = Young Mania Rating Scale.

spontaneous switching rate(s) in patients with complex presentations remains unknown, results of pharmacological TEM from open-label or naturalistic studies without a placebo arm will be difficult to interpret.

NONPHARMACOLOGICAL TREATMENT-EMERGENT MANIA/HYPOMANIA

NONPHARMACOLOGICAL SOMATIC TREATMENTS

ECT

Electroconvulsive therapy (ECT) TEM has been reported in patients with bipolar depression or treatment-refractory MDD (see Table 30.1), but high-quality data are still lacking. An early retrospective study reported that about 12% of patients with endogenous depression (both bipolar and unipolar) switched to mania/hypomania during ECT treatment, and 10% of patients with psychotic unipolar depression switched to hypomania in those who received ECT versus 3.6% in those who did not receive ECT. However, the switch rates in psychotic bipolar depression did not significantly differ between patients receiving ECT (30%) and those who did not receive ECT treatment (32%; Angst, Angst, Baruffol, & Meinherz-Surbeck, 1992). In contrast, another study reported that 22 of 57 depressed bipolar patients successfully treated with ECT experienced subsequent mild hypomania (Koukopoulos et al., 1980). Moreover, there are reports suggesting that the concurrent use of lithium or anticonvulsants are effective to prevent ECT-induced mania/hypomania.

VNS/rTMS

Vagal nerve stimulation (VNS) has been approved for treatment-refractory depression. There have been case reports of VNS-induced mania/hypomania in patients with epilepsy or depression although it is considered rare. TEM during repetitive transcranial magnet stimulation (rTMS) treatment was observed in patients with BPD or MDD. In a review of 10 randomized sham or ECT controlled clinical trials, the overall rate of TEM was not significantly different between active treatment (0.84%) and sham control (0.73%; Xia et al., 2007). However, in a total of 65 bipolar patients, the switching rate in the active rTMS treatment group was estimated to be 3.1%. The switching rate for MDD was 0.34%.

Among 16 cases of rTMS TEM, 10 of them had a previous diagnosis of BPD; 3 had recurrent MDD, and 3 suffered from unspecified depression. Overall, rates of TEM with these physical treatments appear low and may just resemble the natural course of illness in individuals experiencing TEM.

Light therapy

Manic/hypomanic switching after therapeutic sleep deprivation in bipolar depression has been reported (Colombo, Benedetti, Barbini, Campori, & Smeraldi, 1999). Similarly, in a case series, three of four women with bipolar I or II depression treated with morning bright light therapy developed mixed states even with concomitant use of mood stabilizer(s) (Sit, Wisner, Hanusa, Stull, & Terman, 2007). In contrast, none of five patients who received midday light therapy developed manic symptoms.

So far, all nonpharmacological TEM data are from retrospective studies, case reports, or case series. A causal relationship between these treatments and TEM cannot be established. Large, prospective, longitudinal, controlled studies are warranted to support or refute a risk of TEM with those treatment modalities.

PSYCHOSOCIAL INTERVENTIONS

There is convincing evidence that psychosocial interventions can speed up recovery from depressive episodes and delay episode recurrences (Miklowitz et al., 2007). For the same reason, there is a possibility that a subgroup of patients may switch to mania/hypomania with or without a euthymic period during psychosocial interventions for depression. Such a potential switch may be related to personality and temperament, life events, and impaired family psychosocial dynamics (Miklowitz & Johnson, 2009). Some data support that patients with BPD are highly sensitive to reward and excessive goal pursuit after goal attainment events. Goal attainment events have been shown to be associated with the onset of mania/hypomania. One mechanism for life events related mania/hypomania is through sleep disruption. In normal human subjects, sleep deprivation can increase dopamine release in the striatum and thalamus (Volkow et al., 2008). The "sensitized" dopamine system in bipolar patients may lead to an increased release of dopamine following sleep deprivation. Subsequently, manic/hypomanic symptoms may emerge. Previous studies have demonstrated that sleep deprivation can trigger manic symptoms in 10% of patients with bipolar depression (Miklowitz & Johnson,

2009). It is reasonable to speculate that during psychological interventions, a subgroup of patients may be overly involved in goal attainment or highly rewarded activities after the improvement of depressive symptoms. Subsequently, TEM may occur even when a stable dose(s) of pharmacological treatments is maintained. Interpersonal and social rhythm therapy is as effective as cognitive-behavioral therapy and family-focused therapy for bipolar depression (Miklowitz & Johnson, 2009). A balanced combination of these therapies may be useful for preventing TEM.

PHARMACOLOGICAL TREATMENT-EMERGENT DEPRESSION

Antipsychotics

The earliest reference to the putative "depressogenic" properties of antipsychotic agents stems from studies of flupenthixol in mania (Ahlfors et al., 1981; Gao, Gajwani, Elhaj, & Calabrese, 2005). Patients treated with flupenthixol spent more time in depression but less time in mania. Patients augmented with placebo did significantly better compared to those augmented with flupenthixol according to an affective morbidity index. In a double-blind discontinuation study of perphenazine in recent mania, patients given perphenazine were significantly more likely to discontinue the study due to relapse into depression, to have shorter times to relapse into depression, and to discontinue the study for any reason (Zarate & Tohen, 2004). Moreover, a 12-week, double-blind study of olanzapine and haloperidol in acute mania found that haloperidol-treated patients switched to depression significantly earlier than those treated with olanzapine, although the rate was not significantly different. A recent meta-analysis of randomized, placebo-controlled trials of antipsychotics (apripiprazole, olanzapine, quetiapine, risperidone, ziprasidone, and haloperidol) in acute mania found that treatment of acute mania with atypicals was associated with a 42% lower risk of switch to depression than with haloperidol (Goikolea et al., 2013). However, individually, each atypical antipsychotic was not significantly different from haloperidol, although a trend was observed favoring olanzapine, quetiapine, and ziprasidone over haloperidol.

Lithium

Hypofunction of the thyroid gland during lithium treatment is a common side effect. An early study showed that during lithium treatment, a low level of free T4 was associated with more affective episodes and greater severity of depression (Frye et al., 1999). The relationship between lithium treatment-emergent depression and thyroid hypofunction is further supported by a recent post hoc analysis of two maintenance treatment studies of lamotrigine and lithium in bipolar I disorder (Frye et al., 2009). Lithium-treated patients who required an intervention for a depressive episode had a significantly higher adjusted mean TSH level (4.4 μIU/ml) compared with those lithium-treated patients who did not require intervention for a depressive episode (2.4 μIU/ml).

Lamotrigine

A study of suicide-related events in a cohort of more than 5 million patients treated with antiepileptic drugs found that anticonvulsants were associated with decreased risk for suicide-related events in patients with epilepsy only but associated with increased risk for suicide-related events in patients with depression only (Arana, Wentworth, Ayuso-Mateos, & Arellano, 2010). However, there was no significant association between anticonvulsant use and the risk of suicide-related events in patients with BPD only, patients with epilepsy and depression, and patients with epilepsy and BPD. There is no report whether lamotrigine has any direct or indirect effect on treatment-emergent depression. However, lamotrigine treatment- emergent depression may occur through drug-to-drug interactions and a subsequent loss of efficacy. Any medication that increases the enzymatic activity of the glucuronidation processes in the liver can reduce the efficacy of lamotrigine. Since lamotrigine is more efficacious for depressive symptoms and depression-relapse prevention, the treatment-emergent mood switch is more likely a switch to depression instead of to mania/hypomania. Medications increasing the metabolism of lamotrigine and reducing its efficacy include contraceptives and antiretroviral agents, lopinavir/ritonavir. There are consistent reports that co-administration of oral contraceptives, especially those containing estradiol, could reduce lamotrigine serum level by about 50%. Pregnancy also increases the metabolism of lamotrigine. Lopinavir (800 mg/day)/ritonavir (200 mg/day) could reduce lamotrigine plasma concentration by more than 50% in healthy subjects.

Factors associated with switching from mania to depression

A large observational study, the European Mania in Bipolar Longitudinal Evaluation of Medication (EMBLEM), observed that 120 of 2,390 (5%) manic patients switched to depression within the first 12 weeks. Factors associated with greater switching to depression were the number of previous depressive episodes, a history of substance abuse, greater overall illness severity, and the use of benzodiazepines (Vieta et al., 2009). The use of benzodiazepine associated with an increased risk of switching to depression is consistent with previous findings that co-occurrence of anxiety disorders or anxiety symptoms in bipolar patients predicted depressive relapses (Otto et al., 2006; Perlis et al., 2006).

PHARMACOLOGICAL TREATMENT-EMERGENT CYCLE ACCELERATION

Like TEM, the controversy on the causal relationship between antidepressant use and cycle acceleration has never been settled. After a systematic review of the early data prior to the middle of 1980s, Wehr and Goodwin (1987) concluded that antidepressants could precipitate mania and hypomania and decrease cycle length in patients with BPD. The controversy of antidepressant-induced mania and cycle acceleration was revisited by using life-charting methodology in patients with BPD who were treated at the National Institute of Mental Health (Altshuler et al., 1995). The researchers found that in 35% of patients who had a manic episode, these episodes were rated as likely being antidepressant-induced. Cycle acceleration was likely to be associated with antidepressant treatments in 26% of patients. However, longitudinal data of patients who were hospitalized before and after the introduction of antidepressants did not show changes in cycle length (Angst & Sellaro, 2000).

PHARMACOLOGICAL TREATMENT-EMERGENT RAPID CYCLING

A possible outcome of repeated TEM is rapid cycling. Antidepressant-induced rapid cycling was first described in 1956 in a tuberculosis patient treated with iproniazid. Tricyclic antidepressant–induced rapid cycling was reported in late 1970s and early 1980s (Koukopoulos et al., 1980; Wehr & Goodwin, 1979). A rapid cycling course can be the natural course of illness or a presentation of cycle acceleration triggered by external factors (Koukopoulos et al., 2003). While receiving tricyclics, five patients cycled nearly four times more rapidly between mania and

depression compared to periods when they were not receiving the drugs (Wehr & Goodwin, 1979). The mean cycle length during tricyclic treatments was 33 ± 14 days versus 127 ± 50 days during the periods without antidepressants. In a later study, Wehr and Goodwin (1987) showed again that tricyclic antidepressants induced reversible rapid cycling between mania and depression in some patients. Among the patients with rapid cycling, there were about 20% of patients who had shortened cycle lengths during the periods of antidepressant treatments compared to the periods without antidepressant (Wehr, Sack, Rosenthal, & Cowdry, 1988).

Seemingly, there is some evidence supporting that a subgroup of patients with BPD are vulnerable to have antidepressant TEM, cycle acceleration, and/or rapid cycling. However, in a report from the National Institute of Mental Health Collaborative Depression Study, only about 20% cases of bipolar patients with rapid cycling had a rapid cycling course that lasted more than two years after its onset, and its resolution was not associated with a decrease in the use of tricyclic antidepressants (Coryell et al., 2003). The use of tricyclic antidepressants in patients prone to rapid cycling was also not more frequent in the weeks preceding shifts from depression to mania/hypomania compared to its overall use during periods of depression.

These data suggest that even among patients with rapid cycling, the course of illness and the vulnerability to antidepressant-induced switching is not homogenous (Gao et al., 2008). However, the magnitude of this variance is difficult to determine. The inconsistency and conflicting reports of TEM and cycle acceleration could be due to different populations studied in the previous studies. A recent international study of rapid cycling BPD in the community supported ethnic differences in terms of the course of bipolar illness (Lee et al., 2010). In three countries (Bulgaria, Japan, and the Indian territory of Pondicherry) of this study, there was a zero prevalence of rapid cycling BPD. The SLC6A4 (5HTTLPR polymorphism), catechol-O-methyltransferase, brain-derived neurotrophic factor, CYR2 (chryptochrome 2), and P2RX7 genes have been reported to be associated with rapid cycling (Backlund et al., 2012). However, their relationships with antidepressant-induced mood switching are yet to be determined.

CONCLUSION

There are several pharmacological and nonpharmacological factors with a potential to cause mood instability, especially manic/hypomanic switches. A distinct yet insufficiently characterized group of patients with BPD has a higher vulnerability to develop TEM. Although some factors such as bipolar I type, history of SUD, rapid cycling course, or previous history of treatment-emergent mood switching may predict future TEM, a single reliable marker for predicting TEM is still lacking. At the current stage, strategies to prevent treatment-emergent mood instability should include screening for known risk factors by thorough diagnostic assessment and extensive evaluation of previous treatment history, close monitoring, psychoeducation, and initiating an antimanic agent(s) including lithium, valproate, and/or some antipsychotics prior to potential manic-provoking agents.

Disclosure statement: Dr. Gao is on a speaker's bureau of Sunovion. He receives research grant support from the Brain & Behavior Research Foundation and Cleveland Foundation. To his knowledge, all of Dr. Heize Grunze's possible conflicts of interest, financial or otherwise, including direct or indirect financial or personal relationships, interests, and affiliations, whether or not directly related to the subject of the chapter, are as follows: Grant support: National Institute for Health Research United Kingdom, Medical Research Council United Kingdom, Northumberland, Tyne & Wear National Health Service Foundation Trust, Otsuka Pharmaceuticals; receipt of honoraria or consultation fees: Gedeon-Richter, Desitin, Lundbeck, Hofmann-LaRoche; participation in a company-sponsored speaker's bureau: Astra Zeneca, Bristol-Myers Squibb, Otsuka, Lundbeck, Servier. Dr. Renwong Wu and Dr. Calabrese have not disclosed any conflicts of interest.

REFERENCES

Ahlfors, U. G., Baastrup, P. C., Dencker, S. J., Elgen, K., Lingjaerde, O., Pedersen, V.,...Aaskoven, O. (1981). Flupenthixol decanoate in recurrent manic-depressive illness: A comparison with lithium. *Acta Psychiatrica Scandinavica, 64*(3), 226–237.

Altshuler, L. L., Post, R. M., Leverich, G. S., Mikalauskas, K., Rosoff, A., & Ackerman, L. (1995). Antidepressant-induced mania and cycle acceleration: A controversy revisited. *American Journal of Psychiatry, 152*(8), 1130–1138.

Amsterdam, J. D., & Shults, J. (2010). Efficacy and safety of long-term fluoxetine versus lithium monotherapy of bipolar II disorder: A randomized, double-blind, placebo-substitution study. *American Journal of Psychiatry, 167*(7), 792–800.

Angst, J., Angst, K., Baruffol, I., & Meinherz-Surbeck, R. (1992). ECT-induced and drug-induced hypomania. *Convulsive Therapy, 8*(3), 179–185.

Angst, J., & Sellaro, R. (2000). Historical perspectives and natural history of bipolar disorder. *Biological Psychiatry, 48*(6), 445–457.

Angst, J., Gerber-Werder, R., Zuberbühler, H. U., & Gamma, A. (2004). Is bipolar I disorder heterogeneous? *European Archives of Psychiatry and Clinical Neurosciences, 254*(2), 82–91.

Applebaum, J., Bersudsky, Y., & Klein, E. (2007). Rapid tryptophan depletion as a treatment for acute mania: A double-blind, pilot-controlled study. *Bipolar Disorders, 9*(8), 884–887.

Arana, A., Wentworth, C. E., Ayuso-Mateos, J. L., & Arellano, F. M. (2010). Suicide-related events in patients treated with antiepileptic drugs. *New England Journal of Medicine, 363*(6), 542–551.

Arnsten, A. F. (2007). Catecholamine and second messenger influences on prefrontal cortical networks of "representational knowledge": A rational bridge between genetics and the symptoms of mental illness. *Cerebral Cortex, 17*(1), 6–15.

Austin, M., & Tan, Y. C. (2012). Mania associated with infliximab. *Australia and New Zealand Journal of Psychiatry, 46*(7), 684–685.

Backlund, L., Lavebratt, C., Frisén, L., Nikamo, P., HukicSudic, D., Träskman-Bendz, L.,...Schalling, M. (2012). P2RX7: Expression responds to sleep deprivation and associates with rapid cycling in bipolar disorder type 1. *PLoS One, 7*(8), e43057.

Bauer, M., London, E. D., Rasgon, N., Berman, S. M., Frye, M. A., Altshuler, L. L.,...Whybrow, P. C. (2005). Supraphysiological doses of levothyroxine alter regional cerebral metabolism and improve mood in bipolar depression. *Molecular Psychiatry, 10*(5), 456–469.

Berk, M., Dodd, S., Kauer-Sant'Anna, M., Malhi, G. S., Bourin, M., Kapczinski, F., & Norman, T. (2007). Dopamine dysregulation syndrome: Implications for a dopamine hypothesis of bipolar disorder. *Acta Psychiatrica Scandinavica, 434*(Suppl.), 41–49.

Biber, K., Fiebich, B. L., Gebicke-Härter, P., & van Calker, D. (1999). Carbamazepine-induced upregulation of adenosine A1-receptors in astrocyte cultures affects coupling to the phosphoinositol signaling pathway. *Neuropsychopharmacology, 20*(3), 271–278.

Biernacka, J. M., McElroy, S. L., Crow, S., Sharp, A., Benitez, J.,...Frye, M. A. (2012). Pharmacogenomics of antidepressant induced mania: A review and meta-analysis of the serotonin transporter gene (5HTTLPR) association. *Journal of Affective Disorders, 136*(1–2), e21–29.

Bishop, L. C., Bisset, A. D., & Benson, J. I. (1987). Mania and indomethacin. *Journal of Clinical Psychopharmacology, 7*(3), 203–204.

Bottlender, R., Rudolf, D., Strauss, A., & Möller, H. J. (2000). Are low basal serum levels of the thyroid stimulating hormone (b-TSH) a risk factor for switches into states of expansive syndromes (known in Germany as "maniform syndromes") in bipolar I depression? *Pharmacopsychiatry, 33*(2), 75–57.

Bottlender, R., Sato, T., Kleindienst, N., Strauss, A., & Möller, H. J. (2004). Mixed depressive features predict maniform switch during treatment of depression in bipolar I disorder. *Journal of Affective Disorders, 78*(2), 149–152.

Bond, D. J., Noronha, M. M., Kauer-Sant'Anna, M., Lam, R. W., & Yatham, L. N. (2008). Antidepressant-associated mood elevations in bipolar II disorder compared with bipolar I disorder and major depressive disorder: A systematic review and meta-analysis. *Journal of Clinical Psychiatry, 69*(10), 1589–1601.

Brambilla, P., Perez, J., Barale, F., Schettini, G., & Soares, J. C. (2003). GABAergic dysfunction in mood disorders. *Molecular Psychiatry, 8*(8), 721–737, 715.

Calabrese, J. R., Frye, M. A., Yang, R., Ketter, T. A., Armodafinil Treatment Trial Study Network. (2014). Efficacy and safety of adjunctive armodafinil in adults with major depressive episodes associated with bipolar I disorder: a randomized, double-blind, placebo-controlled, multicenter trial. *Journal of Clinical Psychiatry, 75*(10), 1054–1061.

Calabrese, J. R., Huffman, R. F., White, R. L., Edwards, S., Thompson, T. R., Ascher, J. A.,...Leadbetter, R. A. (2008). Lamotrigine in the acute treatment of bipolar depression: Results of five double-blind, placebo-controlled clinical trials. *Bipolar Disorders, 10*(2), 323–233.

Calabrese, J. R., Keck, P. E. Jr., Macfadden, W., Minkwitz, M., Ketter, T. A., Weisler, R. H.,...Mullen, J.(2005). A randomized, double-blind, placebo-controlled trial of quetiapine in the treatment of bipolar I or II depression. *American Journal of Psychiatry, 162*, 1351–1360.

Calabrese, J. R., Ketter, T. A., Youakim, J. M., Tiller, J. M., Yang, R., & Frye, M. A. (2010). Adjunctive armodafinil for major depressive episodes associated with bipolar I disorder: A randomized, multicenter, double-blind, placebo-controlled, proof-of-concept study. *Journal of Clinical Psychiatry, 71*(10), 1363–1370.

Chen, J., Fang, Y., Kemp, D. E., Calabrese, J. R., & Gao, K. (2010). Switching to hypomania and mania: Differential neurochemical, neuropsychological, and pharmacologic triggers and their mechanisms. *Current Psychiatry Reports, 12*(6), 512–521.

Colombo, C., Benedetti, F., Barbini, B., Campori, E., & Smeraldi, E. (1999). Rate of switch from depression into mania after therapeutic sleep deprivation in bipolar depression. *Psychiatry Research, 86*(3), 267–270.

Coryell, W., Solomon, D., Turvey, C., Keller, M., Leon, A. C., Endicott, J.,…Mueller, T. (2003). The long-term course of rapid-cycling bipolar disorder. *Archives of General Psychiatry, 60*(9), 914–920.

Curtin, F., & Schulz, P. (2004). Clonazepam and lorazepam in acute mania: A Bayesian meta-analysis. *Journal of Affective Disorders, 78*(3), 201–208.

Daray, F. M., Thommi, S. B., & Ghaemi, S. N. (2010). The pharmacogenetics of antidepressant-induced mania: A systematic review and meta-analysis. *Bipolar Disorders, 12*(7), 702–706.

Findling, R. L., Short, E. J., McNamara, N. K., Demeter, C. A., Stansbrey, R. J., Gracious, B. L.,…Calabrese, J. R. (2007). Methylphenidate in the treatment of children and adolescents with bipolar disorder and attention-deficit/hyperactivity disorder. *Journal of the American Academy of Child & Adolescent Psychiatry, 46*(11), 1445–1153.

Fountoulakis, K. N., Siamouli, M., Panagiotidis, P., Magiria, S., Kantartzis, S., Iacovides, A., & Kaprinis, G. S. (2008). Ultra short manic-like episodes after antidepressant augmentation with modafinil. *Progress in Neuro-Psychopharmacology & Biological Psychiatry, 32*(3), 891–892.

Frye, M. A., Denicoff, K. D., Bryan, A. L., Smith-Jackson, E. E., Ali, S. O., Luckenbaugh, D.,…Post, R. M. (1999). Association between lower serum free T4 and greater mood instability and depression in lithium-maintained bipolar patients. *American Journal of Psychiatry, 156*(12), 1909–1914.

Frye, M. A., Helleman, G., McElroy, S. L., Altshuler, L. L., Black, D. O., Keck, P. E. Jr.,…Suppes, T. (2009). Correlates of treatment-emergent mania associated with antidepressant treatment in bipolar depression. *American Journal of Psychiatry, 166*(2), 164–172.

Frye, M. A., Yatham, L., Ketter, T. A., Goldberg, J., Suppes, T., Calabrese, J. R.,…Adams, B. (2009). Depressive relapse during lithium treatment associated with increased serum thyroid-stimulating hormone: Results from two placebo-controlled bipolar I maintenance studies. *Acta Psychiatrica Scandinavica, 20*(1), 10–13.

Gao, K., Gajwani, P., Elhaj, O., & Calabrese, J. R. (2005). Typical and atypical antipsychotics in bipolar depression. *Journal of Clinical Psychiatry, 66*(11), 1376–1385.

Gao, K., Kemp, D. E., Ganocy, S. J., Muzina, D. J., Xia, G., Findling, R. L., & Calabrese, J. R. (2008). Treatment-emergent mania/hypomania during antidepressant monotherapy in patients with rapid cycling bipolar disorder. *Bipolar Disorders, 10*(8), 907–915.

Gao, K., Wang, Z., Chen, J., Kemp, D. E., Chan, P. K., Conroy, C. M.,…Calabrese, J. R. (2013). Should an assessment of Axis I comorbidity be included in the initial diagnostic assessment of mood disorders? Role of QIDS-16-SR total score in predicting number of Axis I comorbidity. *Journal of Affective Disorders, 148*(2–3), 256–264.

Gerner, R. H., Fairbanks, L., Anderson, G. M., Young, J. G., Scheinin, M., Linnoila, M.,…Cohen, D. J. (1984). CSF neurochemistry in depressed, manic, and schizophrenic patients compared with that of normal controls. *American Journal of Psychiatry, 141*(12), 1533–1540.

Goikolea, J. M., Colom, F., Torres, I., Capapey, J., Valentí, M., Undurraga, J.,…Vieta, E. (2013). Lower rate of depressive switch following antimanic treatment with second-generation antipsychotics versus haloperidol. *Journal of Affective Disorders, 144*(3), 191–198.

Goldberg, J. F., & Truman, C. J. (2003). Antidepressant-induced mania: An overview of current controversies. *Bipolar Disorders, 5*(6), 407–420.

Goldsmith, M., Singh, M., & Chang, K. (2011). Antidepressants and psychostimulants in pediatric populations: Is there an association with mania? *Paediatric Drugs, 13*(4), 225–243.

Koukopouplos, A., Reginaldi, D., Laddomada, G., Floris, G., Serra, G., & Tondo, L. (1980). Course of the manic-depressive cycle and changes caused by treatments. *Pharmakopsychiatr Neuropsychopharkol, 13,* 156–167.

Koukopoulos, A., Sani, G., Koukopoulos, A. E., Minnai, G. P., Girardi, P., Pani, L.,…Reginaldi, D. (2003). Duration and stability of the rapid-cycling course: A long-term personal follow-up of 109 patients. *Journal of Affective Disorders, 73*(1–2), 75–85.

Lee, S., Tsang, A., Kessler, R. C., Jin, R., Sampson, N., Andrade, L.,…Petukhova, M. (2010). Rapid-cycling bipolar disorder: Cross-national community study. *British Journal of Psychiatry, 196*(3), 217–225.

Leverich, G. S., Altshuler, L. L., Frye, M. A., Suppes, T., McElroy, S. L., Keck, P. E. Jr.,…Post, R. M. (2006). Risk of switch in mood polarity to hypomania or mania in patients with bipolar depression during acute and continuation trials of venlafaxine, sertraline, and bupropion as adjuncts to mood stabilizers. *American Journal of Psychiatry, 163*(2), 232–239.

Loebel, A., Cucchiaro, J., Silva, R., Kroger, H., Hsu, J., Sarma, K., & Sachs, G. (2014). Lurasidone monotherapy in the treatment of bipolar I depression: a randomized, double-blind, placebo-controlled study. *The American Journal of Psychiatry, 171*(2), 160–168.

Losekam, S., Kluge, I., Nittel, K. S., Kircher, T., & Konrad, C. (2013). Shopping frenzy induced by naltrexone—A paradoxical effect in bipolar disorder. *Psychological Medicine, 43*(4), 895.

Maj, M., Ariano, M. G., Arena, F., & Kemali, D. (1984). Plasma cortisol, catecholamine and cyclic AMP levels, response to dexamethasone suppression test and platelet MAO activity in manic-depressive patients: A longitudinal study. *Neuropsychobiology, 11*(3), 168–173.

McElroy, S. L., Weisler, R. H., Chang, W., Olausson, B., Paulsson, B., Brecher, M.,…EMBOLDEN II (Trial D1447C00134) Investigators. (2010). A double-blind, placebo-controlled study of quetiapine and paroxetine as monotherapy in adults with bipolar depression (EMBOLDEN II). *Journal of Clinical Psychiatry, 71*(2), 163–174.

Merikangas, K. R., Akiskal, H. S., Angst, J., Greenberg, P. E., Hirschfeld, R. M., Petukhova, M., & Kessler, R. C. (2007). Lifetime and 12-month prevalence of bipolar spectrum disorder in the National Comorbidity Survey replication. *Archives of General Psychiatry, 64*(5), 543–552.

Micale, V., Di Marzo, V., Sulcova, A., Wotjak, C. T., & Drago, F. (2013). Endocannabinoid system and mood disorders: Priming a target for new therapies. *Pharmacology & Therapeutics, 138*(1), 18–37.

Miklowitz, D. J., Otto, M. W., Frank, E., Reilly-Harrington, N. A., Kogan, J. N., Sachs, G. S.,…Wisniewski, S. R. (2007). Intensive psychosocial intervention enhances functioning in patients with bipolar depression: Results from a 9-month randomized controlled trial. *American Journal of Psychiatry, 164*(9), 1340–1347.

Miklowitz, D. J., & Johnson, S. L. (2009). Social and Familial Factors in the Course of Bipolar Disorder: Basic Processes and Relevant Interventions. *Clinical Psychology (New York), 16*(2), 281–296.

Möller, H. J., & Grunze, H. (2000). Have some guidelines for the treatment of acute bipolar depression gone too far in the restriction of antidepressants? *European Archives of Psychiatry and Clinical Neuroscience, 250*(2), 57–68.

Monteleone, P., Bifulco, M., Maina, G., Tortorella, A., Gazzerro, P., Proto, M. C.,…Maj, M. (2010). Investigation of CNR1 and FAAH endocannabinoid gene polymorphisms in bipolar disorder and major depression. *Pharmacological Research, 61*(5), 400–404.

Mosholder, A. D., Gelperin, K., Hammad, T. A., Phelan, K., & Johann-Liang, R. (2009). Hallucinations and other psychotic symptoms associated with the use of attention-deficit/hyperactivity disorder drugs in children. *Pediatrics, 123*(2), 611–616.

Ostacher, M. J., Perlis, R. H., Nierenberg, A. A., Calabrese, J., Stange, J. P., Salloum, I.,…STEP-BD Investigators. (2010). Impact of substance use disorders on recovery from episodes of depression in bipolar disorder patients: Prospective data from the Systematic Treatment Enhancement Program for Bipolar Disorder (STEP-BD). *American Journal of Psychiatry, 167*(3), 289–297.

Otto, M. W., Simon, N. M., Wisniewski, S. R., Miklowitz, D. J., Kogan, J. N., Reilly-Harrington, N. A.,…STEP-BD Investigators. (2006). Prospective 12-month course of bipolar disorder in out-patients with and without comorbid anxiety disorders. *British Journal of Psychiatry, 189,* 20–25.

Pacchiarotti, I., Bond, D. J., Baldessarini, R. J., Nolen, W. A., Grunze, H., Licht, R. W.,…Vieta, E. (2013). The International Society for Bipolar disorder (ISBD) Task-Force report on antidepressant use in bipolar disorder. *American Journal of Psychiatry, 170*(11), 1249–1262.

Pacchiarotti, I., Valentí, M., Colom, F., Rosa, A. R., Nivoli, A. M., Murru, A.,…Vieta, E. (2011). Differential outcome of bipolar patients receiving antidepressant monotherapy versus combination with an antimanic drug. *Journal of Affective Disorders, 129*(1–3), 321–326.

Peet, M. (1994). Induction of mania with selective serotonin re-uptake inhibitors and tricyclic antidepressants. *British Journal of Psychiatry, 164*(4), 549–550.

Perlis, R. H., Ostacher, M. J., Goldberg, J. F., Miklowitz, D. J., Friedman, E., Calabrese, J.,…Sachs, G. S. (2010). Transition to mania during treatment of bipolar depression. *Neuropsychopharmacology, 35*(13), 2545–2552.

Perlis, R. H., Ostacher, M. J., Patel, J. K., Marangell, L. B., Zhang, H., Wisniewski, S. R.,…Thase, M. E. (2006). Predictors of recurrence in bipolar disorder: Primary outcomes from the Systematic Treatment Enhancement Program for Bipolar Disorder (STEP-BD). *American Journal of Psychiatry, 163*(2), 217–224.

Post, R. M., Altshuler, L. L., Leverich, G. S., Frye, M. A., Nolen, W. A., Kupka, R. W.,…Mintz, J. (2006). Mood switch in bipolar depression: Comparison of adjunctive venlafaxine, bupropion and sertraline. *British Journal of Psychiatry, 189,* 124–131.

Ricke, A. K., Snook, R. J., & Anand, A. (2011). Induction of prolonged mania during ketamine therapy for reflex sympathetic dystrophy. *Biological Psychiatry, 70*(4), e13–14.

Roy, A., Pickar, D., Linnoila, M., Doran, A. R., Ninan, P., & Paul, S. M. (1985). Cerebrospinal fluid monoamine and monoamine metabolite concentrations in melancholia. *Psychiatry Research, 15*(4), 281–292.

Salvadore, G., Quiroz, J. A., Machado-Vieira, R., Henter, I. D., Manji, H. K., & Zarate, C. A. Jr. (2010). The neurobiology of the switch process in bipolar disorder: A review. *Journal of Clinical Psychiatry, 71*(11), 1488–1501.

Scheffer, R. E., Kowatch, R. A., Carmody, T., & Rush, A. J. (2005). Randomized, placebo-controlled trial of mixed amphetamine salts for symptoms of comorbid ADHD in pediatric bipolar disorder after mood stabilization with divalproex sodium. *American Journal of Psychiatry, 162*(1), 58–64.

Schildkraut, J. J. (1965). The catecholamine hypothesis of affective disorders: A review of supporting evidence. *Journal of Neuropsychiatry & Clinical Neurosciences, 7*(4), 524–533.

Shiah, I. S., & Yatham, L. N. (2000). Serotonin in mania and in the mechanism of action of mood stabilizers: A review of clinical studies. *Bipolar Disorders, 2*(2), 7–92.

Sit, D., Wisner, K. L., Hanusa, B. H., Stull, S., & Terman, M. (2007). Light therapy for bipolar disorder: A case series in women. *Bipolar Disorders, 9*(8), 918–927.

Spijker, A. T., van Rossum, E. F., Hoencamp, E., DeRijk, R. H., Haffmans, J., Blom, M.,…Zitman, F. G. (2009). Functional polymorphism of the glucocorticoid receptor gene associates with mania and hypomania in bipolar disorder. *Bipolar Disorders, 11*(1), 95–101.

Strakowski, S. M., DelBello, M. P., Fleck, D. E., Adler, C. M., Anthenelli, R. M., Keck, P. E. Jr.,…Amicone, J. (2005). Effects of co-occurring alcohol abuse on the course of bipolar disorder following a first hospitalization for mania. *Archives of General Psychiatry, 62*(8), 851–858.

Strakowski, S. M., DelBello, M. P., Fleck, D. E., Adler, C. M., Anthenelli, R. M., Keck, P. E. Jr.,…Amicone, J. (2007). Effects of co-occurring cannabis use disorders on the course of bipolar disorder after a first hospitalization for mania. *Archives of General Psychiatry, 64*(1), 57–64.

Suppes, T., Datto, C., Minkwitz, M., Nordenhem, A., Walker, C., & Darko, D. (2010). Effectiveness of the extended release formulation of quetiapine as monotherapy for the treatment of acute bipolar depression. *Journal of Affective Disorders, 121*(1–2), 106–115.

Swann, A. C., Secunda, S., Davis, J. M., Robins, E., Hanin, I., Koslow, S. H., & Maas, J. W. (1983). CSF monoamine metabolites in mania. *American Journal of Psychiatry, 140*(4), 396–400.

Swann, A. C., Stokes, P. E., Casper, R., Secunda, S. K., Bowden, C. L., Berman, N.,…Robins, E. (1992). Hypothalamic-pituitary-adrenocortical function in mixed and pure mania. *Acta Psychiatrica Scandinavica, 85*(4), 270–274.

Thase, M. E., Jonas, A., Khan, A., Bowden, C. L., Wu, X., McQuade, R. D.,…Owen, R. (2008). Aripiprazole monotherapy in non-psychotic bipolar I depression: Results of 2 randomized, placebo-controlled studies. *Journal of Clinical Psychopharmacology, 28*(1), 13–20.

Thase, M. E., Macfadden, W., Weisler, R. H., Chang, W., Paulsson, B., Khan, A.,…BOLDER II Study Group. (2006). Efficacy of quetiapine monotherapy in bipolar I and II depression: A double-blind, placebo-controlled study (the BOLDER II study). *Journal of Clinical Psychopharmacology, 26*(6), 600–609.

Tohen, M., Vieta, E., Calabrese, J., Ketter, T. A., Sachs, G., Bowden, C.,…Breier, A. (2003). Efficacy of olanzapine and olanzapine-fluoxetine combination in the treatment of bipolar depression. *Archives of General Psychiatry, 60,* 1079–1088.

van Laar, M., van Dorsselaer, S., Monshouwer, K., & de Graaf, R. (2007). Does cannabis use predict the first incidence of mood and anxiety disorders in the adult population? *Addiction, 102*(8), 1251–1260.

Valentí, M., Pacchiarotti, I., Bonnín, C. M., Rosa, A. R., Popovic, D., Nivoli, A. M.,…Vieta, E. (2012). Risk factors for antidepressant-related switch to mania. *Journal of Clinical Psychiatry, 73*(2), e271–276.

Vieta, E., Martinez-Arán, A., Goikolea, J. M., Torrent, C., Colom, F., Benabarre, A., & Reinares, M. (2002). A randomized trial comparing paroxetine and venlafaxine in the treatment of bipolar depressed patients taking mood stabilizers. *Jounal of Clinical Psychiatry, 63*(6), 508–512.

Vieta, E., Angst, J., Reed, C., Bertsch, J., Haro, J. M, & EMBLEM advisory board. (2009). Predictors of switching from mania to depression in a large observational study across Europe (EMBLEM). *Journal of Affective Disorders, 118*(1–3), 118–1123.

Volkow, N. D., Wang, G. J., Telang, F., Fowler, J. S., Logan, J., Wong, C.,…Jayne, M. (2008). Sleep deprivation decreases binding of [11C]raclopride to dopamine D2/D3 receptors in the human brain. *Journal of Neuroscience, 28*(34), 8454–8461.

Watson, S., Gallagher, P., Ritchie, J. C., Ferrier, I. N., & Young, A. H. (2004). Hypothalamic-pituitary-adrenal axis function in patients with bipolar disorder. *British Journal of Psychiatry, 184,* 496–502.

Wehr, T. A., & Goodwin, F. K. (1979). Rapid cycling in manic-depressives induced by tricyclic antidepressants. *Archives of General Psychiatry, 36*(5), 555–559.

Wehr, T. A., & Goodwin, F. K. (1987). Can antidepressants cause mania and worsen the course of affective illness? *American Journal of Psychiatry, 144*(11), 1403–1411.

Wehr, T. A., Sack, D. A., Rosenthal, N. E., & Cowdry, R. W. (1988). Rapid cycling affective disorder: Contributing factors and treatment responses in 51 patients. *American Journal of Psychiatry*, *145*(2), 179–184.

Wolf, J., Fiedler, U., Anghelescu, I., & Schwertfeger, N. (2006). Manic switch in a patient with treatment-resistant bipolar depression treated with modafinil. *Journal of Clinical Psychiatry*, *67*(11), 1817.

Xia, G., Gajwani, P., Muzina, D. J., Kemp, D. E., Gao, K., Ganocy, S. J., & Calabrese, J. R. (2007). Treatment-emergent mania in unipolar and bipolar depression: Focus on repetitive transcranial magnetic stimulation. *International Journal of Neuropsychopharmacology*, *11*(1), 119–130.

Young, A. H., Gallagher, P., Watson, S., Del-Estal, D., Owen, B. M., & Ferrier, I. N. (2004). Improvements in neurocognitive function and mood following adjunctive treatment with mifepristone (RU-486) in bipolar disorder. *Neuropsychopharmacology*, *29*(8), 1538–1545.

Young, A. H., McElroy, S. L., Bauer, M., Philips, N., Chang, W., Olausson, B.,...EMBOLDEN I (Trial 001) Investigators. (2010). A double-blind, placebo-controlled study of quetiapine and lithium monotherapy in adults in the acute phase of bipolar depression (EMBOLDEN I). *Journal of Clinical Psychiatry*, *71*(2), 150–162.

Zarate, C. A. Jr., & Manji, H. K. (2008). Bipolar disorder: Candidate drug targets. *Mount Sinai Journal of Medicine*, *75*(3), 226–247.

Zarate, C. A. Jr., Payne, J. L., Singh, J., Quiroz, J. A., Luckenbaugh, D. A., Denicoff, K. D.,...Manji, H. K. (2004). Pramipexole for bipolar II depression: A placebo-controlled proof of concept study. *Biological Psychiatry*, *56*(1), 54–60.

Zarate, C. A., & Tohen, M. (2004). Double-blind comparison of the continued use of antipsychotic treatment versus its discontinuation in remitted mania patients. *American Journal of Psychiatry*, *161*, 169–171.

PART IV

PSYCHOTHERAPY

31.

COGNITIVE BEHAVIORAL THERAPY AND PSYCHOEDUCATION

Dina Popovic, Jan Scott, and Francesc Colom

OVERVIEW OF PSYCHOLOGICAL INTERVENTIONS IN BIPOLAR DISORDER

A number of psychological interventions are currently available to help clinicians and patients manage several aspects of bipolar disorders (BDs). However, it is worth mentioning, that evidence-based interventions have largely become available in the past 15 years and that before that the quality of research in this field was poor—just a bit less than a marasmus—and the benefits of psychological approaches were much debated. Specifically, in 1998 there was not a single well-designed randomized controlled trial on the efficacy of a psychological approach for BDs (Colom, Vieta, Martínez, Jorquera, & Gastó, 1998).Fortunately, this situation was about to change in 1999, when the very first well-designed, randomized, controlled trial was published in the *British Medical Journal* of a brief, six-hour relapse-prevention intervention (Perry, Tarrier, Morriss, McCarthy, & Limb, 1999). This represented a simple and user-friendly psychoeducation intervention. Sixty-nine patients with BDs who had experienced a relapse within the previous 12 months were randomized to receive either standard care alone or standard care plus 7 to 12 individual sessions that taught them to identify early symptoms of relapse and to seek prompt treatment from their health-care providers. Those who received the relapse prevention program showed a significantly longer time to first manic relapse (25th percentile, 65 weeks vs. 17 weeks; $p = .008$), as well as a 30% decrease in the number of manic episodes over 18 months ($p = .013$). However, time to first depressive relapse and number of depressive relapses were unaffected. Overall, social functioning and employment over 18 months were significantly improved with the additional treatment sessions. Thus teaching patients to recognize the early symptoms of manic relapse yielded important clinical gains.

This seminal paper was almost immediately followed by a number of well-designed studies showing the efficacy of group psychoeducation (Colom et al., 2003), cognitive-behavioral therapy (CBT; Lam et al., 2003), family-focused psychoeducation (Miklowitz, George, Richards, Simoneau, & Suddath, 2003; Reinares et al., 2008), and interpersonal social-rhythm therapy (IPSRT; Frank et al., 2005). However, all of these studies were undertaken with euthymic patients and/or recruited samples from specialist affective disorders clinics. The medical Research Council in the United Kingdom therefore funded a pragmatic effectiveness trial that aimed to examine if CBT could be effective in routine clinical practice with patients with more overt instability or comorbidity and/or in an acute episode. This study clearly suggested that there are limits to the benefits of CBT, with a subgroup of patients (about 20% of the total sample) benefiting from the approach, but those cases with more illness episodes, greater levels or comorbidity, and so on failing to show gains over those cases receiving usual treatment (Scott et al., 2006). Since then, both efficacy and effectiveness studies have shown the potential gains but also some of the limitations of the other therapies available (Lobban et al., 2010; Meyer & Hautzinger, 2012; Torrent et al., 2013). Such research highlights the importance of continuing to test the benefits of these therapies across the clinical spectrum (Miklowitz & Scott, 2009) and avoiding a publication bias toward positive studies (Colom & Vieta, 2011).

The development of this field is also shown from the existence of one of the longest existing follow-ups for a psychological intervention (five years; Colom et al., 2009) and several comprehensive studies on the health economics of using these therapies in BDs (Scott et al., 2009; Simon, Ludman, Bauer, Unutzer, & Operskalski, 2006). There are also some interesting papers on mediators of response (Miklowitz & Scott, 2009; Reinares et al., 2010).

Despite advances in our understanding of psychological therapies, the first-line treatment for the long term management of BD is, and will remain, pharmacological treatment (Yatham et al., 2009). However, the far-from-satisfactory outcome, even among patients prescribed medications, is a concern, as relapse rates range from 40% to 60% (Tohen et al., 2003; Tohen et al., 2006; Vieta et al., 2011). These data have led to the development of several adjunctive psychological interventions aimed at delaying recurrences, preventing relapses and reducing episode length (Judd et al., 2008; Popovic et al., 2013).

The targets of different psychological interventions may vary, although the boundaries are blurred and often include similar ingredients. Important differences exist as to the content and structure of various psychological interventions, and this chapter aims to present up-to date data regarding psychoeducation and CBT for BDs. In particular, we explore the essential ingredients of psychoeducation and CBT, how these are being applied to BD, and the future directions for research and randomized controlled trials.

PSYCHOEDUCATION

PSYCHOEDUCATION: THE STATE OF THE ART

Psychoeducation evolves from research into health belief models and their influence on the prognosis of a range of chronic physical disorders. It is a cornerstone of the psychological management of diabetes, asthma, and cancer (Bultz et al., 2000; Durna & Ozcan, 2003; Olmsted et al., 2002) and was initially introduced into psychiatry as a strategy to help individuals with schizophrenia (Pekkala & Merinder, 2004). Psychological interventions based on psychoeducation and those that include psychoeducation as an essential component have proved helpful in improving outcomes in BD (Benyon et al., 2008; Scott, Colom, & Vieta, 2007).

The parallels between chronic physical disorders and severe mental disorders help explain why psychoeducation is a core clinical approach. Bipolar disorder is a lifelong, potentially treatable psychiatric disorder with substantial morbidity and mortality (Swann, 2006). Despite advances in pharmacological treatments to ameliorate the biological instability that drives the illness, episodes can be precipitated by psychosocial factors, and the disorder has psychological and social consequences both for the patient and the family (Reinares et al., 2006). These findings, together with

the large "efficacy–effectiveness" gap in treatment benefits and medication adherence problems, highlight the urgent need to augment the available treatments for BDs with evidence-based psychological approaches.

Central to this integrated treatment approach is the recognition that individuals with BD need information about their illness and its treatment and need skills that enable them to participate actively in the management of their illness, as well as ways of minimizing the stigma associated with the disorder. Psychoeducation is a core element of all adjunctive psychological interventions that have proven efficacy in improving outcomes in BD. Despite the different theoretical models that are promoted to explain the phases of BD and the relative emphasis on different strategies, all of the approaches acknowledge the importance of psychoeducation (e.g., CBT, family-focused therapy, IPSRT, and collaborative care approaches; Colom & Lam, 2005).

PRINCIPLES OF PSYCHOEDUCATION

Psychoeducation is an attitudes and aptitudes behavioral training (Colom, in press) aimed at adjusting lifestyle to cope with BD for improved outcome, including enhancement of illness awareness, treatment adherence, early detection of relapse, and avoidance of potentially harmful factors such as drugs misuse and sleep deprivation, rather than mere transmission of information regarding the disorder.

On the other hand, psychoeducation is not the same as the approach promoted in self-help groups. Colom (in press) suggests that, despite the fact that self-help groups may play a role in the management of BDs, their role is rather complementary to psychoeducation, and self-help is not a substitute for psychoeducation as their goals are in fact slightly different. Colom argues that health professionals rather than patient advocates should implement psychoeducation because (a) the degree of clinical training required demands a professional and (b) psychoeducation is a highly structured and targeted intervention that may quite often require a highly directive style from the therapist. Hence, psychoeducation is an intervention that involves good medical practice and seeks to empower patients with tools allowing them to be more active in their treatment. Through this approach, psychoeducation provides an appropriate therapeutic alliance relying on collaboration, information-sharing, and trust.

Psychoeducation may be aimed both at patients and caregivers, as they both could be crucial in reinforcing "healthy" behaviors by the patient.

THE CORE INGREDIENTS OF PSYCHOEDUCATION

The Barcelona Psychoeducation Program consists of 21 sessions, as shown in Table 31.1. The sessions were initially derived from clinical experience and the problems identified by patients and clinicians. The same components are present in most therapeutic packages for BD worldwide, and they have proven to be efficacious in the prevention of recurrences of mood episodes in BD.

The main areas covered in psychoeducation for BD include illness awareness, treatment adherence, early warning signs identification, avoidance of substance misuse, and regulation of habits.

Table 31.1. SESSIONS INCLUDED IN BARCELONA BIPOLAR DISORDERS PSYCHOEDUCATION PROGRAM

SESSION NUMBER	TITLE
1	Introduction
2	What is bipolar illness?
3	Causal and triggering factors
4	Symptoms (I): Mania and hypomania
5	Symptoms (II): Depression and mixed episodes
6	Course and outcome
7	Treatment (I): Mood stabilizers
8	Treatment (II): Antimanic agents
9	Treatment (III): Antidepressants
10	Serum levels: Lithium, carbamazepine, and valproate
11	Pregnancy and genetic counseling
12	Psychopharmacology vs alternative therapies
13	Risks associated with treatment withdrawal
14	Alcohol and street drugs: Risks in bipolar illness
15	Early detection of manic and hypomanic episodes
16	Early detection of depressive and mixed episodes
17	What to do when a new phase is detected
18	Regularity of habits
19	Stress-management techniques
20	Problem-solving techniques
21	Final session: Farewell

Illness awareness

More than half of patients with BD exhibit inadequate insight into their illness, and denial of the disorder or of its severity is quite common, representing one of the main barriers to starting treatment. Although there is evidence of an association between lack of insight and neuropsychological impairment, other factors such as social stigma increase the risk that the diagnosis will initially be rejected by patient.

On the other hand, the attitudes of clinicians and the language they use does not always help the patient move toward acceptance of the diagnosis and the illness. This is why several sessions are devoted to illness acceptance before moving to other essential issues such as symptom management or medication adherence. Thus it is not by chance that "illness awareness" is a key target in the early stages of therapy. This first component of therapy introduces concepts that are drawn on repeatedly during the group program. Consequently, a large number of sessions should be devoted to this topic, helping to refocus the patient on the importance of understanding the biological nature of the disorder and the need for pharmacological treatment. The fact that during psychoeducation a psychiatrist or a psychologist starts the course of therapy by stressing that BD is a medical condition and initially prioritizes psychobiological over psychosocial elements may, at first, be surprising for some patients who expect that therapy is synonymous with the mind rather than the brain. However, such a presentation can open up important avenues for discussion and also emphasizes that the psychoeducation sessions have a clear strategic approach and should not be confused with less cogent, more nebulous (and untested) therapy models.

Adherence enhancement

Improving adherence to treatment must be one of the main objectives of any psychological intervention in BDs, since the problem of poor adherence is certainly a driver of poor outcome in many patients. Poor adherence can be defined as the inability of the patient to engage in health-promoting behaviours or habits, which can include failure to take prescribed medications or follow medical advice. However, nonadherence is a complex phenomenon with many different facets, and it also shows variability over time, with patients being vulnerable to stopping medication at different points in the illness cycle (e.g., when they feel well—and think there is no need to take the medication as they are asymptomatic).

Harm avoidance

Harm avoidance or *reduction* is the term commonly applied to clinical interventions that target substance misuse. The largest study on co-occurrence of BDs and substance use disorders was conducted as part of the National Epidemiologic Survey on Alcohol and Related Conditions, which assessed more than 40,000 people in the United States. According to that study, there was a lifetime prevalence for co-occurring alcohol use disorders of almost 60% of bipolar I patients, and a 38% lifetime prevalence of any drug use disorder, a finding that is supported in general by all of the existing literature. According to the Epidemiologic Catchment Area data, nearly half of bipolar II patients have a comorbid substance use disorder. Thus the risk that a bipolar patient will have a coexisting substance-related problem is six times higher than that of a member of the general population. Alcohol seems to be the most frequently used substance among older bipolar patients, with younger patients also using illicit drugs (particularly cannabis and, less often, amphetamines). Substance use in any age group is associated with a poorer outcome of BD, including increased episodes of depression, adherence problems, and delayed symptomatic recovery. Data from the Systematic Treatment Enhancement Program for Bipolar Disorder (STEP-BD) suggest also that substance-related disorders are strongly associated with an increased number of hospitalizations, and suicide attempts are more frequent among patients with such comorbidity. Furthermore, many patients who do not meet the criteria for substance abuse or dependence consume substances in quantities that are sufficient to trigger new episodes.

Although patients with severe comorbid substance abuse or dependence may need a specific program that tackles this dual pathology, it is very important that any therapy for BD aims to reduce the regular use of substances with psychotropic effects. To achieve this objective, it may be useful not only to focus on alcohol and street drugs but also on apparently "harmless" or socially accepted substances such as caffeine, as these may act as direct triggers of episodes or act indirectly via the impact on the quality of sleep. The importance of "harm reduction" to improve prognosis (by avoiding substance use or other unhealthy behaviors) is reinforced throughout the program, although usually there is only one session specifically devoted to the topic.

Detection of early warning signs

The detection of early warning signs is one of the key elements of a psychoeducation program and probably requires a higher level of therapist skill from the patient than most of the other interventions used in psychoeducation. Identifying early signs consists of three steps. The first and second are generally discussed during the group program, while the third step usually requires individual intervention (although this may not be essential in all cases). The first step consists of *providing information* regarding the most frequently recognized signs of relapse for depression and (hypo)mania. The goal of the second step is to *personalize* these warning signs (i.e., adapt the information from Step 1 to each individual group member). This step allows the group members to identify the warning signs that appear regularly prior to each type of episode that they experience. The third step is referred to as *specialization*. In this step the patient learns to recognize the signals that precede the warning signs identified—that is, the "warnings of warnings." These are typically behavioral or cognitive alterations, or qualitatively different perceptions (such as colors appearing "brighter" at the start of hypomania). These changes might not be pathological in every patient, as they may not cause alarm in another individual. However, these factors are highly specific and thus very important for an individual patient.

Lifestyle regularity

Regular habits and stress management are extremely important in BD and are purported to play a significant role in preventing relapses. Moreover, improving the regularity of day-to-day activities and habits constitute a core ingredient of IPSRT, and many therapies have adopted elements of the social-regulation approach advocated in this therapy. Psychoeducation encourages patients to implement healthy habits through an emphasis on managing sleeping habits/circadian rhythms and also encouraging healthy diet and adequate physical exercise.

Ending psychoeducation

The final sessions of psychoeducation focus on *stress control techniques*, highlighting the importance of stress as a trigger of relapses and as a mechanism to introduce various psychological techniques that can help patients to better cope with stress and anxiety. Problem-solving strategies are discussed, and, finally, the last session offers a summary of the work done during the course of therapy.

OTHER APPROACHES: FAMILY-FOCUSED THERAPY

There is evidence that a stressful family environment (characterized by negative affect and high levels of critical comments) are often associated with exacerbations of BD, and expressed emotion is an important predictor of symptom severity. However, the illness may represent a significant psychological burden for family members and other caregivers. Thus these family problems may represent a cause or a consequence of BD and logically led to the development of a family-orientated psychoeducation and problem-solving approach.

Family-focused therapy was adapted for bipolar patients from a behavioral family therapy intervention that was initially created for patients with psychosis. It usually consists of three broad components: psychoeducation about BD, communication enhancement training, and problem-solving skills training. It is administered in 21 one-hour sessions. It has shown its efficacy, mainly in the prevention of depressive relapses, and is particularly useful for families who demonstrate high levels of expressed emotion at initial clinical assessment.

LONG-TERM OUTCOME OF PSYCHOEDUCATION

Psychological interventions in BD claim to be a maintenance tool. But, by definition, any maintenance tool must show its efficacy in the long term. Unfortunately, most studies of psychological interventions offer a maximum follow-up of two-years. As such, little is known about the longer term benefits of such treatments.

There is long-term follow-up (five years) data supporting the efficacy of group psychoeducation. It has been shown that, at five-year follow-up, psychoeducated patients showed a longer time to recurrence and had fewer recurrences than patients allocated to an unstructured group intervention (Colom et al., 2009).

Furthermore, psychoeducated patients spent much less time acutely ill than patients allocated to the unstructured group, a difference mainly accounted for by the significant difference in time spent depressed. This is likely to be clinically very important, as the number of days spent in depression was a strong predictor of recurrences in the STEP-BD study (Miklowitz et al., 2007).

The number of hospitalizations in psychoeducated patients (mean 0.24) was less than half that observed in the control group (mean 0.59). For each hospitalized patient, the mean duration of admission was also significantly lower for psychoeducated patients (mean

31.7 days; $SD = 16.4$) compared with the control group (mean 68.3 days; $SD = 65.1$).

Although psychoeducated patients did not participate in any "booster" group sessions, they were more likely than the control-group patients to seek out additional therapy during the five-year follow-up. Furthermore, psychoeducated patients were more likely to attend follow-up appointments, to take more prescribed medications, and to take higher doses of prescribed treatments; they were also less likely to need emergency appointments. Thus it appears a time-limited single intervention (of about 30 hours) is associated with clinically and statistically significant improvements on a range of outcomes in cases BDs and that benefits persist for at least at five years postintervention. It is reasonable to suggest that group psychoeducation may promote behavioral and attitudinal changes that in turn led to these improvements.

LIMITATIONS OF PSYCHOEDUCATION

Any efficacious treatment may have drawbacks or limitations. Psychoeducation too has its limits. For example, like most therapies, it is not recommended as a monotherapy, which means that it should always be considered as an adjunct to pharmacotherapy. Another limitation (again shared with many therapies) is that there is no direct replication of the original study, which may be viewed as undermining the validity. Also, randomized controlled treatment trials that focus on efficacy by definition select homogenous, well-defined samples, which may limit the generalizability of the findings. Likewise, there is evidence that it may be less efficacious in those with multiple episodes and/or neuropsychological impairments. Finally, another limitation of psychoeducation is that is not effective in treating acute episodes, and indeed the target population is euthymic patients (as the goal is to prevent episodes).

COGNITIVE BEHAVIOR THERAPY IN BIPOLAR DISORDERS

This section highlight aspects of CBT that differ from some of the general techniques common to all therapies. Because group CBT shares elements of psychoeducation, this section describes individual CBT. Also, we do not review all the outcome data (some of which has already been discussed), save to say that CBT for BDs shows a mixed pattern of benefits. It is useful in treating acute bipolar depression, and, when provided to euthymic patients, it can prevent depressive relapses for up to two years (with less effect on mania). However, in some studies the benefits of CBT were not substantially greater than other therapy models (e.g., Meyer et al., 2013), and data from a large scale effectiveness study indicate that the early introduction of CBT (i.e., targeting the early stages of illness) is most likely to be helpful, with little evidence of significant benefits in complex cases with multiple physical and mental comorbidities.

INDIVIDUAL THERAPY

In individual CBT, the therapy should begin with a cognitive formulation of the individual's specific problems related to BD. In particular, emphasis is placed on the role of core maladaptive beliefs that underpin and determine the content of dysfunctional automatic thoughts and drive patterns of behaviour. These will guide the choice of interventions and the stage of therapy when to employ it for each individual patient. Although each individual will define a specific set of problems, there are common themes that tend to arise across patient groups with BD.

The main aims of therapy are to facilitate adjustment to BD and its treatment, to enhance medication adherence, to improve self-esteem and self-image, and to reduce maladaptive or high-risk behaviors. Furthermore, CBT aims to recognize and modify psycho-biosocial factors that destabilize the individuals day-to-day functioning and mood state; help the individual recognize and manage psychosocial stressors and interpersonal problems; teach strategies to cope with the symptoms of depression, hypomania, and any cognitive and behavioral problems; teach early recognition of relapse symptoms and to develop effective coping techniques; to identify and modify dysfunctional automatic thoughts and underlying maladaptive beliefs; and, finally, to improve self-management by the means of homework assignments (Basco & Rush, 2005; Lam, Jones, Hayward, & Bright, 1999; Newman et al., 2001; Scott, 2000).

At the beginning of the therapy, individuals are encouraged to tell their story and to identify problem areas through the use of a life chart. Current difficulties are then classified into *intrapersonal* (e.g., low self-esteem, cognitive-processing biases), *interpersonal* (e.g., lack of social network), and *basic problems* (e.g., symptom severity, difficulties coping with work). These issues are explored in about 20 to 25 sessions of cognitive therapy that are held weekly until about Week 15 and then with gradually reducing frequency. A few "booster sessions" are used to review the skills and techniques learned. The overall cognitive therapy program comprises four stages.

Stage A: Socialization into the cognitive therapy model and development of an individualized formulation and treatment goals

Therapy begins with an exploration of the patients' understanding of BD and a detailed discussion of previous episodes focusing on identification of prodromal signs, events or stressors associated with onset of previous episodes, typical cognitive and behavioral concomitants of both manic and depressive episodes, and an exploration of interpersonal functioning (e.g., family interactions). A diagram illustrating the cycle of change in BD is used to allow the individual to explore how changes in all aspects of functioning may arise. Early sessions include development of an understanding of key issues identified in the life chart, education about BD, facilitation of adjustment to the disorder by identifying and challenging negative automatic thoughts, and developing behavioral experiments particularly focused on ideas about stigmatization and fragile self-esteem. Other sessions further develop an individualized formulation of the patient's problems, which takes into account underlying maladaptive beliefs.

Stage B: Cognitive and behavioral approaches to symptom management and dysfunctional automatic thoughts

These sessions aim to teach the individual self-monitoring and self-regulation techniques, which enhance self-management of depressive and hypomanic symptoms, and to explore skills for coping with depression and mania. For example, this involves establishing regular activity patterns, daily routines, regular sleep patterns, developing coping skills, time management, use of support, and recognizing and tackling dysfunctional automatic thoughts about self, world, and future using automatic thought diaries.

Stage C: Dealing with cognitive and behavioral barriers to treatment adherence and modifying maladaptive beliefs

Problems with adherence to medication and other aspects of treatment are tackled, for example, through exploration of barriers (challenging automatic thoughts about drugs, beliefs about BD, excessive self-reliance, or exploring attitudes to authority and control) and using behavioral and cognitive techniques. This, together with the data from previous sessions, are used to help the patient identify their maladaptive assumptions and underlying core beliefs and to commence work on modifying these beliefs.

Stage D: Anti-relapse techniques and belief modification

Recognition of early signs of relapse and coping techniques (fortnightly sessions) are addressed. Features include identifying possible prodromal features (the "relapse signature"), developing a list of "at-risk situations" (e.g., exposure to situations that activate specific personal beliefs) and high-risk behaviors (e.g., increased alcohol intake), combined with a hierarchy of coping strategies for each and planning how to cope and self-manage problems after discharge from cognitive therapy. Sessions also include typical cognitive therapy approaches to the modification of maladaptive beliefs, which may otherwise increase vulnerability to relapse.

CONCLUSION AND FUTURE DIRECTIONS

As with any work in progress, the field of psychological interventions for BDs exists on a continuum between well-established evidence of benefits (relapse prevention, adherence enhancement, early warning signs identification) and largely unexplored territories and/or uncertainty that require research in the oncoming years. These include the following.

THE TREATMENT OF BIPOLAR DEPRESSION

From a clinician's perspective, there is a great need for efficacious therapies for bipolar depression, especially given the risks associated with the use of antidepressants (without co-prescription of mood stabilizers) and the limited benefits of antidepressants (Valentí et al., 2012) and of other agents (Pacchiarotti et al., 2009). Although STEP-BD indicated the acute treatment of bipolar depression was facilitated by IPSRT, CBT, or family-focused treatment, we do not have long-term follow-up data from that study. Furthermore, Scott and Etain (2011) note that the depression-prevention effects of different therapies vary significantly, and, apart from the study of Swartz et al (2012), we have limited data on whether some BDs/spectrum disorders (e.g., bipolar II or not otherwise specified, cyclothymia) might be treatable with therapy alone. Such information would be important for cases in which the indications for the use of medication are less clear-cut or the presence of multiple comorbid physical disorders or other issues prevent the optimal use of medications. Also, given advances in our therapy interventions for depression in general, it would be important to know whether new models, such as rumination-focused therapies, are applicable to bipolar cases, or indeed if they have any adverse effects or contra-indications.

COGNITIVE IMPAIRMENT

Cognitive deficits in established cases of BD persist across phases of illness and show a similar pattern, although of a lesser magnitude to those seen in psychosis, with executive functioning, episodic memory, verbal memory, psychomotor speed, and sustained attention most consistently impaired (Andreou & Bozikas, 2013; Martínez-Arán et al., 2004). Given the importance of cognitive functioning for psychosocial outcomes in BD, the development of psychotherapeutic interventions targeting cognitive dysfunction are imperative for improving recovery rates and quality of life in patients. Neurocognition is a potential predictor of response to evidence-based psychosocial interventions (Goetz et al., 2007), and so one aspect of future research in this area will be to determine which patients should receive neurocognitive interventions and which may do best with other psychological therapies. Pooled data from studies that included cases of bipolar, unipolar, and schizoaffective disorders showed that cognitive remediation can be beneficial in affective disorders and probably is at least as effective as in nonaffective psychosis (Anaya et al., 2012). Evidence on the positive effects of broader-based therapies, such as integrated psychological therapy, shows gains in the domains of neurocognition, social cognition, psychosocial functioning, and negative symptoms in psychosis, and the model appears adaptable to BD (Roder, Mueller, & Schmidt, 2011). Overall, functional remediation (Martínez-Arán et al., 2011) is therefore an approach that needs to be examined internationally, especially given the promising data from the multicenter study undertaken across Spain (Torrent et al., 2013).

BIPOLAR DISORDER AT THE "EXTREMES" OF THE AGE RANGE

Increasingly, researchers are examining how to prevent disease progression in BDs and/or whether it is conceivable to prevent a first episode of mania in high-risk individuals. A recent evidence-mapping study by Vallarino and Scott (2014) has shown that there are 15 studies of psychological approaches that target young people at risk of or in the early stages of BD. However, there are only a few randomized trails, so this is an area where data from pilot studies is likely to be followed by larger scale clinical trials.

STUDIES IN THE ELDERLY

Most of the existing psychotherapy trials exclude individuals aged above 65. However, grant-giving bodies recognize that globally we have an aging population, with more adults surviving into old age. As such, it is important to consider what approaches may be most suitable for older (sometimes termed "graduate" bipolar patients). For example, a pilot study of Medication Adherence Skills Training for older adults (Depp et al., 2007) showed improvement in medication adherence and ability to self-manage medications, depressive symptoms, and selected indices of health-related quality of life. Notwithstanding the study limitations (small sample size, absence of comparator, and lack of follow-up data), this promising preliminary data justify further work in this area, and the need for interventions designed for BD patients in later life remains unmet. This paucity of therapies for this age group is alarming particularly if we consider that given the progressive average aging of the whole population, the number of older adults suffering from a severe psychiatric condition is expected to grow progressively in the next few years.

COMORBIDITIES

Physical health

Patients with severe mental illnesses, including BD, are reported to have a 20% (~13–30 years) reduction in their life expectancy compared to members of the general population. The high rate of mortality in patients with severe mental illnesses is mostly attributable to premature cardiovascular and cerebrovascular deaths, which may be a consequence of lifestyle, high rates of smoking, obesity, and metabolic syndrome (De Hert et al., 2011). Rates of obesity (defined as a body mass index ≥30) and metabolic syndrome in BD are reported as 68% and 22% to 30%, respectively (De Hert et al., 2011). Although some of the most widely used medications are associated with weight gain as a side effect, this alone does not explain the excess morbidity and mortality (Torrent et al., 2008). There are CBT and psychoeducation studies underway in the United States, United Kingdom, and Australia that target physical well-being by encouraging regular exercise and dietary changes (and that monitor body mass index, waist circumference, blood sugar, and lipids). The goals are to increase not only quality of life but also expectancy in patients with BD (see Vallarino & Scott, 2013 for a review).

Substance use

Given the prevalence and prognostic significance of substance misuse in patients with BD, we need to revise and evaluate interventions that target these cases more specifically. This is especially important as the models that exist so far have shown missed results (e.g., with reduced alcohol intake not being accompanied by change in outcome in BDs in terms of symptom levels or relapses). This suggests more basic research is required in the reasons and patterns for substance use across time and phases of the disorder in order to develop a more sophisticated model of intervention.

Anxiety disorders

Anxiety disorders represent the most frequent comorbidity of BD (Merikangas et al., 2007). A review examining the effect of psychosocial treatments in this population conducted by Provencher, Hawke, and Thienot (2011) highlighted a surprising paucity of studies that more specifically addressed this topic, and those that existed were all small-scale and/or exploratory. The review suggested that the most promising option was sequential treatment with CBT followed by mindfulness-based therapy and relaxation training. However, it is clear the models of therapy and best methods for delivery warrant further exploration.

These recommendations identify those areas where it is obvious that more research would be helpful. However, given that BDs is both highly heritable and has a peak age at onset in early adulthood, cause can also be made for more research in women of child bearing age. For example, the potential role of preventive psychotherapy in women who may not be taking medication over a period of time.

In summary, the field of evidence-based psychological therapies for BDs is only in its adolescence (having existed for about 15 years). It is entering a critical phase of development, but hopefully it will mature and graduate with flying colors over the next decade.

Disclosure statement: Dr. Popovic's work is supported by a Sara Borrell postdoctoral grant CD13/00149, provided by Carlos III Institute, Spanish Ministry of Health. She has served as speaker for Bristol-Myers Squibb, Merck Sharp & Dohme, and Janssen-Cilag. Prof. Scott has served as advisory or speaker for the following companies (lifetime): Astra Zeneca, BSM-Otsuka, Eli-Lilly, Glaxo-Smith-Kline, Janssen Cilag, Lundbeck, Pfizer, Sanofi-Aventis, and Servier. The University of Newcastle has received independent investigator grants from Astra Zeneca and Janssen Cilag for Scott's research on training in and the evaluation of a psychological intervention to enhance medication adherence in BDs. Dr. Francesc Colom has served as advisory or speaker for the following companies (lifetime): Adamed, Astra Zeneca, Bristol-Myers, Eli-Lilly, Glaxo-Smith-Kline, Lundbeck, MSD-Merck, Otsuka, Pfizer Inc, Rovi, Sanofi-Aventis, Shire and Tecnifar. He has received copyright fees from: Cambridge University Press, Igaku-Shoin Ltd, Solal Ed., Ars Médica, Giovani Fioriti Ed., Medipage, La Esfera de Los Libros, Morales i Torres Ed, Panamericana, Mayo Ed., and Columna.

REFERENCES

Anaya, C., Martinez Aran, A., Ayuso-Mateos, J. L., Wykes, T., Vieta, E., & Scott J. (2012). A systematic review of cognitive remediation for schizo-affective and affective disorders. *Journal of Affective Disorders, 142,* 13–21.

Andreou, C., & Bozikas, V. P. (2013). The predictive significance of neurocognitive factors for functional outcome in bipolar disorder. *Current Opinion in Psychiatry, 26*(1), 54–59.

Basco, M. R., & Rush, J. A. (2005). *Cognitive-behavioral therapy for bipolar disorder* (2nd ed.). New York: Guilford Press.

Beynon, S., Soares-Weiser, K., Woolacott, N., Duffy, S., & Geddes, J. R. (2008). Psychosocial interventions for the prevention of relapse in bipolar disorder: A systematic review of controlled trials. *British Journal of Psychiatry, 192,* 5–11.

Bultz, B. D., Speca, M., Brasher, Geggie, P. H., & Page, S. A. (2000). A randomized controlled trial of a brief psychoeducational support group for partners of early stage breast cancer patients. *Psycho-Oncology, 9,* 303–313.

Colom, F. (2014). The evolution of psychoeducation: From lithium clinics to integrative psychoeducation. *World Psychiatry, 13*(1), 90–92.

Colom, F., & Lam, D. (2005). Psychoeducation: Improving outcomes in bipolar disorder. *European Psychiatry, 20,* 359–364.

Colom, F., & Vieta, E. (2011). The need for publishing the silent evidence from negative trials. *Acta Psychiatrica Scandinavica, 123,* 91–94.

Colom, F., Vieta, E., Martínez, A., Jorquera, A., & Gastó, C. (1998). What is the role of psychotherapy in the treatment of bipolar disorder? *Psychotherapy and Psychosomatics, 67*(1), 3–9.

Colom, F., Vieta, E., Martínez-Arán, A., Reinares, M., Goikolea, J. M., Benabarre, A.,…Corominas, J. (2003). A randomized trial on the efficacy of group psychoeducation in the prophylaxis of recurrences in bipolar patients whose disease is in remission. *Archives of General Psychiatry, 60,* 402–407.

Colom, F., Vieta, E., Sánchez-Moreno, J., Palomino-Otianiano, R., Reinares, M., Goikolea, J. M.,…Martínez-Arán, A. (2009). Group psychoeducation for stabilised bipolar disorders: 5-year outcome of a randomised clinical trial. *British Journal of Psychiatry, 194,* 260–265.

De Hert, M., Correll, C. U., Bobes, J., Cetkovich-Bakmas, M., Cohen, D., Asai, I.,…Leucht, S. (2011). Physical illness in patients with severe mental disorders: I. Prevalence, impact of medications and disparities in health care. *World Psychiatry, 10*(1), 52–77.

Depp, C. A., Lebowitz, B. D., Patterson, T. L., Lacro, J. P., & Jeste, D. V. (2007). Medication adherence skills training for middle-aged and elderly adults with bipolar disorder: Development and pilot study. *Bipolar Disorders, 9,* 636–645.

Durna, Z., & Ozcan, S. (2003). Evaluation of self-management education for asthmatic patients. *Journal of Asthma, 40,* 631–643.

Frank E., Kupfer, D. J., Thase, M. E., Mallinger, A. G., Swartz, H. A., Fagiolini, A. M.,…Monk, T. (2005). Two-year outcomes for interpersonal and social rhythm therapy in individuals with bipolar I disorder. *Archives of General Psychiatry, 62,* 996–1004.

Goetz, I., Tohen, M., Reed, C., Lorenzo, M., Vieta, E., & EMBLEM Advisory Board. (2007). Functional impairment in patients with mania: Baseline results of the EMBLEM study. *Bipolar Disorders, 9*(1–2), 45–52.

Judd, L. L., Schettler, P. J., Akiskal, H. S., Coryell, W., Leon, A. C., Maser, J. D., &Solomon, D. A. (2008). Residual symptom recovery from major affective episodes in bipolar disorders and rapid episode relapse/recurrence. *Archives of General Psychiatry, 65,* 386–394.

Lam, D. H., Jones, S., Hayward, P., & Bright, J. (1999). *Cognitive therapy for bipolar disorder: A therapist's guide to the concept, methods and practice.* Chichester, UK: John Wiley.

Lam, D. H., Watkins, E. R., Hayward, P., Bright, J., Wright, K., Kerr, N.,…Sham, P. (2003). A randomized controlled study of cognitive therapy for relapse prevention for bipolar affective disorder: Outcome of the first year. *Archives of General Psychiatry, 60,* 145–152.

Lobban, F., Taylor, L., Chandler, C., Tyler, E. Kinderman, P., Kolamunnage-Dona, R.,…Morriss, R. K. (2010). Enhanced relapse prevention for bipolar disorder by community mental health teams: Cluster feasibility randomised trial. *British Journal of Psychiatry, 196*(1), 59–63.

Martínez-Arán, A., Torrent, C., Solé, B, Bonnín, C. M., Rosa, A. R., Sánchez-Moreno, J., & Vieta, E. (2011). Functional remediation for bipolar disorder. *Clinical Practice and Epidemiology in Mental Health, 7,* 112–116.

Martínez-Arán, A., Vieta, E., Reinares, M., Colom, F., Torrent, C., Sánchez-Moreno, J.,…Salamero, M. (2004). Cognitive function across manic or hypomanic, depressed, and euthymic states in bipolar disorder. *American Journal of Psychiatry, 161,* 262–270.

Merikangas, K. R., Akiskal, H. S., Angst, J., Greenberg, P. E., Hirschfeld, R. M., Petukhova, M., Kessler, R. C. (2007). Lifetime and 12-month prevalence of bipolar spectrum disorder in the National Comorbidity Survey replication. *Archives of General Psychiatry, 64,* 543–552.

Meyer, T. D., & Hautzinger, M. (2012). Cognitive behaviour therapy and supportive therapy for bipolar disorders: Relapse rates for treatment period and 2-year follow-up. *Psychological Medicine, 42,* 1429–1439.

Miklowitz, D. J., & Scott, J. (2009). Psychosocial treatments for bipolar disorder: Cost-effectiveness, mediating mechanisms, and future directions. *Bipolar Disorders, 11*(2), 110–122.

Miklowitz, D. J., George, E. L., Richards, J. A., Simoneau, T. L., & Suddath, R. L. (2003). A randomized study of family-focused psychoeducation and pharmacotherapy in the outpatient management of bipolar disorder. *Archives of General Psychiatry, 60,* 904–912.

Miklowitz, D. J., Otto, M. W., Frank, E., Reilly-Harrington, N. A., Wisniewski, S. R., Kogan, J. N.,…Sachs, G. S. (2007). Psychosocial treatments for bipolar depression: A 1-year randomized trial from the Systematic Treatment Enhancement Program. *Archives of General Psychiatry, 64*(4), 419–426.

Newman, C. F., Leahy, R. L., Beck, A. T., Reilly- Harrington, N. A., & Gyulai, L. (2001). *Bipolar disorder: A cognitive therapy approach.* Washington, DC: American Psychological Association.

Olmsted, M. P., Daneman, D., Rydall, A. C., Lawson, M. L., & Rodin, G. (2002). The effects of psychoeducation on disturbed eating attitudes and behaviour in young women with type 1 diabetes mellitus. *International Journal of Eating Disorders, 32,* 230–239.

Pacchiarotti, I., Mazzarini, L., Colom, F., Sanchez-Moreno, J., Girardi, P., Kotzalidis, G. D., & Vieta, E. (2009). Treatment-resistant bipolar depression: Towards a new definition. *Acta Psychiatrica Scandinavica, 120,* 429–440.

Pekkala, E., & Merinder, L. (2004). *Psychoeducation for schizophrenia* (Cochrane Review). The Cochrane Library 1. Chichester, UK: John Wiley.

Perry, A., Tarrier, N., Morriss, R., McCarthy, E., & Limb, K. (1999). Randomised controlled trial of efficacy of teaching patients with bipolar disorder to identify early symptoms of relapse and obtain treatment. *BMJ, 318*(7177), 149–153.

Popovic, D., Reinares, M., Scott, J., Nivoli, A., Murru, A., Pacchiarotti, I.,...Colom F. (2013). Polarity index of psychological interventions in maintenance treatment of bipolar disorder. *Psychotherapy and Psychosomatics, 82*(5), 292–298.

Provencher, M. D., Hawke, L. D., & Thienot, E. (2011). Psychotherapies for comorbid anxiety in bipolar spectrum disorders. *Journal of Affective Disorders, 133*, 371–380.

Reinares, M., Colom, F., Rosa, A. R., Bonnín, C. M., Franco, C., Solé B.,...Vieta, E. (2010). The impact of staging bipolar disorder on treatment outcome of family psychoeducation. *Journal of Affective Disorders, 123*(1–3), 81–86.

Reinares, M., Colom, F., Sánchez-Moreno, J., Torrent, C., Martínez-Arán, A., Comes M.,...Vieta, E. (2008). Impact of caregiver group psychoeducation on the course and outcome of bipolar patients in remission: A randomized controlled trial. *Bipolar Disorders, 10*(4), 511–519.

Reinares, M., Vieta, E., Colom, F., Martínez-Arán, A., Torrent, C., Comes, M.,...Sanchez-Moreno, J. (2006). What really matters to bipolar patients' caregivers: Sources of family burden. *Journal of Affective Disorders, 94*, 157–163.

Roder, V., Mueller, D. R., & Schmidt, S. J. (2011). Effectiveness of integrated psychological therapy (IPT) for schizophrenia patients: A research update. *Schizophrenia Bulletin, 37*(2), S71–79.

Scott, J. (2000). *Overcoming mood swings*. London: Constable Robinson.

Scott, J., & Etain, B. (2011). Which psychosocial interventions in bipolar depression? *Encephale, 37*(3), S214–217.

Scott, J., Colom, F., & Vieta, E. (2007). A meta-analysis of relapse rates with adjunctive psychological therapies compared to usual psychiatric treatment for bipolar disorders. *International Journal of Neuropsychopharmacology, 10*, 123–129.

Scott, J., Colom, F., Popova, E., Benabarre, A., Cruz, N., Valenti, M.,...Vieta, E. (2009). Long-term mental health resource utilization and cost of care following group psychoeducation or unstructured group support for bipolar disorders: A cost-benefit analysis. *Journal of Clinical Psychiatry, 70*(3), 378–386.

Scott, J., Paykel, E., Morriss, R., Bentall, R., Kinderman, P., Johnson, T.,...Hayhurst, H. (2006). Cognitive-behavioural therapy for severe and recurrent bipolar disorders: Randomised controlled trial. *British Journal of Psychiatry, 188*, 313–320.

Simon, G. E., Ludman, E. J., Bauer, M. S., Unutzer, J., & Operskalski, B. (2006). Long-term effectiveness and cost of a systematic care management program for bipolar disorder. *Archives of General Psychiatry, 63*, 500–508.

Swann, A. C. (2006). What is bipolar disorder? *American Journal of Psychiatry, 163*, 177–179.

Swartz, H. A., Frank, E., & Cheng, Y. (2012). A randomized pilot study of psychotherapy and quetiapine for the acute treatment of bipolar II depression. *Bipolar Disorders, 14*, 211–216.

Tohen, M., Calabrese, J. R., Sachs, G. S., Banov, M. D., Detke, H. C., Risser, R., & Bowden, C. L. (2006). Randomized, placebo-controlled trial of olanzapine as maintenance therapy in patients with bipolar I disorder responding to acute treatment with olanzapine. *American Journal of Psychiatry, 163*, 247–256.

Tohen, M., Zarate, C. A. Jr., Hennen, J., Khalsa, H. M., Strakowski, S. M., Gebre-Medhin, P.,...Baldessarini, R. J. (2003). The McLean-Harvard First-Episode Mania Study: Prediction of recovery and first recurrence. *American Journal of Psychiatry, 160*, 2099–2107.

Torrent, C., Amann, B., Sánchez-Moreno, J., Colom, F., Reinares, M., Comes, M.,...Vieta, E. (2008). Weight gain in bipolar disorder: Pharmacological treatment as a contributing factor. *Acta Psychiatrica Scandinavica, 118*, 4–18.

Torrent, C., Bonnin Cdel, M., Martínez-Arán, A., Valle, J., Amann, B. L., González-Pinto, A.,...Vieta E. (2013). Efficacy of functional remediation in bipolar disorder: A multicenter randomized controlledstudy. *American Journal of Psychiatry, 170*(8), 852–859.

Valentí, M., Pacchiarotti, I., Bonnín, C. M., Rosa, A. R., Popovic, D., Nivoli, A. M.,...Vieta, E. (2012). Risk factors for antidepressant-related switch to mania. *Journal of Clinical Psychiatry, 73*(2), 271–276.

Vallarino, M., & Scott, J. (2014). State of the art: psychotherapies for individuals at risk, or experiencing a first episode, of bipolar disorder. *Clinical Insights: Mental Health in Adolescents: Bipolar Disorder, 127*–143.

Vieta, E., Günther, O., Locklear, J., Ekman, M., Miltenburger, C., Chatterton, M. L.,...Paulsson, B. (2011): Effectiveness of psychotropic medications in the maintenance phase of bipolar disorder: A meta-analysis of randomized controlled trials. *International Journal of Neuropsychopharmacology, 14*, 1029–1049.

Yatham, L. N., Kennedy, S. H., Schaffer, A., Parikh, S. V., Beaulieu, S., O'Donovan, C.,...Kapczinski, F. (2009). Canadian Network for Mood and Anxiety Treatments (CANMAT) and International Society for Bipolar Disorders (ISBD) collaborative update of CANMAT guidelines for the management of patients with bipolar disorder: Update 2009. *Bipolar Disorders, 11*, 225–255.

32.

FAMILY-FOCUSED THERAPY, INTERPERSONAL AND SOCIAL RHYTHM THERAPY, AND DIALECTICAL BEHAVIORAL THERAPY

Noreen A. Reilly-Harrington, Stephanie Roberts, and Louisa G. Sylvia

INTRODUCTION

This chapter focuses on three psychosocial approaches to the treatment of bipolar disorder: family-focused therapy (FFT), interpersonal and social rhythm therapy (IPSRT), and dialectical behavioral therapy (DBT). We present an overview of each approach, including underlying theoretical bases, targets for treatment, and a description of therapeutic interventions. We also summarize the current empirical support for each modality in the treatment of bipolar disorder.

FAMILY-FOCUSED THERAPY

RATIONALE FOR FAMILY-FOCUSED THERAPY

Expressed emotion (EE) is a construct drawn from the schizophrenia literature that refers to critical, hostile, or emotionally overinvolved (overprotectiveness, extreme self-sacrifice) attitudes that caregivers exhibit toward mentally ill family members and has been shown to increase risk of relapse (Hooley, 2007). EE is assessed by conducting a clinical interview with the familial caregivers of patients who are suffering from an acute episode. Much research has found that bipolar patients whose familial caregivers express high levels of EE are more likely to have high rates of relapse and/or poor symptomatic outcomes over nine-month to two-year follow-up, as compared to patients with low EE caregivers (e.g., Miklowitz, Goldstein, Neuchterlein, Snyder, & Mintz, 1988). These findings form the theoretical basis for the development of FFT, as it targets the modification of these familial interaction patterns,

with the goal of both aiding in recovery and relapse prevention (Miklowitz, 2008).

ELEMENTS OF TREATMENT

FFT is typically delivered in 21 sessions over a nine-month period (weekly for three months, biweekly for three months, and monthly for three months). A thorough assessment is conducted prior to treatment, in which the emotional attitudes and communication patterns between the patient and family members are carefully evaluated.

The treatment consists of three modules, the first of which is psychoeducation (about seven sessions). During this module patients and their family members learn a great deal of information about bipolar disorder. They discuss symptoms, causes, and treatment of bipolar disorder. Medication compliance is emphasized and the vulnerability-stress model is explained. Patients and their families learn that the course of bipolar disorder is affected by both biological and environmental factors. Coping mechanisms for dealing with stress are developed, and family members are taught to discern personality traits from mood symptoms. They also work together to formulate a relapse-prevention plan by specifying early warning signs of relapse. Stigma and the emotional impact of bipolar disorder on all family members is explored and discussed.

The second module focuses on communication skills (7 to 10 sessions). Using a role-playing/behavioral-rehearsal format, patients and caregivers are taught strategies for coping with intrafamilial stress and improving face-to-face verbal and nonverbal communication. Exercises focus on improving active listening skills, delivering positive/negative feedback, and respectfully requesting changes in behavior. Specific homework assignments reinforce these skills.

Finally, the third module targets problem-solving (four to five sessions). Patients learn to define specific problems related to bipolar disorder and to brainstorm, evaluate, and implement solutions. Typical problems addressed in this module concern medication noncompliance, social-occupational impairment, housing issues, and damage due to previous episodes. Crisis intervention is provided on an as-needed basis throughout FFT and treatment is flexible to address specific life events and early warning signs of episodes, with the goal of preventing relapse.

EMPIRICAL SUPPORT IN TREATMENT OF ADULTS

Numerous randomized controlled trials, as well as several open trials, have supported the effectiveness of FFT for adults with bipolar disorder (see Miklowitz, 2012, for a review). Table 32.1 summarizes the results of the four randomized controlled trials in adults.

In an early study of FFT, 101 adult patients were randomized following an acute manic, mixed, or depressive episode to 21 sessions of FFT plus pharmacotherapy or to 2 sessions of family-based crisis management plus pharmacotherapy (Miklowitz, George, Richards, Simoneau, & Suddath, 2003). At two years, patients undergoing FFT had a greater likelihood of survival without disease relapse (52%) than patients in crisis management (17%). Patients undergoing FFT also showed greater reductions in mood symptoms and better medication adherence than patients in crisis management.

Another early randomized controlled trial of FFT compared FFT plus pharmacotherapy to individual therapy plus pharmacotherapy in 53 patients recently discharged from the hospital following a manic episode (Rea et al., 2003). While the groups did not differ in rates of relapse or rehospitalization during the first year of treatment, patients in FFT showed lower rehospitalization rates and symptomatic relapse than patients in individual therapy at one- to two-year posttreatment follow-up.

The Systematic Treatment Enhancement Program for Bipolar Disorder (STEP-BD) was conducted at 15 US sites and compared up to 30 sessions of intensive therapy: FFT, IPSRT (Frank, 2005), or cognitive-behavioral therapy (Otto, Reilly-Harrington, Kogan, Henin, & Knauz, 2008) with three sessions of a brief psychoeducational approach (collaborative care [CC]) in 293 acutely depressed patients with bipolar I or II disorder. All three of the intensive therapies were associated with higher one-year recovery rates (105/163, or 64.4%) than CC (67/130 or 51.5%). Adding intensive psychotherapy to medication management speeded recovery by an average of 110 days during the study year (Miklowitz, Otto, Frank, Reilly-Harrington, Wisniewski, et al., 2007). Furthermore, patients in intensive treatment were 1.58 times more likely to be well in any month of the one-year study than patients in CC. Patients in intensive therapy also reported better total functioning, relationship functioning, and life satisfaction than patients in CC (Miklowitz, Otto, Frank, Reilly-Harrington, Kogan et al., 2007).

Table 32.1. RANDOMIZED CONTROLLED TRIALS OF FFT COMBINED WITH PHARMACOTHERAPY IN ADULTS WITH BIPOLAR DISORDER

STUDY	SAMPLE SIZE	MOOD STATE	CONTROL GROUP	OUTCOME
Miklowitz et al. (2003)	101	Depressive, mixed, or manic episode in past 3 mos.	CM	FFT, 52% survival rate CM, 17% Survival rate FFT: Greater reduction in mood symptoms and better medication adherence
Rea et al. (2003)	53	Manic episode in past 3 mos.	IT	FFT, 12% Rehospitalization IT, 60% Rehospitalization
Miklowitz et al. (2007)	293	Currently in major depressive episode	3 Educational sessions—CC	Intensive Treatment (FFT, CBT, or IPSRT) 64% Recovered and greater social functioning/life satisfaction CC, 52% Recovered
Perlick et al. (2010)	46 caregivers of adults with BD	Various mood states	HE via videotapes	Both caregivers and patients in FFT had greater reduction in depressive symptoms than in HE

NOTE. FFT = family-focused therapy; CM = crisis management; IT = individual therapy; CC = collaborative care; IPSRT = interpersonal and social rhythm therapy; HE = health education; BD = bipolar disorder.

FFT has also been adapted and tested for use with the caregivers of patients with bipolar disorder (Perlick et al., 2010). This form of FFT (known as FFT–health promoting intervention [HPI]) aims to reduce symptoms of bipolar disorder by enhancing caregivers' illness management and self-care. Perlick et al. (2010) randomly assigned the primary caregivers of 46 patients with bipolar disorder to receive either 12 to15 sessions of a modified version of FFT-HPI or an 8- to 12-session health education intervention delivered via videotapes. Randomization to FFT-HPI was associated with significant decreases in both caregivers' and patients' depressive symptoms.

APPLICATION OF FAMILY-FOCUSED THERAPY TO YOUTH WITH BIPOLAR DISORDER AND THOSE AT RISK

While FFT was initially developed for the treatment of adults with bipolar disorder, it has more recently been studied in adolescents and children with bipolar disorder (Miklowitz et al., 2008), as well as modified for youth who are genetically at risk for bipolar disorder (Miklowitz et al., 2013). Strong empirical support has been found for the use of FFT in hastening and sustaining recovery from depressive symptoms in adolescents with bipolar disorders and in those at high risk for bipolar disorders. Longer term follow-up will examine whether early FFT delays or prevents the development of full manic episodes in those at high genetic risk for bipolar disorder.

INTERPERSONAL AND SOCIAL RHYTHM THERAPY

RATIONALE FOR INTERPERSONAL AND SOCIAL RHYTHM THERAPY

Ehlers, Frank, and Kupfer (1988) proposed that depressive symptoms arise as a consequence of life events disturbing social *zeitgebers* (or external cues that function to entrain biological rhythms), which, in turn, derail social and biological rhythms. According to this social *zeitgeber* theory, disruptions in these rhythms influence somatic symptoms (e.g., sleep propensity), which, in vulnerable individuals, can lead to a major depressive episode (see Figure 32.1).

This theory begins with the concept that life events can trigger depressive episodes, but it has been proposed that they may also trigger manic episodes (Frank, 2005; Grandin, Alloy, & Abramson, 2006). For example, several studies have found that elevated levels of life stress precede

(hypo)manic symptoms and episodes (Hammen & Gitlin, 1997; Johnson & Miller, 1997). More specifically, the social *zeitgeber* theory (Figure 32.1) suggests that life events affect symptomatology by disrupting circadian rhythms. For example, research indicates that life events that disrupt one's social rhythms are associated with manic episodes (Malkoff-Schwartz et al., 2000). Another study found that social rhythm disruption due to jet lag and working the night shift tends to lead naturally to dysphoria, which most often develops into depression (Jones, 2001). In addition, improving the regularity of one's social and/or biological cues reduces the negative effect of social rhythm disruptions (Frank, Swartz, & Kupfer, 2000; Howland & Thase, 1999). Moreover, individuals with bipolar disorder tend to have less-regular daily schedules than matched normal controls, and this predicted prospectively a greater likelihood of depressive and (hypo)manic episodes (Shen, Alloy, & Abramson, 2005). These studies suggest, as proposed by the social *zeitgeber* theory (Figure 32.1), that bipolar individuals may be particularly susceptible to disruptions in their daily routines and that these disruptions may be triggers of their symptoms and affective episodes.

Given these data, Frank (2005) developed IPSRT specifically to help patients with bipolar disorder improve their circadian rhythms as a way to improve their course of illness. IPSRT includes components of interpersonal therapy (Klerman, Weissman, Rousaville, & Chevron, 1984), as Frank proposed that improving a patient's daily social routines, or rhythms, requires improving one's interpersonal effectiveness.

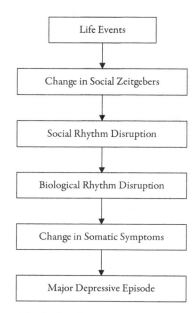

Figure 32.1 The social *zeitgeber* theory

DESCRIPTION OF INTERPERSONAL AND SOCIAL RHYTHM THERAPY

IPSRT has four phases of treatment (Frank, 2005). The first phase, or the initial treatment phase, consists of a focused review of the patient's history in order to understand the impact of social routines and interpersonal relationships on the patient's bipolar episodes. This phase is typically three to five sessions. An Interpersonal Inventory (Klerman et al., 1984) is conducted to assess the quality of patient's previous relationships, as well as the Social Rhythm Metric (Monk, Flaherty, Frank, Hoskinson, & Kupfer, 1990) to determine the regularity of a patient's daily social routines. Finally, a participant selects an interpersonal problem area (i.e., unresolved grief, role transitions, interpersonal role disputes, interpersonal deficits, grief of the loss of the healthy self) to be the initial focus of their therapy.

The second, or intermediate, phase of treatment aims to improve patient's daily social routines or rhythms by improving the selected interpersonal problem area. It is hypothesized that making desired interpersonal changes may have a positive impact on social rhythm regularity, as well as act as a buffer against potentially harmful, future interpersonal relations. This phase can vary in length, as resolving one of these interpersonal problem areas could take several years. For example, the interpersonal problem area of unresolved grief, or individuals still in mourning, may involve teaching patients about the normal process of grief, providing guidance on how to express emotions, and offering support for experiencing grief. The interpersonal therapy manual describes these strategies in greater detail (Klerman et al, 1984). In support of the IPSRT model, evidence suggests that grieving individuals are more likely to have difficulty maintaining a regular routine (Brown et al., 1996), and thus IPSRT seeks to improve daily social rhythms by assisting with this potentially problematic interpersonal area.

IPSRT is also flexible in using other strategies to help individuals establish and maintain stable social rhythms. For example, monitoring medication adherence, effectively managing medication side effects, reducing use of alcohol or drugs, improving one's exercise and nutrition, and involving support (e.g., family, friends, peer support groups, professional help) may all be employed in IPSRT to create a better daily routine for patients. The IPSRT model also focuses on therapy-interfering behaviors, such as seasonal changes, poor therapeutic rapport, or countertransference, and aims to address them accordingly. In short, IPSRT does not suggest that the modification of daily rhythms occurs in isolation but instead requires a good therapeutic relationship and the minimization of other confounding issues that could disrupt one's daily routine.

The third, or continuation/maintenance phase, works to establish patients' confidence in their ability to maintain regular daily schedules and interpersonal relationships. This involves continued effort in problem-solving obstacles to maintaining a regular schedule, such as ongoing issues related to their interpersonal problem area or addressing a secondary interpersonal problem area (i.e., unresolved grief, role transitions, interpersonal role disputes, interpersonal deficits, grief of the loss of the healthy self).

The final phase of treatment is the process of termination with the patient. This phase may last three to five months and consist of monthly or near monthly visits. This phase is focused on healthy termination of the therapeutic relationship with the patient while offering tips for adhering to the goals in the first three phases of IPSRT.

EMPIRICAL EVIDENCE OF INTERPERSONAL AND SOCIAL RHYTHM THERAPY

One hundred seventy-five acutely ill patients with bipolar I disorder were randomized to one of four treatment strategies: (a) IPSRT in the acute phase, followed by an intensive clinical management (ICM) in the preventative phase (IPSRT/ICM); (b)ICM in the acute phase, followed by IPSRT in the preventative phase(ICM/IPSRT); (c) IPSRT in the acute phase, followed by IPSRT in the preventative phase(IPSRT/IPSRT); or (d) ICM in the acute phase, followed by ICM in the preventative phase (ICM/ICM; Frank et al., 1999, 2005). All patients also received psychopharmacological treatment. The ICM control group offered nonspecific support, review of symptoms and side effects, and education about bipolar disorder, medications, and sleep hygiene. The ICM and IPSRT sessions were both administered weekly in the acute phase and then tapered to biweekly and monthly in the preventative phase, but the ICM sessions were half as long as the IPSRT sessions (20 vs. 45 minutes).

After two years of follow-up in the preventative phase, participants treated with IPSRT, as opposed to ICM, in the acute phase experienced longer episode-free periods and were more likely to remain well, irrespective of preventative treatment assignment (Frank et al., 2005) Further, this association was mediated by increased social rhythm regularity for participants receiving IPSRT. Interestingly, IPSRT was more effective for patients who were in better physical health or who had lower levels of medical burden. While the IPSRT group did not initially reach a stable or almost symptom-free state faster than the ICM group, these results provide support for the use of IPSRT in managing bipolar I disorder, particularly with regard to the prevention of new episodes (Frank et al., 2005).

One pilot study conducted with adolescents who had bipolar spectrum disorders found that IPSRT was well tolerated and significantly improved participants' manic, depressive, and general psychiatric symptoms and global functioning over 20 weeks of treatment (Hlastala, Kotler, McClellan, & McCauley, 2010). Effect sizes ranged from medium-large to large. While this study did not use a control group or report findings on whether social rhythm regularity mediated the positive outcomes, it suggests promise for the application of IPSRT in adolescent bipolar populations.

Another recent pilot study compared IPSRT to quetiapiane for the acute treatment of bipolar II depression (Swartz, Frank, & Cheng, 2012). Twenty-five unmedicated, depressed patients with bipolar II disorder were randomly assigned to weekly sessions of IPSRT monotherapy or to quetiapine (flexibly dosed) and followed for 12 weeks. Both groups showed significant decreases in depression and mania scores; however, there were no significant differences between treatment groups. While this was a small sample and conclusions are limited, the authors raise the controversial question of whether pharmacotherapy may be necessary for all individuals with bipolar II disorder. Moreover, these preliminary data suggest the potential utility of IPSRT for individuals with bipolar II disorder for whom pharmacotherapy is contraindicated or intolerable.

In summary, IPSRT is a promising adjunctive psychotherapy for bipolar disorder. It offers a solid rationale, the social *zeitgeber* theory, as to why it may be particularly helpful for patients with bipolar disorder who generally lack regularity in social rhythms. Moreover, IPSRT may be one of the few psychosocial approaches that might be helpful when bipolar patients are in episode or acute phases of treatment and may also reduce risk of relapse. However, similar to most psychotherapies developed to date, future work is needed to elucidate its mediators. For example, further studies should clarify whether social rhythm regularity is responsible for the improvements in bipolar symptoms and functioning in patients treated with IPSRT. Future studies should also more closely examine promising applications of IPSRT for adolescents and patients with bipolar II disorder.

DIALECTICAL BEHAVIOR THERAPY

RATIONALE FOR DIALECTICAL BEHAVIOR THERAPY

DBT was originally developed specifically to treat individuals with borderline personality disorder. Studies of DBT have found it to be the most effective psychosocial treatment for borderline personality disorder (Bohus et al., 2000; Linehan, Armstrong, Suarez, Allmon, & Heard, 1991, 1993). DBT is a principle-driven therapy (Van Dijk, 2012) based on a dialectical worldview (Linehan, 1993). This worldview has three primary characteristics. First, it considers all behaviors to be interrelated. Second, reality is viewed as a number of internal opposing forces, such that it is necessary to integrate differing and opposite views. The third characteristic of the dialectical worldview is that the nature of reality is a process of continuous change, and therefore it is essential to become comfortable with change.

Linehan (1993), the founder of DBT, posits in her biosocial theory that the core disorder in borderline personality disorder is emotion dysregulation. This dysregulation manifests in afflicted individuals as a combination of an overly active and sensitive emotional response system coupled with a failure to moderate the strong emotions and behaviors that follow.

ELEMENTS OF DIALECTICAL BEHAVIOR THERAPY

The main target in DBT is emotion dysregulation. Consequently, DBT is designed to teach a number of strategies that will replace ineffective and maladaptive behavior with skillful responses. These strategies are divided into four core skills areas: mindfulness, distress tolerance, emotional regulation, and interpersonal effectiveness (see Figure 32.2). Mindfulness teaches people to become more aware of their emotions, behaviors, and thoughts. In doing so, they improve their self-control and their ability to manage upsetting emotions and thoughts. Distress-tolerance skills are crisis survival skills that help people identify alternative ways of responding to overwhelming urges like the urge to physically harm oneself or to use alcohol or drugs. Emotion-regulation skills help people manage their emotions more effectively by teaching them to validate their feelings before they become too strong. Individuals also learn to engage in behaviors opposite to their emotions to prevent emotional escalation. Interpersonal effectiveness

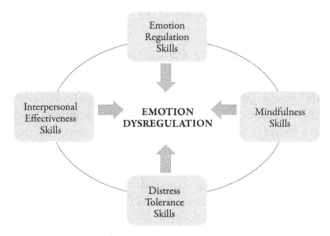

Figure 32.2 Elements of DBT

skills primarily teach assertiveness strategies that can improve relationships and reduce interpersonal disorder.

Throughout the course of DBT treatment, acceptance and validation of current behavior is emphasized. The focus on acceptance comes from a blend of Eastern spirituality and Western treatment approaches. Unlike standard cognitive-behavioral therapies, DBT focuses on balancing acceptance and change. Thoughts, feelings, and behaviors are not considered "distorted" or "wrong" but rather are accepted nonjudgmentally before changes are considered. In DBT, there is also an emphasis on the importance of "therapy-interfering behaviors." Such behaviors are comparable to transference and countertransference from psychodynamic theories. In addition, in DBT the nature of the therapeutic relationship is highly valued and considered critical in order to make meaningful therapeutic progress.

Typically DBT consists of two components for clients: weekly individual therapy sessions and weekly group skills-training sessions, which are held over the course of about one year. In the group sessions, participants are taught the four core skills, and in the individual sessions participants discuss the application of these skills, as well as any issues that have arisen that week. Neither component is intended to be used alone but rather to complement each other. Telephone contact with the individual therapist in between sessions is also a part of DBT procedures (Linehan, 1993), as is a therapy or consultation team that meets regularly and consists of all of the therapists involved in a DBT clinic.

APPLICATIONS TO BIPOLAR DISORDER

Like borderline personality disorder, bipolar disorder is characterized primarily by mood instability. Furthermore,

both conditions are characterized by impulsivity, suicidality, interpersonal difficulties, and treatment nonadherence. Given these similarities, it would seem appropriate that the DBT skills (i.e., mindfulness, distress tolerance, emotion dysregulation, and interpersonal effectiveness) that have been found to be effective in treating borderline personality disorder would also be effective in treating bipolar disorder. However, to date, only a limited number of studies have investigated the effectiveness of DBT in treating bipolar disorder: there are two published studies examining the use of all four core DBT skills and four studies that examined only the DBT core skill of mindfulness. These studies are reviewed next.

EMPIRICAL SUPPORT FOR DIALECTICAL BEHAVIOR THERAPY

Goldstein, Axelson, Birmaher, and Brent (2007) treated 10 adolescents with bipolar disorder and a high degree of illness severity in an open pilot trial of DBT. This intervention was delivered over the course of one year and was divided into two modalities: family skills training (conducted with the family unit) and individual therapy. For the first six months, sessions were held weekly and alternated between the two modalities. There were 12 additional sessions in the final six months to total 18 hours of skills training and 18 hours of individual therapy in the one-year period. In addition, the therapist was available between sessions via pager for coaching. Feasibility and acceptability of the treatment was high. In addition, results indicated that significant improvement was made in reducing suicidality, self-harming behaviors, emotional dysregulation, and depressive symptoms in this adolescent population.

In the only randomized, controlled study of DBT in a sample of individuals with bipolar disorder, Van Dijk, Jeffrey, and Katz (2013) randomized 26 adults with bipolar I or II to intervention or wait-list control. The intervention consisted of twelve 90-minute sessions of which two provided information on bipolar disorder, one on medications used to treat bipolar disorder, and one on self-care skills. The remaining eight sessions were devoted to teaching the three core DBT skills: distress tolerance skills, emotion regulation, and interpersonal effectiveness. The last core DBT skill, mindfulness, was emphasized throughout the 12 weeks. Results indicated that DBT skills reduced depressive symptoms and improved affective control and mindfulness self-efficacy.

In a currently unpublished study, Eisner, Gironde, Nierenberg, and Deckersbach (2013) examined the DBT components of emotion regulation, distress tolerance, and mindfulness in 37 individuals with bipolar disorder over the course of 12 weeks. Overall, this open intervention was well received, and participants showed improvements in general functioning and in the skill areas. Clinician-rated levels of depression and mania did not change over the course of treatment; however, they were relatively low to begin with in this sample, and self-reported depression scores did decrease from pre- to posttreatment. Collectively, these three studies suggest that DBT is well tolerated by individuals with bipolar disorder and may improve mood symptoms, as well as other symptoms related to the disorder (e.g., suicidality).

Mindfulness is unique among the four DBT skill areas because it is emphasized throughout the course of DBT treatment. Therefore, in reviewing studies of DBT and bipolar disorder, it also makes sense to examine studies that have been conducted using mindfulness to treat bipolar disorder. Segal, Williams, and Teasdale (2002) developed a mindfulness-based cognitive therapy for depression, which is a psychotherapy that combines mindfulness practices with psychoeducation about depression. Typically, this course of therapy is eight weeks long. Several studies have applied MBCT in the treatment of bipolar disorder: to date, there have been four studies. The first, conducted by Williams and colleagues (2008), used mindfulness-based cognitive therapy to examine symptoms of depression and anxiety, a common comorbid condition in bipolar disorder, in a group of people with bipolar disorder in remission. In this study, data from a pilot randomized trial of MBCT for 14 people with bipolar disorder, who also had a history of suicidal ideation or behavior, was examined. Participants were randomly assigned to MBCT group or a wait-list control condition. The MBCT classes were led by two experienced therapists and consisted of 12 to 15 participants who met weekly for two hours over a period of eight weeks. Results showed reductions in residual depressive symptoms, as well as significant effects of MBCT in reducing anxiety overtime.

The second study examining the use of mindfulness as a treatment for bipolar disorder was a feasibility trial conducted by Weber and colleagues (2010). In this open study, 15 individuals with various subtypes of bipolar disorder met weekly for two hours over a period of eight weeks. No improvement in symptoms was found, but MBCT was found to be feasible and well perceived among participants. In addition, self-report surveys indicated that MBCT improved participants' ability to cope with emotions.

Deckersbach and colleagues (2012) examined MBCT in 12 nonremitted individuals with bipolar disorder with high levels of residual mood symptoms. In this open trial, MBCT for bipolar disorder consisted of twelve, 120-minute group treatment sessions conducted weekly over the course of three months. At the end of treatment and at three-month follow-up, participants showed increased mindfulness, lower residual mood symptoms, less attentional difficulties, and increased emotion-regulation abilities, psychological well-being, positive affect, and psychological functioning.

Perich, Manicavasager, Mitchell, Ball, and Hadzi-Pavlovic (2013) conducted the only randomized controlled trial of MBCT in individuals with bipolar disorder. This trial examined compared the efficacy of MBCT plus treatment as usual or treatment as usual in 95 participants with bipolar disorder over a one-year period. The MBCT treatment was an adaptation of the eight-week MCBT course developed by Segal and colleagues (2002). Although MBCT did not reduce time to relapse of depression or mania/hypomania or the total number of episodes or mood symptom severity at 12-month follow-up, the results suggested that there was a significant effect for reducing anxiety comorbid with bipolar disorder. This finding is consistent with the findings of Williams et al. (2008) for anxiety.

In summary, DBT, and mindfulness in particular, appear to be a potentially effective adjunctive treatment for bipolar disorder, as well as comorbid anxiety. Since bipolar disorder is characterized by mood dysregulation and all four DBT core skills target emotion dysregulation, it makes logical sense that DBT would be useful in treating this disorder. The proposed mechanisms are as follows: the mindfulness skills teach individuals with bipolar disorder to be more aware of their thoughts, feelings, and behaviors so that they have better control and management of them. The distress-tolerance skills provide alternative ways to cope with the impulsivity that often accompanies bipolar disorder. Emotion-regulation skills teach individuals effective methods of managing emotions before they become overwhelming as they do in episodes of depression or mania/hypomania. Finally, the interpersonal effectiveness skills help restore and maintain interpersonal relationships, an important skill, as, due to the nature of the moods and behaviors in bipolar disorder, problems in interpersonal relationships are common.

However, despite the logic that DBT would be effective in treating bipolar disorder, there are only a few studies to date. The core DBT skill of mindfulness has received the most attention, as evidenced by the development of MBCT, but there are only two published studies to date that examine all four DBT skill areas, and only one of those was a randomized control trial. Although results from these studies are promising, further randomized controlled trials are needed to evaluate the efficacy of DBT in individuals with bipolar disorder. In particular, it may be beneficial to compare DBT to other known effective treatments for bipolar disorder.

Disclosure statement: Dr. Noreen A. Reilly-Harrington was a shareholder in Concordant Rater Systems and serves a consultant for Clintara and Bracket. She receives royalties from the American Psychological Association, New Harbinger, and Oxford University Press. Stephanie Roberts serves as a consultant Clintara and receives monetary compensation from them for services rendered but has no other conflicts to disclose. Dr. Sylvia was a shareholder in Concordant Rater Systems and serves as a consultant for United Biosource Corporation and Clintara. She receives grant funding from National Institute of Mental Health and American Foundation of Suicide and royalties from New Harbinger.

REFERENCES

Bohus, M., Haaf, B., Stiglmayr, C., Pohl, U., Bohme, R., & Linehan, M. (2000). Evaluation of inpatient dialectical-behavioral therapy for borderline personality disorder: A prospective study. *Behavior Research and Therapy, 36*, 3–15.

Brown, L. F., Reynolds, C. F., Monk, T. H., Prigerson, H. G., Dew, M. A., Houck, P. R.,...Kupfer, D. J. (1996). Social rhythm stability following late-life spousal bereavement: Associations with depression and sleep impairment. *Psychiatry Research, 62*, 161–169.

Deckersbach, T., Holzel, B. K, Eisner, L. R, Stange, J. P, Peckham, A. D, Dougherty, D. D,...Nierenberg, A. A. (2012).Mindfulness-based cognitive therapy for nonremitted patients with bipolar disorder. *CNS Neuroscience and Therapeutics, 18*(2), 133–141.

Ehlers, C. L., Frank, E., & Kupfer, D. J. (1988). Social zeitgebers and biological rhythms. *Archives of General Psychiatry, 45*, 948–952.

Eisner, L., Gironde, S., Nierenberg, A. A., & Deckersbach, T. (2013, June). Enhancing emotion regulation in bipolar disorder. Paper presented at the the10th annual meeting of the International Society for Bipolar Disorders, Miami Beach, FL.

Frank, E. (2005). *Treating bipolar disorder: A clinician's guide to interpersonal and social rhythm therapy*. New York: The Guilford Press.

Frank, E., Kupfer, D. J., Thase, M. E., Mallinger, A. G., Swartz, H. A., Fagiolini, A. M.,...Monk, T. (2005). Two-year outcomes for interpersonal and social rhythm therapy in individuals with bipolar I disorder. *Archives of General Psychiatry, 62*, 996–1004.

Frank, E., Swartz, H. A., & Kupfer, D. J. (2000). Interpersonal and social rhythm therapy: Managing the chaos of bi polar disorder. *Biological Psychiatry, 48*, 593–604.

Frank, E., Swartz, H. A., Mallinger, A. G., Thase, M. E., Weaver, E. V., & Kupfer, D. J. (1999). Adjunctive psychotherapy for bipolar disorder: Effects of changing treatment modality. *Journal of Abnormal Psychology, 108*, 579–587.

Grandin, L. D., Alloy, L. B., & Abramson, L. Y. (2006). The social zeitgeber theory, circadian rhythms, and mood disorders: Review and evaluation. *Clinical Psychology Review, 26*, 679–694.

Goldstein, T. R., Axelson, D. A., Birmaher, B., & Brent, D. A. (2007). Dialectical behavior therapy for adolescents with bipolar disorder: A 1-year open trial. *Journal of the American Academy of Child & Adolescent Psychiatry, 46*, 820–830.

Hammen, C., & Gitlin, M. (1997). Stress reactivity in bipolar patients and its relation to prior history of disorder. *The American Journal of Psychiatry, 154*, 856–857.

Hlastala, S. A., Kotler, J. S., McClellan, J. M., & McCauley, E. A. (2010). Interpersonal and social rhythm therapy for adolescents with bipolar disorder: Treatment development and results from an open trial. *Depression and Anxiety, 27*, 457–464.

Hooley, J. M. (2007). Expressed emotion and relapse of psychopathology. *Annual Review of Clinical Psychology, 3*, 329–352.

Howland, R. H., & Thase, M. E. (1999). *Affective disorders: Biological aspects*. London: Oxford University Press.

Johnson, S. L., & Miller, I. (1997). Negative life events and time to recovery from episodes of bipolar disorder. *Journal of Abnormal Psychology, 106*, 449–457.

Jones, S. E. (2001). Circadian rhythms, multilevel models of emotion and bipolar disorder- An initial step towards integration? *Clinical Psychology Review, 21*, 1193–1209.

Klerman, G. L., Weissman, M. M., Rousaville, B. J., & Chevron, E. S. (1984). *Interpersonal psychotherapy for depression*. New York: Basic Books.

Linehan, M. M., Armstrong, H. E., Suarez, A., Allmon, D., & Heard, H. (1991). Cognitive-behavioral treatment of chronically parasuicidal borderline patients. *Archives of General Psychiatry, 48*, 1060–1064.

Linehan, M. M., Armstrong, H. E., Suarez, A., Allmon, D., & Heard, H. (1993). Naturalistic follow-up of a behavioral treatment for chronically parasuicidal patients. *Archives of General Psychiatry, 50*, 971–974.

Linehan, M. M. (1993). *Skills training manual for treating borderline personality disorder*. New York: Guilford Press.

Malkoff-Schwartz, S., Frank, E., Anderson, B. P., Hlastala, S. A., Luther, J. F., Sherril, J. T.,...Kupfer, D. J. (2000).Social rhythm disruption and stressful life events in the onset of bipolar and unipolar episodes. *Psychological Medicine, 30*, 1005–1016.

Miklowitz, D. J. (2008). *Bipolar disorder: A family-focused treatment approach* (2nd ed.). New York: Guilford Press.

Miklowitz, D. J. (2012). Family-focused treatment for children and adolescents with bipolar disorder. *The Israel Journal of Psychiatry and Related Sciences, 49*, 95–103.

Miklowitz, D. J., Axelson, D. A., Birmaher, B., George, E. L., Taylor, D. O., Schneck, C. D.,...Brent, D. A. (2008). Family-focused treatment for adolescents with bipolar disorder: Results from a 2-year randomized trial. *Archives of General Psychiatry, 65*, 1053–1061.

Miklowitz, D. J., George, E. L., Richards, J. A., Simoneau, T. L., & Suddath, R. L. (2003). A randomized study of family-focused psychoeducation and pharmacotherapy in the outpatient manangement of bipolar disorder. *Archives of General Psychiatry, 60*, 904–912.

Miklowitz, D. J., Goldstein, M. J., Nuechterlein, K. H., Snyder, K. S., & Mintz, J. (1988) Family factors and the course of bipolar affective disorder. *Archives of General Psychiatry, 45*, 225–231.

Miklowitz, D. J., Otto, M. W., Frank, E., Reilly-Harrington, N. A., Kogan, J. N., Sachs, G. S.,...Wisniewski, S. R. (2007). Intensive psychosocial intervention enhances functioning in patients with bipolar depression: Results from a 9-month randomized controlled trial. *The American Journal of Psychiatry, 164*, 1–8.

Miklowitz, D. J., Otto, M. W., Frank, E., Reilly-Harrington, N. A., Wisniewski, S. R., Kogan, J. N.,...Sachs, G. S. (2007). Psychosocial treatments for bipolar depression: A 1-year randomized trial from the Systematic Treatment Enhancement Program. *Archives of General Psychiatry, 64*, 419–427.

Miklowitz, D. J., Schneck, C. D., Singh, M. K., Taylor, D. O., George, E. L., Cosgrove, V. E.,...Chang, K. D. (2013). Early intervention for symptomatic youth at risk for bipolar disorder: A randomized trial of family-focused therapy. *Journal of the American Academy of Child & Adolescent Psychiatry, 52*, 121–131.

Monk, T. H., Flaherty, J. F., Frank, E., Hoskinson, K., & Kupfer, D. J. (1990). The Social Rhythm Metric: An instrument to quantify the daily rhythms of life. *Journal of Nervous and Mental Disease, 178*, 120–126.

Otto, M. W., Reilly-Harrington, N. A., Kogan, J. N., Henin, A., & Knauz, R. O. (2008). *Managing bipolar disorder: A cognitive behavior treatment program therapist guide*. New York: Oxford University Press.

Perich, T., Manicavasager, V., Mitchell, P. D., Ball, J. R., & Hadzi-Pavlovic, D. (2013). A randomized control trial of mindfulness-based cognitive therapy for bipolar disorder. *Acta Psychiatrica Scandinavica, 127*, 333–343.

Perlick, D. A., Miklowitz, D. J., Lopez, N., Chou, J., Kalvin, C., Adzhiashvili, V., & Aronson, A. (2010). Family-focused treatment for caregivers of patients with bipolar disorder. *Bipolar Disorders, 12*, 627–637.

Rea, M. M., Thompson, M., Miklowitz, D. J., Goldstein, M. J., Hwang, S., & Mintz, J. (2003). Family focused treatment versus individual treatment for bipolar disorder: Results of a randomized clinical trial. *Journal of Consulting and Clinical Psychology, 71*, 482–492.

Segal, Z. V., Williams, J. M. G., & Teasdale, J. D. (2002). *Mindfulness-based cognitive therapy for depression: A new approach to preventing relapse*. New York: Guilford Publications.

Shen, G. H., Alloy, L. B., & Abramson, L. Y. (2005). Examining social rhythm regularity to predict affective episodes in bipolar spectrum individuals. *Bipolar Disorders, 5*(1), 39–40.

Swartz, H. A., Frank, E., & Cheng, Y. (2012). A randomized pilot study of psychotherapy and quetiapine for the acute treatment of bipolar II depression. *Bipolar Disorders, 14*, 211–216.

Van Dijk, S. (2012). *DBT made simple*. Oakland, CA: New Harbinger Publications.

Van Dijk, S., Jeffrey, J., & Katz, M. R. (2103). A randomized, controlled, pilot study of dialectical behavior therapy skills in a psychoeducational group for individuals with bipolar disorder. *Journal of Affective Disorders, 145*(3), 386–393.

Weber, B., Jermann, F., Gex-Fabry, M., Nallet, A., Bondolfi, G., & Aubry, J. M. (2010). Mindfulness-based cognitive therapy for bipolar disorder: A feasibility trial. *European Psychiatry, 25*, 334–337.

Williams, J. M, Alatiq, Y., Crane, C., Barnhofer, T., Fennell, M. J., Duggan, D. S.,…Goodwin, G. M. (2008). Mindfulness-based cognitive therapy (MBCT) in bipolar disorder: Preliminary evaluation of immediate effects on between-episode functioning. *Journal of Affective Disorders, 107*, 275–279.

PART V

COMORBIDITY

33.

NATURE AND MANAGEMENT OF CO-OCCURRING PSYCHIATRIC ILLNESSES IN BIPOLAR DISORDER PATIENTS

FOCUS ON ANXIETY SYNDROMES

Gustavo H. Vázquez, Leonardo Tondo, and Ross J. Baldessarini

Those who make many species are the "splitters," and those who make few are the "lumpers." (DARWIN, 1857)

INTRODUCTION

CONCEPT OF "COMORBIDITY"

The term "comorbidity" was coined by Feinstein (1970) to indicate the co-occurrence of more than one clinical condition meeting diagnostic criteria for distinct diagnoses, whether or not one illness is considered of primary interest. Bipolar disorders very commonly present clinically with evidence of other, co-occurring major psychiatric, substance-abuse, or personality disorders. In addition, cardiovascular and other general medical disorders occur at higher rates than in persons without bipolar disorder and can lead to excess mortality, especially in older patients (Crump, Sundquist, Winkleby, & Sundquist, 2013; Goodwin & Jamison, 2007; Krishnan, 2005; Kupfer, 2005; Ösby, Brandt, Correia, Ekbom, & Sparén, 2001; Strakowski et al., 1998). The term "comorbidity" in psychiatric disorders is not universally accepted, due largely to its conceptual and semantic ambiguity arising from overlapping symptoms between syndromes, particularly of anxiety and mood disorders (Maj, 2005; National Institute of Mental Health, 2009; van Praag, 1996, 1999; Winokur, 1990; Wittchen, 1996; Zimmerman & Mattia, 1999).

Differentiation of clinical features as representing one or more than one disorder in the same person is not a mere academic quibble. Controversy and uncertainty arise from the question of how to understand the significance of symptoms of more than one disorder, even if sufficient to meet conventional, categorical, diagnostic criteria that describe a syndrome or "disorder." Are these to be understood as the presence of separate disorders or, instead, as manifestations of the potential range of clinical features of one disorder? This question is particularly important for bipolar disorders, which are both complex and changeable over time, as well as having unusually high rates of apparently "comorbid" conditions (Goodwin & Jamison, 2007; Krishnan, 2005).

Indeed, the theoretical limits of bipolar disorder have been a fundamental issue for at least two millennia, since Aretæus of Cappadocia reported "mania" and "melancholia" in the same persons at different times (Adams, 1856). This pattern has been often understood as representing dissimilar symptomatic manifestations of a single illness. The view of a single disorder incorporating features of mania and melancholia continued to develop over the ensuing centuries (Falret, 1854; Pérez, Baldessarini, Cruz, Salvatore, & Vieta, 2011; Pichot, 2004; Sedler, 1983). The topic became more complex when Weygandt, then a protégé of Kraepelin's, realized in 1895 that components of both mania and melancholia could be observed in the same person at the same time, or in rapid succession (Salvatore et al., 2002). By the end of the 19th century, Kraepelin proposed that an unprecedently broad range of essentially major affective disorders could be gathered, at least tentatively, into his concept of "manic-depressive" illness (Trede et al., 2005). Following a century of efforts to separate bipolar and mainly recurrent depressive illnesses and even subtypes within the Kraepelinian manic-depressive category, broader concepts are again being considered. Currently under discussion is a range of types of bipolar disorders, based on descriptive subtypes (types I and II), as well as depression-prone versus mania-prone, familial versus sporadic, and with different degrees of illness severity or other potential subdivisions (Baldessarini, 2000; Baldessarini, Tondo, et al., 2012; Baldessarini, Undurraga, et al., 2012; Phelps, Angst, Katzow, & Sadler, 2008; Salvatore et al., 2009, 2011). In addition, bipolar-like or "bipolar spectrum" disorders, usually conceived as falling between type I bipolar disorder and recurrent major depressive disorder, have been explored (Akiskal, 2007; Angst & Gamma, 2008; Angst et al., 2003; Benazzi, 2007; Mitchell, 2012; Zimmermann et al., 2009).

Questions about the theoretical basis of comorbidity lie at the conceptual heart of psychiatric nosology, which reflects the very ancient tension between "lumping and splitting" throughout medicine (McKusick, 1969). That is, many natural phenomena, and certainly psychiatric illnesses, can be organized into relatively few or into many subgroups. In modern psychiatry, the era preceding the *Diagnostic and Statistical Manual of Mental Disorders* (third edition [*DSM-III*]; American Psychiatric Association, 1980) era included proposals to limit diagnostic categories to a handful of relatively clearly characterized entities, largely for research applications (Feighner et al., 1972; Woodruff, Goodwin, & Guze, 1974). However, since 1980, psychiatric "disorders" have proliferated to several hundreds (American Psychiatric Association, 2013; World Health Organization, 1994, 2014). The implicit hope that some of these would be placed on a sound scientific basis with a clear etiology has not been realized. The decision by the major international nosological systems to follow a *categorical* diagnostic scheme virtually guarantees proliferation of increasing numbers of entities, regardless of how well established they may be clinically or scientifically (American Psychiatric Association, 2013; World Health Organization, 1994, 2013). Their conceptualization as "disorders" further forces recognition of multiple conditions in the same person, even though such classifications may not be warranted. Given the limited realms in which psychopathology can be expressed (as anomalies of thinking, sensation, mood, or behavior), it would not be surprising for such systems to recognize entities without clear borders and distinctions and with overlapping features. An extreme position, supported by psychoanalytic views, would be to argue that each individual psychiatric patient is a diagnostic entity unto himself, or that even tentative efforts to group similar patients and illnesses is not worthwhile without further scientific justification. Although such "splitting" would hardly serve to support most research or clinical needs, many examples of extraordinarily broad

and surely heterogeneous psychiatric (and general medical) entities exist (Baldessarini, 2000; Dulac & Guerrini, 2001; Klein, 2005; Mack, Forman, Brown, & Frances, 1994; McKusick, 1969, 2006). Proposed alternative or supplemental classifications of psychiatric disorders using dimensional models may also be problematic (Helzer, Kraemer, & Krueger, 2006; Narrow & Kuhl, 2011). For instance, if the dimension of *mood* in bipolar disorder were described as a continuum between melancholia and manic excitation, the decision about where to place a border between normality and psychopathology would be uncertain and subjective.

The upshot of these circumstances is that comorbidities are almost inevitable if currently descriptive and tentative diagnostic criteria for "disorders" are taken literally and as valid, as well as reliable. Moreover, we suggest that meeting conventional lists of diagnostic criteria for multiple disorders does not clarify whether a given patient has multiple illnesses or one disease with a wide range of symptomatic expression. Finally, to further complicate the issue, it seems likely that a condition as complex as bipolar disorder may well have *both* broad symptomatic variations, as well as risks of co-occurring conditions at rates well above their prevalence in the general population. As an example that avoids the problem of potentially overlapping psychiatric symptoms, bipolar disorder patients appear to be at increased risk of certain general medical disorders (McIntyre et al., 2006, 2007; Weber, Fisher, Cowan, & Niebuhr, 2011), as is discussed elsewhere in this volume.

In addition to its theoretical challenges, the concept of comorbidity also presents practical problems for diagnosis, treatment, and research. For example, it is not uncommon to overlook the presence of bipolar disorder, especially when it is not fully or typically expressed, among persons presenting with depression, anxiety, substance-use, or medical disorders that command clinical attention (Baldessarini et al., 2013; Krishnan, 2005; Yatham et al., 2013). In particular, identification of hypomania is especially challenging, since such a state of elation is often considered by affected individuals as part of their ordinary or even optimal mood and performance. In addition, it is typically unclear how to treat complex clinical presentations—especially when to rely primarily on mood-stabilizing treatments for a range of psychopathological symptoms in bipolar disorder patients and when to engage in polytherapy directed at symptoms considered as manifestations of separate illnesses or conditions in need of separate treatments (Baldessarini, 2013; Krishnan, 2005). Additional complications can arise when effects of the treatments themselves produce symptoms that can resemble or add to those of the condition(s) being treated. Examples include the mania-inducing actions of antidepressants and depression-resembling effects of antipsychotic agents (Baldessarini, 2013; Goikolea et al., 2013; Tondo, Vázquez, & Baldessarini, 2010). The concept of hierarchical diagnosis and the principle of parsimony call for limiting the number of diagnoses to a minimum that account for clinical observed symptoms (Surtees & Kendell, 1979; Walter-Ryan & Fahs, 1987). Moreover, limiting the number of diagnoses can limit use of multiple treatments, especially when evidence of their necessity, efficacy, efficiency, cost-effectiveness, and safety when combined usually is lacking.

For research, it is virtually a truism that most standard psychiatric syndromes based on descriptions of signs and symptoms are clinically and biologically heterogeneous. This circumstance greatly complicates both biological and experimental therapeutic research, given the range of clinical types among which to select and to match across experimental conditions, especially in an illness as complex as bipolar disorder. For treatment trials, randomization can limit risks of systematic biases but cannot solve the problem of the wide range of phenotypic expressions to be studied (Ghaemi & Thommi, 2010; Ioannidis, 2005). Even clinical selections among apparently similarly effective treatments can be influenced by emphasis on particular symptomatic features of an illness (e.g., aroused mood and activity vs. psychotic thinking in mania; Bourin & Thibaut, 2013).

DISTINGUISHING MULTIPLE- VERSUS SINGLE-ILLNESS HYPOTHESES

Means of distinguishing between a single disorder versus multiple illnesses in bipolar disorder patients considered to have other disorders are limited and unsatisfactory, especially when supposedly comorbid conditions can overlap symptomatically with bipolar disorder itself (Krishnan, 2005; Parker et al., 2010). Simply meeting diagnostic criteria for more than one disorder, based on conventional, descriptive criteria in a diagnostic system that requires a categorical diagnosis, does not resolve the question.

Family studies in which distinct disorders are present in different family members can be taken either as evidence of separate disorders or as support for the view that phenotypic expression of complex illnesses, including bipolar disorder, can be broad and varied among affected individuals and their relatives, as well as over time (Baldessarini, Tondo, et al., 2012; Doughty, Wells, Joyce, Olds, & Walsh, 2004; Lee & Dunner, 2008; MacKinnon, McMahon, Simpson, McInnis, & DePaulo, 1997; Wozniak, Biederman, Monuteaux, Richards, & Faraone, 2002). Notably, it is common to find cases of apparent unipolar major depression, as well as of types I and II bipolar disorders, in different

persons within the same pedigree, and diagnosis of depressive illnesses as unipolar when hypomania or mania have not been identified or have not yet occurred is commonplace, especially in relatively young patients (Axelson et al., 2011; Baldessarini, Faedda, Vázquez, Offidani, & Tondo, 2013; Birmaher et al., 2009).

An alternative strategy might be to consider antecedents to bipolar disorder, which include anxiety and subsyndromal, as well as major depressive disorders, substance abuse, attention disorders, and others, often before clear manifestations of major episodes of depression, mania, hypomania, or mixed states (Baldessarini, Faedda, et al., 2013; Salvatore, Baldessarini, Khalsa, Vázquez, et al., 2014). Again, such temporal evolution does not adequately distinguish single versus multiple, separate disorders.

Another possible means of addressing the question of single or multiple disorders would be to compare therapeutic responses in comorbid bipolar disorder patients versus those without the comorbidity, as well as versus those with the second condition alone as a primary disorder. For example, finding that treatment with lithium or a mood-altering anticonvulsant was effective for anxiety symptoms, as well as manic or depressive features in comorbid bipolar disorder patients, but not in patients with an anxiety disorder alone, might suggest that anxiety features were part of the range of phenotypic expressions of bipolar disorder. Antidepressants are effective in anxiety disorders, as well as major depressive disorders, but given the lack of agreement on the effects of antidepressants in bipolar disorder, interpretation of their possible clinical value in anxiety associated with bipolar disorder as a means of clarifying the single versus multiple disorder question remains ambiguous (Pacchiarotti et al., 2013; Vázquez, Tondo, Undurraga, & Baldessarini, 2013). In general, such treatment studies are rare (Provencher, Guimond, & Hawke, 2012). Some indicate poorer responses in supposedly comorbid bipolar disorder patients, including those with features of anxiety disorders (Lee & Dunner, 2008; Simon et al., 2003; Singh & Zarate, 2006; Yatham et al., 2013) or alcohol abuse (Farren, Hill, & Weiss, 2012), perhaps owing to more severe illnesses. On the other hand, responses to antipsychotic drugs differed little among manic or mixed-state bipolar disorder patients with or without substance abuse, and, moreover, the substance abuse improved with this treatment (Sani et al., 2013).

Findings based on treatment response leave uncertain whether separate disorders are involved, whether having more complex bipolar disorder can sometimes lead to inferior treatment response, or whether different forms of apparent comorbidity may have different relationships to bipolar disorder and to its treatment. In short, none of the preceding approaches to testing the single- versus multiple-diagnosis hypothesis leads to unambiguous conclusions. A fundamental problem is the current general lack of independent validating measures to support diagnoses in psychiatry. It is reasonable to hope that advances in genetic and other biological studies may eventually help to clarify relationships among bipolar disorder and its apparent comorbidities (Juli, Juli, & Juli, 2012; Lim et al., 2013; Sullivan, Daly, & O'Donovan, 2012).

AIMS OF THIS CHAPTER

Despite the fundamental theoretical uncertainties regarding the phenomenon, "comorbidity" is a widely employed expression to indicate co-occurrence in the same patient of symptoms of more than one clinical condition meeting conventional diagnostic criteria of a standard nosological system, such as the *Diagnostic and Statistical Manual of Mental Disorders* (fifth edition [*DSM-5*]; American Psychiatric Association, 2013) or *International Statistical Classification of Diseases and Related Health Problems* (tenth edition [ICD-10]) (World Health Organization, 2014). Presumed comorbid disorders may fall into various categories, such as mood, anxiety, psychotic, substance-use, or personality disorders, or may involve general medical conditions. Often implicitly, one disorder may be considered of more primary interest (usually bipolar disorder in psychiatric settings or a major medical disorder in general medical settings) and others (such as anxiety or substance-use disorders), secondary.

Anxiety symptoms and syndromes are especially prevalent in bipolar disorder patients, but other psychiatric syndromes that have been associated with bipolar disorder include attention, conduct, and eating disorders; abuse of alcohol or drugs; personality characteristics; and general medical disorders. Some of these—including conduct and personality disorders, as well as proposals that other forms of affective illness including major depression and dysthymia can be "comorbid" with bipolar disorder—seem especially closely related to characteristics of bipolar disorder itself. Most of these conditions are addressed in detail in other chapters of this volume. Others (e.g., attention and eating disorders) are less prevalent than anxiety disorders and are not included here. In this chapter, we focus on anxiety-related symptoms or syndromes found in patients meeting diagnostic criteria for types I or II bipolar disorder, either during major affective episodes or separately. The anxiety features are prevalent clinical phenomena; they are considered here to be of unknown theoretical or biomedical significance and

as arising largely by application of conventional, categorical, diagnostic criteria to support more than one diagnosis.

ANXIETY DISORDERS AND BIPOLAR DISORDER

PREVALENCE IN BIPOLAR DISORDER

There is strong evidence of elevated prevalence of symptoms sufficient to support diagnoses of anxiety disorders in bipolar disorder patients compared to general population

Table 33.1. LIFETIME RISKS OF ANXIETY DISORDERS AMONG PATIENTS WITH BIPOLAR DISORDERS

STUDY	DISORDER TYPE	PREVALENCE (%)
Young et al., 1993	GAD	32.0
Kessler et al., 1997	panic + phobias	80.3
Chen and Dilsaver, 1995b	panic + phobias	41.9
Keck et al., 1995	OCD + PTSD	29.0
Krüger et al., 1995	OCD	35.0
Dilsaver et al., 1997	any	62.3
Kessler et al., 1997	panic + phobias	80.3
Pini et al., 1997	any	89.0
Szadoczky et al., 1998	any	48.9
McElroy et al., 2001	any	42.4
Henry et al., 2003	any	24.0
Simon et al., 2004	any	51.2
Faravelli et al., 2006	GAD + panic	40.0
Mantere et al., 2006	any	44.5
Benedetti et al., 2007	any	68.5
Brieger et al., 2007	any	16.0
Albert et al., 2008	any	41.0
Tondo, 2015*	any	42.6
Mean **(95% CI)**	various	46.4 (36.5–56.3)

NOTE: GAD =, generalized anxiety disorder; *OCD*, obsessive-compulsive disorder; *PTSD*, post-traumatic stress disorder; *RR*, relative risk. Estimates based on only some anxiety disorders may underestimate total risks. Note that risks were similar in men and women (RR = 0.96; Benedetti et al., 2007), but much higher in depressive than manic episodes (RR = 1.95; Mantere et al., 2006). (*) Previously unreported data for this review.

samples. A high prevalence of anxiety symptoms and syndromes is also present in unipolar major depressive disorder, but they may be even more prevalent among bipolar disorder patients (Chen & Disalver, 1995a; Simon et al., 2003). High rates of diagnosable anxiety disorders among bipolar disorder patients have been found in both epidemiological (Angst 1998; Chen & Disalver, 1995a, 1995b; Goodwin & Hoven, 2002; Kessler, Rubinow, Holmes, Abelson, & Zhao, 1997; Merikangas et al., 2007, 2008, 2011; Sala et al., 2012; Schaffer et al., 2010) and clinical studies (Angst et al., 2010, 2011; Boylan et al., 2004; Henry et al., 2003; Kauer-Sant'Anna, Kapczinski, & Vieta, 2009; Kessler, Brandenburg, et al., 2005; Kessler, Chiu, Demler, & Walters, 2005; McElroy et al., 2001; Perlis et al., 2004; Pini et al., 1997; Simon et al., 2004). Approximately 40% to 60% of bipolar disorder patients have met standard diagnostic criteria for at least one anxiety disorder at some time (Perlis et al., 2004; Sala et al., 2012; Simon et al., 2004; Table 33.1). Types of syndromes associated with bipolar disorder include panic disorder, social and specific phobias, generalized anxiety, obsessive-compulsive disorder, and posttraumatic stress syndrome (Goldberg & Fawcett, 2012; Table 33.2; Figure 33.1).

Risks of anxiety syndromes appear to be similar among women and men diagnosed with bipolar disorder (Table 33.3). Several studies (Cassano, Pini, Saettoni, & Dell'Osso, 1999; Doughty et al., 2004; Henry et al., 2003; Perugi et al., 1999; Pini et al., 1997), but not all (Sala et al., 2012; Simon et al., 2004), have found anxiety disorders more often among bipolar II than bipolar I disorder patients. In our review of research reports and our own previously unpublished data, we did not find a difference in the overall prevalence of anxiety disorders between bipolar disorders type I and II (Table 33.4). However, when particular anxiety disorders were considered separately, phobias, as well as obsessive-compulsive disorders, were identified significantly more often among type I than type II bipolar disorder patients (Table 33.5).

Anxiety symptoms or syndromes also are prevalent antecedents of bipolar disorders, sometimes years earlier

Table 33.2. ANXIETY DISORDERS CO-OCCURRING WITH BIPOLAR DISORDERS

STUDY	PANIC	PHOBIAS	GAD	PTSD	OCD
Fogarty et al., 1994	—	18.4	—	—	—
Chen and Dilsaver 1995a and 1995b	20.8	—	—	—	21.0
Kessler et al., 1997	32.9	58.6	42.4	38.8	—
Angst, 1998	35.6	12.6	—	—	5.19
McElroy et al., 2001	20.1	12.5	3.13	3.13	4.86
Rihmer et al., 2001	8.43	14.0	12.6	—	—
Goodwin and Hoven, 2002	35.0	—	—	—	—
Simon et al., 2004	17.5	30.3	18.3	17.1	9.89
Grant et al., 2005	19.0	21.8	21.8	—	—
Faravelli et al., 2006	16.0	—	24.0	—	—
Mantere et al., 2006	24.1	27.8	15.2	10.5	2.09
Benedetti et al., 2007	40.0	—	—	—	48.0
Merikangas et al., 2007	28.0	36.5	37.8	32.8	22.8
Albert et al., 2008	10.5	6.67	16.2	—	13.3
Tondo et al., 2013	33.4	1.66	7.41	0.39	4.87
Mean (95% CI)	24.4 (18.7–30.1)	21.9 (11.1–32.6)	19.9 (11.0–28.7)	17.1 (0.62–33.6)	14.7 (3.2–25.8)

NOTE: GAD = generalized anxiety disorder; *OCD* = obsessive-compulsive disorder; *PTSD* = posttraumatic stress disorder; CI = confidence interval.

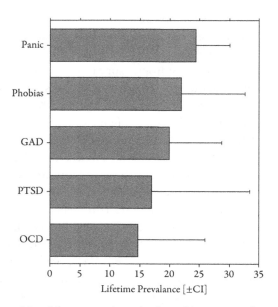

Figure 33.1 Mean lifetime prevalence (with confidence interval) of anxiety disorders co-occurring with bipolar disorders. GAD = generalized anxiety disorder; PTSD = posttraumatic stress disorder; OCD = obsessive-compulsive disorder. Based on data summarized in Table 33.2.

and in youth (Salvatore, Baldessarini, Khalsa, Vázquez, et al., 2014). In addition, rates of newly emerging mania or hypomania in placebo-controlled trials of antidepressant treatment for juvenile anxiety disorders are at least as high as in trials for juvenile depression (Offidani, Fava, Tomba, & Baldessarini, 2013). This finding might suggest that anxiety, as well as depression, may sometimes precede clinical expression of typical bipolar disorder; alternatively, the mood switches involved may sometimes be due to adverse effects of antidepressant treatment (Tondo et al., 2010). In addition, first episodes of bipolar disorder often include admixtures of anxiety, depression, and sleep disturbances (McElroy et al., 2001;

Table 33.3. COMPARISON OF CO-OCCURRENCE OF ANXIETY SYNDROMES IN MOOD DISORDERS: MEN VERSUS WOMEN

DIAGNOSIS	MEN	WOMEN	RELATIVE RISK
BD-I	50/115 (43.5%)	66/144 (45.8%)	0.95
BD-II	39/92 (42.4%)	46/121 (38.0%)	1.16
All BD	89/207 (43.0%)	112/265 (42.3%)	1.02
UP-MDD	99/186 (53.2%)	191/346 (55.2%)	0.96

NOTE: Unpublished data, provided by Tondo (2015).

Table 33.4. LIFETIME RISKS OF ALL CO-OCCURRING ANXIETY DISORDERS WITH BIPOLAR DISORDERS, TYPE I VERSUS TYPE II

STUDY OR SYNDROME	PREVALENCE (%) (N)		I/II RISK RATIO
	BIPOLAR I	BIPOLAR II	
Kessler et al., 1997	92.9 (29)	—	—
Angst, 1998	—	57.6 (59)	—
McElroy et al., 2001	41.8 (239)	44.9 (49)	0.93
Simon et al., 2004	52.8 (360)	46.1 (115)	1.15
Mantere et al., 2006	35.6 (90)	52.5 (101)	0.68
Merikangas et al., 2007	86.7 (82)	89.2 (102)	0.97
Albert et al., 2008	40.9 (44)	41.0 (61)	1.00
Tondo, 2015[a]	44.8 (259)	39.9 (213)	1.13
Weighted Average (N) (95% CI)	**50.2 (1103)** (31.0–69.4)	**51.9 (700)** (36.3–67.2)	**0.97** (0.74–1.21)

NOTE: Random effects meta-analysis also indicated no significant difference by diagnostic subtype (RR = 0.999; 95% CI: 0.871–1.12).

[a] Previously unreported data provided for this review.

Salvatore, Baldessarini, Khalsa, Indic, et al., 2013). Episodes of anxiety syndromes, as well as of mania, depression, and mixed states, can recur episodically over time among bipolar disorder patients (Strakowski et al., 1998). Sometimes, in bipolar disorder patients followed longitudinally, anxiety syndromes may be more prominent than other typical features of bipolar disorder (Freeman, Freeman, & McElroy, 2002; McIntyre et al., 2007, 2012; Yatham et al., 2013). However, as discussed previously, such findings do not necessarily clarify whether the anxiety features are part of the spectrum of manifestations of bipolar disorder or an indication of the presence of two distinct disorders. Moreover, quantification of the distribution of particular anxiety features with or independently of other typical components of bipolar disorder remains to be studied.

There is a basis of clinical suspicion that anxiety symptoms are more likely during depressive or mixed manic-depressive episodes than in mania or hypomania, but such associations have rarely been studied systematically. However, a recent prospective study found

Table 33.5. PREVALENCE OF SPECIFIC ANXIETY SYNDROMES IN BIPOLAR I AND BIPOLAR II PATIENTS

DISORDER	BIPOLAR I ($N = 992$)	BIPOLAR II ($N = 539$)	I/II RISK RATIO	X^2	P VALUE
Phobias	21.2 (0.71 to 41.7)	13.2 (0.41 to 26.0)	1.61	14.9	<0.0001
Obsessive-compulsive disorder	8.56 (4.57 to 12.5)	5.75 (0.04 to 11.5)	1.49	3.96	0.047
Posttraumatic stress disorder[a]	9.38 (−5.53 to 24.3)	6.71 (−2.42 to 15.8)	1.40	2.97	0.085
Panic disorder	23.3 (9.10 to 37.5)	24.1 (11.6 to 36.6)	0.97	0.67	0.413
Generalized anxiety disorder	10.1 (−3.20 to 20.2)	9.64 (1.42 to 17.9)	1.05	0.07	0.787

NOTE: For specific syndromes: data from McElroy et al. (2001); Simon et al. (2004); Mantere et al. (2006); Albert et al. (2008); Tondo (2013). Data are for lifetime risk except Mantere et al. (2006) reported point-prevalence during bipolar depressive episodes.

[a] Total numbers for posttaumatic stress syndrome are 948 bipolar I and 478 bipolar II subjects since Albert et al. (2008) did not report on its prevalence.

that anxiety symptoms were more strongly associated with depressive than manic phases of bipolar disorder (Mantere et al., 2010). This observation is consistent with an association of anxiety symptoms (but not disorders) with greater long-term depressive morbidity in bipolar disorder patients (Coryell et al., 2009). There was also a strong association of excesses of later anxiety and depression among bipolar disorder patients whose first-lifetime episode was anxiety or depression (Baldessarini, Tondo, & Visioli, 2013). These observations may suggest some nonindependence of the mood disorder and anxiety symptoms. On the other hand, some bipolar disorder patients never meet diagnostic criteria for an anxiety disorder, and most anxiety disorder patients lack features typical of bipolar disorder. That is, at least some cases of bipolar disorder and anxiety disorders seem to represent separate illnesses (Kessler, Brandenburg, et al., 2005; Simon et al., 2004).

As most population-based studies report lifetime or 12-month prevalence rather than current status (point prevalence), they may lead to inflated impressions of overall comorbid risks, particularly considering that current morbidity in bipolar disorder is markedly dissimilar at different times (Parker, 2010) and that the proportion of time in specific anxious states in bipolar disorder patients remains to be studied longitudinally. Conversely, since *DSM* diagnostic criteria for some anxiety syndromes, such as generalized anxiety disorder, require at least six months of symptoms, whereas major affective episodes require only two weeks, it is possible to underestimate associations of anxiety symptoms and major mood disorders (Goldberg & Fawcett, 2012). A basic point, again, is that proportions of time with anxiety versus other symptoms in bipolar disorder subtypes, considered longitudinally, are not clearly established.

EFFECTS OF ANXIETY ON COURSE AND OUTCOME IN BIPOLAR DISORDER

It is widely accepted that comorbid anxiety symptoms and disorders (and other comorbidities) in bipolar disorder patients are typically associated with slower or inferior treatment responses and a worse overall prognosis, as reflected in greater morbidity and costs associated with mania as well as depression, and increased risk of substance abuse and of suicide (Albert, Rosso, Maina, & Bogetto, 2008; Feske et al., 2000; Gao, Chan, et al., 2010; Gaudiano & Miller 2005; Goldberg & Fawcett, 2012; Judd et al., 2003; Keck, Kessler, & Ross, 2008; Keck et al., 1995; Mantere et al., 2010). Among 500 bipolar I and II disorder patients, onset age was younger and clinical outcomes were generally poorer among those with anxiety features than among otherwise similar patients lacking such features (Simon et al., 2004). Children diagnosed with bipolar disorder with prominent anxiety symptoms had an earlier age of onset and more hospitalizations than those without anxiety (Dickstein et al., 2005), leaving uncertain whether the relevant factor was early onset or the reported comorbidity.

ANXIETY AND SUICIDAL RISK

Of particular public health significance, several studies have found that anxiety symptoms accompanying bipolar disorder or major depressive disorder were associated with substantially increased risks of suicidal ideation, attempted suicide, and suicide (Goldberg & Fawcett 2012; Goldstein et al., 2012; MacKinnon, Zandi, & Gershon, 2003; Simon, Hunkeler, Fireman, Lee, & Savarino, 2007). Epidemiological studies in North America and Europe have also found higher rates of suicide attempts and suicides, as well as a more severe course, among bipolar disorder patients with anxiety symptoms or disorders (Angst, Angst, Gerber-Werder, & Gamma, 2005; Angst et al. 2010; Merikangas, 2011; Sala et al., 2012). Such findings leave uncertain whether suicidal risks are related to anxiety specifically or to more severe or complex bipolar illness.

TREATMENT OF ANXIETY SYNDROMES OCCURRING IN BIPOLAR DISORDER PATIENTS

GENERAL ISSUES

Therapeutics research for anxiety syndromes occurring in bipolar disorder patients remains severely underdeveloped (Rakofsky & Dunlop, 2011; Singh & Zarate, 2006; Yatham et al., 2013). Recent reviews have noted that there are very few randomized, controlled trials of either pharmacotherapies or psychotherapies directed at any type of anxiety morbidity in bipolar disorder patients, and virtually none directed at specific anxiety syndromes or at anxiety in particular phases (depression, mixed states, mania/hypomania, euthymia) or types (I vs. II) of bipolar disorder.

An alternative approach has been to consider trials of medicines commonly used in the treatment of bipolar disorders for their effects on apparently primary anxiety disorders (Singh & Zarate, 2006; Yatham et al., 2013). These treatments include lithium, antimanic or mood-stabilizing anticonvulsants, antipsychotic drugs, and antidepressants. With few exceptions, this strategy also has yielded limited evidence and very little arising from randomized, controlled trials. Moreover, there is an unresolved question of whether anxiety symptoms and syndromes encountered in association with bipolar disorder are entirely equivalent to those associated with primary anxiety disorders. Similar concerns pertain to comparisons of the characteristics and treatment of bipolar and nonbipolar forms of major depression (Baldessarini, Vieta, Calabrese, Tohen, & Bowden, 2010; Vázquez et al., 2013). Moreover, the still poorly defined natural course of anxiety symptoms and syndromes in bipolar disorder has obvious implications for planning for their long-term treatment and clinical management.

TREATMENT OF PRIMARY ANXIETY DISORDERS WITH DRUGS USED FOR BIPOLAR DISORDER

There is some information concerning mood-stabilizing, antimanic, or antidepressant medicines in the treatment of primary anxiety disorders. Antidepressants, including tricyclics, monoamine oxidase inhibitors, and modern serotonin-reuptake inhibitors and serotonin-norepinephrine-reuptake inhibitors, are standard treatments for a range of anxiety disorders, as are benzodiazepines. However, their application for anxiety syndromes in bipolar disorder remains unstudied, at least in part owing to concern for potential mood- and behavior-destabilizing actions of antidepressants (Baldessarini, 2013; Tondo et al., 2010). Lithium appears to lack useful anxiolytic activity, although it has been studied only rarely and in few types of anxiety disorder, including as an adjunct to other treatments for obsessive-compulsive disorder (McDougle, Price, Goodman, Charney, & Heninger, 1991; Pigott et al., 1991; Singh & Zarate, 2006). An alternative suggestion is that subtle anxiolytic effects of lithium may occur in mood disorders (Phelps & Manipod, 2012).

Among anticonvulsants with antimanic or mood-stabilizing effects, carbamazepine was found to be ineffective in primary panic disorder (Uhde, Stein, & Post, 1988), lamotrigine has some evidence of benefit for posttraumatic stress disorder and perhaps obsessive-compulsive disorder (Hertzberg et al., 1999; Keck et al., 2006; Mula, Pini, & Cassano, 2007; van Ameringen, Mancini, Pipe, & Bennett, 2004), gabapentin may have some benefits in primary social phobia but perhaps not in panic disorder (Keck et al., 2006; Mula et al., 2007; Pande et al., 1999, 2000; van Ameringen et al., 2004), and pregabalin may be effective in social phobia and probably is effective in generalized anxiety disorder (Keck et al., 2006; Mula et al., 2007; Strawn & Geracioti, 2007; van Ameringen et al., 2004). Valproate is poorly studied as a treatment for primary anxiety disorders (Bowden 2007; Singh & Zarate 2006; van Ameringen et al., 2004; Yatham et al., 2013) but may have beneficial effects in generalized anxiety disorder and possibly in panic disorder (Aliyev & Aliyev, 2008; Keck et al., 2006; Rakofsky & Dunlop, 2011). Again, systematic assessments of lithium or mood-stabilizing anticonvulsants for effects on anxiety features in bipolar disorder patients are yet to be carried out.

There are a few studies of antipsychotic drugs for anxiety, usually involving modern, second-generation agents. They have yielded inconsistent effects on particular types of primary anxiety disorders (Rakofsky & Dunlop, 2011; Singh & Zarate, 2006; Vulink, Figee, & Denys, 2011; Yatham et al., 2013). For example, risperidone has supportive evidence of efficacy in several controlled trials for primary obsessive-compulsive disorder and posttraumatic stress disorder (Bartzokis, Lu, Turner, Mintz, & Saunders, 2005; Li et al., 2005; Reich, Winternitz, Hennen, Watts, & Stanculescu, 2004). Olanzapine has shown inconsistent effects in obsessive-compulsive disorder (Bystritsky et al.,

2004; Shapira et al., 2004) and has some evidence of efficacy in posttraumatic stress disorder (Butterfield et al., 2001; Stein, Kline, & Matloff, 2002). Aripiprazole appeared to be effective for some forms of anxiety in open trials, including patients with anxiety syndromes associated with major depression (Katzman, 2011), consistent with the strong epidemiological overlap of anxiety disorders and depressive disorders (Kessler et al., 2003). Quetiapine has shown inconsistent or weak effects in obsessive-compulsive disorder (Altmaca, Kuloglu, Tezcan, & Gecici, 2002; Denys, de Geus, van Megen, & Westenberg, 2004; Fineberg, Sivakumaran, Roberts, & Gale, 2005) but has been promising in generalized anxiety disorder (Gao, Sheehan, & Calabrese, 2009). Of note, most of these applications have been for otherwise treatment-unresponsive cases or as adjunctive treatments with other anxiolytic agents.

TREATMENTS FOR ANXIETY SYNDROMES IN BIPOLAR DISORDER PATIENTS

Very few trials have been reported concerning treatment of anxiety symptoms or syndromes in bipolar disorder patients. Generally, some second-generation antipsychotics may have beneficial effects against anxiety symptoms in these patients (Rakofsky & Dunlop, 2011). Risperidone has been reported to be ineffective against panic or obsessive-compulsive disorders associated with bipolar disorder (Rakofsky & Dunlop, 2011; Sheehan et al., 2009). Olanzapine added to lithium was more effective against anxiety symptoms than was lamotrigine, and olanzapine was effective in depressed bipolar disorder patients with anxiety symptoms, even when given as a monotherapy (Tohen et al., 2007). Quetiapine, which has beneficial effects in mania and bipolar depression, was found to be effective in depressed bipolar I or II disorder patients (Hirschfeld, Weisler, Raines, & Macfadden, 2006), and, in a recent controlled trial, it was more effective than valproate or placebo against generalized anxiety or even panic in bipolar disorder patients (Sheehan et al., 2013).

Mood-stabilizing anticonvulsants have rarely been studied in the treatment of anxiety disorders co-occurring with bipolar disorder. However, at least one trial found valproate to be effective for panic disorder in bipolar disorder patients, even for those who had responded poorly to antidepressants (Perugi et al., 2010). There is also an observation of greater risk of anxiety disorder morbidity among bipolar disorder patients who had received less mood-stabilizer treatment, but cause-and-effect relationships in this association are not clear (Gao, Kemp, et al., 2010).

Studies of psychosocial treatments for coexisting anxiety disorders and bipolar disorder also remain rare. Nevertheless, there is some evidence that cognitive-behavioral methods may be effective and possibly even more effective than interpersonal psychotherapy, family therapy, or psychoeducational programs (Provencher, Hawke, & Thienot, 2011).

EXPERIMENTAL TREATMENTS FOR ANXIETY DISORDERS

Another potential source of treatments to be tested for anxiety disorders associated with bipolar disorder are a growing number of experimental treatments for various primary anxiety disorders. Promising preliminary findings for the treatment of anxiety symptoms have been reported for such diverse treatments as the antiglutamate agent *riluzole* (Pittenger et al., 2008; Zarate & Manji, 2008), the *N*-methyl-D-aspartate glutamate receptor antagonist *memantine* developed to treat dementia (Sani et al., 2012), and intranasal *ketamine* in juvenile bipolar disorder with prominent fears of harm (Papolos, Teicher, Faedda, Murphy, & Mattis, 2013). Among nonpharmacological methods, repeated transcranial magnetic stimulation, recently Food and Drug Administration–approved for treatment of major depression, has been considered for treatment of anxiety disorders, so far with very limited success (George et al., 2009; Paes et al., 2011; Prasko et al., 2007). Finally, it is important to underscore that none of these experimental approaches has been tested in anxiety syndromes associated with bipolar disorder.

CONCLUSION

This overview indicates that anxiety syndromes are highly prevalent among bipolar disorder patients, affecting perhaps half of them at some time. The prevalence of specific anxiety disorders in bipolar disorder patients has ranked: panic ≥ various phobias > generalized anxiety > posttraumatic stress disorder ≥ obsessive-compulsive disorder (Table 33.2). Risks appear to be similar among women and men, as well as in types I and II bipolar disorder (Tables 33.3 and 33.4). Type II bipolar disorder may carry a higher risk of phobias and possibly of obsessive-compulsive disorder than type I disorder (Table 33.5). Specific details of the longitudinal distribution of anxiety symptoms over time in bipolar disorder patients, and of their possible association with particular components of bipolar disorder, require clarification. Well-designed therapeutic trials for particular anxiety syndromes co-occurring with specific types of bipolar disorder are lacking, although some suggestive findings are emerging. A fundamental remaining riddle is whether anxiety syndromes co-occurring in bipolar disorder represent separate illnesses ("disorders") or represent the range of symptomatic-phenotypic expression of bipolar disorder.

ACKNOWLEDGMENTS

This chapter was supported in part by a research award from the Aretæus Foundation of Rome and by the Lucio Bini Private Donors Research Fund to Leonardo Tondo, and by a grant from the Bruce J. Anderson Foundation and the McLean Private Donors Research Fund to Ross J. Baldessarini.

Disclosure statement: No author or immediate family member has relationships with corporate or other commercial entities that might represent potential conflicts of interest with the material reported.

REFERENCES

Adams, F. (Ed.). (1856). *The extant works of Aretæus, the Cappadocian*. London: Sydenham Society.

Akiskal, H. S. (2007). Emergence of the bipolar spectrum: Validation along clinical-epidemiologic and familial-genetic lines. *Psychopharmacology Bulletin, 40*, 99–115.

Albert, U., Rosso, G., Maina, G., & Bogetto, F. (2008). Impact of anxiety disorder comorbidity on quality of life in euthymic bipolar disorder patients: Differences between bipolar I and II subtypes. *Journal of Affective Disorders, 15*, 297–303.

Aliyev, N. A., & Aliyev, Z. N. (2008). Valproate (depakine-chrono) in the acute treatment of outpatients with generalized anxiety disorder without psychiatric comorbidity: Randomized, double-blind placebo-controlled study. *European Psychiatry, 23*, 109–114.

Altmaca, M., Kuloglu, M., Tezcan, E., & Gecici, O. (2002). Quetiapine augmentation in patients with treatment resistant obsessive-compulsive disorder: Single-blind, placebo-controlled study. *Internatinal Clinical Psychopharmacology, 17*, 115–119.

American Psychiatric Association. (1980). *Diagnostic and statistical manual of mental disorders* (3rd ed.). Washington, DC: Author.

American Psychiatric Association. (1994). *Diagnostic and statistical manual of mental disorders* (4th ed.). Washington, DC: Author.

American Psychiatric Association. (2013). *Diagnostic and statistical manual of mental disorders* (5th ed.). Washington, DC: Author.

Angst, J. (1998). The emerging epidemiology of hypomania and bipolar II disorder. *Journal of Affective Disorders, 50*, 143–151.

Angst, J., Angst, F., Gerber-Werder, R., & Gamma, A. (2005). Suicide in 406 mood-disorder patients with and without long-term medication: A 40 to 44 years' follow-up. *Archives of Suicide Research, 9*, 279–300.

Angst, J., Azorin, J.-M., Bowden, C. L., Perugi, G., Vieta, E., Gamma, A., & Young, A. H. (2011). Prevalence and characteristics of undiagnosed bipolar disorder in patients with major depressive episode. *Archives of General Psychiatry, 68*, 791–799.

Angst, J., Cui, L., Swendsen, J. J., Rothen, S., Cravchik, A., Kessler, R., & Merikangas, K. (2010). Major depressive disorder with sub-threshold bipolarity in the national comorbidity survey replication. *American Journal of Psychiatry, 167*, 1194–1201.

Angst, J., & Gamma, A. (2008). Diagnosis and course of affective psychoses: Was Kraepelin right? *European Archives of Psychiatry and Clinical Neuroscience, 258*(2), 107–110.

Angst, J., Gamma, A., Benazzi, F., Ajdacic, V., Eich, D., & Rossler, W. (2003). Toward a re-definition of subthreshold bipolarity: Epidemiology and proposed criteria for bipolar-II, minor bipolar disorders and hypomania. *Journal of Affective Disorders, 73*, 133–146.

Axelson, D., Birmaher, B., Strober, M. A., Goldstein, B. I., Ha, W., Gill, M. K.,…Keller, M. B. (2011). Course of subthreshold bipolar disorder in youth: Diagnostic progression from bipolar disorder not otherwise specified. *Journal of the American Academy of Child & Adolescent Psychiatry, 50*, 1001–1016.

Baldessarini, R. J. (2000). Plea for the integrity of the bipolar disorder concept. *Bipolar Disorders, 2*, 3–7.

Baldessarini, R. J. (2013). *Chemotherapy in psychiatry* (3rd ed.). New York: Springer.

Baldessarini, R. J., Faedda, G. L., Vázquez, G. H., Offidani, E., & Tondo, L. (2013). Rate of new-onset mania or hypomania in patients diagnosed with unipolar major depression. *Journal of Affective Disorders, 148*, 129–135.

Baldessarini, R. J., Tondo, L., Vázquez, G. H., Bolzani, L., Khalsa, H.-M. K., Lai, M.,…Tohen, M. (2012). International study of functional and symptomatic outcome versus onset-age in 1437 bipolar-I disorder patients. *World Psychiatry, 11*, 40–46.

Baldessarini, R. J., Tondo, L., & Visioli, C. (2014). First-episode types in bipolar disorder: Predictive associations with later illness. *Acta Psychiatrica Scandinavica 129*(5), 383–392.

Baldessarini, R. J., Undurraga, J., Vázquez, G. H., Tondo, L., Salvatore, P., Ha, K.,…Vieta, E. (2012). Predominant recurrence polarity among 928 adult international bipolar-I disorder patients. *Acta Psychiatrica Scandinavica, 125*, 293–302.

Baldessarini, R. J., Vieta, E., Calabrese, J. R., Tohen, M., & Bowden, C. (2010). Bipolar depression: Overview and commentary. *Harvard Review of Psychiatry, 18*, 143–157.

Bartzokis, G., Lu, P. H., Turner, J., Mintz, J., & Saunders, C. S. (2005). Adjunctive risperidone in the treatment of chronic combat-related post-traumatic stress disorder. *Biological Psychiatry, 57*, 474–479.

Benazzi, F. (2007). Is there a continuity between bipolar and depressive disorders? *Psychotherapy and Psychosomatics, 76*, 70–76.

Benedetti, A., Fagiolini, A., Casamassima, F., Mian, M. S., Adamovit, A., Musetti, L.,…Cassano, G. B. (2007). Gender differences in bipolar disorder type I: 48 week prospective follow-up of 72 patients treated in an Italian tertiary care center. *Journal of Nervous and Mental Disease, 195*, 93–96.

Birmaher, B., Axelson, D., Goldstein, B., Strober, B., Gill, M. K., Hunt, J.,…Keller, M. (2009). Four-year longitudinal course of children and adolescents with bipolar spectrum disorder: The Course and Outcome of Bipolar Youth (COBY) Study. *American Journal of Psychiatry, 166*, 795–804.

Bourin, M., & Thibaut, F. (2013). How to assess drugs in the treatment of acute bipolar mania? *Frontiers in Pharmacology, 29*(4), 4.

Bowden, C. L. (2007). Spectrum of effectiveness of valproate in neuropsychiatry. *Expert Review of Neurotherapeutics, 7*, 9–16.

Boylan, K. R., Bieling, P. J., Marriott, M., Begin, H., Young, L. T., & MacQueen, G. M. (2004). Impact of comorbid anxiety disorders on outcome in a cohort of patients with bipolar disorder. *Journal of Clinical Psychiatry, 65*, 1106–1113.

Brieger, P., Rottig, S., Rottig, D., Marneros, A., & Priebe, S. (2007). Dimensions underlying outcome criteria in bipolar I disorder. *Journal of Affective Disorders, 99*, 1–7.

Butterfield, M. I., Becker, M. E., Connor, K. M., Sutherland, S., Churchill, L. E., & Davidson, J. R. (2001). Olanzapine in the treatment of post-traumatic stress disorder: Pilot study. *International Clinical Psychopharmacology, 16*, 197–203.

Bystritsky, A., Ackerman, D. L., Rosen, R. M., Vapnik, T., Gorbis, E., Maidment, K. M., & Saxena, S. (2004). Augmentation of serotonin-reuptake inhibitors in refractory obsessive-compulsive disorder using adjunctive olanzapine: Placebo controlled trial. *Journal of Clinical Psychiatry, 65*, 565–568.

Cassano, G. B., Pini, S., Saettoni, M., & Dell'Osso, L. (1999). Multiple anxiety disorder comorbidity in patients with mood spectrum disorders with psychotic features. *American Journal of Psychiatry, 156*, 474–476.

Chen, Y.-W., & Dilsaver, S. C. (1995a). Comorbidity for obsessive-compulsive disorder in bipolar and unipolar disorders. *Psychiatry Research, 59*, 57–64.

Chen, Y.-W., & Dilsaver, S. C. (1995b). Comorbidity of panic disorder in bipolar illness: Evidence from the Epidemiology Catchment Area survey. *American Journal of Psychiatry, 152*, 280–282.

Coryell, W., Solomon, D. A., Fiedorowicz, J. G., Endicott, J., Schettler, P. J., & Judd, L. L. (2009). Anxiety and outcome in bipolar disorder. *American Journal of Psychiatry, 166*, 1238–1243.

Crump, C., Sundquist, K., Winkleby, M. A., & Sundquist, J. (2013). Comorbidities and mortality in bipolar disorder: A Swedish national cohort study. *JAMA Psychiatry, 70*(9), 931–939.

Darwin, C. (1857). Letter to J. D. Hooker. Retrieved from https://en.wikipedia.org/wiki/Lumpers_and_splitters

Denys, D., de Geus, F., van Megen, H. J., & Westenberg, H. G. (2004). Double-blind, randomized, placebo-controlled trial of quetiapine addition in patients with obsessive-compulsive disorder refractory to serotonin reuptake inhibitors. *Journal of Clinical Psychiatry, 65*, 1040–1048.

Dickstein, D. P., Rich, B. A., Binstock, A. B., Pradella, A. G., Towbin, K. E., Pine, D. S., & Leibenluft, E. (2005). Comorbid anxiety in phenotypes of pediatric bipolar disorder. *Journal of Child and Adolescent Psychopharmacology, 15*, 534–548.

Dilsaver, S. C., Chen, Y. W., Swann, A. C., Shoaib, A. M., Tsai-Dilsaver, Y., & Krajewski, K. J. (1997). Suicidality, panic disorder and psychosis in bipolar depression, depressive-mania and pure-mania. *Psychiatry Research, 73*, 47–56.

Doughty, C. J., Wells, J. E., Joyce, P. R., Olds, R. J., & Walsh, A. E. (2004). Bipolar-panic disorder comorbidity within bipolar disorder families: A study of siblings. *Bipolar Disorders, 6*, 245–252.

Dulac, O., & Guerrini, R. (2001). Seizure types and syndromes: Lumping or splitting. *Epilepsy Research, 45*, 37–40.

Falret, J.-P. (1854). Mémoire sur la folie circulaire. *Bulletin de L'Academie Imperiale de Médecine, 19*, 382–400.

Faravelli, C., Rosi, S., Alessandra, S. M., Lampronti, L., Amedei, S. G., & Rana, N. (2006). Threshold and subthreshold bipolar disorders in the Sesta Fiorentino Study. *Journal of Affective Disorders, 94*, 111–119.

Farren, C. K., Hill, K. P., & Weiss, R. D. (2012). Bipolar disorder and alcohol use disorder: A review. *Current Psychiatry Reports, 14*, 659–666.

Feighner, J. P., Robins, E., Guze, S. B., Woodruff, R. A., Winokur, G., & Munoz, R. (1972). Diagnostic criteria for use in psychiatric research. *Archives of General Psychiatry, 26*, 57–63.

Feinstein, A. R. (1970). Pre-therapeutic classification of comorbidity in chronic disease. *Journal of Chronic Diseases, 23*, 455–468.

Feske, U., Frank, E., Mallinger, A. G., Houck, P. R., Fagiolini, A., Shear, M. K.,…Kupfer, D. J. (2000). Anxiety as a correlate of response to acute treatment of bipolar 1 disorder. *American Journal of Psychiatry, 157*, 956–962.

Fineberg, N. A., Sivakumaran, T., Roberts, A., & Gale, T. (2005). Adding quetiapine to SRI in treatment-resistant obsessive-compulsive disorder: Randomized controlled treatment study. *International Clinical Psychopharmacology, 20*, 223–226.

Fogarty, F., Russell, J. M., Newman, S. C., & Bland, R. C. (1994). Epidemiology of psychiatric disorders in Edmonton. *Acta Psychiatrica Scandinavica, 376*(Suppl.), 16–23.

Freeman, M. P., Freeman, S. A., & McElroy, S. L. (2002). The comorbidity of bipolar and anxiety disorders: Prevalence, psychobiology, and treatment issues. *Journal of Affective Disorders, 68*, 1–23.

Gao, K., Chan, P. K., Verduin, M. L., Kemp, D. E., Tolliver, B. K., Ganocy, S. J.,…Calabrese, J. R. (2010). Independent predictors for lifetime and recent substance use disorders in patients with rapid-cycling bipolar disorder: Focus on anxiety disorders. *American Journal on Addictions, 19*, 440–449.

Gao, K., Kemp, D. E., Conroy, C., Ganocy, S. J., Findling, R. L., & Calabrese, J. R. (2010). Comorbid anxiety and substance use disorders associated with a lower use of mood-stabilizers in patients with rapid-cycling bipolar disorder: Descriptive analysis of cross-sectional data of 566 patients. *International Journal of Clinical Practice, 64*, 336–344.

Gao, K., Sheehan, D. V., & Calabrese, J. R. (2009). Atypical antipsychotics in primary generalized anxiety disorder or comorbid with mood disorders. *Expert Review of Neurotherapeutics, 9*, 1147–1158.

Gaudiano, B. A., & Miller, I. W. (2005). Anxiety disorder comorbidity in bipolar I disorder: Relationship to depression severity and treatment outcome. *Depression and Anxiety, 21*, 71–77.

George, M. S., Padberg, F., Schlaepfer, T. E., O'Reardon, J. P., Fitzgerald, P. B., Nahas, Z. H., & Marcolin, M. A. (2009). Controversy: Repetitive transcranial magnetic stimulation or transcranial direct current stimulation shows efficacy in treatment psychiatric diseases (depression, mania, schizophrenia, obsessive-compulsive disorder, panic, posttraumatic stress disorder). *Brain Stimulation, 2*, 14–21.

Ghaemi, S. N., & Thommi, S. B. (2010). Death by confounding: bias and mortality. *International Journal of Clinical Practice, 64*, 1009–1014.

Goikolea, J. M., Colom, F., Torres, I., Capapey, J., Valentí, M., Undurraga, J.,…Vieta, E. (2013). Lower rate of depressive switch following antimanic treatment with second-generation antipsychotics vs. haloperidol. *Journal of Affective Disorders, 144*, 191–198.

Goldberg, D., & Fawcett, J. (2012). The importance of anxiety in both major depression and bipolar disorders. *Depression and Anxiety, 29*, 471–478.

Goldstein, T. R., Ha, W., Axelson, D. A., Goldstein, B. I., Liao, F., Gill, M. K.,…Birmaher, B. (2012). Predictors of prospectively examined suicide attempts among youth with bipolar disorder. *Archives of General Psychiatry, 69*, 1113–1122.

Goodwin, F. K., & Jamison, K. R. (2007). *Manic-depressive illness* (2nd ed.). New York: Oxford University Press.

Goodwin, R. D., & Hoven, C. W. (2002). Bipolar-panic comorbidity in the general population: Prevalence and associated morbidity. *Journal of Affective Disorders, 70*, 27–33.

Grant, B. F., Stinson, F. S., Hasin, D. S., Dawson, D. A., Chou, S. P., Ruan, W. J., & Huang, B. (2005). Prevalence, correlates, and comorbidity of bipolar I disorder and axis I and II disorders: Results from the National Epidemiologic Survey on Alcohol and Related Conditions. *Journal of Clinical Psychiatry, 66*, 1205–1215.

Helzer, J. E., Kraemer, H. C., & Krueger, R. F. (2006). Feasibility and need for dimensional psychiatric diagnoses. *Psychological Medicine, 36*, 1671–1680.

Henry, C., van den Bulke, D., Bellivier, F., Etain, B., Rouillon, F., & Leboyer, M. (2003). Anxiety disorders in 318 bipolar patients: prevalence and impact on illness severity and response to mood stabilizer. *Journal of Clinical Psychiatry, 64*, 331–335.

Hertzberg, M. A., Butterfield, M. I., Feldman, M. E., Beckham, J. C., Sutherland, S. M., Connor, K. M., & Davidson, J. R. (1999). Preliminary study of lamotrigine for the treatment of posttraumatic stress disorder. *Biological Psychiatry, 45*, 1226–1229.

Hirschfeld, R. M. A., Weisler, R. H., Raines, S. R., & Macfadden, W. (2006). Quetiapine in the treatment of anxiety in patients with bipolar I or II depression: Secondary analysis from a randomized, double-blind, placebo-controlled study. *Journal of Clinical Psychiatry, 67*, 355–362.

Ioannidis, J. P. A. (2005). Why most published research findings are false. *PLoS Medicine, 2*, e124-0696–e124-0701.

Judd, L. L., & Akiskal, H. S. (2003). The prevalence and disability of bipolar spectrum disorders in the US population: Re-analysis of the

ECA database taking into account sub-threshold cases. *Journal of Affective Disorders, 73,* 123–131.

Juli, G., Juli, M. R., & Juli, L. (2012). Involvement of genetic factors in bipolar disorders: Current status. *Psychiatria Danubina, 24*(Suppl), S112–S116.

Katzman, M. A. (2011). Aripiprazole: clinical review of its use for the treatment of anxiety disorders and anxiety as a comorbidity in mental illness. *Journal of Affective Disorders, 128*(Suppl), S11–S20.

Kauer-Sant'Anna, M., Kapczinski, F., & Vieta, E. (2009). Epidemiology and management of anxiety in patients with bipolar disorder. *CNS Drugs, 23,* 953–964.

Keck, P. E. Jr., Kessler, R. C., & Ross, R. (2008). Clinical and economic effects of unrecognized or inadequately treated bipolar disorder. *Journal of Psychiatric Practice, 14*(2), 31–38.

Keck, P. E. Jr., McElroy, S. L., Strakowski, S. M., West, S. A., Hawkins, J. M., Huber, T. J.,...DePriest, M. (1995). Outcome and comorbidity in first- compared with multiple-episode mania. *Journal of Nervous and Mental Disease, 183,* 320–324.

Keck, P. E. Jr., Strawn, J. R., & McElroy, S. L. (2006). Pharmacologic treatment considerations in co-occurring bipolar and anxiety disorders. *Journal of Clinical Psychiatry, 67*(1), 8–15.

Kessler, R. C., Berglund, P., Demler, O., Jin, R., Joretz, D., Merikangas, K. R.,...Wang, P. S. (2003). Epidemiology of major depressive disorder: Results from the National Comorbidity Survey Replication (NCS-R). *JAMA, 289,* 3095–3105.

Kessler, R. C., Brandenburg, N., Lane, M., Roy-Byrne, P., Stang, P. D., Stein, D. J., & Wittchen, H. U. (2005). Rethinking the duration requirement for generalized anxiety disorder: Evidence from the National Comorbidity Survey Replication. *Psychological Medicine, 35,* 1073–1082.

Kessler, R., Chiu, W. T., Demler, O., & Walters, E. F. (2005). Prevalence severity and comorbidity of 12 month DSM-IV disorders in the National Comorbidity Survey Replication. *Archives of General Psychiatry, 62,* 617–627.

Kessler, R. C., Rubinow, D. R., Holmes, C., Abelson, J. M., & Zhao, S. (1997). Epidemiology of DSM-III-R bipolar I disorder in a general population survey. *Psychological Medicine, 27,* 1079–1089.

Klein, C. (2005). Movement disorders: Classifications. *Journal of Inherited Metabolic Disease, 28,* 425–439.

Krishnan, K. R. (2005). Psychiatric and medical comorbidities of bipolar disorder. *Psychosomatic Medicine, 67,* 1–8.

Krüger, S., Cooke, R. G., Hasey, G. M., Jorna, T., & Persad, E. (1995). Comorbidity of obsessive compulsive disorder in bipolar disorder. *Journal of Affective Disorders, 34,* 117–120.

Kupfer, D. J. (2005). The increasing medical burden in bipolar disorder. *JAMA, 293,* 2528–2530.

Lee, J. H., & Dunner, D. L. (2008). Effect of anxiety disorder comorbidity on treatment resistant bipolar disorder. *Depression and Anxiety, 25,* 91–97.

Li, X., May, R. S., Tolbert, L. C., Jackson, W. T., Flournoy, J. M., & Baxter, L. R. (2005). Risperidone and haloperidol augmentation of serotonin reuptake inhibition in refractory obsessive-compulsive disorders: Crossover study. *Journal of Clinical Psychiatry, 66,* 736–743.

Lim, C. S., Baldessarini, R. J., Vieta, E., Yucil, M., Bora, E., & Sim, K. (2013). Longitudinal neuroimaging and neuropsychological changes in bipolar disorder patients: Review of the evidence. *Neuroscience & Biobehavioral Reviews, 37,* 418–435.

Mack, A. H., Forman, L., Brown, R., & Frances, A. (1994). Brief history of psychiatric classification: From the ancients to DSM-IV. *Psychiatric Clinics of North America, 17,* 515–523.

MacKinnon, D. F., McMahon, F. J., Simpson, S. G., McInnis, M. G., & DePaulo, J. R. (1997). Panic disorder with familial bipolar disorder. *Biological Psychiatry, 42,* 90–95.

MacKinnon, D. F., Zandi, P. P., & Gershon, E. (2003). Rapid switching of mood in families with multiple cases of bipolar disorder. *Archives of General Psychiatry, 60,* 921–928.

Maj, M. (2005). "Psychiatric comorbidity": An artefact of current diagnostic systems? *British Journal of Psychiatry, 186,* 182–184.

Mantere, O., Isometsä, E., Ketokivi, M., Kiviruusu, O., Suominen, K., Valtonen, H. M.,...Leppämäki, S. (2010). A prospective latent analyses study of psychiatric comorbidity of DSM-IV bipolar I and II disorders. *Bipolar Disorders, 12,* 271–284.

Mantere, O., Melartin, T. K., Suominen, K., Rytsälä, H. J., Valtonen, H. M., Arvilommi, P.,...Isometsä, E. T. (2006). Differences in Axis I and II comorbidity between bipolar I and II disorders and major depressive disorder. *Journal of Clinical Psychiatry, 67,* 584–593.

McDougle, C. J., Price, L. H., Goodman, W. K., Charney, D. S., & Heninger, G. R. (1991). Controlled trial of lithium augmentation in fluvoxamine-refractory obsessive-compulsive disorder: Lack of efficacy. *Journal of Clinical Psychopharmacology, 11,* 175–184.

McElroy, S. L., Altshuler, L., Suppes, T., Keck, P. E. Jr., Frye, M. A., Denicoff, K. D.,...Post, R. M. (2001). Axis I psychiatric comorbidity and its relationship to historical illness variables in 288 patients with bipolar disorder. *American Journal of Psychiatry, 158,* 420–426.

McIntyre, R. S., Konarski, J. Z., Soczynska, J. K., Wilkins, K., Panjwani, G., Bouffard, B.,...Kennedy, S. H. (2006). Medical comorbidity in bipolar disorder: Implications for functional outcomes and health service utilization. *Psychiatric Services, 57,* 1140–1144.

McIntyre, R. S., Rosenbluth, M., Ramasubbu, R., Bond, D., Taylor, V. H., Beaulieu, S., & Schaffer, A. (2012). Managing medical and psychiatric comorbidity in individuals with major depressive disorder and bipolar disorder. *Annals of Clinical Psychiatry, 24,* 163–169.

McIntyre, R. S., Soczynska, J. K., Beyer, J. L., Woldeyohannes, H. O., Law, C. W., Miranda, A.,...Kennedy, S. H. (2007). Medical comorbidity in bipolar disorder: Re-prioritizing unmet needs. *Current Opinion in Psychiatry, 20,* 406–416.

McKusick, V. A. (1969). On lumpers and splitters, or the nosology of genetic disease. *Perspectives in Biology and Medicine, 12,* 298–312.

McKusick, V. A. (2006). A 60-year tale of spots, maps, and genes. *Annual Review of Genomics and Human Genetics, 7,* 1–27.

Merikangas, K. R., Akiskal, H. S., Angst, J., Greenberg, P. E., Hirschfeld, R. M., Petukhova, M., & Kessler, R. C. (2007). Lifetime and 12-month prevalence of bipolar spectrum disorder in the National Comorbidity Survey replication. *Archives of General Psychiatry, 64,* 543–352.

Merikangas, K. R., Jin, R., He, J. P., Kessler, R. C., Lee, S., Sampson, N. A.,...Zarkov, Z. (2011). Prevalence and correlates of bipolar spectrum disorder in the world mental health survey initiative. *Archives of General Psychiatry, 68,* 241–251.

Mitchell, P. B. (2012). Bipolar disorder: The shift to overdiagnosis. *Canadian Journal of Psychiatry, 57,* 659–665.

Mula, M., Pini, S., & Cassano, G. B. (2007). Role of anticonvulsant drugs in anxiety disorders: Critical review of the evidence. *Journal of Clinical Psychopharmacology, 27,* 263–272.

Narrow, W. E., & Kuhl, E. A. (2011). Dimensional approaches to psychiatric diagnosis in DSM-5. *Journal of Mental Health Policy and Economics, 14,* 197–200.

National Institute of Mental Health. (2009). Bipolar Disorder Research (Publication No. 09-3679). Retrieved from http://www.nimh.nih.gov/health/publications/bipolar-disorder/index.shtml.

Offidani, E., Fava, G. A., Tomba, E., & Baldessarini, R. J. (2013). Excessive mood-elevation with juvenile antidepressant treatment in depressive versus anxiety disorders: Systematic review. *Psychotherapy and Psychosomatics, 82,* 132–141.

Ösby, U., Brandt, L., Correia, N., Ekbom, A., & Sparén, P. (2001). Excess mortality in bipolar and unipolar disorder in Sweden. *Archives of General Psychiatry, 58,* 844–850.

Pacchiarotti, I., Bond, D. J., Baldessarini, R. J., Nolen, W. A., Grunze, H., Licht, R. W.,...Vieta, E. (2013). International Society for Bipolar Disorders (ISBD) task-force report on antidepressant use in bipolar disorders. *American Journal of Psychiatry, 170*(11), 1249–1262.

Paes, F., Machado, S., Arias-Carrión, O., Velasques, B., Teixeira, S., Budde, H.,...Nardi, A. E. (2011). Value of repetitive transcranial magnetic stimulation (rTMS) for the treatment of anxiety disorders: Integrative review. *CNS & Neurological Disorders: Drug Targets, 10*, 610–620.

Pande, A. C., Davidson, J. R., Jefferson, J. W., Janney, C. A., Katzelnick, D. J., Weisler, R. H.,...Sutherland, S. M. (1999). Treatment of social phobia with gabapentin: Placebo-controlled study. *Journal of Clinical Psychopharmacology, 19*, 341–348.

Pande, A. C., Pollack, M. H., Crockett, J., Greiner, M., Chouinard, G., Lydiard, R. B.,...Shiovitz, T. (2000). Placebo-controlled study of gabapentin treatment of panic disorder. *Journal of Clinical Psychopharmacology, 20*, 467–471.

Papolos, D., Teicher, M. H., Faedda, G. L., Murphy, P., & Mattis, S. (2013). Clinical experience using intranasal ketamine in the treatment of pediatric bipolar disorder/fear of harm phenotype. *Journal of Affective Disorders, 147*, 431–436.

Parker, G. (2010). Comorbidities in bipolar disorder: Models and management. *Medical Journal of Australia, 193*(4), S18–S20.

Pérez, J., Baldessarini, R. J., Cruz, N., Salvatore, P., & Vieta, E. (2011). Andrés Piquer-Arrufat (1711–1772): Contributions of an eighteenth-century Spanish physician to the concept of manic-depressive illness. *Harvard Review of Psychiatry, 19*, 68–77.

Perlis, R. H., Miyahara, S., Marangell, L. B., Wisniewski, S. R., Ostacher, M., DelBello, M. P.,...Nierenberg, A. A. (2004). Long-term implications of early onset in bipolar disorder: Data from the first 1000 participants in the systematic treatment enhancement program for bipolar disorder (STEP-BD). *Biological Psychiatry, 55*, 875–881.

Perugi, G., Akiskal, H. S., Ramacciotti, S., Nassini, S., Toni, C., Milanfranchi, A., & Musetti, L. (1999). Depressive comorbidity of panic, social phobic, and obsessive-compulsive disorders re-examined: Is there a bipolar II connection? *Journal of Psychiatric Research, 33*, 53–61.

Perugi, G., Frare, F., Toni, C., Tusini, G., Vannucchi, G., & Akiskal, H. S. (2010). Adjunctive valproate in panic disorder patients with comorbid bipolar disorder or otherwise resistant to standard antidepressants: A 3-year "open" follow-up study. *European Archives of Psychiatry and Clinical Neuroscience, 260*, 553–560.

Phelps, J., Angst, J., Katzow, J., & Sadler, J. (2008). Validity and utility of bipolar spectrum models. *Bipolar Disorders, 10*(1 Pt. 2), 179–193.

Phelps, J., & Manipod, V. (2012). Treating anxiety by discontinuing antidepressants: Case series. *Medical Hypotheses, 79*, 338–341.

Pichot, P. (2004). 50ème anniversaire de la Folie Circulaire (Circular insanity, 150 years on (French)). *Bulletin de L'Academie Nationale de Medecine, 188*, 275–284.

Pigott, T. A., Pato, M. T., L'Heureux, F., Hill, J. L., Grover, G. N., Bernstein, S. E., & Murphy, D. L. (1991). Controlled comparison of adjuvant lithium carbonate or thyroid hormone in clomipramine-treated patients with obsessive-compulsive disorder. *Journal of Clinical Psychopharmacology, 11*, 242–248.

Pini, S., Cassano, G. B., Simonini, E., Savino, M., Russo, A., & Montgomery, S. A. (1997). Prevalence of anxiety disorders comorbidity in bipolar depression, unipolar depression and dysthymia. *Journal of Affective Disorders, 42*, 145–153.

Pittenger, C., Coric, V., Banasr, M., Bloch, M., Krystal, J. H., & Sanacora, G. (2008). Riluzole in the treatment of mood and anxiety disorders. *CNS Drugs, 22*, 761–786.

Prasko, J., Zálesky, R., Bares, M., Horácek, J., Kopecek, M., Novák, T., & Pasková, B. (2007). Effect of repetitive transcranial magnetic stimulation (rTMS) added on to serotonin reuptake inhibitors in patients with panic disorder: Randomize, double-blind, sham-controlled study. *Neuroendocrinology Letters, 1*, 33–38.

Provencher, M. D., Guimond, A. J., & Hawke, L. D. (2012). Comorbid anxiety in bipolar spectrum disorders: A neglected research and treatment issue? *Journal of Affective Disorders, 137*, 161–164.

Provencher, M. D., Hawke, L. D., & Thienot, E. (2011). Psychotherapies for comorbid anxiety in bipolar spectrum disorders. *Journal of Affective Disorders, 133*, 371–380.

Rakofsky, J. J., & Dunlop, B. W. (2011). Treating nonspecific anxiety and anxiety disorders in patients with bipolar disorder: Review. *Journal of Clinical Psychiatry, 72*, 81–90.

Reich, D. B., Winternitz, S., Hennen, J., Watts, T., & Stanculescu, C. (2004). Preliminary study of risperidone in the treaetment of post-traumatic stress disorder related to childhood abuse in women. *Journal of Clinical Psychiatry, 65*, 1601–1606.

Rihmer, Z., Szádóczky, E., Füredi, J., Kiss, K., & Papp, Z. (2001). Anxiety disorders comorbidity in bipolar I, bipolar II and unipolar major depression: Results from a population-based study in Hungary. *Journal of Affective Disorders, 67*, 175–179.

Sala, R., Goldstein, B., Morcillo, C., Liu, S.-M., Castellanos, M., & Blanco, C. (2012). Course of comorbid anxiety disorders among adults with bipolar disorder in the U.S. population. *Journal of Psychiatric Research, 46*, 865–872.

Salvatore, P., Baldessarini, R. J., Centorrino, F., Egli, S., Albert, M., Gerhard, A., & Maggini, C. (2002). Weygandt's *The Manic-Depressive Mixed States*: A translation and commentary on its significance in the evolution of the concept of bipolar manic-depressive disorder. *Harvard Review of Psychiatry, 10*, 255–275.

Salvatore, P., Baldessarini, R. J., Khalsa, H.-M. K., Indic, P., Maggini, C., & Tohen, M. (2013). Negative affective features in 516 cases of first psychotic disorder episodes: Relationship to suicidal risk. *Journal of Depression & Anxiety, 27*, 2.

Salvatore, P., Baldessarini, R. J., Khalsa, H.-M. K., Vázquez, G. H., Pérez, J., Maggini, C., & Tohen, M. (2014). McLean-Harvard International First Psychotic episode study: Antecedents in 263 bipolar I disorder patients. *Acta Psychiatrica Scandinavica, 129*(4), 275–285.

Salvatore, P., Baldessarini, R. J., Tohen, M., Khalsa, H.-M. K., Sanchez-Toledo, J. P., Zarate, C. A. Jr.,...Maggini, C. (2009). McLean-Harvard International First-Episode Project: Two-year stability of DSM-IV diagnoses in 500 first-episode psychotic disorder patients. *Journal of Clinical Psychiatry, 70*, 458–466.

Salvatore, P., Baldessarini, R. J., Tohen, M., Khalsa, H.-M. K., Sanchez-Toledo, J. P., Zarate, C. A. Jr.,...Maggini, C. (2011). McLean-Harvard International First-Episode Project: Two-year stability of ICD-10 diagnoses in 500 first-episode psychotic disorder patients. *Journal of Clinical Psychiatry, 72*, 183–193.

Sani, G., Kotzalidis, G. D., Vöhringer, P., Pucci, D., Simonetti, A., Manfredi, G.,...Ghaemi, S. N. (2013). Effectiveness of short-term olanzapine in patients with bipolar I disorder, with or without comorbidity with substance use disorder. *Journal of Clinical Psychopharmacology, 33*, 231–235.

Sani, G., Serra, G., Kotzalidis, G. D., Romano, S., Tamorri, S. M., Manfredi, G.,...Girardi, P. (2012). Role of memantine in the treatment of psychiatric disorders other than the dementias: Review of current preclinical and clinical evidence. *CNS Drugs, 26*, 663–690.

Schaffer, A., Cairney, J., Veldhuizen, S., Kurdyak, P., Cheung, A., & Levitt, A. (2010). Population-based analysis of distinguishers of bipolar disorder from major depressive disorder. *Journal of Affective Disorders, 125*, 103–110.

Sedler, M. J. (1983). Falret's discovery: The origin of the concept of bipolar affective illness. *American Journal of Psychiatry, 140*, 1127–1133.

Shapira, N. A., Ward, H. E., Mandoki, M., Murphy, T. K., Yang, M. C., Blier, P., & Goodman, W. K. (2004). Double-blind, placebo-controlled trial of olanzapine addition in fluoxetine-refractory obsessive-compulsive disorder. *Biological Psychiatry, 55*, 553–555.

Sheehan, D. V., Harnet-Sheehan, K., Hidalgo, R. B., Janavs, J., McElroy, S. L., Amado, D., & Suppes, T. (2013). Randomized, placebo-controlled trial of quetiapine-XR and divalproex-ER monotherapies in the treatment of the anxious bipolar patient. *Journal of Affective Disorders, 145*, 83–94.

Sheehan, D. V., McElroy, S. L., Harnett-Sheehan, K., Keck, P. E. Jr., Janavs, J., Rogers, J., ... Suppes, T. (2009). Randomized placebo-controlled trial of risperidone for acute treatment of bipolar anxiety. *Journal of Affective Disorders, 115*, 376–385.

Simon, G. E., Hunkeler, E., Fireman, B., Lee, J. Y., & Savarino, J. (2007). Risk of suicide attempt and suicide death in patients treated for bipolar disorder I. *Bipolar Disorders, 9*, 526–530.

Simon, N. M., Otto, M. W., Wisniewski, S. R., Fossey, M., Sagduyu, K., Frank, E., ... Pollack, M. H. (2004). Anxiety disorder comorbidity in bipolar disorder patients: Data from the first 500 participants in the systematic treatment enhancement program for bipolar disorder (STEP-BD). *American Journal of Psychiatry, 161*, 2222–2229.

Simon, N. M., Smoller, J. W., Fava, M., Sachs, G., Racette, S. R., Perlis, R., ... Rosenbaum, J. F. (2003). Comparing anxiety disorders and anxiety-related traits in bipolar disorder and unipolar depression. *Journal of Psychiatric Research, 37*, 187–192.

Singh, J. B., & Zarate, C. (2006). Pharmacological treatment of psychiatric comorbidity in bipolar disorder: A review of controlled trials. *Bipolar Disorders, 8*, 696–709.

Stein, M. B., Kline, N. A., & Matloff, J. L. (2002). Adjunctive olanzapine for SSRI-resistant combat-related PTSD: Double-blind, placebo-controlled study. *American Journal of Psychiatry, 159*, 1777–1779.

Strakowski, S. M., Sax, K. W., McElroy, S. L., Keck, P. E. Jr., Hawkins, J. M., & West, S. A. (1998). Course of psychiatric and substance abuse syndromes co-occurring with bipolar disorder after a first psychiatric hospitalization. *Journal of Clinical Psychiatry, 59*, 465–471.

Strawn, J. R., & Geraciotti, T. D. Jr. (2007). Treatment of generalized anxiety disorder with pregabalin, an atypical anxiolytic. *Neuropsychiatric Disease and Treatment, 3*, 237–243.

Surtees, P. G., & Kendell, R. E. (1979). Hierarchy model of psychiatric symptomatology: An investigation based on present state examination ratings. *British Journal of Psychiatry, 135*, 438–443.

Szadoczky, E., Papp, Z. S., Vitrai, J., Ríhmer, Z., & Füredi, J. (1998). Prevalence of major depressive and bipolar disorders in Hungary: Results from a national epidemiologic survey. *Journal of Affective Disorders, 50*, 153–162.

Sullivan, P. F., Daly, M. J., & O'Donovan, M. (2012). Genetic architectures of psychiatric disorders: The emerging picture and its implications. *Nature Reviews Genetics, 13*, 537–551.

Tohen, M., Calabrese, J. R., Vieta, E., Bowden, C. L., González-Pinto, A., Lin, D., ... Corya, S. (2007). Effect of comorbid anxiety on treatment response in bipolar depression. *Journal of Affective Disorders, 104*, 137–146.

Tondo, L., Vázquez, G. H., & Baldessarini, R. J. (2010). Mania associated with antidepressant-treatment: Comprehensive meta-analytic review. *Acta Psychiatrica Scandinavica, 121*, 404–414.

Tondo, L., & Baldessarini, R. (2013). "Clinical Characteristics of Bipolar Disorders in Sardinia (Italy)". Presented as a plenary lecture at the V IberoAmerican Meeting on Affective Disorders, organized by the Argentine Society for Affective Disorders. July 25–27, Buenos Aires, Argentina.

Trede, K., Salvatore, P., Baethge, C., Gerhard, A., Maggini, C., & Baldessarini, R. J. (2005). Manic-depressive illness: Evolution in Kraepelin's textbook, 1883-1926. *Harvard Review of Psychiatry, 13*, 155–178.

Uhde, T. W., Stein, M. B., & Post, R. M. (1988). Lack of efficacy of carbamazepine in the treatment of panic disorder. *American Journal of Psychiatry, 145*, 1104–1109.

van Ameringen, M., Mancini, C., Pipe, B., & Bennett, M. (2004). Antiepileptic drugs in the treatment of anxiety disorders: role in therapy. *Drugs, 64*, 2199–2220.

van Praag, H. M. (1996). Comorbidity (psycho)analysed. *British Journal of Psychiatry, 168*(30), 129s–134s.

van Praag, H. M. (1999). Impact of classification on psychopharmacology and biological psychiatry. *Dialogues in Clinical Neuroscience, 1*, 141–151.

Vázquez, G. H., Tondo, L., Undurraga, J., & Baldessarini, R. J. (2013). Overview of antidepressant treatment in bipolar depression: Critical commentary. *International Journal of Neuropsychopharmacology, 22*, 1–13.

Vulink, N. C. C., Figee, M., & Denys, D. (2011). Review of atypical antipsychotics in anxiety. *European Neuropsychopharmacology, 21*, 429–449.

Walter-Ryan, W. G., & Fahs, J. J. (1987). The problem with parsimony: Mania and hyperthyroidism. *Journal of Clinical Psychiatry, 48*, 289–290.

Weber, N. S., Fisher, J. A., Cowan, D. N., & Niebuhr, D. W. (2011). Psychiatric and general medical conditions comorbid with bipolar disorder in the National Hospital Discharge Survey. *Psychiatric Services, 62*, 1152–1158.

Winokur, G. (1990). The concept of secondary depression and its relationship to comorbidity. *Psychiatric Clinics of North America, 13*, 567–583.

Wittchen, H. U. (1996). Critical issues in the evaluation of comorbidity of psychiatric disorders. *British Journal of Psychiatry, 168*(30), 9s–16s.

Woodruff, R. A. Jr., Goodwin, D. W., & Guze, S. B. (1974). *Psychiatric diagnosis.* New York: Oxford University Press.

World Health Organization. (1994). *International statistical classification of diseases and related health problems* (10th ed.). Geneva.

World Health Organization. (2014). *International statistical classification of diseases and related health problems* (11th ed.). Geneva: Author.

Wozniak, J., Biederman, J., Monuteaux, M. C., Richards, J., & Faraone, S. V. (2002). Parsing the comorbidity between bipolar disorder and anxiety disorders: Familial risk analysis. *Journal of Child and Adolescent Psychopharmacology, 12*, 101–111.

Yatham, L. N., Kennedy, S. H., Parikh, S. V., Schaffer, A., Beaulieu, S., Alda, M., ... Berk, M. (2013). Canadian Network for Mood and Anxiety Treatments (CANMAT) and International Society for Bipolar Disorders (ISBD) collaborative update of CANMAT guidelines for the management of patients with bipolar disorder. *Bipolar Disorders, 15*, 1–44.

Young, L. T., Cooke, R. G., Robb, J. C., Levitt, A. J., & Joffe, R. T. (1993). Anxious and non-anxious bipolar disorder. *Journal of Affective Disorders, 29*, 49–52.

Zarate, C. A. Jr., & Manji, H. K. (2008). Riluzole in psychiatry: Systematic review of the literature. *Expert Opinion on Drug Metabolism & Toxicology, 4*, 1223–1234.

Zimmermann, P., Bruckl, T., Nocon, A., Pfister, H., Lieb, R., Wittchen, H. U., ... Angst, J. (2009). Heterogeneity of DSMIV major depressive disorder as a consequence of sub-threshold bipolarity. *Archives of General Psychiatry, 66*, 1341–1352.

Zimmerman, M., & Mattia, J. I. (1999). Psychiatric diagnosis in clinical practice: Is comorbidity being missed? *Comprehensive Psychiatry, 40*, 182–191.

34.

MANAGEMENT OF CYCLOTHYMIA AND COMORBID PERSONALITY DISORDERS

Giulio Perugi and Giulia Vannucchi

INTRODUCTION

The relationship between severe melancholic and manic states and attenuated or subclinical and temperamental forms of mood disorders has been recognized since antiquity. In modern psychiatry, the term *cyclothymia* was introduced by Hecker in 1877 (Koukopoulos, 2003); his accurate clinical characterizations make him the forerunner of modern descriptions of cyclothymic and bipolar II disorders. Kraepelin included within manic-depressive illness the "attenuated depressive conditions alternated with episodes of manic excitement of lower intensity" and described long-lasting, stable depressive, manic (hyperthymic), cyclothymic, or irritable temperamental traits (which he referred to as basic states).

Since the 1960s, the broader Kraepelinian concept of manic-depressive illness has been replaced by the unipolar–bipolar distinction introduced by Leonhard, Angst, and Winokur. This has probably contributed to relegate subsyndromal chronic affective forms in the context of the so-called personality disorders, as suggested in the second revision of the *Diagnostic and Statistical Manual of Mental Disorders* (2nd ed., American Psychiatric Association, 1968), the Research Diagnostic Criteria, and the ninth revision of the *International Statistical Classification of Diseases* (World Health Organization, 1975). Mostly thanks to the contribution of Hagop S. Akiskal (Akiskal, Djenderedjian, Rosenthal, & Khani, 1977), during the past century, the unipolar–bipolar dichotomy revealed did not fit the clinical reality, and the diagnosis of "cyclothymic disorder" was included in the third edition of the *Diagnostic and Statistical Manual of Mental Disorders* (3rd ed. [*DSM-III*]; American Psychiatric Association, 1980) in the chapter on "Mood Disorders". Subsequently the *International Statistical Classification of Diseases and Related Health Problems* (10th ed. [ICD-10];

World Health Organization, 1994) has followed this trend, and cyclothymia received a large empirical validation as a bipolar spectrum disorder. For this reason it remained in the fourth (*DMS-IV*) and fifth (*DSM-5*) editions of the *Diagnostic and Statistical Manual of Mental Disorders* (American Psychiatric Association, 1994, 2013).

Epidemiological data largely confirmed the spectrum model of mood disorders: it is estimated that the 4% to 5% of the general population suffers from predominantly depressive manifestations associated with short-lasting and attenuated hypomanic symptoms (Angst & Marneros, 2001). Based on these observations, the four-days duration threshold required for the *DSM* hypomania diagnosis has been criticized: this definition does not permit proper identification of cyclothymic forms, which present short hypomanic episodes and result as the most common phenotypes of mood disorder in the general population (Angst et al., 2010).

Despite its epidemiological relevance, cyclothymia remains understudied from clinical and therapeutic points of view, and most of the research on bipolar disorder (BPD) is focused on bipolar I manic and depressive episodes. This is partly due to the fact that in current classifications specific symptoms for cyclothymia are not provided, except for the reduced intensity of mood episodes and protracted duration (more than two years). In the *DSM-5,* diagnostic criteria for cyclothymic disorder included "numerous period of" hypomanic and depressive "symptoms that do not met criteria for hypomania and major depressive episode." No specific type or cut-off number of symptoms is required. This definition is likely to increase the overlap with Cluster B personality disorders. However, the fact that coexistence of lifetime manic, hypomanic, and depressive episodes does not permit the diagnosis of cyclothymic disorder is highly questionable. In clinical practice, most cyclothymic patients are or have been referred for major affective episodes. Finally, in *DSM-5,* like in previous editions, the link between cyclothymia and the other bipolar spectrum disorders is not appropriately underlined and the continuity with temperament and personality dispositions is not mentioned.

These conceptual limitations have negatively affected the research on cyclothymia. Some authors, however, continuing the most "classic" sense of the disorder, define it as a "temperamental style," present during the largest part of the life beginning in childhood or adolescence (Akiskal, 1981; Koukopoulos, 2003). Particularly Akiskal has developed the temperamental perspective of cyclothymia, incorporating Kraepelian concept of "basic states" as constitutional expression of manic-depressive illness. The criteria for cyclothymic temperament proposed by Akiskal et al. (1998) reflect the classic descriptions of sudden mood swings and require three out of five opposed conditions of each of the following two sets. The first set includes (a) hypersomnia versus decreased need for sleep; (b) introverted self-absorption versus uninhibited people-seeking; (c) taciturn versus talkative; (d) unexplained tearfulness versus buoyant jocularity; and (e) psychomotor inertia versus restless pursuit of activities. The second set includes (a) lethargy and somatic discomfort versus eutonia; (b) dulling of senses versus keen perceptions; (c) slow-witted versus sharpened thinking; (d) shaky self-esteem alternating between low self-confidence and overconfidence; and (e) pessimistic brooding versus optimism and carefree attitudes. The bipolar nature of cyclothymic temperament is supported by a series of studies that have highlighted the strong propensity of these subjects to switch toward hypomania and/or mania when treated with antidepressants and to have a positive family history for BPD (Angst & Marneros, 2001; Koukopoulos, 2003).

A source of diagnostic difficulties is derived from the fact that some of the core characteristics of cyclothymia, such as affective instability, mood reactivity, and extreme emotionality, are reported in *DSM-IV* as in *DSM-5* among the criteria of a dramatic cluster of personality disorders. Many criteria proposed by the manual for histrionic and borderline personality disorders seem to describe some aspects of cyclothymia from a different perspective and favor the misdiagnosis of many patients, especially in the early phases of the disorders. Moreover, the tendency to include many of the characteristics of cyclothymia in personality disorders limits the probability of understanding the existing relationship among stable temperamental

dysregulations, problematic behaviors in bipolar patients, and major mood episodes.

EPIDEMIOLOGICAL AND CLINICAL ASPECTS

Among mood disorders, cyclothymia is the one that has received less attention in epidemiological studies, and only recently prevalence rates in the general population have become available. This is surprising given the frequency of the disorder in clinical practice. Recent studies conducted in Switzerland reported high lifetime prevalence rates of mood instability and cyclothymic traits ranging from 4% to 6% of the general population, with a preponderance of about 2:1 among women. The lifetime prevalence rates ranged from 5% to 8% for short episodes of hypomania associated with recurrent brief depression and from 6% to 13% for subsyndromal bipolarity (Angst et al., 2010; Angst & Marneros, 2001).

The prevalence of cyclothymia in clinical populations is even higher: more than 30% of depressed outpatients (Hantouche et al., 1998) and 50% of those suffering from obsessive-compulsive disorder present a cyclothymic temperament (Hantouche et al., 2003). This figure was also confirmed in general practice settings, where it is assumed that observed cases are less severe (Manning, Haykal, Connor, & Akiskal, 1997).

The clinical presentation of cyclothymia is particularly rich in psychopathological manifestations, which are mainly expressed as behavioral disorders and impaired interpersonal relationships. In this sense, the *DSM-IV* description, essentially based on the presence of mood symptoms, can be misleading. This is the main limitation of current diagnostic classifications, which result in a generalized tendency to underestimate cyclothymia and its clinical relevance.

The intensity of mood swings is generally limited, although in many cases major affective episodes of both polarities may be present. Cyclothymic subjects have continuous and irregular "highs" and "lows" of mood for extended periods of time; mood switches are often abrupt, while interposed periods of relative mood stability are infrequent. The unpredictability of mood swings is a major cause of distress, as it weakens self-esteem and produces considerable instability in terms of vocation, behavior, and personal relations.

Mood reactivity expressed as extreme sensitivity to physical, chemical, and psychological stimulations, often associated with the tendency to amplify emotional reactions in terms of intensity and duration, is a stable characteristic present since adolescence. Exaggerated positive and negative emotional reactions can be triggered by any sort of external stimuli, either psychological (e.g., falling in love vs. sentimental disappointments), environmental (e.g., meteorological changes or changes of time zone), physical (e.g., immobility vs. hyperactivity), or chemical (e.g., medications and alcohol or drugs).

The cyclothymics react to favorable events with joy, enthusiasm, initiative, and dynamism that sometimes turn into excessive euphoria and impulsiveness. In the case of negative events (real or experienced as such) they become distressed and experience feelings of deep prostration, sadness, and extreme fatigue. They can become tactless and hostile, or in many cases they have explosions of rage following minor disputes, although subjectively amplified, which have the effect of triggering "avalanche" reactions with destructive consequences on their interpersonal life. In these circumstances even minor adversity and frustrations may precipitate clamorous reactions or self-harming gestures. These features show that the interpersonal relationships domain is usually the most impaired in cyclothymia. In this context, the hypomanic episodes are not easily identifiable, especially keeping in mind the four-days' duration criteria requested by *DSM*. Indeed, in many cases elated phases last for one or two days or even less, and they can easily be confused with a state of "normal" excitement. The mood swings may assume a circadian component with biphasic characteristics, such as lethargy alternated with euphoria, reduced verbal productivity alternated with excessive loquacity, or low self-esteem alternated with excessive trust in their own abilities.

Mood reactivity is closely related to interpersonal sensitivity, defined as the peculiar disposition to misperceive elements of personal deficiency and weak self-esteem, resulting in high sensitivity to judgment, criticism, and rejection by others. Mood reactivity and interpersonal sensitivity seem to represent the affective and cognitive aspects of the same psycho(patho)logical dimension, respectively. Mood instability of the cyclothymic type is strongly related to mood reactivity and interpersonal sensitivity, suggesting the existence of a common background (Perugi, Toni, Travierso, & Akiskal, 2003) The main psychological consequences of cyclothymia are summarized in Box 34.1..

In many cyclothymic subjects, susceptibility to rejection and disapproval by others is a major source of distress. They are promptly offended and sensitive to the possibility of being wounded, with feelings of hostility and anger toward those who evocate these reactions and who are considered responsible for their sufferance. When emotional reactions are very intense, the sensitivity may favor the onset of more or less transient tendency to interpretation and overvalued ideas. The fear of being rejected, turned away, and disapproved of may heighten the tendency to want to please others with submissive behaviors and excessive dedication, even resulting in hyperempathy and "pathological altruism." The oscillation between complacency and excessive feelings of anger/hostility, between inhibition and behavioral disinhibition, results in stormy, unstable, and difficult to manage relational, familial, working, and emotional patterns. Individuals with such a mood reactivity, when switching toward exhilaration, often seek sentimental and interpersonal relationships; on the contrary, dysphorics tend to isolate themselves from the others. Indeed, the youth of many of these patients can be a continuous succession of tempestuous short and intense sentimental relations with often unsuitable or unlikely partners. What appears to most afflict these patients is their periodic swinging between behavioral inhibition and activation, which prompts them toward interpersonal relations, situations in which they respond afterward with an avalanche of hardly manageable emotional reactions, creating a path full of existential dramas and tragedies.

The other great dimension of cyclothymia is impulsiveness, which is also closely related to mood reactivity. Impulsivity determines sensation/novelty-seeking and self-stimulation behaviors, which amplifies during elated phases (Perugi & Akiskal, 2002). In many cases this is the starting ground for the development of true impulse control disorders such as pathological gambling and compulsive sexuality in men and compulsive buying and binge eating in women. Cyclothymia also represents a fertile ground for drug abuse (Maremmani, Perugi, Pacini, & Akiskal,

---

Box 34.1 PSYCHOLOGICAL ASPECTS OF CYCLOTHYMIA

Sensitivity to rejection
Sensitivity to separation and affective dependency
Pathological jealousy
Excessive need to please others
Sensitivity to judgment and criticism
Compulsive need for compliments and emotional rewards
Tendency to test and exceed limits in interpersonal relationships
Novelty seeking mixed with harm avoidance
Hypercontrol
Compulsive and impulsive behaviors
Lack of future projection
Shaky self-esteem, from low self-confidence to overconfidence

2006). Sensation-seeking behavior and a high sensitivity to substances encourage the use of alcohol, stimulants, and cocaine, as well as hypnotics and sedatives. In some subjects, for environmental reasons, mood instability and impulsivity combined with substance abuse can favor the emergence of antisocial conduct with legal problems.

Due to this great variety of pathological behaviors and to the coexistence of contradictory psychopathological elements such as anxiety and impulsiveness, cyclothymic subjects often meet the *DSM* criteria for cluster B "dramatic" or "emotional" personality disorders. Histrionic, narcissistic, and borderline disorders have broad symptomatic areas in common with cyclothymia, such as "emotional instability" and excessive "mood reactivity". Also, personality disorders are defined by behavioral and emotional patterns with onset during adolescence or early adulthood, so severe as to condition impairment in several areas. In many cases, the distinction between cyclothymia and histrionic or borderline personality disorders mainly depends on the perspective and moment of observation rather than on real clinical differences (Levitt, Joffe, Ennis, MacDonald, & Kutcher, 1990).

CYCLOTHYMIA AND PERSONALITY DISORDERS

Defining cyclothymia simply as the succession of "numerous depressive and hypomanic symptoms" for a period of two years is a bit like defining a storm as the mere combination and rapid mixing of air and water for a period of hours. Affective instability, impulsivity, emotional lability, and hyperreactivity and their psychological consequences such as interpersonal rejection and separation sensitivity can be misinterpreted as the result of character disturbances or personality problems rather than as specific cyclothymic features. This is the main source of debate about the syndromal and behavioral overlap between cyclothymia and Cluster B personality disorders, otherwise described as "dramatic," "amplifying-emotional," "fickle," or "unpredictable."

Very few data are available on the co-occurrence of cyclothymia and personality disorders. In fact, the majority of the studies have evaluated personality traits during depressive episodes or in major depressive or BPD patients. In a study by Alnæs and Tæorgensen (1989), cyclothymics with a major depressive episode were compared with purely depressed patients: cyclothymia in depressive patients was highly associated with Cluster B and C personality disorders according to *DSM-III* criteria, particularly borderline (28% vs. 10%), avoidant (83% vs. 53%), histrionic (28%

vs. 10%), and passive-aggressive (21% vs. 7%), and less frequently with narcissistic (7% vs. 0%).

Recently, a large, multinational, cross-sectional study (Angst et al., 2011: BRIDGE) was conducted on 5,635 patients with major depressive episode, recruited and evaluated by community and hospital-based psychiatrists. A descriptive, bottom-up approach to assess validity of different definitions of hypomania was applied (Angst et al., 2011). The validity of *DSM-IV* BPDs diagnosis was compared with a "bipolar specifier." This latter was defined on the basis of the presence of hyperactivity/increased energy as entrance criteria for hypomania, together with elated or irritable mood, the elimination of the duration criteria, and the inclusion of drugs/substance-induced episodes. The specifier definition resulted more associated than *DSM-IV* to all the explored external validators of bipolarity such as family history of BPDs, history of switches with antidepressants, early age at onset, number of previous episodes, presence of mixed features, and comorbidity with other mental disorders. In this sample, 9.3% of the patients showed current comorbidity with BPD; they reported more frequently than patients without comorbid BPD a diagnosis of bipolar specifier (72.6% vs. 44.5%, *p* < .0001; Perugi et al., 2013a, 2013b). Bipolar disorder rates were significantly different—also utilizing a more restrictive definition of bipolar specifier with at least a two-day (respectively, 67.4% vs. 42.3%, *p* < .0001) or at least a four-day (respectively, 55.2% vs. 36.7%, *p* < .0001) duration of hypomania. A diagnosis of bipolar specifier was strongly and independently predicted by the presence of specific *Diagnostic and Statistical Manual of Mental Disorders* (fourth edition, text revision [*DSM-IV-TR*]; American Psychiatric Association, 2000) criteria for BPD: unstable and intense interpersonal relationships; impulsivity in at least two areas potentially self-damaging; affective instability owing to a marked reactivity of mood; and inappropriate, intense anger or difficulty controlling anger. The two groups showed statistically significant differences with regard to early age at onset; family history of BPD; history of antidepressant-induced hypomanic switches; seasonality of mood episodes; history of suicide attempts; prior mood episodes (≥4); rates of current psychiatric comorbidity; and presence of current psychotic symptoms, mixed states, atypical features, and resistance to treatment. All of these features can be considered reliable external validators of bipolarity and were more common in depressive patients with than in those without comorbid BPD. These findings suggest a strong correlation between BPD and BPD in patients with major depressive episode, with important clinical and therapeutic implications. Specific and clinical features of cyclothymia are highlighted in Box 34.2

DSM-5 diagnostic criteria for borderline, narcissistic, and histrionic personality disorders describe some aspects of the cyclothymic picture from a different perspective. In particular, the histrionic profile is characterized by changeability, superficiality, and exasperated emotional expressiveness, while borderline personality criteria include sensitivity to separation, affective instability, emotional reactivity, unjustified anger and hostility, impulsivity, instability of interpersonal relationships, and suicidal tendencies. DSM-5 borderline, narcissistic, and histrionic personality disorders criteria are summarized in Box 34.3

In the past decades the debate has mainly involved the relationships between bipolar spectrum and BPD. The term *borderline* represents the interface between the psychiatric tradition and psychoanalysis (Stone, 2006). Used for the first time in the late 19th century to indicate conditions difficult to place between psychosis and neurotic disorders, in the 1920s it was adopted in the field of psychoanalysis for those conditions not easily treatable with psychotherapy but neither clearly refractory. In other words, these pathological conditions were considered "borderline" in relation to psychosis. Hypersensitivity to criticism, tendency to depression, ego weakness, infantilism, tantrums, and impulsivity were described among the first characteristics of the disorder. Kernberg (1967) coined the description of "borderline personality organization," meaning the term *personality* as a peculiar organization of psychic life of the self. He proposed a distinction between a higher level of mental organization or "neurotic" type, in which the sense of self-identity and reality testing were preserved, and a lower or "psychotic" type in which both were grossly compromised. According to this distinction, the borderline personality organization would be characterized on one hand by the reality-testing conservation, except for a tendency to

overestimate judgments loaded with emotional meanings ("overvalued or prevailing ideas"), and on the other hand for a weakening of the sense of self-identity.

Later the term *borderline* was used to indicate multiple ideas: (a) secondary manifestation to a developmental arrest in the phase of separation-individuation; (b) a particularly "difficult" patient; (c) different types of patients, in a range including individuals with near-psychosis to those with analytical depression and excellent functioning; (d) a peculiar narcissistic insult; and (e) a personality disorder defined by more objective and easily measurable operational criteria (Gunderson & Singer, 1975).

This concept of BPD became one of the two matrices (the other was represented by the Kernberg [1967] borderline personality organization) from which the description of BPD officially entered in 1980 into the Axis II of the *DSM-III*. The influence of Kernberg and later that of Gunderson (Gunderson & Singer, 1975) is the main reason for BPD inclusion among Axis II disorders, rather than Axis I, despite its diagnostic criteria referring more to symptoms than to temperamental and character traits. Indeed, BPD shows a peculiarity regarding to its diagnostic definition codified by the nine *DSM-IV* criteria (one more than in *DSM-III*). A personality trait is assumed to represent a stable and usual pattern of psychological functioning. It should be noted that only three of the nine *DSM-IV* criteria for BPD respect this assumption: impulsivity, affective instability, and anger. These traits are defined as describing strongly symptomatic behaviors as well. This is a difference between BPD and other personality disorders, for which the diagnostic criteria refer to proper personality traits. One of the consequences of the choice of defining a personality disorder through the symptoms rather than the traits is it exposes it to a certain interpretation variability: the diagnostic criteria of BPD characterize nonspecific manifestations that are strongly related to mood disorders in general and to cyclothymia in particular, such as (a) separation anxiety, (b) stormy lifestyle, (c) impulsive behaviors, (d) suicidal threats or conduct, (e) unprovoked and intense anger, (f) mood reactivity and instability, and (g) brief psychotic episodes developed on affective and paranoid backgrounds, not typically schizophrenic.

This description makes BPD an extremely heterogeneous entity; therefore it is not surprising that it is regularly associated with several other mental and personality disorders. Among the Axis I disorders, depression, BPD, eating disorders, anxiety disorders, substance abuse, dissociative disorders, posttraumatic stress disorder, and impulsive aggressiveness are more frequently found in association with BPD. Cyclothymia, not surprisingly, shares this pattern of comorbidity.

To date, the question of the relationship between BPD and bipolar spectrum remains unresolved. Some of the BPD diagnostic criteria really show a strong affective connotation: unprovoked anger, affective instability, suicidal tendencies, unstable relationships. High prevalence of cyclothymia and/or attenuated bipolar spectrum disorders has been documented in different series of borderline patients and, vice versa, the prevalence of borderline personality traits is very high among cyclothymic patients (Levitt et al., 1990; Stone, 1990).

In a German study that rigorously evaluated "subaffective personality disorders," BPD patients and those with cyclothymic-irritable temperament presented considerably overlapping clinical pictures (Sass, Herpertz, & Steinmeyer, 1993). In addition, the borderline personality has been demonstrated to be a predictive factor for antidepressant-induced hypomania (Levy, Kimhi, Barak, Aviv, & Elizur, 1998; Stone, 2006). Even long-term follow-up studies suggested a close relationship between BPD and mood disorders, considering the great number of young borderline patients who developed, over the years, a frank bipolar I or, more frequently, bipolar II disorder or recurrent depression.

On the basis of these data, Akiskal suggested that the BPD psychopathological core would be represented by a defective "mood regulation," at least for many patients. In such a patient, the disorder would be so stable and long-lasting to provoke "character" manifestations similar to pathological traits and marked maladjustment. In this perspective the chronic affective disorder would be considered as primary and the maladaptive traits and behaviors cluster that address the diagnosis of BPD would be secondary.

Essential elements of BPD affective dysregulation are the extreme reactivity and mood lability that, together with interpersonal sensitivity, may be the substrate for some of the common elements among cyclothymia, hysteroid dysphoria, atypical depression, and BPD. In fact, interpersonal conflicts, sexual promiscuity, poor job performance, working and geographical instability, substance abuse, sociorelational mismatch, antisocial conduct and possible legal problems, economic vagaries, financial troubles, and self-harming tendencies could be interpreted as the result of long-term rapid emotional swings and excessive mood reactivity (Akiskal, Khani, & Scott-Strauss, 1979). The recurrent suicide attempts and other self-harm acts may reflect despair and hopelessness; unstable and tumultuous relationships may result from low self-esteem and excessive impulsiveness. In this context, Akiskal et al. (1977) suggested that many forms of minor social deviance may actually originate from attenuated, unrecognized, or masked, potentially treatable affective disorders.

However, it should be noted that many authors with great experience in this area minimize the affective component in BPD and ascribe the extreme emotional and behavioral derangement to physical and psychological abuse. In summary, several hereditary, biological, and environmental factors contribute in various ways to determine this process. Examining different and opposite points of view, authors can be divided into two groups: on the one hand are those who give priority to constitutional factors, and on the other are those who attribute the disease to characterological development-related events.

Donald Klein proposed a broad hypothesis arguing the centrality of affective processes underlying the characterological pathology of some borderline patients. He and his collaborators described the "emotionally unstable character disorder" (EUCD), indicating the extreme expression of character pathology of some patients with atypical depression, which he regarded as outside the bipolar spectrum (Rifkin, Levitan, Galewski, & Klein, 1972). According to this perspective, patients with EUCD would be characterized by a "poorly developed conscience" and exhibit antisocial and irresponsible behavior, while cyclothymic patients would be considered more syntonic and friendly individuals, able to pursue socially acceptable objectives. However, clinical experience suggests that these two poles are due to a greater or lesser severity of affective and impulsive symptoms and to the presence or absence of an adequate "goodness of fit" rather than belonging to two distinct categories. By *goodness of fit* we mean the possibility that some elements of the environment, as well as expectations and demands, comply with the personality, temperamental characteristics, and lifestyle of the individual. In this perspective, it is perhaps easier to understand how cyclothymia and its variants may represent the background for antisocial and psychopathic behaviors at one end and the extraordinary qualities of adaptability, creativity, and leadership attitude at the other end. This is partly due to variables not related to mood disorder, such as skills, talents, and intelligence, but also opportunities, luck, and external influences.

COURSE

In cyclothymic subjects, short-lasting hypomanic and depressive symptomatology alternates beginning in adolescence, in most cases in a highly unstable way. This complex course may often be complicated by the lack of clear-cut episodes, extremely rich comorbidity, early onset, and overlap with personality disorders.

Usually the depressive phases dominate the clinical presentation, with the interposition of periods of relative stability, irritability, or occasional hypomania; cyclothymics most frequently seek physicians' aid for depressive symptoms. Depression frequently shows atypical features such as mood reactivity, hypersomnia, hyperfagia, and marked fatigue (leaden paralysis), responsible for significant functional impairment (Benazzi, 1999; Davidson, Miller, Turnbull, & Sullivan, 1982; Perugi et al., 1998; Perugi

et al., 2003). Severe manifestations such as psychotic symptoms and serious psychomotor disorders are generally rare.

Although cyclothymia can be observed in some patients with full-blown manic-depressive disorder (bipolar I), it is more commonly associated with the bipolar type II pattern. In a French study on major depression, 88% of subjects with cyclothymic characteristics belonged to the bipolar II subtype (Hantouche et al., 1998). Akiskal and Pinto (1999) defined major depression in a cyclothymic background as bipolar II ½ disorder, in order to distinguish it from the bipolar II disorder characterized by major depressive episodes alternating with protracted hypomania and free intervals (*DSM-IV* bipolar II disorder).

The National Institute of Mental Health study (Akiskal et al., 1995) on originally unipolar patients who switched to bipolar II during a long-term perspective follow-up provided some important information. The variables that characterized at entry the patients with subsequent hypomanic switches were early age at onset, recurrent depression, high rates of divorce or separation, high rates of scholastic and/ or job maladjustment, isolated "antisocial acts," and drug abuse. In addition, the index of depressive episode was characterized by such features as phobic anxiety, interpersonal sensitivity, separation anxiety, obsessive-compulsive symptoms, somatization (subpanic symptoms), worsening in evening, self-pity, subjective or overt anger, jealousy, suspiciousness, and ideas of reference. This pattern points to a broad array of cyclothymic and atypical depressive symptoms with comorbid anxious and impulsive features. Finally, some temperamental attributes of mood lability, energy activity, and daydreaming, already described by Kretschmer for "cycloid temperament," have been proven specific to unipolar depressives who switched to hypomania. Some of these features also broadly overlap with Cluster B and C personality descriptions.

Cyclothymia seems to be the basic state of many bipolar II depressions, in which mood instability is supported by an intrinsic temperamental deregulation. Unfortunately, the major diagnostic systems (ICD-10 and *DSM-IV*) are oriented primarily on symptomatology and do not recognize the role of traits and temperamental dispositions.

A series of follow-up studies conducted since the 1980s on BPD inpatients provided useful information on the long-term course of cyclothymia (Stone, 1990). Many of these patients showed clinical presentations compatible with the diagnosis of bipolar II disorder or cyclothymia and, along the course of the illness, reported mild cross-sectional symptoms disproportionate with respect to significantly impaired interpersonal relationships. From 3% to 9% of the sample had committed suicide. Higher rates of suicide correlated with earlier age at initial assessment. Favorable prognostic factors were represented by high intelligence, artistic talent, and, in the case of patients who had comorbid alcohol abuse, ability to follow rehabilitative treatments. On the contrary, negative prognostic factors, with high risk of suicide, were represented by physical or sexual abuse by family members, the combination of antisocial traits, and marked impulsiveness.

In several studies, the suicidal rates of cyclothymic patients are analogous to patients with BDP or schizophrenia (Rihmer & Pestality, 1999), which indicates the seriousness of the disorder. However, most cases present a better long-term prognosis than that of major psychosis. In fact, many subjects begin to improve after passing the age threshold of 40 years. This observation is another element in common with data on BPD.

Many studies have explored the possible role of comorbid personality disorders on the course of mood disorders, particularly depression. Axis II comorbidity has been correlated with premature relapse after remission (Grilo et al., 2010), less complete or delayed response to pharmacotherapy alone or to pharmacotherapy and psychotherapy together (Bschor, Canata, Muller-Oerlinghausen, & Bauer, 2001; Rothschild & Zimmerman, 2004; Shea, Widiger, & Klein, 1992), and, more generally, decreased propensity to respond to the treatment for chronic depression (Howland & Thase, 2005). However, there is no consensus regarding these findings, with several studies not supporting these data or even showing opposite results (Rosenbluth, Macqueen, McIntyre, Beaulieu, & Schaffer, 2012).

TREATMENT STRATEGIES AND PRACTICAL MANAGEMENT

Treatment of cyclothymic and bipolar II depression is surprisingly understudied, especially in comparison with mania and unipolar depression. This is incredible, mostly considering depressive and hypomanic symptoms are usually severe and highly subjected to recurrence. Moreover, in cyclothymics risk of suicide, substance abuse and pejorative impact on functioning are also significantly augmented. These are only few of the reasons why cyclothymia, especially when personality disorder traits complicate the clinical picture, requires more sophisticated and integrated treatment than classical bipolar forms.

Agents such as lithium, valproate, and carbamazepine have been studied much more thoroughly in bipolar I. Similarly, only a few controlled studies have focused on the efficacy of antidepressants in monotherapy. The relative risk of (hypo)manic switches or of rapid cycles induction further complicates the treatment of cyclothymic depression.

In the literature, the reported rates of (hypo)manic switches among bipolar depressives treated with antidepressants range from 10% to 70% (Moller & Grunze, 2000; Thase & Sachs, 2000). The extreme variability of these estimates is due to the heterogeneity of study designs (sampling, settings, symptoms evaluation, randomized controlled vs. naturalistic, monotherapy vs. combined). In this perspective it would seem reasonable to limit the risk assessment of antidepressant-induced (hypo)mania to randomized, placebo-controlled trials. However, this approach shows several limitations: such trials are not primarily designed to assess these issues but are mainly designed to assess efficacy. Depression rating scales are not sensitive to correctly detect hypomanic symptoms, especially if mild and soft, until the paradox of misidentifying them as response or remission. Furthermore, side effects are frequently underestimated in clinical trials because of numerous exclusion criteria that screen out those with risk factors for serious side effects. For example, some potential risk factors, such as substance abuse or BPD itself (Goldberg & Whiteside, 2002), are common exclusion criteria, which could lead to a worrisome underestimation. Therefore, for a more comprehensive examination, data derived from case reports, case series, and observational studies that report follow-up should be considered too. The literature is rich with reports that antidepressants may worsen the course of all forms of bipolarity, both acutely and long term, causing polarity changes, mixed states, suicidality, and cycle acceleration.

New-generation antidepressants as selective serotonin reuptake inhibitors (SSRIs), serotonin–norepinephrine reuptake inhibitors (SNRIs), and bupropion are claimed to be less likely prone to induce (hypo)manic "switches" than tricyclic antidepressants (TCAs). However, this conclusion mostly derives from pooled analysis of adverse events reported in randomized clinical trials (Peet, 1994). In this context, a switch rate of 4% with SSRIs versus 12% with TCAs and 4% with placebo has been reported. Randomized trials included almost only unipolar patients and only a limited number of bipolar II/soft bipolar patients. Moreover, we know from the experience with SSRI-related sexual dysfunction that this approach can seriously underestimate the prevalence of side effects due to measurement bias. It is likely that hypomania, very frequent with SSRIs and SNRIs in clinical practice, may be recorded as full remission instead of adverse reaction in a significant proportion of cases.

In contrast with these findings, the contemporary literature is extremely rich in case reports and series describing (hypo)manic switches with SSRIs, not only in patients with major depression but also in those treated for dysthymia, anxiety, eating disorders, and impulse control disorders (Perugi & Akiskal, 2002). Although in clinical practice when a bipolar diathesis is identified mood stabilizers are recommended, this aid does not seem sufficient to completely prevent antidepressant-induced (hypo)mania (Bottlender, Rudolf, Strauss, & Moller, 1998).

Antidepressants can also worsen bipolar illness in the long term by causing rapid cycling or cycle acceleration. These conditions represent a serious worsening of the course of the illness, often with longer, more frequent, and more complicated depressive episodes. Usually randomized settings are not adequate to catch the long-term complex nature of the illness and definitively assess cycle acceleration. In fact, to our knowledge there is only one sufficiently prolonged study that has attempted to do so (Wehr, Sack, Rosenthal, & Cowdry, 1988), and it supports an association between antidepressant use and cycle acceleration. Observational evidence can be cited both for and against this association, as is the case with observational evidence for many topics.

With this background, some conclusions seem reasonable. Antidepressants may be acutely effective in cyclothymics, but long-term continuation might be ineffective at best and harmful at worst. These conclusions lead to the recommendation of limiting as much as possible the use of antidepressants to the short-term treatment of major depressive episodes, with rapid (perhaps within two to six months) discontinuation after recovery. Indeed, this was the suggestion of the American Psychiatric Association's (2006) treatment guidelines for BPD, severely criticized by some clinicians in Europe (Moller & Grunze, 2000).

The biggest source of concern is the not-infrequent report of depressive relapse after antidepressants discontinuation (Altshuler et al., 2001). Actually, the two possibilities are not contradictory, but this represents a major dilemma for clinicians: how to identify patients who, with long-term use of antidepressants, develop an increasing frequency of episodes and rapid cycling and those who, when antidepressant medications are discontinued, tend to produce depressive recurrences. The strongest predictor of antidepressant-induced switch is a history of past switching: for such patients antidepressants should be avoided.

In practice, mood stabilizers should be preferred and antidepressants chosen for nonresponders. In particular, lithium and lamotrigine appear to have antidepressant properties. Lithium is indisputably superior in the treatment of (hypo)manic phases and for their prevention, but there are also several experiences suggesting its effectiveness for both acute depression (even as monotherapy) and the prevention of relapse. The data supporting the use of lamotrigine are more limited, particularly because of its little utility in acute phases, although it is the only drug with a Food and Drug Administration indication for the prophylaxis of depressive relapses. In our experience, the use of this anticonvulsant might be circumscribed because it may cause a transient worsening of anxiety, mostly when a panic disorder is associated with the mood disorder. In those cyclothymics with depressive symptoms, history of panic attacks, and prominence of anxiety, valproate is the alternative of choice. There are also some reports, in anxious cyclothymic patients, of an antidepressant action of valproate; it is also effective in the long term as continuation and maintenance therapy (Perugi et al., 2010).

Predictors of lithium response are the clear cyclic course (especially with the pattern excitement–depression–free interval and no more than two episodes per year), "euphoric" connotation of the elated phase, alternation between acceleration and retardation, shorter duration of illness, absence of anxiety disorders, family history of mood disorders, and responsiveness to lithium (Young, Cooke, Robb, Levitt, & Joffe, 1993). The predictors of valproate response are the mixture of manic and depressive symptoms (mixed states), "dysphoric" connotation of mood, comorbid anxiety disorders (e.g., panic attacks), rapid cycling (at least four affective episodes per year), long duration of the disease, late onset, substance abuse (alcohol, cocaine, sedatives, polyabuse), history of migraine, associated head trauma, or neurological abnormalities (Bowden, 2004; Calabrese, Woyshville, Kimmel, & Rapport, 1993; McElroy, Keck, Pope, & Hudson, 1992; Swann et al., 1997; Vigo & Baldessarini, 2009).

An alternative or additional possible option is represented by quetiapine, which has been reported to be effective in the treatment of acute bipolar I and II depression (Hirschfeld, Weisler, Raines, & Macfadden, 2006; Thase et al., 2006). Long-term efficacy and side effects, such as sedation and weight gain, might limit its utility in the treatment of cyclothymia. Antidepressants should be added only in the most severe or resistant forms, always in combination with mood stabilizers; high dosages of antidepressants and their presumably synergistic combination should be avoided. Their long-term use is justified in rare cases only with mood stabilizers. Even in those studies supporting long-term antidepressant use (Altshuler et al., 2003), only about 15% of bipolar depressive patients appeared to benefit. In many patients it is advisable to combine two mood stabilizers (lithium plus valproate, lithium plus olanzapine, lamotrigine plus quetiapine) before adding an antidepressant. With this approach, the acute depressive symptoms of most patients can be treated and mood-stabilizing combination continued in the long term. Anticipated use of antidepressants may be necessary in the most severe or hospitalized patients, in which more rapid recovery is desired.

The treatment of cyclothymic patients is often complicated by the presence of comorbidity. In many cases the concomitant anxiety, lack of impulse control, or eating disorders represent the major complaints and require specific treatment. Most of the controlled trials on bipolar and depressive disorders exclude patients with such comorbidities; as a consequence, the empirical basis for treating these subtypes of patients are almost exclusively derived from open clinical experience. This is a deplorable situation, because the most common patients treated in everyday clinical practice are cyclothymic-bipolar II with complex comorbidity. The "pure" BPD is an abstract concept rarely encountered in real world.

Antidepressant-induced (hypo)manic symptoms have been reported to occur in the course of the treatment of virtually all anxiety disorders, including obsessive-compulsive, panic disorder/agoraphobia, and social phobia (Himmelhoch, 1998; Sholomskas, 1990). When treating comorbid bipolar and anxiety disorders, it is imperative to begin treatment with a mood stabilizer at first.

As already said, in the treatment of comorbid cyclothymia and panic disorder/agoraphobia (Calabrese & Delucchi, 1990; Perugi et al., 2010), it appears reasonable to utilize as first choice mood stabilizers that have been shown to possess some antipanic efficacy, such as valproate. In patients with persistent and disabling anxiety, combination with small dosages of SSRI or TACs (i.e., paroxetine or trimipramine) can be considered. Paroxetine, although not free from the concern of other antidepressants, may be considered an optimal choice, because it is effective in all anxiety disorders as well as major depression and in addition has proven efficacy in bipolar II depression in combination with mood stabilizers (Young et al., 2000).

Less information is available for comorbid cyclothymia and social phobia. A small positive study on gabapentin in social phobia suggests the possible efficacy of this drug for both mood and anxiety disorders (Pande et al., 1999). The combination of mood stabilizers with SSRIs, reversible inhibitors of monoamine oxidase A, or monoamine oxidase inhibitors might reduce the number of switches in these patients, although data on long-term outcome of patients treated with drug combinations for comorbid BPD and social anxiety are substantially lacking.

Patients with cyclothymia and comorbid obsessive-compulsive disorder are among the most difficult to treat. While no mood stabilizer has been shown to exert any anti-obsessive-compulsive activity, highly effective anti-obsessive pharmacological treatments (e.g., high doses of clomipramine or SSRIs) are likely to trigger (hypo)manic switches and mixed states (Akiskal et al., 2003; Perugi et al., 2003). A combination of different mood stabilizers (e.g., lithium plus anti-epileptics) is often necessary. However, many of these patients present residual obsessive-compulsive symptomatology and very severe manic or mixed episodes (aggressive, hostile mood) that may require hospitalization. In some cases, SSRI augmentation with low dose of atypical antipsychotics (e.g., risperidone, olanzapine, aripiprazole) can be considered on an empirical basis.

Short-term benzodiazepines—such as clonazepam—can be useful both for the management of comorbid anxiety symptoms and acute mood phases when other treatments are not yet functioning. Benzodiazepines are relatively safe and well tolerated, but their use may be problematic due to the development of tolerance, physical dependence, and withdrawal phenomena, which are particularly likely in such cyclothymic patients with prominent impulsivity, sensation-seeking, and high potential for addiction. Gabapentin could be helpful when anxiety disorders or alcohol abuse are comorbid (Perugi & Akiskal, 2002) and when benzodiazepine withdrawal is necessary and/or difficult.

In the literature, the management of comorbid mood and personality disorders is a complicated and unresolved issue, mostly due to the lack of specific studies. Patients with prominent personality disorders are usually excluded from trials. Merging the literature on pharmacotherapy for mood disorders and personality disorders results in indirect comparisons of unknown validity. However, some conclusions might be reached and compared with clinical experience. Certain personality traits have negative implications for medication response, particularly through poor adherence and difficult doctor–patient relationship (Ekselius, Bengtsson, & von Knorring, 2000; Kennedy, Farvolden, Cohen, Bagby, & Costa, 2005; Sirey et al., 2001). In a three-year follow-up study on bipolar (I and II) patients, Axis II dimensional features predicted a poor long-term outcome (Bieling et al., 2003). These considerations are largely applicable to bipolar patients with a cyclothymic background.

National Institute for Health and Clinical Excellence guidelines do not recommend use of medications for BPD, suggesting that the efficacy demonstrated in several trials is only partial, often due to the treatment of a comorbid condition and not specific for the core dimensions of the disorder. This line is sustained by the fact that few trials and, if possible, even fewer comparative effectiveness studies have been conducted; some of them suggest benefits with second-generation antipsychotics (SGAs), mood stabilizers, and omega-3 fatty acids. Evidence on the use of antidepressants for BPD alone is insufficient. No study suggests total severity of BPD is influenced by any medication or the superiority of a medication or class compared to others (Stoffers et al., 2010). These indications seem to be largely arbitrary; in fact the evidence of efficacy of mood stabilizers and SGA is not inferior to that of other psychological treatments. On the contrary, some core BPD domains seem to benefit from a psychopharmacological treatment, especially with mood stabilizers and SGA. Valproate and lamotrigine have been demonstrated to be effective as first-line treatments, particularly for those symptoms pertaining to affective dysregulation and impulsivity-dyscontrol dimensions. Aripiprazole and olanzapine, such as first-generation haloperidol, may be effective for treating cognitive-perceptual symptoms. Despite the expectations, SSRIs lack strong evidence of effectiveness in BPD (Lieb, Vollm, Rucker, Timmer, & Stoffers, 2010). Considering these data and the large overlap between cyclothymia and BPD, pharmacotherapy should therefore be considered and targeted at specific symptoms. Combining the evidence regarding the treatment of cyclothymia and BPD and considering the potential side-effect burden of atypical antipsychotics, mood stabilizers seem to be a reasonable first-choice treatment when these conditions coexist.

Several studies demonstrate both for cyclothymia and BPD a greater efficacy when medications are combined with nonpharmacological interventions: cognitive-behavioral therapy and interpersonal therapy have been particularly tested (Bellino, Rinaldi, & Bogetto, 2010; Swartz, Pilkonis, Frank, Proietti, & Scott, 2005), but a psychoeducational intervention might also be useful. Cyclothymia should be considered a distinct form of bipolarity that requires a specific approach, particularly because it does not match with the disorder model proposed for bipolar I. An appropriate "format" based on an adapted model is needed. In these patients, free intervals and long-lasting remissions are very rare, and for this reason the psychoeducational intervention should start as soon as possible. It should be focused on becoming an "expert" on cyclothymia, becoming familiar with its resulting psychological dysfunction and behavioral problems, and developing self-skills to reduce them and the illness impact. At the moment, the correct evaluation of the role and effectiveness of this type of nonpharmacological intervention requires better-designed prospective observations.

General principles in the practical management of patients with cyclothymia are summarized in Box 34.4. In a hierarchical perspective, outcome measures should consider first hypomania, avoiding the frequent error of considering depression everything that is not typical (hypo)mania. In addition, cyclothymic patients often show complaints regarding not being "hypomanic," because of the lost ability of recognizing and accepting euthymia. The therapeutic intervention should focus not only on major affective episodes but also on the basic mood dysregulation that underlies most of the psychological dysfunctions and behavioral problems in these patients. Both the pharmacological and psychoeducational interventions should target specific goals such as excitement, depression, comorbidity, impulsivity, hostility, mood reactivity, interpersonal sensitivity, and risk-taking behavior. Moreover, in order to increase treatment adherence, psychoeducation should be started

---

Box 34.4 PRACTICAL MANAGEMENT OF CYCLOTHYMIA

Refine diagnosis:
 - Primacy of hypomania
 - Systematic error: "everything that is not typical (hypo) mania is depression"
 - Excitement, irritability, inner agitation, and impulsivity are fundamental dimensions of soft bipolarity
Conception of the basic illness
 - Episodes are probably the "wings" emerging from temperaments that could be the "roots"
 - Mood episodes, psychological dysfunctions, and behavioral problems result from a "clash" between basic temperament and environment (importance of "patient's life systems")
Focus treatment on specific clinical targets
 - Depression
 - Comorbidity
 - Specific dimensions: impulsivity, hostility, hyperreactivity, interpersonal sensitivity, risk-taking behavior, excitement, inner tension
Start psychoeducation from the beginning
Use mood stabilizers or antimanic drugs before antidepressants
Be vigilant when using antidepressants
 - Hypomanic switches
 - Cycle acceleration
 - Prolonged excitement (protracted mixed states)

from the beginning. Finally, concerning the pharmacological approach, mood stabilizers or antimanic drugs should be used before antidepressants, and, when the latter are utilized, particular attention should be paid to the possibility of hypomanic switches or cycle acceleration (Hantouche & Trybou, 2011).

CONCLUSION

Cyclothymia continues to be underestimated and is frequently misdiagnosed and inappropriately treated, despite the evidence that it affects 30% to 50% of patients referred for depression, anxiety, or impulsivity-related behavioral problems in clinical settings. The proportion of depressed patients who can be classified as cyclothymic grows significantly if the threshold and the exclusion criteria for the hypomanic episode proposed by the *DSM-IV* are reconsidered and probably if *DSM-5* criteria are utilized.

Many patients receive correct diagnosis and treatments after many years of illness, when the superposition of many complications reduces the possibility of complete remission. The diagnostic delay may be due to several factors, such as the lack of consensus on the definition of bipolar spectrum and subsequent difficulties in identifying hypomania, especially in its broader definition. Other obstacles that could contribute include a discrepancy between a complex clinical picture characterized by behavioral rather than cross-sectional/state symptoms, lack of clear-cut episodes, frequent and abundant comorbidity, early onset, and extensive overlap with personality disorders criteria. Complicated patient–doctor relationships and weak response to conventional approaches produce further difficulties in the recognition of cyclothymia, and, even when properly identified, there is no consensus on its treatment.

Cyclothymia should be considered the common denominator of a complex clinical picture with a combination of mood, anxiety, and impulse-control disorders, with early onset and protracted course, often becoming dysfunctional and invalidating from the beginning of adult life. Such a complex and variable clinical picture requires an elaborate approach to the pharmacological treatment of subthreshold presentations of bipolarity (typical and atypical ups and downs). This approach should be accounted not only for cyclothymia and personality problems but also for other aspects of the complex clinical syndromes characterized by depression, psychic excitement, anxiety, impulse control, substance use, and attention deficit disorders (Perugi & Akiskal, 2002; Perugi, Fornaro, & Akiskal, 2011; Skirrow, McLoughlin, Kuntsi, & Asherson, 2009).

The first objective of such an approach is the early recognition of illness: this should permit the early start of specific multiple interventions. Specific psychological techniques and psychoeducation, focused not only on the prevention of the mood episode but also on the complex comorbidity and the basic temperamental dysregulation, have been demonstrated to be particularly helpful. Best results are obtained when such an approach is applied to children and young patients who are drug naïve (Hantouche & Trybou, 2011).

An appropriate approach to correctly manage cyclothymia is also needed to reduce complications and risks. Unnecessary exposure to antidepressants is the most dangerous and, unfortunately, the most frequent issue for a large number of patients suffering from cyclothymic disorder. Mood stabilizers should be considered as the first-line treatment, with the addition of antidepressants only in the most resistant cases. SGAs, in particular olanzapine, aripiprazole, or quetiapine, should be accounted in nonresponders or when psychotic, mixed, or impulsivity-dyscontrol features are present. Besides classical mood stabilizers, such as lithium, carbamazepine, and valproate, the use of which is sometimes limited by side effects, lamotrigine has shown a great balance between tolerability and efficacy in preventing rapid cycling and depressive recurrences. The use of psychotropic combinations is often necessary to treat syndromic complexity due to the frequent coexistence of cyclothymia and anxiety, impulse control, and eating and substance use disorders.

Some major challenges concerning medical education, clinical, pharmacological, psychological, and genetic researches are still open (Greenwood, Akiskal, Akiskal, & Kelsoe, 2012; Tomba, Rafanelli, Grandi, Guidi, & Fava, 2012; Van Meter, Moreira, & Youngstrom, 2011). From a mere clinical point of view, the most important issue is represented by the improvement of recognition in early phases of the illness, especially in youth.

Disclosure statement: Prof. Giulio Perugi has acted as consultant of Sanofi Aventis, Astra Zeneca, Eli Lilly, and Lundbeck; received grant/research support from Eli Lilly, Astra Zeneca, and Lundbeck; and is on the speaker/advisory board of Sanofi Aventis, Astra Zeneca, Eli Lilly, Jannsen-Cilag, and Lundbeck. Dr. Giulia Vannucchi has no conflict of interest

REFERENCES

Akiskal, H. S. (1981). Subaffective disorders: Dysthymic, cyclothymic and bipolar II disorders in the "borderline" realm. *Psychiatric Clinics of North America, 4*(1), 25–46.

Akiskal, H. S., Djenderedjian, A. M., Rosenthal, R. H., & Khani, M. K. (1977). Cyclothymic disorder: Validating criteria for inclusion in the bipolar affective group. *The American Journal of Psychiatry, 134*(11), 1227–1233.

Akiskal, H. S., Hantouche, E. G., Allilaire, J. F., Sechter, D., Bourgeois, M. L., Azorin, J. M.,...Lancrenon, S. (2003). Validating antidepressant-associated hypomania (bipolar III): A systematic comparison with spontaneous hypomania (bipolar II). *Journal of Affective Disorders, 73*(1–2), 65–74.

Akiskal, H. S., Khani, M. K., & Scott-Strauss, A. (1979). Cyclothymic temperamental disorders. *Psychiatric Clinics of North America, 2*, 527–554.

Akiskal, H. S., Maser, J. D., Zeller, P. J., Endicott, J., Coryell, W., Keller, M.,...Goodwin, F. (1995). Switching from "unipolar" to bipolar II: An 11-year prospective study of clinical and temperamental predictors in 559 patients. *Archives of General Psychiatry, 52*(2), 114–123.

Akiskal, H. S., & Pinto, O. (1999). The evolving bipolar spectrum: Prototypes I, II, III, and IV. *Psychiatric Clinics of North America, 22*(3), 517–534.

Akiskal, H. S., Placidi, G. F., Maremmani, I., Signoretta, S., Liguori, A., Gervasi, R.,...Puzantian, V. R. (1998). TEMPS-I: Delineating the most discriminant traits of the cyclothymic, depressive, hyperthymic and irritable temperaments in a nonpatient population. *Journal of Affective Disorders, 51*(1), 7–19.

Alnaes, R., & Torgensen, S. (1989). Personality and personality disorders among patients with major depression in combination with dysthymic or cyclothymic disorders. *Acta Psychiatrica Scandinavica, 79*(4), 363–369.

Altshuler, L., Kiriakos, L., Calcagno, J., Goodman, R., Gitlin, M., Frye, M., & Mintz, J. (2001). The impact of antidepressant discontinuation versus antidepressant continuation on 1-year risk for relapse of bipolar depression: A retrospective chart review. *Journal of Clinical Psychiatry, 62*(8), 612–616.

Altshuler, L., Suppes, T., Black, D., Nolen, W. A., Keck, P. E. Jr., Frye, M. A.,...Post, R. (2003). Impact of antidepressant discontinuation after acute bipolar depression remission on rates of depressive relapse at 1-year follow-up. *The American Journal of Psychiatry, 160*(7), 1252–1262.

American Psychiatric Association. (1968). *Diagnostic and statistical manual of mental disorders* (2nd ed.). Washington, DC: Author.

American Psychiatric Association. (1980). *Diagnostic and statistical manual of mental disorders* (3rd ed.). Washington, DC: Author.

American Psychiatric Association. (1994). *Diagnostic and statistical manual of mental disorders* (4th ed.). Washington, DC: Author.

American Psychiatric Association. (2000). *Diagnostic and statistical manual of mental disorders* (4th ed., text rev.). Washington, DC: Author.

American Psychiatric Association. (2006). *American Psychiatric Association practice guidelines for the treatment of psychiatric disorders compendium*. Washington, DC: Author.

American Psychiatric Association. (2013). *Diagnostic and statistical manual of mental disorders* (5th ed.). Washington, DC: Author.

Angst, J., Azorin, J. M., Bowden, C. L., Perugi, G., Vieta, E., Gamma, A.,...BRIDGE Study Group. (2011). Prevalence and characteristics of undiagnosed bipolar disorders in patients with a major depressive episode: The BRIDGE study. *Archives of General Psychiatry, 68*(8), 791–798.

Angst, J., Cui, L., Swendsen, J., Rothen, S., Cravchik, A., Kessler, R. C., & Merikangas, K. R. (2010). Major depressive disorder with subthreshold bipolarity in the National Comorbidity Survey Replication. *The American Journal of Psychiatry, 167*(10), 1194–1201.

Angst, J., & Marneros, A. (2001). Bipolarity from ancient to modern times: Conception, birth and rebirth. *Journal of Affective Disorders, 67*(1–3), 3–19.

Bellino, S., Rinaldi, C., & Bogetto, F. (2010). Adaptation of interpersonal psychotherapy to borderline personality disorder: A comparison of combined therapy and single pharmacotherapy. *Canadian Journal of Psychiatry, 55*(2), 74–81.

Benazzi, F. (1999). Prevalence of bipolar II disorder in atypical depression. *European Archives of Psychiatry and Clinical Neurosciences, 249*(2), 62–65.

Bieling, P. J., MacQueen, G. M., Marriot, M. J., Robb, J. C., Begin, H., Joffe, R. T., & Young, L. T. (2003). Longitudinal outcome in patients with bipolar disorder assessed by life-charting is influenced by DSM-IV personality disorder symptoms. *Bipolar Disorders, 5*(1), 14–21.

Bottlender, R., Rudolf, D., Strauss, A., & Moller, H. J. (1998). Antidepressant-associated maniform states in acute treatment of patients with bipolar-I depression. *European Archives of Psychiatry and Clinical Neurosciences, 248*(6), 296–300.

Bowden, C. L. (2004). The effectiveness of divalproate in all forms of mania and the broader bipolar spectrum: Many questions, few answers. *Journal of Affective Disorders, 79*(1), S9–14.

Bschor, T., Canata, B., Muller-Oerlinghausen, B., & Bauer, M. (2001). Predictors of response to lithium augmentation in tricyclic antidepressant-resistant depression. *Journal of Affective Disorders, 64*(2–3), 261–265.

Calabrese, J. R., & Delucchi, G. A. (1990). Spectrum of efficacy of valproate in 55 patients with rapid-cycling bipolar disorder. *The American Journal of Psychiatry, 147*(4), 431–434.

Calabrese, J. R., Woyshville, M. J., Kimmel, S. E., & Rapport, D. J. (1993). Predictors of valproate response in bipolar rapid cycling. *Journal of Clinical Psychopharmacology, 13*(4), 280–283.

Davidson, J. R., Miller, R. D., Turnbull, C. D., & Sullivan, J. L. (1982). Atypical depression. *Archives of General Psychiatry, 39*(5), 527–534.

Ekselius, L., Bengtsson, F., & von Knorring, L. (2000). Non-compliance with pharmacotherapy of depression is associated with a sensation seeking personality. *International Clinical Psychopharmacology, 15*(5), 273–278.

Goldberg, J. F., & Whiteside, J. E. (2002). The association between substance abuse and antidepressant-induced mania in bipolar disorder: A preliminary study. *Journal of Clinical Psychiatry, 63*(9), 791–795.

Greenwood, T. A., Akiskal, H. S., Akiskal, K. K., & Kelsoe, J. R. (2012). Genome-wide association study of temperament in bipolar disorder reveals significant associations with three novel Loci. *Biological Psychiatry, 72*(4), 303–310.

Grilo, C. M., Stout, R. L., Markowitz, J. C., Sanislow, C. A., Ansell, E. B., Skodol, A. E.,...McGlashan, T. H. (2010). Personality disorders predict relapse after remission from an episode of major depressive disorder: A 6-year prospective study. *Journal of Clinical Psychiatry, 71*(12), 1629–1635.

Gunderson, J. G., & Singer, M. T. (1975). Defining borderline patients: An overview. *The American Journal of Psychiatry, 132*(1), 1–10.

Hantouche, E. G., Akiskal, H. S., Lancrenon, S., Allilaire, J. F., Sechter, D., Azorin, J. M.,...Châtenet-Duchêne, L. (1998). Systematic clinical methodology for validating bipolar-II disorder: Data in mid-stream from a French national multi-site study (EPIDEP). *Journal of Affective Disorders, 50*(2–3), 163–173.

Hantouche, E. G., Angst, J., Demonfaucon, C., Perugi, G., Lancrenon, S., & Akiskal, H. S. (2003). Cyclothymic OCD: A distinct form? *Journal of Affective Disorders, 75*(1), 1–10.

Hantouche, E. G., & Trybou, T. (2011). *Live happily with ups and downs*. Paris: Odile Jacob.

Himmelhoch, J. M. (1998). Social anxiety, hypomania and the bipolar spectrum: Data, theory and clinical issues. *Journal of Affective Disorders, 50*(2–3), 203–213.

Hirschfeld, R. M., Weisler, R. H., Raines, S. R., & Macfadden, W. (2006). Quetiapine in the treatment of anxiety in patients with bipolar I or II depression: A secondary analysis from a randomized, double-blind, placebo-controlled study. *Journal of Clinical Psychiatry, 67*(3), 355–362.

Howland, R. H., & Thase, M. E. (2005). Refractory and chronic depression: The role of axis II disorders in assessment and treatment. In M. Rosenbluth, S. H. Kennedy, & R. M. Bagby (Eds.), *Depression and personality: Conceptual and clinical challenges* (pp. 157–187). Arlington, VA: American Psychiatric Publishing.

Kennedy, S. H., Farvolden, P., Cohen, N. L., Bagby, R. M., & Costa, P. T. (2005). The impact of personality on pharmacological treatment of depression. In M. Rosenbluth, S. H. Kennedy, & R. M. Bagby (Eds.), *Depression and personality: Conceptual and clinical challenges* (pp. 97–121). Arlington, VA: American Psychiatric Publishing.

Kernberg, O. (1967). Borderline personality organization. *Journal of the American Psychoanalytic Association, 15*(3), 641–685.

Koukopoulos, A. (2003). Ewald Hecker's description of cyclothymia as a cyclical mood disorder: Its relevance to the modern concept of bipolar II. *Journal of Affective Disorders, 73*(1–2), 199–205.

Levitt, A. J., Joffe, R. T., Ennis, J., MacDonald, C., & Kutcher, S. P. (1990). The prevalence of cyclothymia in borderline personality disorder. *Journal of Clinical Psychiatry, 51*(8), 335–339.

Levy, D., Kimhi, R., Barak, Y., Aviv, A., & Elizur, A. (1998). Antidepressant-associated mania: A study of anxiety disorders patients. *Psychopharmacology, 136*(3), 243–246.

Lieb, K., Vollm, B., Rucker, G., Timmer, A., & Stoffers, J. M. (2010). Pharmacotherapy for borderline personality disorder: Cochrane systematic review of randomised trials. *The British Journal of Psychiatry, 196*(1), 4–12.

Manning, J. S., Haykal, R. F., Connor, P. D., & Akiskal, H. S. (1997). On the nature of depressive and anxious states in a family practice setting: The high prevalence of bipolar II and related disorders in a cohort followed longitudinally. *Comprehensive Psychiatry, 38*(2), 102–108.

Maremmani, I., Perugi, G., Pacini, M., & Akiskal, H. S. (2006). Toward a unitary perspective on the bipolar spectrum and substance abuse: Opiate addiction as a paradigm. *Journal of Affective Disorders, 93*(1–3), 1–12.

McElroy, S. L., Keck, P. E. Jr., Pope, H. G. Jr., & Hudson, J. I. (1992). Valproate in the treatment of bipolar disorder: Literature review and clinical guidelines. *Journal of Clinical Psychopharmacology, 12*(1), 42S–52S.

Moller, H. J., & Grunze, H. (2000). Have some guidelines for the treatment of acute bipolar depression gone too far in the restriction of antidepressants? *European Archives of Psychiatry and Clinical Neuroscience, 250*(2), 57–68.

Pande, A. C., Davidson, J. R., Jefferson, J. W., Janney, C. A., Katzelnick, D. J., Weisler, R. H.,…Sutherland, S. M. (1999). Treatment of social phobia with gabapentin: A placebo-controlled study. *Journal of Clinical Psychopharmacology, 19*(4), 341–348.

Peet, M. (1994). Induction of mania with selective serotonin re-uptake inhibitors and tricyclic antidepressants. *The British Journal of Psychiatry, 164*(4), 549–550.

Perugi, G., & Akiskal, H. S. (2002). The soft bipolar spectrum redefined: Focus on the cyclothymic, anxious-sensitive, impulse-dyscontrol, and binge-eating connection in bipolar II and related conditions. *Psychiatric Clinics of North America, 25*(4), 713–737.

Perugi, G., Akiskal, H. S., Lattanzi, L., Cecconi, D., Mastrocinque, C., Patronelli, A.,…Bemi, E. (1998). The high prevalence of "soft" bipolar (II) features in atypical depression. *Comprehensive Psychiatry, 39*(2), 63–71.

Perugi, G., Angst, J., Azorin, J. M., Bowden, C., Vieta, E., & Young, A. H. (2013a). Is comorbid borderline personality disorder in patients with major depressive episode and bipolarity a developmental subtype? Findings from the international BRIDGE study. *Journal of Affective Disorders, 144*(1–2), 72–78.

Perugi, G., Angst, J., Azorin, J. M., Bowden, C., Vieta, E., & Young, A. H. (2013b). The bipolar-borderline personality disorders connection in major depressive patients. *Acta Psychiatrica Scandinavica, 128*(5), 376–383.

Perugi, G., Fornaro, M., & Akiskal, H. S. (2011). Are atypical depression, borderline personality disorder and bipolar II disorder overlapping manifestations of a common cyclothymic diathesis? *World Psychiatry, 10*(1), 45–51.

Perugi, G., Frare, F., Toni, C., Tusini, G., Vannucchi, G., & Akiskal, H. S. (2010). Adjunctive valproate in panic disorder patients with comorbid bipolar disorder or otherwise resistant to standard antidepressants: A 3-year "open" follow-up study. *European Archives of Psychiatry and Clinical Neuroscience, 260*(7), 553–560.

Perugi, G., Toni, C., Travierso, M. C., & Akiskal, H. S. (2003). The role of cyclothymia in atypical depression: Toward a data-based reconceptualization of the borderline-bipolar II connection. *Journal of Affective Disorders, 73*(1–2), 87–98.

Rifkin, A., Levitan, S. J., Galewski, J., & Klein, D. F. (1972). Emotionally unstable character disorder—A follow-up study: I. Description of patients and outcome. *Biological Psychiatry, 4*(1), 65–79.

Rihmer, Z., & Pestality, P. (1999). Bipolar II disorder and suicidal behavior. *Psychiatric Clinics of North America, 22*(3), 667–673.

Rosenbluth, M., Macqueen, G., McIntyre, R. S., Beaulieu, S., & Schaffer, A. (2012). The Canadian Network for Mood and Anxiety Treatments (CANMAT) task force recommendations for the management of patients with mood disorders and comorbid personality disorders. *Annals of Clinical Psychiatry, 24*(1), 56–68.

Rothschild, L., & Zimmerman, M. (2004). Interface between personality and depression. In J. E. Alpert & M. Fava (Eds.), *Handbook of chronic depression* (pp. 19–48). New York: Marcel Dekker.

Sass, H., Herpertz, S., & Steinmeyer, E. M. (1993). Subaffective personality disorders. *International Clinical Psychopharmacology, 8*(1), 39–46.

Shea, M. T., Widiger, T. A., & Klein, M. H. (1992). Comorbidity of personality disorders and depression: Implications for treatment. *Journal of Consulting and Clinical Psychology, 60*(6), 857–868.

Sholomskas, A. J. (1990). Mania in a panic disorder patient treated with fluoxetine. *The American Journal of Psychiatry, 147*(8), 1090–1091.

Sirey, J. A., Bruce, M. L., Alexopoulos, G. S., Perlick, D. A., Friedman, S. J., & Meyers, B. S. (2001). Stigma as a barrier to recovery: Perceived stigma and patient-rated severity of illness as predictors of antidepressant drug adherence. *Psychiatric Services, 52*(12), 1615–1620.

Skirrow, C., McLoughlin, G., Kuntsi, J., & Asherson, P. (2009). Behavioral, neurocognitive and treatment overlap between attention-deficit/hyperactivity disorder and mood instability. *Expert Review of Neurotherapeutics, 9*(4), 489–503.

Stoffers, J., Vollm, B. A., Rucker, G., Timmer, A., Huband, N., & Lieb, K. (2010). Pharmacological interventions for borderline personality disorder. *Cochrane Database of Systematic Reviews, 6*, CD005653.

Stone, M. H. (1990). *The fate of borderline patients: Successful outcome and psychiatric practice.* New York: Guilford.

Stone, M. H. (2006). Relationship of borderline personality disorder and bipolar disorder. *The American Journal of Psychiatry, 163*(7), 1126–1128.

Swann, A. C., Bowden, C. L., Morris, D., Calabrese, J. R., Petty, F., Small, J.,…Davis, J. M. (1997). Depression during mania: Treatment response to lithium or divalproex. *Archives of General Psychiatry, 54*(1), 37–42.

Swartz, H. A., Pilkonis, P. A., Frank, E., Proietti, J. M., & Scott, J. (2005). Acute treatment outcomes in patients with bipolar I disorder and co-morbid borderline personality disorder receiving medication and psychotherapy. *Bipolar Disorders, 7*(2), 192–197.

Thase, M. E., Macfadden, W., Weisler, R. H., Chang, W., Paulsson, B., Khan, A.,…BOLDER II Study Group. (2006). Efficacy of quetiapine monotherapy in bipolar I and II depression: A double-blind, placebo-controlled study (the BOLDER II study). *Journal of Clinical Psychopharmacology, 26*(6), 600–609.

Thase, M. E., & Sachs, G. S. (2000). Bipolar depression: Pharmacotherapy and related therapeutic strategies. *Biological Psychiatry, 48*(6), 558–572.

Tomba, E., Rafanelli, C., Grandi, S., Guidi, J., & Fava, G. A. (2012). Clinical configuration of cyclothymic disturbances. *Journal of Affective Disorders, 139*(3), 244–249.

Van Meter, A. R., Moreira, A. L., & Youngstrom, E. A. (2011). Meta-analysis of epidemiologic studies of pediatric bipolar disorder. *Journal of Clinical Psychiatry, 72*(9), 1250–1256.

Vigo, D. V., & Baldessarini, R. J. (2009). Anticonvulsants in the treatment of major depressive disorder: An overview. *Harvard Review of Psychiatry, 17*(4), 231–241.

Wehr, T. A., Sack, D. A., Rosenthal, N. E., & Cowdry, R. W. (1988). Rapid cycling affective disorder: Contributing factors and treatment responses in 51 patients. *The American Journal of Psychiatry, 145*(2), 179–184.

World Health Organization. (1975). *International statistical classification of diseases and related health problems* (9th ed.). Geneva: Author.

World Health Organization. (1994). *International statistical classification of diseases and related health problems* (10th ed.). Geneva: Author.

Young, L. T., Cooke, R. G., Robb, J. C., Levitt, A. J., & Joffe, R. T. (1993). Anxious and non-anxious bipolar disorder. *Journal of Affective Disorders, 29*(1), 49–52.

Young, L. T., Joffe, R. T., Robb, J. C., MacQueen, G. M., Marriott, M., & Patelis-Siotis, I. (2000). Double-blind comparison of addition of a second mood stabilizer versus an antidepressant to an initial mood stabilizer for treatment of patients with bipolar depression. *The American Journal of Psychiatry, 157*(1), 124–126.

35.

MANAGEMENT OF COMORBID SUBSTANCE OR ALCOHOL ABUSE

Ihsan Salloum and Pedro Ruiz

INTRODUCTION

Bipolar disorder has the highest rate of associated substance use disorders (SUD) as compared to any other major psychiatric disorders with the exception of antisocial personality disorder (Regier et al., 1990). SUD comorbidity has significant impact on the identification, diagnosis, and treatment of bipolar disorder. Management of this comorbidity is often complicated by the presence of other psychiatric and medical disorders comorbidities. The chronic course of both bipolar disorder and SUD increase the complexity of management of this condition with potential recurrences and relapses requiring a longitudinal approach with focus on symptomatic and functional recovery.

The aims of this chapter are to briefly review the public health and clinical significance of bipolar disorder with comorbid SUD, including diagnostic and treatment implications. We also review empirical studies of pharmacotherapy and psychosocial interventions proposed specifically to address this comorbidity.

SIGNIFICANCE OF THE PROBLEM

Comorbid bipolar and SUD is highly frequent in clinical and community settings; it is associated with multiple clinical challenges and often presents as multi-comorbid conditions rather than "dual diagnosis." Furthermore, this comorbidity is likely to develop early in life, thus exacting significant impairment in social and occupational functioning.

Substance abuse are highly prevalent among patients with bipolar disorder. The high rate of association between bipolar disorder and SUD has been consistently reported by large epidemiological surveys and clinical studies (Conway, Compton, Stinson, & Grant, 2006; Grant et al., 2004; Regier et al., 1990). For example, a large, population-based, epidemiological survey of a representative sample of the US population (Grant et al., 2004) highlighted the very high association between mania and drug or alcohol dependence during a 12-month period. That study reported that the odds ratio of having drug dependence over the past year in responders with mania was 14, and the odds ratio of having alcohol dependence was 6. On the other hand, data from the same survey also pointed to a higher-than-expected rate of lifetime mania and hypomania in those with SUD as well (Conway et al., 2006). The lifetime prevalence of the major drugs of abuse in decreasing frequency include alcohol (up to 61%), cannabis (up to 46%), cocaine (up to 24%), and opioid (up to 8.5%; reviewed in Cerullo & Strakowski, 2007). However, tobacco dependence is the most frequent SUD in bipolar disorder with an estimated lifetime rate of over 82% and an estimated current smoker's rate of 68% (Lasser et al., 2000).

Comorbidity of bipolar disorder with SUDs represents significant clinical challenges. SUDs impact negatively on symptom presentation, manifestation, and course of bipolar disorder and on treatment adherence. Severe clinical presentations in these comorbid patients are often characterized by increased impulsive and suicidal behavior. Suicide rate in this population is among the highest in psychiatry. This heightened severity in symptoms presentation often leads to increased costly hospitalizations as well (Frye & Salloum 2006; Kupfer et al., 2002; Salloum, Douaihy, & Williams, 2008; Weiss et al., 2005).

Comorbidity of bipolar disorder with SUDs is more of a "multi-comorbidity" rather than a "dual-diagnosis" condition. Multi-comorbidity is often the rule in these patients with additional psychiatric and medical disorders, in addition to major psychosocial issues (Salloum et al., 2008). Anxiety disorders are the most frequently reported psychiatric comorbidity in bipolar disorder. These include generalized anxiety disorder, social phobia, panic disorder, and posttraumatic stress disorder. Very high rates have been reported in bipolar I disorder, which ranged from 86% to 92%, with social phobia estimated at up to 52% (El-Mallakh & Hollifield 2008). High rates of anxiety disorders have been reported in large clinical samples as well (Krishnan, 2005; Simon et al., 2004). The recently published *Diagnostic and Statistical Manual of Mental Disorders* (fifth edition [*DSM-5*]; American Psychiatric Association, 2013) considers anxiety symptoms an aspect of bipolar disorder, which are assessed dimensionally. Anxiety symptoms appear to impart poor prognosis with decreased response to treatment and greater likelihood of suicide attempts (Frank et al., 2002; McIntyre et al., 2006; Otto et al., 2006; Simon et al., 2004; Sharma 2003). Obsessive-compulsive disorder also reported frequently in bipolar disorder with an estimated lifetime rate of 30% (Otto et al., 2006). Further complicating the diagnostic picture is the reported additional psychiatric comorbidity that may overlap with symptoms of bipolar disorder such as impulse control disorder, including pathological gambling and personality disorders.

Medical disorders comorbidity are also highly frequent in this population and reflect conditions that have been associated with bipolar disorder in general, as well as conditions that are likely to occur as a consequence of SUDs. Frequently reported medical conditions in bipolar disorder include chronic cardiovascular and metabolic diseases and certain respiratory diseases such as sleep apnea. Conditions related to increased exposure because of substance abuse include tobacco- and cannabis-smoking related disorders. Other conditions include chronic infectious diseases frequently associated with addictive disorders such as hepatitis A, B, and C and HIV infection (Salloum et al., 2008).

Comorbidity of bipolar disorder and SUD have an early age of onset and may result in significant psychosocial impairments. Both bipolar and SUDs have a peak age of onset in teenage years to early adulthood (Salloum & Thase, 2000). Teenage-onset bipolar disorder is reported to be a risk factor for SUD. Teenage-onset bipolar disorder appears to have over 8 times increased risk of developing SUD compared to childhood-onset bipolar disorder (Wilens et al., 1999). The consequences on social and occupational functioning of this comorbid condition during this formative period are significant, especially with the current lack of specifically tailored effective preventative and therapeutic interventions.

MANAGEMENT OF BIPOLAR DISORDER WITH COMORBID SUBSTANCE USE DISORDERS

Management of bipolar disorder with comorbid SUD presents specific challenges that increase the complexity of the care plan. Case recognition and diagnostic ascertainment of the bipolar disorder in the presence of SUD and the adoption of adequate care model along with the availability of effective interventions tailored to meet the treatment needs of this population remains key management issues. In this section we address first diagnostic challenges raised by the presence of SUD. We then cover general treatment issues raised by the presence of comorbidity and review psychotherapeutic and pharmacological interventions designed to specifically address this comorbidity.

DIAGNOSTIC ASCERTAINMENT

The presence of substance abuse complicates an already challenging diagnostic process of bipolar disorder. While the diagnosis of a prototypical acute manic episode is relatively straightforward, the recognition of more subtle syndrome or of atypical or mixed presentation could be challenging. Most patients with bipolar disorder seek help during a depressive episode, and it has been documented that it may take up to 10 years to correctly identify bipolar disorder (Hirschfeld & Vornik, 2004). Substance abuse increases the complexity and challenges in recognizing and ascertaining the presence of bipolar disorder. Substances of abuse can alter the symptom presentation by producing symptoms that mimic, overlap, exacerbate, or obscure the symptoms of bipolar disorder. For example, stimulants intoxication can mimic, overlap, and exacerbate a manic, irritable, and paranoid state. Stimulant withdrawal, on the other hand, can mimic, overlap, or exacerbate a depressive state. Alcohol and other depressants abuse can also induce a depressive state that mimics, overlaps, and exacerbates a depressive episode. Alcohol and depressant use can also potentially suppress and mask manic symptoms, while alcohol and other depressants withdrawal can produce severe anxiety and agitation that can interfere with the diagnostic picture. Hallucinogen intoxication may be confused with affective psychosis as well. Complicating further the diagnostic ascertainment is the reported high rate of mixed bipolar subtype in comorbid substance abuse, where symptoms of dysphoria, irritability, and hyperactivity predominate (Salloum et al., 2008).

Untangling the diagnostic picture on a cross-sectional evaluation in the absence of objective biomarkers relies on presenting symptoms and on historical and anamnestic information, although at times the diagnosis can be ascertained only on longitudinal follow-up.

In the recently published *DSM-5* (American Psychiatric Association, 2013), a substance-induced bipolar disorder develops during or soon after substance intoxication or withdrawal; the effect of the substance involved should be capable of producing the symptoms. Indicators of a primary bipolar disorder would include the presence of symptoms preceding the onset of the substance abuse or symptoms that persist for about a month after the cessation of the symptoms of intoxication or withdrawal. Another indicator suggestive of an independent bipolar disorder is the presence of reliable history of such disorder.

Usually the type and duration of symptoms that occur during either intoxication or withdrawal reflect the specific pharmacodynamics and pharmacokinetic profile of the substance involved. While the guidance to observe persistent psychiatric symptoms for about 30 days in the absence of substance abuse is a useful general rule, evidence from studies of patients with alcohol dependence and major depression reported that while depressive symptoms decreased during the acute withdrawal state (i.e., over the first 7 to 10 days after cessation of alcohol use), further decrease in these symptoms was minimal beyond this period (Cornelius et al., 1997; Salloum & Jones, 2008). Thus treatment could be initiated earlier than four weeks if symptoms persist beyond the pharmacologic and pharmacokinetic properties of the substance of abuse involved. This is more apparent in the case of cocaine abuse; the half-life of cocaine is very short, and symptoms due to intoxication or withdrawal are not expected to last longer than three to four days. Other useful historical information includes significant worsening of symptoms despite stable pattern of substance abuse, documented history of bipolar disorder during a relatively protracted period of abstinence, history of adolescence-onset severe depressive disorder, and first-degree relatives with bipolar disorder.

Screening and assessment instruments may improve identification and diagnostic ascertainment; however, tested instruments to detect mood disorders in the context of substance abuse are very scarce. For example, the Altman-Self Rating Mania Scale (Altman, Hedeker, Peterson, & Davis, 1997) is suggested as a Level 2 self-report instrument to further screen for mania in *DSM-5* (American Pscyhiatric Association, 2013); however, its usefulness in screening for bipolar disorder in the context of SUD is unclear. The Mood Disorder Questionnaire (Hirschfeld et al., 2000) screens broadly for manic and depressive symptoms. The usefulness of this instrument in those with SUD is also unclear. The Symptom Checklist (Franken & Hendriks, 2001) reportedly has shown high sensitivity and moderate specificity for detecting mood disorders in patients with substance abuse. Objective rating scales that require a trained evaluator, such as the Young Mania Rating Scale (Young, Biggs, Ziegler, & Meyer Biggs, 1978) and the Bech-Rafaelsen Mania Scale (Bech, Bolwig, Kramp, & Rafaelse, 1979), as well as structured diagnostic interviews (Hasin et al., 1996; Sheehan et al., 1998), may be helpful in confirming the symptoms cluster consistent with bipolar disorder.

Screening for alcohol and other drugs of abuse in psychiatric settings is enhanced by the systematic use of validated screening instruments such as the Alcohol Use Disorders Identification Test (Allen, Litten, Fertig, & Babor, 1997) and the Drug Abuse Screening Test (Cocco & Carey, 1998).

TREATMENT CONSIDERATIONS

Treatment of comorbid bipolar disorder and SUD includes attention to special general considerations that impact on the treatment process. It also involves the selection of adequate model of care and the use of specific interventions tailored to meet the needs of this high risk population.

GENERAL CONSIDERATIONS IN APPROACHING SUBSTANCE ABUSE AND BIPOLAR COMORBIDITY

Attitudinal issues, stigma, and treatment adherence are salient problems, especially related to the treatment of addictive and psychiatric disorders in general that could have a significant impact on treatment. Attitudinal issues, whether on the part of the provider, the community, or the patient and families, could hamper efforts at treatment. *Stigmatization* involving the health-care provider, the family, and the patient still exists and may be expressed in multiple ways. For example, persistent pessimistic attitude, often expressed as therapeutic nihilism by health-care providers feeling that "no matter what is done, there is little hope of treatment response," influence providers' enthusiasm and efforts in providing optimal care for these patients. Health-care providers using different rationales such as thinking the treatment is unsafe in the context of substance abuse, or that one problem should be cleared before the other condition can be treated, or even that patient is not ready to be treated may withheld or delay treatment for the bipolar disorder. On the part of patients or their families there may be resistance to taking medications and receiving treatment for either the bipolar disorder or the addictive disorder. Within the self-help community, certain self-help groups still discourage the use of medications for psychiatric problems, which are pejoratively labeled as "mind-altering" drugs. Furthermore, the fear of being doubly labeled and stigmatized for having SUD and bipolar disorder ("double stigma") may drive patients to deny the problems or avoid seeking care.

Treatment adherence is a major challenge that besets chronic disease treatment in general and is particularly pronounced in this patient population. Bipolar disorder, as well as SUDs, are known to impair insight into the illness, and denial is considered a typical behavior for a substantial number of people affected with these conditions. Furthermore, active substance abuse interferes significantly with adherence to treatment and medication in bipolar disorder, leading to poor treatment response and persistent residual mood symptoms with increased likelihood of relapse to full mood episode (Judd, Schettler, et al., 2008).

On the other hand, an unstable bipolar disorder, with either manic or depressive symptoms, may impair patients' ability to adhere to a recovery program or participate in self-help groups. Persistent and untreated depressive symptoms were found to be associated with early relapse to alcohol abuse (Greenfield et al., 1998).

INTEGRATED CARE MODEL

A chronic disease–integrated model of care is currently considered the treatment model of choice for these complex conditions. This model emphasizes continuity of care, relapse prevention, recovery, and health restoration ideally involving multiple stakeholders, including patients and their families or significant others and community support. Multiple factors related to comorbid bipolar disorder and SUD dictate the need for an integrated care model. Both bipolar disorder and SUDs are chronic, relapsing conditions that require ongoing treatment. Both disorders have a parallel trajectory of treatment need, from acute stabilization to achieving remission to preventing relapse and achieving symptomatic and functional recovery.

Furthermore, the course of bipolar disorder and SUDs are intertwined with reciprocal or bidirectional negative impact, which may lead to a pernicious cycle of relapses, acute episodes, and chronicity. The negative interaction between these two disorders leads to a worsening course of each of the disorders. Mood symptoms (mania or depression) may worsen substance abuse or precipitate relapse, while substance abuse interferes with medication adherence and medication effects and may induce mood symptoms

and precipitate a bipolar episode. Traditionally there has been a split between services for addictive disorders and those for mental health, which resulted in difficult access to needed care and inadequate treatment for either disorder depending on which service was involved. Thus the need for integrated care that addresses both disorders simultaneously is crucial. Integrated care involves addressing patients' presenting problems in the same setting by the same treatment provider and employing integrated treatment strategies effective for the comorbid disorder.

The emphasis on integrated care in addressing chronic and complex conditions in general is highlighted by the advent of the "medical care home" refocusing care from diseases-based interventions to person- and patient-centered care (Fisher, 2008; Mezzich et al., 2010; Salloum & Mezzich, 2011).

ADDRESSING SUBSTANCE WITHDRAWAL STATES IN BIPOLAR DISORDER

Treatment of substances of abuse withdrawal states in bipolar disorder are often required. Alcohol/depressants withdrawal and opioid withdrawal syndromes are the main withdrawal syndromes that may need medical detoxification. Withdrawal from multiple substances has also become more frequent in recent years. Depression due to stimulants withdrawal, such as cocaine withdrawal, may be accompanied with severe depressive symptoms and suicidal risk that require inpatient monitoring (Salloum, Daley, Cornelius, Kirisci, & Thase, 1996).

Primary goals in the treatment of the drug withdrawal syndromes are to prevent withdrawal complications, alleviate the specific symptoms of the withdrawal state, and use this period as a "window of opportunity" to introduce the patient to the treatment and the long-term goal of sobriety and recovery. In the management of withdrawal states the use of objective rating scales and symptoms-triggered medication dosing has become the preferred treatment model.

Alcohol withdrawal is the most frequent withdrawal syndrome that requires medical detoxification in these patients. The symptom-triggered approach to the treatment of alcohol withdrawal is commonly guided by the use of the Clinical Institute Withdrawal Assessment–Revised (Sullivan, Sykora, Schneiderman, Naranjo, & Sellers, 1989). Studies have shown that symptoms-triggered treatment reduces the likelihood of either under- or overuse of medication when compared to the standard medical detoxification methods (Saitz et al., 1994).

Long-acting benzodiazepines such as diazepam may present an advantage over shorter-acting medications because of the self-tapering properties of these medications. Short-acting medications require repeated dosing and are associated with marked fluctuation in blood levels and possible breakthrough of withdrawal symptoms. Few studies have focused on the optimal management of psychoactive substance withdrawal in bipolar disorder or other severe psychopathology. An early model in the treatment of alcohol withdrawal in psychiatric population is the use of the diazepam loading-dose (Salloum, Cornelius, Daley, & Thase, 1995) described by Sellers and colleagues (1983). An inpatient study of 125 acutely ill hospitalized patients with severe mood, anxiety, and related disorders found this method to be effective with a minimum complications rate (Salloum et al., 1995).

The symptoms-triggered approach is also used for the management of the opioid withdrawal syndrome. The Short Opiate Withdrawal Scale has been extensively used (Gossop, 1990) as an assessment instrument to evaluate the severity of the opioid withdrawal syndrome and to guide buprenorphine dosing and induction of maintenance treatment.

SPECIFIC INTERVENTIONS FOR COMORBID BIPOLAR AND SUBSTANCE USE DISORDERS

There is a paucity of information about interventions for comorbid bipolar disorder and SUD, and few clinical trials have been carried out in this population. While trials testing interventions for bipolar disorder, as well as those for alcoholism, have regularly excluded comorbid conditions, conducting studies in this comorbid population has also proven very challenging. Therefore, only a few studies have been conducted to test targeted pharmacologic agents in this population, and, similarly, even fewer studies have tested specific psychosocial interventions.

Psychotherapies for comorbid bipolar disorder and substance use disorder

Psychotherapy is essential in the management of bipolar disorder with comorbid SUD to enhance treatment alliance and adherence and to help patients develop coping skills to optimize their disease management skills/relapse prevention for both disorders and recovery efforts. While there are several, empirically tested, effective therapies for noncomorbid bipolar disorder and a substantial menu of similarly empirically tested effective therapies for addictive disorders, there are a very limited number of psychotherapies specifically tailored for patients with bipolar disorder with comorbid SUD.

Integrated Group Therapy (IGT). IGT (Weiss et al., 2007, 2009) is an empirically tested group therapy developed specifically for the treatment of comorbid bipolar and addictive disorders. IGT had an advantage over standard group drug counseling in two randomized-controlled trials. IGT significantly decreased number of days of substance use during treatment and follow-up compared to standard group counseling. Key elements in the IGT compared to drug counseling is the integration of therapeutic interventions simultaneously addressing the bipolar disorder and the SUD.

Early Recovery Adherence Therapy (ERAT). ERAT (Salloum et al., 2006) is an integrated, manual-guided individual therapy for patients with bipolar disorder and comorbid alcoholism. It focuses on the early phases of recovery from an acute episode and utilizes a motivational approach integrating principles and techniques from several therapies used in these conditions such as motivational enhancement therapy, relapse prevention, and educational and disease management approaches. ERAT was tested in a pilot, randomized trial and found to be superior to 12-step facilitation therapy on decreasing the quantity of alcohol use and on decreasing depressive symptoms in patients with bipolar disorder and comorbid alcoholism (Salloum et al., 2008).

Interestingly, the integrated interventions (IGT and ERAT) in this population had a better outcome on substance abuse compared to the interventions designed to address only the substance abuse, such as the standard group counseling and the 12-step facilitation therapy. This effect may be expected, as the integrated interventions may have provided better understanding and enhanced coping skills to deal with mood states and substance abuse and their potential interactions and impact on the individual's health.

Pharmacotherapies

Guidance in choosing effective pharmacotherapy for bipolar disorder with comorbid SUD is still limited due to the lack of large-scale clinical trials demonstrating definite advantage for one intervention over placebo or over other existing treatments. To date, there have been few published randomized, double-blind, placebo-controlled trials, mostly conducted at one site with limited sample size (Brown, Garza, & Carmody, 2008; Brown, Gorman, & Hynan, 2007; Brown et al., 2009; Geller et al., 1998; Salloum, Cornelius, Daley, et al., 2005; Tolliver, Desantis, Brown, Prisciandaro, & Brady, 2012) in addition to several open-label trials (Salloum et al., 2008).

Tested medications included medications used in bipolar disorder such as the anticonvulsants sodium valproate and lamotrigine, the atypical antipsychotic quetiapine, the mood stabilizer lithium carbonate, and medications used in alcoholism including naltrexone, disulfiram, and acamprosate. Additionally, there is also a trial of the cognitive enhancer citicoline.

STUDIES OF MEDICATIONS USED IN BIPOLAR DISORDER

ANTICONVULSANTS

Anticonvulsants with GABAergic and glutamatergic activities have been tested for their efficacy in the treatment of addictive disorders (Brady, Myrick, Henderson, & Coffey, 2002; Brady, Sonne, et al., 2002; Johnson, Ait-Daoud, Akhtar, & Javors, 2005; Mueller et al., 1997). Several open-label pilot studies have pointed to the potential usefulness of sodium valproate (Albanese, Clodfelter, & Khantzian, 2000; Brady, Sonne, Anton, & Ballenger, 1995; Salloum et al., 2007) and lamotrigine (Brown, Perantie, et al., 2006) in the treatment of cocaine or alcohol abuse in bipolar disorder.

Sodium valproate is still the only empirically tested medication that has shown efficacy in decreasing heavy alcohol use in bipolar disorder with comorbid alcoholism. Salloum, Cornelius, Daley, et al. (2005) compared divalproex sodium as an add-on to lithium carbonate versus placebo add-on to lithium carbonate in a six-month, double-blind, placebo-controlled trial in bipolar I disorder and alcohol dependence. Divalproex sodium was found superior to placebo in decreasing the proportion of heavy drinking days, as well as the number of standard alcohol drinks per heavy drinking days and on relapse to sustained heavy drinking. Those who were assigned to placebo reported on average 10 standard drinks per heavy drinking day while those who were assigned to divalproex sodium reported an average of 5 drinks per heavy drinking day (a heavy drink day is defined as four or more standard drinks for females or five or more standard drinks for males). Those assigned to divalproex sodium had significantly lower gamma glutamyl transpeptidase, an indirect objective measure of alcohol consumption, compared to placebo. Decrease in alcohol use inversely correlated with valproate blood levels (maintained within a range between 50 and 100 µg/mL). In a secondary analyses of this randomized trial, divalproex sodium was also found to have an advantage over placebo in decreasing cocaine use in subjects with bipolar disorder and alcoholism

who also had cocaine abuse (Salloum, Cornelius, Douaihy, et al., 2005).

Lamotrigine was tested in a randomized, double-blind, placebo-controlled trial in 120 patients with bipolar disorder (depressed or mixed phase) and cocaine dependence (Brown, Sunderajan, Hu, Sowell, & Carmody, 2012). Lamotrigine was started at 25 mg per day and titrated up to 200 mg/day over five weeks, although an increase to 400 mg/day was allowed. Lamotrigine was not superior to placebo on the study's primary outcome measure, urine drug screens, or self-reported number of cocaine use days. However, lamotrigine had an advantage over placebo on self-report of money spent on cocaine. There was also a strong correlation between changes in mood symptoms, especially depression and changes in self-reported cocaine use.

Some related studies have tested *atypical antipsychotics*. The largest studies to dates in patients with comorbid bipolar disorder and alcoholism have been conducted testing the atypical antipsychotic quetiapine. *Quetiapine* is very appealing medication to test in this population as it was proven effective in the treatment of both the depressive and the manic episode of bipolar disorder (Calabrese et al., 2005).

One promising pilot study (Brown, Nejtek, Perantie, & Bobadilla, 2002) and two relatively large clinical trials have been published to date testing the efficacy of quetiapine as an add-on medication for patients with bipolar disorder and alcoholism. (Brown et al., 2008; Stedman et al., 2010). Brown and colleagues conducted a 12-week trial of add-on quetiapine (titrated to 600 mg/day) in 115 patients with bipolar disorder and alcoholism with 82% of the sample in the depressive phase. The results of that study showed that the quetiapine group did not differ from the group assigned to placebo on improvement in alcohol abuse outcome. Steadman and colleagues (2010) reported on the results of a multisite, 12-week trial of quetiapine, added on to either lithium carbonate or valproate, in 362 patients with bipolar I disorder and alcohol dependence. The results of that multisite, largest conducted trial in this population also did not find a difference between quetiapine and placebo. Thus the results of these two studies do not support the efficacy of quetiapine in decreasing alcohol abuse among patients with bipolar disorder.

Lithium carbonate was tested in a small, six-week, double-blind, placebo-controlled pilot study of adolescents with bipolar I or bipolar II disorders (Geller et al., 1998). Lithium was found significantly better than placebo on negative urine drug screen (mostly marijuana) and on improved scores of the Global Clinical Impression. It is noteworthy that this was not an add-on study, thus the placebo group in this study did not have any other medication to stabilize their mood.

STUDIES OF MEDICATIONS USED IN SUBSTANCE USE DISORDERS

Currently, there are four medications approved by the US Food and Drug Administration (FDA) for the treatment of alcohol dependence: disulfiram, naltrexone hydrochloride, oral formulation and monthly intramuscular formulation, and acamprosate. Of the approved medications, trials have been conducted with oral naltrexone, acamprosate, and disulfiram.

Naltrexone hydrochloride is a pure opiate antagonist that decreases alcohol use and relapse by decreasing the positive reinforcing effects of alcohol. It was tested in pilot studies and in a small randomized-controlled pilot trial as well as with a Veterans Affairs population who had psychopathology, which included bipolar disorder. Oral naltrexone (50 mg/day dose), as an-add on medication was studied in a double-blind, placebo-controlled trial of 50 patients (Brown, Beard, Dobbs, & Rush, 2006; Brown et al., 2009). Naltrexone showed a trend toward advantage over placebo in greater decrease in drinking days and alcohol craving (Brown et al., 2009). A small, open-label, randomized-assignment pilot study tested naltrexone added to valproate compared to valproate alone found a significant decrease in alcohol use in those on the naltrexone added to valproate group (Salloum et al., 2006). A large Veterans Affairs–based study compared disulfiram with naltrexone and their combination in a sample of comorbid psychiatric disorder (Petrakis et al., 2005). Although that study did not specifically perform subgroup analysis based on psychiatric diagnosis, it did report that naltrexone or disulfiram, used alone or in combination, were tolerated by this population. Patients on these medications had significantly more consecutive weeks of abstinence and less craving than those treated with placebo, although the combination of disulfiram and naltrexone was not superior to either medication alone.

Acamprosate is classified as a modulator of glutamate neurotransmission, and it presumably acts by alleviating the negative reinforcing effects of alcohol withdrawal. Acamprosate did not show an advantage over placebo on drinking outcomes in a recently published, eight-week, randomized, double-blind, placebo-controlled trial in 33 patients with bipolar I or bipolar II disorder and alcohol dependence (Tolliver et al., 2012). Patients were randomized to add-on acamprosate (1,998 mg/day) or placebo.

A post hoc analysis of that study found an advantage of acamprosate over placebo on clinical global impression in Weeks 7 and 8 of the study.

Citicoline, a cognitive enhancer that also modulates phospholipids metabolism, was tested in a 12-week, randomized-controlled trial as an add-on medication in 44 outpatients with comorbid bipolar disorder and cocaine dependence (Brown et al., 2007). The results of that study indicated that the citicoline group was significantly less likely to have cocaine-positive urine compared to the placebo group. They also reported significantly improved declarative memory compared to the placebo group.

Currently there are no published pharmacotherapy trials for the treatment of opioid dependence or tobacco dependence in bipolar disorder. Opioid substitution pharmacotherapy (methadone and buprenorphine/naloxone) and naltrexone hydrochloride (oral and monthly injectable formulations) are the current available medications to treat opioid dependence. The availability of methadone maintenance, however, is limited to specialized addiction treatment settings. The recent introduction of office-based treatment with buprenorphine/naloxone for opioid maintenance treatment (Cowan, 2007) presents a distinct advantage in opening access to this effective treatment to a broader population, including those with bipolar disorder.

Tobacco dependence, as the most frequent SUD in bipolar disorder, represents a serious health hazard. *Varenicline*, the most effective medication for smoking cessation, has become of interest in helping these patients quit smoking. Varenicline, an FDA-approved medication for smoking cessation classified as an α-4, β 2 nicotinic acetylcholine receptor partial agonist, has shown by small case series to decrease smoking among patients with bipolar disorder (Frye et al., 2013). This is encouraging, although there have been a number of case reports of varenicline-induced manic episodes (Francois, Odom, & Kotbi, 2011; Hussain, Kayne, Guwanardane, & Petrides, 2011; Knibbs & Tsoi 2011). A number of treatment options are clinically available as well to address smoking in this population. These include, in addition to varenicline, the different formulations of nicotine replacement therapies and other pharmacotherapies such as bupropion hydrochloride (Johnson, 2006).

CONCLUSION

Patients with bipolar disorder are more likely to develop SUD. The presence of this comorbidity complicates the clinical picture and may lead to increase in negative consequences, including worsening symptoms severity, increased suicide risk, and inpatient hospitalization in addition to increased medical morbidity and social problems. Treatment needs for this comorbid condition is still largely unmet, with few empirical data to support effective psychosocial and pharmacotherapy treatments. The challenges of diagnostic ascertainment of bipolar disorder in the context of substance abuse as well as the suboptimal treatment adherence and impediments to accessing adequate treatment services still hinder interventions for these patients. Integrated chronic disease treatment approach is the preferred intervention strategy with a focus on achieving and maintaining sobriety, symptoms, and episode remission, along with enhancing recovery and health restoration. Integrated psychotherapeutic interventions seem promising, although larger studies in diverse settings are still needed. Anticonvulsants and medications used for alcoholism, such as naltrexone, have also shown promise for this population and indicate the need for larger, multisite studies to establish their efficacy.

Disclosure statement: Dr. Ihsan Salloum and Dr. Pedro Ruiz have not disclosed any conflicts of interest.

REFERENCES

Albanese, M. J., Clodfelter, R. C. J., & Khantzian, E. J. (2000). Divalproex sodium in substance abusers with mood disorder. *Journal of Clinical Psychiatry, 61*(12), 916–921.

Allen, J. P., Litten, R. Z., Fertig, J. B., & Babor, T. (1997). A review of research on the Alcohol Use Disorders Identification Test (AUDIT). *Alcoholism: Clinical & Experimental Research, 21*(4), 613–619.

Altman, E. G., Hedeker, D., Peterson, J. L., & Davis, J. M. (1997). The Altman Self-Rating Mania Scale. *Biological Psychiatry, 42,* 948–955.

American Psychiatric Association. (2013). *Diagnostic and statistical manual of mental disorders* (5th ed.). Washington, DC: Author.

Bech, P., Bolwig, T. G., Kramp, P., & Rafaelsen, O. J. (1979). The Bech-Rafaelsen Mania Scale and the Hamilton Depression Scale. *Acta Psychiatrica Scandinavica, 59,* 420–430.

Brady, K. T., Myrick, H., Henderson, S., & Coffey, S. F. (2002). The use of divalproex in alcohol relapse prevention: a pilot study. *Drug and Alcohol Dependence, 67*(3), 323–330.

Brady, K. T., Sonne, S. C., Anton, R., & Ballenger, J. C. (1995). Valproate in the treatment of acute bipolar affective episodes complicated by substance abuse: A pilot study. *Journal of Clinical Psychiatry, 56*(3), 118–121.

Brady, K. T., Sonne, S. C., Malcolm, R. J., Randall, C. L., Dansky, B. S., Simpson, K.,…Brondino, M. (2002). Carbamazepine in the treatment of cocaine dependence: Subtyping by affective disorder. *Experimental & Clinical Psychopharmacology, 10*(3), 276–285.

Brown, E. S., Beard, L., Dobbs, L., & Rush, A. J. (2006). Naltrexone in patients with bipolar disorder and alcohol dependence. *Depression and Anxiety, 23*(8), 492–495.

Brown, E. S., Carmody, T. J., Schmitz, J. M., Caetano, R., Adinoff, B., Swann, A. C., & Rush, A. J. (2009). A randomized, double-blind, placebo-controlled pilot study of naltrexone in outpatients with bipolar disorder and alcohol dependence. *Alcohol: Clinical and Experimental Research, 33*(11), 1863–1869.

Brown, E. S., Garza, M., & Carmody, T. J. (2008). A randomized, double-blind, placebo-controlled add-on trial of quetiapine in outpatients with bipolar disorder and alcohol use disorders. *Journal of Clinical Psychiatry, 69*(5), 701–705.

Brown, E. S., Gorman, A. R., & Hynan, L. S. (2007). A randomized, placebo-controlled trial of citicoline add-on therapy in outpatients with bipolar disorder and cocaine dependence. *Journal of Clinical Psychopharmacology, 27*(5), 498–502.

Brown, E. S., Nejtek, V. A., Perantie, D. C., & Bobadilla, L. (2002). Quetiapine in bipolar disorder and cocaine dependence. *Bipolar Disorders, 4*(6), 406–411.

Brown, E. S., Perantie, D. C., Dhanani, N., Beard, L., Orsulak, P., & Rush, A. J. (2006). Lamotrigine for bipolar disorder and comorbid cocaine dependence: A replication and extension study. *Journal of Affective Disorders, 93*(1–3), 219–222.

Brown, E. S., Sunderajan, P., Hu, L. T., Sowell, S. M., & Carmody, T. J. (2012). A randomized, double-blind, placebo-controlled, trial of lamotrigine therapy in bipolar disorder, depressed or mixed phase and cocaine dependence. *Neuropsychopharmacology, 37*(11), 2347–2354.

Calabrese, J. R., Keck, P. E. Jr., Macfadden, W., Minkwitz, M., Ketter, T. A., Weisler, R. H.,…Mullen, J. (2005). A randomized, double-blind, placebo-controlled trial of quetiapine in the treatment of bipolar I or II depression. *The American Journal of Psychiatry, 162*(7), 1351–1360.

Cerullo, M., & Strakowski, S. (2007). The prevalence and significance of substance use disorders in bipolar type I and II disorder. *Substance Abuse Treatment, Prevention, and Policy, 2*(1), 29.

Cocco, K. M., & Carey, K. B. (1998). Psychometric properties of the drug abuse screening test in psychiatric outpatients. *Psychological Assessment, 10*(4), 408–414.

Conway, K. P., Compton, W., Stinson, F. S., & Grant, B. F. (2006). Lifetime comorbidity of DSM-IV mood and anxiety disorders and specific drug use disorders: Results from the National Epidemiologic Survey on Alcohol and Related Conditions. *Journal of Clinical Psychiatry, 67*(2), 247–257.

Cornelius, J. R., Salloum, I. M., Ehler, J. G., Jarrett, P. J., Cornelius, M. D., Perel, J. M.,…Black, A. (1997). Fluoxetine in depressed alcoholics: A double-blind, placebo-controlled trial. *Archives of General Psychiatry, 54*(8), 700–705.

Cowan, A. P. (2007). Buprenorphine: The basic pharmacology revisited. *Journal of Addiction Medicine, 1*(2), 68–72.

El-Mallakh, R. S., & Hollifield, M. (2008). Comorbid anxiety in bipolar disorder alters treatment and prognosis. *Psychiatric Quarterly, 79*(2), 139–150.

Fisher, E. S. (2008). Building a medical neighborhood for the medical home. *New England Journal of Medicine, 359*(12), 1202–1205.

Francois, D., Odom, A., & Kotbi, N. (2011). A case of late-life onset mania during Varenicline assisted smoking cessation. *International Journal of Geriatric Psychiatry, 26*(6), 658–659.

Frank, E., Cyranowski, J. M., Rucci, P., Shear, M. K., Fagiolini, A., Thase, M. E.,…Kupfer, D. J. (2002). Clinical significance of lifetime panic spectrum symptoms in the treatment of patients with bipolar I disorder. *Archives of General Psychiatry, 59*(10), 905–911.

Franken, I. H., & Hendriks, V. M. (2001). Screening and diagnosis of anxiety and mood disorders in substance abuse patients. *American Journal on Addictions, 10*(1), 30–39.

Frye, M. A., Ebbert, J. O., Prince, C. A., Lineberry, T. W., Geske, J. R., & Patten, C. A. (2013). A feasibility study of varenicline for smoking cessation in bipolar patients with subsyndromal depression. *Journal of Clinical Psychopharmacology, 33*(6), 821–823.

Frye, M. A., & Salloum, I. M. (2006). Bipolar disorder and comorbid alcoholism: Prevalence rate and treatment considerations. *Bipolar Disorders, 8*(6), 677–685.

Geller, B., Cooper, T. B., Sun, K., Zimerman, B., Frazier, J., Williams, M., & Heath, J. (1998). Double-blind and placebo-controlled study of lithium for adolescent bipolar disorders with secondary substance dependency. *Journal of the American Academy of Child & Adolescent Psychiatry, 37*(2), 171–178.

Gossop, M. (1990). The development of a Short Opiate Withdrawal Scale (SOWS). *Addictive Behaviors, 15*(5), 487–490.

Grant, B. F., Stinson, F. S., Dawson, D. A., Chou, S. P., Dufour, M. C., Compton, W.,...Kaplan, K. (2004). Prevalence and co-occurrence of substance use disorders and independent mood and anxiety disorders: Results from the National Epidemiologic Survey on Alcohol and Related Conditions. *Archives of General Psychiatry, 61*(8), 807–816.

Greenfield, S. F., Weiss, R. D., Muenz, L. R., Vagge, L. M., Kelly, J. F., Bello, L. R., & Michael, J. (1998). The effect of depression on return to drinking: A prospective study. *Archives of General Psychiatry, 55*(3), 259–265.

Hasin, D. S., Trautman, K. D., Miele, G. M., Samet, S., Smith, M., & Endicott, J. (1996). Psychiatric Research Interview for Substance and Mental Disorders (PRISM): Reliability for substance abusers. *The American Journal of Psychiatry, 153*, 1195–1201.

Hirschfeld, R. M., & Vornik, L. A. (2004). Recognition and diagnosis of bipolar disorder. *Journal of Clinical Psychiatry, 65*(15), 5–9.

Hirschfeld, R. M., Williams, J. B., Spitzer, R. L., Calabrese, J. R., Flynn, L., Keck, P. E. Jr.,...Zajecka, J. (2000). Development and validation of a screening instrument for bipolar spectrum disorder: The Mood Disorder Questionnaire. *The American Journal of Psychiatry, 157*(11), 1873–1875.

Hussain, S., Kayne, E., Guwanardane, N., & Petrides, G. (2011). Varenicline induced mania in a 51-year-old patient without history of bipolar illness. *Progress in Neuro-Psychopharmacology & Biological Psychiatry, 35*(4), 1162–1163.

Johnson, B. A. (2006). New weapon to curb smoking: No more excuses to delay treatment. *Archives of Internal Medicine, 166*(15), 1547–1550.

Johnson, B. A., Ait-Daoud, N., Akhtar, F. Z., & Javors, M. A. (2005). Use of oral topiramate to promote smoking abstinence among alcohol-dependent smokers: A randomized controlled trial. *Archives of Internal Medicine, 165*(14), 1600–1605.

Judd, L. L., Schettler, P. J., Akiskal, H. S., Coryell, W., Leon, A. C., Maser, J. D., & Solomon, D. A. (2008). Residual symptom recovery from major affective episodes in bipolar disorders and rapid episode relapse/recurrence. *Archives of General Psychiatry, 65*(4), 386–394.

Knibbs, N., & Tsoi, D. T. (2011). Varenicline induces manic relapse in bipolar disorder. *General Hospital Psychiatry, 33*(6), 641–642.

Krishnan, K. R. (2005). Psychiatric and medical comorbidities of bipolar disorder. *Psychosomatic Medicine, 67*(1), 1–8.

Kupfer, D. J., Frank, E., Grochocinski, V. J., Cluss, P. A., Houck, P. R., & Stapf, D. A. (2002). Demographic and clinical characteristics of individuals in a bipolar disorder case registry. *Journal of Clinical Psychiatry, 63*(2), 120–125.

Lasser, K., Boyd, J. W., Woolhandler, S., Himmelstein, D. U., McCormick, D., & Bor, D. H. (2000). Smoking and mental illness: A population-based prevalence study. *JAMA, 284*, 2606–2610.

McIntyre, R. S., Soczynska, J. K., Bottas, A., Bordbar, K., Konarski, J. Z., & Kennedy, S. H. (2006). Anxiety disorders and bipolar disorder: A review. *Bipolar Disorders, 8*(6), 665–676.

Mezzich, J. E., Salloum, I. M., Cloninger, C. R., Salvador-Carulla, L., Kirmayer, L. J., Banzato, C. E. M.,...Botbol, M. (2010). Person-centred integrative diagnosis: Conceptual bases and structural model. *Canadian Journal of Psychiatry/Revue Canadienne de Psychiatrie, 55*(11), 701–708.

Mueller, T. I., Stout, R. L., Rudden, S., Brown, R. A., Gordon, A., Solomon, D. A., & Recupero, P. R. (1997). A double-blind, placebo-controlled pilot study of carbamazepine for the treatment of alcohol dependence. *Alcoholism: Clinical & Experimental Research, 21*(1), 86–92.

Otto, M. W., Simon, N. M., Wisniewski, S. R., Miklowitz, D. J., Kogan, J. N., Reilly-Harrington, N. A.,...STEP-BD Investigators. (2006). Prospective 12-month course of bipolar disorder in out-patients with and without comorbid anxiety disorders. *The British Journal of Psychiatry, 189*, 20–25.

Petrakis, I. L., Poling, J., Levinson, C., Nich, C., Carroll, K., Rounsaville, B., & MIRECC Study Group. (2005). Naltrexone and disulfiram in patients with alcohol dependence and comorbid psychiatric disorders. *Biological Psychiatry, 57*(10), 1128–1137.

Regier, D. A., Farmer, M. E., Rae, D. S., Locke, B. Z., Keith, S. J., Judd, L. L., & Goodwin, F. K. (1990). Comorbidity of mental disorders with alcohol and other drug abuse: Results from the Epidemiologic Catchment Area (ECA) Study. *JAMA, 264*, 2511–2518.

Saitz, R., Mayo-Smith, M. F., Roberts, M. S., Redmond, H. A., Bernard, D. R., & Calkins, D. R. (1994). Individualized treatment for alcohol withdrawal: A randomized double-blind controlled trial. *JAMA, 272*(7), 519–523.

Salloum, I. M., Cornelius, J. R., Daley, D. C., Kirisci, L., Himmelhoch, J. M., & Thase, M. E. (2005). Efficacy of valproate maintenance in patients with bipolar disorder and alcoholism: A double-blind placebo-controlled study. *Archives of General Psychiatry, 62*(1), 37–45.

Salloum, I. M., Cornelius, J. R., Daley, D. C., & Thase, M. E. (1995). The utility of diazepam loading in the treatment of alcohol withdrawal among psychiatric inpatients. *Psychopharmacology Bulletin, 31*(2), 305–310.

Salloum, I. M., Cornelius, J. R., Douaihy, A., Daley, D. C., Kirisci, L., Kelly, T. M., & Thase, M. E. (2005). Divalproex reduces cocaine use in patients with bipolar disorder and comorbid alcoholism. *Alcoholism: Clinical & Experimental Research, 29*(5), 79A.

Salloum, I. M., Daley, D. C., Cornelius, J. R., Kirisci, L., & Thase, M. E. (1996). Disproportionate lethality in psychiatric patients with concurrent alcohol and cocaine abuse. *The American Journal of Psychiatry, 153*(7), 953–955.

Salloum, I. M., Douaihy, A., Cornelius, J. R., Daley, D. C., Kelly, T. M., & Kirisci, L. (2006). Open label randomized pilot study of combined naltrexone and valproate in bipolar alcoholics. *Alcoholism: Clinical & Experimental Research, 30*, 104A.

Salloum, I. M., Douaihy, A., Cornelius, J. R., Kirisci, L., Kelly, T. M., & Hayes, J. (2007). Divalproex utility in bipolar disorder with co-occurring cocaine dependence: A pilot study. *Addictive Behaviors, 32*(2), 410–415.

Salloum, I., Douaihy, A., & Williams, L. (2008). Diagnostic and treatment considerations: Bipolar patients with comorbid substance use disorders. *Psychiatric Annals, 38*(11), 716.

Salloum, I. M., & Jones, Y. O. (2008). Efficacy of pharmacotherapy for comorbid major depression and substance use disorders: A review. *Current Psychiatry Reviews, 4*(1), 14–27.

Salloum, I. M., & Mezzich, J. E. (2011). Outlining the bases of person-centred integrative diagnosis. *Journal of Evaluation in Clinical Practice, 17*(2), 354–356.

Salloum, I. M., & Thase, M. E. (2000). Impact of substance abuse on the course and treatment of bipolar disorder. *Bipolar Disorders, 2*(3), 269–280.

Sellers, E. M., Naranjo, C. A., Harrison, M., Devenyi, P., Roach, C., & Sykora, K. (1983). Diazepam loading: Simplified treatment of alcohol withdrawal. *Clinical Pharmacology & Therapeutics, 34*(6), 822–826.

Sharma, V. (2003). Atypical antipsychotics and suicide in mood and anxiety disorders. *Bipolar Disorders, 5*(Suppl. 2), 48–52.

Sheehan, D. V., Lecrubier, Y., Sheehan, K., Amorim, P., Janavs, J., Weiller, E.,...Dunbar, G. C. (1998). The Mini-International Neuropsychiatric Interview (M.I.N.I): The development and validation of a structured diagnostic psychiatric interview for DSM-IV and ICD-10. *Journal of Clinical Psychiatry, 59*(20), 22–33.

Simon, N. M., Otto, M. W., Wisniewski, S. R., Fossey, M., Sagduyu, K., Frank, E., ... Pollack, M. H. (2004). Anxiety disorder comorbidity in bipolar disorder patients: Data from the first 500 participants in the Systematic Treatment Enhancement Program for Bipolar Disorder (STEP-BD). *The American Journal of Psychiatry, 161*(12), 2222–2229.

Stedman, M., Pettinati, H. M., Brown, E. S., Kotz, M., Calabrese, J. R., & Raines, S. (2010). A double-blind, placebo-controlled study with quetiapine as adjunct therapy with lithium or divalproex in bipolar I patients with coexisting alcohol dependence. *Alcoholism: Clinical & Experimental Research, 34*(10), 1822–1831.

Sullivan, J. T., Sykora, K., Schneiderman, J., Naranjo, C. A., & Sellers, E. M. (1989). Assessment of alcohol withdrawal: The revised clinical institute withdrawal assessment for alcohol scale (CIWA-Ar). *British Journal of Addiction, 84*(11), 1353–1357.

Tolliver, B. K., Desantis, S. M., Brown, D. G., Prisciandaro, J. J., & Brady, K. T. (2012). A randomized, double-blind, placebo-controlled clinical trial of acamprosate in alcohol-dependent individuals with bipolar disorder: A preliminary report. *Bipolar Disorders, 14*(1), 54–63.

Weiss, R. D., Ostacher, M. J., Otto, M. W., Calabrese, J. R., Fossey, M., Wisniewski, S. R., ... Sachs, G. H. (2005). Does recovery from substance use disorder matter in patients with bipolar disorder? *Journal of Clinical Psychiatry, 66*(6), 730–735; quiz 808–739.

Weiss, R. D., Griffin, M. L., Kolodziej, M. E., Greenfield, S. F., Najavits, L. M., Daley, D. C., ... Hennen, J. A. (2007). A randomized trial of integrated group therapy versus group drug counseling for patients with bipolar disorder and substance dependence.[see comment]. *American Journal of Psychiatry, 164*(1), 100–107.

Weiss, R. D., Griffin, M. L., Jaffee, W. B., Bender, R. E., Graff, F. S., Gallop, R. J., & Fitzmaurice, G. M. (2009). A "community-friendly" version of integrated group therapy for patients with bipolar disorder and substance dependence: A randomized controlled trial. *Drug and Alcohol Dependence, 104*(3), 212–219.

Wilens, T. E., Biederman, J., Millstein, R. B., Wozniak, J., Hahesy, A. L., & Spencer, T. J. (1999). Risk for substance use disorders in youths with child- and adolescent-onset bipolar disorder. *Journal of the American Academy of Child & Adolescent Psychiatry, 38*(6), 680–685.

Young, R. C., Biggs, J. T., Ziegler, V. E., & Meyer, D. A. (1978). A rating scale for mania: Reliability, validity, and sensitivity. *The British Journal of Psychiatry, 133*, 429–435.

36.

MEDICAL COMORBIDITY IN BIPOLAR DISORDER

Jelena Vrublevska and Konstantinos N. Fountoulakis

INTRODUCTION

General medical comorbidity is an important problem for psychiatric patients, leading to increased mortality among sufferers (Alstrom, 1942; Babigian & Odoroff, 1969). In this framework, it is important to note that bipolar disorder (BD) patients are less likely to receive proper diagnosis and care for their somatic problems, and this, together with their own lack of cooperation, are largely responsible for a worse overall outcome (Morriss & Mohammed, 2005). It has been reported that psychiatric patients in general (including BD patients) have a life expectancy of 25 to 30 years less than expected, with premature mortality primarily due to cardiovascular problems (Colton & Manderscheid, 2006). In this frame, it is embarrassing that some pharmacological interventions, although effective in ameliorating psychiatric symptomatology, eventually put the patient at a higher risk for the manifestation of specific somatic disorders.

Depending on the study sample, from one-fifth to more than two-thirds of BD patients are reported to manifest some kind of somatic comorbidity, with cardiovascular, endocrinological, gastrointestinal disorders, and pain being the most prevalent (Castelo et al., 2012; Feldman, Gwizdowski, Fischer, Yang, & Suppes, 2012; Kemp et al., 2013; Krishnan 2005; Magalhaes et al., 2012; McIntyre et al., 2006, 2007; Oreski, Jakovljevic, Aukst-Margetic, Orlic, & Vuksan-Cusa, 2012; Perron et al., 2009; Strakowski, MeElroy, Keck, & West, 1994; Strakowski et al., 1992; Subramaniam, Abdin, Vaingankar, & Chong, 2013; Weber, Fisher, Cowan, & Niebuhr, 2011). Multiple somatic comorbidity seems to be the rule rather than the exception with BD patients suffering from an average of 2.7 or more medical conditions (Kilbourne et al., 2009; McIntyre et al., 2006; Soreca, Frank, & Kupfer, 2009). This high medical comorbidity eventually leads to a worse overall long-term course and outcome (McIntyre et al., 2006; Thompson, Kupfer, Fagiolini, Scott, & Frank, 2006) and to a significantly greater disability (Perron et al., 2009).

OBESITY

Overweight and obesity are both important public health problems, and their prevalence is increasing in the general population. Its magnitude is even greater in psychiatric patients, including BD patients. Technically, the US National Heart, Lung and Blood Institute (1998) defined overweight as body mass index (BMI) $\geq 25 \text{kg/m}^2$ but $< 30 \text{ kg/m}^2$ and obesity as BMI $> 30 \text{ kg/m}^2$. The prevalence of obesity in BD patients is 20% to 49% (Elmslie, Silverstone, Mann, Williams, & Romans, 2000; McElroy et al., 2002), probably higher in comparison to the 18% reported in the general US population (Fagiolini et al., 2002). There are a number of possible causes for obesity, including sedentary lifestyle, medication exposure, neuroendocrine disorder, comorbid eating disorders, and genetic predisposition, among others.

Frequently patients who receive pharmacologic treatment for BD gain weight. Atypical antipsychotic medications are specifically associated with central obesity, with the main localization of body fat occurring around the abdomen (Elmslie et al., 2000). It is interesting that a retrospective study of 50 consecutive patients with BD type I revealed that the weight gain occurred during the acute treatment rather than during maintenance treatment (Fagiolini et al., 2002).

BD is frequently comorbid with substance use disorders and binge-eating disorder, which both result in increased weight (McIntyre et al., 2007). BD patients may also be particularly vulnerable to the appetite-stimulating effects of some substances of abuse. The association between depressive episodes and weight gain may be due to biological and behavioral changes because of depression, as well as the result of appetite-stimulating effects occurring with use of some psychotropics.

There is growing evidence that obesity in patients with BD leads to higher morbidity and mortality than expected, and in interaction with specific clinical features of BD, leads to poorer prognosis and outcome of BD itself. It has been reported that obese BD patients experienced a greater number of lifetime manic and depressive episodes than non-obese BD patients and are more likely to manifest recurrence, particularly of depressive episodes. It has also been suggested that increased obesity in BD patients is related to an increased risk of suicidal ideation and suicidal acts. BD patients with overweight have also been reported to manifest more frequent subthreshold social and generalized anxiety disorders, diabetes mellitus type II, and hypertension. (Alciati, Gesuele, Rizzi, Sarzi-Puttini, & Foschi, 2011).

CARDIOVASCULAR RISK FACTORS AND DISEASE

The most common cause of death associated with physical disorders for people with severe mental illness is cardiovascular disease. In a population-based cohort study of 4.6 million persons born in Denmark followed up for 13 years, the heart disease admissions and the rates of mortality from heart disease were estimated. The incidence rate ratio of heart disease contacts in persons with severe mental illness to that of nonpsychiatric population was 1.11 (95% confidence interval [CI]: 1.08–1.14). The psychiatric patient's excess mortality risk ratio from heart disease was 2.90 (95% CI: 2.71–3.10). Within five years of a first contact due to a somatic disease, the risk of dying from a heart disease was 8.26% for persons with severe mental illness who are aged <70 years, compared to the rate of 2.86% in patients with a heart disease but without psychiatric comorbidity. Furthermore, in the population with psychiatric comorbidity the rate of invasive procedures were considerably lower, and survival after the first contact for heart disease was reduced (Laursen, Munk-Olsen, Agerbo, Gasse, & Mortensen, 2009).

The fact that cardiovascular disease is the most common cause of death is not radically different from the general population; however, psychiatric patients convey higher risk to develop cardiovascular disease at an earlier age and with greater severity. It is well known that risk factors for cardiovascular diseases are multifactorial and comprises some genetic and lifestyle components, as well as some disease-specific treatment related effects, which in the case of psychiatric patients are some specific psychotropic agents, including some new generation antipsychotics and antidepressants. Opposing to this increased risk, many patients with severe mental disorders have limited access to health care and as such with less opportunity for cardiovascular risk screening and prevention relative to the general population (De Hert et al., 2009). For patients with access to heath care main clinical focus is often psychiatric illness and clinician neglect for mental disease- and/or treatment-induced modifiable risk factors further contributes to increased cardiovascular death rates. To exemplify weight gain during acute and maintenance treatment is a well-established side effect of antipsychotics and affects 15% to 72% of BD patients. Antidepressants and mood-stabilizing drugs, such as lithium and valproate, may also induce weight gain (De Hert et al., 2009). It is also well known that weight gain may induce or worsen hypertension as such cardiovascular diseases. As a result, bipolar patients are at a particularly high risk to develop a cardiovascular disease in comparison to patients with other psychiatric illnesses. In a retrospective study in which the data were collected from hospital records, the prevalence of comorbid diagnoses were compared between schizophrenia and BD. Patients with BD had more somatic (67.1% vs. 50.6%) and psychiatric (29.9% vs. 10.9%) comorbid conditions in comparison to patients with schizophrenia. More interesting was the finding that the most prevalent somatic comorbidity in patients with BD was cardiovascular disease (22.6%; Oreski et al., 2012). Another study in 1,379 patients with BD who were treated from 2001 to 2002 in outpatient psychiatric clinics reported that the most common somatic diseases were cardiovascular and, most specifically, hypertension, affecting 10.7% of that population. As expected, risk of medical comorbidities and cardiovascular diseases increased with patients' age. The baseline rate was also staggeringly high, with 30% of BD patients suffering from at least one medical condition already in their 20s. (Beyer, Kuchibhatla, Gersing, & Krishnan, 2005). A retrospective study of administrative claims confirmed this by revealing that the average age of BD patients was 39 years, indicating that medical conditions are prevalent at a very young age (Carney & Jones 2006). A four-year cross-sectional survey among Taiwanese BD patients showed the highest relative risk for the development of ischemic heart disease and hypertension (relative risk = 4.74. and 4.08, respectively) was in the age group under 20 years. The lowest relative risk for developing ischemic heart disease and hypertensive disorder were observed in the age group equal or older than 65 years. There was no significant gender difference in the cardiovascular disease prevalence rates among the study participants. Also, these findings are consistent with those that have indicated that males and females with mood disorders shared a similar level of risk for developing cardiovascular diseases in contrast to what is observed in the general population (Huang, Su, Chen, Chou, & Bai, 2009).

From a reverse point of view, a retrospective cohort study analyzed administrative data from 21,745 inpatients admitted with an acute myocardial infarction. Psychiatric comorbidity was identified using secondary inpatient diagnosis codes from the index of hospitalization and diagnosis or from one or more outpatient encounters during the 12 months prior to admission. In total, 0.9% of cases from the index inpatient admissions and 2.0% from the prior outpatient visits confirmed a comorbid diagnosis of BD. The results also suggested that patients with psychiatric comorbidity were younger and had lower mean laboratory severity scores. However, the rates of psychiatric comorbidity differed depending on the identification approach and were substantially more frequent when using diagnostic codes from prior outpatient encounters instead of secondary diagnostic codes from inpatient admissions. The patients with psychiatric comorbidity identified on the basis of prior outpatient encounters had a modestly elevated risk of both 30- and 365-day adjusted mortality rates, whereas patients identified on the basis of secondary inpatient diagnosis codes had similar 30- and 365-day adjusted mortality rates compared to the patients without such codes (Abrams, Vaughan-Sarrazin, & Rosenthal, 2009). A retrospective study of administrative claims revealed that cardiovascular conditions were more common among BD patients, ranging from a 23% increase in hypertension to a 185% increase in stroke. That particular study suggests that the increased odds for cardiovascular disease may be the result of weight gain, nicotine use, or unhealthy diet among subjects with BD (Carney & Jones 2006). While several studies have suggested that BD elevates risk of cardiovascular disease, few studies have examined the specific relationship of mania and hypomania with cardiovascular disease. In one study, the history of manic and hypomanic episodes was associated with a 2.5 to 3 times higher odds of cardiovascular disease in comparison to individuals without a history of hypomanic/manic or depressive episodes. The reasons behind this correlation are unclear; however, it is likely that manic or hypomanic episodes elevate the risk for the development of a cardiovascular disease through a multifactorial pathway. It is known that the increased severity of illness, worse treatment outcome, and less time spent in a recovered state are associated with negative health behaviors in BD, which in turn increase the risk for cardiovascular disease and start a vicious cycle (Ramsey, Leoutsakos, Mayer, Eaton, & Lee, 2010). The study by Cassidy and Carroll

(2002), which reviewed the records of 366 BD patients, reported that late-onset mania patients did demonstrate an increased frequency of current vascular risk factors compared with early-onset mania subjects. However, that study included 228 BD inpatients for which the medical comorbidity was quantified using referral as the criterion. In that sample, the most common medical condition was arterial hypertension, and severe active comorbidity prolonged hospital stay (Douzenis et al., 2012).

Overall, the literature suggests that BD patients are at a higher risk in comparison both to the general population and to other psychiatric patients to develop some type of cardiovascular disease. They are also at a higher risk to develop a more severe form of the disease and at an earlier age. When they are physically healthy, BD patients have limited access to screening and preventive programs, and after such a condition develops they have inadequate treatment and care. All of these factors result in poorer outcome of both BD and somatic disorder, higher disability, as well as an increased overall mortality because of cardiovascular disease resulting in a shorter average lifespan.

ENDOCRINE DISORDERS

The increased risk of metabolic side effects in patients with severe mental illness including BD has received much attention because of the high mortality manifested in these patients due to physical illness and especially to the combination of diabetes mellitus, obesity, hypertension, and cardiovascular disease (De Hert at al., 2011). A number of studies have revealed that metabolic syndrome is two to three times more common in patients with severe mental disorders compared to the general population (Ohaeri & Akanji, 2011). A study of 345 hospitalized BD patients reported that the prevalence of diabetes was 9.9%, significantly greater than expected from national norms (3.4%; Cassidy, Ahearn, & Carroll, 1999). This higher prevalence seems to concern all age groups under 60 years and both sexes; it is more pronounced in low-income individuals and among residents living in urban rather than rural areas (Chien, Chang, Lin, Chou, & Chou, 2010). The patients with comorbid diabetes mellitus are reported to have significantly more lifetime psychiatric hospitalizations than the nondiabetic subjects, although the age at first hospitalization and duration of psychiatric disorder were similar in the two groups (Cassidy et al., 1999). Another study that examined clinical data from 222 patients with BD (26 diabetic and 196 nondiabetic) found that diabetic BD patients were significantly older than nondiabetic patients

($p < .001$), had higher rates of rapid cycling ($p = .02$) and chronic course of BD ($p = .006$), and were more often on disability benefit because of BD ($p < .001$; Ruzickova et al., 2003). Additionally, the patients with comorbid diabetes mellitus had significantly more lifetime psychiatric hospitalizations than the nondiabetic subjects, although the age at first hospitalization and duration of psychiatric disorder were similar in the two groups (Cassidy et al., 1999).

This more complex clinical picture and course brings forward the fact that antipsychotic treatment is associated with a higher prevalence of diabetes in persons with BD. Although there are some disputes on how strong this contribution of antipsychotic treatment is on the development of diabetes mellitus, the literature supports this correlation (Chien et al., 2010; Ruzickova et al., 2003; Weber et al., 2011). From a reverse angle, a nationwide, population-based, prospective 10-year study reported that patients with BD were at an increased risk of initiation of antidiabetic (10.1% vs. 6.3%, $p = .012$; Hazard Ratio = 1.702, 95% CI: 1.155–2.507) and anti-hyperlipidemia medications (15.8% vs. 10.5%, $p = 0.004$; HR = 1.506, 95% CI: 1.107–2.047) in comparison to controls (Bai, Su, Chen, Chen, & Chang, 2013).

Another possible cause for this higher-than- expected comorbidity might be a shared genetic susceptibility. The tyrosine hydroxylase-INS-insulin-like growth factor II gene cluster on the short arm of chromosome 11 has been implicated as a susceptibility locus for diabetes mellitus, and although initial reports of the INS gene being a susceptibility locus for BD were subsequently discounted after a reanalysis of a larger sample, tyrosine hydroxylase markers might still be an area deserving further research (Meloni et al., 1995). The two diseases may also affect similar systems or areas of the brain. For example, the suprachiasmatic nucleus of the hypothalamus has been implicated both in disturbances of the sleep–wake cycle noted during mania and in the regulation of glucose metabolism. The other probable causatory factors include sedentary lifestyle, especially concerning unhealthy eating habits and lack of exercise, nicotine dependency, and of course treatment with antipsychotics, lithium, and antiepileptics (Correll, Frederickson, Kane, & Manu, 2008; Grandjean & Aubry, 2009; Martin, Han, Anton, Greenway, & Smith, 2009; Newcomer, 2007).

Some data suggest that abnormalities in thyroid function are more prevalent in patients with mood disorders than in the general population and may interfere with treatment responsiveness. Although overt hyper- or hypothyroidism may present, mood disorders are more frequently associated with more subtle dysfunction of the hypothalamic-pituitary-thyroid axis (Hendrick, Altshuler, & Whybrow, 1998). A study on general medical comorbidity of all BD hospital discharges ($n = 27,054$) in the United States in the period from 1979 to 2006 showed higher proportions of some medical conditions, including acquired hypothyroidism (proportional morbidity ratio = 2.6; Weber et al., 2011).

Some studies have reported that overt or subclinical hypothyroidism was more prevalent in BD patients with a rapid cycling course, although others did not find such an association. Lithium has antithyroid effects that may lead to clinical or subclinical hypothyroidism in up to 23% of patients (Kleiner, Altshuler, Hendrick, & Hershman, 1999). Lithium interferes with the synthesis and release of thyroid hormones through various mechanisms, and it has been suggested that it induces or exacerbates the development of autoimmune thyroiditis.

Asymptomatic autoimmune thyroiditis with a euthyroid state and a mildly increased level of circulating antibodies is not uncommon and occurs in 5% to 15% of the normal population, predominantly in women; the prevalence increases with age (Rapoport & McLachlan, 1996). In a recent study on a large sample of outpatients with BD, the prevalence of autoimmune thyroiditis (as evidenced by a higher prevalence of antithyroid antibodies) and of thyroid failure (as evidenced by a raised serum thyroid-stimulating hormone) was found to be higher than in the general population and other control patient groups (Kupka et al., 2002). The higher prevalence of autoimmune thyroiditis in BD patients cannot be attributed to lithium exposure alone. It should be noted that there are no differences in the prevalence rates of autoimmune thyroiditis between euthymic BD patients and patients in an acute manic or depressive episode. A study in monozygotic and dizygotic bipolar twins and matched control twins found that autoimmune thyroiditis is related not only to BD itself but also to the genetic vulnerability to develop the disorder. Thus, autoimmune thyroiditis, with thyroperoxidase antibodies serving as marker, is a possible endophenotype for BD (Vonk, van der Schot, Kahn, Nolen, & Drexhage, 2007).

HIV/AIDS

The prevalence of human immunodeficiency virus (HIV) among the general population of adults in the United States has been estimated to be 0.3% to 0.4% (HIV Surveillance Report, 2011). However, the risk of HIV was found to be increased in outpatients with mental disorders. More specifically, patients with BD are at a significantly higher risk of HIV infection in comparison to the general adult US population and at a greater risk even in comparison to the rest of psychiatric patients. They represent a rarely recognized and infrequently studied subgroup of HIV-infected patients (Beyer, Taylor, Gersing, & Krishnan, 2007). In the study of Beyer et al. (2005), from 1,379 patients who were treated for BD from 2001 to 2002 in outpatient psychiatric clinics, 2.8% were diagnosed with HIV. Although any direct comparison is difficult, this is much higher than anticipated. In the same database, only 46 of 4,509 (1.0%) unipolar depressed outpatients were diagnosed with HIV, and this is much lower than the respected rate observed in the bipolar population. These findings might suggest that bipolar patients may be at an increased risk of exposure to life-threatening infection, possibly due to impulsive behaviors such as substance abuse and unsafe sexual activity.

In another study on 194 HIV-infected adult outpatients, the diagnosis of BD was confirmed in 8.1% ($N = 16$) of the sample. There was an almost four times higher prevalence of BD among the HIV-infected patients (8.1%) than in the US general population (2.1%). The prevalence of BD type I in the HIV patients was 5.6% ($N = 11$), which is almost six times higher than the respective rate in the US general population (1%; Merikangas et al., 2007). The variables associated with the diagnoses of BD were younger age at first sexual intercourse, sex with prostitute partners, sex outside the primary relationship, alcohol use disorder, and illicit drug abuse (de Sousa Gurgel et al., 2013). Even though it cannot be established whether these behaviors occurred independently of BD, previous studies have associated manic states with risky sexual behavior, and BD is strongly associated with alcohol and substance abuse (Ramrakha et al., 2000). In another study, longitudinal analysis was used to explore the relationship between diagnosis of serious mental illness and subsequent new diagnoses of HIV. Logistic regression was used to predict HIV/AIDS diagnoses among beneficiaries ($N = 6,417,676$) who were without HIV. After substance abuse or dependence was longitudinally controlled for, no independent association between serious mental illness and the risk of new HIV diagnoses was found (Prince, Walkup, Akincigil, Amin, & Crystal, 2012). In a chart review ($N = 162$) study at a hospital AIDS clinic, it was estimated that manic syndromes affected 8% ($N = 9$) of patients who had AIDS. Of the patients with manic episodes, those without a family or personal history of mood disorder developed mania later in the course of HIV infection and had a higher prevalence of comorbid dementia (Lyketsos et al., 1993). In the study by Carney and Jones (2006), the odds for HIV/AIDS in inpatient and

outpatient claims submitted by a health-care provider were 9.53 times higher than expected.

There are several issues concerning the treatment of HIV-infected persons in general, including lack of access to treatment, social support, and medication side effects. Patients with HIV and psychiatric comorbidity have been reported to have more favorable admission characteristics and have been less likely to be discharged or to die. They might be admitted earlier in their disease course for reasons not exclusively due to HIV infection (Goulet, Molde, Constantino, Gaughan, & Selwyn, 2000).

One of the important factors that appears to negatively affect anti-HIV medication adherence is co-occurrence of a serious mental disorder. The estimated adherence rates can vary greatly when assessing HIV positive individuals with comorbid BD, while among HIV positive persons without BD, self-reported antiretroviral medication adherence measures were reported to correlate significantly with objective assessments of medication adherence (Medication Event Monitoring System). It is interesting that correlations between self-reported and objective measures were not significant in dually affected patients. Among participants reporting adherence on self-report measures but classified as nonadherent based on the objective assessment, 94% had a diagnosis of BD (Badiee et al., 2012).

HEPATITIS C

The prevalence of hepatitis C (HCV) is higher in certain populations, and often HCV infection coexists with HIV and other infections. The presence of multiple comorbidities may potentially provide additional reasons for treatment failure and lack of treatment adherence in this population. In this framework, the presence of psychiatric comorbid conditions is among the leading reasons for lack of treatment of HCV in infected persons. In BD patients, the increased risk may come from participation in high-risk behaviors including intermittent/episodic drug use or indiscriminate hypersexuality when manic. In addition, alcohol use disorders are relatively common in BD patients and may increase the likelihood of high-risk behaviors, as well as the risk of liver disease in those patients with comorbid alcohol use and HCV.

A retrospective study on 325,410 patients seen between 1998 and 2004 found that the relative risk for a patient having HCV if he or she had BD (with or without a substance use disorder) was 3.6 (Matthews, Huckans, Blackwell, & Hauser, 2008). Another study of HCV infected ($N = 5,737$) persons on dialysis reported a prevalence of 1.5% in persons with BD with the odds ratio (OR) equal to 1.19 (95% CI: 0.92–1.59; Butt, Evans, Skanderson, & Shakil, 2006).

Screening, testing, and appropriately treating HCV in the bipolar population may reduce the progression of liver disease and decrease liver-related side effects of medications used to treat BD.

CANCER

Although cancer is the second-leading cause of death among the overall population, evidence on cancer risk varies among persons with severe mental disorders. In a retrospective cohort study that used administrative data to examine cancer incidence by diagnosis, race, and cancer site, the total cancer risk in the study cohort with severe mental illnesses versus a population-based register risk was 2.6 higher for persons with schizophrenia and BD.

The lung cancer incidence among patients with schizophrenia or BD was more than four times higher than the respected based on population-based registries data. The incidence of colorectal cancer was similarly elevated with standardized incidence ratios (SIRs) of 4.0 for persons with BD. Female participants had heightened risk of breast cancer with an SIR equal to 1.9. There was no increased risk for prostate cancer. The study cohort showed no racial effect on cancer risk (McGinty et al., 2012). In another retrospective study of 3,557 subjects with BD and administrative claims, elevated ORs were found for cancers concerning all organ systems. Lymphoma and metastatic cancer were the only conditions less likely to occur in persons with BD (Carney & Jones, 2006).

The risk factors are disproportionally prevalent in mental health patients and increase the risk for the developing of certain types of cancer, but not cancer in general. High rates of smoking in the population with serious mental illness probably contributes to the increased lung cancer incidence. The possible but inconclusive elevated risk of breast cancer may be due to the low childbirth rate and to the elevated prolactin levels caused by treatment with specific antipsychotics. The high risk of colon cancer (SIRs = 4.0) might be related to smoking, sedentary lifestyle, or diet high in fat and low in fruits and vegetables.

MIGRAINE

The estimates of annual prevalence of migraine in the general population range from 3.3% to 21.9% for women and from 0.7% to 16.1% for men (Lipton & Bigal, 2005).

However, migraine is a common problem in psychiatric patients, and it is characterized by the recurrence of painful and nonpainful episodic phenomena and a variety of neurological manifestations (Antonaci et al., 2011). Migraine is up to four times more common in females than in males, with its peak incidence occurring between ages 25 and 44 years old (Lipton et al., 2002).

Several authors have reported migraine prevalence rates as high as 39% among those with BD (Nancy, du Fort, & Cervantes, 2003). The Canadian Community Health Survey, with a sample of 36,964 subjects, reported the presence of a significant association between migraine and BD, with migraine subjects suffering from BD twice as often as those without migraine. Migraine and BD were common in those with the lowest and lower middle income and was less frequent in those who were married (Jette, Patten, Williams, Becker, & Wiebe, 2008). Similar results were reported by a large study in a population-based sample (Ratcliffe et al., 2009). Another large, population-based study confirmed that the odds of having migraine were significantly increased in subjects with both manic and depressive episodes in comparison to either episodes alone (OR = 1.5 vs. manic episodes alone; 1.8 vs. depressive episodes alone). Additionally, migraine comorbidity in BD patients was associated with an earlier onset of mental illness, while in subjects with either manic or depressive episodes alone migraine comorbidity was associated with increased suicidality and anxiety (Nguyen & Low, 2013). A number of studies have found higher prevalence of migraine particularly in those with BD type II, as well as higher rates of suicidal behavior, panic disorder, generalized anxiety disorder, obsessive-compulsive disorder, and social phobia (Ortiz et al., 2010).

Migraine and BD share several characteristics, such as an episodic course, an increased vulnerability to stress, response to specific antiepileptic drugs, and family history for both migraine and mood disorders. The two main theories that have been proposed are that a common etiologic factor (environmental or genetic) influences both conditions and a causal relationship exists between mental disorders and migraine. Furthermore, Dilsaver, Benazzi, Oedegaard, Fasmer, and Akiskal (2009) reported that having a first-degree relative with BD increases the likelihood of having migraine among patients with unipolar depression (OR = 4.3) and BD (OR = 2.9). Serotoninergic dopaminergic and glutamate systems abnormalities (D'Andrea, Welch, Riddle, Grunfeld, & Joseph, 1989; Goodwin & Jamison, 2007; Peroutka, Wilhoit, & Jones, 1997) have been implicated in the pathogenesis of migraine, as well as in the pathogenesis of mood disorders. It has been suggested that the low platelet monoamine oxidase activity observed in patients with migraine could serve as an indicator of increased vulnerability for the development of psychiatric disorders (Littlewood et al., 1989).

GASTROENTEROLOGICAL DISORDERS

Studies that have included patients with mood disorders have reported significantly higher rates of gastrointestinal problems in comparison to the general population. More specifically, community-based studies have demonstrated an association between peptic ulcer disease and mood disorders among adults. BDs were reported to be robustly associated with peptic ulcer disease (OR = 2.91), although nicotine and alcohol dependence might play a substantial role in explaining the link of BD with peptic ulcer disease (Goodwin, Keyes, Stein, & Talley, 2009). Studies have shown that smoking reduces the amount of bicarbonate in the duodenum, which causes problems in the neutralization of acid (Ainsworth, Hogan, Koss, & Isenberg, 1993). In addition, smoking decreases the gastroduodenal mucosal synthesis of prostaglandin, an important factor in regulation of mucosal defense, including the stimulation of duodenal mucosal bicarbonate secretion (Fletcher, Shulkes, & Hardy, 1985).

In patients with BD, studies suggest that over 50% of patients have one or more past or present alcohol and substance use disorders. This increased presence of substance and alcohol use disorders in BD patients in turn increases the risk of chronic liver disease. In the retrospective electronic chart review of the Veterans Integrated Services Network, the patients with BD ($N = 5,319$) had a higher prevalence of liver disease (21.5% vs. 3.5%; OR = 7.58); HCV (15.5% vs. 2.1%; OR = 8.60), and alcohol-related liver cirrhosis (1.6% vs. 0.4%; OR = 3.82) in comparison to matched controls (Fuller et al., 2011).

COMORBID ENCEPHALOPATHY

While white matter hyperintensities are not usually seen in young subjects, deep white matter hyperintensities have been reported in up to 25% of young patients with BD, and they seem to be stable over time (Dupont et al., 1990). The clinical implications of MRI findings in patients with BD are not well understood. Only in a late-onset BD with concomitant organic (usually of cerebrovascular origin) substrate can this relationship be easily understood. Ahearn et al. (1998) obtained MRIs from 21 members of a family with a strong history of BD. Eight of them were suffering from BD, and one had symptoms of BD but did not meet the full *Diagnostic and Statistical Manual of Mental Disorders* criteria. Four of these nine subjects also had deep white matter lesions, and eight had lesions in the subcortical gray nuclei. It is highly probable that the presence of white matter hyperintensities is suggestive of the presence of some comorbid medical condition (e.g., migraine, cerebrovascular disease, or multiple sclerosis) and do not relate directly to BD per se.

CONCLUSION

Overall, the literature is conclusive concerning the high rate of medical comorbidity in BD patients and its adverse effect on overall outcome. However, it is rather inconclusive concerning specific diseases and rates. This is because of differences in study samples (e.g., inpatients, outpatients, registered and covered by insurance, which by definition might suffer from a less severe bipolar, etc.) and assessment methods. In spite of these problems in the literature, a robust conclusion is that complex multiple comorbidity seems to be very frequent.

The treatment of these multiple somatic comorbidities is difficult, and several principles exist to manage the increasingly complex problems. Central to the proper strategic design of the treatment are correct diagnosis, risk assessment, determining the appropriate setting for treatment, and determining the sequence of treatments since simultaneous treatments might be problematic. Following these, the planning for the long-term management and detailed assessment of the different facets of the outcome with the use of psychometric and neuropsychological tools and laboratory testing are also of prime importance (McIntyre et al., 2012; Ramasubbu, Beaulieu, Taylor, Schaffer, & McIntyre, 2012; Soreca et al., 2008).

Disclosure statement: Dr. Fountoulakis has received support to attend congresses from Eli Lilly, Pfizer, Astra Zeneca, Janssen and others. He receives research grant support from Pfizer Foundation. Dr. Jelena Vrublevska has no conflicts to disclose.

REFERENCES

Abrams, T. E., Vaughan-Sarrazin, M., & Rosenthal, G. E. (2009). Psychiatric comorbidity and mortality after acute myocardial infarction. Circulation. *Cardiovascular Quality and Outcomes, 2,* 213–220.

Ahearn, E. P., Steffens, D. C., Cassidy, F., Van Meter, S. A., Provenzale, J. M., Seldin, M. F.,...Krishnan, K. R. (1998). Familial leukoencephalopathy in bipolar disorder. *The American Journal of Psychiatry, 155*, 1605–1607.

Ainsworth, M. A., Hogan, D. L., Koss, M. A., & Isenberg, J. I. (1993). Cigarette smoking inhibits acid-stimulated duodenal mucosal bicarbonate secretion. *Annals of Internal Medicine, 119*, 882–886.

Alciati, A., Gesuele, F., Rizzi, A., Sarzi-Puttini, P., & Foschi, D. (2011). Childhood parental loss and bipolar spectrum in obese bariatric surgery candidates. *International Journal of Psychiatry in Medicine, 41*, 155–171.

Alstrom, C. (1942). Mortality in mental hospitals. *Acta Psychiatrica and Neurologica, 17*, 1–42.

Antonaci, F., Nappi, G., Galli, F., Manzoni, G. C., Calabresi, P., & Costa, A. (2011). Migraine and psychiatric comorbidity: A review of clinical findings. *Journal of Headache and Pain, 12*, 115–125.

Babigian, H. M., & Odoroff, C. L. (1969). The mortality experience of a population with psychiatric illness. *The American Journal of Psychiatry, 126*(4), 470–480.

Badiee, J., Riggs, P. K., Rooney, A. S., Vaida, F., Grant, I., Atkinson, J. H., & Moore, D. J. (2012). Approaches to identifying appropriate medication adherence assessments for HIV infected individuals with comorbid bipolar disorder. *AIDS Patient Care and STDs, 26*, 388–394.

Bai, Y. M., Su, T. P., Chen, M. H., Chen, T. J., & Chang, W. H. (2013). Risk of developing diabetes mellitus and hyperlipidemia among patients with bipolar disorder, major depressive disorder, and schizophrenia: A 10-year nationwide population-based prospective cohort study. *Journal of Affective Disorders, 150*, 57–62.

Beyer, J. L., Taylor, L., Gersing, K. R., & Krishnan, K. R. (2007). Prevalence of HIV infection in a general psychiatric outpatient population. *Psychosomatics, 48*, 31–37.

Beyer, J., Kuchibhatla, M., Gersing, K., & Krishnan, K. R. (2005). Medical comorbidity in a bipolar outpatient clinical population. *Neuropsychopharmacology, 30*, 401–404.

Butt, A. A., Evans, R., Skanderson, M., & Shakil, A. O. (2006). Comorbid medical and psychiatric conditions and substance abuse in HCV infected persons on dialysis. *Journal of Hepatology, 44*, 864–868.

Carney, C. P., & Jones, L. E. (2006). Medical comorbidity in women and men with bipolar disorders: A population-based controlled study. *Psychosomatic Medicine, 68*, 684–691.

Cassidy, F., Ahearn, E., & Carroll, B. J. (1999). Elevated frequency of diabetes mellitus in hospitalized manic-depressive patients. *The American Journal of Psychiatry, 156*, 1417–1420.

Cassidy, F., & Carroll, B. J. (2002). Vascular risk factors in late onset mania. *Psychological Medicine, 32*, 359–362.

Castelo, M. S., Hyphantis, T. N., Macedo, D. S., Lemos, G. O., Machado, Y. O., Kapczinski, F.,...Carvalho, A. F. (2012). Screening for bipolar disorder in the primary care: A Brazilian survey. *Journal of Affective Disorders, 143*(1–3), 118–124. doi:10.1016/j.jad.2012.05.040 S0165-0327(12)00395-3 [pii]

Centers for Disease Control and Prevention. (2011). *HIV surveillance report.* Atlanta, GA: Author.

Chien, I. C., Chang, K. C., Lin, C. H., Chou, Y. J., & Chou, P. (2010). Prevalence of diabetes in patients with bipolar disorder in Taiwan: A population-based national health insurance study. *General Hospital Psychiatry, 32*, 577–582.

Colton, C. W., & Manderscheid, R. W. (2006). Congruencies in increased mortality rates, years of potential life lost, and causes of death among public mental health clients in eight states. *Preventing Chronic Disease, 3*(2), A42. doi:A42 [pii]

Correll, C. U., Frederickson, A. M., Kane, J. M., & Manu, P. (2008). Equally increased risk for metabolic syndrome in patients with bipolar disorder and schizophrenia treated with second-generation antipsychotics. *Bipolar Disorders, 10*, 788–797.

D'Andrea, G., Welch, K. M., Riddle, J. M., Grunfeld, S., & Joseph, R. (1989). Platelet serotonin metabolism and ultrastructure in migraine. *Archives of Neurology, 46*, 1187–1189.

De Hert, M., Correll, C. U., Bobes, J., Cetkovich-Bakmas, M., Cohen, D., Asai, I.,...Leucht, S. (2011). Physical illness in patients with severe mental disorders: I. Prevalence, impact of medications and disparities in health care. *World Psychiatry, 10*, 52–77.

De Hert, M., Dekker, J. M., Wood, D., Kahl, K. G., Holt, R. I. G., & Moller, H. J. (2009). Cardiovascular disease and diabetes in people with severe mental illness position statement from the European Psychiatric Association (EPA), supported by the European Association for the Study of Diabetes (EASD) and the European Society of Cardiology (ESC). *European Psychiatry, 24*, 412–424.

de Sousa Gurgel, W., da Silva Carneiro, A. H., Barreto Reboucas, D., Negreiros de Matos, K. J., do Menino Jesus Silva Leitao, T., & de Matos e Souza, F. G. (2013). Prevalence of bipolar disorder in a HIV-infected outpatient population. *AIDS Care, 25*, 1499–1503.

Dilsaver, S. C., Benazzi, F., Oedegaard, K. J., Fasmer, O. B., & Akiskal, H. S. (2009). Is a family history of bipolar disorder a risk factor for migraine among affectively ill patients? *Psychopathology, 42*, 119–123.

Douzenis, A., Seretis, D., Nika, S., Nikolaidou, P., Papadopoulou, A., Rizos, E. N.,...Lykouras, L. (2012). Factors affecting hospital stay in psychiatric patients: The role of active comorbidity. *BMC Health Services Research, 12*, 166.

Dupont, R. M., Jernigan, T. L., Butters, N., Delis, D., Hesselink, J. R., Heindel, W., & Gillin, J. C. (1990). Subcortical abnormalities detected in bipolar affective disorder using magnetic resonance imaging: Clinical and neuropsychological significance. *Archives of General Psychiatry, 47*, 55–59.

Elmslie, J. L., Silverstone, J. T., Mann, J. I., Williams, S. M., & Romans, S. E. (2000). Prevalence of overweight and obesity in bipolar patients. *Journal of Clinical Psychiatry, 61*, 179–184.

Fagiolini, A., Frank, E., Houck, P. R., Mallinger, A. G., Swartz, H. A., Buysse, D. J.,...Kupfer, D. J. (2002). Prevalence of obesity and weight change during treatment in patients with bipolar I disorder. *Journal of Clinical Psychiatry, 63*, 528–533.

Feldman, N. S., Gwizdowski, I. S., Fischer, E. G., Yang, H., & Suppes, T. (2012). Co-occurrence of serious or undiagnosed medical conditions with bipolar disorder preventing clinical trial randomization: A case series. *Journal of Clinical Psychiatry, 73*(6), 874–877. doi:10.4088/JCP.11m07331

Fletcher, D. R., Shulkes, A., & Hardy, K. J. (1985). The effect of cigarette smoking on gastric acid secretion and gastric mucosal blood flow in man. *Australian and New Zealand Journal of Medicine, 15*, 417–420.

Fuller, B. E., Rodriguez, V. L., Linke, A., Sikirica, M., Dirani, R., & Hauser, P. (2011). Prevalence of liver disease in veterans with bipolar disorder or schizophrenia. *General Hospital Psychiatry, 33*, 232–237.

Goodwin, F., & Jamison, K. (2007). *Manic-depressive illness: Bipolar disorders and recurrent depression.* New York: Oxford University Press.

Goodwin, R. D., Keyes, K. M., Stein, M. B., & Talley, N. J. (2009). Peptic ulcer and mental disorders among adults in the community: The role of nicotine and alcohol use disorders. *Psychosomatic Medicine, 71*, 463–468.

Goulet, J. L., Molde, S., Constantino, J., Gaughan, D., & Selwyn, P. A. (2000). Psychiatric comorbidity and the long-term care of people with AIDS. *Journal of Urban Health: Bulletin of the New York Academy of Medicine, 77*, 213–221.

Grandjean, E. M., & Aubry, J. M. (2009). Lithium: Updated human knowledge using an evidence-based approach: Part III: Clinical safety. *CNS Drugs, 23*, 397–418.

Hendrick, V., Altshuler, L., & Whybrow, P. (1998). Psychoneuroendocrinology of mood disorders: The hypothalamic-pituitary-thyroid axis. *Psychiatric Clinics of North America, 21*, 277–292.

Huang, K. L., Su, T. P., Chen, T. J., Chou, Y. H., & Bai, Y. M. (2009). Comorbidity of cardiovascular diseases with mood and anxiety disorder: A population based 4-year study. *Psychiatry & Clinical Neurosciences, 63*, 401–409.

Jette, N., Patten, S., Williams, J., Becker, W., & Wiebe, S. (2008). Comorbidity of migraine and psychiatric disorders—A national population-based study. *Headache, 48*, 501–516.

Kemp, D. E., Sylvia, L. G., Calabrese, J. R., Nierenberg, A. A., Thase, M. E., Reilly-Harrington, N. A.,...Iosifescu, D. V. (2013). General medical burden in bipolar disorder: Findings from the LiTMUS comparative effectiveness trial. *Acta Psychiatrica Scandinavica.* doi:10.1111/acps.12101

Kilbourne, A. M., Perron, B. E., Mezuk, B., Welsh, D., Ilgen, M., & Bauer, M. S. (2009). Co-occurring conditions and health-related quality of life in patients with bipolar disorder. *Psychosomatic Medicine, 71*(8), 894–900. doi:10.1097/PSY.0b013e3181b49948 PSY.0b013e3181b49948 [pii]

Kleiner, J., Altshuler, L., Hendrick, V., & Hershman, J. M. (1999). Lithium-induced subclinical hypothyroidism: Review of the literature and guidelines for treatment. *Journal of Clinical Psychiatry, 60*, 249–255.

Krishnan, K. R. (2005). Psychiatric and medical comorbidities of bipolar disorder. *Psychosomatic Medicine, 67*, 1–8.

Kupka, R. W., Nolen, W. A., Post, R. M., McElroy, S. L., Altshuler, L. L., Denicoff, K. D.,...Drexhage, H. A. (2002). High rate of autoimmune thyroiditis in bipolar disorder: Lack of association with lithium exposure. *Biological Psychiatry, 51*, 305–311.

Laursen, T. M., Munk-Olsen, T., Agerbo, E., Gasse, C., & Mortensen, P. B. (2009). Somatic hospital contacts, invasive cardiac procedures, and mortality from heart disease in patients with severe mental disorder. *Archives of General Psychiatry, 66*, 713–720.

Lipton, R. B., & Bigal, M. E. (2005). Migraine: Epidemiology, impact, and risk factors for progression. *Headache, 45*, 3–13.

Lipton, R. B., Scher, A. I., Kolodner, K., Liberman, J., Steiner, T. J., & Stewart, W. F. (2002). Migraine in the United States: Epidemiology and patterns of health care use. *Neurology, 58*, 885–894.

Littlewood, J., Prasad, A., Gibb, C., Glover, V., Sandler, M., Joseph, R., & Rose, F. C. (1989). Psychiatric morbidity, platelet monoamine oxidase and tribulin output in headache. *Psychiatry Research, 30*, 95–102.

Lyketsos, C. G., Hanson, A. L., Fishman, M., Rosenblatt, A., McHugh, P. R., & Treisman, G. J. (1993). Manic syndrome early and late in the course of HIV. *The American Journal of Psychiatry, 150*, 326–327.

Magalhaes, P. V., Kapczinski, F., Nierenberg, A. A., Deckersbach, T., Weisinger, D., Dodd, S., & Berk, M. (2012). Illness burden and medical comorbidity in the Systematic Treatment Enhancement Program for Bipolar Disorder. *Acta Psychiatrica Scandinavica, 125*(4), 303–308. doi:10.1111/j.1600-0447.2011.01794.x

Martin, C. K., Han, H., Anton, S. D., Greenway, F. L., & Smith, S. R. (2009). Effect of valproic acid on body weight, food intake, physical activity and hormones: Results of a randomized controlled trial. *Journal of Psychopharmacology, 23*, 814–825.

Matthews, A. M., Huckans, M. S., Blackwell, A. D., & Hauser, P. (2008). Hepatitis C testing and infection rates in bipolar patients with and without comorbid substance use disorders. *Bipolar Disorders, 10*, 266–270.

McElroy, S. L., Frye, M. A., Suppes, T., Dhavale, D., Keck, P. E. J., Leverich, G. S.,...Post, R. M. (2002). Correlates of overweight and obesity in 644 patients with bipolar disorder. *Journal of Clinical Psychiatry, 63*, 207–213.

McGinty, E. E., Zhang, Y., Guallar, E., Ford, D. E., Steinwachs, D., Dixon, L. B.,...Daumit, G. L. (2012). Cancer incidence in a sample of Maryland residents with serious mental illness. *Psychiatric Services, 63*(7), 714–717. doi:10.1176/appi.ps.201100169 1204715 [pii]

McIntyre, R. S., Konarski, J. Z., Soczynska, J. K., Wilkins, K., Panjwani, G., Bouffard, B.,...Kennedy, S. H. (2006). Medical comorbidity in bipolar disorder: Implications for functional outcomes and health service utilization. *Psychiatric Services, 57*(8), 1140–1144. doi:57/8/1140 [pii] 10.1176/appi.ps.57.8.1140

McIntyre, R. S., McElroy, S. L., Konarski, J. Z., Soczynska, J. K., Bottas, A., Castel, S.,...Kennedy, S. H. (2007). Substance use disorders and overweight/obesity in bipolar I disorder: Preliminary evidence for competing addictions. *Journal of Clinical Psychiatry, 68*, 1352–1357.

McIntyre, R. S., Rosenbluth, M., Ramasubbu, R., Bond, D. J., Taylor, V. H., Beaulieu, S., & Schaffer, A. (2012). Managing medical and psychiatric comorbidity in individuals with major depressive disorder and bipolar disorder. *Annals of Clinical Psychiatry, 24*(2), 163–169. doi:acp_2402g [pii]

McIntyre, R. S., Soczynska, J. K., Beyer, J. L., Woldeyohannes, H. O., Law, C. W., Miranda, A.,...Kennedy, S. H. (2007). Medical comorbidity in bipolar disorder: Re-prioritizing unmet needs. *Current Opinion in Psychiatry, 20*(4), 406–416. doi:10.1097/YCO.0b013e3281938102 00001504-200707000-00017 [pii]

Meloni, R., Leboyer, M., Bellivier, F., Barbe, B., Samolyk, D., Allilaire, J. F., & Mallet, J. (1995). Association of manic-depressive illness with tyrosine hydroxylase microsatellite marker. *Lancet, 345*, 932.

Merikangas, K. R., Akiskal, H. S., Angst, J., Greenberg, P. E., Hirschfeld, R. M. A., Petukhova, M., & Kessler, R. C. (2007). Lifetime and 12-month prevalence of bipolar spectrum disorder in the National Comorbidity Survey replication. *Archives of General Psychiatry, 64*, 543–552.

Morriss, R., & Mohammed, F. A. (2005). Metabolism, lifestyle and bipolar affective disorder. *Journal of Psychopharmacology, 19*(6), 94–101. doi:19/6_suppl/94 [pii] 10.1177/0269881105058678

Nancy, C. P. L., du Fort, G. G., & Cervantes, P. (2003). Prevalence, clinical correlates, and treatment of migraine in bipolar disorder. *Headache, 43*, 940.

National Heart, Lung, and Blood Institute, Obesity Task Force. (1998). *Clinical guidelines on the identification, evaluation, and treatment of overweight and obesity in adults: The evidence report.* Bethesda, MD: National Institutes of Health.

Newcomer, J. W. (2007). Metabolic considerations in the use of antipsychotic medications: A review of recent evidence. *Journal of Clinical Psychiatry, 68*(1), 20–27.

Nguyen, T. V., & Low, N. C. (2013). Comorbidity of migraine and mood episodes in a nationally representative population-based sample. *Headache, 53*, 498–506.

Ohaeri, J. U., & Akanji, A. O. (2011). Metabolic syndrome in severe mental disorders. *Metabolic Syndrome and Related Disorders, 9*, 91–98.

Oreski, I., Jakovljevic, M., Aukst-Margetic, B., Orlic, Z. C., & Vuksan-Cusa, B. (2012). Comorbidity and multimorbidity in patients with schizophrenia and bipolar disorder: Similarities and differencies. *Psychiatria Danubina, 24*, 80–85.

Ortiz, A., Cervantes, P., Zlotnik, G., van de Velde, C., Slaney, C., Garnham, J.,...Alda, M. (2010). Cross-prevalence of migraine and bipolar disorder. *Bipolar Disorders, 12*, 397–403.

Peroutka, S. J., Wilhoit, T., & Jones, K. (1997). Clinical susceptibility to migraine with aura is modified by dopamine D2 receptor (DRD2) NcoI alleles. *Neurology, 49*, 201–206.

Perron, B. E., Howard, M. O., Nienhuis, J. K., Bauer, M. S., Woodward, A. T., & Kilbourne, A. M. (2009). Prevalence and burden of general medical conditions among adults with bipolar I disorder: Results from the National Epidemiologic Survey on Alcohol and Related Conditions. *Journal of Clinical Psychiatry, 70*(10), 1407–1415. doi:10.4088/JCP.08m04586yel

Prince, J. D., Walkup, J., Akincigil, A., Amin, S., & Crystal, S. (2012). Serious mental illness and risk of new HIV/AIDS diagnoses: An analysis of Medicaid beneficiaries in eight states. *Psychiatric Services, 63*, 1032–1038.

Ramasubbu, R., Beaulieu, S., Taylor, V. H., Schaffer, A., & McIntyre, R. S. (2012). The CANMAT task force recommendations for the management of patients with mood disorders and comorbid medical conditions: Diagnostic, assessment, and treatment principles. *Annals of Clinical Psychiatry, 24*(1), 82–90. doi:acp_2401h [pii]

Ramrakha, S., Dickson, N., Paul, C., Caspi, A., Moffitt, T. E., & Bennett, Bauman. (2000). Psychiatric disorders and risky sexual behaviour in young adulthood: Cross sectional study in birth cohort. *BMJ: British Medical Journal (International Edition), 321,* 263.

Ramsey, C. M., Leoutsakos, J. M., Mayer, L. S., Eaton, W. W., & Lee, H. B. (2010). History of manic and hypomanic episodes and risk of incident cardiovascular disease: 11.5 year follow-up from the Baltimore Epidemiologic Catchment Area Study. *Journal of Affective Disorders, 125*(1–3), 35–41. doi:10.1016/j.jad.2009.12.024 S0165-0327(10)00003-0 [pii]

Rapoport, B., & McLachlan, S. M. (1996): Thyroid peroxidase autoantibodies. In J. B. Peter & Y. Schoenfeld (Eds.), *Autoantibodies* (pp. 816–821). Amsterdam: Elsevier Science.

Ratcliffe, G. E., Enns, M. W., Jacobi, F., Belik, S. L., & Sareen, J. (2009). The relationship between migraine and mental disorders in a population-based sample. *General Hospital Psychiatry, 31,* 14–19.

Ruzickova, M., Slaney, C., Garnham, J., & Alda, M. (2003). Clinical features of bipolar disorder with and without comorbid diabetes mellitus. *Canadian Journal of Psychiatry, 48,* 458–461.

Soreca, I., Fagiolini, A., Frank, E., Houck, P. R., Thompson, W. K., & Kupfer, D. J. (2008). Relationship of general medical burden, duration of illness and age in patients with bipolar I disorder. *Journal of Psychiatric Research, 42*(11), 956–961. doi:S0022-3956(07)00183-5 [pii] 10.1016/j.jpsychires.2007.10.009

Soreca, I., Frank, E., & Kupfer, D. J. (2009). The phenomenology of bipolar disorder: What drives the high rate of medical burden and determines long-term prognosis? *Depression and Anxiety, 26*(1), 73–82. doi:10.1002/da.20521

Strakowski, S. M., McElroy, S. L., Keck, P. W. Jr., & West, S. A. (1994). The co-occurrence of mania with medical and other psychiatric disorders. International *Journal of Psychiatry in Medicine, 24*(4), 305–328.

Strakowski, S. M., Tohen, M., Stoll, A. L., Faedda, G. L., & Goodwin, D. C. (1992). Comorbidity in mania at first hospitalization. *The American Journal of Psychiatry, 149*(4), 554–556.

Subramaniam, M., Abdin, E., Vaingankar, J. A., & Chong, S. A. (2013). Prevalence, correlates, comorbidity and severity of bipolar disorder: Results from the Singapore Mental Health Study. *Journal of Affective Disorders, 146*(2), 189–196. doi:10.1016/j.jad.2012.09.002 S0165-0327(12)00621-0 [pii]

Thompson, W. K., Kupfer, D. J., Fagiolini, A., Scott, J. A., & Frank, E. (2006). Prevalence and clinical correlates of medical comorbidities in patients with bipolar I disorder: Analysis of acute-phase data from a randomized controlled trial. *Journal of Clinical Psychiatry, 67*(5), 783–788.

Vonk, R., van der Schot, A. C., Kahn, R. S., Nolen, W. A., & Drexhage, H. A. (2007). Is autoimmune thyroiditis part of the genetic vulnerability (or an endophenotype) for bipolar disorder? *Biological Psychiatry, 62,* 135–140.

Weber, N. S., Fisher, J. A., Cowan, D. N., & Niebuhr, D. W. (2011). Psychiatric and general medical conditions comorbid with bipolar disorder in the National Hospital Discharge Survey. *Psychiatric Services, 62*(10), 1152–1158. doi:10.1176/appi.ps.62.10.1152 62/10/1152 [pii]

PART VI

SUICIDALITY

37.

CLINICAL MANAGEMENT OF SUICIDAL RISK

Leonardo Tondo and Ross J. Baldessarini

INTRODUCTION

Suicide remains a major, unsolved problem for modern medicine and psychiatry. A ubiquitous international phenomenon, recognized cases of suicide account for at least 800,000 fatalities worldwide annually, but many cases are undiagnosed or unreported (sometimes for cultural or religious reasons or lack of systematic ascertainment) or may be considered "accidents." The study of suicide is challenging for several reasons. Until recently, there seemed to be some doubt that suicide is not only a personal tragedy and sociological problem but also a medical condition with a strong association with psychiatric disorders. Moreover, the concept that suicide risk might be altered (in either direction) by application of medical treatments has been very slow to emerge and be accepted, and only in recent years (Baldessarini & Jamison, 1999). Therapeutic investigations have been particularly uncommon. To date only one treatment—the antipsychotic drug clozapine—has regulatory recognition as having some long-term ability to reduce suicidal risk, but only for patients diagnosed with schizophrenia (Meltzer et al., 2003). For other treatments, with the possible exception of long-term use of lithium salts in major mood disorders, there is only suggestive evidence (Baldessarini et al., 2006). Other plausible treatments that might be of value include antidepressants or electroconvulsive treatment (ECT), as well as various forms of psychotherapy, emergency hospitalization, and others. However, all of these methods remain inadequately tested or their research assessments are inconsistent and inconclusive, even though they are widely employed empirically.

Limitations to research on treatments aimed at reducing suicidal risk include obvious clinical and ethical problems when an inactive or ineffective treatment, such as a placebo condition, would be compared to an experimental intervention. In addition, the infrequency of suicide, even among psychiatrically ill persons, has encouraged reliance for research on surrogate outcome measures such as self-injurious acts, threats so compelling as to require intervention, or even elusive and subjective thoughts of suicide or death. However, although a suicidal act necessarily includes previous ideation, the relationships of such surrogate measures to suicide are not close.

In the general population the reported ratio of attempts to suicides (A/S, proposed as an index of "lethality") is 30 to 50, and the ratio of identified "suicidal ideation" to attempts is about 6 (Kessler, Berglund, Borges, Nock, & Wang, 2005), with a proportion of nearly 180 cases involving putative suicidal ideation for every suicide in the United States, based on a national suicide rate of 0.011% per year (Table 37.1). However, the definitions and prevalence of nonfatal suicide-related behaviors ("attempts," "gestures") and suicidal thoughts ("plans," "ideation") are much less reliable than for suicides and certainly are underreported, as well as highly variable in suicidal intent and in the seriousness or potential lethality of methods involved (Kessler et al., 2005; Tondo, Isacsson, & Baldessarini, 2003). It is important to note that, in mood-disorder patients, these ratios shift substantially from the general population: the A/S ratio is only 5 to 10 (lower with greater intent to die), the ratio of identified suicidal ideation to attempts is about 3, and the ratio of ideation to suicides is about 20 to 25 (Nordstrom, Samuelsson, & Åsberg, 1995; Tondo & Baldessarini, 2007). These considerations indicate that relationships among levels of suicidal risk (thoughts, acts, deaths) are not close quantitatively and that suicidal ideation as an outcome measure bears only a distant relationship to suicide, even among psychiatric patients at risk. Moreover, suicidal ideation is a self-reported and subjective measure of uncertain reliability that can range from weariness of life to explicit, self-destructive plans. Nevertheless, ideation is the first step toward a possible suicide act and, appropriately, is carefully considered in clinical and research assessments of suicidal risk, particularly in patients diagnosed with a major mood

Table 37.1. REPORTED INTERNATIONAL SUICIDE RATES FOR MALES AND FEMALES

COUNTRY	YEAR	SUICIDE RATES (PER 100,000 PERSON-YEARS)			
		OVERALL	MALES	FEMALES	SEX RATIO (M/F)
Africa					
Egypt	2009	0.1	0.1	0.0	—
Mauritius	2008	6.8	11.8	1.9	6.21
South Africa	2007	0.9	1.4	0.4	3.50
Zimbabwe	1990	7.9	10.6	5.2	2.04
Africa mean	(*n* = 4)	3.92 ± 3.99	5.97 ± 6.08	1.88 ± 2.36	3.92 ± 2.12
North America					
Canada	2004	11.3	17.3	5.4	3.20
USA	2005	11.0	17.7	4.5	3.93
North America mean	(*n* = 2)	11.2 ± 0.21	17.5 ± 0.28	4.95 ± 0.64	3.56 ± 0.52
Central America & Caribbean					
Costa Rica	2009	6.1	10.2	1.9	5.37
Cuba	2008	12.3	19.0	5.5	3.46
Guatemala	2008	3.6	5.6	1.7	3.29
Mexico	2008	4.2	7.0	1.5	4.67
Nicaragua	2006	5.8	9.0	2.6	3.46
Panama	2008	5.5	9.0	1.9	4.74
Puerto Rico	2005	7.4	13.2	2.0	6.60
Central America mean	(*n* = 7)	6.41 ± 2.88	10.0 ± 4.48	2.44 ± 1.39	4.51 ± 1.22
South America					
Argentina	2008	7.7	12.6	3.0	4.20
Belize	2008	3.7	6.6	0.7	9.43
Brazil	2008	4.8	7.7	2.0	3.85
Chile	2007	11.1	18.2	4.2	4.33
Colombia	2007	4.9	7.9	2.0	3.95
Ecuador	2009	7.1	10.5	3.6	2.92
Guyana	2006	26.4	39.0	13.4	2.91
Paraguay	2008	3.6	5.1	2.0	2.55
Peru	2007	1.4	1.9	1.0	1.90
Suriname	2005	14.4	23.9	4.8	4.98
Trinidad	2006	10.7	17.9	3.8	4.71
Uruguay	2004	15.8	26.0	6.3	4.13
Venezuela	2007	3.2	5.3	1.2	4.42
South America mean	(*n* = 13)	8.83 ± 6.91	14.0 ± 10.6	3.69 ± 3.34	4.18 ± 1.82

(continued)

Table 37.1. CONTINUED

COUNTRY	YEAR	SUICIDE RATES (PER 100,000 PERSON-YEARS)			
		OVERALL	MALES	FEMALES	SEX RATIO (M/F)
Middle East					
Bahrain	2006	3.8	4.0	3.5	1.14
Iran	1991	0.2	0.3	0.1	3.00
Israel	2007	4.3	7.0	1.5	4.67
Jordan	2008	0.1	0.2	0.0	—
Kuwait	2009	1.8	1.9	1.7	1.12
Syria	1985	0.1	0.2	0.0	—
Middle-East mean	(*n* = 6)	1.72 ± 1.93	2.27 ± 2.76	1.13 ± 1.39	2.48 ± 1.70
Western Europe					
Austria	2010	15.0	23.7	6.8	3.48
Belgium	2005	19.4	28.8	10.3	2.80
Cyprus	2008	4.5	7.4	1.7	4.35
Denmark	2006	11.9	17.5	6.4	2.73
Finland	2009	19.3	29.0	10.0	2.90
France	2007	16.3	24.7	8.5	2.91
Germany	2010	12.3	18.6	6.1	3.05
Greece	2009	3.5	6.0	1.0	6.00
Iceland	2008	11.9	16.5	7.0	2.36
Ireland	2009	11.8	19.0	4.7	4.04
Italy	2008	6.5	10.3	2.9	3.55
Luxembourg	2008	9.6	16.1	3.2	5.03
Malta	2008	3.4	5.9	1.0	5.90
Netherlands	2009	9.3	13.1	5.5	2.38
Norway	2009	11.9	17.3	6.5	2.66
Portugal	2009	9.6	15.6	4.0	3.90
Spain	2008	7.6	11.9	3.4	3.50
Sweden	2010	12.1	17.9	6.4	2.80
Switzerland	2007	18.0	24.8	11.4	2.18
UK	2009	6.9	10.9	3.0	3.63
West Europe mean	(*n* = 19)	10.8 ± 4.91	16.4 ± 6.94	5.42 ± 3.10	3.51 ± 1.13
Eastern Europe					
Albania	2003	4.0	4.7	3.3	1.42
Armenia	2008	1.9	2.8	1.1	2.54

(*continued*)

Table 37.1. CONTINUED

COUNTRY	YEAR	SUICIDE RATES (PER 100,000 PERSON-YEARS)			
		OVERALL	MALES	FEMALES	SEX RATIO (M/F)
Austria	2010	15.0	23.7	6.8	3.48
Azerbajan	2007	0.6	1.0	0.3	3.33
Belarus	2009	28.4	49.6	9.8	5.06
Bosnia & Herzegovina	1991	11.8	20.3	3.3	6.15
Bulgaria	2008	12.3	18.8	6.2	3.03
Croatia	2009	17.8	28.9	7.5	3.85
Czech Republic	2009	14.0	23.9	4.4	5.43
Estonia	2008	18.1	30.6	7.3	4.19
Georgia	2009	4.3	7.1	1.7	4.18
Hungary	2009	24.6	40.0	10.6	3.77
Latvia	2009	22.9	40.0	8.2	4.88
Lithuania	2009	34.1	61.3	10.4	5.89
Poland	2008	14.9	26.4	4.1	6.44
Moldova	2008	17.4	30.1	5.6	5.38
Romania	2009	12.0	21.0	3.5	6.00
Russian Federation	2006	30.1	53.9	9.5	5.67
Serbia	2009	18.8	28.1	10.0	2.810
Slovakia	2005	12.6	22.3	3.4	6.56
Slovenia	2009	21.9	34.6	9.4	3.68
Macedonia	2003	6.8	9.5	4.0	2.38
Ukraine	2009	21.2	37.8	7.0	5.40
East Europe mean	(*n* = 23)	15.9 ± 8.91	26.8 ± 16.0	5.97 ± 3.15	4.41 ± 1.45
Asia					
China	1999	13.9	13.0	14.8	0.88
India	2009	10.5	13.0	7.8	1.67
Hong Kong	2009	14.6	19.0	10.7	1.78
Kazakhstan	2008	25.6	43.0	9.4	4.57
Kyrgystan	2009	8.8	14.1	3.6	3.92
Maldives	2005	0.3	0.7	0.0	—
Sri Lanka	1991	31.0	44.6	16.8	2.66
South Korea	2009	31.0	39.9	22.1	1.80
Tajikistan	2001	2.6	2.9	2.3	1.26
Thailand	2002	7.8	12.0	3.8	3.16

(*continued*)

Table 37.1. CONTINUED

COUNTRY	YEAR	SUICIDE RATES (PER 100,000 PERSON-YEARS)			
		OVERALL	MALES	FEMALES	SEX RATIO (M/F)
Turkmenistan	1998	8.6	13.8	3.5	3.94
Uzbekistan	2005	4.7	7.0	2.3	3.04
Asia mean	(*n* = 12)	13.3 ± 10.5	18.6 ± 15.3	8.09 ± 6.86	2.61 ± 1.22
Pacific					
Australia	2006	8.2	12.8	3.6	3.56
Japan	2009	24.4	36.2	13.2	2.74
New Zealand	2007	11.7	18.1	5.5	3.29
Philippines	1993	2.1	2.5	1.7	1.47
Singapore	2006	10.3	12.9	7.7	1.68
Pacific mean	(*n* = 5)	11.3 ± 8.17	16.5 ± 12.4	6.34 ± 4.43	2.55 ± 0.94
Overall					
Overall Means [95% CI]	(*N* = 91)	10.9 [9.22–12.6]	17.2 [14.4–19.9]	5.04 [4.19–5.89]	3.73 [3.41–4.05]

NOTE: Regional means are with ± standard deviations. Data from World Health Organization (2013). CI = confidence interval.

disorder. In general, nonfatal suicide-related behaviors (attempts, violent and nonviolent self-injurious acts, "gestures," and ideation) vary in definition and potential lethality, can be unreliable or unfeasible outcome measures, and surely are underreported (Kessler et al., 2005; Tondo et al., 2003). Assessment of suicide-related behaviors is further complicated by generally relatively higher rates of suicide attempts among women and of suicides among men, and with increasing age in both sexes (Simon & Hales, 2012).

In short, it is not surprising that experimental therapeutics research on interventions aimed at suicide prevention is difficult conceptually, ethically, clinically, technically, and quantitatively. It follows that even widely employed, seemingly plausible methods of treating suicidal persons are not adequately supported by empirical research evidence, leaving tension between the obligation to intervene clinically, often rapidly, despite a paucity of clear empirical evidence about how best to do it.

EPIDEMIOLOGY OF SUICIDE

INTERNATIONAL SUICIDE RATES

The worldwide annual rate of reported suicide averages approximately 11/100,000 (0.011% per year; Table 37.1), with wide variation among and even within regions (the lowest reported rates are in the Middle East and the highest in Eastern Europe). Average rates are consistently much higher for men than women (by an average of 3.7-fold), with the notable exception of China, are very low in children, and relatively high among elderly men (Simon & Hales, 2012; World Health Organization, 2013; Table 37.1, Figure 37.1). The marked differences in reported rates among world regions probably reflect differences attributable to genetic predisposition (Baldessarini & Hennen, 2004) and availability of health-care services (Tondo, Albert, & Baldessarini, 2006), among other factors but also, importantly, to case identification and reporting procedures (Diekstra, 1993; Simon & Hales, 2012; World Health Organization, 2013). Even among countries with relatively reliable data, suicide rates vary markedly by world region, being extraordinarily high in Eastern Europe and relatively low in Latin America and Southern Europe (Table 37.1; Figure 37.1). In the United States, there were 38,400 identified suicides in 2010 for an annual rate of 12.4 per 100,000 population (Centers for Disease Control and Prevention, 2012), consistently higher in men than women, especially over age 65, with marked differences among ethnic groups (Native Americans > Caucasians > African-Americans ≥ Latinos) and far higher in Alaska, the Southwest, and the Intermountain West than on the East or West Coasts. Reported rates are lower in states with higher population and clinician densities, higher average socioeconomic status,

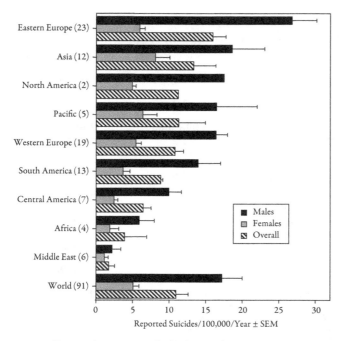

Figure 37.1 Reported international suicide rates (per 100,000 persons/year) ± SEM among males and females, and overall, in nine world regions (with numbers of reporting countries in parentheses), ranked in descending order by overall rates across 9 world regions involving 91 countries (World Health Organization, 2013).

and greater average availability of health insurance (Centers for Diseases Control and Prevention, 2013; Simon & Hales, 2012; Tondo et al., 2006).

Internationally, suicide rates have shifted by relatively small amounts up or down, more less at random, over the past half-century, with increases reported in about half of reporting nations and moderate decreases found in another half, including in northern Europe and North America (Baldessarini et al., 2007; World Health Organization, 2013). Reported decreases have been proposed to reflect improved diagnosis and treatment of mood disorders in recent years (American Psychiatric Association, 2003; Baldessarini et al., 2006, 2007; Nordstrom et al., 1995; Oquendo, Chaudhury, & Mann, 2005; Simon & Hales, 2012; Tondo et al., 2006). Paradoxically, increases in suicide rates in some regions may reflect improvements in case-finding and reporting.

ASSOCIATIONS OF SUICIDE WITH PSYCHIATRIC DISORDERS

Some studies indicate that perhaps 90% of suicides occur by persons with at least one clinically diagnosable psychiatric disorder (Goldsmith, Pellmar, Kleinman, & Bunney, 2002; Harris & Barraclough, 1998), nearly half of which (48.5%) are mood disorders (Simon & Hales, 2012). Major mood

disorders have the highest standardized mortality risk as a ratio to the general population, ranking: bipolar disorders ≥ severe major depressive disorder with hospitalization > moderate depression among outpatients (Harris & Barraclough, 1998; Simon & Hales, 2012). Risk factors for suicide, aside from previous suicide attempts (the strongest predictor), include the presence of a major mood disorder with hopelessness, especially if complicated by co-occurring abuse of alcohol or illicit drugs and social isolation (Kessler et al., 2005; Tondo et al., 1999). Risk is especially high among young, impulsive-aggressive men and older, unmarried or socially isolated men (American Psychiatric Association, 2003; Simon & Hales, 2012), although all of these factors may be confounded by the presence of a mental disorder.

According to US federal statistical data for 2010, 42% of persons considered to have committed suicide were currently depressed, 45% had a diagnosable psychiatric disorder, and 33% abused alcohol or drugs, but only 32% were receiving any treatment (Murphy, Xu, & Kochanek, 2012). Women were more than twice as likely as men to have a history of suicide attempt (34% vs. 16%) and 1.6 times more likely to be diagnosed with a psychiatric illness (62% vs. 40%). However, women also were 1.8 times more likely than men to receive treatment for it (50% vs. 27%), which may contribute to their lower rate of suicide than in men.

The unusually high risk of suicide among mood-disorder patients was supported by our review of the medical records of over 2,800 outpatients with major mood disorders evaluated and treated at the Lucio Bini Mood Disorders Research Center in Cagliari, Sardinia (Tondo & Baldessarini, 2007). We also found substantially greater suicide risks among bipolar disorder patients than in those with recurrent, unipolar major depressive disorder. The risk of suicides was similar among 843 types I and II bipolar disorder patients, averaging 150/100,000 per year, or 14 times greater than the average international rate in the general population (at 11/100,000 per year; Table 37.1, Figure 37.1), more than 10 times higher than in the general population of Sardinia, and 3 times greater than among 1,983 outpatients diagnosed with unipolar depression. These rates suggest a risk of dying by suicide among bipolar disorder patients of approximately 10% and among unipolar depressive patients of over 3%, considering potential risk exposure of approximately 60 years. However, among severly ill unipolar depressed patients, standardized mortality risk can be 20 times over general population suicide rates, or similar to risks among bipolar disorder patients (Harris & Barraclough, 1998; Simon & Hales, 2012), and risk is approximately 3 times greater among ever-hospitalized unipolar patients than those treated only as outpatients and with less severe current symptom ratings (Tondo, Lepri, & Baldessarini, 2008). In general, the most frequent condition associated with suicide has been currently depressed mood or agitated-dysphoric states in both bipolar and unipolar mood-disorder patients (Isometsä et al., 1994; Rihmer, Gonda, Balazs, & Faludi, 2008; Tondo & Baldessarini, 2007). We found the rate of suicide attempts to average 1.26% per year among bipolar disorder patients, and 25% of these acts were violent (Baldessarini et al., 2006). In contrast, the risk of attempts was 2.6 times less (0.48% per year) in unipolar than bipolar cases, and only 12.5% of suicidal acts among unipolar patients were considered violent. For comparison, rates of suicide attempts in the general population average 0.2% to 0.6% per year, or approximately 36 times the average international suicide rate (Goldsmith et al., 2002; Kessler et al., 2005). A more than three times lower ratio (A/S) of attempts to suicide indicates higher lethality among mood-disorder patients than in the general population. We found A/S ratios of 8.6 in bipolar disorder patients and 9.6 in unipolar depressive patients, or 3.6 to 4.1-times lower that the ratio of approximately 35 in the general population (Baldessarini et al., 2006; Kessler et al., 2005; Tondo et al., 2003). A particularly notable observation was that more than one-third of all suicidal acts occurred within the first few years from onset of major mood disorders, and before bipolar disorder is recognized (Baldessarini et al., 2006). Given this timing, and as suicidal concerns or acts may be the initial basis for seeking psychiatric treatment, the need for early diagnosis and intervention in patients diagnosed with major mood disorders is underscored.

Not only is the ratio of A/S much lower among mood-disorder patients (greater lethality) than in the general population (Baldessarini et al., 2006; Kessler et al., 2005; Tondo & Baldessarini, 2007), but this ratio is half as great in men as in women (12 vs. 23), consistent with greater lethality of suicide attempts in men (Nordstrom et al., 1995). In addition, risk of later suicide was somewhat lower among men aged above versus below a median of 35 years (7.0% vs. 9.7%) but 2.4 times *greater* in older than younger women (6.0% vs. 2.5%; Nordstrom et al., 1995). Accordingly, the relative risk of suicide among younger men was four times higher than in younger women (9.7% vs. 2.5%), whereas risks in older men and women scarcely differed (7.0% vs. 6.0%). These findings indicate that the lethality of suicidal behavior in women over age 35 approached that of men of similar age and that risks of suicidal behaviors ranked: men ≥ older women > younger women.

In bipolar disorder patients, suicide risk is high despite the growing variety of treatments with putative mood-stabilizing effects. This disparity almost certainly reflects the great difficulty of treating bipolar depressive and mixed manic-depressive states effectively (Baldessarini, Vieta, Calabrese, Tohen, & Bowden, 2010b; Rihmer et al., 2008; Saunders & Hawton, 2013). Indeed, approximately three-quarters of the surprisingly high proportion (about 40%–50%), of weeks ill during follow-up, even from illness onset) of unresolved morbidity in bipolar disorder is depressive or dysphoric (Baldessarini, Salvatore, Khalsa, et al., 2010a; De Dios, Ezquiaga, Garcia, Soler, & Vieta, 2010; Forte et al., 2015; Judd et al., 2002).

PHARMACOLOGICAL TREATMENTS AIMED AT REDUCING SUICIDAL RISKS

The high level of unsolved depressive morbidity in treated bipolar disorder patients, as well as substantial levels of unresolved or recurring depression among treated unipolar depressed patients, strongly encourage high rates of both short- and long-term use of psychotropic medicines and other interventions for their treatment. Treatment interventions are further encouraged by the very plausible hypothesis that reduced symptomatic severity or time in depression should reduce suicidal risk. However, the research supporting the efficacy and safety of all available psychiatric treatments—medicinal and psychosocial—as a means of reducing risk of suicide is meager, inconsistent, and largely inconclusive, often resting on rare, relatively small, often inadequately controlled trials that do not consistently involve patients diagnosed with a major mood disorder. Nevertheless, we next consider available evidence pertaining to particular psychiatric treatments and their association with suicidal risks.

PHARMACOLOGICAL TREATMENTS AND SUICIDAL RISKS

Effects of treatments on suicidal risk currently are of intense clinical and research interest. Evidence that modern psychiatric treatments reduce long-term suicide risk is very limited for most treatments, including methods as diverse as psychotherapy, rapid hospitalization, and even ECT, which can be lifesaving, in the short term and in acute emergencies (American Psychiatric Association, 2003; Goldsmith et al., 2002; Simon & Hales, 2012; Weinger 2000). Even though many patients at risk for suicide receive various treatments, the magnitude of effects of specific interventions on suicide risk remains uncertain. Moreover, fewer than one-third of persons committing suicide have received *any* clinical care at the time of their deaths, suggesting that identification of suicidal persons and their enrollment or retention in treatment programs has had limited success (Centers for Disease Control and Prevention, 2013; Ernst, Bird, Goldberg, & Ghaemi, 2010). Evidence pertaining to potential antisuicidal effects of treatment with particular classes of psychotropic drugs, let alone specific agents, has been strikingly limited, as well as often inconsistent and inconclusive.

Antidepressants

Relatively high levels of unresolved depressive and agitated-dysphoric morbidity in patients with both bipolar disorder and unipolar depression make short- and long-term treatment with antidepressants an attractive option (Baldessarini, 2013). However, such treatment is not explicitly approved by regulatory bodies for use with bipolar depression, and evidence of long-term prophylactic effects of antidepressant treatment is lacking in bipolar disorder and is only tentative in unipolar major depression (Baldessarini, 2013; Ghaemi, Hsu, Soldani, & Goodwin, 2003; Khan, Warner, & Brown, 2000; Möller, 2006; Søndergård, Kvist, Lopez, Andersen, & Kessing, 2006; Tondo et al., 2003). Studies of antidepressant treatment have yielded inconsistent evidence concerning suicides or attempts. They have employed various methods, including randomized, placebo-controlled trials, clinical cohort studies, and epidemiological or ecological studies of associations between general usage of antidepressants and regional or national suicide rates (Baldessarini et al., 2007; Barbui, Esposito, & Cipriani, 2009; Hammad, Laughren, & Racoosin, 2006; Zisook et al., 2009). A specific limitation in most such research is that suicidal outcomes, even defined by objective behaviors, usually are not an explicit outcome measure.

Lack of anticipated, robust associations of effective treatment for depression with reduced suicidal risk suggests that additional psychopathological and behavioral conditions are required for suicidal behaviors to occur and these may be potential therapeutic targets. Such conditions are likely to include agitation, dysphoria, restlessness, irritability, anger, and insomnia, as well as a degree of behavioral disinhibition, often associated with substance abuse—all leading to aggressive, commonly impulsive suicidal acts (Akiskal, Benazzi, Perugi, & Rihmer, 2005; Koukopoulos & Koukopoulos, 1999; Maj, Pirozzi, Magliano, Fiorillo, & Bartoli, 2006; Pacchiarotti et al., 2013; Simon & Hales, 2012; Tondo et al., 1999). Such features are particularly prevalent among types I and II bipolar disorder patients, and sometimes are worsened by antidepressant treatment in both bipolar and unipolar mood-disorder patients (Pacchiarotti et al., 2013). In addition, effects of antidepressants on suicidal risks may

be significantly age-dependent, with selective benefits in older adults (Hammad et al., 2006; Figure 37.2).

Evidence that antidepressant treatment may be associated with reductions in risk of suicides or attempts is mixed. It includes data from correlative or "ecological," pharmacoepidemiological studies that compare suicide rates by regions or years with concurrent rates of prescriptions for antidepressant drugs (not necessarily in the same people; Baldessarini et al., 2007). In some Nordic countries and the United States, modern, less-toxic antidepressants emerged in the 1990s to dominate clinical practice, and their massive market penetration was associated with moderate decreases in some but not other regional suicide rates that varied among sex and age groups as well as regions (Reseland, Bray, & Gunnell, 2006; Søndergård et al., 2006; Tondo et al., 2003). However, in the United States and Sweden, at least, similar trends toward declining suicide rates were in evidence at least a decade before the introduction of fluoxetine as the first clinically successful modern antidepressant (Baldessarini et al., 2007; Tondo et al., 2003).

Other sources of information concerning antidepressants include large cohorts of depressed patients from general practice or health-maintenance organization data sources, relatively large, case-control comparisons of subgroups varying in exposure to antidepressants, and clinical

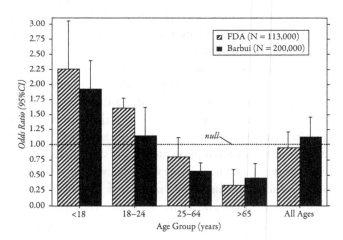

Figure 37.2 Meta-analytic compilations of observed rates of suicidal ideation or behaviors as odds ratios (OR), with their 95% confidence intervals (CI); (ORs <1.0 [null] indicate reduced suicidal risk) for patients in various age-groups treated with an antidepressant. Data are derived from post hoc analyses conducted by the US FDA of data from 396 short-term, placebo-controlled trials of antidepressants involving 113,000 subjects (striped bars; Laughren, 2006), as well as from a compilation of eight large, long-term, clinical cohort and case-control studies involving 200,000 subjects treated with a serotonin-reuptake inhibitor (shaded bars) (Barbui, et al., 2009). Reprinted with permission from *Canadian Medical Association Journal*).

cohort studies. Many of these studies were not designed to test for suicidal behavior as an explicit outcome measure and considered findings on a post hoc basis to test for *greater* hypothesized suicidal risks with modern antidepressants compared to older agents or other treatments; they have yielded inconsistent and inconclusive findings (Möller, 2006; Tondo et al., 2003). Moreover, interpretation of findings from such studies is severely compromised by their risk of confounding by morbidity or by indication. That is, medical treatments, in general, are more likely to be sought, given to, and taken by more severely ill patients at higher risk of suicide. Medicines with relatively low risks of toxic effects or lethality on acute overdosing (such as the modern antidepressants) are more likely to be selected clinically than more toxic agents (such as older tricyclic antidepressants) to treat patients considered to be at increased risk for suicide. Nonrandomized, clinically selected treatment in many such studies can severely distort observed associations between greater suicidal risk and use of particular treatments.

Randomized controlled trials (RCTs) should, theoretically, be the best source of data on effects of antidepressant treatment on suicidal risks, and hundreds of such trials have supported the licensing and clinical applications of antidepressants for depressive and anxiety disorder patients since the 1950s (Baldessarini, 2013). However, individual trials are unlikely to include enough patients for sufficiently long times as to identify suicidal acts, and, moreover, almost none has defined suicidal behaviors as an explicit, a priori, outcome measure with well-validated methods of ascertainment. Even pooling of data across multiple RCTs, such as by use of meta-analytic methods, has proved difficult to provide substantial numbers of suicidal behaviors and mainly involves unverifiable suicidal ideation. It is notable that, even with efforts to exclude suicidal subjects from controlled trials, rates of suicidal behaviors may be at least as high in controlled trials involving acutely depressed patients as in clinical samples of depressive-disorder patients at widely varying levels of current morbidity. For example, suicide rates pooled across several recent large meta-analyses of modern and older antidepressants or placebo were similar with all treatments and averaged 862/100,000 per year (Acharya et al., 2006; Khan et al., 2000; Khan, Khan, Kolts, & Brown, 2003), or 78 times above the approximate average international general population rate of 11/100,000 per year (Table 37.1) and perhaps 17 times above rates in outpatients diagnosed with a depressive disorder, of about 50/100,000 (Tondo & Baldessarini, 2007)! In addition, to considerable extent, the high observed rates of suicidal behaviors in controlled trials for the treatment of depression reflect exaggeration arising from annualizing observed rates based on relatively brief exposure times (typically 6–12 weeks) in most trials in acute depression, and early in the course of treatment, as well as high variance owing to the paucity of suicidal outcomes in even relatively large trials.

Several meta-analyses have found only minor differences in rates of suicidal behaviors between depressed patients treated with modern antidepressants, other types antidepressants, or a placebo. Some analyses have detected indications of greater risks with antidepressants versus placebo controls. However, such findings have included increased risks in juveniles and young adults but decreased risks in older adults, and most have relied on unreliable, elusive suicidal ideation as a surrogate outcome measure (Hammad et al., 2006; Laughren, 2006; Figure 37.2). These analyses also assume that the trials analyzed remained well randomized through their duration, despite substantial dropout rates, which are assumed (questionably) to be at random, and that temporal exposures in both drug and placebo arms remained well-balanced throughout the duration of the trials. They also assume that surrogate measures of suicidal ideation or even minor self-injurious behaviors are fairly and comparably ascertained in different treatment groups and that they have important predictive value for suicide itself. All of these are questionable assumptions. Moreover, no such study has been based on explicit and validated outcome measures pertinent to suicide. Instead, indications of the imprecise concept "suicidality," like other treatment-associated, emerging "adverse events," almost always have been ascertained passively and incidentally rather than by direct inquiry and adequate assessment.

One of the largest studies based on post hoc meta-analysis reviewed 295 placebo-controlled trials of 11 modern antidepressants in nearly 77,000 depressed or anxious subjects to compare the antidepressant drugs versus placebos for "suicidal risks" as nonlethal adverse events in trials lasting an average of eight weeks, submitted to the US Food and Drug Administration (FDA) for licensing purposes. These included subject risks of only 0.010% for suicides and an average of 0.17% for suicide attempts—both similar to risks in the general population (Laughren, 2006). There was no overall difference in risk of suicidal acts (suicides were rare) between antidepressant treatments (76/39,729 = 0.19%) and placebo controls (46/27,164 = 0.17%), based on pooling by meta-analysis. However, secondary post hoc analyses, based on stratifying by age groups, suggested increased risk of broadly defined "suicidality" (again, mainly ideation) with modern antidepressants versus placebo at ages below 25 years but possible beneficial effects in older adults. An even larger sampling from FDA analyses yielded similar impressions (Figure 37.2). A meta-analytic review of large cohort and case-control studies of antidepressants found closely similar results as the FDA analyses, in that younger patients experienced increased risk of suicides or attempts, whereas older adults had lower risks associated with antidepressant treatment (Barbui et al., 2009). These post hoc meta-analyses show remarkably similar risks versus age that require prospective and controlled assessment (Figure 37.2).

Even though these meta-analyses of data from placebo-controlled trials or clinical cohort studies found no evidence of overall (all ages pooled) alterations of rates of suicides, attempts, or ideation during antidepressant treatment, many placebo-controlled antidepressant trials in depressed adults have found substantial reductions in average ratings of suicidal ideation with antidepressants compared to placebo, usually based on suicide-related items of standard depression symptom rating scales (Acharya et al., 2006; Beasley et al., 1991; Tollefson et al., 1994). However, these findings are subjective and based on post hoc assessments of individual items on standard depression symptom-rating scales, which may be influenced by impressions of overall clinical improvement. Again, studies with antidepressants that explicitly consider suicidal ideation and behaviors as outcome measures remain to be carried out, if ethical and clinically acceptable study designs can be developed.

To recapitulate, it is important to emphasize that even RCTs have limitations that can lead to artifacts and uncertainties. They include potential unreliability of essentially incidental, passive reporting of suicidal thoughts or behaviors in most RCTs, based on currently typical "adverse event reporting" systems under conditions not designed explicitly to detect and assess suicidal events. In addition, the relatively short duration of most trials of treatments for acute depression is unlikely to provide an adequate basis for evaluating potential effects of treatment on rare suicidal behaviors, comparable to the long-term trials available for clozapine, lithium, and anticonvulsants, as discussed later. Moreover, much of what has been reported involves suicidal ideation of highly uncertain clinical significance and very limited quantitative relationship to actual life-threatening behaviors. Also as noted, another potential source of bias is that initial randomization in RCTs can break down during the conduct of trials. Premature, and potentially nonrandom, dropping out, owing usually to lack of perceived benefit or emergence of intolerable but sometimes undocumented adverse effects of treatment, is encountered routinely in controlled trials. More specifically, observed rates of "suicidal events"

rarely are corrected for actual exposure times for individual patient-subjects given specific treatments. Such correction to observed adverse-event rates (events/person-weeks) can be important if *actual* exposures are not closely matched between trial treatment arms, and particularly when rare events such as suicides and attempts are involved (Schalkwijk et al., 2015). For example, earlier dropping out of a trial arm involving ineffective placebo treatment can paradoxically limit observable suicidal risk with placebo, artifactually making active drug treatment seem "riskier" than placebo. The emergence of new suicidal behaviors among adults treated with sustained antidepressant treatment in clinical settings is very uncommon, involving perhaps 5/1,000 patients within a year, excluding patients whose treatment was altered earlier due to emerging suicidal tendencies (Tondo et al., 2008).

Findings suggesting worsening of suicidal risks in some, especially young, antidepressant-treated patients further suggest potential scientifically and clinically important developmental differences in affective and behavioral responses to antidepressants that require further study, especially with respect to risks of actual suicidal behavior. Such reactions, also possible in adults, are especially likely to arise among depressed juveniles previously not recognized as having a bipolar disorder, as well as others with particular behavioral sensitivities to mood-elevating agents that can include increased agitation, irritability, and insomnia. Such responses might contribute to the reported excess of suicidal ideation in young patients treated with modern antidepressants (Hammad et al., 2006) but are important to monitor early in the initiation of antidepressant treatment at any age.

Anxiolytics and sedatives

Suicide rates are surprisingly high among persons diagnosed with anxiety disorders (Diefenbach, Woolley, & Goethe., 2009; Harris & Barraclough, 1998; Khan, Leventhal, Khan, & Brown, 2002), including in controlled trials, and have been as high as 193/100,000 person-years (Khan et al., 2002), possibly reflecting their frequent co-occurrence with mood or substance-use disorders. Such associations might suggest that treatments effective for anxiety disorders may also reduce suicidal risks. However, the limited evidence available does not support the hypothesis that antianxiety agents alter suicidal risk either short or long term in patients with an anxiety disorder or other psychiatric illnesses (Yerevanian & Choi, 2013). A meta-analysis found little evidence of different risks of suicides or attempts among patients diagnosed with anxiety-related disorders (panic, social phobia, generalized anxiety, posttraumatic stress, or obsessive-compulsive disorders), comparing either active agents to placebo or specific medicines (Khan et al., 2002). On the other hand, discontinuation of benzodiazepine treatment, especially rapidly, is a stressor that may increase suicidal risk (Gaertner, Gilot, Heidrich, & Gaertner, 2002). Moreover, behavioral disinhibition associated with benzodiazepine use might increase impulsive and aggressive behaviors, especially in combination with alcohol, and in personality-disordered patients (Gaertner et al., 2002).

Lithium

Association of reduced suicidal risk with long-term lithium treatment in bipolar disorder patients is supported consistently by many (Angst, Angst, Gerber-Werder, & Gamma, 2005; Baldessarini et al., 2006; Baldessarini & Tondo, 2008; Müller-Oerlinghausen, Ahrens, & Felber, 2006) but not all studies (Marangell et al., 2008; Oquendo et al., 2011). Support for this association includes meta-analyses and reviews, as well as several randomized, placebo-controlled efficacy trials not specifically designed to test for effects on suicide risk (Angst et al., 2005; Baldessarini et al., 2006; Cipriani, Pretty, Hawton, & Geddes, 2005; Khan et al., 2011; Lauterbach et al., 2008; Tondo, Hennen, & Baldessarini, 2001). In meta-analyses of data from nearly three dozen trials (10 randomized, with placebo or active-alternative treatments as controls), we considered suicidal behavior in patients treated long term with lithium, usually for bipolar disorder or other recurrent mood disorders, and involving more than 110,000 person-years of risk. The results indicated five- or six-fold lower risks of suicides and attempts during treatment with lithium among patients with recurrent mood disorders or bipolar disorder, respectively (Baldessarini et al., 2006; Baldessarini & Tondo, 2008). We also estimated a number needed to treat (22.6; 95% confidence interval [CI]: 21.0–24.6), which suggests that about 23 patients would need to be treated with lithium to avoid one life-threatening or fatal suicidal act more than by a chance—a relatively large number that in part probably reflects the low incidence of suicidal acts. Notably, in one of the studies analyzed (Tondo et al., 1998), rates of suicidal acts increased by 20-fold within several months after discontinuing lithium maintenance treatment and were twice greater with abrupt or rapid versus gradual (over ≥2 weeks) discontinuation, later returning to levels encountered before lithium treatment had started. In addition, in data meta-analytically pooled from eight studies of patients diagnosed with recurrent unipolar depression (at risk a total of 2,434 patient-years), we found

evidence of a substantial (four-fold) reduction of risk of suicide and attempts with lithium versus alternatives that included anticonvulsants (Guzzetta, Tondo, Centorrino, & Baldessarini, 2007).

Since our initial meta-analysis (Tondo et al., 2001), additional studies have provided more data. One is a rare RCT (Lauterbach et al., 2008), which found a substantial but statistically nonsignificant difference in rates of suicidal acts between patients treated for 12 months with lithium compared to others randomized to placebo (adjusted hazard ratio: 0.52; 95% CI: 0.18–1.43, favoring lithium). However, the three suicides were associated with placebo treatment. In another randomized comparison of lithium versus placebo added to citalopram treatment for four weeks, suicidal behavior and ideation were rated explicitly with the Montgomery-Åsberg Depression Rating Scale, Sheehan-Suicidality Tracking Scale, Beck Suicide Scale, and Beck Hopelessness Scale. No suicides or attempts occurred in either group in this brief trial, but all of the suicidal rating scale scores decreased significantly more with the combination of citalopram and lithium than with citalopram plus placebo (Khan et al., 2011). In addition, a study based on retrospective data from 161 bipolar disorder patients found that nonlethal suicide-related events were fewer during long-term lithium treatment than with other mood-stabilizers given alone or with first- or second-generation antipsychotic drugs (Koek, Yerevanian, & Mintz, 2012). Based on all of these studies, a recent review (Lewitzka, Bauer, Felber, & Müller-Oerlinghausen, 2013) and a report by the European Psychiatric Association (Wasserman et al., 2012) recommended the use of long-term lithium treatment to reduce risk of suicidal behavior in bipolar disorder patients.

A curious and provocative finding is that rates of suicide and other violent behaviors have sometimes been lower in populations from different world regions with drinking water containing relatively high, trace concentrations of lithium salts (Kapusta et al., 2011; Ohgami, Terao, Shiotsuki, Ishii, & Iwata, 2009; Vita, De Peri, & Sacchetti, 2014), whereas other studies reported a lack of association (Kabacs, Memon, Obinwa, Stochl, & Perez, 2011) or an association only in specific subgroups or with particular types of analysis (Blüml, Regier, Hlavin, et al., 2013; Sugawa, Yasui-Furukori, Ishii, et al., 2013). The significance of these improbable findings is far from clear, especially as the lithium exposures were very low (less than 0.064 mEq/day at a daily drinking-water intake of about 2 L) by comparison to up to 600 times higher clinical doses of 8 to 40 mEq of lithium ion (in 300–1,500 mg/day of lithium carbonate). Nevertheless, it is conceivable that lifelong exposure to even low concentrations of lithium may have unrecognized biological effects.

Despite these several findings, a direct role of lithium treatment in decreasing suicide risk is not securely demonstrated. A major limitation is that support for lower suicidal risk during long-term treatment with lithium derives almost entirely from incidental findings in studies designed for other therapeutic purposes but not addressing suicidal behavior as an explicit outcome measure. In contrast, the single, remarkable, pivotal trial largely responsible for establishing antisuicidal effects of clozapine in schizophrenia was designed to test for effects on suicide-related behaviors and events (not suicide itself) after randomizing to clozapine versus olanzapine (Meltzer et al., 2003). An additional potential limitation to studies of lithium—and, indeed, of all studies of therapeutic effects—is that patients who accept, tolerate, and sustain long-term treatment with particular treatments may well be self-selected and not entirely representative of the full spectrum of clinically encountered patients. Moreover, sex, marital status, educational level and employment status, personality traits, lack of obvious losses or other stressors, and being less severely ill for less time, as well as relative improvement of depressive symptoms with treatment and limited adverse effects, all appear to decrease suicidal risk (Simon & Hales, 2012). Such factors can confound interpretation of observed effects of lithium without randomization to treatment versus an alternative condition (placebo is rarely an ethical option). On the other hand, in testing for long-term effects of *any* treatment, only patients who accept and tolerate it can be considered for analysis.

The apparent effectiveness of lithium treatment in preventing suicide is likely to be associated with reduction of risk or severity of recurrences of depression or dysphoric-agitated, mixed states in bipolar disorder and probably also with reduced impulsivity and aggressiveness in various mood disorders, which may be mediated by enhancing the function of the central serotonin system (Bschor & Bauer, 2006; Kovacsics, Fawcett 2001; Gottesman, & Gould, 2009; Manchia, Hajek, O'Donovan, et al., 2013; Müller-Oerlinghausen & Lewitzka, 2010; Saunders & Hawton, 2009). Some experts have suggested that lithium may have specific effects against suicide independent of its of mood-stabilizing actions, based on reductions of suicidal risk even among patients whose primary mood symptoms had not responded well to lithium (Müller-Oerlinghausen & Lewitzka, 2010).

Long-term treatment with lithium (and clozapine) requires closer monitoring of patients than with most other psychotropic drugs. The added level of clinical care itself might facilitate identification of emerging symptoms associated with suicidal behavior, including suicidal ideation and early agitation, dysphoria, or anger, or otherwise provide supportive influences that may add a protective effect. Nevertheless, additional clinical contact and close supervision may not be critical, given the results of the InterSePT trial for schizophrenia patients, in which contact time with clinicians was very similar between treatment options (Meltzer et al., 2003). A detailed history of research on lithium, including its role in suicide prevention is provided in a recent book chapter (Tondo & Baldessarini, 2014).

Anticonvulsants

There is limited research that directly compares suicidal risks during treatment with proved or putative mood-stabilizers other than lithium (Oquendo et al., 2011; Søndergård, Lopez, Andersen, & Kessing, 2008), but at least two studies found nearly three-fold lower average risks of suicidal behavior with lithium than with carbamazepine or valproate among bipolar or schizoaffective disorder patients (Goodwin et al., 2003; Thies-Flechtner, Müller-Oerlinghausen, Seibert, Walther, & Greil, 1996). Nevertheless, anticonvulsants may have some beneficial effects on suicidal behavior (Gibbons, Hur, Brown, & Mann, 2009; Smith, Søndergård, Lopez, Andersen, & Kessing, 2009; Yerevanian, Koek, & Mintz, 2007). In a meta-analysis (Baldessarini & Tondo, 2009), we compared protective effects against suicidal behavior of lithium versus several mood-stabilizing anticonvulsants (mainly valproate and some use of carbamazepine or lamotrigine) in six direct comparisons including more than 30,000 patients who were at risk longer with lithium than with an anticonvulsant (31 vs. 19 months). Half of the trials involved randomized assignment to treatments. The observed rate of suicidal acts averaged 0.3% per year during treatment with lithium versus 0.9% per year with anticonvulsants, to yield a meta-analytically pooled risk ratio of 2.86 (95% CI: 2.29–3.57; $p < 0.0001$), or nearly three-fold superiority favoring lithium over the few anticonvulsants that have been tested in this way.

The FDA (2008) conducted a meta-analysis of placebo-controlled trials involving 11 anticonvulsants used to treat epileptic patients. This analysis found that suicidal ideation and behaviors were *more* prevalent with anticonvulsants than with placebo. The finding led to a warning about possible suicide risk–promoting effects of some antiepileptic drugs. However, this association was not found for psychiatric applications of anticonvulsants (US Food and Drug Administration, 2008; Gibbons et al., 2009), was not confirmed by a recent study from the Task Force of the Commission on Neuropsychobiology of the International League against Epilepsy (Mula, Kanner, Schmitz, & Schachter, 2013), and recently was reviewed critically (Siamouli, Samara, & Fountoulakis, 2014).

A recent study on this topic from the US Veteran Administration system on more than 1,300 veterans diagnosed with bipolar disorder found that incidence rates for attempted suicide ranked: lithium plus divalproex (0.63) < divalproex alone (7.0) ≤ lithium alone (7.7 attempts/10,000 person-months of exposure; Ahearn et al., 2013). It remains unclear whether this study supports the hypothesis that both valproate and lithium exert similar antisuicidal effects or simply is inconclusive.

Antipsychotics

Most studies of associations between antipsychotic treatment and suicidal risk involve patients with schizophrenia or schizoaffective disorder. First-generation neuroleptic drugs are little studied for effects on suicidal behavior, unlike modern, atypical antipsychotic agents (Simon & Hales, 2012). A study based on more than 10,000 psychotic patients found no statistical difference in relatively short-term risk of suicides and attempts during treatment with modern or older antipsychotics versus placebo (Khan, Khan, Leventhal, & Brown, 2001). However, a large study found that mortality, including due to suicide, was more prevalent among psychotic-disorder patients *not* treated with antipsychotic drugs (Tiihonen et al., 2006).

The first US FDA-approved treatment of any kind with an antisuicide indication was clozapine for schizophrenia patients. This regulatory approval in 2003 was based largely on a single, remarkable, randomized trial (InterSePT) that compared clozapine with olanzapine among not necessarily treatment-resistant schizophrenia patients at high suicidal risk (Meltzer et al., 2003), as well as other supportive evidence (Hennen & Baldessarini, 2005). The InterSePT trial found greater prolongation of time to interventions for emerging suicidal risk and reduced rates of suicide attempts but *not* reduction of mortality, compared to treatment with olanzapine, based on very few suicides with either treatment. The beneficial effect of clozapine in schizophrenia patients was later supported by a clinical comparison with risperidone or quetiapine, as well as olanzapine (Haukka, Tiihonen, Härkänen, & Lönnqvist, 2008). It is not known whether clozapine may exert antisuicidal effects in other major psychiatric disorders.

PSYCHOSOCIAL INTERVENTIONS

PSYCHOLOGICAL ASPECTS OF TREATING SUICIDAL PATIENTS

Intense suicidal risk is a leading basis of psychiatric hospitalization, and suicidal ideation is often a reason for seeking consultation with a mental-health professional. Various types of psychosocial interventions have been employed to assist patients at risk for suicide, although it is usual clinical practice to combine psychotherapy with pharmacological interventions. Most studies of psychotherapy and suicidal risk are clinical and not well controlled, so evidence-based support for effective reduction of suicidal risk by such interventions remains very limited. Clinical interventions intended to reduce suicidal risk have included individual (cognitive-behavioral, interpersonal, or psychodynamic), group, and family psychotherapies. The aim of such interventions is to decrease agitation and dysphoric anguish associated with current thoughts of death, to support efforts to cope with them, and to improve problem-solving and dealing with personal and environmental challenges.

It is also important to consider that psychotherapies can have adverse effects in some suicidal patients if interventions are excessively provocative and stressful. When self-destructive preoccupations appear during ongoing psychotherapy, the therapeutic method often is modified to a relatively supportive, directive, counseling, and reassuring form. In addition, it may help to advise or assist suicidal patients in avoiding social isolation and in maintaining daily activities. It also may be beneficial to explain that suicidal ideation represents a symptom of a depressive illness, which can be treated effectively (Acharya et al., 2006; Birtchnell 1996; Hawton et al., 1998; Hendin 1996; Rosenberg 1993). It is also important to understand the meaning of suicidal ideation in the lives of individual patients and in relation to their treatment. However, attempts to encourage suicidal patients to prefer life over death, such as by thinking of their family and friends, risk reinforcing their conviction that living for others contributes to their ineffectual and suicidal feelings. Clinicians should help to rebuild the patient's network of relationships and interests by putting themselves at the center of these connections through direct and honest communication and avoid division of clinical responsibility among cooperating specialists by taking responsibility for combining medical and psychotherapeutic aspects of treatment. Arranging such integrated treatment can be challenging in the current era of common separation of clinicians prescribing psychotropic medicines and those providing psychotherapy. Useful psychotherapeutic strategies can be based on clinical observations indicating that the more a clinician respects a patient's right to take his own life, the more he may be open to discussing suicidal thoughts with someone perceived as accepting, interested, and understanding.

Clinicians need to consider their own reactions toward suicide. These may include (a) anxiety about the outcome of treatment and fear of professional criticism or legal liability; (b) increased interest in the patient's life that was not present previously; (c) efforts to restrain patients with inadequate explanation; (d) anger about suicidal ideation or acts they could not prevent; (e) denying, minimizing, or not dealing directly with suicidal concerns for fear of increasing risk of suicide, and potentially contributing to the patient's guilt for having suicidal thoughts; and (f) diminished connection with the patient for any or all of these reactions. Even if such reactions by clinicians do not become explicit, patients may sense them and give them more importance if they are not expressed and discussed. Resulting responses by patients may include (a) distrust and fear of rejection or abandonment; (b) increased fear of dealing with suicidal preoccupations; (c) further inhibition of free emotional expression; (d) increased ambivalence toward treatment; (e) aggressive or provocative tendencies, including threats, aimed at testing the tolerance of the clinician; (f) anger and even lower self-esteem; and (g) hopelessness. Moreover, clinicians may experience the ambivalence of seeming to have enormous power in handling a life-and-death situation but also being manipulated by threats by patients to kill themselves. In such circumstances, the clinician may sense failure and respond with anger or rejection of the patient, with further intensification of the suicidal thoughts.

According to Shneidman (1996), the most relevant feature of a suicidal person is *psychache* (mental pain), a state of discomfort with agitation that increases lethality. He advised that the aim of psychotherapy should be to decrease lethality through decreased intensity of psychic pain and aimed at improving understanding of suicide with a series of aphorisms (Shneidman, 1984). Notable points included his views that suicide (a) is not a desire of death but rather avoidance of intolerable pain, (b) needs to be evaluated more on the grounds of perturbation and lethality than as a diagnostic category, and (c) is not a rational act but rather a reaction to frustrated psychological needs. His recommendations included that the purpose of psychotherapy with potentially suicidal patients is to deal with their elevated level of perturbation, which should be "mollified sufficiently so as to drop below the lethal threshold of suicidal action."

Psychodynamic treatments explore patients' internal psychology and conflicts (Gabbard, 2005). Psychodynamic treatment of suicidal patients typically includes consideration of (a) possible unconscious meanings of suicide, (b) unconscious motivations contributing to suicidal thoughts as a form of "resistance" to treatment, and (c) transference of ideas or feelings from patient to clinician as well as counter-transference of anger or rescue fantasies from clinician to patient. One traditional psychodynamic hypothesis considers a psychological struggle between an "internal executioner" and his victim, from which suicide is considered to have the potential to help restore internal harmony (Gabbard, 2012). Gabbard also recommends seven steps in the treatment of suicidal patients: (a) establishing a therapeutic alliance, (b) differentiating between the fantasy and the act of suicide, (c) discussing the limits of treatment frankly, (d) investigating precipitating events, (e) exploring fantasies about the interpersonal impact of suicide, (f) establishing the level of suicidal risk present initially, and (g) monitoring transference and countertransference.

Research on psychosocial interventions for suicide

Controlled research trials of psychotherapy or other psychosocial interventions for suicidal patients are rare. Case reports on the topic usually describe only positive outcomes, suggesting reluctance to report on failed efforts, contributing to a lack of balanced, critical assessments. In addition, data on psychotherapies are difficult to collect and are limited by major methodological pitfalls (Arensman et al., 2001). As noted, an important limitation to research on effects of any treatment on suicidal behavior is the rarity of suicidal acts in time-limited studies with moderate numbers of subjects.

A notable review based on 20 RCTs involved 2,460 subjects considered clinically to be acutely suicidal and 10 different treatment conditions (1–6 trials per treatment; Hawton et al., 1998). Based on random-effects meta-analyses, only one form of intervention (adding the antipsychotic agent flupenthixol) was highly (71%) statistically superior to a control treatment ($p = 0.003$), based on a single, small, placebo-controlled trial with 30 subjects. The only psychosocial intervention that appeared to be significantly superior to standard aftercare (by 56%; $p = 0.03$, with 39 subjects) was a dialectical form of behavior therapy for borderline disorder patients with repeated self-injurious behaviors, again in a single trial. Six treatments did not differ significantly from their control conditions, including (a) giving patients a card with an emergency referral versus standard care (one trial; $p = 0.06$); (b) problem-solving versus standard care (four trials; $p = 0.24$); (c) behavior therapy versus insight-oriented psychotherapy in hospital (one trial, $p = 0.62$); (d) antidepressant treatment versus placebo (two trials, $p = 0.68$); (e) admission to a general hospital or not (two trials; $p = 0.72$); and (f) long-term versus brief psychotherapy ($p = 1.0$). Moreover, two forms of treatment were or tended to be *less* effective than their controls: (a) retaining the current clinician versus referral to another clinician (one trial; $p = 0.02$) and (b) intensive outreach versus standard care (six trials; $p = 0.86$). The outcomes did not appear to be related to the length of follow-up, although longer exposure times would probably tend to increase the risk of recurring suicidal status.

A rare, randomized study of acutely suicidal patients recruited in an emergency service compared interpersonal psychodynamic therapy based on four home visits versus a treatment-as-usual control condition, typically involving referral back to a primary-care physician (Guthrie et al., 2003). It found more reduction of suicidal ideation up to six months with the psychotherapy. However, the subjects were only moderately depressed and had no history of self-harm or current alcohol abuse, and the treatment itself might have affected later ascertainment of subjective states.

Cognitive behavioral therapy (CBT) has become a popular method of psychological treatment, based on strong research support and well-defined procedures. With modifications specific for suicidal patients, CBT aimed at improving cognitive and behavioral skills may be helpful to limit suicidal risk in clinical crises (Simon & Hales, 2012) and perhaps longer term. This form of treatment attempts to identify relevant risk factors associated with suicidal crises and to encourage strategies of coping. One controlled study of 120 patients found 43% fewer suicide attempts (24% vs. 42%) within 18 months among patients randomized to CBT versus enhanced usual care (Brown et al., 2005). Linehan's dialectical behavior therapy—a combination of cognitive therapy and Buddhism-like, meditative acceptance-based strategies tested mainly in persons diagnosed with borderline syndrome—may be a particularly effective approach in suicidal patients, perhaps including those with bipolar disorder (Chesin & Stanley, 2013; Linehan, Armstrong, Suarez, Allmon, & Heard, 1991). In addition, Rucci and colleagues (2002) studied risks of suicidal behaviors among 175 bipolar disorder patients receiving mood-stabilizing treatments (mainly lithium) who were randomized to either interpersonal therapy or intensive clinical management; there was a significantly greater reduction of suicidal behavior among those randomized to interpersonal psychotherapy.

As already noted, some interventions have been associated with no reduction or even suggestions of *worse* suicidal outcomes than with comparison treatments assigned at random (Hawton et al., 1998). That such outcomes can occur with psychotherapy is further suggested by a study (Möller, 1992) involving 218 patients with a variety of psychiatric disorders and a recent history of attempted suicide by overdose who were randomized to follow-up treatment options for 12 months after index hospitalization. Treatments included routine clinical care with involvement of suicide specialists (152 cases) or supplementation with brief outpatient psychotherapy ($n = 66$). Risks of suicidal behavior during follow-up were somewhat higher among patients randomized to receive psychotherapy ($12/66 = 18.2\%$) than others ($17/152 = 11.2\%$), but the difference was not significant ($\chi^2 = 1.95$, $p = 0.16$). This finding is congruent with the studies reviewed by Hawton and colleagues (1998) indicating lack of efficacy in reducing suicidal risks with treatments that included intensive outreach, giving patients an emergency referral, problem-solving therapy, admission to a general hospital, behavior therapy in hospital, retaining or changing clinicians, long-term psychotherapy, or antidepressant treatment.

In addition, some recent reviews have been skeptical about the efficacy of psychotherapeutic interventions for preventing suicide, although they found evidence of reduced hopelessness (Chesin & Stanley, 2013; Cuijpers et al., 2013). Despite lack of consistent and compelling evidence of effectiveness of some psychotherapeutic interventions, prudent clinical practice usually includes giving suicidal patients psychological support, addressing their suicidal thinking directly, and contacting other clinicians involved as well as family members (American Psychiatric Association, 2003).

MISCELLANEOUS TREATMENTS

Additional options for clinical management of suicidal patients usually are empirical and lack formal testing but are often based on decades of accumulated practical experience, though largely limited to acute suicidal risk. A good example is the use of ECT, which often appears to be lifesaving in suicidal emergencies but lacks evidence of sustained antisuicidal efficacy (Fink, Kellner, & McCall, 2014). Other methods of external electrical or magnetic stimulation of the brain, vagal nerve stimulation, or deep brain stimulation are being investigated or introduced for the treatment of otherwise treatment-resistant depression but remain to be tested for specific effects on suicidal behavior.

Table 37.2. SUMMARY OF RESULTS FROM PHARMACOLOGICAL AND PSYCHOTHERAPEUTIC INTERVENTIONS

INTERVENTION	TIMING	FINDINGS	LIMITATIONS
Antidepressants	Short- and long-term effects not established	Inconclusive and inconsistent findings in controlled and uncontrolled trials; may increase risk of nonlethal suicidality in juveniles	Frequent lack of exposure times; suicidality usually assessed incidentally
Antipsychotics	May have short-term benefits; clozapine may be effective long term	Clozapine is the only FDA-recognized "antisuicidal" treatment. Other antipsychotics have yielded inconsistent or negative research findings	Clozapine's status based on one controlled trial with no effect on mortality
Anxiolytics and sedatives	Most likely to be beneficial short term	Very limited and inconclusive research	Potential disinhibition with increased suicidal risk
Anticonvulsants	Short- and long-term effects not established	Valproate is most studied. Anticonvulsants may be less effective vs. suicide than lithium	Outcomes have been incidental. Some anticonvulsants may increase suicidal risks in epileptic patients
Lithium	Probably effective long term	Consistent decrease of suicide risk in uncontrolled studies and a few placebo-controlled trials	Incidentally identified outcomes. Risk of self-selection by acceptance and tolerance of long-term treatment
Psychotherapies	Short- and long-term effects not established, but widely assumed empirically	Inconsistent results from research. Many expert favor dialectic and cognitive-behavioral methods, which have been relatively better studied	Acceptance of psychotherapy implies self-selection

Additional interventions include emergency hospitalization, and acute suicidal risk remains a prevalent indication for inpatient psychiatric care that almost surely has practical, short-term value but is less likely to have long-lasting effectiveness against future suicidal risk. Some apparently widely employed techniques of clinical management, including "contracts for safety" as a means of encouraging suicidal patients to avoid self-harm and to seek help when in danger, are of unproved value and might even increase suicidal risk if clinical vigilance is reduced. A summary tabulation of proposed treatments aimed at reducing suicidal risk is provided in Table 37.2.

CONCLUSION

More than most psychiatric disorders, mood disorders are associated with major increases of suicidal behavior in association with depressed mood. Risks are especially high in mixed, dysphoric-agitated states, and perhaps also with anger, aggression, or impulsivity—all of which are particularly prevalent in bipolar disorder patients and probably contribute to their unusually high suicide risk. In such conditions, antidepressants have not been proved to exert beneficial effects and may even increase suicide risk, at least temporarily early in treatment, and especially in young patients who may become more agitated, irritable, and sleepless. It is important when antidepressant treatment is initiated that clinicians monitor for early indications of worsening or emerging agitation, dysphoria, restlessness, and psychotic symptoms, including mixed states in bipolar disorder patients. In contrast, long-term treatment with lithium salts may be a more effective component of comprehensive clinical management aimed at suicide prevention. Altered suicidal risk also may be obtained with some modern antipsychotic and anticonvulsant drugs commonly used to treat psychiatric patients whose illnesses are likely to present increased suicidal risks. However, clozapine remains the only treatment with regulatory recognition for reducing suicidal behaviors, and only in patients diagnosed with schizophrenia. Long-term use of lithium appears to reduce risk of suicide and attempts, at least in bipolar disorder patients, although its short-term value is doubtful.

It is important to identify alternative treatments that may reduce suicidal risk and can reasonably be used as comparison treatments in controlled trials without recourse to placebo controls, which are clinically and ethically problematic. Potentially feasible experimental therapeutic studies can include randomized assignment to specific treatment conditions, ideally for prolonged periods, and should involve reliable and validated outcome measures specific to suicidal behavior. So far, however, trials that compare, for example, lithium to an anticonvulsant or antipsychotic agent, or even a placebo, are rare and almost never continued for more than several months or involve explicit suicide-related outcome measures. Moreover, head-to-head comparisons of different drug products are unlikely to be favored by manufacturers of one of them. In addition to possible specific antisuicidal actions of some treatments, a more general component of suicide reduction is suggested by correlations of regional suicide rates and various measures that may reflect better access to clinical care, such as greater population and clinician density, higher economic status, and availability of medical insurance.

Finally, the preceding overview leads to the conclusion that research support for specific therapeutic interventions aimed at reducing suicidal risk remains very limited. Treatments with evidence of value, including use of clozapine in schizophrenia or lithium for major mood disorders, are not proven to be effective short term or in clinical emergencies, as ECT and rapid hospitalization may be. Nevertheless, the need for effective clinical management of suicidal patients makes it essential to rely on clinical experience, with skillful and sensitive application of direct and supportive personal interventions in as protective an environment as possible.

ACKNOWLEDGMENTS

The writing of this chapter was supported in part by a research award from the Aretæus Association of Rome and the Lucio Bini Private Donors Research Fund (to Leonardo Tondo), and by a grant from the Bruce J. Anderson Foundation and the McLean Private Donors Research Fund (to Ross J. Baldessarini).

Disclosure statement: No author or immediate family member has relationships with corporate or other commercial entities that might represent potential conflicts of interest with the material reported.

REFERENCES

Acharya, N., Rosen, A. S., Polzer, J. P., D'Souza, D. N., Perahia, D. G., Cavazzoni, P. A., & Baldessarini, R. J. (2006). Duloxetine: Meta-analyses of suicidal behaviors and ideation in clinical trials for major depressive disorder. *Journal of Clinical Psychopharmacology, 26*(6), 587–594.

Ahearn, E. P., Chen, P., Hertzberg, M., Cornette, M., Suvalsky, L., Cooley-Olson, D.,…Krahn, D. (2013). Suicide attempts in veterans with bipolar disorder during treatment with lithium, divalproex, and atypical antipsychotics. *Journal of Affective Disorders, 145*(1), 77–82.

Akiskal, H. S., Benazzi, F., Perugi, G., & Rihmer, Z. (2005). Agitated "unipolar" depression re-conceptualized as a depressive mixed state: Implications for the antidepressant-suicide controversy. *Journal of Affective Disorders, 85*(3), 245–258.

American Psychiatric Association. (2003). Practice guideline for the assessment and treatment of patients with suicidal behaviors. *The American Journal of Psychiatry, 160*(11), 1–60.

Angst, J., Angst, F., Gerber-Werder, R., & Gamma, A. (2005). Suicide in 406 mood-disorder patients with and without long-term medication: 40 to 44 years' follow-up. *Archives of Suicide Research, 9,* 279–300.

Arensman, E., Townsend, E., Hawton, K., Bremner, S., Feldman, E., Goldney, R.,…Träskman-Bendz, L. (2001). Psychosocial and pharmacological treatment of patients following deliberate self-harm: The methodological issues involved in evaluating effectiveness. *Suicide and Life-Threatening Behavior, 31*(2), 169–180.

Baldessarini, R. J. (2013). *Chemotherapy in psychiatry* (3rd ed.). New York: Springer.

Baldessarini, R. J., & Hennen, J. (2004). Genetics of suicide: An overview. *Harvard Review of Psychiatry, 12*(1), 1–13.

Baldessarini, R. J., & Jamison, K. R. (1999). Effects of medical interventions on suicidal behavior: Summary and conclusions. *Journal of Clinical Psychiatry, 60*(2), 117–122.

Baldessarini, R. J., Salvatore, P., Khalsa, H. M., Gebre-Medhin, P., Imaz, H., González-Pinto, A., Pérez, J., Cruz, N., Maggini, C., & Tohen, M. (2010a). Morbidity in 303 first-episode bipolar I disorder patients. *Bipolar Disorders, 12*(3), 264–270.

Baldessarini, R. J., & Tondo, L. (2008). Lithium and suicidal risk. *Bipolar Disorders, 10*(1), 114–115.

Baldessarini, R. J., & Tondo, L. (2009). Suicidal risks during treatment of bipolar disorder patients with lithium versus anticonvulsants. *Pharmacopsychiatry, 42*(2), 72–75.

Baldessarini, R. J., Tondo, L., Davis, P., Pompili, M., Goodwin, F. K., & Hennen, J. (2006). Decreased suicidal risk during long-term lithium treatment: Meta-analysis. *Bipolar Disorders, 8*(5), 625–639.

Baldessarini, R. J., Tondo, L., Strombom, I., Dominguez, S., Fawcett, J., Oquendo, M., Tohen, M. (2007). Analysis of ecological studies of relationships between antidepressant utilization and suicidal risk. *Harvard Review of Psychiatry, 15*(4), 133–145.

Baldessarini, R. J., Vieta, E., Calabrese, J. R., Tohen, M., & Bowden, C. L. (2010b). Bipolar depression: Overview and commentary. *Harvard Review of Psychiatry, 18*(3), 143–157.

Barbui, C., Esposito, E., & Cipriani, A. (2009). Selective serotonin reuptake inhibitors and risk of suicide: Systematic review of observational studies. *CMAJ, 180*(3), 291–297.

Beasley, C. M. Jr., Dornseif, B. E., Bosomworth, J. C., Sayler, M. E., Rampey, A. H. Jr., Heiligenstein, J. H., Masica, C. N. (1991). Fluoxetine and suicide: Meta-analysis of controlled trials of treatment for depression. *BMJ, 303*(6804), 685–692.

Birtchnell, J. (1996). Psychotherapeutic considerations in the management of the suicidal patient. In J. T. Maltsberger & M. J. Goldblatt (Eds.), *Essential papers on suicide* (pp. 463–479). New York: New York University Press.

Blüml, V., Regier, M. D., Hlavin, G., Rockett, I. R., König, F., Vyssoki, B.,…Kapusta, N. D. (2013). Lithium in the public water supply and suicide mortality in Texas. *Journal of Psychiatric Research, 47*(3), 407–411.

Brown, G. K., Ten Have, T., Henriques, G. R., Xie, S. X., Hollander, J. E., & Beck, A. T. (2005). Cognitive therapy for the prevention of suicide attempts: A randomized controlled trial. *JAMA, 294*(5), 563–570.

Bschor, T., & Bauer, M. (2006). Efficacy and mechanisms of action of lithium augmentation in refractory major depression. *Current Pharmaceutical Design, 12*(23), 2985–2992.

Centers for Disease Control and Prevention. (2012). Injury Prevention & Control: Data & Statistics (WISQARS™). Retrieved from http://www.cdc.gov/injury/wisqars/index.html

Chesin, M., & Stanley, B. (2013). Risk assessment and psychosocial interventions for suicidal patients. *Bipolar Disorders, 15*(5), 584–593.

Cipriani, A., Pretty, H., Hawton, K., & Geddes, J. R. (2005). Lithium in the prevention of suicidal behavior and all-cause mortality in patients with mood disorders: Systematic review of randomized trials. *The American Journal of Psychiatry, 162*(10), 1805–1819.

Cuijpers, P., De Beurs, D. P., van Spijker, B. A., Berking, M., Andersson, G., & Kerkhof, A. J. (2013). Effects of psychotherapy for adult depression on suicidality and hopelessness: Systematic review and meta-analysis. *Journal of Affective Disorders, 144*(3), 183–190.

De Dios, C., Ezquiaga, E., Garcia, A., Soler, B., & Vieta, E. (2010). Time spent with symptoms in a cohort of bipolar disorder outpatients in Spain: Prospective, 18-month follow-up study. *Journal of Affective Disorders, 125*(1–3), 74–81.

Diefenbach, G. J., Woolley, S. B., & Goethe, J. W. (2009). The association between self-reported anxiety symptoms and suicidality. *Journal of Nervous and Mental Disease, 197*(2), 92–97.

Diekstra, R. F. W. (1993). Epidemiology of suicide and parasuicide. *Acta Psychiatrica Scandinavica, 371*(Suppl.), 9–20.

Ernst, C. L., Bird, S. A., Goldberg, J. F., & Ghaemi, S. N. (2010). Prescription of psychotropic medications for patients discharged from a psychiatric emergency service. *Journal of Clinical Psychiatry, 67*(5), 720–726.

Fawcett, J. (2001). Treating impulsivity and anxiety in the suicidal patient. *Annals of the New York Academy of Sciences, 932*, 94–102.

Fink, M., Kellner, C. H., & McCall, W. V. (2014). Role of ECT in suicide prevention. *The Journal of ECT, 30*(1), 5–9.

Forte, A., Baldessarini, R. J., Tondo, L., Vázquez, G. H., Pompili, M., & Girardi, P. (2015). Long-term morbidity in bipolar I, and bipolar II, and major depressive disorders. *Journal of Affective Disorders*, in press.

Gabbard, G. O. (2005). *Psychodynamic psychotherapy in clinical practice* (4th ed.). Washington, DC: American Psychiatric Press.

Gabbard, G. O. (2012). Psychodynamic treatment. In R. I. Simon & R. E. Hales (Eds.), *Textbook of suicide assessment and management* (2nd ed., pp. 221–234). Washington, DC: American Psychiatric Press.

Gaertner, I., Gilot, C., Heidrich, P., & Gaertner, H. J. (2002). Case control study on psychopharmacotherapy before suicide committed by 61 psychiatric inpatients. *Pharmacopsychiatry, 35*(2), 37–43.

Ghaemi, S. N., Hsu, D. J., Soldani, F., & Goodwin, F. K. (2003). Antidepressants in bipolar disorder: The case for caution. *Bipolar Disorders, 5*(6), 421–433.

Gibbons, R. D., Hur, K., Brown, C. H., & Mann, J. J. (2009). Relationship between antiepileptic drugs and suicide attempts in patients with bipolar disorder. *Archives of General Psychiatry, 66*(12), 1354–1360.

Goldsmith, S. K., Pellmar, T. C., Kleinman, A. M., & Bunney, W. E. Jr. (Eds.). (2002). *Reducing suicide*. Washington, DC: Institute of Medicine of the US National Academies of Science.

Goodwin, F. K., Fireman, B., Simon, G. E., Hunkeler, E. M., Lee, J., & Revicki, D. (2003). Suicide risk in bipolar disorder during treatment with lithium and divalproex. *JAMA, 290*(11), 1467–1473.

Guthrie, E., Kapur, N. E., Mackway-Jones, K., Chew-Graham, C., Moorey, J., Mendel, E., … Boddy, G. (2003). Predictors of outcome following brief psychodynamic-interpersonal therapy for deliberate self-poisoning. *Australian & New Zealand Journal of Psychiatry, 37*(5), 532–536.

Guzzetta, F., Tondo, L., Centorrino, F., & Baldessarini, R. J. (2007). Lithium treatment reduces suicidal risk in recurrent major depressive disorder. *Journal of Clinical Psychiatry, 68*(3), 380–383.

Harris, E. C., & Barraclough, B. (1998). Excess mortality of mental disorder. *British Journal of Psychiatry, 173*, 11–53.

Hammad, T. A., Laughren, T. P., & Racoosin, J. A. (2006). Suicide rates in short-term randomized controlled trials of newer antidepressants. *Journal of Clinical Psychopharmacology, 26*(2), 203–207.

Haukka, J., Tiihonen, J., Härkänen, T., & Lönnqvist, J. (2008). Association between medication and risk of suicide, attempted suicide and death in nationwide cohort of suicidal patients with schizophrenia. *Pharmacoepidemiology and Drug Safety, 17*(7), 686–696.

Hawton, K., Arensman, E., Townsend, E., Bremner, S., Feldman, E., Goldney, R., … Träskman-Bendz, L. (1998). Deliberate self harm: Systematic review of efficacy of psychosocial and pharmacological treatments in preventing repetition. *BMJ, 317*(7156), 441–447.

Hendin, H. (1996). Psychotherapy and suicide. In J. T. Maltsberger & M. J. Goldblatt (Eds.), *Essential papers on suicide* (pp. 427–441). New York: New York University Press.

Hennen, J., & Baldessarini, R. J. (2005). Suicidal risk during treatment with clozapine: Meta-analysis. *Schizophrenia Research, 73*(2–3), 139–145.

Isometsä, E. T., Henriksson, M. M., Aro, H. M., Heikkinen, M. E., Kuoppasalmi, K. I., & Lönnqvist, J. K. (1994). Suicide in major depression. *The American Journal of Psychiatry, 151*(4), 530–536.

Judd, L. L., Akiskal, H. S., Schettler, P. J., Endicott, J., Maser, J., Solomon, D. A., … Keller, M. B. (2002). Long-term natural history of the weekly symptomatic status of bipolar I disorder. *Archives of General Psychiatry, 59*(6), 530–537.

Kabacs, N., Memon, A., Obinwa, T., Stochl, J., & Perez, J. (2011). Lithium in drinking water and suicide rates across the East of England. *The British Journal of Psychiatry, 198*(5), 406–407.

Kapusta, N. D., Mossaheb, N., Etzersdorfer, E., Hlavin, G., Thau, K., Willeit, M., … Leithner-Dziubas, K. (2011). Lithium in drinking water and suicide mortality. *The British Journal of Psychiatry, 198*(5), 346–350.

Kessler, R. C., Berglund, P., Borges, G., Nock, M., & Wang, P. S. (2005). Trends in suicide ideation, plans, gestures, and attempts in the United States, 1990–1992 to 2001–2003. *JAMA, 293*(20), 2487–2495.

Khan, A., Khan, S. R., Hobus, J., Faucett, J., Mehra, V., Giller, E. L., & Rudolph, R. L. (2011). Differential pattern of response in mood symptoms and suicide risk measures in severely ill depressed patients assigned to citalopram with placebo or citalopram combined with lithium: Role of lithium levels. *Journal of Psychiatric Research, 45*(11), 1489–1496.

Khan, A., Khan, S., Kolts, R., & Brown, W. A. (2003). Suicide rates in clinical trials with SRIs, other antidepressants, and placebo: Analysis of FDA reports. *The American Journal of Psychiatry, 160*(4), 790–792.

Khan, A., Khan, S. R., Leventhal, R. M., & Brown, W. A. (2001). Symptom reduction and suicide risk among patients treated with placebo in antipsychotic clinical trials: An analysis of the Food and Drug Administration database. *The American Journal of Psychiatry, 158*(9), 1449–1454.

Khan, A., Leventhal, R. M., Khan, S., & Brown, W. A. (2002). Suicide risk in patients with anxiety disorders: Meta-analysis of the FDA database. *Journal of Affective Disorders, 68*(2–3), 183–190.

Khan, A., Warner, H. A., & Brown, W. A. (2000). Symptom reduction and suicide risk in patients treated with placebo in antidepressant clinical trials: Analysis of the FDA database. *Archives of General Psychiatry, 57*(4), 311–317.

Koek, R. J., Yerevanian, B. I., & Mintz, J. (2012). Subtypes of antipsychotics and suicidal behavior in bipolar disorder. *Journal of Affective Disorders, 143*(1–3), 27–33.

Koukopoulos, A., & Koukopoulos, A. (1999). Agitated depression as a mixed state and the problem of melancholia. *Psychiatric Clinics of North America, 22*(3), 547–564.

Kovacsics, C. E., Gottesman, I. I., & Gould, T. D. (2009). Lithium's antisuicidal efficacy: Elucidation of neurobiological targets using endophenotype strategies. *Annual Review of Pharmacology and Toxicology, 49*, 175–198.

Laughren, T. P. (2006). Meeting of the Psychopharmacology Drug Advisory Committee (PDAC) concerning suicidal risk in trials of antidepressant drugs in juvenile and adult patients. Retrieved from http://www.fda.gov/ohrms/dockets/ac/06/briefing//2006-4272b1-01-fda.pdf

Lauterbach, E., Felber, W., Müller-Oerlinghausen, B., Ahrens, R., Brinisch, T., Meyer, T., Hohagen, F. (2008). Adjunctive lithium treatment in the prevention of suicidal behavior in depressive disorders: Randomized, placebo-controlled, 1-year trial. *Acta Psychiatrica Scandinavica, 118*(6), 469–479.

Lewitzka, U., Bauer, M., Felber, W., & Müller-Oerlinghausen, B. (2013). Antisuicidal effect of lithium: Current state of research and its clinical implications for the long-term treatment of affective disorders. *Nervenärzt, 84*(3), 294–306.

Linehan, M. M., Armstrong, H. E., Suarez, A., Allmon, D., & Heard, H. L. (1991). Cognitive-behavioral treatment of chronically parasuicidal borderline patients. *Archives of General Psychiatry, 48*(12), 1060–1064.

Maj, M., Pirozzi, R., Magliano, L., Fiorillo, A., & Bartoli, L (2006). Agitated "unipolar" major depression: Prevalence, phenomenology, and outcome. *Journal of Clinical Psychiatry, 67*(5), 712–719.

Manchia, M., Hajek, T., O'Donovan, C., Deiana, V., Chillotti, C., Ruzickova, M., Del Zompo, M., & Alda, M. (2013). Geneti& c risk of suicidal behavior in bipolar spectrum disorder: analysis of 737 pedigrees. *Bipolar Disorders, 15*(5), 496–506.

Marangell, L. B., Dennehy, E. B., Wisniewski, S. R., Bauer, M. S., Miyahara, S., Allen, M. H., & Thase, M. E. (2008). Case-control analyses of the impact of pharmacotherapy on prospectively observed suicide attempts and completed suicides in bipolar disorder. *Journal of Clinical Psychiatry, 69*(6), 916–922.

Meltzer, H. Y., Alphs, L., Green, A. I., Altamura, A. C., Anand, R., Bertoldi, A., & Potkin, S. (2003). Clozapine treatment for suicidality in schizophrenia: International Suicide Prevention Trial (InterSePT). *Archives of General Psychiatry, 60*(1), 82–91.

Möller, H. J. (1992). Attempted suicide: Efficacy of different aftercare strategies. *International Clinical Psychopharmacology, 6*(6), 58–69.

Möller, H. J. (2006). Is there evidence for negative effects of antidepressants on suicidality in depressive patients? Systematic review. *European Archives of Psychiatry and Clinical Neuroscience, 256*(8), 476–496.

Mula, M., Kanner, A. M., Schmitz, B., & Schachter, S. (2013). Antiepileptic drugs and suicidality: An expert consensus statement from the Task Force on Therapeutic Strategies of the ILAE Commission on Neuropsychobiology. *Epilepsia, 54*(1), 199–203.

Müller-Oerlinghausen, B., Ahrens, B., & Felber, W. (2006). Suicide-preventive and mortality-reducing effect of lithium. In M. Bauer, P. Grof, & B. Müller-Oerlinghausen (Eds.), *Lithium in neuropsychiatry* (pp. 79–192). London: Informa Healthcare.

Müller-Oerlinghausen, B., & Lewitzka, U. (2010). Lithium reduces pathological aggression and suicidality: Mini-review. *Neuropsychobiology, 62*(1), 43–49.

Murphy, S. L., Xu, J., & Kochanek, K. D. (2012). Deaths: Preliminary data for 2010. *National Vital Statistics Reports, 60*(4), 1–51. Retrieved from http://www.cdc.gov/nchs/data/nvsr/nvsr60/nvsr60_04.pdf

Nordstrom, P., Samuelsson, M., & Åsberg, M. (1995). Survival analysis of suicide risk after attempted suicide. *Acta Psychiatrica Scandinavica, 91*(5), 336–340.

Ohgami, H., Terao, T., Shiotsuki, I., Ishii, N., & Iwata, N. (2009). Lithium levels in drinking water and risk of suicide. *The British Journal of Psychiatry, 194*(5), 464–465.

Oquendo, M. A., Chaudhury, S. R., & Mann, J. J. (2005). Pharmacotherapy of suicidal behavior in bipolar disorder. *Archives of Suicide Research, 9*(3), 237–250.

Oquendo, M. A., Galfalvy, H. C., Currier, D., Grunebaum, M. F., Sher, L., Sullivan, G. M., Mann, J. J. (2011). Treatment of suicide attempters with bipolar disorder: Randomized clinical trial comparing lithium and valproate in the prevention of suicidal behavior. *The American Journal of Psychiatry, 168*(10), 1050–1056.

Pacchiarotti, I., Bond, D. J., Baldessarini, R. J., Nolen, W. A., Grunze, H., Licht, R. W., ... Vieta, E. (2013) The International Society for Bipolar Disorders (ISBD) Task-Force report on antidepressant use

in bipolar disorders. *The American Journal of Psychiatry, 170*(11), 1249–1262.

Reseland, S., Bray, I., & Gunnell, D. (2006). Relationship between antidepressant sales and secular trends in suicide rates in the Nordic countries. *The British Journal of Psychiatry, 188*, 354–358.

Rihmer, A., Gonda, X., Balazs, J., & Faludi, G. (2008) Importance of depressive mixed states in suicidal behaviour. *Neuropsychopharmacol Hung, 10*(1), 45–49.

Rosenberg, N. K. (1993). Psychotherapy of the suicidal patient. *Acta Psychiatrica Scandinavica, 371*(Suppl.), 54–56.

Rucci, P., Frank, E., Kostelnik, B., Fagiolini, A., Mallinger, A. G., Swartz, H. A., ... Kupfer, D. J. (2002). Suicide attempts in patients with bipolar I disorder during acute and maintenance phases of intensive treatment with pharmacotherapy and adjunctive psychotherapy. *The American Journal of Psychiatry, 159*(7), 1160–1164.

Saunders, K. E., & Hawton, K. (2009). Role of psychopharmacology in suicide prevention. *Epidemiol Psychiatr Soc, 18*(3), 172–178.

Saunders, K. E., & Hawton, K. (2013). Clinical assessment and crisis intervention for the suicidal bipolar disorder patient. *Bipolar Disorders, 15*(5), 575–583.

Schalkwijk, S., Undurraga, J., Tondo, L., & Baldessarini, R. J. (2015). Declining efficacy in controlled trials of antidepressants: Effects of placebo dropout, *International Journal of Neuropsychopharmacology, 17*(8), 1343–1352.

Shneidman, E. S. (1984). Aphorisms of suicide and some implications for psychotherapy. *The American Journal of Psychotherapy, 38*(3), 319–328.

Shneidman, E. S. (1996). Psychotherapy with suicidal patients. In J. T. Maltsberger & M. J. Goldblatt (Eds.), *Essential papers on suicide* (pp. 417–426). New York: New York University Press.

Siamouli, M., Samara, M., & Fountoulakis, K. N. (2014). Is antiepileptic-induced suicidality a data-based class effect or an exaggeration? A comment on the literature. *Harvard Review of Psychiatry, 22*(6), 379–381.

Simon, R. I., & Hales, R. E. (Eds.). (2012). *Textbook of suicide assessment and management* (2nd ed.). Washington, DC: American Psychiatric Press.

Smith, E. G., Søndergård, L., Lopez, A. G., Andersen, P. K., & Kessing, L. V. (2009). Association between consistent purchase of anticonvulsants or lithium and suicide risk: A longitudinal cohort study from Denmark, 1995–2001. *Journal of Affective Disorders, 117*(3), 162–167.

Søndergård, L., Kvist, K., Lopez, A. G., Andersen, P. K., & Kessing, L. V. (2006). Temporal changes in suicide rates for persons treated and not treated with antidepressants in Denmark during 1995–1999. *Acta Psychiatrica Scandinavica, 114*(3), 168–176.

Søndergård, L., Lopez, A. G., Andersen, P. K., & Kessing, L. V. (2008). Mood-stabilizing pharmacological treatment in bipolar disorders and risk of suicide. *Bipolar Disorders, 10*(1), 87–94.

Sugawara, N., Yasui-Furukori, N., Ishii, N., Iwata, N., & Terao, T. (2013). Lithium in tapwater and suicide in Japan. *International Journal of Environmental Research and Public Health, 10*(11), 6044–6048.

Thies-Flechtner, K., Müller-Oerlinghausen, B., Seibert, W., Walther, A., & Greil, W. (1996). Effect of prophylactic treatment on suicide risk in patients with major affective disorders: Data from a randomized prospective trial. *Pharmacopsychiatry, 29*(3), 103–107.

Tiihonen, J., Wahlbeck, K., Lönnqvist, J., Klaukka, T., Ioannidis, J. P., Volavka, J., & Haukka, J. (2006). Effectiveness of antipsychotic treatments in a nationwide cohort of patients in community care after first hospitalization due to schizophrenia and schizoaffective disorder: Observational follow-up study. *BMJ, 333*(7561), 224–229.

Tollefson, G. D., Rampey, A. H. Jr., Beasley, C. M. Jr., Enas, G. G., & Potvin, J. H. (1994). Absence of a relationship between adverse events and suicidality during pharmacotherapy for depression. *Journal of Clinical Psychopharmacology, 14*(3), 163–169.

Tondo, L., Albert, M., & Baldessarini, R. J. (2006). Suicide rates in relation to health-care access in the United States. *Journal of Clinical Psychiatry, 67*(4), 517–523.

Tondo, L., & Baldessarini, R. J. (2007). Suicidal risks among 2826 major affective disorder patients. Acta Psychiatrica Scandinavica, *116*(6), 419–428.

Tondo, L., & Baldessarini, R. J. (2014). Reduction of suicidal behavior in bipolar disorder patients during long-term treatment with lithium. In S. H. Koslow, P. Ruiz, & C. B. Nemeroff (Eds.), *Concise guide to understanding suicide: Epidemiology pathophysiology and prevention* (pp 217–228). Cambridge, UK: Cambridge University Press.

Tondo, L., Baldessarini, R. J., Hennen, J., Floris, G., Silvetti, F., & Tohen, M. (1998). Lithium treatment and risk of suicidal behavior in bipolar disorder patients. *Journal of Clinical Psychiatry, 59*(8), 405–414.

Tondo, L., Baldessarini, R. J., Hennen, J., Minnai, G. P., Salis, P., Scamonatti, L.,...Mannu, P. (1999). Suicide attempts in major affective disorder patients with comorbid substance use disorders. *Journal of Clinical Psychiatry, 60*(2), 63–69.

Tondo, L., Hennen, J., & Baldessarini, R. J. (2001). Reduced suicide risk with long-term lithium treatment in major affective illness: Meta-analysis. *Acta Psychiatrica Scandinavica, 104*(3), 163–172.

Tondo, L., Isacsson, G., & Baldessarini, R. J. (2003). Suicide in bipolar disorder: Risk and prevention. *CNS Drugs, 17*(7), 491–511.

Tondo, L., Lepri, B., & Baldessarini, R. J. (2008). Suicidal status during antidepressant treatment in 789 Sardinian patients with major affective disorder. *Acta Psychiatrica Scandinavica, 118*(2), 106–115.

US Food and Drug Administration. (2008). *Statistical review and evaluation antiepileptic drugs and suicidality.* Retrieved from http://www.fda.gov/2008-4372b1-01.pdf.

Vita, A., De Peri, L., & Sacchetti, E. (2014). Lithium in drinking water and suicide: a review. *International Clinical Psychopharmacology,* in press.

Wasserman, D., Rihmer, Z., Rujescu, D., Sarchiapone, M., Sokolowski, M., Titelman, D.,...Carli, V. (2012). European Psychiatric Association (EPA) guidance on suicide treatment and prevention. *European Psychiatry, 27*(2), 129–141.

Weinger, R. D. (Ed.) (2000). *Practice of electroconvulsive therapy: Recommendations for treatment, training, and privileging: Task Force Report of the American Psychiatric Association* (2nd ed.). Washington, DC: American Psychiatric Press.

World Health Organization. (2013). International suicide rates. Retrieved from http://www.who.int/mental_health/prevention/suicide/country_reports/en/index.html

Yerevanian, B. I., & Choi, Y. M. (2013). Impact of psychotropic drugs on suicide and suicidal behaviors. *Bipolar Disorders, 15*(5), 594–621.

Yerevanian, B. I., Koek, R. J., & Mintz, J. (2007). Bipolar pharmacotherapy and suicidal behavior: Lithium, divalproex and carbamazepine. *Journal of Affective Disorders, 103*(1–3), 23–28.

Zisook, S., Trivedi, M. H., Warden, D., Lebowitz, B., Thase, M. E., Stewart, J. W.,...Rush, A. J. (2009). Clinical correlates of the worsening or emergence of suicidal ideation during SSRI treatment of depression. *Journal of Affective Disorders, 117*(1–2), 63–73.

PART VII

PREGNANCY AND LACTATION

38

MANAGEMENT OF BIPOLAR DISORDER DURING PREGNANCY AND LACTATION

Julie Hyman and D. Jeffrey Newport

INTRODUCTION

Pregnancy and lactation pose unique challenges in the management of bipolar disorder (BD). Clinicians must consider the risks, both to mother and child, posed by the illness, as well as those posed by available treatments. Moreover, sound decision making is clouded by the limited volume and inconsistent quality of data regarding the reproductive safety of psychotropic drugs.

Despite these challenges, a rational approach to the perinatal management of BD can be derived from the extant data. In this chapter, we first present an overview of the reproductive safety profiles for medications often used in the treatment of BD. We then summarize general principles that serve to guide the formulation of a perinatal treatment plan and conclude the chapter with a review of pertinent factors to consider at each step in the process: preconception, early gestation, late gestation, and the postpartum (PP) period.

MEDICATION SAFETY PROFILES

The five category US Food and Drug Administration (FDA) pregnancy rating system (cf. Table 38.1), often viewed as the definitive authority for determining reproductive safety, upon closer inspection, is plagued with numerous shortcomings. First, among medications with the same FDA safety rating, the frequency and severity of reported adverse outcomes can vary widely. Similarly, the volume and quality of the research data underlying the rating can be highly variable. Newer agents, which have been subjected to little scrutiny, should not be given a presumption of safety regardless the FDA pregnancy rating; instead, an absence or paucity of data should carry a presumption of risk. In addition, the FDA rating does not elucidate the window of risk for a

particular outcome linked to a medication. Furthermore, FDA review of the reproductive safety of individual medications is not regularly scheduled but often occurs sporadically, triggered by events such as the manufacturer seeking approval for a new indication. Finally, neurodevelopmental outcomes, important when considering psychotropic safety profiles, are seldom factored into FDA classifications.

Thomas Hales' *Medications and Mothers Milk* (2014), now in its 16th edition, has emerged as the standard reference for lactation safety ratings (cf. Table 38.1). Hale also uses a five-category system, rating medications from L1 (Safest) to L5 (Contraindicated). The entry for each medication includes a list of complications reported in nursing infants and a quantitative index of lactation exposure level, called relative infant dose (RID). Expressed as a percentage, the RID is calculated by dividing the total daily ingestion of a medication by an exclusively breastfed infant (mg/kg infant body weight) by the mother's daily dose of the medication (mg/kg maternal body weight). Hale advises that a RID less than 10% can be considered safe; however, this recommendation has never been objectively verified.

Sound decision making requires a more comprehensive knowledge of the risk profiles than provided by pregnancy or lactation risk categories. This includes understanding the level of offspring exposure in addition to the potential consequences of exposure, such as structural teratogenesis, obstetrical complications, neonatal or nursing complications, and neurodevelopmental sequelae. The reproductive safety profiles for mood stabilizers, including lithium, antiepileptic drugs (AEDs), and second generation antipsychotics (SGAs), are reviewed here.

LITHIUM

The risk of cardiac malformations, particularly Ebstein's anomaly, a tricuspid valve malformation, with lithium

Table 38.1. REPRODUCTIVE SAFETY RATINGS OF MOOD STABILIZERS

US FOOD & DRUG ADMINISTRATION PREGNANCY CATEGORIES		HALE'S *MEDICATIONS AND MOTHER'S MILK*	
		LACTATION CATEGORIES	RELATIVE INFANT DOSE
A	Adequate studies have failed to demonstrate risk in the 1st trimester. There is no evidence of risk in later trimesters.	L1 SAFEST	
	None	None	
B	Animal studies have failed to demonstrate risk. There are no adequate studies in pregnant women.	L2 SAFER	
	Clozapine	Carbamazepine	3.8%–5.9%
	Lurasidone	Olanzapine	0.3%–1.2%
		Quetiapine	0.07%–0.1%
		Ziprasidone	0.07%–1.2%
C	Animal studies have shown an adverse effect. There are no adequate studies in humans, but potential benefits may warrant use in pregnancy despite risks.	L3 MODERATELY SAFE	
	Aripiprazole	Aripiprazole	1.0%
	Asenapine	Asenapine	Not Reported
	Iloperidone	Clozapine	1.4%
	Lamotrigine	Iloperidone	Not Reported
	Olanzapine	Lamotrigine	9.2%–18.3%
	Paliperidone	Lithium	12%–30.1%
	Quetiapine	Lurasidone	Not Reported
	Risperidone	Paliperidone	Not Reported
	Ziprasidone	Risperidone	Not Reported
		Valproic Acid	1.4%–1.7%
D	There is evidence of risk based on investigational or marketing experience or studies in humans, but potential benefits may warrant use in pregnancy despite risks.	L4 POSSIBLY HAZARDOUS	
	Carbamazepine	None	
	Lithium		
	Valproic acid		
X	Studies in animals or humans have demonstrated fetal abnormalities and/or there is positive evidence of human fetal risk based on adverse reaction data from investigational or marketing experience, and the risks in pregnancy clearly outweigh potential benefits.	L5 CONTRAINDICATED	
	None	None	

exposure has been long reported. Early estimates suggested a 400-fold increase in the risk for Ebstein's anomaly; however, a subsequent review estimated a much lower 20-fold increase, rising from 1:20,000 to 1:1000 (Altshuler et al., 1996). A recent meta-analysis of lithium teratogenicity did not observe statistically significant risk estimates for cardiac defects; however, the authors concluded that "the upper confidence limit is consistent with a clinically significant increase in risk" (p. 727) (McKnight et al., 2012). At present, it should be assumed that lithium exposure does increase heart defect risk, albeit at lower rates than once believed. Polyhydramnios, as a consequence of

lithium-induced fetal nephrogenic diabetes insipidus, and fetal goiter have also been reported.

Lithium rapidly equilibrates across the placenta with neonatal concentrations uniformly equivalent to maternal concentrations at delivery. The high level of fetal exposure coupled with lithium's low therapeutic index warrants concern for neonatal toxicity. Indeed, a pooled analysis indicated that the prevalence of numerous neonatal complications, including cardiac arrhythmias, hypoglycemia, hypothyroidism, and flaccidity, was greater among neonates with higher lithium concentrations (Newport et al., 2005).

The neurodevelopmental consequences of prenatal lithium exposure have yet to be comprehensively examined. Preclinical studies have raised concerns regarding neurobehavioral outcomes, but the only clinical study reported no adverse sequelae among lithium-exposed school-age children (Schou, 1976).

Lithium was long contraindicated in lactation; however, it has been upgraded to the L3 (Moderately Safe) category in recent editions of Hale's lactation reference (Hale & Rowe, 2014). Despite its upgraded safety rating, lithium use during lactation should be approached with considerable caution given its low therapeutic index, high level of excretion into breast milk (reported RID 12%–30%), and numerous reports of adverse events among nursing infants, including hypotonia, hypothermia, hypothyroidism, electrocardiograph changes, and frank toxicity.

ANTIEPILEPTIC DRUGS

Valproic acid

Valproic acid (VPA) exposure is associated with numerous congenital malformations, including neural tube, craniofacial, cardiovascular, and limb anomalies. The neural tube defect (NTD) rate of 1% to 2%, 10 to 20 times higher than the general population, rises to 3.8% when the VPA daily dose exceeds 1,000 mg. It is important to note that neural tube closure occurs during the fourth week of gestation, before most women have recognized they are pregnant. A fetal VPA syndrome, characterized by stereotypical facial features, including bifrontal narrowing, midface hypoplasia, a broad nasal bridge, a short nose with anteverted nares, epicanthal folds, micrognathia, a shallow philtrum, and a thin upper and thick lower lip, has been described.

Folate antagonism by VPA may underlie the risk for both NTDs and fetal VPA syndrome. A case-control study of fetal AED syndromes reported a significantly higher rate of homozygosity for a key folate metabolic enzyme (Dean et al., 1999) among children exhibiting fetal AED syndromes.

Neurodevelopmental outcomes associated with VPA are especially concerning. Studies have consistently reported higher rates of cognitive delay among children exposed to VPA during pregnancy compared to those exposed to other AEDs (Palac & Meador, 2011), with developmental delay evident in as many as 20% of VPA-exposed children. Furthermore, fetal VPA syndrome has been associated with both cognitive delay and autism.

Like lithium, VPA readily crosses the placenta with neonatal concentrations equaling or surpassing maternal levels. However, there is greater variability in neonate-to-maternal concentration ratios, likely as a consequence of placental efflux transporters that help regulate VPA, but not lithium, placental transmission. Neonatal toxicities, including hepatotoxicity, coagulopathies, and hypoglycemia, have been reported.

Hale (2014) downgraded VPA's lactation rating from L2 (Safer) to L3 (Moderately Safe) in recent versions of his reference. Reassuring is VPA's low RID (1.4%–1.7%) and the fact that only one adverse event (thrombocytopenia) has been reported in a nursing infant. Clinicians should be cautioned, however, that hepatic complications are possible, and the neurodevelopmental effects of VPA exposure via nursing have not been investigated.

Carbamazepine

A meta-analysis indicated that carbamazepine (CBZ) exposure is associated with an increased risk of NTDs, orofacial clefts, and cardiovascular and urinary tract anomalies (Matalon et al., 2002). A fetal CBZ syndrome manifested by a short nose, long philtrum, epicanthal folds, hypertelorism, upslanting palpebral fissures, and fingernail hypoplasia has also been described. The teratogenic risks of CBZ exposure in many respects parallel those seen with VPA, typically occurring, however, with lower frequency or less severity. For example, the NTD risk attributable to CBZ exposure, 0.5% to 1.0%, is approximately one-half the VPA-associated risk. A study reporting a lower NTD rate for CBZ-treated women receiving periconceptional folate supplements (Hernandez-Diaz et al., 2001) contributed to blanket recommendations to administer high-dose (4–5 mg daily) folic acid supplementation to all AED-treated women of reproductive capacity.

The placental transfer of CBZ, with umbilical cord-maternal plasma ratios equaling 0.5 to 0.8, is lower than other AEDs. Hepatotoxicity is the only neonatal complication of CBZ exposure reported to date; however, neonatal blood dyscrasias are plausible.

Data regarding the neurodevelopmental sequelae of fetal CBZ exposure have been mixed. Some early studies reported developmental delay in CBZ-exposed children; however, many later systematic studies demonstrated no evidence of developmental delay. Of note, one recent study reported an association between prenatal CBZ exposure and poorer verbal performance in school-aged children (Meador et al., 2011).

The database regarding CBZ safety in lactation is large relative to other psychotropic agents, likely contributing to its surprisingly favorable L2 (Safer) lactation safety rating

(Hale & Rowe, 2014). Despite the L2 rating, the RID of CBZ in lactation (3.8%–5.9%) is considerably higher than VPA, and hepatic dysfunction has been reported among several CBZ-exposed infants.

Lamotrigine

Reproductive safety data for lamotrigine (LTG) has rapidly accrued and compares favorably to other mood stabilizers. Overall, the available evidence has not demonstrated an association between LTG exposure and NTDs or other major malformations (cf. Moore and Aggarwal, 2012, for review). One study did report a high rate (0.89%) of orofacial clefts; however, the collective rate (0.10%) of clefts among seven other prospective studies is consistent with the general population rate, and a large European case-control study reported an adjusted odds ratio of 0.67 for orofacial clefts following LTG exposure.

Placental passage studies indicate that neonatal concentrations of LTG are approximately equal to maternal concentrations. Despite readily crossing the placenta, there have been no reports of acute adverse events observed in LTG-exposed neonates. Of note, there have been no reports of rash among neonates exposed to LTG during gestation.

The neurodevelopmental effects of fetal exposure to LTG, like VPA and CBZ, have been subject to a series of systematic investigations. Results of these studies have been reassuring with no evidence of adverse developmental sequelae (Palac & Meador, 2011).

Unique to LTG has been the extensive investigation of clearance alterations across gestation, which heightened attention to LTG as a consequence of its unique metabolic profile. Unlike most psychotropics, which are primarily metabolized by cytochrome P450 oxidation, LTG is almost exclusively metabolized via conjugation by the UDP-glucuronosyltransferase 1A4 (UGT1A4) enzyme. Because estradiol induces UGT1A4 activity, LTG clearance can rapidly escalate during pregnancy, leading some to recommend serial monitoring of LTG levels and requisite dose adjustments in response to declining levels across gestation (Pennell et al., 2008).

Hale (2014) has assigned LTG an L3 (Moderately Safe) lactation category. This less favorable rating, relative to CBZ, is presumably a consequence of LTG's higher RID (9.2%–18.3%) coupled with concerns that nursing infants may be unable to metabolize LTG (because glucuronide enzymes are not yet fully active in human neonates). Yet, despite the higher RID, the level of LTG exposure incurred by an exclusively breastfed neonate equals approximately 1 mg/kg/day, considerably lower than the 2 to 3 mg/kg/day

administered to treat infant febrile seizures. One adverse event, an apneic episode, has been reported in association with LTG exposure via nursing.

Olanzapine

The reproductive safety profile for olanzapine, as for all SGAs, is derived from a limited volume of data (Brunner, Falk, Jones, Dey, & Shatapathy, 2013). Rates of malformation, miscarriage, and preterm delivery are generally consistent with population norms; however, the number of pregnancies studied remains too low to derive definitive conclusions. Studies encompassing approximately 400 pregnancies collectively report a 4.4% rate of major malformations.

A recent study reported the risk of gestational diabetes is doubled among women receiving antipsychotic therapy (Boden, Lundgren, Brandt, Reutfors, & Kieler, 2012). Olanzapine was the most frequent antipsychotic exposure in this study, comprising nearly one-third of exposures, but risk ratios were not reported for individual agents.

The mean neonate-to-maternal concentration ratio for olanzapine is 72% (Newport et al., 2007). An increased prevalence of low birth weight has been reported among olanzapine-exposed neonates (Boden et al., 2012); however, statistical adjustment indicates this may be attributable to concomitant exposures, in particular tobacco.

There are no available data regarding the neurodevelopmental effects of olanzapine exposure during pregnancy or lactation.

Olanzapine, which produces a RID of 0.3% to 1.2% in lactation, carries an L2 (Safer) lactation rating (Hale, 2012). No adverse events have been reported in nursing infants.

SECOND-GENERATION ANTIPSYCHOTICS

Risperidone

Prospective reports regarding the reproductive safety of risperidone encompass approximately 150 pregnancies. Rates of malformations and miscarriages are within population norms, but again, these data are too limited to derive definitive recommendations.

The placental passage rate reported for risperidone equals 49% (Newport et al., 2007), a relatively low rate among psychotropic compounds. No neonatal complications have been reported among the few studies published to date.

There are no reports, to our knowledge, regarding the neurodevelopment sequelae of prenatal exposure to risperidone.

Risperidone, which produces a RID of 2.3% to 4.7% in lactation, carries an L3 (Moderately Safe) lactation risk (Hale & Rowe, 2014).

Quetiapine

The reproductive safety profile for quetiapine is derived from fewer than 100 pregnancies. Though limited, these data have been reassuring with no reports of major malformations. However, quetiapine was the second most highly represented medication (18%) in the previously cited report of heightened risk for gestational diabetes in association with antipsychotic exposure (Boden et al., 2012).

The placental passage rate for quetiapine (23%) is to our knowledge the lowest rate ever reported for a psychotropic agent (Newport et al., 2007).

There are no available data regarding the neurodevelopmental effects of quetiapine exposure during pregnancy.

Quetiapine carries a lactation safety rating of L2 (Safer; Hale, 2012), producing a RID of 0.07% to 0.1% via lactation with no reported complications among nursing infants.

Other agents

As the first SGA introduced to the US market, reproductive data accrued for *clozapine* prior to the arrival of the other agents in this class. However, due to the significant medical risks associated with clozapine, in particular agranulocytosis, it is difficult to justify administering clozapine during pregnancy despite its favorable pregnancy category B designation.

The reproductive safety profiles for the remaining SGAs, including *aripiprazole, asenapine, iloperidone, lurasidone, paliperidone*, and *ziprasidone*, have accrued little or no prenatal safety data. No neurodevelopmental data has been reported following prenatal exposure to any of these compounds. Nevertheless, favorable outcomes in animal studies did secure a pregnancy category B designation for lurasidone.

Ziprasidone (RID: 0.07%–1.2%) has been assigned an L2 (Safer) lactation safety rating (Hale & Rowe, 2014). An L3 (Moderately Safe) rating has been assigned to aripiprazole (RID: 0.9%), asenapine, clozapine (RID: 1.4%), iloperidone, lurasidone, and paliperidone (Hale & Rowe, 2014).

GUIDING PRINCIPLES FOR PERINATAL DECISION MAKING

When approaching the management of a pregnant or breast-feeding patient with BD, the risks to mother and child posed by the illness must be weighed against those posed by psychotropic exposure. Unfortunately, no risk-free alternative exists, other than choosing not to conceive. Thus there are numerous overarching concerns to be confronted no matter what pharmacotherapy, if any, is under consideration. These concerns form the basis for delineating general principles to guide perinatal treatment planning for BD. These principles are perhaps best conveyed through a series of questions commonly encountered during childbearing.

IS IT SAFE TO TAKE MEDICATION WHILE PREGNANT?

Patients, and many clinicians, often reduce the risk assessment to this sole question, seeking an answer devoid of ambiguity. However, any recommendation predicated upon this sole question is wholly inadequate. First, the question ignores the risk posed by the illness. Second, there is no psychotropic medication for which all potential risks have been exhaustively examined. Consequently, no psychotropic medication can be categorically deemed safe during pregnancy or lactation. Third, when posed in this manner, the question inexorably leads to an assumption that maternal well-being competes with fetal well-being. This so-called fetal–maternal conflict should be avoided, as it is a sure path to self-recrimination for any expectant mother faced with decisions regarding management of a mental disorder.

As no psychotropic can be guaranteed safe during pregnancy, this question must be reframed so that it does not place the expectant mother in conflict with her baby. The better question is, "What will provide this expectant mother *and* her baby the best chance of a safe, healthy pregnancy?" This more appropriate question, however, opens the door to a series of additional questions.

WHAT RISK DOES BIPOLAR DISORDER POSE TO MOTHER AND INFANT?

This question is not unique to BD. In fact, it is not unique to mental disorders. It is encountered whenever a pregnant or nursing mother has a medical or psychiatric condition requiring pharmacotherapy. If an illness poses little risk to mother and/or infant (e.g., allergic rhinitis), then little pharmacological risk can be justified. However, considerable pharmacological risk may be acceptable when an illness poses great risk to expectant mother and/or infant (e.g., epilepsy, HIV).

There are considerable data regarding the impact of maternal depression during pregnancy. Prenatal depression has been associated with aberrant maternal health behaviors resulting in poorer compliance with obstetrical care and greater use of medications, prescription and nonprescription, and various habit-forming substances (Newport et al., 2012). Depression during pregnancy has also been associated with numerous adverse obstetrical and neonatal outcomes, including poor maternal weight gain and greater risk for preeclampsia, preterm delivery, low birth weight, small for gestational age neonate, and reduced neonate head circumference (Marcus, 2009). Finally, prenatal depression has been associated with adverse neurodevelopmental effects on child cognition, language, and motor activity (Kingston, Tough, & Whitfield, 2012). Because it is unclear how much of this data is derived from depressive episodes of BD versus major depressive disorder, it remains widely assumed that the risks attributable to major depressive disorder and bipolar depression are equivalent.

To our knowledge, no studies have examined the effect of mania or hypomania on pregnancy outcome. The impaired judgment characterizing manic episodes arguably leads to maternal risk-taking that would jeopardize the well-being of both mother and infant. Whether maternal hypomania poses a risk for obstetrical or infant outcome remains obscure.

Postpartum episodes of BD may also convey considerable risk. Studies of postpartum depression have shown a wide range of detrimental effects on children, including impaired attachment (Lovejoy, Graczyk, O'Hare, & Neuman, 2000) and problems with cognitive, language, and emotional development (Grace, Evindar, & Stewart, 2003; Weissman et al., 2006). Postpartum psychosis, frequently a consequence of BD (Brockington et al., 1981), is considered a psychiatric emergency.

HOW LIKELY IS A BIPOLAR DISORDER RECURRENCE DURING PREGNANCY IF MOOD STABILIZER THERAPY IS DISCONTINUED?

In an ideal scenario, an expectant mother would remain well despite stopping psychotropic treatment, sparing mother and child the risks attributable to both illness and pharmacological exposure. Unfortunately, most evidence indicates this is unlikely. The most extensive study to date reported an 86% BD recurrence rate among pregnant women who discontinued mood stabilizer treatment versus 37% of those who continued pharmacotherapy, with especially rapid recurrence among those who abruptly stopped treatment (Viguera et al., 2007).

Unfortunately, existing research has not yet identified the characteristics of the subset of women with BD who remain well during pregnancy without treatment. Nevertheless, our experience suggests that clinicians may also consider the individual patient's psychiatric history when trying to determine whether a temporary cessation of treatment is advisable. Pertinent questions include: How many previous BD episodes has she experienced? How severe were the earlier episodes? What was the polarity? Were psychotic symptoms present? Has she previously had a period of sustained euthymia after stopping treatment? Did previous recurrences arise gradually or abruptly? With resumption of treatment, how quickly did the episodes resolve? And finally, has she experienced a BD recurrence during or following a previous pregnancy?

HOW EFFECTIVE ARE NONPSYCHOTROPIC TREATMENTS?

It is axiomatic that pharmacotherapy is a necessary component of BD treatment. Yet nonpharmacological interventions may augment treatment, helping to avoid dose increases or addition of other psychotropic agents, though no data exists, as yet, to demonstrate this. Because psychotherapy carries minimal risk during gestation and has demonstrated benefit for BD, it should be routinely recommended to pregnant women with BD. Standard psychotherapies during pregnancy include interpersonal and cognitive-behavioral therapies.

Complementary treatments of low risk, such as daily exercise, prenatal yoga, and meditation, may also be included. However, naturopathic supplements (e.g., St. John's wort, Rhodiola rosea, saffron, lavender, maharishi amrit kalash, mentat, etc.) are not recommended during pregnancy because they are not subject to FDA scrutiny and reproductive safety data is sparse.

WHAT MEDICATION(S) SHOULD BE RECOMMENDED?

Pregnancy is not a time to experiment with novel treatments; thus, choosing the best treatment from the outset is critical. The ideal medication balances safety and efficacy. All too often, understandably preoccupied with the safety profiles of available medications, clinicians lose sight of the need for an efficacious treatment. Doing so often leads to ill-advised decisions. If the justification for administering a medication during pregnancy is to protect mother and infant from illness-associated risks, then a medication is only advisable if there is a reasonable expectation of protective benefit.

The efficacy of particular mood-stabilizer agents during pregnancy and the PP period has, to our knowledge, received limited scrutiny. Thus the considerable volume of data regarding the respective efficacies of various agents for BD outside of pregnancy is applied to the perinatal context. That information is reviewed extensively elsewhere in this volume.

Equally important to anticipating the perinatal efficacy of available treatments is reviewing the patient's treatment history. Even a medication with a favorable reproductive safety profile is difficult to justify if the patient has previously failed an adequate trial of it. Obtaining a comprehensive treatment history, documenting the efficacy, tolerability, dose, and treatment duration for each agent is instrumental in narrowing the list of viable medication choices. Particularly important is the utility of a medication during or immediately following a previous pregnancy.

After identifying medications with a reasonable likelihood of efficacy, safety considerations enter the decision-making process. It is important to review the reproductive safety profiles of agents deemed likely to provide therapeutic efficacy, taking into consideration the gestational timing when the decision is being made.

The ideal medication regimen lies at the intersection of the efficacy and safety survey. If multiple agents remain under consideration, then the choice can be further refined by considering potential tolerability during gestation. The scope of tolerability includes selecting agents that are less likely to contribute to pregnancy-related conditions such as gestational diabetes.

PRECONCEPTION DECISION-MAKING

BEGINNING AT PUBERTY

It is vital to consider the possibility of conception when treating women of reproductive potential, long before conception is being planned. One-half of all pregnancies in the United States are unplanned. In such cases, women are typically in the sixth week of gestation or later before recognizing they are pregnant. By this time, neural tube closure and the beginning of cardiogenesis have occurred.

Even when pregnancy is planned, couples seldom seek consultation for perinatal treatment recommendations until just before trying to conceive. If safety considerations dictate a treatment change, then the patient is faced with the unwelcome prospect of postponing conception to

ensure the new agent is likely to be effective or, alternatively, entering pregnancy treated with a newly introduced medication with uncertain efficacy.

CONTRACEPTION

Method of contraception should be documented at every clinical visit. Clinicians should be aware of the potential impact of drug interactions upon contraceptive reliability. In particular, CBZ and other enzyme-inducing AEDs reduce the effectiveness of hormonal contraceptives. Thus barrier methods of contraception are preferred for women treated with these agents.

There is also a drug interaction between estrogen-containing contraceptives and LTG. Because estradiol induces the UGT1A4 enzyme that metabolizes LTG, coadministering the two may reduce the circulating concentrations of LTG and thereby limit its effectiveness.

PREGNANCY PLANNING

Preconception planning should begin with maternal health behavior counseling. Women should be advised to start prenatal vitamins and reminded to avoid alcohol, tobacco, caffeine, and herbal remedies. They should be encouraged to consume eight 8-ounce glasses of water daily and to engage in moderate daily exercise unless otherwise directed by their obstetrician. Those taking AEDs should be prescribed an additional 4 mg folate supplement.

When considering pregnancy, the initial decision faced by a woman with BD is whether to conceive at all, remembering that the only risk-free option is choosing not to conceive. If she opts to proceed with conception, the patient may discontinue pharmacotherapy, continue her current regimen, switch the regimen, or temporarily suspend treatment. These options can be applied to particular agents as detailed below and summarized in Box 38.1.

Lithium

Lithium-treated women wishing to conceive have the option of postponing conception to switch to an alternative agent, proceeding with conception and accepting the risk of lithium exposure in order to protect mother and infant from the risks of untreated BD, or temporarily suspending lithium treatment to avoid exposure during cardiogenesis (Weeks 5–12 of gestation). Due to the inherent risks of lithium therapy during lactation, switching to an alternative agent should be considered by women for whom breast-feeding is important.

Prior to conceiving, a laboratory evaluation, including lithium, creatinine, and thyroid-stimulating hormone serum concentrations, should be completed. The lithium level will serve as a target concentration should dose adjustments be required during pregnancy.

When electing to suspend therapy, lithium administration is ideally discontinued before conception and not resumed until the 14th week of gestation or later. It is wise to decide on a contingency plan should the patient experience a recurrence before cardiogenesis is complete. Alternatives, when illness recurs before the conclusion of cardiogenesis, include resumption of lithium despite the teratogenic risk, institution of electroconvulsive therapy (ECT), and switching to an alternative agent.

Valproic acid

The only preconception option, other than not conceiving, available to VPA-treated women is to switch treatment. Recognizing the severity and frequency of adverse consequences associated with VPA exposure, continuing VPA is not viable. Because the safety concerns attributable to VPA traverse the entirety of gestation, temporary suspension of VPA is also not an alternative.

When switching the mood-stabilizer regimen prior to conception, we empirically recommend postponing the attempt to conceive for six months. The postponement of conception is advised in an effort to ensure the new regimen will offer sustained efficacy. Should conception occur immediately after switching treatment, there remains a heightened risk that the newly introduced treatment may fail.

It is important to evaluate the VPA-treated patient to rule out polycystic ovarian syndrome. VPA treatment has been associated with the development of polycystic ovarian syndrome (Bilo & Meo, 2008), the most common endocrine cause of infertility.

Lamotrigine

The only viable preconception alternatives for women receiving LTG therapy are to continue or discontinue the medication. Switching treatment is unreasonable as there are no alternative agents with a safety profile that compares favorably to LTG. Treatment suspension is also inadvisable due to the protracted titration schedule necessary when resuming LTG. Given the high risk of BD recurrence during pregnancy, most women treated effectively with LTG are best advised to continue the medication. A 4 mg folic acid supplement should be instituted and continued throughout gestation.

Carbemazepine

Due to risk for numerous birth defects, CBZ should be avoided from conception through the 16th week of gestation. Because some studies, though not all, indicate that CBZ also carries adverse neurodevelopmental consequences, avoiding it throughout the entirety of gestation may also be advisable. In rare instances, when alternative agents have proven ineffective, patients may elect to continue CBZ therapy while taking a high dose (4 mg) folic acid supplement.

Second-Generation Antipsychotics

The reproductive safety profiles for these agents remains limited; thus, there is insufficient evidence to conclude that any are definitively safer than others. Previous treatment response is therefore the key discriminator when selecting among the SGAs as a component of the treatment regimen. It may, however, be advisable to switch patients at risk for gestational diabetes from one agent (e.g., olanzapine) to another (e.g., ziprasidone) within this class if the metabolic syndrome profile can be improved by doing so. Otherwise, prior to conception, the options available to patients treated with these medications include discontinuing the medication, switching to LTG (the only alternative with a clearly superior reproductive safety profile), or continuing the medication, accepting its risk in an effort to protect mother and infant from the risks attributable to BD.

If the patient is taking a SGA that is likely to cause hyperprolactinemia, such as risperidone, a serum prolactin level should be checked to ensure that the medication will not interfere with the patient's ability to conceive.

EARLY PREGNANCY DECISION-MAKING

Many patients fail to seek reproductive safety counseling until already pregnant. This imposes a sense of urgency on the clinical evaluation as offspring exposure is actively unfolding while clinical decisions are being deliberated and executed. Yet, in many respects, because fetal drug exposure has already occurred, decisions prove simpler than during preconception planning. In particular, switching treatments is often a less attractive option at this juncture.

Key considerations to inform early pregnancy decision-making include recognizing that fetal drug exposure has already occurred and understanding that the window of risk for some outcomes has already passed. In addition, treatment recommendations at this juncture are informed both by whether the pregnant patient has already discontinued mood-stabilizer therapy and whether she is already experiencing a BD recurrence. Refer to Box 38.2 for a summary of early pregnancy clinical pearls.

WHEN MOOD STABILIZER HAS NOT BEEN DISCONTINUED

In this scenario, the fetus has already been exposed to one or more psychotropic medications and the window of risk for certain birth defects has already commenced. Furthermore, switching medications is problematic in that it exposes the baby to yet another drug while increasing the likelihood of BD recurrence when switching to a treatment unfamiliar to the patient. Medication-specific recommendations are as follows.

Lithium

When a pregnant patient presents for consultation, cardiogenesis, in all likelihood, is already underway. By the time lithium can be tapered and allowed to clear the circulation, heart formation will be virtually complete. Because the opportunity for protecting the child from a lithium-induced cardiac malformation has essentially passed, it may be advisable to continue lithium, thereby protecting mother and child from the risks of BD recurrence.

Discontinuing lithium at this juncture should be reserved for those whose treatment history suggests there is a viable chance of remaining euthymic throughout gestation without treatment. When that option is taken, contingency plans for managing an early illness recurrence should be decided in advance. Treatment choices for recurrence during early pregnancy include ECT, resumption of lithium, or institution of another agent.

Valproic Acid and Carbamazepine

The window to protect the child from a NTD will have already passed; however, there may still be an opportunity to offer protection from other birth defects (e.g., orofacial clefts) or neurodevelopmental effects of exposure to these medications. Thus switching VPA to an alternative medication is always recommended, and CBZ-treated patients are encouraged to consider switching. As with lithium, treatment discontinuation should be reserved for the patient whose history indicates she has a reasonable chance of remaining euthymic during gestation without treatment.

Box 38.1 CLINICAL PEARLS: PRECONCEPTION

- The preconception period begins not when a pregnancy is being contemplated; preconception starts at puberty.

- All women of reproductive capacity should be considered potentially pregnant, at any moment.

- Avoid prescribing medications that you would feel obligated to discontinue at knowledge of conception to women of reproductive capacity.

- Administer folic acid 4 mg daily to all women of reproductive capacity who are being treated with an antiepileptic drug or benzodiazepine. Do not wait until knowledge of conception to do so.

- Start a prenatal vitamin before conception.

- When treating women of reproductive capacity, prescribe valproic acid only as a medication of last resort and never as a first-line agent.

- Because carbamazepine interferes with the efficacy of hormonal contraception, barrier contraceptives are recommended for women receiving carbamazepine (and other enzyme-inducing antiepileptic drugs).

- Lithium-treated women who wish to breastfeed should be counseled to switch to an alternative agent prior to conception.

Immediate institution of high dose (4 mg) folic acid, which may protect offspring not only from NTDs but from orofacial clefts and perhaps neurodevelopmental effects of exposure, is always recommended.

Lamotrigine

A patient whose BD is effectively managed with LTG is advised to continue taking this agent when pregnant. If she is not yet receiving a folic acid supplement, one should be initiated immediately.

Because estrogen-induced changes in LTG metabolism can cause unpredictable changes in the drug's metabolism at any time during pregnancy, frequent visits for symptom monitoring and dose titration, when warranted, is advised.

Second-Generation Antipsychotics

When a patient conceives during treatment with a SGA, the alternatives for most patients are to continue or discontinue the medication. As noted previously, this decision is predicated on an assessment of the likelihood that she will remain euthymic without treatment. Most are best advised to continue treatment given the high rate of recurrence following discontinuation.

Switching from a SGA during pregnancy is generally ill advised. LTG is the only mood stabilizer with a clearly superior reproductive safety profile; however, the utility of LTG as a replacement is limited by the protracted titration schedule that is required. There is insufficient

evidence to justify attempts to improve reproductive safety by switching from one SGA to another; however, this may be considered for patients at heightened risk for gestational diabetes who are treated with agents carrying the highest risk for metabolic syndromes (e.g., olanzapine).

WHEN MOOD STABILIZER HAS BEEN DISCONTINUED

In this setting, although the patient is no longer receiving treatment, it is important to remember that the baby has already been exposed to psychotropic medication. Frequently, the patient will have already experienced a recurrence of BD prior to her clinical evaluation. The risks to mother and child alike attributable to BD illness warrant a resumption of treatment. The remaining decision is whether to resume the previous treatment or switch to an alternative. Less often, despite having discontinued treatment, the mother will remain euthymic at the time of consultation. When this occurs, it is important to determine when treatment should be resumed.

Lithium

For the patient whose BD has been most effectively managed with lithium, a recurrence before cardiogenesis is complete requires thoughtful consideration. One option is to postpone resumption of lithium until heart formation is complete. If the patient remains euthymic despite stopping lithium, this is the best course of action. Many patients will opt to postpone a resumption of lithium therapy until a fetal echocardiogram can be completed (at around 19 weeks gestation) to document cardiogenesis is complete.

If, however, the patient is already experiencing a recurrence of illness, postponing treatment resumption should be discouraged unless cardiogenesis is nearing completion or the symptoms remain mild. Resuming lithium may be considered despite the fact that cardiogenesis is not yet complete. This option is often preferable when numerous alternative treatments have previously failed.

Finally, the decision can be made to switch to an alternative treatment either for the remainder of gestation or at least until organogenesis is complete. Viable alternatives include ECT and any of the SGAs. The safety concerns of VPA and CBZ preclude them from consideration, and the protracted titration schedule required for LTG limits its usefulness in this context.

Valproic Acid and Carbamazepine

The window of risk for many well-documented adverse effects of VPA and CBZ, including neurodevelopmental sequelae, will not have passed. Therefore, it is best to avoid resuming these agents, replacing them with an alternative treatment (e.g., ECT or a SGA) during pregnancy.

Lamotrigine

Recognizing its favorable reproductive safety profile, resuming LTG is advisable. Even if the patient remains euthymic, resumption of LTG is preferred as its greatest utility is as a prophylactic agent. However, due to the lengthy titration schedule or paucity of data to support the utility of LTG as a treatment for an acute BD episode, it may be necessary to coadminister another mood stabilizer as an acute treatment providing a clinical bridge to the prophylactic benefit of LTG.

Second-Generation Antipsychotics

If the patient remains euthymic at presentation, then the timing of resumption of treatment is largely dictated by the likelihood, potential severity, and rapidity of onset of a recurrence later in pregnancy. When the decision is made to restart SGA therapy, it is best to resume the previously effective SGA, to which the baby has already been exposed, titrating to the previously effective dose.

LATE PREGNANCY DECISION-MAKING

The treatment issues encountered in later pregnancy include symptom monitoring to identify the need for dose adjustments and maximizing neonatal safety as delivery approaches. Refer to Box 38.3 for a summary of late pregnancy clinical pearls.

Numerous pharmacokinetic changes during pregnancy, including increases in hepatic metabolism, renal clearance, and blood volume, combine to lower medication concentrations. Anecdotal evidence suggests declining medication levels may dictate dose increases to maintain efficacy and that this is most likely to occur during the late second or early third trimester. When a dose adjustment is needed, a single stepwise dose increment is typically sufficient to sustain patient well-being. Because LTG clearance is subject to vast increases at any point in pregnancy, dose increases may be necessary in early pregnancy as well. For most mood stabilizers, dose adjustments can be accomplished without serum monitoring of medication concentrations; however, due to lithium's low therapeutic index, regular monitoring of levels across gestation is advised.

LITHIUM

Many of the numerous neonatal complications attributable to lithium are linked to the level of infant exposure at delivery (Newport et al., 2005). To minimize the risk for delivery and neonatal complications, the following guidelines are proposed: (a) monitor lithium levels regularly, particularly during late gestation when glomerular filtration rate dramatically rises, maintaining a target concentration at the minimal effective level for the patient; (b) avoid medications that might predispose the patient and her child to lithium toxicity, including diuretics, calcium channel blockers, and nonsteroidal inflammatory drugs; (c) lower the lithium dose in the event of obstetrical complications such as preeclampsia or polyhydramnios that may predispose the patient or her child to lithium toxicity; (d) suspend lithium therapy 24 to 48 hours before a scheduled delivery or at the onset of labor in the event of a spontaneous delivery; and (e) check the patient's lithium level when she presents for delivery and administer oral or intravenous hydration throughout labor and delivery. This brief suspension of treatment coupled with hydration during labor and delivery can dramatically lower maternal and fetal lithium concentration at delivery improving neonatal well-being.

Finally, it is important to frequently remind the patient to advise her obstetrical care provider that she cannot be treated with nonsteroidal anti-inflammatory drugs following delivery.

VALPROIC ACID AND CARBAMAZEPINE

Typically, these medications will have been discontinued earlier in gestation. In the rare circumstance that they have been resumed during late pregnancy, it is important to resume coadministration of a high dose folic acid supplement with these agents.

LAMOTRIGINE AND SECOND-GENERATION ANTIPSYCHOTICS

There are no particular late pregnancy concerns unique to these agents other than coadministration of folic acid with LTG.

POSTPARTUM DECISION MAKING

Two key clinical concerns arise following delivery: (a) potential illness exacerbation and (b) the safety of the mood-stabilizer regimen during lactation. These two concerns are interrelated, in that treatment adjustments necessitated by clinical deterioration may alter the lactation safety profile. Refer to Box 38.4 for a summary of postpartum and lactation clinical pearls.

POSTPARTUM EXACERBATION OF ILLNESS

Historical interest in the PP course of BD dates to Kraepelin (1921), who noted that episodes of mania or melancholia were common in pregnancy but even more so following childbirth. The PP period is a window of risk for women with BD, marked by high recurrence rates (30%–50%) and severe episodes, often requiring hospitalization. Of greatest concern are numerous lines of evidence linking BD and PP

psychosis (Chaudron & Pies 2003). Moreover, the onset of PP psychosis can occur rapidly, often arising within days of delivery (Brockington et al., 1981).

Unpublished data from our group indicates that women who, following delivery, were not taking the same medication(s) that they had previously reported as their most effective BD regimen were nearly twice as likely (40% vs. 23%) to experience a PP recurrence. Unfortunately, women with BD often switch from the most effective regimen during pregnancy in an effort to improve reproductive safety. An unintended consequence of safety-motivated treatment modifications may be a heightened risk for recurrence of illness following delivery. Consequently, pregnant women who, for safety reasons, have switched from the mood-stabilizer regimen that was previously most effective may consider returning to that previously effective regimen immediately following delivery. Arguably, those who have experienced BD symptoms during gestation should be encouraged to do so.

LACTATION SAFETY

When a PP recurrence of BD necessitates the introduction of medication(s) not used during pregnancy, the advisability of lactation is brought into question. In such cases, a patient may opt to discontinue breast-feeding to avoid the incremental risk of additional medication exposure(s).

However, when an effective medication regimen used during pregnancy is continued into the PP period, there is often little reason to discourage breast-feeding. In such cases, nursing only continues an exposure that the infant has experienced during pregnancy, at levels that are consistently a small fraction of the exposure levels incurred during gestation and at a time when the child's central nervous system is presumably less sensitive to untoward developmental effects.

If a nursing infant exhibits a concerning symptom that is suspected to be due to medication exposure via breast milk, then lactation should be immediately discontinued. When this occurs, with the exception of lithium, there is no reason to check the nursing infant's medication level. Deciding whether to discontinue the medication is predicated on the index of suspicion that the medication is the causative agent regardless of the infant's medication level.

Lithium

Breast-feeding during lithium therapy should be approached with extreme caution and discouraged for all but the most adherent patients. The key concern is that infant hydration status is subject to rapid shifts, particularly during febrile syndromes, when ibuprofen has emerged as a first-line treatment. This combination can easily produce dangerous lithium toxicity in a nursing infant.

Lithium-treated women who are nursing should be reminded, at every clinical encounter, to regularly monitor their infants' hydration status and to avoid using nonsteroidal anti-inflammatory drugs, both for themselves and their babies. In addition, the prescribing physician should perform periodic laboratory monitoring of both mother and nursing infant, evaluating serum levels of lithium, creatinine, and thyroid-stimulating hormone. It cannot be assumed that the pediatric care provider will order laboratory monitoring for the breast-fed infant.

Valproic Acid and Carbamazepine

Contrary to the dire warnings assigned to these agents during pregnancy, both have favorable lactation safety ratings (Hale & Rowe, 2014). Nevertheless, hepatic complications and blood dyscrasias are possible and have been reported in infants exposed to these agents during lactation. Moreover, it is possible that nursing infants remain susceptible to adverse neurodevelopment effects of exposure to VPA or CBZ.

Caution is therefore advised when breast-feeding is being considered during VPA or CBZ therapy, even when the infant was already exposed to one of these agents during gestation. The prescribing physician should perform periodic laboratory monitoring, for both mother and nursing infant, of both liver enzymes and blood counts. Finally, women nursing during CBZ therapy should be cautioned that febrile illness in their infants warrants an emergent evaluation to rule out CBZ-induced leukopenia.

Lamotrigine and Second-Generation Antipsychotics

When infants have been exposed to LTG or SGAs during pregnancy, there is little justification for discouraging mothers who are taking them from breast-feeding. Women who are continuing therapy with these agents from pregnancy into the PP period can be encouraged to breast-feed as the exposure level via lactation is considerably lower than the exposure level already incurred during gestation. However, women nursing during clozapine therapy should be cautioned that febrile illness in their infants warrants an emergent evaluation to rule out drug-induced leukopenia.

Disclosure statement: Dr. Newport has received research support from Eli Lilly, GlaxoSmithKline, Janssen, the National Alliance for Research on Schizophrenia and Depression, the National Institutes of Health, and Wyeth. He has served on speakers' bureaus and/or received honoraria from Astra-Zeneca, Eli Lilly, GSK, Pfizer, and Wyeth. He has served on advisory boards for GlaxoSmithKline. He has never served as a consultant to any biomedical or pharmaceutical corporations. Neither he nor family members have ever held equity positions in biomedical or pharmaceutical corporations.
Dr. Hyman has no conflicts to disclose.

REFERENCES

Altshuler, L. L., Cohen, L. S., Szuba, M. P., Burt, V. K., Gitlin, M. J., & Mintz, J. (1996). Pharmacologic management of psychiatric illness in pregnancy: Dilemmas and guidelines. *The American Journal of Psychiatry, 153*, 592–606.

Bilo, L., & Meo, R. (2008). Polycystic ovary syndrome in women using VPA: A review. *Gynecological Endocrinology, 24*(10), 562–570.

Boden, R., Lundgren, M., Brandt, L., Reutfors, J., & Kieler, H. (2012). Antipsychotics during pregnancy: Relation to fetal and maternal metabolic effects. *Archives of General Psychiatry, 69*(7), 715–721.

Brockington, I. F., Cernik, K. F., Schofield, E. M., Downing, A. R., Francis, A. F., & Keelan, C. (1981). Puerperal psychosis: Phenomena and diagnosis. *Archives of General Psychiatry, 38*(7), 829–833.

Brunner, E., Falk, D. M., Jones, M., Dey, D. K., & Shatapathy, C. C. (2013). Olanzapine in pregnancy and breastfeeding: A review of data from global safety surveillance. *BMC Pharmacology and Toxicology, 14*, 38.

Chaudron, L. H., & Pies, R. W. (2003). The relationship between postpartum psychosis and bipolar disorder: A review. *Journal of Clinical Psychiatry, 64*, 1284–1292.

Dean, J. C. S., Moore S. J., Osborne, A., Howe, J., Tumpenny, P. D. (1999). Fetal anticonvulsant syndrome and mutation in the maternal MTHFR gene. *Clinical Genetics, 56*, 216–220.

Grace, S. L., Evindar, A., & Stewart, D. E. (2003). The effect of postpartum depression on child cognitive development and behavior: A review and critical analysis of the literature. *Archives of Women's Mental Health, 6*(4), 263–274.

Hale, T. W., Rowe, H. E. (2014). *Medications and mother's milk 2014: A manual of lactational pharmacology.* Amarillo, TX: Hale.

Hernandez-Diaz, S., Werler, M. M., Walker, A. M., & Mitchell, A. A. (2001). Neural tube defects in relation to use of folic acid antagonists during pregnancy. *American Journal of Epidemiology, 153*, 961–968.

Kingston, D., Tough, S., & Whitfield, H. (2012). Prenatal and postpartum maternal psychological distress and infant development: A systematic review. *Child Psychiatry & Human Development, 43*(5), 683–714.

Kraepelin, E. (1921). *Manic-depressive insanity and paranoia.* Edinburgh, UK: E&S Livingstone.

Lovejoy, M. C., Graczyk, P. A., O'Hare, E., & Neuman, G. (2000). Maternal depression and parenting behavior: A meta-analytic review. *Clinical Psychology Review, 20*(5), 561–592.

Marcus, S. M. (2009). Depression during pregnancy: Rates, risks and consequences—Motherisk Update 2008. *Canadian Journal of Clinical Pharmacology, 16*(1), e15–e22.

Matalon, S., Schechtman, S., Goldzweig, G., & Ornoy, A. (2002). The teratogenic effect of carbamazepine: a meta-analysis of 1255 exposures. *Reproductive Toxicology, 16,* 9–17.

McKnight, R. F., Adida, M., Budge, K., Stockton, S., Goodwin, G. M., & Geddes, J. R. (2012). Lithium toxicity profile: A systematic review and meta-analysis. *Lancet, 379,* 721–728.

Meador, K. J., Baker, G. A., Browning, N., Cohen, M. J., Clayton-Smith, J., Kalayjian, L. A., Kanner, A., Liporace, J. D., Pennell, P. B., Privitera, M., Loring, D. W., NEAD Study Group. (2011). Foetal antiepileptic drug exposure and verbal versus non-verbal abilities at three years of age. *Brain, 134*(Pt 2), 396–404.

Moore, J. L., & Aggarwal, P. (2012). Lamotrigine use in pregnancy. *Expert Opinion on Pharmacotherapy, 13*(8), 1213–1216.

Newport, D. J., Calamaras, M. R., DeVane, C. L., Knight, B. T., Gibson, B. B., Viguera, A. C.,…Stowe, Z. N. (2007). Atypical antipsychotic administration during late pregnancy: Placental passage and obstetrical outcomes. *The American Journal of Psychiatry, 164,* 1214–1220.

Newport, D. J., Ji, S., Long, Q., Knight, B. T, Zach, E. B., Smith, E. N., & Stowe, Z. N. (2012). Maternal depression and anxiety differentially impact fetal exposures during pregnancy. *Journal of Clinical Psychiatry, 73*(2), 247–251.

Newport, D. J., Viguera, A. C., Beach, A. J., Ritchie, J. C., Cohen, L. S., & Stowe, Z. N. (2005). Lithium placental passage and obstetrical outcome: Implications for clinical management during late pregnancy. *The American Journal of Psychiatry, 162*(11), 2162–2170.

Palac, S., & Meador, K. J. (2011). Antiepileptic drugs and neurodevelopment: An update. *Current Neurology and Neuroscience Reports, 11*(4), 423–427.

Pennell, P. B., Peng, L., Newport, D. J., Ritchie, J. C., Koganti, A., Holley, D. K.,…Stowe, Z. N. (2008). Lamotrigine in pregnancy: Clearance, therapeutic drug monitoring, and seizure frequency. *Neurology, 70,* 2130–2136.

Schou, M. (1976). What happened later to the lithium babies? Follow-up study of children born without malformations. *Acta Psychiatrica Scandinavica, 54,* 193–197.

Viguera, A. C., Whitfield, T., Baldessarini, R. J., Newport, D. J., Stowe, Z., Reminick, A., & Cohen, L. S. (2007). Risk of recurrence in women with bipolar disorder during pregnancy: Prospective study of mood stabilizer discontinuation. *The American Journal of Psychiatry, 164*(12), 1817–1824.

Weissman, M. M., Wickramaratne, P., Nomura, Y., Warner, V., Pilowsky, D., & Verdeli, H. (2006). Offspring of depressed parents: 20 years later. *The American Journal of Psychiatry, 163*(6), 1001–1008.

PART VIII

CHILDREN AND ADOLESCENTS

39.

MANAGEMENT OF BIPOLAR DISORDER IN CHILDREN AND ADOLESCENTS

Luis R. Patino, Nina R. McCune, and Melissa P. DelBello

INTRODUCTION

The first step in treating children and adolescents with bipolar disorder is making an accurate diagnosis. This remains a significant challenge even for the most experienced clinicians. As established in previous chapters, there are still controversies regarding phenomenological presentation and the validity of applying adult-derived criteria to children and adolescents. Beyond establishing an accurate diagnosis, well-established developmental differences in the presentation between youth and adults further complicate the treatment and management (Axelson et al., 2006). One example is that adults exhibit distinct episodes of depression and mania, whereas the pattern of illness observed in young people is often characterized by mixed or dysphoric mood states accompanied by irritability (Chang, 2007). Moreover, children and adolescents seem to experience more symptomatic periods and may be more susceptible to rapid cycling (Geller et al., 2004). Most patients with pediatric bipolar disorder also have comorbid or co-occurring conditions, most commonly attention deficit hyperactivity disorder (ADHD; (Joshi & Wilens, 2009). Furthermore, there is a large gap between the data available regarding medication safety and efficacy in adults and children with bipolar disorder. There is growing evidence suggesting that merely extrapolating from adults is insufficient.

In the midst of the challenges of recognizing and managing bipolar disorder in children and adolescents, it is also clear that children and adolescents with bipolar disorder require prompt treatment to ameliorate symptoms and to prevent (or at least reduce) the psychosocial morbidity that accompanies the illness. In fact, early detection and treatment seems paramount since earlier onset and longer duration of illness is associated with poor rates of recovery (Birmaher et al., 2006).

Treatment of pediatric bipolar disorder requires a multimodal approach that includes pharmacologic and psychosocial interventions. Although medication is the cornerstone of any treatment approach, adjunctive psychosocial approaches are critical. This chapter reviews the empirical evidence available regarding the efficacy and safety for both pharmacological and psychosocial interventions for bipolar disorder in children and adolescents.[1]

EMPIRICAL EVIDENCE OF THE PHARMACOLOGICAL TREATMENT OF BIPOLAR DISORDER IN CHILDREN AND ADOLESCENTS WITH MANIC EPISODES

SECOND-GENERATION ANTIPSYCHOTICS

Aripiprazole

Aripiprazole is a second-generation antipsychotics with US Food and Drug Administration (FDA) approval for the treatment of mixed or manic mood episodes in patients age ≥10 years. Empirical evidence of the efficacy and safety of aripiprazole is available in several reports, including retrospective chart reviews (Barzman et al., 2004), open-label studies (Biederman, Mick, Spencer, Doyle, et al., 2007; Tramontina, Zeni, Pheula, de Souza, & Rohde, 2007), and two double-blind, placebo controlled trials (Findling et al., 2012; Tramontina et al., 2009). In both double-blind, placebo-controlled trials, aripiprazole was significantly superior to placebo in decreasing manic symptoms scores, response rates, and remission rates. Response rates were 44.8% in the 10-mg group (effect size $d = 0.46$), 63.6% in the 30-mg (effect size $d = 0.88$) group, and 88.9% in the flexible-dose (effect size $d = 1.1$) study. Remission was achieved by 25% of the 10-mg group (effect size $d = 0.97$), 47.5% of the patients in the 30-mg group (effect size $d = 1.52$), and in 72% of the patients in the flexible-dose study (effect size d = 0.94).

Common adverse events reported in these studies included sedation, gastrointestinal complaints, cold symptoms, headache, extrapyramidal symptoms, and akathisia.

Clozapine

There are no randomized, controlled trials of clozapine use in children and adolescents with bipolar disorder. The limited data regarding the utility of clozapine in pediatric bipolar disorder comes from three retrospective case series involving a pool of 27 cases (Kant et al., 2004; Kowatch, Suppes, & Gilfillin, 1995; Masi, Mucci, & Millepiedi, 2002). These reports suggest that clozapine may improve symptoms for adolescents with treatment-refractory manic or mixed episodes. However, data are limited, making it difficult to assess efficacy. Concerns regarding the use of clozapine stems from the association of clozapine with neutropenia and agranulocytosis (Idänpään-Heikkilä, Alhava, Olkinuora, & Palva, 1975). Other common side effects include hypersalivation, sedation, incontinence, weight gain, cardiac side effects such as electrocardiogram abnormalities (QT prolongation, orthostatic hypotension, tachycardia, and rarely endocarditis), abnormal electroencephalographic activity and/or lowered seizure threshold, akathisia, and metabolic changes. Due to the lack of evidence, clozapine should be reserved for use in patients who have demonstrated resistance to multiple other medication regimens.

Olanzapine

Olanzapine is currently FDA-approved for use for mania in adolescents age ≥13 years. The empirical evidence of olanzapine's efficacy in the treatment of children and adolescents with bipolar disorder in acute mania comes from four open-label studies (Biederman, Mick, Hammerness, et al., 2005; DelBello, Cecil, Adler, Daniels, & Strakowski, 2006; Frazier et al., 2001; Wozniak et al., 2009), and a randomized, double-blind, placebo-control clinical trial (Tohen et al., 2007). Response rates for olanzapine were 74%, 61%, 33%, and 47%, in the open-label studies. In the double-blind, placebo-controlled trial olanzapine proved to be superior to placebo with a response rate of 45% (vs. 22% for placebo) and a remission rate of 35% (vs. 11.1% for placebo).

Common side effects included sedation and appetite increase. However, weight gain and metabolic changes remain the most prominent concern of olanzapine use in children and adolescents. In the three-week period of the randomized, double-blind, placebo-controlled trial, subjects displayed a significantly higher weight gain than placebo. Specifically, adolescents increased an average of 4 kg, and 42% increased 7% or more from their baseline bodyweight. Subjects also displayed mean baseline-to-endpoint changes in prolactin, fasting glucose, fasting total cholesterol, uric acid, and the hepatic enzymes aspartate transaminase and alanine transaminase.

Age-related differences in weight gain and metabolic changes have been observed. Adolescents gained an average of 7.4 kg compared to 3.2 kg in adults. Children appear more sensitive to the prolactin-increasing effects of olanzapine (55.5%) than adults (29.0%). In contrast, adolescents had fewer adverse metabolic changes than adults, with 3% of young and 11.8% of older patients moving from normal or impaired glucose to high blood glucose, and 17% to 21% of adolescents compared to 31% to 38% of adults developing borderline dyslipidemias (Singh, Ketterm, & Chang, 2010).

Paliperidone

To date there are limited data regarding the efficacy and safety of paliperidone in the treatment of acute mania in youth. An eight-week open-label study examined paliperidone monotherapy for acute manic, mixed, or hypomanic episode in pediatric patients ($n = 15$; 6–17 years of age) with bipolar spectrum disorders (Joshi et al., 2013). At the end of follow-up period, 11 subjects (73%) completed the study; treatment with paliperidone was associated with a 60% response rate (50% decrease in the Young Mania Rating Scale [YMRS]) and 40% remission (YMRS <12). However, treatment with paliperidone was associated with an increase in body weight (mean increase 2 kg ± 2.5 kg), and in total 40% of subjects developed clinically significant weight gain following paliperidone trial (≥7% weight gain).

Quetiapine

Quetiapine is approved by the FDA for manic episodes as monotherapy or adjunctive therapy in bipolar youth (age > 10 years). Quetiapine was shown to be safe and effective in children and adolescents with mania in retrospective chart reviews (Marchand, Wirth, & Simon, 2004), at least two open-label studies (Duffy, Milin, & Grof, 2009; Joshi et al., 2012), and three randomized, controlled studies

(DelBello, Kowatch, Adler, Stanford, Welge, Barzman, Nelson, Strakowski, 2006; DelBello, Schwiers, Rosenberg, & Strakowski, 2002; Pathak et al., 2013). Quetiapine has shown to be effective in reducing manic symptoms and maintaining stabilization through 48 weeks (Duffy et al., 2009). In randomized, controlled trails, quetiapine was shown to be superior to valproate combined with placebo (DelBello et al., 2002), superior to valproate as monotherapy (DelBello, Kowatch, Adler, Stanford, Welge, Barzman, Nelson, Strakowski, 2006), and superior to placebo as monotherapy (Pathak et al., 2013). Response rates for quetiapine in these studies ranged from 58% to 87%. Treatment with quetiapine revealed a statistically significant separation from placebo within the first week of treatment (Pathak et al., 2013). Adverse events associated with quetiapine were mostly mild to moderate in intensity and were broadly consistent with the known profile of quetiapine in adults with bipolar disorder (Fraguas et al., 2011). More commonly sedation, gastrointestinal upset, and weight gain were reported. Weight increase for quetiapine was on average 1.7kg in three weeks and 3.4 kg in eight weeks. None of these studies reported statistically significant differences in metabolic parameters.

Youth with bipolar disorder tolerate a rapid titration with quetiapine starting at 100 mg and increasing by 100 mg a day to a target dose of 400–600 mg (Scheffer, Tripathi, Kirkpatrick, & Schultz, 2010). Of note, the half-life for quetiapine may be significantly shorter in pediatric patients compared to adults (3 hours vs. 6 hours); an extended-release formulation of quetiapine is available, albeit no studies have established that it yields additional benefits over the immediate-release formulation (Findling et al., 2006).

Risperidone

Risperidone was the first second-generation antipsychotic approved by the FDA for a psychiatric disorder in youth (originally for the treatment of irritability associated with autistic disorder in children and adolescents age 5–16 years). Later on, this SGA received approval for the treatment of acute manic or mixed episodes in youth. Evidence of its efficacy in pediatric bipolar disorder comes from three open-label studies (Biederman, Mick, Wozniak, et al., 2005; Pavuluri, Henry, et al., 2004, 2006), one retrospective chart review (Frazier et al., 1999) and a randomized, double-blind, placebo-controlled trial (Haas et al., 2009). Subjects in the randomized, double-blind, placebo-controlled trial were assigned to either low-dosage (0.5–2.5 mg/day) or high-dosage (3.0–6.0 mg/day)

risperidone or placebo. In both active medication groups, treatment with risperidone significantly decreased manic symptom. Response rates in the low-dose (59%) and high-dose (63%) groups were superior to placebo (26%). There was a dose-dependent increase in the frequency of side effects. The results of this study suggest that low-dosage risperidone is just as effective as larger dosages but better tolerated.

Additionally, risperidone has been compared to valproate in two head-to-head randomized, double-blind trials (Geller et al., 2012; Pavuluri et al., 2010) and one with lithium (Geller et al., 2012). Risperidone was shown to be superior to both valproate and lithium in achieving response and in remission rates. It has also been shown to be effective as augmentation therapy in lithium nonresponders (Pavuluri et al., 2006).

Side-effect profile of risperidone in youth is similar to those in adults. Most commonly, risperidone is associated with fatigue, dizziness, dystonia, Parkinsonian symptoms, akathisia, abdominal pain, dyspepsia, nausea, vomiting, and diarrhea. Risperidone has also been associated with weight gain, diabetes, and hyperprolactinemia in pediatric populations. Special care should be taken about the possibility of hyperprolactinemia in pediatric populations since this adverse effect might affect bone development and bring about undesirable menstrual abnormalities (Fraguas et al., 2011).

Ziprasidone

Recent studies of ziprasidone support its use in pediatric bipolar disorder (Biederman, Mick, Spencer, Dougherty, et al., 2007; DelBello, Versavel, Ice, Keller, & Miceli, 2008; Findling, Cavuş, Pappadopulos, Vanderburg, Schwartz, Gundapaneni, DelBello, 2013). In an eight-week open-label study, ziprasidone was evaluated as monotherapy in 21 patients (age 6–17 years) with significant manic symptoms; this study found a response rate of 33% with a drop-out rate of 33% (DelBello et al., 2008). A larger (n = 237) four-week double-blind, placebo-controlled study of ziprasidone in pediatric mania revealed that subjects treated with ziprasidone improved significantly compared to those treated with placebo Findling, Cavuş, Pappadopulos, Vanderburg, Schwartz, Gundapaneni, DelBello (2013). Separation of ziprasidone from placebo reached statistical significance as early as Week 1, and the overall response rate was 53% (22% in placebo arm). An important finding in this study was that subjects weighing less than 45 kg did not show a significant improvement compared to placebo.

Ziprasidone is well tolerated in children and adolescents, with no significant weight increases or metabolic changes. The most commonly occurring adverse effects (i.e., sedation, dizziness, and somnolence) were similar to what has been reported in adults. Although QTc prolongations have been noted with ziprasidone use, they are typically minimal and not clinically significant (Correll et al., 2011; Findling et al., 2013).

Ziprasidone is available in both oral and short-acting intramuscular forms. Oral administration without food significantly decreases its absorption (Sallee et al., 2006). Ziprasidone appears to have a lower risk of being associated with metabolic syndrome than the other SGA and may be a more appropriate agent for patients who appear to be at risk of developing metabolic syndrome or those who already suffer from it.

Ziprasidone has recently been approved in Europe for the treatment of moderately manic or mixed episodes associated with bipolar disorder in children and adolescents age 10–17 to years.

LITHIUM

Lithium salts have been used since the late 19th century, initially as part of popular tonics such as the "Bib-Label Lithiated Lemon-Lime Soda," better known under the name of 7UP. The first publication of lithium's use in adults with bipolar disorder dates back more than 60 years ago (Cade, 1949) and studies of lithium use in psychiatrically ill children started to emerge in the medical literature 50 years ago (van Krevelen & van Voorst, 1959). However, given the historical difficulties in diagnostic consensus for pediatric bipolar disorder, initial reports of its use in pediatric population are characterized by a clinically heterogeneous group. The first publication of lithium use in children appeared in 1959; van Krevelen and van Voorst describe the successful treatment of 14-year-old boy who suffered from "periodic psychosis with longer manic and shorter depressive phases"; several case reports and case series that included a mix of patients with and without potential bipolar disorder followed thereafter. In the late 1970s and early 1980s a handful of double-blind, placebo-controlled, randomized, cross-over trials in children and adolescents tested lithium's use in patients with a mélange of vaguely defined clinical syndromes that may or may not have been pediatric bipolar disorder (i.e. "severely hyperactive children with mood swings"; Greenhill, Rieder, Wender, Buchsbaum, & Zhan, 1973; "episodic mood and behavior disturbance"; Lena, Surtees, & Maggs, 1978; "behaviorally disordered children of parents who are lithium responders"; McKnew

et al., 1981). Although many of these studies yielded positive results, the diagnostic ambiguity limits the conclusions that can be drawn. Despite the limited data, the FDA approved lithium for the treatment of mania in children 12 years and older.

More recent open-label studies, with more homogeneously defined diagnostic criteria, have suggested that patients treated with lithium achieve a response rate between 38% and 55% as monotherapy and 82% when used in combination with SGAs (e.g., risperidone; Geller et al., 2012; Kowatch et al., 2000; Pavuluri et al., 2006). In an open-label lithium study of 100 adolescents (12–18 years of age) with an acute manic episode, 63% achieved response and 26% remission (Kafantaris, Coletti, Dicker, Padula, & Kane, 2003). Furthermore, in a double-blind, randomized, placebo-controlled discontinuation study, 62% of patients who initially responded to lithium and switched to placebo experienced clinically significant exacerbation of symptoms, while 53% of those who responded and remained on lithium had symptomatic relapse; this difference was not statistically significant (Kafantaris et al., 2004).

Recently, the multisite Collaborative Lithium Trials (CoLT) developed protocols aimed at (a) establishing evidence-based dosing strategies for lithium, (b) characterizing the pharmacokinetics and biodisposition of lithium, (c) examining the acute efficacy of lithium in pediatric bipolar disorder, (d) investigating the long-term effectiveness of lithium treatment, and (e) characterizing the short- and long-term safety of lithium. In December of 2006, enrollment into the first of these studies began across seven sites. Updates on CoLT indicate a 58% response rate to lithium as monotherapy in the eight-week open-label phase for acute mania (ClinicalTrials.gov identifiers: NCT01166425 and NCT00442039; Findling et al., 2013). Furthermore, patients in this trial that displayed at least a partial response to 8 weeks of open-label treatment with lithium were eligible to receive open-label lithium for an additional 16 weeks. In this continuation postacute phase, 68.3% of patients met a priori criteria for response, with 53.7% considered to be in remission. These data suggest that patients who initially responded to lithium maintained mood stabilization during continuation treatment, but partial responders did not experience further improvement. Results from CoLT's randomized, double-blind, placebo-controlled trial are still pending.

Furthermore, there is some evidence suggesting that lithium response may run in families (Duffy et al., 2002) and that lithium may be particularly effective in preventing suicidal behavior (Cipriani, Hawton, Stockton, & Geddes, 2013; Cipriani, Pretty, Hawton & Geddes, 2005).

Common adverse effects associated with lithium include nausea, headache, acne, weight gain, thyroid dysfunction, diabetes insipidus, and tremor. Baseline complete blood counts, thyroid panels, blood urea nitrogen, creatinine, serum calcium, urinalysis, and pregnancy test are recommended prior to initiation of lithium, as well as every three to six months thereafter.

ANTIEPILEPTIC MEDICATIONS

Carbamazepine

Despite its track record in adults, carbamazepine has been studied in only a few open-label trials in youth with bipolar disorder. A six-week open-label comparison of carbamazepine with valproate and lithium showed a modest response rate of 38% for carbamazepine, 38% for lithium, and 53% for valproate; these differences were statistically not significant (Kowatch et al., 2000). Another open-label study evaluated carbamazepine extended release and showed a similar response rate of 44% (Joshi et al., 2010). To date there are no double-blind, randomized, placebo-controlled trials of carbamazepine for the treatment of pediatric bipolar disorder.

The most common adverse events with carbamazepine include nausea and sedation (Evans, Clay, & Gualtieri 1987). A baseline complete blood count and follow-up measurements should be obtained since carbamazepine has been associated with agranulocytosis and aplastic anemia (Seetharam & Pellock, 1991) In addition, carbamazepine carries a risk of Stevens-Johnson syndrome in patients of Asian ancestry; therefore, it is recommended that such patients should be screened for the HLA-B* 1502 allele, which has been associated with an increased risk of developing this syndrome (Chong et al., 2013).

Oxcarbazepine

Despite initial case reports that hinted at oxcarbazepine's positive tolerability and its effect in treatment of pediatric mania (Davanzo et al., 2004; Teitelbaum, 2001), its efficacy has not been proven in controlled studies. In a double-blind, placebo-controlled trial, no significant difference between oxcarbazepine and placebo was detected in any of the efficacy measures. Remarkably, the study had a very high dropout rate (66% oxcarbazepine and 60% placebo). There were more adverse events in the oxcarbazepine group, including dizziness, nausea, somnolence, diplopia, fatigue, and rash (Wagner et al., 2006).

Topiramate

There are limited data available for the use of topiramate in pediatric acute mania. Although studies in adults do not support efficacy of topiramate as monotherapy in acute mania or mixed episodes (Kushner, Khan, Lane, & Olson, 2006), there are some data to suggest that topiramate might have some effect on pediatric mania. Two retrospective studies suggested that adjunctive topiramate reduces the severity of bipolar mania in pediatric patients in both inpatients and outpatients (Barzman et al., 2005; DelBello et al., 2002). A four-week, double-blind, placebo-controlled trial of topiramate in pediatric mania was conducted but was prematurely terminated by the sponsor based on negative results in adults (DelBello et al., 2005). This study showed at least a statistically significant steeper slope of improvement in the topiramate group, tentatively suggesting that improvement may have been more rapid in this group. Common adverse effects reported in these studies included decreased appetite, nausea, and weight loss.

Topiramate use has also been explored in preventing weight gain associated with certain SGAs. An eight-week open-label study of olanzapine monotherapy compared to olanzapine plus topiramate showed that both treatments were capable of reducing symptom scores and that those patients with topiramate plus olanzapine combination had lower weight gain than the group only treated with olanzapine (Wozniak et al., 2009). Of caution, there is at least one case report of hyperthermia and rhabdomyolysis in a 14-year-old patient with the combination of olanzapine and topiramate (Strawn, Adler, Strakowski, & DelBello, 2008).

Lamotrigine

There have been only two open-label studies of lamotrigine monotherapy in pediatric acute mania (Biederman et al., 2010; Pavuluri et al., 2009). In an open-label 14-week study, 46 children (age 6–17 years) received lamotrigine, which was slowly uptitrated for eight weeks. In this study, lamotrigine appeared to be effective in maintaining symptom control of manic symptoms in pediatric bipolar disorder with a response rate of 72% and a remission rate of 56%. In another open-label study, lamotrigine was found to produce a response rate of 54%. Common adverse effects reported in this study included gastrointestinal symptoms, headaches, and skin rashes. A serious concern found lamotrigine use to be related to Stevens-Johnson syndrome. Of note, in the two pediatric studies mentioned, report rates differed slightly. In one study a benign rash was noted in 6.4% of patients (Pavuluri et al., 2009), while in the other study 38% of patients developed some form of skin reaction; of these, six required the medication be stopped and none were reported to have developed Stevens-Johnson syndrome (Biederman et al., 2010).

Valproate

Despite traditionally being considered a first-line agent, recent data suggest that valproate may be less effective than SGAs when used for the treatment of pediatric mania. Several open-label studies have evaluated the effectiveness of valproate in pediatric patients with bipolar disorder; these studies indicated response rate for valproate was between 53% to 75% (Papatheodorou et al., 1995; Wagner et al., 2002; West et al., 1994).

However, more recent reports have come to question the overall efficacy of valproate in the treatment of acute mania in pediatric bipolar disorder. Three double-blind studies of valproate sodium exemplify these questions. One study compared valproate immediate release against quetiapine and showed that quetiapine was markedly superior to valproate (DelBello, Kowatch, Adler, Stanford, Welge, Barzman, Nelson, Strakowski,2006). Patients receiving quetiapine showed larger mania response (84% vs. 56% $p < .05$) and manic remission rates (60% vs. 28%).

A second study suggested risperidone is superior and better tolerated than valproate (Pavuluri et al., 2010). In this double-blind, randomized trial, risperidone showed superior response (78.1% for risperidone vs. 45.5% for valproate, $p < .01$) and remission rates (62.5% vs. 33.3%, $p < .05$). Also, subjects in the valproate group had higher drop-out due to adverse events (48% vs. 24%), with irritability being the most common reported cause).

The third double-blinded study failed to separate valproate extended release from placebo (Wagner et al., 2009). In this well-powered study, no significant differences in YMRS change from baseline, nor response (24% vs. 23%) or remission rates (16% vs. 19%), were detected between placebo and valproate.

Common side effects of valproate include gastrointestinal symptoms, sedation, and weight gain. Pancreatitis, hepatotoxicity, alopecia, thrombocytopenia, and polycystic ovary syndrome have also been associated with this medication. Recommendations for laboratory monitoring include obtaining complete blood counts, liver function tests, and pregnancy screening at baseline and every six months thereafter, as well as careful monitoring of menstrual cycles in girls who are prescribed valproate sodium.

SUMMARY

Data regarding efficacy of pharmacologic agents for the treatment of acute mania in youth is scarce, compared to the findings available for adults with mania. However, data is slowly accumulating with new studies being published in peer-reviewed journals. Election of a pharmacological agent to treat an acute manic episode should take into consideration the available empirical evidence suggesting its efficacy and also balance the latent harm

Table 39.1. EFFICACY MEASURES OF ANTIPSYCHOTICS AND MOOD STABILIZERS VERSUS PLACEBO IN CONTROLLED TRIALS IN PEDIATRIC PATIENTS WITH BIPOLAR I DISORDER

	YMRS	RESPONSE[a]	REMISSION[b]
	ES 95%CI	NNT 95%CI	NNT 95%CI
Aripiprazole	0.69 (0.44–0.94)	3.6 (2.6–5.9)	3.2 (2.5–4.3)
Olanzapine	0.75 (0.41–1.08)	3.8 (2.4–8.5)	4.1 (2.7–8.3)
Quetiapine	0.60 (0.35–0.86)	4.2 (2.8–8.4)	4.2 (3.1–11.0)
Risperidone	0.81 (0.48–1.14)	2.8 (2.0–5.1)	3.7 (2.4–6.8)
Ziprasidone	0.48 (0.21–0.76)	3.8 (2.5–7.5)	N/A
Divalproex	0.28 (0.01–0.54)	7.4 (3.9–82.7)	N/A
Lithium	0.31 (0.12–0.73)	8.4 (3.1–12.5)	N/A

NOTE: YMRS = Young Mania Rating Scale; ES = effect size; CI = confidence interval; NNT = number needed to treat

[a] Response defined as ≥50% reduction in YMRS.

[b] Remission defined as YMRS ≤ 12.

Table 39.2. SUMMARY OF SIDE EFFECT PROFILE MEASURES OF SECOND-GENERATION ANTIPSYCHOTICS IN THE TREATMENT OF BIPOLAR DISORDER

	SOMNOLENCE	AKATHISIA	EXTRAPIRAMIDAL SIDE EFFECTS	WEIGHT GAIN	>7% WEIGHT GAIN
	NNH (95% CI)	NNH (95% CI)	NNH (95% CI)	ES (95% CI)	NNH (95% CI)
Aripiprazole	5.1 (3.8–7.7)	13.3 (7.9–37.6)	4.1	0.17 (0–0.4)	27.8 (–37–11)
Olanzapine	4.6 (3.2–8.4)	107.5 (N/A)	N/A	1.65 (1.3–2.6)	2.5 (2.0–3.3)
Quetiapine	5.0 (3.4–9.0)	(N/A)	38.5	0.63 (0.4–0.8)	8.2 (6.1–13.6)
Risperidone	3.3 (2.3–6.3)	8.7 (5.0–47.0)	8.7	0.46 (0.1–0.8)	14.7 (–58–6.8)
Ziprasidone	5.9 (3.9–12.6)	N/A	N/A	–0.04 (0.3–0.2)	46.1

NOTE: CI = confidence interval; NNH = number needed to harm.

induced by the potential side effects. Tables 39.1 and 39.2 offer a summary of the available data. Overall, SGAs seem to be more effective than lithium and mood stabilizers for acute mania in children and adolescents with bipolar disorder. Indeed, two recent meta-analysis determined that SGAs are more effective than lithium and mood stabilizers when considering effect sizes, likelihood of achieving remission, and number needed to treat (Correll, Sheridan, DelBello, 2010; Liu et al., 2011). In the near future, results from ongoing pediatric mania studies of medications that have been previously shown to be effective for mania in adults may become available (e.g., asenepine, tamoxifen). Still, research and data collection on those pharmacological agents already available should not be abandoned so that definite recommendations can ultimately be made.

EMPIRICAL EVIDENCE OF THE PHARMACOLOGICAL TREATMENT OF BIPOLAR DEPRESSION IN CHILDREN AND ADOLESCENTS

Youth with bipolar disorder may experience full depressive episodes or subsyndromal depressive symptomatology. Overall, as in adults, depression in children and adolescents with a bipolar spectrum disorder is a primary source of burden; youth suffering from bipolar disorders spend nearly 40% of the time with impairing depressive symptoms (Geller et al., 2004). Furthermore, prospective studies have demonstrated that after remitting from a manic episode, children and adolescents may be more likely to relapse into a major depressive episode than into hypomanic, manic, or mixed episodes (Birmaher, Axelson, & Goldstein, 2009). Unfortunately, there is a paucity of controlled data regarding pharmacotherapy for depression among youth with bipolar disorder.

OLANZAPINE/FLUOXETINE COMBINATION

An eight-week randomized, double-blind, placebo-controlled trial involving 255 children ages 10 to 17 years (170 olanzapine/fluoxetine combination [OFC], 85 placebo) evaluated the efficacy of this combination strategy in patients with bipolar depression. On average patients in active treatment showed a significantly larger decrease in symptomatology (–28 vs. –23, $p = .003$), a larger proportion of them achieved remission (59% vs. 43%, $p = .03$) and response (78% vs. 59%, $p = .003$). There was no difference in treatment-emergent suicidal ideation/behavior and on worsening of manic symptoms between placebo and OFC. Roughly 20% of participants in the OFC treatment arm had weight gain (on average slightly more than 4 kg), and they experienced worsening of fasting cholesterol and triglycerides. To date OFC is the only FDA-approved treatment for bipolar depression in children and adolescents (ClinicalTrials.gov identifier NCT00844857).

LITHIUM

Lithium has an established efficacy in adults with bipolar disorder and in treatment-resistant depression. However, to date the only published study exploring lithium efficacy is an open-label study conducted in 27 adolescents with bipolar depression (Patel et al., 2006). This study showed a rather large effect size ($d = 1.7$), a response rate of 48%, and a remission of 30%. Lithium was well tolerated and did not lead to an abnormally high attrition rate. More studies exploring lithium's efficacy are needed to confirm its robust properties in pediatric bipolar depression.

LAMOTRIGINE

Lamotrigine has emerged as a first-line agent for adult bipolar depression. In pediatric bipolar depression, several case reports describe successful use of lamotrigine for periods of up to eight months (Bildik et al., 2006; Soutullo, Diez-Suarez, & Figueroa-Quintana, 2006). Also, in a study of 46 adolescents with manic or mixed episodes, lamotrigine successfully reduced depressive symptoms during the study's maintenance phase (Pavuluri et al., 2009). In an open-label study of depressed adolescents with a pediatric bipolar spectrum disorders diagnosis, lamotrigine as monotherapy or adjunctive therapy (mean dose of 131 ± 31 mg/day) was well tolerated and resulted in a response rate of 63% and a remission rate of 58% (Chang, Saxena, & Howe, 2006).

QUETIAPINE

Quetiapine is a well-established treatment for adults with bipolar depression; however, in a double-blind, placebo-controlled, randomized clinical trial in adolescents with bipolar depression, response rates did not differ from placebo (DelBello et al., 2009). This was a small study of 32 adolescents conducted in two sites. Quetiapine seemed to be well tolerated with some reports of mild gastrointestinal side effects and increased levels of triglycerides. The response rate in this study was 71% for quetiapine and 67% for placebo (difference was not statistically significant). In another large, double-blind, placebo-controlled, randomized clinical trial of 193 youths with bipolar depression, subjects on quetiapine displayed a 63% response rate, while those on placebo showed a 55% response rate; the difference was not statistically significant (ClinicalTrials.gov identifier NCT00811473).

High placebo responses are not uncommon in pediatric depression studies, which may imply the need for different designs like placebo or psychosocial lead-in designs (Cohen et al., 2010).

ANTIDEPRESSANTS

Antidepressants are effective and well tolerated for the treatment of unipolar depression in children and adolescents (Henry, Kisicki, & Varley, 2012); however, their use in bipolar depression has not been thoroughly examined. In fact, their role in depressed adults with bipolar disorder remains unclear; two meta-analyses suggest divergent findings regarding their efficacy and ability to induce manic episodes (Gijsman, Geddes, Rendell, Nolen, & Goodwin, 2004; Sidor & Macqueen, 2011). Much less empirical data is available in children and adolescents. Retrospective chart reviews suggest the use of antidepressants may be effective; however, those on antidepressants were three times more likely to develop treatment-emergent mania (Thomas, Stansifer, & Findling, 2011).

The risk of potentially inducing mania as a result of treatment with selective serotonin reuptake inhibitors (SSRIs) or other antidepressants must be weighed against the potential therapeutic benefits, as well as the very real suicide risk that often accompanies severe depression. Given the scarce data available, caution is indicated when considering the use of antidepressants in depressed patients with bipolar disorder.

SUMMARY

OFC to date is the only FDA-approved treatment for bipolar depression in children and adolescents; hence it is an obvious first option. However, a careful consideration of the potential side effects should be examined. Both lithium and lamotrigine have shown to be feasible options in the treatment of pediatric bipolar depression. However, double-blind, placebo-controlled trials for both these medications are needed to give a definite recommendation. On the other hand, quetiapine failed to separate from placebo on a randomized, double-blind, placebo-controlled study; however, given its track record with adult bipolar depression and the fact that in that study there was a large placebo response, its use cannot be entirely discarded, but clinicians who might consider its use should take note of these findings. Antidepressants can be considered an option only after carefully considering the risks of treatment-emergent mania and after other options have been explored. Given the high response rates and the evidence of its efficacy in unipolar depression, psychosocial intervention, particularly those with a cognitive-behavioral component, should be considered. In fact, in certain cases, particularly those with milder depression, psychosocial intervention may be the first-line option for pediatric bipolar depression.

TREATMENT-RESISTANT BIPOLAR DISORDER

Despite documented efficacy of several pharmacological agents in the treatment of bipolar disorder in children and adolescents, empirical evidence shows that a substantial proportion of patients fail to achieve an adequate response or remission of symptoms. Indeed, longitudinal studies suggest pediatric bipolar disorder is associated with a more prolonged and treatment-refractory course, more subsyndromal interepisodic symptoms, and reduced interepisode recovery compared to adults with mania (Geller et al., 2004). Given these factors, children and adolescents are at an increased risk of receiving polypharmacy or to continue to suffer functional impairment from persistent clinically significant symptoms (Toteja et al., 2013).

When evaluating patients with persistent mood symptoms, it may be instructive to consider whether symptoms persist as a result of inadequate response to treatment or as an expected response to inadequate treatment. For this reason, our experience suggests that a set of steps should be taken when evaluating children and adolescents with bipolar disorder and a poor treatment response.

1. Assess whether the patient was been *adequately evaluated* and whether the diagnosis is accurate. The use of semistructured (e.g., Kiddie Schedule for Affective Disorders and Schizophrenia; Chambers et al., 1985) or structured (i.e., Mini International Neuropsychiatry Interview for Children; Sheehan et al., 2010) diagnostic interviews are useful resources not only in the research setting but also as a tool clinicians can use to verify patients meet criteria for bipolar disorder and evaluate comorbid conditions and/ or that the symptoms are not better accounted by other conditions (i.e., medical conditions, substance induced). Obtaining baseline measures of symptom frequency and intensity is of paramount importance when evaluating whether or not the patient is responding to treatment. Standard rating scales (i.e. YMRS, Children Depression Rating Scale–Revised) can help quantify improvement (Ponzanski & Mokros, 1996; Young, Biggs, Ziegler, & Meyer, 1978).

2. A common source of treatment nonresponse is *poor medication compliance*. In an observational study, adolescent self-reports revealed that only about one-third of patients (34%) were fully compliant (Coletti, Leigh, Gallelli, & Kafantaris, 2005). Evaluating patient's adherence to treatment is essential before assuming a patient is treatment resistant. Multisource information and an open, nonjudgmental conversation with the patient is a good starting point. Several psychosocial interventions (see later) utilize psychoeducational elements aimed at improving adherence to treatment and should be considered when clinicians suspect medication adherence is a problem.

3. Consider *discontinuation of potential destabilizing elements*. Antidepressants are commonly used in pediatric patients with bipolar disorder. Studies suggest that antidepressants are at least poorly tolerated, can induce manic symptoms, or can lead to rapid cycling (Biederman, Mick, Spencer, Wilens, & Faraone, 2000; Strawn et al., 2013). Carefully evaluating the necessity of antidepressant use should be an important step in the evaluation of patients who have been nonresponsive to treatment.

Discontinuing GABAergic medications like benzodiazepines, gabapentin, pregabalin, and zolpidem may be helpful in this group of patients. Although GABA-ergic agents may temporarily be useful in select circumstances and patients, continued use in children and adolescents may induce disinhibition symptoms (Barnett & Riddle, 2003).

Moreover, given the frequency of comorbid ADHD, the use of stimulants in patients with bipolar disorder is frequent. The use of stimulants in patients at risk for bipolar disorder may also be problematic (Faedda, Baldessarini, Glovinsky, & Austin, 2004). Specifics about the treatment of comorbid ADHD are discussed later.

Substance use, even if not at a level of dependence or abuse, has generally been associated with poor treatment compliance and mood destabilization (DelBello et al., 2007; Lagerberg et al., 2010; Strakowski et al., 2007). Evaluating substance use in adolescents is of vital importance. Epidemiological studies show that at least 25% of adolescents (age 12–17 years) have experimented with psychotropic substances, and, of those subjects, 32% consume it regularly without meeting criteria for a substance use disorder (Fryar, Merino, Hirsch, & Porter, 2009). Adolescents with bipolar disorder are five times more likely to consume psychotropic substances and develop a substance use disorder than healthy comparison subjects (Wilens et al., 1999; Wilens et al., 2004).

4. Conduct an *evaluation of treatment history and ensure optimization of current medication*. Often, subtherapeutic doses are erroneously prescribed for pediatric patients or trials are too short lived (Scheffer, Tripathi, Kirkpatrick, & Schultz, 2011); when evaluating patients that have "failed to respond" an accurate history of previous medication doses and duration of treatment is of extreme importance. When assessing nonresponse to current treatment regime, it is essential to optimize pharmacologic agents as much as patients can tolerate them, making sure they are within the therapeutic window. In patients treated with lithium and/ or valproate, serum guidelines showed be followed; with other agents recommended dosage range should be reached (Kowatch et al., 2005).

5. *Attempt to use the minimal amount of medications* at any given time, ensuring they are given at an adequate dose and for a reasonable duration of time. Although monotherapy is optimal, unfortunately a modest polypharmacy is usually the norm.

COMBINATION TREATMENTS

A handful of studies have empirically evaluated combination treatments; however, they comprise a mixture of acute mania studies and continuation/maintenance treatment studies. There have been eight studies evaluating combination therapy: six open-label and two double-blind studies. These studies have evaluated mainly the combination of SGA with mood stabilizers.

A study comparing quetiapine with valproate to valproate alone (DelBello et al., 2002) found that response rates were higher in the combination group compared to monotherapy (87% vs. 53%). However, subjects in the combination gained more weight (4.2 ± 3.2 kg vs. 2.5 ± 2.1 kg).

The combination of risperidone and lithium has been tested in two studies. In one study subjects received a combination of risperidone plus lithium or valproate (Pavuluri, Henry, et al., 2004). The other study was a one-year open-label study for subjects who did not respond adequately to eight weeks of lithium monotherapy (Pavuluri et al., 2006). Patients on risperidone plus lithium combination achieved an average response rate of 84% and a remission rate of 60%. Overall, weight gain was significant in this combination strategy and dropout rates were high (approximately 35%).

An eight-week open-label study compared olanzapine monotherapy with the combination of olanzapine and topiramate in youths with pediatric bipolar disorders in mixed or manic episodes (Wozniak et al., 2009). The combination of topiramate and olanzapine was associated with less weight gain but not with greater symptom improvement compared to olanzapine monotherapy.

The combination of lithium and valproate has been examined in an open-label trial (N = 90), in a 20-week period in youth with pediatric bipolar disorder and a manic or hypomanic episode within the three months preceding enrollment (Findling, McNamara, et al., 2003). There was a significant reduction in manic and depressive symptoms at Week 8 and at the end of the study, and 47% met criteria for clinical remission. However, in this study the concomitant use of antipsychotics was allowed if needed and subjects who had experienced a manic episode while on therapeutic lithium or valproate levels were excluded; this likely enhanced the sample for treatment responsiveness.

The empirical evidence seems to support the use of combination therapy when monotherapy is unsuccessful; however, a paucity of data precludes a definite recommendation. Polypharmacy, despite the fact that it might be very prevalent, should be addressed with caution. The use of multiple pharmacological agents increases the likelihood of adverse events that may be a factor affecting treatment adherence. As stated earlier, an adequate evaluation of treatment history and adherence is paramount. In those selected patients who are truly treatment resistant, a combination of two antimanic agents may be warranted.

PSYCHOSOCIAL INTERVENTIONS IN THE TREATMENT OF BIPOLAR DISORDER

The development of bipolar disorder during childhood or adolescence disrupts ongoing developmental processes, including academic, social, and family functioning. Therefore, a comprehensive, multimodal treatment approach that combines psychopharmacology with adjunctive psychosocial therapies is almost always indicated for children and adolescents with bipolar disorder (McClellan, Kowatch, & Findling, 2007). However, there is little research on how psychosocial treatment used in conjunction with medication might enhance treatment, prevent poor outcomes, and improve the quality of life for patients and their families.

Many therapeutic elements are common across treatments, such as the central role of psychoeducation for the family and affect regulation for the child (Weinstein, West, & Pavuluri, 2013). Although the existing treatments are in differing stages of empirical validation, they nonetheless assist with delineating the features that are critical to the effective multimodal treatment of pediatric bipolar disorder (Miklowitz, 2006).

MULTIFAMILY PSYCHOEDUCATION GROUPS

Multifamily psychoeducation groups (MFPG) consist of eight 90-minute group sessions that occur separately but simultaneously for parents and children (Fristad, Goldberg-Arnold, & Gavazzi, 2002). The treatment is highly structured, with the specific content and skills to be practiced and outlined for each session. The goals of MFPG include teaching children and parents about the patient's illness, its treatment, symptom management, and also improving problem-solving and communications skills. This psychosocial intervention offers direct education to parents in how to become more involved with their child's treatment and serve as an effective advocate. It also teaches coping skills for children through the identification of pleasant and relaxing activities in four categories (creative, physical, social, and relaxing) that can be used to combat negative emotional states. Participants of MFPG receive support, both from other group members and from professionals who understand the disorder. The MFPG intervention has been empirically tested in a randomized, control-comparing treatment as usual (TAU) plus MFPG with TAU + waiting list control (Fristad et al., 2009). This study involved 165 children, 70% of whom had a bipolar spectrum diagnosis. Children receiving MFPG + TAU had a significant improvement in mood symptom severity compared with waiting list control + TAU over one-year follow-up.

FAMILY-FOCUSED TREATMENT FOR ADOLESCENTS

Family-focused therapy (FFT), a treatment originally developed for adults with bipolar disorder, has been adapted by Miklowitz and colleagues (2000) for use with adolescents (FFT-A). The FFT-A intervention lasts nine months and consists of 21 (12 weekly, 6 biweekly, and 3 monthly) 50-minute sessions. This treatment involves the parents, any available siblings, and the adolescent with bipolar disorder. The goal of FFT-A is to reduce symptoms through the development of an increased awareness of how to cope with the disorder, promote a reduction in the levels of expressed emotion from caregivers, and foster the family's problem-solving and communication skills. FFT-A relies on three main treatment components: psychoeducation, communication enhancement training, and problem-solving skills training. The psychoeducation component focuses on the family developing a common understanding of the symptoms, etiology, and course of the disorder. The communication enhancement training component includes role-playing and rehearsal to assist with the development of skills for active listening, providing positive feedback, delivering constructive criticism, or requesting changes in another person's behavior. Finally, the problem-solving component involves teaching participants how to identify problems in daily life, generate solutions, and implement those solutions.

Evidence of FFT-A's efficacy comes from a two-site randomized, control trial with a two-year follow up (Miklowitz et al., 2008). Adolescents with bipolar spectrum disorders ($n = 58$) were randomized to receive FFT-A in combination

with regular pharmacotherapy or enhanced care and regular pharmacotherapy. Outcome measures were assessed by blind evaluators. Completion and adherence rates were fair and did not differ between groups. There were no differences between FFT-A and enhanced care in rates of recovery from index episode; however, patients in the FFT-A group recovered faster from depressive episodes. The groups also did not differ in time to recurrence of depression or mania, but patients in FFT-A spent fewer weeks in depressive episodes and had a more favorable trajectory of depression symptoms for two years. A subsequent analysis revealed that there may be moderators for FFT-A's efficacy; adolescents in families that rated high for expressed emotion showed greater reductions in depressive and manic symptoms in FFT-A than in enhanced care (Miklowitz et al., 2009).

INTERPERSONAL AND SOCIAL RHYTHM THERAPY FOR ADOLESCENTS

Interpersonal and social rhythm therapy (IPSRT) is a manual-based psychotherapy founded on the theory that at least one aspect of the biological diathesis to bipolar disorder is a vulnerability of the circadian system and the neurotransmitter systems involved in its regulation (Hlastala & Frank, 2006). In this model, psychosocial stressors are hypothesized to precipitate and/or exacerbate bipolar episodes through their ability to disrupt social and sleep routines. In vulnerable individuals, social routine disruption leads to a desynchronization of circadian systems; this in turn may result in new episodes of mania or depression. Observational studies support this theoretical framework by elucidating the effects that stressful life events, social support, social routine disruption, and sleep disturbances have in the onset and maintenance of mania and depression (for a review see Milhiet, Etain, Boudebesse, & Bellivier, 2011). Evidence from adults with bipolar disorder has shown that individuals with high amounts of psychosocial stress remit significantly slower and relapse quicker (Post et al., 2006). In addition, life events characterized by social rhythm disruptions (e.g., transmeridian air travel, sleep deprivation with birth of a child) have been found to precipitate manic episodes (Boland et al., 2012).

IPSRT attempts to address three interrelated pathways to symptom exacerbation in bipolar patients: medication nonadherence, disruptions in social and sleep routines, and psychosocial stressors. IPSRT addresses the interplay between the interpersonal and the biological spheres by helping patients see how psychosocial stressors and social role transitions can disrupt the daily routines that are important to the maintenance of circadian integrity. Specifically, IPSRT focuses on clarifying the patient's understanding of the relationship between psychosocial stressors and mood fluctuations, the importance of maintaining regular daily rhythms, the identification of potential precipitants of rhythm dysregulation, and the identification and management of affective symptoms.

Hlastala, Kotler, McClellan, and McCauley (2010) developed an adapted version of interpersonal and social rhythm therapy for adolescents (IPSRT-A) with bipolar disorder. IPSRT-A consists of 16 to 18 sessions delivered over 20 weeks, most of which are with the adolescent alone, aside from two to three family psychoeducation sessions and familial involvement as needed. In an open pilot study of 12 adolescents diagnosed with bipolar spectrum disorders, feasibility and acceptability of IPSRT-A were high; IPSRT-A participants experienced significant decreases in manic, depressive, and general psychiatric symptoms over the 20 weeks of treatment. Participants' global functioning increased significantly, and effect sizes ranged from medium-large to large.

DIALECTICAL BEHAVIOR THERAPY FOR ADOLESCENTS

Dialectical behavior therapy (DBT) is an evidence-based psychotherapy designed for adults with borderline personality disorder; its primary focus is to reduce emotional dysregulation. DBT has been adapted for the treatment of adolescents with bipolar disorder; the intervention consists of six months of weekly, 60-minute psychotherapy sessions followed by another six months of bimonthly sessions and has the aim of increasing and maintaining individual and family skills (MacPherson, Cheavens, & Fristad, 2013). Family skills training includes psychoeducation about bipolar disorder, as well as teaching coping skills (i.e., mindfulness, distress tolerance, emotion regulation, interpersonal effectiveness, and walking the middle path skills). Individual therapy sessions address target behaviors outlined in the DBT hierarchy (i.e., life-threatening, treatment interfering, and quality-of-life interfering behaviors skills development) by employing problem-solving strategies within a validating environment.

A small open trial of DBT in 10 adolescents with bipolar disorder indicated that the treatment is feasible and acceptable for this patient population (Goldstein, Axelson, Birmaher, & Brent, 2007). Overall retention throughout this long intervention was good. Participants who received DBT exhibited decreased suicidality, nonsuicidal self-injury,

emotional dysregulation, and depression symptoms following treatment. There were no significant improvements in mania or interpersonal functioning, and no differences in number of medications prescribed.

COGNITIVE-BEHAVIORAL THERAPY FOR PEDIATRIC BIPOLAR DISORDER

Cognitive behavioral therapy (CBT) has been studied in single-family settings (Pavuluri, Graczyk, et al., 2004), multiple-family settings (West et al., 2009), and individual settings (with limited familial involvement; Feeny, Danielson, Schwartz, Youngstrom, & Findling, 2006). Child- and family-focused CBT (CFF-CBT; Pavuluri, Graczyk, et al., 2004) was adapted from FFT and developed as an adjunctive psychosocial intervention for children age 8 to 12 with bipolar spectrum disorders and their families. CFF-BT consists of 12 sessions that integrate psychoeducational, cognitive-behavioral, and interpersonal techniques; focus on psychosocial factors influencing course of illness (e.g., expressed emotion, stressful life events); and teach coping, CBT, communication, and problem-solving skills. An open trial using CFF-CBT plus pharmacotherapy in 34 youths ages 5 to 17 with bipolar spectrum disorders found the intervention feasible and showed significant improvements in ADHD, aggression, mania, psychosis, depression, sleep disturbance, and global functioning posttreatment. Participation in the CFF-CBT maintenance phase was associated with preservation of improvements in symptoms and functioning over a three-year follow-up (West, Henry, & Pavuluri, 2007).

A multiple-family adaptation of CFF-CBT consisting of 12 concurrent parent and child group sessions was examined in an open trial with 26 children ages 6 to 12 with bipolar disorder and their families (West et al., 2009). Multiple-family CFF-CBT was deemed feasible and acceptable to parents; it also revealed significant improvement in children's manic symptoms and psychosocial functioning and nonsignificant improvement in parents' knowledge and perceived self-efficacy in coping.

A program of CBT for adolescents with bipolar disorder spectrum diagnoses has also been developed and tested. It consists of 12 weekly sessions of acute-phase treatment (i.e., individual therapy, two to four parent and child sessions, one parent session) followed by 6 to 10 biweekly sessions and biannual booster sessions (Feeny, Danielson, Schwartz, Youngstrom, & Findling, 2006). Treatment involves psychoeducation about symptoms and course of bipolar disorder, medication compliance, mood monitoring, anticipating stressors and problem-solving, identifying and modifying unhelpful thinking, sleep regulation and relaxation, family communication and assertiveness, and relapse prevention, with optional modules for substance abuse, social skills, anger management, and contingency management. A pilot study compared eight youths ages 10 to 17 with bipolar spectrum disorders who received acute CBT with eight matched historical controls. CBT showed no significant between-group differences posttreatment or at eight-week follow-up; between-group effect sizes favored CBT for depressive and manic symptoms. The CBT group reported nonsignificant improvement in depression and mania at both time points. Parents of CBT adolescents also reported significant posttreatment improvement in youths' depression and mania; however, significant improvements were maintained only for depression.

COMPLEMENTARY MEDICINE

OMEGA-3 FATTY ACIDS

Omega-3 fatty acids are long-chain polyunsaturated fatty acids (LC-PUFAs) and are named due to the position of the last double bond in their chemical structures. Omega-3 are essential LC-PUFA, meaning they are obtained only from diet sources, as mammals are unable to synthesize them de novo and can only elongate and desaturate them (i.e., changing plant-based alpha-linoleic acid into marine-based eicosapentanoic acid [EPA] and EPA into docosahexaenoic acid [DHA]; Lapillonne & Carlson, 2001). Omega-3 LC-PUFAs have recently gained attention for their role in the management of depressive symptoms and ADHD (McNamara & Strawn, 2013). Their use in bipolar disorder has grown; however, data concerning its overall efficacy is still lacking.

To date, two published studies for omega-3 use exist in the literature. The first is an eight-week open-label trial of combined EPA/DHA as monotherapy (starting at 1,125 mg EPA/165 mg DHA, with flexible dosing up to EPA 1,290 mg/DHA 4,300 mg) in 20 children and adolescents with bipolar I, II, or not otherwise specified, and a YMRS score of >15 (Wozniak et al., 2007). Symptom reduction at study endpoint was noted, along with 50% ($n = 10$) of subjects with a 30% reduction in baseline YMRS scores and 35% ($n = 7$) with a 50% reduction in baseline YMRS scores; depressive symptoms also improved. The other study is a pilot randomized, controlled trial of flax oil up to 12,000 mg/day in children and adolescents with BP I and II disorder for 16 weeks; it found no difference for primary mood measures but moderate effects for clinician-rated

global improvement and severity of overall illness in those who displayed decreases in arachidonic acid and increases in alpha-linoleic acid and EPA (Gracious et al., 2010). This study suggests the importance of change in blood biomarkers as measures of compliance and outcome. Ongoing and future research into omega-3 LC-PUFA should take biologic marker changes into account in analyses as determinants of compliance and downstream metabolism in PUFA pathways and should also determine whether dietary intake data can predict outcome.

Omega-3 supplementation may also positively benefit attention in the more than half of youth with bipolar disorder who also have comorbid ADHD. DHA supplementation in healthy boys has been found to increase activity in attention networks in the prefrontal cortex during sustained attention tasks (McNamara et al., 2010). The side-effect profile for omega-3 LC-PUFA administration is typically benign, with gastrointestinal disturbance including transient nausea or diarrhea the most common concern, especially in younger children. Although typically well tolerated, rare cases of bleeding have been reported for concomitant use with aspirin and anticoagulants, especially when taken in exceptionally large doses (Larson et al., 2008).

To our knowledge there are no studies describing the efficacy or safety of other complementary treatment options (St. John's wort, inositol, S-adenosyl-L-methionine, acupuncture) in youth with bipolar disorder.

PSYCHOPHARMACOLOGICAL TREATMENT OF BIPOLAR DISORDER WITH COMORBID CONDITIONS

ATTENTION DEFICIT HYPERACTIVITY DISORDER

AHDH is the most common comorbid psychiatric disorder in youth with bipolar disorder (Joshi & Wilens, 2009). The presence of ADHD in a patient with pediatric bipolar disorder poses special treatment considerations. Patients with pediatric bipolar disorder and ADHD are less likely to respond to treatment and may be at increased risk of substance use disorders. Furthermore, conventional first-line agents in the treatment of ADHD have been associated with treatment-emergent mania and worsening of symptoms; approximately 2.5% to 10% of patients treated with stimulants or atomoxetine (adjunctive to mood-stabilizing medication) experience psychiatric adverse events (i.e., hypo/mania and/or suicidality).

Specifically, the American Academy of Child and Adolescent Psychiatry treatment guidelines advise that symptoms of bipolar disorder should be stabilized first, and if impairing symptoms of ADHD persist, they may be judiciously treated, with stimulants as first-line treatment. Few trials for antimanic agents have reported their efficacy in treating ADHD symptoms. In patients ages 6 to 17 years, these studies have found ADHD rates of response of 33% for ziprasidone (Biederman et al., 2007), 30% for risperidone (Biederman et al., 2008), and 60% for aripiprazole (Tramontina et al., 2007, 2009).

When significant symptoms of ADHD persist despite mood stabilization, adding a medication for ADHD may be warranted. Both mixed amphetamine and methylphenidate have been studied in controlled trials in stabilized pediatric bipolar patients. In a study of 30 pediatric patients with bipolar disorder and ADHD who were stabilized on valproate and then randomized to placebo or mixed amphetamine salts, patients who were in the active arm showed significant reduction of ADHD symptoms and no statistically significant side effects or worsening of manic symptoms (Scheffer, Kowatch, Carmody, & Rush, 2005). Methylphenidate has been studied in youth with bipolar disorder in two studies, one with prior stabilization with valproate and/or lithium (Findling et al., 2007) and the other with bipolar disorder patients previously stabilized with aripiprazole (Zeni, Tramontina, Ketzer, Pheula, & Rohde, 2009). In both studies, patients had significantly improved symptoms of ADHD without any significant worsening of manic symptoms.

Atomoxetine has been studied in a retrospective chart review (Hah et al., 2005) and an open-label study (Chang, Nayar, Howe, & Rana, 2009) and appears to be effective in lowering ADHD symptoms without a significant worsening of mood symptoms. However, future studies evaluating other treatments less likely to cause mood destabilization (e.g., alpha-2 agonists) are needed.

ANXIETY

Anxiety disorders are very common in pediatric bipolar disorder (Joshi & Wilens, 2009), and patients with comorbid anxiety disorders are at increased risk for poor treatment response and treatment-emergent episodes. Despite this, we know of no clinical trials that have explicitly studied the treatment of comorbid anxiety in pediatric bipolar disorder. Both SSRIs and cognitive behavior therapy are efficacious for pediatric anxiety in the absence of bipolar disorder. Concerns regarding the potential for treatment-emergent mania/hypomania and the absence

of empirical data regarding safety and efficacy of SSRIs for comorbid anxiety in pediatric bipolar disorder suggest psychosocial treatments should be considered before an SSRI is initiated. However, the lack of data strongly implies a great need for pharmacologic and psychosocial studies for the treatment of anxiety in pediatric bipolar disorder.

SUBSTANCE USE DISORDERS

As noted earlier, substance use and substance use disorders are common among adolescents with bipolar disorder. However, few clinical trials have specifically examined the effective pharmacological treatments when comorbid substance use disorders are present. In a six-week randomized, placebo-controlled study using lithium for pediatric bipolar spectrum disorders with secondary substance dependence, subjects were less likely to test positive for a urine drug assay after six weeks and had significantly greater improvement on the Children's Global Assessment Scale (Geller et al., 1998). A 16-week, randomized, double-blind, placebo-controlled study examined the efficacy of topiramate (average dose 175 mg/day) versus placebo, adjunctive to quetiapine, in 75 manic adolescents with co-occurring cannabis use disorders (ClinicalTrials.gov identifier: NCT00393978). There was a significantly greater reduction in cannabis use in the topiramate group versus the placebo group. There was also significantly less weight gain, greater reduction in appetite, and greater rate of excitement as side effects of topiramate versus placebo.

The optimal treatment of adolescents with substance abuse and bipolar disorder involves an integration of treatment modalities rather than merely consecutive treatments with a specific focus on either substance abuse or bipolar disorder. Psychosocial interventions that target some of the known risk and perpetuating factors for substance use (e.g., parental alcoholism or other substance abuse, poor parent–child relationships, low parental support, inconsistent or ineffective discipline, and poor parent supervision) may be useful.

CONCLUSION

The reviewed literature to date supports the existence of effective treatments available for pediatric bipolar disorder, in manic/mixed or depressed phase. Data so far support several conclusions regarding the treatment options for pediatric bipolar disorder. SGAs are highly efficacious for the treatment of acute manic/mixed episodes, although tolerability remains a major concern. The evidence regarding the traditional mood stabilizers (e.g., valproate) suggests that they may be less efficacious than SGAs among youth; however, this conclusion remains tentative pending additional placebo-controlled trials.

Furthermore, it is obvious that additional evidence for the pharmacological and nonpharmacological treatments of pediatric bipolar disorder is still needed. In addition, because it is highly unlikely that any given medication will be proven universally effective in youths with bipolar disorder (or in any age group for that matter), more studies searching for adequate predictors of treatment response is of vital importance to achieve individualized treatment strategies. These predictors can be anywhere from demographic characteristics, symptomatic clusters, family history, pharmacogenetic markers, and cognitive deficits to neuroimaging traits. Moreover, given that no single study will be sufficiently powered to detect predictors of treatment response to all available treatment options, efforts should be taken to have an available pool of data to collectively search for those predictors. Systematic data collection, similar data designs, and uniform rater reliability in efficacy measurements should be the initial steps in this endeavor. Vigorous and concerted efforts to address these and other questions will ensure that the momentum of progress in the treatment of pediatric bipolar disorder is sustained over the coming years.

Disclosure statement: Dr. Luis R. Patino, Dr. Melissa P. DelBello, and Nina R. McCune have not disclosed any conflicts of interest.

REFERENCES

Axelson, D., Birmaher, B., Strober, M., Gill, M. K., Valeri, S., Chiappetta, L.,...Keller, M. (2006). Phenomenology of children and adolescents with bipolar spectrum disorders. *Archives of General Psychiatry*, 63(10), 1139–1148.

Barnett, S. R., & Riddle, M. A. (2003). Anxiolytics: Benzodiazapines, buspirone, and others. In A. Martin, L. Scahill, S. D. Charney, & F. J. Leckman (Eds.), *Pediatric psychopharmacology* (p. 345). New York: Oxford University Press.

Barzman, D. H., DelBello, M. P., Kowatch, R. A., Gernert, B., Fleck, D. E., Pathak, S.,...Strakowski, S. M. (2004). The effectiveness and tolerability of aripiprazole for pediatric bipolar disorders: A retrospective chart review. *Journal of Child and Adolescent Psychopharmacology*, 14(4), 593–600.

Barzman, D. H., DelBello, M. P., Kowatch, R. A., Warner, J., Rofey, D., Stanford, K.,...Strakowski, S. M. (2005). Adjunctive topiramate in hospitalized children and adolescents with bipolar disorders. *Journal of Child and Adolescent Psychopharmacology*, 15(6), 931–937.

Biederman, J., Hammerness, P., Doyle, R., Joshi, G., Aleardi, M., & Mick, E. (2008). Risperidone treatment for ADHD in children and adolescents with bipolar disorder. *Neuropsychiatric Disease and Treatment*, 4(1), 203–207.

Biederman, J., Joshi, G., Mick, E., et al. (2010). A prospective open-label trial of lamotrigine monotherapy in children and adolescents with bipolar disorder. *CNS Neuroscience & Therapeutics*, 16, 91–102.

Biederman, J., Mick, E., Hammerness, P., Harpold, T., Aleardi, M., Dougherty, M., & Wozniak, J. (2005). Open-label, 8-week trial of olanzapine and risperidone for the treatment of bipolar disorder in preschool-age children. *Biological Psychiatry*, 58(7), 589–594.

Biederman, J., Mick, E., Spencer, T., Dougherty, M., Aleardi, M., & Wozniak, J. (2007). A prospective open-label treatment trial of ziprasidone monotherapy in children and adolescents with bipolar disorder. *Bipolar Disorders*, 9(8), 888–894.

Biederman, J., Mick, E., Spencer, T., Doyle, R., Joshi, G., Hammerness, P.,...Wozniak, J. (2007). An open-label trial of aripiprazole monotherapy in children and adolescents with bipolar disorder. *CNS Spectrums*, 12, 683–689.

Biederman, J., Mick, E., Spencer, T. J., Wilens, T. E., & Faraone, S. V. (2000). Therapeutic dilemmas in the pharmacotherapy of bipolar depression in the young. *Journal of Child and Adolescent Psychopharmacology*, 10(3), 185–192.

Biederman, J., Mick, E., Wozniak, J., Aleardi, M., Spencer, T., & Faraone, S. V. (2005). An open-label trial of risperidone in children and adolescents with bipolar disorder. *Journal of Child and Adolescent Psychopharmacology*, 15(2), 311–317.

Bildik, T., Tamar, M., Korkmaz, S., et al. (2006). Lamotrigine add-on therapy to venlafaxine treatment in adolescent-onset bipolar II disorder: A case report covering an 8-month observation period. *International Journal of Clinical Pharmacology and Therapeutics*, 44(5), 198–206.

Birmaher, B., Axelson, D., & Goldstein, B. (2009). Four-year longitudinal course of children and adolescents with bipolar spectrum disorders: The Course and Outcome of Bipolar Youth (COBY) Study. *The American Journal of Psychiatry*, 166, 795–804.

Birmaher, B., Axelson, D., Strober, M., et al. (2006). Clinical course of children and adolescents with bipolar spectrum disorders. *Archives of General Psychiatry*, 63, 175–183.

Boland, E. M., Bender, R. E., Alloy, L. B., Conner, B. T., Labelle, D. R., & Abramson, L. Y. (2012). Life events and social rhythms in bipolar spectrum disorders: An examination of social rhythm sensitivity. *Journal of Affective Disorders*, 139(3), 264–272.

Cade, J. F. (1949). Lithium salts in the treatment of psychotic excitement. *Medical Journal of Australia*, 2(10), 349–352.

Chambers, W. J., Puig-Antich, J., Hirsch, M., Paez, P., Ambrosini, P. J., Tabrizi, M. A., & Davies, M. (1985). The assessment of affective disorders in children and adolescents by semistructured interview: Test–retest reliability of the schedule for affective disorders and schizophrenia for school-age children, present episode version. *Archives of General Psychiatry*, 42(7), 696–702.

Chang, K. (2007). Adult bipolar disorder is continuous with pediatric bipolar disorder. *Canadian Journal of Psychiatry*, 52, 418–425.

Chang, K., Nayar, D., Howe, M., & Rana, M. (2009). Atomoxetine as an adjunct therapy in the treatment of co-morbid attention-deficit/hyperactivity disorder in children and adolescents with bipolar I or II disorder. *Journal of Child and Adolescent Psychopharmacology*, 19(5), 547–551.

Chang, K., Saxena, K., & Howe, M. (2006). An open-label study of lamotrigine adjunct or monotherapy for the treatment of adolescents with bipolar depression. *Journal of the American Academy of Child & Adolescent Psychiatry*, 45(3), 298–304.

Chong, K. W., Chan, D. W., Cheung, Y. B., Ching, L. K., Hie, S. L., Thomas, T.,...Tan, E. C. (2013). Association of carbamazepine-induced severe cutaneous drug reactions and HLA-B*1502 allele status, and dose and treatment duration in paediatric neurology patients in Singapore. *Archives of Disease in Childhood*, 2013 epub: Nov 13.

Cipriani, A., Hawton, K., Stockton, S., & Geddes, J. R. (2013). Lithium in the prevention of suicide in mood disorders: Updated systematic review and meta-analysis. *BMJ*, 346, f3646.

Cipriani, A., Pretty, H., Hawton, K., & Geddes, J. R. (2005). Lithium in the prevention of suicidal behavior and all-cause mortality in patients with mood disorders: A systematic review of randomized trials. *The American Journal of Psychiatry, 162*(10), 1805–1819.

Cohen, D., Consoli, A., Bodeau, N., Purper-Ouakil, D., Deniau, E., Guile, J. M., & Donnely, C. (2010). Predictors of placebo response in randomized controlled trials of psychotropic drugs for children and adolescents with internalizing disorders. *Journal of Child and Adolescent Psychopharmacology, 20*(1), 39–47.

Coletti, D. J., Leigh, E., Gallelli, K. A., & Kafantaris, V. (2005). Patterns of adherence to treatment in adolescents with bipolar disorder. *Journal of Child and Adolescent Psychopharmacology, 15*(6), 913–917.

Correll, C. U., Lops, J. D., Figen, V., Malhotra, A. K., Kane, J. M., & Manu, P. (2011). QT interval duration and dispersion in children and adolescents treated with ziprasidone. *Journal of Clinical Psychiatry, 72*(6), 854–860.

Correll, C. U., Sheridan, E. M., DelBello, M. P. (2010). Antipsychotic and mood stabilizer efficacy and tolerability in pediatric and adult patients with bipolar I mania: a comparative analysis of acute, randomized, placebo-controlled trials. *Bipolar Disord, 12*(2), 116–141.

Davanzo, P., Nikore, V., Yehya, N., et al. (2004). Oxcarbazepine treatment of juvenile-onset bipolar disorder. *Journal of Child and Adolescent Psychopharmacology, 14*(3), 344–345.

DelBello, M. P., Cecil, K. M., Adler, C. M., Daniels, J. P., & Strakowski, S. M. (2006) Neurochemical effects of olanzapine in first-hospitalization manic adolescents: A proton magnetic resonance spectroscopy study. *Neuropsychopharmacology, 31*(6), 1264–1273.

DelBello, M. P., Chang, K., Welge, J. A., et al. (2009). A double-blind, placebo-controlled pilot study of quetiapine for depressed adolescents with bipolar disorder. *Bipolar Disorders, 11*(5), 483–493.

Delbello, M. P., Findling, R. L., Kushner, S., Wang, D., Olson, W. H., Capece, J. A.,…Rosenthal, N. R. (2005). A pilot controlled trial of topiramate for mania in children and adolescents with bipolar disorder. *Journal of the American Academy of Child & Adolescent Psychiatry, 44*(6), 539–547.

DelBello, M. P., Hanseman, D., Adler, C. M., Fleck, D. E., & Strakowski, S. M. (2007). Twelve-month outcome of adolescents with bipolar disorder following first hospitalization for a manic or mixed episode. *The American Journal of Psychiatry, 164*(4), 582–590.

DelBello, M. P., Kowatch, R. A., Adler, C. M., Stanford, K. E., Welge, J. A., Barzman, D. H.,…Strakowski, S. M. (2006). A double-blind randomized pilot study comparing quetiapine and divalproex for adolescent mania. *Journal of the American Academy of Child & Adolescent Psychiatry, 45*(3), 305–313.

DelBello, M. P., Kowatch, R. A., Warner, J., Schwiers, M. L., Rappaport, K. B., Daniels, J. P.,…Strakowski, S. M. (2002). Adjunctive topiramate treatment for pediatric bipolar disorder: A retrospective chart review. *Journal of Child and Adolescent Psychopharmacology, 12*(4), 323–330.

DelBello, M. P., Schwiers, M. L., Rosenberg, H. L., & Strakowski, S. M. (2002). A double-blind, randomized, placebo-controlled study of quetiapine as adjunctive treatment for adolescent mania. *Journal of the American Academy of Child & Adolescent Psychiatry, 41*, 1216–1223.

DelBello, M. P., Versavel, M., Ice, K., Keller, D., & Miceli, J. (2008). Tolerability of oral ziprasidone in children and adolescents with bipolar mania, schizophrenia, or schizoaffective disorder. *Journal of Child and Adolescent Psychopharmacology, 18*(5), 491–499.

Duffy, A., Alda, M., Kutcher, S., Cavazzoni, P., Robertson, C., Grof, E., & Grof, P. (2002). A prospective study of the offspring of bipolar parents responsive and nonresponsive to lithium treatment. *Journal of Clinical Psychiatry, 63*(12), 1171–1178.

Duffy, A., Milin, R., & Grof, P. (2009). Maintenance treatment of adolescent bipolar disorder: Open study of the effectiveness and tolerability of quetiapine. *BMC Psychiatry, 9*, 4.

Evans, R. W., Clay, T. H., & Gualtieri, C. T. (1987). Carbamazepine in pediatric psychiatry. *Journal of the American Academy of Child & Adolescent Psychiatry, 26*(1), 2–8.

Faedda, G. L., Baldessarini, R. J., Glovinsky, I. P., & Austin, N. B. (2004). Treatment-emergent mania in pediatric bipolar disorder: a retrospective case review. *Journal of Affect Disorders, 82*(1), 149–158.

Feeny, N. C., Danielson, C. K., Schwartz, L., Youngstrom, E. A., & Findling, R. L. (2006). Cognitive-behavioral therapy for bipolar disorders in adolescents: A pilot study. *Bipolar Disorders, 8*, 508–515.

Findling, R. L., Cavuş, I., Pappadopulos, E., Vanderburg, D. G., Schwartz, J. H., Gundapaneni, B. K., & Delbello, M. P. (2013). Efficacy, long-term safety, and tolerability of ziprasidone in children and adolescents with bipolar disorder. *Journal of Child and Adolescent Psychopharmacology, 23*(8), 545–557.

Findling, R. L., Correll, C. U., Nyilas, M., Forbes, R. A., McQuade, R. D., Jin, N.,…Carlson, G. A. (2013). Aripiprazole for the treatment of pediatric bipolar I disorder: A 30-week, randomized, placebo-controlled study. *Bipolar Disorders, 15*(2), 138–149.

Findling, R. L., Frazier, J. A., Kafantaris, V., Kowatch, R., McClellan, J., Pavuluri, M.,…Taylor-Zapata, P. (2008). The Collaborative Lithium Trials (CoLT): specific aims, methods, and implementation. *Child and Adolescent Psychiatry and Mental Health, 2*(1), 21.

Findling, R. L., McNamara, N. K., Gracious, B. L., Youngstrom, E. A., Stansbrey, R. J., Reed, M. D.,…Calabrese, J. R. (2003). Combination lithium and divalproex sodium in pediatric bipolarity. *Journal of American Academy of Child & Adolescent Psychiatry, 42*(8), 895–901.

Findling, R. L., Reed, M. D., O'Riordan, M. A., et al. (2006). Effectiveness, safety, and pharmacokinetics of quetiapine in aggressive children with conduct disorder. *Journal of the American Academy of Child & Adolescent Psychiatry, 45*(7), 792–800.

Findling, R. L., Short, E. J., McNamara, N. K., Demeter, C. A., Stansbrey, R. J., Gracious, B. L.,…Calabrese, J. R. (2007). Methylphenidate in the treatment of children and adolescents with bipolar disorder and attention-deficit/hyperactivity disorder. *Journal of the American Academy of Child & Adolescent Psychiatry, 46*(11), 1445–1453.

Findling, R. L., Youngstrom, E. A., McNamara, N. K., et al. (2012). Double-blind, randomized, placebo-controlled long-term maintenance study of aripiprazole in children with bipolar disorder. *Journal of Clinical Psychiatry, 73*(1), 57–63.

Fraguas, D., Correll, C. U., Merchán-Naranjo, J., Rapado-Castro, M., Parellada, M., Moreno, C., & Arango, C. (2011). Efficacy and safety of second-generation antipsychotics in children and adolescents with psychotic and bipolar spectrum disorders: Comprehensive review of prospective head-to-head and placebo-controlled comparisons. *European Neuropsychopharmacology, 21*(8), 621–645.

Frazier, J. A., Biederman, J., Tohen, M., Feldman, P. D., Jacobs, T. G., Toma, V.,…Nowlin, Z. M. (2001). A prospective open-label treatment trial of olanzapine monotherapy in children and adolescents with bipolar disorder. *Journal of Child and Adolescent Psychopharmacology, 11*(3), 239–250.

Frazier, J. A., Meyer, M. C., Biederman, J., et al. (1999). Risperidone treatment for juvenile bipolar disorder: A retrospective chart review. *Journal of the American Academy of Child & Adolescent Psychiatry, 38*(8), 960–965.

Fristad, M. A., Goldberg-Arnold, J. S., & Gavazzi, S. M. (2002). Multifamily psychoeducation groups (MFPG) for families of children with bipolar disorder. *Bipolar Disorders, 4*(4), 254–262.

Fryar, C. D., Merino, M. C., Hirsch, R., & Porter, K. S. (2009). Smoking, alcohol use, and illicit drug use reported by adolescents aged 12-17 years: United States, 1999–2004. *National Health Statistics Report, 15*, 1–23.

Geller, B., Cooper, T. B., Sun, K., Zimerman, B., Frazier, J., Williams, M., & Heath, J. (1998). Double-blind and placebo-controlled study of lithium for adolescent bipolar disorders with secondary substance dependency. *Journal of the American Academy of Child & Adolescent Psychiatry, 37*(2), 171–178.

Geller, B., Luby, J. L., Joshi, P., Wagner, K. D., Emslie, G., Walkup, J. T.,...Lavori, P. (2012). A randomized controlled trial of risperidone, lithium, or divalproex sodium for initial treatment of bipolar I disorder, manic or mixed phase, in children and adolescents. *Archives of General Psychiatry, 69*(5), 515–528.

Geller, B., Tillman, R., Craney, J. L., et al. (2004). Four-year prospective outcome and natural history of mania in children with a prepubertal and early adolescent bipolar disorder phenotype. *Archives of General Psychiatry, 61*, 459–467.

Gijsman, H. J., Geddes, J. R., Rendell, J. M., Nolen, W. A., & Goodwin, G. M. (2004). Antidepressants for bipolar depression: A systematic review of randomized, controlled trials. *The American Journal of Psychiatry, 161*(9), 1537–1547.

Goldstein, T. R., Axelson, D. A., Birmaher, B., & Brent, D. A. (2007). Dialectical behavior therapy for adolescents with bipolar disorder: A 1-year open trial. *Journal of the American Academy of Child & Adolescent Psychiatry, 46*(7), 820–830.

Gracious, B. L., Chirieac, M. C., Costescu, S., Finucane, T. L., Youngstrom, E. A., & Hibbeln, J. R. (2010). Randomized, placebo-controlled trial of flax oil in pediatric bipolar disorder. *Bipolar Disorders, 12*(2), 142–154.

Greenhill, L. L., Rieder, R. O., Wender, P. H., Buchsbaum, M., & Zhan, T. P. (1973). Lithium carbonate in the treatment of hyperactive children. *Archives of General Psychiatry, 28*(5), 636–640.

Haas, M., Delbello, M. P., Pandina, G., et al. (2009). Risperidone for the treatment of acute mania in children and adolescents with bipolar disorder: A randomized, double-blind, placebo-controlled study. *Bipolar Disorders, 11*(7), 687–700.

Hah, M., & Chang, K. (2005). Atomoxetine for the treatment of attention-deficit/hyperactivity disorder in children and adolescents with bipolar disorders. *Journal of Child and Adolescent Psychopharmacology, 15*(6), 996–1004.

Henry, A., Kisicki, M. D., & Varley, C. (2012). Efficacy and safety of antidepressant drug treatment in children and adolescents. *Molecular Psychiatry, 17*(12), 1186–1193.

Hlastala, S. A., & Frank, E. (2006). Adapting interpersonal and social rhythm therapy to the developmental needs of adolescents with bipolar disorder. *Development and Psychopathology, 18*(4), 1267–1288.

Hlastala, S. A., Kotler, J. S., McClellan, J. M., & McCauley, E. A. (2010). Interpersonal and social rhythm therapy for adolescents with bipolar disorder: Treatment development and results from an open trial. *Depression and Anxiety, 27*(5), 457–464.

Idänpään-Heikkilä, J., Alhava, E., Olkinuora, M., & Palva, I. (1975). Letter: Clozapine and agranulocytosis. *Lancet, 2*(7935), 611.

Joshi, G., Petty, C., Wozniak, J., Faraone, S. V., Doyle, R., Georgiopoulos, A.,...Biederman, J. (2012). A prospective open-label trial of quetiapine monotherapy in preschool and school age children with bipolar spectrum disorder. *Journal of Affective Disorders, 136*(3), 1143–1153.

Joshi, G., Petty, C., Wozniak, J., Faraone, S. V., Spencer, A. E., Woodworth, K. Y.,...Biederman, J. (2013). A prospective open-label trial of paliperidone monotherapy for the treatment of bipolar spectrum disorders in children and adolescents. *Psychopharmacology, 227*(3), 449–458.

Joshi, G., & Wilens, T. (2009). Comorbidity in pediatric bipolar disorder. *Child & Adolescent Psychiatric Clinics of North America, 18*(2), 291–319.

Joshi, G., Wozniak, J., Mick, E., Doyle, R., Hammerness, P., Georgiopoulos, A.,...Biederman, J. (2010). A prospective open-label trial of extended-release carbamazepine monotherapy in children with bipolar disorder. *Journal of Child and Adolescent Psychopharmacology, 20*(1), 7–14.

Kafantaris, V., Coletti, D., Dicker, R., Padula, G., & Kane, J. M. (2003). Lithium treatment of acute mania in adolescents: A large open trial. *Journal of the American Academy of Child & Adolescent Psychiatry, 42*(9), 1038–1045.

Kafantaris, V., Coletti, D. J., Dicker, R., Padula, G., Pleak, R. R., & Alvir, J. M. (2004). Lithium treatment of acute mania in adolescents: A placebo-controlled discontinuation study. *Journal of the American Academy of Child & Adolescent Psychiatry, 43*(8), 984–993.

Kant, R., Chalansani, R., Chengappa, K. N., et al. (2004). The off-label use of clozapine in adolescents with bipolar disorder, intermittent explosive disorder, or posttraumatic stress disorder. *Journal of Child and Adolescent Psychopharmacology, 14*(1), 57–63.

Kowatch, R. A., Fistad, M., Birmaher, B., et al. (2005). The Child Psychiatric Workgroup on Bipolar Disorder: Treatment guidelines for children and adolescents with bipolar disorder. *Journal of the American Academy of Child & Adolescent Psychiatry, 44*, 213–235.

Kowatch, R. A., Suppes, T., Carmody, T. J., Bucci, J. P., Hume, J. H., Kromelis, M.,...Rush, A. J. (2000). Effect size of lithium, divalproex sodium, and carbamazepine in children and adolescents with bipolar disorder. *Journal of the American Academy of Child & Adolescent Psychiatry, 39*(6), 713–720.

Kowatch, R. A., Suppes, T., & Gilfillin, S. K. (1995). Clozapine treatment of children and adolescents with bipolar disorder and schizophrenia: A clinical case series. *Journal of Child and Adolescent Psychopharmacology, 5*(4), 241–253.

Kushner, S. F., Khan, A., Lane, R., & Olson, W. H. (2006). Topiramate monotherapy in the management of acute mania: Results of four double-blind placebo-controlled trials. *Bipolar Disorders, 8*(1), 15–27.

Lagerberg, T. V., Andreassen, O. A., Ringen, P. A., Berg, A. O., Larsson, S., Agartz, I.,...Melle, I. (2010). Excessive substance use in bipolar disorder is associated with impaired functioning rather than clinical characteristics, a descriptive study. *BMC Psychiatry, 10*, 9.

Lapillonne, A., & Carlson, S. E. (2001). Polyunsaturated fatty acids and infant growth. *Lipids, 36*(9), 901–911.

Larson, M. K., Ashmore, J. H., Harris, K. A., Vogelaar, J. L., Pottala, J. V., Sprehe, M., & Harris, W. S. (2008). Effects of omega-3 acid ethyl esters and aspirin, alone and in combination, on platelet function in healthy subjects. *Thrombosis and Haemostasis, 100*(4), 634–641.

Lena, B., Surtees, S. J., & Maggs, R. (1978). The efficacy of lithium in the treatment of emotional disturbance in children and adolescents. In F. N. Johnson & S. Johnson (Eds.), *Lithium in medical practice* (pp. 79–83). Lancaster, UK: MTP Press.

Liu, H. Y., Potter, M. P., Woodworth, K. Y., Yorks, D. M., Petty, C. R., Wozniak, J. R.,...Biederman, J. (2011). Pharmacologic treatments for pediatric bipolar disorder: a review and meta-analysis. *Journal of American Academy Child Adolescent Psychiatry, 50*(8), 749–762.

MacPherson, H. A., Cheavens, J. S., & Fristad, M. A. (2013). Dialectical behavior therapy for adolescents: Theory, treatment adaptations, and empirical outcomes. *Clinical Child and Family Psychology Review, 16*(1), 59–80.

Marchand, W. R., Wirth, L., & Simon, C. (2004). Quetiapine adjunctive and monotherapy for pediatric bipolar disorder: A retrospective chart review. *Journal of Child and Adolescent Psychopharmacology, 14*(3), 405–411.

Masi, G., Mucci, M., & Millepiedi, S. (2002). Clozapine in adolescent inpatients with acute mania. *Journal of Child and Adolescent Psychopharmacology, 12*(2), 93–99.

McClellan, J., Kowatch, R., & Findling, R. L. (2007). Practice parameter for the assessment and treatment of children and adolescents with bipolar disorder. *Journal of the American Academy of Child & Adolescent Psychiatry, 46*(1), 107–125.

McKnew, D. H., Cytryn, L., Buchsbaum, M. S., Hamovit, J., Lamour, M., Rapoport, J. L., & Gershon, E. S. (1981). Lithium in children of lithium-responding parents. *Psychiatry Research, 4*(2), 171–180.

McNamara, R. K., Able, J., Jandacek, R., Rider, T., Tso, P., Eliassen, J. C.,...Adler, C. M. (2010). Docosahexaenoic acid supplementation increases prefrontal cortex activation during sustained attention in healthy boys: A placebo-controlled, dose-ranging, functional magnetic resonance imaging study. *The American Journal of Clinical Nutrition, 91*(4), 1060–1067.

McNamara, R. K., & Strawn, J. R. (2013). Role of long-chain omega-3 fatty acids in psychiatric practice. *PharmaNutrition, 1*(2), 41–49.

Miklowitz, D. J., Axelson, D. A., Birmaher, B., George, E. L., Taylor, D. O., Schneck, C. D.,…Brent, D. A. (2008). Family-focused treatment for adolescents with bipolar disorder: Results of a 2 year randomized trial. *Archives of General Psychiatry, 65*(9), 1053–1061.

Miklowitz, D. J., Axelson, D. A., George, E. L., Taylor, D. O., Schneck, C. D., Sullivan, A. E.,…Birmaher, B. (2009). Expressed emotion moderates the effects of family-focused treatment for bipolar adolescents. *Journal of the American Academy of Child & Adolescent Psychiatry, 48*(6), 643–651.

Miklowitz, D. J., Simoneau, T. L., George, E. L., Richards, J. A., Kalbag, A., Sachs-Ericsson, N., & Suddath, R. (2000). Family-focused treatment of bipolar disorder: 1-year effects of a psychoeducational program in conjunction with pharmacotherapy. *Biological Psychiatry, 48*(6), 582–592.

Miklowitz, D. J. (2006). A review of evidence-based psychosocial interventions for bipolar disorder. *Journal of Clinical Psychiatry, 67*(11), 28–33.

Milhiet, V., Etain, B., Boudebesse, C., & Bellivier, F. (2011). Circadian biomarkers, circadian genes and bipolar disorders. *Journal of Physiology (Paris), 105*(4–6), 183–189.

Papatheodorou, G., Kutcher, S. P., Katic, M., et al. (1995). The efficacy and safety of divalproex sodium in the treatment of acute mania in adolescents and young adults: An open clinical trial. *Journal of Clinical Psychopharmacology, 15*(2), 110–116.

Patel, N. C., DelBello, M. P., Bryan, H. S., et al. (2006). Open-label lithium for the treatment of adolescents with bipolar depression. *Journal of the American Academy of Child & Adolescent Psychiatry, 45*(3), 289–297.

Pathak, S., Findling, R. L., Earley, W. R., Acevedo, L. D., Stankowski, J., & Delbello, M. P. (2013). Efficacy and safety of quetiapine in children and adolescents with mania associated with bipolar I disorder: A 3-week, double-blind, placebo-controlled trial. Journal of Clinical Psychiatry, *74*(1), e100–109.

Pavuluri, M. N., Graczyk, P. A., Henry, D. B., Carbray, J. A., Heidenreich, J., & Miklowitz, D. J. (2004). Child- and family-focused cognitive-behavioral therapy for pediatric bipolar disorder: Development and preliminary results. *Journal of the American Academy of Child & Adolescent Psychiatry, 43*(5), 528–537.

Pavuluri, M. N., Henry, D. B., Carbray, J. A., Naylor, M. W., & Janicak, P. G. (2005). Divalproex sodium for pediatric mixed mania: A 6-month prospective trial. *Bipolar Disorders, 7,* 266–273.

Pavuluri, M. N., Henry, D. B., Carbray, J. A., Sampson, G., Naylor, M. W., & Janicak, P. G. (2004). Open-label prospective trial of risperidone in combination with lithium or divalproex sodium in pediatric mania. *Journal of Affective Disorders, 82*(1), S103–111.

Pavuluri, M. N., Henry, D. B., Carbray, J. A., Sampson, G. A., Naylor, M. W., & Janicak, P. G. (2006). A one-year open-label trial of risperidone augmentation in lithium nonresponder youth with preschool-onset bipolar disorder. *Journal of Child and Adolescent Psychopharmacology, 16*(3), 336–350.

Pavuluri, M. N., Henry, D. B., Findling, R. L., Parnes, S., Carbray, J. A., Mohammed, T.,…Sweeney, J. A. (2010). Double-blind randomized trial of risperidone versus divalproex in pediatric bipolar disorder. *Bipolar Disorders, 12*(6), 593–605.

Pavuluri, M. N., Henry, D. B., Moss, M., Mohammed, T., Carbray, J. A., & Sweeney, J. A. (2009). Effectiveness of lamotrigine in maintaining symptom control in pediatric bipolar disorder. *Journal of Child and Adolescent Psychopharmacology, 19*(1), 75–82.

Poznanski, E., & Mokros, H. (1996). *Children's Depression Rating Scale–Revised.* Los Angeles: WPS.

Sallee, F. R., Miceli, J. J., Tensfeldt, T., Robarge, L., Wilner, K., & Patel, N. C. (2006). Single-dose pharmacokinetics and safety of ziprasidone in children and adolescents. *Journal of the American Academy of Child & Adolescent Psychiatry, 45*(6), 720–728.

Scheffer, R. E., Kowatch, R. A., Carmody, T., & Rush, A. J. (2005). Randomized, placebo-controlled trial of mixed amphetamine salts for symptoms of comorbid ADHD in pediatric bipolar disorder after mood stabilization with divalproex sodium. *The American Journal of Psychiatry, 162*(1), 58–64.

Scheffer, R. E., Tripathi, A., Kirkpatrick, F. G., & Schultz, T. (2011). Guidelines for treatment-resistant mania in children with bipolar disorder. *Journal of Psychiatric Practice, 17*(3), 186–193.

Scheffer, R. E., Tripathi, A., Kirkpatrick, F. G., & Schultz, T. (2010). Rapid quetiapine loading in youths with bipolar disorder. *Journal of Child and Adolescent Psychopharmacology, 20*(5), 441–445.

Seetharam, M. N., & Pellock, J. M. (1991). Risk-benefit assessment of carbamazepine in children. *Drug Safety, 6*(2), 148–158.

Sheehan, D. V., Sheehan, K. H., Shytle, R. D., Janavs, J., Bannon, Y., Rogers, J. E.,…Wilkinson, B. (2010). Reliability and validity of the Mini International Neuropsychiatric Interview for Children and Adolescents (MINI-KID). *Journal of Clinical Psychiatry, 71*(3), 313–326.

Sidor, M. M., & Macqueen, G. M. (2011). Antidepressants for the acute treatment of bipolar depression: A systematic review and meta-analysis. *Journal of Clinical Psychiatry, 72*(2), 156–167.

Singh, M. K., Ketterm, T. A., & Chang, K. D. (2010). Atypical antipsychotics for acute manic and mixed episodes in children and adolescents with bipolar disorder: Efficacy and tolerability. *Drugs, 70*(4), 433–442.

Soutullo, C. A., Diez-Suarez, A., & Figueroa-Quintana, A. (2006). Adjunctive lamotrigine treatment for adolescents with bipolar disorder: Retrospective report of five cases. *Journal of Child and Adolescent Psychopharmacology, 16*(3), 357–364.

Strakowski, S. M., DelBello, M. P., Fleck, D. E., Adler, C. M., Anthenelli, R. M., Keck, P. E. Jr.,…Amicone, J. (2007). Effects of co-occurring cannabis use disorders on the course of bipolar disorder after a first hospitalization for mania. *Archives of General Psychiatry, 64*(1), 57–64.

Strawn, J. R., Adler, C. M., Strakowski, S. M., & DelBello, M. P. (2008). Hyperthermia and rhabdomyolysis in an adolescent treated with topiramate and olanzapine. *Journal of Child and Adolescent Psychopharmacology, 18*(1), 116–118.

Teitelbaum, M. (2001). Oxcarbazepine in bipolar disorder. *Journal of the American Academy of Child & Adolescent Psychiatry, 40*(9), 993–994.

Thomas, T., Stansifer, L., & Findling, R. L. (2011). Psychopharmacology of pediatric bipolar disorders in children and adolescents. *Pediatric Clinics of North America, 58*(1), 173–187.

Tohen, M., Kryzhanovskaya, L., Carlson, G., Delbello, M., Wozniak, J., Kowatch, R.,…Biederman, J. (2007). Olanzapine versus placebo in the treatment of adolescents with bipolar mania. *The American Journal of Psychiatry, 164*(10), 1547–1556.

Toteja, N., Gallego, J. A., Saito, E., Gerhard, T., Winterstein, A., Olfson, M., & Correll, C. U. (2013). Prevalence and correlates of antipsychotic polypharmacy in children and adolescents receiving antipsychotic treatment. *International Journal of Neuropsychopharmacology, 14,* 1–11.

Tramontina, S., Zeni, C. P., Ketzer, C. R., Pheula, G. F., Narvaez, J., & Rohde, L. A. (2009). Aripiprazole in children and adolescents with bipolar disorder comorbid with attention-deficit/hyperactivity disorder: A pilot randomized clinical trial. *Journal of Clinical Psychiatry, 70,* 756–764.

Tramontina, S., Zeni, C. P., Pheula, G. F., de Souza, C. K., & Rohde, L. A. (2007). Aripiprazole in juvenile bipolar disorder comorbid with attentiondeficit/hyperactivity disorder: An open clinical trial. *CNS Spectrums, 12,* 758–762.

van Krevelen, D., & van Voorst, J. A. (1959). Lithium in der Behandlung einer Psychose unklarer Genese bei einem Jugendlichen. *Acta Paedopsychiatrica, 26,* 148–152.

Wagner, K. D., Kowatch, R. A., Emslie, G. J., Findling, R. L., Wilens, T. E., McCague, K.,...Linden, D. (2006). A double-blind, randomized, placebo-controlled trial of oxcarbazepine in the treatment of bipolar disorder in children and adolescents. *The American Journal of Psychiatry, 163*(7), 1179–1186.

Wagner, K. D., Redden, L., Kowatch, R. A., et al. (2009). A double-blind, randomized, placebo-controlled trial of divalproex extended release in the treatment of bipolar disorder in children and adolescents. *Journal of the American Academy of Child & Adolescent Psychiatry, 48*, 519–532.

Wagner, K. D., Weller, E. B., Carlson, G. A., et al. (2002). An open-label trial of divalproex in children and adolescents with bipolar disorder. *Journal of the American Academy of Child & Adolescent Psychiatry, 41*, 1224–1230.

Weinstein, S. M., West, A. E., & Pavuluri, M. (2013). Psychosocial intervention for pediatric bipolar disorder: Current and future directions. *Expert Review of Neurotherapeutics, 13*(7), 843–850.

West, A. E., Henry, D. B., & Pavuluri, M. N. (2007). Maintenance model of integrated psychosocial treatment in pediatric bipolar disorder: A pilot feasibility study. *Journal of the American Academy of Child & Adolescent Psychiatry, 46*(2), 205–212.

West, A. E., Jacobs, R. H., Westerholm, R., Lee, A., Carbray, J., Heidenreich, J., & Pavuluri, M. N. (2009). Child and family-focused cognitive-behavioral therapy for pediatric bipolar disorder: Pilot study of group treatment format. *Journal of the Canadian Academy of Child and Adolescent Psychiatry, 18*(3), 239–246.

West, S., Keck, P., McElroy, S., et al. (1994). Open trial of valproate in the treatment of adolescent mania. *Journal of Child and Adolescent Psychopharmacology, 4*, 263–267.

Wilens, T. E., Biederman, J., Kwon, A., Ditterline, J., Forkner, P., Moore, H.,...Faraone, S. V. (2004). Risk of substance use disorders in adolescents with bipolar disorder. *Journal of the American Academy of Child & Adolescent Psychiatry, 43*(11), 1380–1386.

Wilens, T. E., Biederman, J., Millstein, R. B., Wozniak, J., Hahesy, A. L., & Spencer, T. J. (1999). Risk for substance use disorders in youths with child- and adolescent-onset bipolar disorder. *Journal of the American Academy of Child & Adolescent Psychiatry, 38*(6), 680–685.

Wozniak, J., Biederman, J., Mick, E., Waxmonsky, J., Hantsoo, L., Best, C.,...Laposata, M. (2007). Omega-3 fatty acid monotherapy for pediatric bipolar disorder: A prospective open-label trial. *European Neuropsychopharmacology, 17*(6–7), 440–447.

Wozniak, J., Mick, E., Waxmonsky, J., Kotarski, M., Hantsoo, L., & Biederman, J. (2009). Comparison of open-label, 8-week trials of olanzapine monotherapy and topiramate augmentation of olanzapine for the treatment of pediatric bipolar disorder. *Journal of Child and Adolescent Psychopharmacology, 19*(5), 539–545.

Young, R. C., Biggs, J. T., Ziegler, V. E., & Meyer, D. A. (1978). A rating scale for mania: Reliability, validity and sensitivity. *British Journal of Psychiatry, 133*, 429–435.

Zeni, C. P., Tramontina, S., Ketzer, C. R., Pheula, G. F., & Rohde, L. A. (2009). Methylphenidate combined with aripiprazole in children and adolescents with bipolar disorder and attention-deficit/hyperactivity disorder: A randomized crossover trial. *Journal of Child and Adolescent Psychopharmacology, 19*(5), 553–561.

Notes1 For the purpose of this chapter, response and remission rates are reported as indicated in the original publications. Definitions for response and remission vary across different studies, however, and differ based on the scale used and/or the cut-off used (e.g., percentage change and absolute score).

PART IX

ELDERLY

40.

BIPOLAR DISORDER IN THE ELDERLY

Elizabeth A. Crocco, Samir Sabbag, and Rosie E. Curiel

INTRODUCTION

The number of older adults in the United States over the age of 65 is projected to almost double from 41 million in 2013 to 80 million by the year 2040 (US Department of Health and Human Services, 2013). Prolonged life expectancy and improved health care are both contributing factors to this growing elderly population. Most notable is the aging of the baby boomers, those born between 1946 and 1964, that began to reach age 65 in 2011 (US Census Bureau, 2010). This substantial rise in the geriatric population will continue to increase the number of elderly individuals living with chronic mental illnesses, including bipolar disorder (BPD).

Developing evidence-based and best practice guidelines in BPD is quite challenging due to the highly complex nature of the disease. Currently, there are clinical limitations to understanding BPD in patients of any age and a dearth of information on older adults. Reasons for this paucity of knowledge in geriatric BPD may include the increased mortality of younger BPD patients, sampling biases from the limited number of research studies, variances across research settings in which patients are studied, and shifts in diagnostic criteria over time (Depp & Jeste, 2004).

Much of our previous knowledge about geriatric BPD is built on information collected from anecdotal evidence, case reports, expert consensus, and a small number of open-label clinical trials. To date, these limitations make it challenging to develop optimal evidence-based diagnostic evaluations and treatments for elderly BPD patients. Elderly patients differ significantly from younger patients in multiple ways, and these differences must be carefully considered in any treatment formulation. In this chapter, we present and synthesize the most recent data available pertaining to geriatric BPD and its treatment.

EPIDEMIOLOGY

In community settings, studies suggest that BPD in the elderly is rare. The Epidemiologic Catchment Area Survey, the most comprehensive psychiatric epidemiological study to date conducted over 20 years ago, indicated that BPD has a prevalence rate of 0.1% in individuals over 65 years of age (Weissman et al., 1988). The lifetime prevalence rate in geriatric BPD was found to be 0.5% to 1% among community dwelling elders. This differs from younger adults with BPD where a community prevalence of 1.4% (Weissman et al., 1988) and a lifetime prevalence of 2.6 to 7.8% was found (Sadock, Kaplan, & Sadock, 2007). Several factors have been ascribed to this age-related decline of BPD in the community. They include a higher mortality at a younger age due to suicide, as well as early death linked to cardiovascular disease in bipolar patients, who die up to nine years prior to those without the illness (Crump, Sundquist, Winkleby, & Sundquist, 2013).

While geriatric BPD appears to be quite rare according to this data, such a generalization could be potentially misleading. The prevalence of BPD in the elderly can reflect the setting in which older adults are studied. In a comprehensive review of the literature, Dols and colleagues (2014) reviewed 188 studies of mania in older adults over the age of 50 years. Eighteen of these studies were then selected because of methodological rigor and indicated that the overall prevalence of late-life mania was 6% among 1,519 psychiatric inpatients. This relatively high prevalence rate can be attributed to the fact that 85% of studies sampling elderly patients with bipolar illness have been performed with information derived from inpatient units (Depp et al., 2004). This is despite the fact that most geriatric patients with mental illness reside in the community and are not often hospitalized (Meeks & Murell, 1997).

Additional studies have found that elderly BPD patients are less likely to utilize psychiatric services when compared to younger BPD adults. Instead, older adults are much more likely to seek out care for psychiatric illness in medical/primary care settings. As compared with geriatric unipolar depressed persons, geriatric BPD individuals are even more likely to sustain substantial medical burden (Gildengers et al., 2008). Subsequently, elderly BPD patients might be less able to reside independently due to disabling physical conditions and/or functional impairments (Depp, Davis, Mittal, Patterson, & Jeste, 2006). There are greater numbers of elderly BPD patients residing in nursing homes and residential care facilities (Depp et al., 2006). These factors may explain the discrepancies in prevalence rates, which do not clearly represent the scope of the illness.

A comprehensive review by Depp and colleagues (2004) reveals that multiple studies have shown gender differences in geriatric BPD. Overall, the female-to-male ratio in this population is 2:1, differing from a younger population where the ratio is more equivalent. This inequality is thought to parallel the gender ratio for the general elderly population, where females predominate (US Census Bureau, 2010). Other studies have suggested that gender ratios are similar in bipolar individuals both young and old (Oostervink, Boomsma, & Nolen, 2009).

CLINICAL FEATURES

Accurately recognizing the clinical features of BPD in the elderly is imperative for proper diagnosis, and it may be difficult given medical and neurological comorbidity. Regardless of the age of onset, in a review of multiple studies the phenomenology of geriatric BPD does appear to be similar to that seen in younger patients with the condition (Depp et al., 2004); both ends of the spectrum are similarly seen in the illness presenting at any age with minor differences. In more recent select studies, the older cohort is less likely to have symptoms such as psychosis and more likely to relapse into depression (Kessing, 2006). Other studies have found psychosis, depression, and manic symptoms across younger and older age groups to be equivalent (Al Jurdi, 2009).

LATE-ONSET BPD

Late-onset BPD is generally defined as the diagnosis of bipolar illness at age 50 or older (Van Gerpen, Johnson, & Winstead, 1999), but there is no current definitive consensus to this classification. Moreover, there is a lack of standardization used to establish disease onset. Common

markers include first hospitalization, first mood episode, or first manic episode. Different etiological factors that influence disease onset may account for the variance found among the young and old in terms of the initial symptomatology. A better understanding of etiological subtypes may impact response to treatment and prognosis.

A record review of several hundred patients with bipolar illness (Moorhead & Young, 2003) indicated that those with a negative family history of psychiatric illness were hospitalized for the first time at an older age. These findings suggest that those diagnosed over 50 were from a different etiological subgroup, implicating medical or neurological origins. This would be consistent with our current knowledge that late-onset mania may be more closely related to neurological factors that may lead to cognitive and functional impairments. Conversely, onset of mania at an earlier age may be more closely linked to genetic factors (McDonald & Nemeroff, 1996).

DIFFERENTIAL DIAGNOSIS AND SECONDARY MANIA

Evaluating symptoms of mania in the bipolar older adult requires a comprehensive evaluation to accurately determine causality. The new onset of bipolar symptoms in later years may represent secondary mania attributable to medical dysfunction, degenerative neurological disorders, or the impact of pharmacological agents. Guidelines for assistance with the differential diagnosis of BPD that have particular relevance to the elderly are provided.

NEURODEGENERATIVE DISEASES

Approximately 4.5% to 19% of elderly individuals with BPD have dementia (Lala & Sajatovic, 2012). Additionally, patients with neurological disorders often have behavioral symptoms that resemble mania. Box 40.1 depicts the most common neurological disorders that may potentially cause manic symptoms. Diagnosing mania is challenging in older adults with severely impaired cognition, as patients who suffer from dementia or delirium are more likely to develop severe behavioral disturbances, similar to the symptoms of mania. In a review of the literature, Trinh and Forester (2007) emphasize that in an elderly patient with comorbid dementia, the onset of a manic episode may be indicated by a rapid decline in cognitive functioning, along with fluctuations in mood, energy, and sleep.

Box 40.1. NEUROLOGICAL CAUSES OF MANIA

Alzheimer's disease

Central nervous system tumors/space-occupying lesions

Creutzfeldt-Jakob disease

Encephalitis due to metabolic disturbances or inflammatory disease

Frontotemporal dementia/Pick's disease

HIV encephalitis

Huntington's disease

Multiple sclerosis

Neurosyphilis

Normal pressure hydrocephalus

Parkinson's disease/Diffuse Lewy body disease

Temporal lobe epilepsy

Traumatic brain injury

Tourette's syndrome

Vascular dementia/stroke

Viral encephalitis

Vitamin deficiencies (B12, Niacin)

Wilson's disease

Adapted from: Mendez (2000).

Neurodegenerative disorders characterized by disinhibition syndromes can also be difficult to distinguish from bipolar illness. For example, behavioral impulsivity and hyper-sexuality may be features of frontotemporal dementia (FTD), Parkinson's disease or Diffuse Lewy Body dementia. In turn, apathy, also a common symptom of FTD and Alzheimer's disease, may be mistaken as depression (Heuristic, 2008).

The following expanded guidelines offered by Trinh and Forrester (2007) may assist clinicians in differentiating mania from a primary neurocognitive disorder:

- In an older adult, a more rapid decline in cognitive functioning, paired with fluctuations in mood, goal-directed energy, and sleep, may indicate the onset of a manic episode.

- Neurodegenerative disorders are typically associated with focal neurological or cognitive deficits, such as aphasia, apraxia, impaired visuospatial functioning, or gait disturbance.

- Individuals with neurodegenerative disorders do not typically demonstrate prominent elevated mood or euphoria, which are the classic hallmark features of bipolar illness.

- BPD elderly do not typically exhibit significant changes in personality, commonly seen in neurodegenerative diseases like FTD.

- If symptoms of nighttime agitation and confusion occur, accompanied by reversal of the sleep–wake cycle, this may be more suggestive of a major neurocognitive disorder or delirium rather than BPD.

- A negative family history of BPD may be unreliable, as family members may have not received an accurate diagnosis before the modern classification system.

MEDICATIONS CAUSING MANIA

Older BPD persons are often prescribed multiple medications due to medical comorbidities. New-onset mania in an older individual may be directly related to medications. Box 40.2 lists the most commonly prescribed medications that have the potential to induce mania. Medications such as corticosteroids, stimulants, and sympathomimetic drugs are well known to induce manic symptoms. Dopaminergic agents that are used to treat Parkinson's disease must be carefully monitored. Antidepressants have the potential to induce mania and may be prescribed for medical reasons. For example, older bipolar individuals who are prescribed the antidepressant duloxetine for diabetic neuropathy may be at higher risk for manic switching.

COMORBIDITIES

The identification of any potentially treatable medical condition that can contribute to manic or depressive symptoms is necessary in the assessment of older adults. This is particularly important where a history of BPD has not been established. Comorbid medical illnesses may interfere with pharmacological treatment response or the attainment of optimal dosages. In an older adult with a history of BPD, a change in baseline mood or functioning suggests a potential decompensation. This may warrant a medical work-up to identify factors that may contribute to or worsen their psychiatric symptoms. Careful assessment

Box 40.2. MEDICATIONS INDUCING MANIA

Angiotensin-converting enzyme inhibitors

Amphetamines/stimulants

Antidepressants

Baclofen

Bronchodilators

Benzodiazepines

Chloroquine

Corticosteroids

Dopaminergic/anti-Parkinson's medications

Estrogen hormones

Isoniazid

Levodopa

Metachlopramide

Phencyclidine

Sympathomametic drugs

Thyroid hormones

Adapted from Peet & Peters (1995)

should aim to gather information to establish a baseline from which to monitor treatment response and/or adverse effects.

It has been reported that elderly individuals with BPD are disproportionally impacted by medical illness (Kilbourne, Post & Nossek, 2008). Lala and Sajatovic (2012) found that a mean of three to four medical conditions appears to be the norm in this population. In particular, cardiovascular disease and cardiovascular risk factors such as hypertension, type II diabetes, and obesity are more common in elderly BPD. It is not clear at times whether these symptoms are truly comorbid, a consequence of treatment regimens, or a combination of both (Gildengers et al., 2008). Additionally, other medical conditions such as chronic obstructive pulmonary disease and endocrine abnormalities are frequently observed.

Psychiatric comorbid conditions differ in the elderly as compared to their younger counterparts. The National Epidemiologic Survey on Alcohol and Related Conditions surveyed a modest sample of elderly patients with BPD (Goldstein, Herrmann, & Shulman) and found that

elderly patients with BPD were less likely to have alcohol use disorders, dysthymia, generalized anxiety disorder, and panic disorder when compared to younger BPD patients. However, in general, anxiety and substance use disorders are more prevalent in older BPD individuals when compared to elders without BPD and warrant consideration (Goldstein et al., 2006; Lala et al., 2012). The presence of comorbid psychiatric conditions is important as it may lead to difficulty in proper diagnosis and resistance to standard treatment.

NEUROIMAGING

Structural brain changes are observed in individuals with BPD. Regardless of age of onset, elderly patients with BPD had reduced total brain volume and decreased caudate volume. Those with late-onset illness in particular were found to have significantly decreased right and total caudate volumes compared to normal controls (Beyer et al., 2004). Regarding white matter differences, a study by Tamashiro and colleagues (2008) compared T2-weighted magnetic resonance imaging data between early-onset and late-onset elderly BPD patients and healthy controls. A greater prevalence of white matter hyperintensities in the deep parietal region and basal ganglia were found in the late-onset BPD group, suggesting a higher risk for vascular disease. This finding supports a neurodegenerative rather than a neuroprogressive disease course. Moreover, Haller et al. (2011) found significant decreases in the ventral part of the corpus callosum. Gray matter concentration was reduced in the anterior limbic areas, along with fiber tract integrity, which was reduced in the corpus callosum of elderly patients with longstanding BPD.

More recently, the neuroprotective effects of lithium have been proposed. Beyer et al. (2004) found geriatric BPD individual treated with lithium had increased left hippocampal volumes. Additionally, Lyoo and colleagues (2010) found that grey matter volume was increased in patients treated with lithium when compared to those treated with valproic acid or healthy older controls. Although the effects of lithium treatment warrant further study, elderly BPD patients at greatest risk for neurodegeneration may receive benefit from lithium's potential protective effects in the long term.

COGNITION AND FUNCTIONAL IMPAIRMENT

In general, cognitive impairment and difficulty performing everyday tasks of daily living is present among 60%

of individuals with bipolar illness, even during euthymic states (Martino et al., 2008). Very few studies in elderly BPD patients have established whether cognitive decline in this population exceeds the decline expected with normal aging (Depp et al., 2005). Schouws and colleagues (2012) examined the neurocognitive performance of older individuals with BPD who performed worse than the comparison group overall. Cognitive decline over a two-year period did not differ. In contrast, Dhingra and Rabins (1991) did find a notable decline in cognition when elderly BPD patients were followed for five to seven years; however, no comparisons were made to healthy controls. Gildengers and colleagues (2009) found that BPD individuals, 60 years and older, who were euthymic at the time of testing performed significantly worse on the Dementia Rating Scale at baseline and at follow-up when compared to healthy peers.

There have been varied hypotheses regarding the potential etiologies of cognitive impairment associated with geriatric BPD. These include neurodevelopmental abnormalities, deterioration from recurrent mood episodes, cerebrovascular disease, substance abuse, and medication side effects (Gildengers et al., 2004). One of the challenges in evaluating the results of neuropsychological testing among those with BPD is to determine whether patients are evaluated when euthymic, depressed, or during a state in which manic symptoms are present. The most powerful studies are those that can evaluate performance longitudinally, effectively using the subject as their own controls. As with other medical conditions, growth models and random effects mixed growth models may be useful to examine those factors that influence group differences in trajectories of cognitive decline over time.

Functionally, Huxley and colleagues (2007) found that compared to the general population, only 19% to 23% of adult BPD patients were married, 19% to 58% resided with relatives, and up to 80% had at least partial vocational disability. A more recent study that analyzed instrumental activities of daily living and cognitive function in an elderly BPD group (Gildengers et al., 2013) found that compared to controls, BPD patients displayed worse cognitive function in all domains and worse performance over a two-year time period on instrumental activities of daily living.

Their findings support long-standing neuroprogressive processes compounded by normal cognitive aging rather than accelerated cognitive loss. In older adults, cognitive dysfunction and accelerated cognitive decline can lead to a reduced level of independence, more reliance on familial and community support, and assisted-living facility placement.

TREATMENT

The treatment of geriatric bipolar disease is complex at multiple levels. BPD patients are typically managed with polypharmacy, and geriatric patients are no exception. Multiple medical comorbidities can lead to worsening of psychiatric symptoms, and the use of multiple psychiatric medications can potentially cause side effects, intolerability, and drug–drug interactions. In evaluating a geriatric BPD patient, a comprehensive examination should include the following: physical and neurological exam, complete metabolic panel, thyroid studies, complete blood count, toxicology, urinalysis, electrocardiogram, and liver studies. Neuroimaging may also be useful in assessing potential neurological conditions such as cerebrovascular disease.

Multiple psychotropic medications are well documented to have unique side effects related to age-associated changes and the potential for interaction with different medications. For instance, elderly patients have a significant decline in cholinergic activity within the brain. Moreover, some individuals may have a more pronounced decrease in the production of acetyl choline and their receptors due to a neurodegenerative disease process. Many psychotropic medications commonly used in BPD have significant anticholinergic properties. This is of particular relevance to the older adult as medications with potent blockade of acetyl choline will more likely lead to serious side effects. Common reactions can include dry mouth, blurred vision, constipation, urinary retention, hypotension, tachycardia, cognitive impairment, and delirium (Cilag & Abbott 2001). Thus it is important to avoid or minimize the dosage of anticholinergic medications used in elderly BPD whenever possible. Table 40.1 depicts medications used in BPD that demonstrate a significant risk of developing anticholinergic side effects and strategies to reduce risk.

In terms of pharmacologic evidence for the treatment of elderly BPD, the data is extremely limited. Gold-standard, placebo-controlled, double-blind trials are sparse. As such, clinicians are required to formulate an individualized approach to treatment, combining available guidelines from geriatrics and BPD in general. The adequate management of BPD patients alone is rarely achieved through monotherapy. The following treatment regimens have gained evidence for use in geriatric BPD treatment. Additionally, those side effects and adverse reactions that are most relevant in the elderly BPD patient are discussed. Table 40.2 lists common medications used in geriatric BPD and their most critical side effects as well as strategies for their cure and prevention in the elderly.

Table 40.1. MEDICATIONS USED IN BIPOLAR DISORDER WITH SIGNIFICANT ANTICHOLINERGIC SIDE EFFECTS

DRUG CLASS	DRUG	CRITICAL SIDE EFFECT(S)	STRATEGY TO REDUCE OR PREVENT SIDE EFFECT
Antidepressants			
Tricyclic Antidepressants	Amitriptyline Clomipramine Desipramine Doxepin Imipramine Nortriptyline Protriptyline Trimipramine Maprotiline	Sedation, seizures, weight gain, orthostatic hypotension, cardiac conduction abnormalities, tachycardia, dry mouth, blurred vision, constipation, urinary retention, memory problems delirium, mania	Prescribe SSRIs or SNRIs for the treatment of bipolar depression for geriatric patients.
SSRI	Paroxetine	Gastrointestinal distress, sexual dysfunction, weight gain, headache, dizziness, insomnia, anxiety, agitation, confusion, suicidal behavior, dry mouth, nausea, constipation, diarrhea	Prescribe SSRI/SNRI with less anticholinergic potency (i.e.,citalopram, sertraline, venlafaxine, buproprion, mirtazapine)
Antipsychotics			
Typical	Chlorpromazine Loxapine Molindone Pimozide Promethazine Thioridazine	Extrapyramidal symptoms, hyperprolactinemia, parkinsonism, tardative dyskinesia, neuroleptic malignancy syndrome, seizure, orthostatic hypotension, agranulocytosis of aplastic anemia, thrombocytopenia, dry mouth, constipation, urinary retention, priapism, leukopenia	Prescribe atypical antipsychotics with less anticholinergic properties such as risperidone and aripripazole. Patients who develop considerable side effects such as gynecomastia or who have significant signs of osteopenia and risks for osteoporosis should when possible be switched to an atypical antipsychotic that is less likely to cause hyperprolactinemia, such as quetiapine or aripiprazole.
Atypical	Clozapine Olanzapine Quetiapine	Headaches, insomnia, sedation, anticholinergic effects, weight gain, orthostatic hypotension, extrapyramidal symptoms	Prescribe less anticholinergic atypical antipsychotics (i.e., risperidone, aripripazole)
Anticonvulsants/Mood Stabilizers			
	Carbamazepine	Hepatic toxicity, leukopenia, agranulocytosis	Prescribe mood stabilizer with less anticholinergic potency (i.e., valproic acid, lamotrigine)
Benzodiazepines			
	Alprazolam Chlordiazepoxide Diazepam Oxazepam Flurazepam	Insomnia, irritability, dizziness, headache, anxiety, confusion, drowsiness, lightheadedness, sedation, semblance, difficulty speaking, impaired coordination, memory impairment, fatigue, depression, suicide, diarrhea, dry mouth, constipation, decreased libido, nervousness, restlessness, nightmares, mania	Avoid all benzodiazepines when possible. If necessary, use shorter-acting agents with less anti cholinergic potency such as lorazepam, and reserve for short-term use only (<3 months).
Other			
	Benztropine Trihexyphenidyl Diphenhydramine	Delirium, seizures, coma, agitation, hallucinations, severe hypotension, supraventricular tachycardia sedation, constipation, nausea, dry mouth, nervousness, hallucinations, urinary retention, fainting	Avoid these highly anticholinergic medications in the elderly when possible.

NOTE: SSRI = serotonin specific reuptake inhibitor; SNRI =serotonin norepinephrine reuptake inhibitor.

Table 40.2. PHARMACOLOGICAL TREATMENTS USED IN ELDERLY BIPOLAR DISORDER

DRUG CLASS	DRUG	DOSE RANGE	SIDE EFFECTS	STRATEGIES TO PREVENT/ TREAT SIDE EFFECTS
Mood Stabilizers/Anticonvulsants	Lithium	Starting dose: 300 mg daily. 900–`1,200 mg daily. Aim for serum level 0.6–0.8 mEq/L	Slowed reaction time, memory difficulties, increased thirst, polyuria, gastrointestinal distress, weight gain, tremors, fatigue, cognitive impairment, parkinsonism, ataxia, dysarthria, nausea, decreased appetite, vomiting, diarrhea, thyroid dysregulation, hyperkalemia, toxicity, decreased renal function, hypercalcemia, hyperparathyroidism	Prescribe mood stabilizers with better tolerability in the elderly (i.e., valproic acid, lamotrigine). Check calcium levels annually. Monitor electrolytes, renal and thyroid function regularly.
	Valproic acid	Starting dose: 250 mg daily. Aim for 4–-100 mg/L serum level	Sedation, tremor, ataxia, hair loss, weight gain, hepatic toxicity, pancreatitis, thrombocytopenia	Monitor liver function tests and complete blood count every three months. Avoid large, fatty meals to prevent increased blood levels. Monitor blood levels when prescribing highly protein-bound medications.
	Carbamazepine	Starting dose: 100–200 mg daily, increase up to 1,000 mg daily	Hepatic toxicity, leukopenia, agranulocytosis, ataxia, dizziness, hyponatremia, cardiac conduction delays, leukopenia, cognitive slowing	Prescribe mood stabilizers with better tolerability in the elderly (i.e., valproic acid, lamotrigine). Monitor electrolytes, electrocardiogram, and complete blood count after initial dosing and every three months.
	Oxcarbazepine	1,200–1,500 mg daily	Hyponatremia, agranulocytosis	Monitor electrolytes and complete blood count after initial dosing and every three months.
	Topiramate	200 mg twice daily	Fatigue, somnolence, anxiety, cognitive slowing	Avoid in renal insufficiency.
	Lamotrigine	Starting dose: 12.5 mg increase by 12.5 mg every week up to 100 mg daily	Nausea/vomiting, upset stomach, dry mouth, tremors, and drowsiness/panic, rash (Stevens-Johnson syndrome)	To prevent rash, titrate slowly.
	Gabapentin	600 mg–800 mg daily	Dizziness, ataxia, fatigue, nystagmus	
Atypical Antipsychotics	Clozapine	6.25–100 mg/day	Weight gain, diabetes, hyperlipidemia, anticholinergic side effects, hypotension, sedation, agranulocytosis, respiratory arrest, seizures	Monitor complete blood count weekly. Monitor BMI, glucose and lipid profile carefully. Prescribe atypical antipsychotic with less risk of the metabolic syndrome.

(continued)

Table 40.2. CONTINUED

DRUG CLASS	DRUG	DOSE RANGE	SIDE EFFECTS	STRATEGIES TO PREVENT/ TREAT SIDE EFFECTS
	Risperidone	Starting dose: 0.5 mg daily and increase to 1.5 mg to 3 mg daily	Hyperprolactinemia, sedation, urinary tract infection, hypotension, extrapyramidal symptoms	Monitor bone density and preventive treatment with exercise, vitamin D, calcium, and bisphosphonates. Patients with gynecomastia, osteopenia or osteoporosis should be switched to an atypical antipsychotic such as quetiapine or aripiprazole.
	Olanzapine	Starting dose: 2.5 mg and increase to 5 mg–10 mg daily	Weight gain, hyperlipidemia, diabetes, extrapyramidal symptoms, anticholinergic side effects	Prescribe atypical antipsychotic with less anticholinergic properties and less risk of the metabolic syndrome.
	Quetiapine	Starting dose: 100 mg daily, increase dose to 400–600 mg	Weight gain, orthostatic hypotension, dry mouth, sedation, anticholinergic side effects	Prescribe atypical antipsychotic with less anticholinergic properties and less risk of the metabolic syndrome.
	Ziprasidone	40–160 mg/day	Cardiac conduction delays, extrapyramidal symptoms	Avoid in patients with cardiac disease.
	Aripriprazole	Starting dose: 5 mg daily (2 mg if frail elderly) increase up to 15 mg daily	Restlessness, insomnia, drooling, diarrhea	
	Lurasidone	40–120 mg/day	Extrapyramidal symptoms, hyperglycemia, diabetes, dyslipidemia, weight gain, hyperprolactinemia	Similar treatment for side effects as risperdone
	Asenepine	5–10 mg twice a day	Extrapyramidal symptoms, diabetes, weight gain, hyperprolactinemia, orthostatic hypotension, syncope, leukopenia, neutropenia, agranulocytosis, QT prolongation, seizures	Avoid in patients with cardiac disease. Similar treatment for side effects as risperdone

LITHIUM AND ANTICONVULSANTS

Although the data is limited, the mood stabilizers lithium and valproic acid are generally considered effective in geriatric BPD. Previous studies have suggested that the standard treatment of mania, such as lithium, may not be as effective in the elderly as in younger patients (Depp & Jeste, 2004, Gildengers et al., 2005). In a recent study examining the longitudinal outcome of a large cohort of outpatients with BPD, Al Jurdi et al. (2008) demonstrated the recovery rate in patients prescribed either lithium or valproic acid was equivalent in older and younger BPD individuals. Additionally, in a systematic review of both open-label trials and case series available, Aziz, Lorberg, & Tampi (2006) found elderly BPD patients outcomes improved on both mood stabilizers.

Lithium treatment may be underutilized in the elderly, despite evidence that it works well in mixed-age BPD. This may be related to its poor tolerability, significant side-effect profile, multiple drug–drug interaction, as well as its narrow therapeutic index and toxicity. Unfortunately, despite its potential usefulness in elderly BPD, there is a paucity of data on how to dose lithium optimally. Side effects such as ataxia, tremor, cognitive slowing, and other forms of neurotoxicity can be daunting in geriatric patients. Both lithium level and the development of side effects should be closely monitored.

The long-term side effects of lithium may be of particular importance in older BPD patients. Conditions such as hypothyroidism and renal insufficiency may worsen in the context of endocrine abnormalities and decreased renal function already present. One naturalistic study by Rej, Herrmann, & Shulman (2012), demonstrated those patients with chronic renal insufficiency who continued to take lithium had changes in their glomerular filtration rate compared to discontinuers. Additionally, lithium can induce hypercalcemia and hyperparathyroidism (Lehmann & Lee, 2012) in geriatric BPD. Clinicians should check calcium levels in their geriatric BPD patients at least on a yearly basis.

Data on the effects of lithium in the brain of patients with BPD has been recently investigated. Gray matter volume is increased in patients treated with lithium when compared to healthy elderly subjects or BPD patients treated with valproic acid (Lyoo et al., 2010). It has been proposed that lithium may decrease the production of amyloid precursor protein and phosphorylated tau through the inhibition of glycogen synthase kinase-3. This can protect against neurodegenerative processes like Alzheimer's disease. One retrospective study demonstrated the continued use of lithium in elderly BPD reduced the risk of developing dementia more so than the use of antipsychotics, antidepressants, and other mood stabilizers (Kessing, Forman, & Andersen, 2010). Additionally, a recent randomized, single-blind, placebo-controlled trial of lithium on patients with Alzheimer's disease demonstrated that subjects on lithium had significant improvements in cognitive performance (Hampel et al., 2009).

Although Depp and Jeste (2004) had found similar use of lithium and valproic acid in older and younger BPD patients, more recent studies demonstrate an increased rate of valproic acid use in comparison to lithium in the elderly population and at lower doses (Al Jurdi et al., 2008). This is most likely due to its reduced potential for toxicity and long-term side effects as compared to lithium, and it has therefore replaced lithium as the preferred mood stabilizer for BPD in the elderly. Valproic acid should have a starting dose of 250 mg daily with a target serum level of 45 to 100 mg/L. A typically accepted clinical standard for dosing with geriatric patients is about half the dose used with younger individuals. Valproic acid is a potent inhibitor of the the cytochrome P450 enzyme system and will inhibit the breakdown of carbamazepine metabolites. The concomitant use of both valproic acid and carbamazepine in the elderly should be avoided as this can lead to significantly increased levels of carbamazepine. As a highly protein-bound compound, valproic acid also competes with fatty acids for albumin-bound intravascular transfer. Large, fatty meals can raise the level of free valproic acid in the blood and lead to toxicity. Valproic acid can also displace

medications such as warfarin and digoxin. Thus patients taking other highly protein-bound medications should be monitored closely and dosages should be adjusted appropriately. In general, side effects and adverse reactions due to valproic acid may include sedation, tremor, ataxia, hair loss, weight gain, hepatic toxicity, and pancreatitis. Bleeding due to thrombocytopenia may occur and lead to the risk of cerebrovascular accident, particularly with elderly patients at risk (Trannel, Ahmed, & Goebert, 2001).

Evidence from a recent open-label trial with lamotrigine demonstrated significant benefit in geriatric BPD patients who are depressed with cardiovascular risk factors (Gildengers et al., 2012). Lamotrigine can be useful in geriatric BPD given its better tolerability profile, such as less cognitive slowing, compared to other mood stabilizers. The side effects experienced by patients taking lamotrigine were nausea/vomiting, upset stomach, dry mouth, tremors, and drowsiness/panic. Potential side effects such as severe rash may be of concern in older individuals; therefore the recommended starting dose is 12.5 mg daily. The drug should be slowly increased by 12.5 mg every week up to a dose of 100 mg daily to prevent Stevens-Johnson syndrome.

Due to their substantial side-effect profile or lack of clinical evidence, mood stabilizers such as carbamazepine, oxcarbazepine, and topiramate are not commonly used as a first-line treatment in BPD in the elderly. Drug interactions, liver toxicity, and/or cognitive slowing may be less tolerable in older individuals. Additionally, clinicians who prescribe these drugs may use lower doses in their older patients, which may not reach therapeutic dosing. Carbamazepine, which is effective in the treatment of mania in BPD, may have significant side effects and risks to the elderly. Starting dose in BPD elderly is 100 to 200 mg daily, and titration up to 1,000 mg daily is recommended. Carbamazepine is a potent inducer of the cytochrome P450 enzyme system and can autometabolizes itself, as well as other drugs. Serious side effects may include hepatic toxicity, leukopenia, agranulocytosis, ataxia, dizziness, hyponatremia, as well as anticholinergic effects and potential cardiac conduction delays. For these reasons, it is not considered a first-line treatment for BPD in the elderly. Oxcarbazepine demonstrates less drug–drug interaction than carbamezapine, as well as fewer side effects. It is, however, both an inducer and inhibitor of select P450 enzymes. Additionally, it also may induce hyponatremia and needs to be used in caution with elderly patients at risk of medical conditions and medications that would lower serum sodium. The target dose of oxcarbazepine in the BPD elderly is in the range of 1,200 to 1,500 mg daily if tolerated. Gabapentin in general may both be better tolerated than other mood stabilizers in the elderly; however, its efficacy in adult BPD has not been well established.

ANTIPSYCHOTICS

The use of typical antipsychotics in acute manic episodes has shown evidence of efficacy in the elderly, although risk of anticholinergic, orthostatic, and extrapyramidal symptoms limits their use. Atypical antipsychotics in general have a better side effect profile, are Food and Drug Administration–indicated for the treatment of acute mania, and should be considered first in the manic elderly. In one recent post hoc analysis of two clinical trials, the use of quetiapine in patients over the age of 55 demonstrated improvement in manic symptoms (Sajatovic et al., 2008). In another study by Sajatovic et al., an open-label trial on elderly BPD patients treated with aripiprazole showed improvement in both depression and mania. Although there is a paucity of data describing the use of antipsychotics in geriatric BPD, these trial data suggest that usefulness in the elderly may be similar to their younger counterparts.

Because atypical antipsychotics are potent treatments in acute mania, in many clinical situations it will seem reasonable to continue them after remission. However, there are very few studies that show antipsychotics being as effective in maintenance of BPD. Quetiapine, olanzapine, aripiprazole, ziprazidone, and long-acting risperidone are Food and Drug Administration–approved for the maintenance of adult BPD, but their efficacy in geriatric BPD is not well documented. Additionally, their tolerability and safety profile has not been well studied in the elderly BPD patient.

Atypical antipsychotics carry less of a risk of extrapyramidal symptoms than typical antipsychotics, but in elderly patients, the long-term risk of neurologic symptoms such as tardive dyskinesia are present and greater than in younger patients (Correll, Leucht, & Kane, 2004). Hyperprolactinemia resulting from the use of atypical antipsychotics with significant dopaminergic D2 receptor antagonism, such as risperidone, can lead to bone density loss with increased risk of osteopenia and osteoporosis. There also may be a link between hyperprolactinemia and increased risk of breast cancer in postmenopausal women (Bostwick, Guthrie, & Ellingrod, 2009). Patients who develop gynecomastia, osteopenia, and/or osteoporosis should, when possible, be switched to an atypical antipsychotic such as quetiapine or aripiprazole, which carry less of a risk. For those patients on risperidone that has a greater D2 affinity, dosing should be no greater than 3 mg daily. Monitoring of bone density and preventive treatment with weight-bearing exercise, vitamin D, and calcium, as well as bisphosphonates, should be recommended. Prolactin-lowering agents/dopamine agonists such as bromocriptine can be used to treat hypoprolactinemia with minimal side effects; however, switching to another agent with lower potential for neurological side effects should be considered first.

In addition to extra-pyramidal side effects, their use warrants particular concern as many atypical antipsychotics, widely used in the treatment of mixed-age patients with BPD, can be associated with changes in metabolic function as described by Lala and Sajatovic (2012). Given the higher rates of metabolic abnormalities in elderly patients with BPD and apparent risk of diabetes, treatments that do not potentially alter endocrine status are preferred in patients with significant vascular disease risks. Risk of death associated with the use of antipsychotic medication in cognitively impaired elderly (Schneider, Dagerman, & Insel, 2005) also precludes their use as select patients with dementia may experience manic symptoms.

ANTIDEPRESSANTS

In comparison to younger patients, older BPD patients are more likely to be on antidepressants (Oostervink, Boomsma, & Nolen, 2009). This is most likely a consequence of having more depressive episodes later in life. Elderly BPD patients who are depressed are more likely to receive antidepressants because they often are on a lower dose of mood stabilizers than required for treatment efficacy. The addition of antidepressants may be necessary to achieve better response to a debilitating depressive episode than the use of mood stabilizers alone.

Tricyclic antidepressants can cause significant adverse reactions due to their anticholineric side effects, cardiac-conduction delays, and orthostatic hypotension due to adrenergic effects. The serotonin specific reuptake inhibitors have a better safety profile and are a better choice, but paroxetine can be problematic as it also has anticholinergic risks. Venlafaxine, buproprion, and mirtazapine may also be considered given their tolerability, safety profile in the elderly, and less likelihood of drug–drug interaction.

BENZODIAZEPINES

There is widespread use of benzodiazepines in the geriatric population despite significant side effects and adverse events. These include sedation, falls, hip fractures, depressed mood, motor vehicle crashes, urinary incontinence, and cognitive impairment. One recent study demonstrated an increased risk of incident dementia with benzodiazepine use (Wu, Wang, Chang, & Lin, 2009). Another study confirmed the increased risk of disability as evidenced by decreased mobility, as well as increased activities of daily living dependence, in patients who use benzodiazepines (Gray et al., 2006). The use of benzodiazepines can be useful in the treatment of BPD, particularly in the treatment of acute mania, sleep disturbances, and agitated depression. However, in situations where the use of benzodiazepines in geriatric bipolar patients is indicated, their use should be closely monitored for potential side effects. Additionally, their use should be, whenever possible, restricted to the short term for the most acute phases of mania or agitated depression. Short-acting agents are indicated, although studies indicate the risks associated with these agents are similar to longer-acting agents with more active metabolites (Wang, Bohn, Glynn, Mogun, & Avorn, 2001). Benzodiazepines with significant anticholinergic effects should be particularly avoided.

ELECTROCONVULSIVE THERAPY

Electroconvulsive therapy (ECT) is a well-documented and effective treatment for BPD. Studies demonstrate that in both manic and depressed states of BPD, ECT has a high rate of response (Loo, 2011). Older patients in particular may benefit ECT because of their inability to tolerate the therapeutic doses and side effects of psychiatric medications. ECT has demonstrated tolerability and safety in the elderly (Van der Wurff et al., 2003). Patients who require rapid response to treatment may derive the most benefit from this form of treatment. These include instances of catatonia, acute suicidal behavior, poor oral intake, severe psychosis, or agitation leading to imminent danger.

PSYCHOTHERAPEUTIC TREATMENT AND PSYCHOSOCIAL INTERVENTIONS

There is a lack of empirical knowledge surrounding non-pharmacological interventions in geriatric BPD, yet psychosocial factors have been found to account for 25% to 30% of the variance in the course of the disease (Hafner & Harrari, 1994). Stress associated with life changes, family conflicts, and limited social support is more likely to be responsive to psychological interventions. Moreover, older depressed adults in general often have better treatment compliance, lower dropout rates, and more positive responses to psychotherapy than younger patients (Nierenberg & McColl, 1996). Studies have demonstrated the efficacy of psychotherapy in preventing relapse of symptoms in bipolar patients by improving medication compliance (Peet & Harvey, 1991), monitoring and managing stress (Frank et al., 1997), and reducing family-related discord (Miklowitz, Otto, Frank, Reilly-Harrington, Wisniewski, 2007). There is limited information however, regarding the improvement of these issues in a geriatric BPD population.

Given the complex medical and psychosocial context that influences the treatment of bipolar older adults, additional interventions such as education (i.e., teaching better coping and adaptation skills), family counseling, participation in bereavement groups, involvement with a senior citizen center, and use of visiting nurse services to help with medication adherence (Birrer et al., 2004) may also essential. Select psychotherapies have gained some evidence in the treatment of geriatric unipolar depressed persons that may be applied to bipolar elderly—for instance, interpersonal therapy, a brief psychotherapy that focuses on the interpersonal context of the depressed individual. Cognitive-behavioral therapy and, more specifically, gero-cognitive behavior therapy has demonstrated promising results by combining a developmental perspective with cognitive interventions (Antognini, 2003). Social rhythm therapy includes preventive strategies, including management of stress, attention to biological rhythms, improved medication compliance, and reparative measures to deal with the interpersonal, social, and practical aftermath of the manic or depressive episode and family-focused interventions that have been found to be more effective than other therapies as an adjunct to medication in individuals with bipolar illness (Miklowitz, 2007).

CONCLUSION AND FUTURE DIRECTIONS

In general, there is very limited data on geriatric BPD. Because of the rapid growth of this population, it is increasingly important to understand the characteristics and best treatment strategies available. The prevalence of geriatric BPD is significantly more common in medical settings than in the community, and studies geared toward BPD patients in acute medical settings and long-term care facilities are warranted. Given the confounding presence of medical and psychiatric comorbidities among elderly patients with BPD, it is critical that treating physicians carefully establish the presence of concurrent conditions and utilize treatments that reduce the likelihood of negatively impacting comorbid conditions. Regarding cognitive and functional status, there is the need to examine the earliest changes among elderly individuals with BPD that may indicate a vascular or neurodegenerative etiology. The lack of randomized control studies supporting evidence for treatment in acute mania, depression, and maintaining remission in BPD is a fertile ground for new research in the field of geriatric psychiatry.

Disclosure statement: Dr. Sabbag has received no financial support from drug companies, a manufacturer, or a publisher. He has no conflict of interest to disclose. Dr. Crocco has received financial grant support from the State of Florida Department of Elder Affairs, the National Institute on Aging and the Health Services Research Administration. Dr. Rosie E. Curiel has not disclosed any conflicts of interest.

REFERENCES

Al Jurdi, R. K., Dixin, L., & Sajatovic, M. (2010). Role of extended release quetiapine in the management of bipolar disorders. *Neuropsychiatric Disease and Treatment, 6*, 29.

Al Jurdi, R. K., Marangell, L. B., Petersen, N. J., Martinez, M., Gyulai, L., & Sajatovic, M. (2008). Prescription patterns of psychotropic medications in elderly compared to younger participants who achieved a "recovered" status in the systematic treatment enhancement program for bipolar disorder (STEP-BD). *American Journal of Geriatric Psychiatry, 16*(11), 922.

Antognini, F. C. (2003). Psychotherapy with depressed older adults. *Medical Psychiatry, 23*, 257–296.

Aziz, R., Lorberg, B., & Tampi, R. R. (2006). Treatments for late-life bipolar disorder. *The American Journal of Geriatric Pharmacotherapy, 4*(4), 347–364.

Beyer, J. L., Kuchibhatla, M., Payne, M. E., Moo-Young, M., Cassidy, F., Macfall, J., & Krishnan, K. R. (2004). Hippocampal volume measurement in older adults with bipolar disorder. *American Journal of Geriatric Psychiatry, 12*(6), 613–620.

Birrer, R. B., & Vemuri, S. P. (2004). Depression in later life: A diagnostic and therapeutic challenge. *American Family Physician, 69*(10), 2375–2382.

Bostwick, J. R., Guthrie, S. K., & Ellingrod, V. L. (2009). Antipsychotic-induced hyperprolactinemia. *Pharmacotherapy, 29*(1), 64–73.

Cilag, J., & Abbott, E. (2001). Anticholinergic effects of medication in elderly patients. *Journal of Clinical Psychiatry, 62*(21), 11–14.

Correll, C. U., Leucht, S., & Kane, J. M. (2004). Lower risk for tardive dyskinesia associated with second-generation antipsychotics: A systematic review of 1-year studies. *The American Journal of Psychiatry, 161*(3), 414–425.

Crump, C., Sundquist, K., Winkleby, M. A., Sundquist, J. (2013). Comorbidities and mortality in bipolar disorder: A Swedish national cohort study. *JAMA Psychiatry, 70*(9), 931–939.

Depp, C. A., Davis, C. E., Mittal, D., Patterson, T. L., & Jeste, D. V. (2006). Health-related quality of life and functioning of middle-aged and elderly adults with bipolar disorder. *Journal of Clinical Psychiatry, 67*(2), 215–221.

Depp, C. A., & Jeste, D. V. (2004). Bipolar disorder in older adults: A critical review. *Bipolar Disorders, 6*(5), 343–367.

Depp, C. A., Lindamer, L. A., Folsom, D. P., Gilmer, T., Hough, R. L., Garcia, P., & Jeste, D. V. (2005). Differences in clinical features and mental health service use in bipolar disorder across the lifespan. *American Journal of Geriatric Psychiatry, 13*(4), 290–298.

Dhingra, U., & Rabins, P. V. (1991). Mania in the elderly: A 5–7 year follow-up. *Journal of the American Geriatrics Society, 39*, 581–583.

Dols, A., Kupka, R. W., Lammeren, A., Beekman, A. T., Sajatovic, M., & Stek, M. L. (2014). The prevalence of late-life mania: a review. *Bipolar Disorders, 16*(2), 113–118.

Frank, E., Hlastala, S., Ritenour, A., Houck, P., Tu, X. M., Monk, T. H.,…Kupfer, D. J. (1997). Inducing lifestyle regularity in recovering bipolar disorder patients: Results from the maintenance therapies in bipolar disorder protocol. *Biological Psychiatry, 41*(12), 1165–1173.

Gildengers, A. G., Butters, M. A., Seligman, K., McShea, M., Miller, M. D., Mulsant, B. H.,…Reynolds, C. F. (2004). Cognitive functioning in late-life bipolar disorder. *The American Journal of Psychiatry, 161*(4), 736–738.

Gildengers, A. G., Chisholm, D., Butters, M. A., Anderson, S. J., Begley, A., Holm, M.,…Mulsant, B. H. (2012). Two-year course of cognitive function and instrumental activities of daily living in older adults with bipolar disorder: Evidence for neuroprogression? *Psychological Medicine, 43*, 801–811.

Gildengers, A. G., Mulsant, B. H., Begley, A., Mazumdar, S., Hyams, A. V., Reynolds, C. F. III, & Butters, M. A. (2009). The longitudinal course of cognition in older adults with bipolar disorder. *Bipolar Disorders, 11*(7), 744–752.

Gildengers, A. G., Mulsant, B. H., Begley, A. E., McShea, M., Stack, J. A., Miller, M. D.,…Reynolds, C. F. (2005). A pilot study of standardized treatment in geriatric bipolar disorder. *The American Journal of Geriatric Psychiatry, 13*(4), 319–323.

Gildengers, A. G., Whyte, E. M., Drayer, R. A., Soreca, I., Fagiolini, A., Kilbourne, A. M., & Mulsant, B. H. (2008). Medical burden in late-life bipolar and major depressive disorders. *American Journal of Geriatric Psychiatry, 16*(3), 194.

Goldstein, B. I., Herrmann, N., & Shulman, K. I. (2006). Comorbidity in bipolar disorder among the elderly: Results from an epidemiological community sample. *The American Journal of Psychiatry, 163*(2), 319–321.

Gray, S. L., LaCroix, A. Z., Hanlon, J. T., Penninx, B. W., Blough, D. K., Leveille, S. G.,…Buchner, D. M. (2006). Benzodiazepine use and physical disability in community-Dwelling older adults. *Journal of the American Geriatrics Society, 54*(2), 224–230.

Haller, S., Xekardaki, A., Delaloye, C., Canuto, A., Lövblad, K. O., Gold, G., & Giannakopoulos, P. (2011). Combined analysis of grey matter voxel-based morphometry and white matter tract-based spatial statistics in late-life bipolar disorder. *Journal of Psychiatry & Neuroscience, 36*(6), 391–401.

Hampel, H., Ewers, M., Burger, K., Annas, P., Mortberg, A., Bogstedt, A.,…Basun, H. (2009). Lithium trial in Alzheimer's disease: A randomized, single-blind, placebo-controlled, multicenter 10-week study. *Journal of Clinical Psychiatry, 70*(6), 922.

Harari, E., & Hafner, J. (1994). *The family in clinical psychiatry.* Oxford: Oxford University Press.

Heuristic. (2008). In frontotemporal dementia. Retrieved from http://memory.ucsf.edu/ftd/overview/ftd/isitftd

Huxley, N., & Baldessarini, R. J. (2007). Disability and its treatment in bipolar disorder patients. *Bipolar Disorders, 9*(1–2), 183–196.

Kessing, L. V. (2006). Differences in diagnostic subtypes among patients with late and early onset of a single depressive episode. *International Journal of Geriatric Psychiatry, 21*(12), 1127–1131.

Kessing, L. V., Forman, J. L., & Andersen, P. K. (2010). Does lithium protect against dementia? *Bipolar Disorders, 12*(1), 87–94.

Kilbourne, A. M., Post, E. P., Nossek, A., et al. (2008). Improving medical and psychiatric outcomes among individuals with bipolar disorder: A randomized controlled trial. *Psychiatric Services, 59*(7), 760–768.

Lala, S. V., & Sajatovic, M. (2012). Medical and psychiatric comorbidities among elderly individuals with bipolar disorder: A literature review. *Journal of Geriatric Psychiatry and Neurology, 25*(1), 20–25.

Lehmann, S. W., & Lee, J. (2012). Lithium-associated hypercalcemia and hyperparathyroidism in the elderly: What do we know? *Journal of Affective Disorders, 146*(1), 151–157.

Loo, C., Katalinic, N., Mitchell, P. B., & Greenberg, B. (2011). Physical treatments for bipolar disorder: A review of electroconvulsive therapy, stereotactic surgery and other brain stimulation techniques. *Journal of Affective Disorders, 132*(1), 1–13.

Lyoo, I. K., Dager, S. R., Kim, J. E., Yoon, S. J., Friedman, S. D., Dunner, D. L., & Renshaw, P. F. (2010). Lithium-induced gray matter volume increase as a neural correlate of treatment response in bipolar disorder: A longitudinal brain imaging study. *Neuropsychopharmacology, 35*(8), 1743–1750.

Martino, D. J., Strejilevich, S. A., Scápola, M., Igoa, A., Marengo, E., Ais, E. D., & Perinot, L. (2008). Heterogeneity in cognitive functioning among patients with bipolar disorder. *Journal of Affective Disorders, 109*(1), 149–156.

McDonald, W. M., & Nemeroff, C. B. (1996). The diagnosis and treatment of mania in the elderly. *Bulletin of the Menninger Clinic, 60*(2), 174–196.

Mendez, M. F. (2000). Mania in neurologic disorders. *Current Psychiatry Reports, 2*(5), 440–445.

Meeks, S., & Murrell, S. A. (1997). Mental illness in late life: Socioeconomic conditions, psychiatric symptoms, and adjustment of long-term sufferers. *Psychology and Aging, 12*(2), 296.

Miklowitz, D. J., Otto, M. W., Frank, E., Reilly-Harrington, N. A., Wisniewski, S. R., Kogan, J. N., & Sachs, G. S. (2007). Psychosocial treatments for bipolar depression: A 1-year randomized trial from the Systematic Treatment Enhancement Program. *Archives of General Psychiatry, 64*(4), 419.

Moorhead, S. R., & Young, A. H. (2003). Evidence for a late onset bipolar-I disorder sub-group from 50 years. *Journal of affective disorders, 73*(3), 271–277.

Nierenberg, A. A., & McColl, R. D. (1996). Management options for refractory depression. *American Journal of Medicine, 101*(6), 45S–52S.

Oostervink, F., Boomsma, M. M., & Nolen, W. A. (2009). Bipolar disorder in the elderly; different effects of age and of age of onset. *Journal of Affective Disorders, 116*(3), 176–183.

Peet, M., & Harvey, N. S. (1991). Lithium maintenance: 1. A standard education programme for patients. *The British Journal of Psychiatry, 158*(2), 197–200.

Peet, M., & Peters, S. (1995). Drug-induced mania. *Drug Safety, 2*, 146–153.

Rej, S., Herrmann, N., & Shulman, K. (2012). The effects of lithium on renal function in older adults—a systematic review. *Journal of Geriatric Psychiatry and Neurology, 25*(1), 51–61.

Sadock, B. J., Kaplan, H. I., & Sadock, V. A. (2007). Mood disorder. In B. J. Sadock & V. A. Sadock (Eds.), *Kaplan & Sadock's synopsis of psychiatry: Behavioral sciences/clinical psychiatry* (10th ed., pp. 527–528). Philadelphia: Wolter Kluwer/Lippincott Williams & Wilkins.

Sajatovic, M., Calabrese, J. R., & Mullen, J. (2008). Quetiapine for the treatment of bipolar mania in older adults. *Bipolar Disorders, 10*(6), 662–671.

Schouws, S. N. T. M., Stek, M. L., Comijs, H. C., Dols, A., & Beekman, A. T. F. (2012). Cognitive decline in elderly bipolar disorder patients: A follow-up study. *Bipolar Disorders, 14*(7), 749–755.

Schneider, L. S., Dagerman, K. S., & Insel, P. (2005). Risk of death with atypical antipsychotic drug treatment for dementia: Meta-analysis of randomized placebo-controlled trials. *JAMA, 294*, 1934–1943.

Tamashiro, J. H., Zung, S., Zanetti, M. V., De Castro, C. C., Vallada, H., Busatto, G. F., & De Toledo Ferraz Alves, T. C. (2008). Increased rates of white matter hyperintensities in late-onset bipolar disorder. *Bipolar Disorders, 10*(7), 765–775.

Trannel, T. J., Ahmed, I., & Goebert, D. (2001). Occurrence of thrombocytopenia in psychiatric patients taking valproate. *The American Journal of Psychiatry, 158*(1), 128–130.

Trinh, N. H., & Forester, B. (2007). Bipolar disorder in the elderly: Differential diagnosis and treatment. *Psychiatric Times, 24*(14), 38–43.

US Census Bureau. (2010). *The next four decades: The older population in the United States: 2010–2050 report*. Washington, DC: Author.

US Department of Health and Human Services, Administration on Aging. (2013). *A profile of older Americans: 2012*. Washington, DC: Author. Retrieved from http://www.aoa.gov/AoARoot/Aging_Statistics/Profile/2012/2.aspx

Van der Wurff, F. B., Stek, M. L., Hoogendijk, W. J., et al. (2003). The efficacy and safety of ECT in depressed older adults: A literature review. *International Journal of Geriatric Psychiatry, 18*(10), 894–904.

Van Gerpen, M. W., Johnson, J. E., & Winstead, D. K. (1999). Mania in the geriatric patient population: A review of the literature. *American Journal of Geriatric Psychiatry, 7*(3), 188–202.

Wang, P. S., Bohn, R. L., Glynn, R. J., Mogun, H., & Avorn, J. (2001). Hazardous benzodiazepine regimens in the elderly: Effects of half-life, dosage, and duration on risk of hip fracture. *The American Journal of Psychiatry, 158*(6), 892–898.

Weissman, M. M., Leaf, P. J., Tischler, G. L., Blazer, D. G., Karno, M., Bruce, M. L., & Florio, L. P. (1988). Affective disorders in five United States communities. *Psychological Medicine, 18*(1), 141–153.

Wu, C. S., Wang, S. C., Chang, I., & Lin, K. M. (2009). The association between dementia and long-term use of benzodiazepine in the elderly: Nested case–control study using claims data. *American Journal of Geriatric Psychiatry, 17*(7), 614–620.

SECTION IV

FUTURE RESEARCH

41

PLACEBO RESPONSE IN CLINICAL TRIALS OF BIPOLAR DISORDER

POTENTIAL CAUSES, POTENTIAL SOLUTIONS

Bret R. Rutherford, Steven P. Roose, and Jane M. Tandler

INTRODUCTION

Placebo response in clinical trials for psychiatric disorders has been a long-standing issue for psychiatric researchers and clinicians, and it has recently captured the attention of the lay public as well. Scientific interest focuses on the influence of placebo response on signal detection in clinical trials and what the physiologic mechanisms of placebo response may reveal about the pathophysiology of the disorder under study. The public would like to know whether responses to psychiatric medications are caused by specific effects of the medications or are "just" placebo effects. Clinicians may alternately view placebo response as a confounding factor in their effort to practice evidence-based medicine and a potential tool to improve patient care. This chapter reviews the data on placebo response in clinical trials for bipolar disorder (BD), presents a model of what causes placebo response in bipolar trials, and then discusses the methodological implications of this model germane to minimizing placebo response in future trials.

THE MAGNITUDE OF PLACEBO RESPONSE IN BIPOLAR DISORDER

Placebo response in clinical trials for BD is more complex than that in major depressive disorder (MDD) or other psychiatric illnesses. There is a potential placebo response in at least three different conditions, including (a) acute response of depressive symptoms to placebo in trials of antidepressant medications for depressive episodes associated with BD, (b) acute response of manic symptoms to placebo in trials of mood-stabilizing medications for manic/mixed episodes associated with BD, and (c) prophylactic effect of placebo for recurrent mood episodes in the maintenance treatment of BD. One might add additional categories for trials primarily enrolling patients diagnosed with BD type II or those having subthreshold symptoms. The magnitude of placebo response may be very different in these different phases of illness and bipolar subtypes.

Whereas it was previously thought that clinical trials of the severe and primarily "biological" mental illnesses such as BD and schizophrenia were immune from the issue of high placebo response, it has been increasingly recognized that clinical trials enrolling BD patients may be associated with high and possibly rising rates of placebo response. Vieta et al. (2010) performed a meta-analysis evaluating the effectiveness of treatments for the depressive phase of BD from 19 double-blind, active comparator or placebo-controlled acute studies. They found that placebo response in these studies was strikingly variable, ranging from 9% to 56% and having a mean of 39.4%.

Consistent with these findings, Sidor and MacQueen (2011) identified six acute clinical trials of antidepressants versus placebo for depressive episodes in patients with BD. Placebo response ranged from 12.5% to 42.0% in these trials, with an overall average of 38.4% across all studies (see Table 41.1). The authors found that antidepressant medications were not associated with a significant decrease in depressive symptoms relative to placebo, nor were they associated with increased frequency of affective switching relative to placebo. This average placebo-response rate compares to an average placebo response of 31% in antidepressant clinical trials for adults with unipolar MDD (compared to a mean medication response of 50%) and placebo response of 46% (compared to a mean medication response of 59%) in pediatric MDD trials (Bridge Birmaher, Iyengar, Barbe, & Brent, 2009). Thus, although the number of

Table 41.1. SELECTION OF RECENT CLINICAL TRIALS OF MONOTHERAPY FOR ACUTE DEPRESSIVE EPISODES IN PATIENTS WITH BIPOLAR DISORDER

AUTHOR	DATE	NITT	GROUPS	LENGTH (WEEKS)	COMPLETERS (%)	CHANGE IN DEPRESSION SCORE (%)	RESPONDERS (%)
Agosti and Stewart	2007	23	Imipramine	6	100	NA	57
		25	Phenelzine		84		52
		22	Placebo		100		23
Calabrese et al.	1999	66	Lamotrigine 50 mg	7	65.2	54.4	45
		63	Lamotrigine 200 mg		71.4	55.4	51
		66	Placebo		71.2	41.1	37
Calabrese et al.	2005	180	Quetiapine 300 mg	8	54.4	54.6	58
		181	Quetiapine 600 mg		66.9	56.0	58
		181	Placebo		59.1	34.7	36
Cohn et al.	1989	30	Fluoxetine	6	57	50.2	86
		30	Imipramine		47	37.3	57
		29	Placebo		34	14.3	38
McElroy et al.	2010	229	Quetiapine 300 mg	8	90.1	59.7	67
		232	Quetiapine 600 mg		87.7	61.5	67
		118	Paroxetine		86.8	50.4	55
		121	Placebo		91.9	46.3	53
Muzina et al.	2008	26	Divalproex ER	6	NA	NA	38
		28	Placebo				11
Nemeroff et al.	2001	39	Paroxetine	10	59.0	50.0	36
		35	Imipramine		71.4	48.8	43
		43	Placebo		62.8	37.4	34.9
Suppes et al.	2010	137	Quetiapine ER Placebo	8	62.1	58.4	65.4
		140			68.6	39.5	43.1
Thase et al.	2006	169	Quetiapine 600 mg	8	53.3	53.5	58.3
		172	Quetiapine 300 mg		58.7	54.5	60.0
		168	Placebo		65.5	40.3	44.7
Thase et al.	2008	187	Aripiprazole	8	58.8	NA	45
		188	Placebo		70.2		44
Thase et al.	2008	186	Aripiprazole	8	53.2	NA	43.2
		188	Placebo		64.9		39
Tohen et al.	2003	370	Olanzapine	8	48.4	46.4	39
		86	Olanzapine-fluoxetine.		64.0	54.3	56
		377	Placebo		38.5	37.9	30
Young et al.	2010	225	Quetiapine 300 mg	8	75.5	54.7	69
		263	Quetiapine 600 mg		76.5	56.9	70
		136	Lithium		75.0	48.1	62
		129	Placebo		72.2	41.4	56
Zarate et al.	2004	10	Pramipexole	6	90.0	47.1	60
		11	Placebo		91.0	12.4	9

NOTE: NITT = Number patients in intent to treat analysis; NA = not available; ER = extended release.

Table 41.2. SELECTION OF RECENT CLINICAL TRIALS OF MOOD-STABILIZING MEDICATIONS FOR ACUTE MANIC OR MIXED EPISODES IN PATIENTS WITH BIPOLAR DISORDER

AUTHOR	DATE	NITT	GROUPS	LENGTH (WEEKS)	COMPLETERS (%)	% CHANGE IN MANIA SCORE	RESPONDERS (%)
Bowden et al.	1994	36	Lithium	3	61.1	23.0	49
		69	Divalproex		47.8	23.4	48
		74	Placebo		63.5	8.9	25
Bowden et al.	2005	107	Quetiapine	3	90.7	14.6	53.3
		98	Lithium		85.7	15.2	53.1
		65	Placebo		69.1	6.7	27.4
Hirschfeld et al.	2004	127	Risperidone	3	56.0	10.6	43.3
		119	Placebo		41.6	4.8	24.4
Janicak et al.	1998	8	Verapamil	3	17.6	1.1	37.5
		12	Placebo		40	1.3	16.7
Keck et al.	2003a	123	Aripiprazole	3	41.5	8.2	39.8
		120	Placebo		21.2	3.4	19.2
Keck et al.	2003b	131	Ziprasidone	3	53.6	12.4	50.4
		66	Placebo		44.3	7.8	34.8
Keck et al.	2009	124	Aripiprazole	3	44.2	12.6	46.8
		125	Lithium		48.8	12.0	45.8
		163	Placebo		47.3	9.0	34.4
Khanna et al.	2005	144	Risperidone	3	89	22.7	74.3
		142	Placebo		70.8	10.5	36.6
Kushner et al.	2006	215	Topiramate 200	3	70.0	6	27.0
		113	+ 400 mg		74.3	12.9	46
		111	Lithium Placebo		73.9	7.7	28
Kushner et al.	2006	115	Topira-	3	87.1	8.2	28
		114	mate 400 mg		81.6	13.8	28
		112	Lithium Placebo		86.6	8.4	28
Kushner et al.	2006	107	Topira-	3	56.0	5.1	27
		106	mate 400 mg Placebo		73.6	6.4	28
Kushner et al.	2006	209	Topiramate 400	3	58.9	8.1	27
		99	+ 600 mg Placebo		72	7.7	28
McIntyre et al.	2005	98	Haloperidal	12	55.1	58.6	70.4
		101	Quetiapine		54.5	51.5	61.4
		100	Placebo		41.6	28.6	39.0
McIntyre et al.	2009	189	Asenapine	3	62.9	13.1	41.3
		188	Olanzapine		79.6	13.9	50.0
		103	Placebo		61.5	7.4	25.2
Pande et al.	2000	59	Lithium and/or	10	53	34.6	37
		58	Valproate + Gabapentin Placebo		64	53.8	47
Pope et al.	1991	15	Valproate	1-3	23.5	11.4	52.9
		19	Placebo		21.1	.2	10.5
Potkin et al.	2005	137	Ziprasidone	3	60.7	11.1	46.7
		65	Placebo		54.5	5.6	29.2

(*continued*)

Table 41.2. CONTINUED

AUTHOR	DATE	NITT	GROUPS	LENGTH (WEEKS)	COMPLETERS (%)	% CHANGE IN MANIA SCORE	RESPONDERS (%)
Sachs et al.	2002	52	Risperidone	3	35	51	53
		53	Haloperidol		53	49.1	50
		51	Placebo		49	41	30
Sachs et al.	2006	136	Aripiprazole	3	54.7	12.5	52.9
		132	Placebo		51.9	7.2	32.6
Smulevich et al.	2005	150	Risperidone	12	90.3	13.9	47.2
		144	Haloperidol		89	15.1	47.7
		138	Placebo		85	9.4	33.3
Tohen et al.	1999	70	Olanzapine	3	61.4	10.3	48.6
		66	Placebo		34.8	4.9	24.2
Tohen et al.	2000	54	Olanzapine	4	61.8	14.8	64.8
		56	Placebo		41.7	8.1	42.9
Tohen et al.	2003	351	Olanzapine	8	48.4	-1.4	39.0
		82	Olanzapine +		64.0	-1.9	56.1
		355	Fluoxetine Placebo		38.5	-.1	30.4
Vieta et al.	2005	208	Quetiapine	12	60.8	40.7	66.8
		195	Placebo		38.9	23.2	40.0
Vieta et al.	2010a	190	Paliperidone	3	82	13.2	44.2
		192	Quetiapine		79	11.7	49.0
		104	Placebo		62	7.4	34.6
Vieta et al.	2010b	176	Ziprasidone	3	66.9	10.4	36.9
		170	Haloperidol		71.3	15.9	54.7
		88	Placebo		50.0	6.1	20.5
Weisler et al.	2004	94	Carbamaze-pine ER	3	49.5	8.7	40.4
		98	Placebo		44.7	5.2	21.4
Weisler et al.	2005	120	Carbamaze-pine ER	3	65.6	15.1	60.8
		115	Placebo		54.7	7.1	28.7
Yildiz et al.	2008	32	Tamoxifen	3	82.9	16.6	43.8
		26	Placebo		67.7	-4.8	3.8
Young et al.	2009	166	Aripiprazole	3	75.4	12.0	47.0
		161	Haloperidol		73.3	12.8	49.7
		152	Placebo		71.2	9.7	38.2
Zarate et al.	2007	8	Tamoxifen	3	50.0	18.3	62.5
		8	Placebo		62.5	-4.7	12.5

NOTE: NITT = Number patients in intent to treat analysis; NA = not available; ER = extended release.

studies available for analysis is much smaller in the case of BD, acute response rates of depressive symptoms to placebo appear similar to or perhaps greater than patients with unipolar MDD.

Two recent meta-analyses provide data on placebo response in clinical trials of mood-stabilizing medications to treat acute manic or mixed states. Yildiz, Vieta, Tohen, & Baldessarini (2011) analyzed 38 placebo-controlled trials for acute mania and reported a placebo response rate of 30.8%, while Sysko and Walsh (2007) found a placebo response rate of 31.2% in 21 clinical trials for bipolar mania. See Table 41.2 for a summary of these studies. In the Sysko et al. (2007) data set, there was a significant association between response rates (as measured by the Young Mania Rating Scale) and year of publication, though this was not corroborated subsequently by Yildiz et al. As a result, it is unclear whether placebo response in randomized controlled trials (RCTs) for BD is rising, as has been shown to be the case in MDD.

The typical placebo-controlled maintenance trial entails open treatment with a mood-stabilizing medication to treat the acute mood episode followed by randomization of responders to continued medication or placebo. Participants are then followed over time (typically one to two years) to determine the rate of relapse on medication compared to placebo (where recurrence is defined as hospitalization, change in medications, or a suprathreshold score on a symptom rating scale). Thus the "placebo response" in these studies is the protective effect of placebo on recurrence rather than acute therapeutic effects on existing mood symptoms.

A recent meta-analysis aggregating data from seven placebo-controlled maintenance trials found that the odds of recurrence at 20 to 24 weeks follow-up for patients receiving placebo were 4.1 times the odds of recurrence on medication (Keck, Welge, Strakowski, Arnold, & Mcelroy, 2000). Relapse rates for patients receiving medication ranged from 24% to 26% at one year compared to relapse rates of 38% to 64% on placebo (see Table 41.3 for a representative selection of such studies). One important factor to keep in mind when evaluating maintenance studies is whether the discontinuation of active treatment was abrupt or tapered over several weeks. Abrupt discontinuation of active treatment may cause increased symptoms among patients treated with placebo and artificially increase relapse rates.

High placebo response reduces medication–placebo differences, in response to which investigators often make methodological modifications (i.e., the use of multiple study sites to increase sample size) that increase measurement error. Both decreased medication–placebo differences and increased measurement error make it more difficult to demonstrate a statistically significant benefit of a medication over placebo. An illustration of this phenomenon has occurred in antidepressant trials for MDD, where the average difference observed between medication and placebo has decreased from an average of 6 points on the Hamilton Rating Scale for Depression (HAM-D) scale in 1982 to 3 points in 2008 (Khan, Bhat, Kolts, Thase, & Brown, 2010). For most currently approved antidepressants, less than half of the efficacy trials filed with the Food and Drug Administration for regulatory approval found active drug superior to placebo (Hooper & Amsterdam, 1998; Khan, Khan, & Brown, 2002). While not all trials that fail to distinguish medication from placebo represent false negatives, meta-analyses of antidepressant trials suggest that high placebo response rather than low medication response explains most of the variability in drug–placebo differences across studies (Bridge et al., 2009). The increasing number of failed trials in recent years has made developing psychiatric medications progressively more time-consuming (average of 13 years to develop a new medication) and expensive (estimates range from $800 million to $3 billion per new agent) compared to medications for non–central nervous system indications (Nutt & Goodwin, 2011). These considerations contributed to recent decisions by several large pharmaceutical companies to reduce or discontinue research and development on medications for brain disorders, prompting warnings of "psychopharmacology in crisis" (Cressey, 2011).

CAUSES OF PLACEBO RESPONSE IN BIPOLAR TRIALS

Placebo response refers to the change in symptoms occurring during a clinical trial in patients randomized to receive placebo. In contrast, the term *placebo effect* can be defined as the therapeutic effect of receiving a substance or undergoing a procedure that is not caused by any inherent powers of the substance or procedure (Stewart-Williams & Podd, 2004). Thus whereas placebo response is directly observed and quantified in a research study, a placebo effect is a theoretical, unobserved construct that is hypothesized to cause placebo response. To clarify this differentiation further, the sources of symptom change in clinical trials can be grouped into categories.

Treatment factors comprise all the interventions and study procedures experienced by a patient in a clinical trial. Placebo effects are one type of treatment factor occurring when a patient takes a pill believed to be an effective treatment for depression. Supportive contacts with study clinicians and undergoing medical tests and procedures may

Table 41.3. **SELECTION OF RECENT CLINICAL TRIALS FOR MAINTENANCE OF EUTHYMIA IN PATIENTS WITH BIPOLAR DISORDER**

AUTHOR	DATE	NITT	GROUPS	LENGTH (WEEKS)	% PLACEBO MANIA RELAPSE	% PLACEBO DEPRESSION RELAPSE
Bowden et al.	2000	91 187 94	Lithium Valproate Placebo	52	22.3	16.0
Bowden et al.	2003	46 59 70	Lithium Lamotrigine Placebo	76	31.4	30
Bowden et al.	2010	127 111	Ziprasidone + Lithium/ Divalproex Placebo	24	12.6	14.4
Calabrese et al.	2003	215 120 119	Lamotrigine Lithium Placebo	72	16	39.5
Keck et al.	2007	77 83	Aripiprazole Placebo	100	27.7	15.7
Macfadden et al.	2009	65 59	Risperidone LAI + treatment as usual Placebo	52	20.3	18.6
Marcus et al.	2011	168 169	Aripiprazole + Lithium/ Divalproex Placebo	52	14.8	13
Prien et al.	1973	101 104	Lithium Placebo	24	51	13.5
Quiroz et al.	2010	336 367	Risperidone LAI Placebo	96	45.9	10.4
Suppes et al.	2009	310 313	Quetiapine + Lithium/ Divalproex Placebo	104	19.5	32.6
Tohen et al.	2004	30 38	Olanzapine + Lithium/ Divalproex Placebo	72	29	39.5
Tohen et al.	2006	225 136	Olanzapine Placebo	48	32.4	39
Vieta et al.	2008a	336 367	Quetiapine + Lithium/ Divalproex Placebo	104	26.2	22.9
Vieta et al.	2008b	26 29	Oxcarbazepine + Lithium Placebo	52	27.6	31
Vieta et al.	2012	131 130 132	Risperidone LAI Olanzapine Placebo	NA	39.4	17.4
Weisler et al.	2008	364 404 404	Lithium Quetiapine Placebo	104	72	46

NOTE: NITT = Number patients in intent to treat analysis; NA = not available; LAI = long-acting injectable.

also have therapeutic elements. Some evidence suggests that expectancy-based placebo effects and effects of the therapeutic setting may be moderated by patient demographic and clinical characteristics. *Measurement factors* represent sources of bias and error inherent in measuring manic and depressive symptoms, and *natural history factors* reflect spontaneous improvement and worsening in the patient's condition that is unrelated to the study procedures. According to this conceptual framework, the symptom change observed in patient receiving placebo in a clinical trial (i.e., placebo response) is caused by the sum effects of these factors and their interactions. While large placebo effects may be one cause of large observed placebo response, it is also possible that high placebo response could be observed even where there are minimal placebo effects operative. This might occur, for example, if there has been substantial improvement resulting from contacts with health-care providers or a structured therapeutic setting, regression to the mean, rater bias, or spontaneous fluctuation in illness severity.

TREATMENT FACTORS

Expectancy-based placebo effects

Data about the influence of patient expectancy primarily come from antidepressant clinical trials for MDD, because fewer studies investigating the components of placebo response are available in patients with BD. The first investigators to document the influence of patient expectancy on were Khan, Kolts, Thase, Krishnan and Brown (2004), who reported that the number of treatment arms in a study was negatively correlated with the "success" of the trial (defined as finding a significant difference between drug and placebo). This finding may be explained by the fact that a greater number of treatment arms entails a greater probability of receiving active medication, which may increase patient expectations and generate higher placebo response. Consistent findings have been observed in meta-analyses comparing medication response in placebo-controlled trials (i.e., one or more medications compared to placebo) and active comparator trials (i.e., one or more medications with no placebo group). In adults and older adults with MDD, mean medication response rates in comparator trials are significantly greater than the mean medication response rates in placebo-controlled trials (Rutherford, Sneed, & Roose 2009; Sneed et al. 2008). Patients in comparator trials know they have a 100% chance of receiving an active medication, which may increase their expectancy of improvement, leading to enhanced placebo effects and greater observed antidepressant response.

Two prospective antidepressant studies for adults with MDD have directly measured patient expectancy, and each reported that higher expectancy predicts greater symptom improvement. In the National Institute of Mental Health Treatment of Depression Collaborative Study, which enrolled 239 outpatients with MDD, higher patient expectation of improvement predicted greater likelihood of depression response and lower final depression scores in all four treatment conditions (cognitive behavior therapy, interpersonal therapy, imipramine, and placebo-clinical management; Meyer et al., 2002). In a single-blind trial of reboxetine for 25 subjects with MDD, subjects with a higher pretreatment expectation of medication effectiveness had a greater likelihood of response: 90% of patients with high expectations of improvement responded compared to 33% of patients with lower expectations (Krell, Leuchter, Morgan, Cook, & Abrams, 2004). Moreover, a recent pilot study experimentally manipulated expectancy in subjects with MDD by randomizing 43 adult outpatients to placebo-controlled (i.e., 50% chance of receiving active drug) or comparator (i.e., 100% chance of receiving active drug) administration of antidepressant medication (Rutherford et al., 2013). Randomization to the comparator condition resulted in significantly increased patient expectancy relative to the placebo-controlled arm of the study, and a trend was observed for higher pretreatment expectancy of improvement to be positively correlated with the change in depressive symptoms observed over the study.

Therapeutic setting

In addition to receiving an expectation of improvement, participants in a clinical trial receive a great deal of supportive care and attention from clinicians. Individuals who may be experiencing social isolation and decreased activity levels as part of their depressive illness enter a behaviorally activating and interpersonally rich new environment. Manic patients enter a calm and structured setting that reinforces a healthy sleep schedule and places limits on impulsive and self-destructive behavior. All clinical trial participants interact with research coordinators and medical staff, receive lengthy clinical evaluations by highly trained professionals, and are provided with diagnoses and psychoeducation that explain their symptoms. Medical procedures are performed, such as blood tests, electrocardiograms, and vital sign measurements. Finally, clinicians meet with patients frequently to listen to their experiences and facilitate compliance by instilling faith in the effectiveness of treatment.

Such supportive care has been shown to positively influence antidepressant treatment of depressive symptoms. Posternak and Zimmerman (2007) investigated the influence of therapeutic contact frequency on antidepressant and placebo response in 41 RCTs of antidepressants for MDD. These investigators calculated the change in HAM-D scores observed over the first six weeks of treatment in patients assigned to antidepressant medication and placebo, comparing studies with more versus fewer numbers of assessment visits. A cumulative therapeutic effect of additional follow-up visits on placebo response was found, such that patients with weekly visits improved 4.24 HAM-D points between Weeks 2 and 6, while those with one less visit improved 3.33 points and those with two fewer visits improved 2.49 points. Additional follow-up visits appeared to explain approximately 50% of the symptom change observed between Weeks 2 and 6 among patients receiving placebo. Interestingly, the relative effect of this increased therapeutic contact on medication response was approximately 50% less than that observed in patients assigned to placebo.

One might expect the influence of supportive care on manic symptoms to be even greater, since most participants in clinical trials for acute mania receive inpatient treatment during the study. The structured environment and health-care provider attention provided in such a setting may have significant therapeutic effects. Acutely ill patients may not have been sleeping overnight owing to their decreased need for sleep, or else they may have been impulsively pursuing self-destructive activities, both of which might be expected to worsen their mood symptoms. For these reasons, being placed in a setting where a regular sleep schedule is instituted and strict limits are placed on impulsive behavior may thus have significant benefits, irrespective of whether medication or placebo is prescribed.

Concomitant medications

Rescue medications such as benzodiazepines may help decrease severity scores on items pertaining to sleep and agitation, and this may be particularly significant in studies of acute mania. In some studies, subjects receiving placebo receive significantly higher average doses of rescue medications compared to those treated with active medication (Chengappa et al., 2000).

MEASUREMENT FACTORS

Error and bias associated with the measurement of psychiatric symptoms affect outcome measurements in clinical trials for BD. For example, regression to the mean is a statistical phenomenon occurring when repeated measurements associated with random error are made on the same subject over time (Barnett, Van Der Pols & Dobson, 2005). If a patient with a "true" HAM-D score of 10 underwent repeated ratings, a normal distribution with a mean of 10 would be obtained due to random error in measurement. If baseline symptom measurement happened to be unusually high (e.g., 14), then the next observed value likely would be closer to the subject's true mean score of 10 based on chance alone. This tendency for the depression scores of some subjects to decrease on repeated measurement may give the appearance of group-level improvement when in fact no true change has occurred.

While random error and regression to the mean can be an important factor in all clinical trials, sources of bias can be more problematic in studies of psychiatric conditions, which often lack objective measurements, such as serum cholesterol or blood pressure. Investigators in bipolar trials assess change in the severity of patient's illness based on symptom changes that are self-reported by patients or elicited by trained raters. Thus these measurements are subject to rater bias, which occurs when an individual's rating of symptom severity in an antidepressant clinical trial is influenced by underlying beliefs or motivations with respect to the treatments under study (Marcus et al. 2006). For example, assessments of eligibility for a clinical trial may be biased toward baseline score inflation when investigators have a financial incentive to recruit patients (Mundt et al., 2007). An increased number of collaborating study sites. Indeed, Yildiz et al. (2011) reported that the number of study sites, which may covary with increased financial incentives to recruit patients and thus with increased rater bias, was significantly associated with placebo response in their meta-analysis ($p < .0001$).

NATURAL HISTORY FACTORS

By definition, BD is a fluctuating disorder in which depressive and manic episodes occur and remit on their own accord. Patients are most likely to seek treatment during periods of symptomatic worsening, so those who enroll in a clinical trial at this time of peak symptomatology may experience natural waning of symptoms or alleviation of the precipitating stressors irrespective of the treatment they are provided. Given the ethical difficulties associated with following the untreated course of BD, few prospective non-intervention studies using modern diagnostic criteria exist that may be used to estimate the magnitude of spontaneous improvement that can be expected in acute depressive and manic episodes. In general, however, one might expect the amount of spontaneous improvement observed to be larger for individuals with rapid-cycling forms of illness, who by definition fluctuate more than the average bipolar patient.

Some information is available regarding the natural course of depressive episodes in unipolar MDD, though the generalizability of this information to BD is unclear. One can examine the change occurring among patients in wait-list control groups within psychotherapy studies for depression to estimate the natural course of the illness. A recent meta-analysis of acute symptom change in wait-list control conditions found that individuals with unipolar MDD experience an average improvement of 4 HAM-D points (Cohen's d effect size = 0.5) over a mean follow-up duration of 10 weeks (Rutherford, Mori, Sneed, Pimontel, & Roose, 2012). Since meta-analyses of medication and placebo response in antidepressant clinical trials report standardized effect sizes of approximately 1.5 for medication conditions and 1.2 for placebo conditions (Kirsch & Sapirstein, 1998), patients in wait-list control conditions appear to experience approximately 33% of the improvement occurring with medication treatment and 40% of the improvement seen with placebo administration. Obviously, wait-list controls are not utilized in studies of acutely manic patients, so it is difficult to estimate the rate of spontaneous improvement occurring in this phase of the illness.

PATIENT-LEVEL MODERATORS OF PLACEBO RESPONSE

Historically, most studies have failed to identify consistent characteristics of patients likely to respond to placebo, giving rise to the term *the elusive placebo reactor* as early as the 1960s (Liberman, 1967). This led many to reject the hypothesis that certain people respond to placebos while others do not, and instead the consensus view arose that most individuals appear capable of being influenced by placebo effects under the appropriate conditions (Doongaji, Vahia, & Bharucha, 1978). While that may be largely true, features of the depressive illness in unipolar MDD have been shown to influence the magnitude of placebo response. Both Kirsch et al. (2008) and Fournier et al. (2010) found that placebo response significantly declined as baseline HAM-D increased (particularly as it exceeded a score of 25). Other studies suggest that patients suffering from psychotic or recurrent MDD have decreased rates of placebo response, as do elderly depressed patients with early-onset

(prior to age 60) depression (Glassman & Roose, 1981, Lesperance et al., 2007; Roose et al., 2004).

In trials enrolling only patients with BD, younger mean patient age, increased percentage of male subjects, and the presence of psychotic symptoms have all been associated with decreased placebo response and increased drug–placebo differences (Yildiz et al., 2011). Additionally, diagnosis with a mixed episode has been reported to decrease drug response while leaving placebo response unaffected, thus having the sum effect of decreasing drug–placebo differences (Yildiz et al., 2011).

METHODS OF MINIMIZING PLACEBO RESPONSE IN BIPOLAR TRIALS

Based on the foregoing conceptual model of the sources of placebo response, as well as patient-level moderators of placebo response that have been identified, a number of methodological suggestions can be made toward the goal of minimizing placebo response. The many failed attempts to deal with the problem of rising placebo response are evidence that finding a balance between excessive placebo response and excessive dropout (for example) is difficult to achieve. Unfortunately, to the extent that many of the following methodological points may reduce placebo response, they may also have a tendency to decrease recruitment or increase noncompliance or attrition.

First, it follows from the treatment factors reviewed here that minimizing patient expectancy may be helpful when the goal is to demonstrate a significant difference between a putative antidepressant or mood-stabilizing agent and placebo. Rather than attempting to modify the behavior of individual study clinicians (i.e., by instructing them to be neutral or pessimistic), a more successful strategy may be to maximize the percentage of patients randomized to placebo in the study design. This suggestion stems from meta-analyses documenting higher medication response in active comparator relative to placebo-controlled trials and higher placebo response as the probability of receiving placebo diminishes. Of note, dealing with expectancy-based placebo effects by conducting single-blind lead-in periods aimed at identifying and excluding participants whose symptoms respond quickly to placebo has generally not been successful in clinical trials for unipolar depression. Multiple analyses have determined that such lead-ins have not been effective in reducing placebo response or improving detection of drug–placebo differences (Trivedi & Rush, 1994).

Second, insofar as it is practicable in terms of maintaining patient safety, there is evidence to suggest placebo response may be diminished by decreasing the amount of supportive care provided in a clinical trial. For outpatient studies, the primary variable to decrease would be visit frequency, since it has been convincingly demonstrated that increasing contact in the form of more frequent visits raises placebo response and decreases drug–placebo differences (Posternak & Zimmerman, 2007). This methodological adjustment may be quite feasible to implement, since no benefit of more frequent visits on decreasing dropout or improving compliance has been demonstrated. With respect to inpatient patient populations, perhaps more attention could be given to limiting the amount of supportive therapeutic contact patients receive. While this contact may be the same for patients receiving medication as well as placebo, there is evidence that therapeutic contact influences placebo response more than medication response, thereby reducing separation between medication and placebo. Similarly, minimizing concurrently administered medications may also be helpful, since placebo-treated patients tend to make more use of rescue medications compared to those on active medication.

Third, conducting clinical trials at multiple sites has been associated with increased placebo response by multiple studies across psychiatric disorders (Bridge et al., 2009). It has been hypothesized that increased financial incentives to recruit participants in large, multicenter studies may result in baseline score inflation and increased placebo response. Addressing this tendency for score inflation among raters with financial incentives may help reduce placebo response. For example, smaller, single-site RCTs for acute mania have actually reported symptom worsening for patients assigned to placebo rather than improvement (Yildiz, Guleryuz, Ankerst, Ongur, & Renshaw, 2008). Single-site studies may reduce financial bias, as well as limit the heterogeneity of the study sample and reduce rater variability. Given that multicenter studies do offer some significant advantages over single-site studies, particularly with respect to feasibility and generalizability of results, making methodological refinements aimed at reducing the impact of rater bias would be advisable. A minimum depression severity score required for enrollment into the study may be specified, but then a higher score threshold may be set a priori for including the subject in the data analysis. Another technique is to blind raters at individual study sites to the timing of baseline assessment so that they are unaware which ratings will be used to ascertain patient eligibility for the study. Finally, many investigators now utilize two separate depression rating scales for clinical trials: one measure to determine subject eligibility and a different scale to serve as the primary outcome measure in analyses.

Using centralized raters to perform the screening and outcome measures in clinical trials is another option. Centralized raters are less prone to bias by virtue of their off-site location and blinding to study entry criteria, patient phase of treatment, and treatment assignment (Kobak, Kane, Thase, & Nierenberg, 2007). This method may help relieve pressure to enroll patients, reduce biases toward baseline score inflation and observing improvement, and eliminate effects of repeated assessments by the same clinician. A relative disadvantage of using centralized raters is the necessity of assessing patients remotely via videoconference or telephone rather than having a face-to-face interview, and this may be a problem for trials of acute mania.

Fourth, some effort could be made to select for patient characteristics that minimize natural history factors as contributors to placebo response. For bipolar depression studies, requiring longer durations of current illness for inclusion (i.e., two to three months vs. two weeks) may be helpful. Multiple baseline assessments prior to actual enrollment of the patient in the study may help ensure that patients are not enrolled at a particular peak of symptom severity. In maintenance trials, enrollment of BD patients who have been in remission for lengthy periods may result in a low recurrence rate and little drug–placebo difference.

Finally, maximizing retention rates may be another useful strategy for decreasing placebo response. Limiting dropout may allow significant worsening over time to be documented in placebo-treated patients, which is not possible in studies having higher dropout rates. More trial completers among patients assigned to active medication has also been shown to increase drug-placebo separation in acute RCTs for mania (Yildiz et al., 2011).

CONCLUSION

In summary, placebo response in bipolar clinical trials is a fascinating and complex phenomenon. Investigating the mechanisms of placebo effects has the potential to illuminate the pathophysiology of BD as well as the active components of clinical trials. Furthermore, knowledge of the contributors to placebo response in bipolar trials may permit the development of strategies to improve signal detection in drug development studies.

Disclosure statements: Dr. Rutherford has received compensation from MedAvante for a grand rounds presentation and has received consulting fees from RCT Logic. Grant Support: National Institutes of Health (K23 MH085236 and R01 MH102293). Dr. Steven P. Roose and Jane M. Tandler have not disclosed any conflicts of interest.

REFERENCES

Agosti, V., & Stewart, J. W. (2007). Efficacy and safety of antidepressant monotherapy in the treatment of bipolar-II depression. *International Clinical Psychopharmacology*, *22*(5), 309–311.

Barnett, A. G., Van Der Pols, J. C., & Dobson, A. J. (2005). Regression to the mean: What it is and how to deal with it. *International Journal of Epidemiology*, *34*(1), 215–220.

Bowden, C. L., Brugger, A. M., Swann, A. C., Calabrese, J. R., Janicak, P. G., Petty, F.,…Small J. G. (1994). Efficacy of divalproex vs lithium and placebo in the treatment of mania. *JAMA*, *271*(12), 918–924.

Bowden, C. L., Calabrese, J. R., Sachs, G., Yatham, L. N., Asghar, S. A., Hompl, M.…Deveaugh-Geiss, J. (2003). A placebo-controlled 18-month trial of lamotrigine and lithium maintenance treatment in recently manic or hypomanic patients with bipolar I disorder. *Archives of General Psychiatry*, *60*(4), 392–400.

Bowden, C. L., Grunze, H., Mullen, J., Brecher, M., Paulsson, B., Jones, M.,…Svensson, K. (2005). A randomized, double-blind, placebo-controlled efficacy and safety study of quetiapine or lithium as monotherapy for mania in bipolar disorder. *Journal of Clinical Psychiatry*, *66*(1), 111–121.

Bowden, C. L., Vieta, E., Ice, K. S., Schwartz, J. H., Wang, P. P., & Versavel, M. (2010). Ziprasidone plus a mood stabilizer in subjects with bipolar I disorder: A 6-month, randomized, placebo-controlled, double-blind trial. *Journal of Clinical Psychiatry*, *71*(2), 130–137.

Bridge, J., Birmaher, B., Iyengar, S., Barbe, R., & Brent, D. (2009). Placebo response in randomized controlled trials of antidepressants for pediatric major depressive disorder. *American Journal of Psychiatry*, *166*(1), 42–49.

Calabrese, J. R., Bowden, C. L., Sachs, G. S., Ascher, J. A., Monaghan, E., & Rudd, G. D. (1999). A double-blind placebo-controlled study of lamotrigine monotherapy in outpatients with bipolar I depression. *Journal of Clinical Psychiatry*, *60*(2), 79–88.

Calabrese, J. R., Bowden, C. L., Sachs, G., Yatham, L. N., Behnke, K., Mehtonen, O. P.…Lamictal Study Group. (2003). A placebo-controlled 18-month trial of lamotrigine and lithium maintenance treatment in recently depressed patients with bipolar I disorder. *Journal of Clinical Psychiatry*, *64*(9), 1013–1024.

Calabrese, J. R., Keck, P. E., Macfadden, W., Minkwitz, M., Ketter, T. A., Weisler, R. H.,…Mullen, J. (2005). A randomized, double-blind, placebo-controlled trial of quetiapine in the treatment of bipolar I or II depression. *American Journal of Psychiatry*, *162*(7), 1351–1360.

Chengappa, K. R., Tohen, M., Levine, J., Jacobs, T., Thase, M. E., Sanger, T. M., & Kupfer, D. J. (2000). Response to placebo among bipolar I disorder patients experiencing their first manic episode. *Bipolar Disorders*, *2*(4), 332–335.

Cohn, J. B., Collins, G., Ashbrook, E., & Wernicke, J. (1989). A comparison of fluoxetine, imipramine and placebo in patients with bipolar depressive disorder. *International Clinical Psychopharmacology*, *4*(4), 313–322.

Cressey, D. (2011). Psychopharmacology in crisis. *Nature News*. doi:10.1038/news.2011.367.20.

Doongaji, D., Vahia, V., & Bharucha, M. (1978). On placebos, placebo responses and placebo responders—A review of psychological, psychopharmacological and psychophysiological factors: II. Psychopharmacological and psychophysiological factors. *Journal of Postgraduate Medicine*, *24*(3), 147–157.

Fournier, J. C., Derubeis, R. J., Hollon, S. D., Dimidjian, S., Amsterdam, J. D., Shelton, R. C., & Fawcett, J. (2010). Antidepressant drug effects and depression severity: A patient-level meta-analysis. *JAMA*, *303*(1), 47–53.

Glassman, A., & Roose, S. P. (1981). Delusional depression: A distinct clinical entity? *Archives of General Psychiatry*, *38*(4), 424–427.

Hirschfeld, R. M., Keck, P. E., Kramer, M., Karcher, K., Canuso, C., Eerdekens, M., & Grossman, F. (2004). Rapid antimanic effect of risperidone monotherapy: A 3-week multicenter, double-blind, placebo-controlled trial. *American Journal of Psychiatry*, *161* (6), 1057–1065.

Hooper, M., & Amsterdam, J. (1998, June). *Do clinical trials reflect drug potential? A review of FDA evaluation of new antidepressants.* Paper presented at the 39th annual NCDEU meeting, Boca Raton, FL.

Janicak, P. G., Sharma, R. P., Pandey, G., & Davis, J. M. (1998). Verapamil for the treatment of acute mania: A double-blind, placebo-controlled trial. *American Journal of Psychiatry*, *155*(7), 972–973.

Keck, P. E. Jr., Calabrese, J. R., Mcintyre, R. S., Mcquade, R. D., Carson, W. H., Eudicone, J. M.,…Sanchez, R. (2007). Aripiprazole monotherapy for maintenance therapy in bipolar I disorder: A 100-week, double-blind study versus placebo. *Journal of Clinical Psychiatry*, *68*(10), 1480–1491.

Keck, P. E. Jr., Welge, J. A., Strakowski, S. M., Arnold, L. M., & Mcelroy, S. L. (2000). Placebo effect in randomized, controlled maintenance studies of patients with bipolar disorder. *Biological Psychiatry*, *47*(8), 756–761.

Keck, P. E., Marcus, R., Tourkodimitris, S., Ali, M., Liebeskind, A., Saha, A.,…Aripiprazole Study Group. (2003). A placebo-controlled, double-blind study of the efficacy and safety of aripiprazole in patients with acute bipolar mania. *American Journal of Psychiatry*, *160*(9), 1651–1658.

Keck, P. E., Versiani, M., Potkin, S., West, S. A., Giller, E., & Ice, K. (2003). Ziprasidone in the treatment of acute bipolar mania: A three-week, placebo-controlled, double-blind, randomized trial. *American Journal of Psychiatry*, *160*(4), 741–748.

Keck, P., Orsulak, P., Cutler, A., Sanchez, R., Torbeyns, A., Marcus, R.,…Carson, W. (2009). Aripiprazole monotherapy in the treatment of acute bipolar I mania: A randomized, double-blind, placebo-and lithium-controlled study. *Journal of Affective Disorders*, *112*(1), 36–49.

Khan, A., Bhat, A., Kolts, R., Thase, M. E., & Brown, W. (2010). Why has the antidepressant-placebo difference in antidepressant clinical trials diminished over the past three decades? *CNS Neuroscience & Therapeutics*, *16*(4), 217–226.

Khan, A., Khan, S., & Brown, W. A. (2002). Are placebo controls necessary to test new antidepressants and anxiolytics? *International Journal of Neuropsychopharmacology*, *5*(3), 193–197.

Khan, A., Kolts, R. L., Thase, M. E., Krishnan, K. R. R., & Brown, W. (2004). Research design features and patient characteristics associated with the outcome of antidepressant clinical trials. *American Journal of Psychiatry*, *161*(11), 2045–2049.

Khanna, S., Vieta, E., Lyons, B., Grossman, F., Eerdekens, M., & Kramer, M. (2005). Risperidone in the treatment of acute mania: Double-blind, placebo-controlled study. *BJP*, *187*, 229–234.

Kirsch, I., & Sapirstein, G. (1998). Listening to Prozac but hearing placebo: A meta-analysis of antidepressant medication. *Prevention & Treatment*, *1*(2), 2–16.

Kirsch, I., Deacon, B. J., Huedo-Medina, T. B., Scoboria, A., Moore, T. J., & Johnson, B. T. (2008). Initial severity and antidepressant benefits: A meta-analysis of data submitted to the food and drug administration. *PLoS Medicine*, *5*(2), 260–268.

Kobak, K. A., Kane, J. M., Thase, M. E., & Nierenberg, A. A. (2007). Why do clinical trials fail? The problem of measurement error in clinical trials: Time to test new paradigms? *Journal of Clinical Psychopharmacology*, 27(1), 1–5.

Krell, H. V., Leuchter, A. F., Morgan, M., Cook, I. A., & Abrams, M. (2004). Subject expectations of treatment effectiveness and outcome of treatment with an experimental antidepressant. *Journal of Clinical Psychiatry*, 65(9), 1174–1179.

Kushner, S. F., Khan, A., Lane, R., & Olson, W. H. (2006). Topiramate monotherapy in the management of acute mania: Results of four double-blind placebo-controlled trials. *Bipolar Disorders*, 8(1), 15–27.

Lesperance, F., Frasure-Smith, N., Koszycki, D., Lalibert'E, M., Van Zyl, L. T., Baker, B.,...CREATE Investigators. (2007). Effects of citalopram and interpersonal psychotherapy on depression in patients with coronary artery disease: The Canadian Cardiac Randomized Evaluation of Antidepressant and Psychotherapy Efficacy (CREATE) trial. *JAMA*, 297(4), 367–379.

Liberman, R. P. (1967) The elusive placebo reactor. *Neuropsychopharmacology*, 5, 557–566.

Macfadden, W., Alphs, L., Haskins, J. T., Turner, N., Turkoz, I., Bossie, C.,...Mahmoud, R. (2009). A randomized, double-blind, placebo-controlled study of maintenance treatment with adjunctive risperidone long-acting therapy in patients with bipolar I disorder who relapse frequently. *Bipolar Disorders*, 11(8), 827–839.

Marcus, R., Khan, A., Rollin, L., Morris, B., Timko, K., Carson, W., & Sanchez, R. (2011). Efficacy of aripiprazole adjunctive to lithium or valproate in the long-term treatment of patients with bipolar I disorder with an inadequate response to lithium or valproate monotherapy: A multicenter, double-blind, randomized study. *Bipolar Disorders*, 13(2), 133–144.

Marcus, S. M., Gorman, J. M., Tu, X., Gibbons, R. D., Barlow, D. H., Woods, S. W., & Katharine Shear, M. (2006). Rater bias in a blinded randomized placebo-controlled psychiatry trial. *Statistics in Medicine*, 25(16), 2762–2770.

Mcelroy, S. L., Weisler, R. H., Chang, W., Olausson, B., Paulsson, B., Brecher, M.,...EMBOLDEN II Investigators. (2010). A double-blind, placebo-controlled study of quetiapine and paroxetine as monotherapy in adults with bipolar depression (EMBOLDEN II). *Journal of Clinical Psychiatry*, 71(2), 163–174.

McIntyre, R. S., Brecher, M., Paulsson, B., Huizar, K., & Mullen, J. (2005). Quetiapine or haloperidol as monotherapy for bipolar mania—A 12-week, double-blind, randomised, parallel-group, placebo-controlled trial. *European Neuropsychopharmacology*, 15(5), 573–585.

McIntyre, R. S., Cohen, M., Zhao, J., Alphs, L., Macek, T. A., & Panagides, J. (2009). Asenapine versus olanzapine in acute mania: A double-blind extension study. *Bipolar Disorders*, 11(8), 815–826.

Meyer, B., Pilkonis, P. A., Krupnick, J. L., Egan, M. K., Simmens, S. J., & Sotsky, S. M. (2002). Treatment expectancies, patient alliance and outcome: Further analyses from the national institute of mental health treatment of depression collaborative research program. *Journal of Consulting and Clinical Psychology*, 70(4), 1051–1055.

Mundt, J. C., Greist, J. H., Jefferson, J. W., Katzelnick, D. J., Debrota, D. J., Chappell, P. B., & Modell, J. G. (2007). Is it easier to find what you are looking for if you think you know what it looks like? *Journal of Clinical Psychopharmacology*, 27(2), 121–125.

Nemeroff, C. B., Evans, D. L., Gyulai, L., Sachs, G. S., Bowden, C. L., Gergel, I. P.,...Pitts, C. D. (2001). Double-blind, placebo-controlled comparison of imipramine and paroxetine in the treatment of bipolar depression. *American Journal of Psychiatry*, 158(6), 906–912.

Nutt, D., & Goodwin, G. (2011). ECNP Summit on the future of CNS drug research in Europe 2011: Report prepared for ECNP by David Nutt and Guy Goodwin. *European Neuropsychopharmacology*, 21(7), 495–499.

Pande, A. C., Crockatt, J. G., Janney, C. A., Werth, J. L., & Tsaroucha, G. (2000). Gabapentin in bipolar disorder: A placebo-controlled trial of adjunctive therapy. *Bipolar Disorders*, 2, 249–255.

Pope, H. G., McElroy, S. L., Keck, E., & Hudson, J. I. (1991). Valproate in the treatment of acute mania: A placebo-controlled study. *Archives of General Psychiatry*, 48(1), 62–68.

Posternak, M. A., & Zimmerman, M. (2007). Therapeutic effect of follow-up assessments on antidepressant and placebo response rates in antidepressant efficacy trials meta-analysis. *BJP*, 190(4), 287–292.

Potkin, S. G., Keck, P. E. Jr., Segal, S., Ice, K., & English, P. (2005). Ziprasidone in acute bipolar mania: A 21-day randomized, double-blind, placebo-controlled replication trial. *Journal of Clinical Psychopharmacology*, 25(4), 301–310.

Prien, R. F., Point, P., Caffey, E. M., & Klett, C. J. (1973). Prophylactic efficacy of lithium carbonate in manic-depressive illness: Report of the Veterans Administration and National Institute of Mental Health collaborative study group. *Archives of General Psychiatry*, 28(3), 337–341.

Quiroz, J. A., Yatham, L. N., Palumbo, J. M., Karcher, K., Kushner, S., & Kusumakar, V. (2010). Risperidone long-acting injectable monotherapy in the maintenance treatment of bipolar I disorder. *Biological Psychiatry*, 68(2), 156–162.

Roose, S. P., Sackeim, H. A., Krishnan, K. R. R., Pollock, B. G., Alexopoulos, G., Lavretsky, H.,...Hakkarainen, H. (2004). Antidepressant pharmacotherapy in the treatment of depression in the very old: A randomized, placebo-controlled trial. *American Journal of Psychiatry*, 161(11), 2050–2059.

Rutherford, B. R., Mori, S., Sneed, J. R., Pimontel, M. A., & Roose, S. P. (2012). Contribution of spontaneous improvement to placebo response in depression: A meta-analytic review. *Journal of Psychiatric Research*, 46(6), 697–702.

Rutherford, B. R., Sneed, J. R., & Roose, S. P. (2009). Does study design influence outcome? *Psychotherapy and Psychosomatics*, 78(3), 172–181.

Rutherford, B., Marcus, S., Wang, P., Sneed, J., Pelton, G., Devan, D....Roose, S. (2013). A randomized, prospective pilot study of patient expectancy and antidepressant outcome. *Psychological Medicine*, 43(5), 975–982.

Sachs, G. S., Grossman, F., Ghaemi, S. N., Okamoto, A., & Bowden, C. L. (2002). Combination of a mood stabilizer with risperidone or haloperidol for treatment of acute mania: A double-blind, placebo-controlled comparison of efficacy and safety. *American Journal of Psychiatry*, 159(7), 1146–1154.

Sachs, G., Sanchez, R., Marcus, R., Stock, E., Mcquade, R., Carson, W.,...Aripiprazole Research Group. (2006). Aripiprazole in the treatment of acute manic or mixed episodes in patients with bipolar I disorder: A 3-week placebo-controlled study. *Journal of Psychopharmacology*, 20(4), 536–546.

Sidor, M. M., & Macqueen, G. M. (2011). Antidepressants for the acute treatment of bipolar depression: A systematic review and meta-analysis. *Journal of Clinical Psychiatry*, 72(2), 156–167.

Smulevich, A. B., Khanna, S., Eerdekens, M., Karcher, K., Kramer, M., & Grossman, F. (2005). Acute and continuation risperidone monotherapy in bipolar mania: A 3-week placebo-controlled trial followed by a 9-week double-blind trial of risperidone and haloperidol. *European Neuropsychopharmacology*, 15(1), 75–84.

Sneed, J. R., Rutherford, B. R., Rindskopf, D., Lane, D. T., Sackeim, H. A., & Roose, S. P. (2008). Design makes a difference: A meta-analysis of antidepressant response rates in placebo-controlled versus comparator trials in late-life depression. *The American Journal of Geriatric Psychiatry*, 16(1), 65–73.

Stewart-Williams, S., & Podd, J. (2004). The placebo effect: Dissolving the expectancy versus conditioning debate. *Psychological Bulletin*, 130(2), 324–340.

Suppes, T., Datto, C., Minkwitz, M., Nordenhem, A., Walker, C., & Darko, D. (2010). Effectiveness of the extended release formulation of quetiapine as monotherapy for the treatment of acute bipolar depression. *Journal of Affective Disorders, 121*(1), 106–115.

Suppes, T., Vieta, E., Liu, S., Brecher, M., Paulsson, B., & Trial 127 Investigators. (2009). Maintenance treatment for patients with bipolar I disorder: Results from a North American study of quetiapine in combination with lithium or divalproex (trial 127). *American Journal of Psychiatry, 166*(4), 476–488.

Sysko, R., & Walsh, B. T. (2007). A systematic review of placebo response in studies of bipolar mania. *Journal of Clinical Psychiatry, 68*(8), 1213–1217.

Thase, M. E., Jonas, A., Khan, A., Bowden, C. L., Wu, X., Mcquade, R. D.,…Owen, R. (2008). Aripiprazole monotherapy in non-psychotic bipolar I depression: Results of 2 randomized, placebo-controlled studies. *Journal of Clinical Psychopharmacology, 28*(1), 13–20.

Thase, M. E., Macfadden, W., Weisler, R. H., Chang, W., Paulsson, B., Khan, A.,…The BOLDER II Study Group. (2006). Efficacy of quetiapine monotherapy in bipolar I and II depression: A double-blind, placebo-controlled study (The BOLDER II Study). *Journal of Clinical Psychopharmacology, 26*(6), 600–609.

Tohen, M., Calabrese, J. R., Sachs, G. S., Banov, M. D., Detke, H., Risser, R.,…Bowden, C. L. (2006). Randomized, placebo-controlled trial of olanzapine as maintenance therapy in patients with bipolar I disorder responding to acute treatment with olanzapine. *American Journal of Psychiatry, 163*(2), 247–256.

Tohen, M., Chengappa, K. R., Suppes, T., Baker, R. W., Zarate, C. A., Bowden, C. L.,…Calabrese J. R. (2004). Relapse prevention in bipolar I disorder: 18-month comparison of olanzapine plus mood stabiliser v. mood stabiliser alone. *BJP, 184*(4), 337–345.

Tohen, M., Jacobs, T. G., Grundy, S. L., Mcelroy, S. L., Banov, M. C., Janicak, P. G.,…Breier, A. (2000). Efficacy of olanzapine in acute bipolar mania: A double-blind, placebo-controlled study. *Archives of General Psychiatry, 57*(9), 841–849.

Tohen, M., Sanger, T. M., Mcelroy, S. L., Tollefson, G. D., Chengappa, K. R., Daniel, D. G.,…The Olanzapine HGEH Study Group. (1999). Olanzapine versus placebo in the treatment of acute mania. *American Journal of Psychiatry, 156*(5), 702–709.

Tohen, M., Vieta, E., Calabrese, J., Ketter, T. A., Sachs, G., Bowden, C.,…Breier A. (2003). Efficacy of olanzapine and olanzapine-fluoxetine combination in the treatment of bipolar I depression. *Archives of General Psychiatry, 60*(11), 1079–1088.

Trivedi, M. H., & Rush, J. (1994). Does a placebo run-in or a placebo treatment cell affect the efficacy of antidepressant medications? *Neuropsychopharmacology, 11*(1), 33–43.

Vieta, E., Montgomery, S., Sulaiman, A. H., Cordoba, R., Huberlant, B., Martinez, L., & Schreiner, A. (2012). A randomized, double-blind, placebo-controlled trial to assess prevention of mood episodes with risperidone long-acting injectable in patients with bipolar I disorder. *European Neuropsychopharmacology, 22*(11), 825–835.

Vieta, E., Nuamah, I. F., Lim, P., Yuen, E. C., Palumbo, J. M., Hough, D. W., & Berwaerts, J. (2010). A randomized, placebo-and active-controlled study of paliperidone extended release for the treatment of acute manic and mixed episodes of bipolar I disorder. *Bipolar Disorders, 12*(3), 230–243.

Weisler, R. H., Calabrese, J. R., Thase, M. E., Arvekvist, R., Stening, G., Paulsson, B., & Suppes, T. (2008). Efficacy of quetiapine monotherapy for the treatment of depressive episodes in bipolar I disorder: A post hoc analysis of combined results from 2 double-blind, randomized, placebo-controlled studies. *Journal of Clinical Psychiatry, 69*(5), 769–782.

Weisler, R. H., Kalali, A. H., & Ketter, T. A. (2004). A multicenter, randomized, double-blind, placebo-controlled trial of extended-release carbamazepine capsules as monotherapy for bipolar disorder patients with manic or mixed episodes. *Journal of Clinical Psychiatry, 65*(4), 478–484.

Weisler, R. H., Keck, P. E. Jr., Swann, A. C., Cutler, A. J., Ketter, T. A., & Kalali, A. H. (2005). Extended-release carbamazepine capsules as monotherapy for acute mania in bipolar disorder: A multicenter, randomized, double-blind, placebo-controlled trial. *Journal of Clinical Psychiatry, 66*(3), 323–330.

Yildiz, A., Guleryuz, S., Ankerst, D. P., Ongur, D., & Renshaw, P. F. (2008). Protein kinase C inhibition in the treatment of mania: A double-blind, placebo-controlled trial of tamoxifen. *Archives of General Psychiatry, 65*(3), 255–263.

Yildiz, A., Vieta, E., Tohen, M., & Baldessarini, R. J. (2011). Factors modifying drug and placebo responses in randomized trials for bipolar mania. *International Journal of Neuropsychopharmacology, 14*(7), 863–875.

Young, A. H., McElroy, S. L., Bauer, M., Philips, N., Chang, W., Olausson, B.,…Brecher, M. (2010). A double-blind, placebo-controlled study of quetiapine and lithium monotherapy in adults in the acute phase of bipolar depression (EMBOLDEN I). *Journal of Clinical Psychiatry, 71*(2), 150–162.

Young, A. H., Oren, D. A., Lowy, A., Mcquade, R. D., Marcus, R. N., Carson, W. H.,…Sanchez, R. (2009). Aripiprazole monotherapy in acute mania: 12-week randomised placebo-and haloperidol-controlled study. *BJP, 194*(11), 40–48.

Zarate, C. A. Jr., Payne, J. L., Singh, J., Quiroz, J. A., Luckenbaugh, D. A., Denicoff, K. D.,…Manji, H. K. (2004). Pramipexole for bipolar II depression: A placebo-controlled proof of concept study. *Biological Psychiatry, 56*(1), 54–60.

Zarate, C. A., Singh, J. B., Carlson, P. J., Quiroz, J., Jolkovsky, L., Luckenbaugh, D. A., & Manji, H. K. (2007). Efficacy of a protein kinase C inhibitor (tamoxifen) in the treatment of acute mania: A pilot study. *Bipolar Disorders, 9*(6), 561–570.

42.

STRATEGIES FOR IMPROVING RANDOMIZED TRIAL EVIDENCE FOR TREATMENT OF BIPOLAR DISORDER

Ayşegül Yildiz, Juan Undurraga, Eduard Vieta, Dina Popovic,

Sarah Wooderson, and Allan H. Young

INTRODUCTION

Presently approved treatments of bipolar disorder are, for the most part, uniformly unable to address the underlying etiology (Baldessarini, 2013; Yildiz, Guleryuz, Ankerst, Ongur, & Renshaw, 2008). Yet contemporary era has witnessed furthermost scientific understanding of the pathophysiological mechanisms underlying bipolar disorder and has led to investigations of specific molecular targets and their neural correlates (Machado-Vieira et al., 2010; Mathew, Manji, & Charney, 2008). However, despite substantial investment for development of target-specific, receptor-oriented central nervous system (CNS) therapeutics, including the ones for bipolar disorder, a very limited number of the investigated compounds have survived to launch in recent years (Hoertel, de Maricourt, & Gorwood, 2013; Kemp et al., 2010). This result does not seem solely to be due to failure of the underlying rationale or ineffectiveness of the candidate compounds, which carried them to Phase I trials but also increased noise encountered in the context of randomized controlled trials (RCTs). For CNS therapeutics only, failure rates at Phase II stage reach 50%, which is about 15% more than the previous decade (Hurko & Ryan, 2005; Kemp et al., 2010; Mallinckrodt, Zhang, Prucka, & Millen, 2010; Tarr, Herbison, de la Barra, & Glue, 2011). Considering $15,000 cost per subject for a Phase II or III trial, it can be appreciated why such high failure rates may discourage investment in CNS drug development research (Kemp et al., 2010; Kobak et al., 2010). From the business perspective, the worst scenario (failure in Phase III of compounds that appeared to work in Phase II) is increasingly common (Vieta et al., 2014). Clearly,

addressing the methodological obstacles that are impeding progress in this critical sector of therapeutic development is warranted.

Regulatory agencies such as the US Food and Drug Administration (FDA) and the European Medicines Agency have taken the position that a true appreciation of an intervention against a major psychiatric illness such as schizophrenia, depression, and bipolar disorder is only possible by employment of a placebo-controlled design (Alphs, Benedetti, Fleischhacker, & Kane, 2012). This perspective has had a tremendous impact on drug development for these common psychiatric disorders (Alphs et al., 2012). For instance, more than two-thirds of the available evidence on antimanic, antipsychotic, and antidepressant treatments are against placebo (Kirsch, 2009; Leucht, Cipriani, et al., 2013; Sidor & MacQueen, 2011; Yildiz, Vieta, Leucht, & Baldessarini, 2011). This may partially be due to the requirement of the drug-regulatory authorities but is also due to preferences of the pharmaceutical industry for testing their new compounds against placebos rather than an active comparator, since the latter necessitates truly more efficacious drugs (Leucht, Heres, & Davis, 2013). Obviously, restricting progress in pharmacology to superiority studies would seriously restrict progress in other matters such as improved safety or tolerability (Vieta & Cruz, 2012), but the use of placebo as the only suitable comparator for registration studies is taking the field to a no-end road. Difficulties in conducting placebo-controlled trials for clinically challenging severe mental disorders with frequently encountered symptomatic exacerbations have likely instigated distinct research populations. The predominantly profit nature of funding with predictable pressure for speedy completion with positive outcomes might have further contributed to the formation of such exclusive trial populations. These placebo-controlled trials-compatible patients are likely to be at the least severe end of the disease spectrum, respond to placebo, and increase attention provided in a research context via the so called "Hawthorne' effect." A population enriched for placebo responders and deprived for true drug responders would lead to shrunken drug–placebo contrasts, which in turn would lead to larger sample sizes and a greater number of study sites and increased variance as well as noise. Such a vicious cycle may be operating since cumulative introduction of "me too" drugs and have led to recent "anti-psychopharmacology" public acts fostered in some scientific reviews (Kirsch, 2009). Considering published, as well as FDA registered and unpublished RCTs, such critical reviews have for instance claimed trivial effect of antidepressant drugs (Kirsch, 2009). In interpretation of such critical evidence synthesis reports, one should take into account the potential effect of failure trials, which have typically failed to detect the true treatment contrasts; potential mediator effect of disease severity; and nature of source data attained in the context of RCTs involving distinct research populations with milder forms of disease presentations. In the context of RCTs it has been previously documented those patients with severer forms of disease manifestation were more likely to benefit from drug treatment (Kirsch, 2009). The real-world clinical samples on the other side, for the most part, uniformly involve patients with higher symptomatic severity so would likely to be enriched for drug responders. However, due to difficulties in conducting placebo-controlled experiments in such patients, clinical trials are typically left to patients with milder disease forms. Indeed, for severe mental illnesses, the RCTs settings may better be perceived as simulation environments; and evidence synthesis reports based on numeric data attained in these circumstances need to be translated to the actual life settings. Further, sometimes even a small actual treatment effect experienced in the real-life settings may have magnified impacts, as in the critical clinical positions involving the line between life and death or delusional acts and insight (Leucht, Hierl, Kissling, Dold, & Davis, 2012). Recent evidence indicates that, as with schizophrenia, there is accelerated aging in bipolar disorder with a consequent shortening in life expectancy of 10 to 13.6 years relative to the general population of same age (Chang et al., 2011; García-Rizo et al., 2014; Laursen, 2011). Evidence also indicates that effective treatment of bipolar disorder is not only important for alleviation of symptomatic exacerbations but also for protection against premature death associated with medical causes related to disturbed immune responses and increased systemic oxidative stress, as well as suicide (Ahrens et al., 1995; Cipriani, Hawton, Stockton, & Geddes, 2013; Drexhage et al., 2011; Leboyer et al., 2012). Considering longitudinal course and lifetime consequences, observed drug–placebo contrasts gain even greater appreciation. However, as with other major psychiatric disorders, there is certainly much room for development of new therapeutics with robust target specific effects and no or minimum undesired effects for treatment and prophylaxis of bipolar disorder. For achieving this goal, identification of the methodological obstacles in design and conduct of RCTs is absolutely warranted.

PLACEBO EFFECT VERSUS PLACEBO RESPONSE

By definition, the placebo *effect* engulfs the psychobiological phenomena attributable to the placebo, which is triggered via the perception or the symbolic meaning of the treatment (Alphs et al., 2012; Kirsch, 2009; Raz, Zigman, & de Jong, 2009). Placebo-like effects may also occur without administration of an actual placebo, highlighting the central role of expectation and suggestion in placebo-related phenomena. Some effects, especially relating to the immune and endocrine systems, are due to conditioning types of processes. For example, Benedetti (2009) discusses studies involving rats showing that a flavored liquid had immunosuppressant effects after being repeatedly coadministered with an immunosuppressant drug. Likewise, administration of a placebo with patient expectation of pain relief typically activates the endogenous opioid system. Conversely, administering active analgesics via hidden administration—that is, without the patient's awareness—significantly reduces their effectiveness (Benedetti, 2009; Raz et al., 2009). Another approach to the placebo effect is associated with the context surrounding the medical encounter (Moerman, 2002). This "meaning model" attempts to explain why red placebos stimulate whereas blue placebos calm, why more placebos work better than few, and why more expensive placebos work better than cheaper ones. Psychological and behavioral evidence points to the powerful and unique role of suggestion and expectation in eliciting placebo effects (Benedetti, 2009; Raz et al., 2009).

Placebo *response*, on the other hand, designates the improvement observed in the placebo arm of a clinical trial, which is produced by the totality of the placebo biological phenomenon combined with other potential factors contributing to symptom amelioration, such as passage of time, spontaneous remission, or natural history of the disorder, regression to the mean, biases, geographical and cultural factors, and/or judgment errors (Alphs et al., 2012; Kirsch, 2009; Raz et al., 2009; Vieta, Pappadopulos, Mandel, Lombardo, 2011). The difference between the placebo response and improvement in a no-treatment control group can be interpreted as the placebo effect (Kirsch, 2009).

As with the actual drug effect, genotype and phenotype related personal codes might determine individual tendencies for the placebo effect. Since expectation and anticipation-based responses are in action, a clear level of consciousness and insight should be preserved for the phenomenon of actual placebo effect. Given that executive functions such as insight, judgment, expectation, and anticipation would often be disturbed in patients experiencing severe mental illnesses, a true placebo effect would hardly be attainable in such patients. Consequently, as also indicated in the previous section, patient populations with more severe expressions of such mental illnesses would likely to be enriched for drug response. Given ethical and clinical concerns, this aspect of true placebo effect that is related with disease severity cannot be fully encountered in the context of clinical trial settings. However, efforts for achieving better simulation environments in the context of clinical trials can be optimized. A wider window for manipulation of the placebo-associated responses can be encountered through the effect of time on the establishment of partial or full remissions, regression to the mean, biases, and judgment errors.

CLINICAL TRIALS OF BIPOLAR MANIA

EFFECT SIZE FOR ANTIMANIC TREATMENTS RELATIVE TO OTHER MEDICAL ILLNESSES

Effective treatments of acute mania yield an absolute difference in responder rates of 17% and a standardized mean difference (SMD), as Hedges' *g* based effect size of 0.41 (Yildiz, Vieta, Leucht, et al., 2011), which is comparable to corresponding values of 18% and 0.51 for second-generation antipsychotics in the acute treatment of schizophrenia (Leucht, Arbter, Engel, Kissling, & Davis, 2009). In a

recent mega-analysis considering 94 meta-analytic reports of 48 drugs in 20 medical diseases and 16 drugs in 8 psychiatric disorders, effect sizes computed for psychotropic agents were compared to general medical drugs (Leucht et al., 2012). This analysis revealed a pooled SMD of 0.54 for antihypertensive treatments; 0.41 for antimigraine treatments; 0.87 for fasting glucose and 0.27 for mortality with antidiabetic treatments; 0.22 for antibiotic treatments of otitis media; 0.44 for treatments of ulcerative colitis; 0.36 for treatments increasing ventilatory volume; and 0.20 for prevention of exacerbations in chronic obstructive pulmonary disease. The authors concluded that antimanic or antipsychotic drugs are not generally less efficacious than average medical drugs (Leucht et al., 2012). Nonetheless, clearly there is much room for the development of more effective therapeutics with better efficacy and safety profiles for patients with bipolar disorder.

IS PLACEBO RESPONSE RISING IN ANTIMANIC TREATMENT TRIALS?

Increasing placebo response is a major concern for antipsychotic drug trials (Alphs et al., 2012; Kemp et al., 2010; Leucht, Heres, et al., 2013). In a comprehensive meta-analysis of 50 placebo-controlled antipsychotic drug trials of schizophrenia spectrum disorders conducted since 1970, Agid and colleagues (2013) reported that placebo response has increased over the past few decades, especially from 1993 to 2010. In this work, a standardized mean change (SMC) of –0.33 (95% confidence interval [CI] = –0.44 to –0.22) from baseline to endpoint for the placebo group was reported. The authors also reported that larger placebo mean improvements were associated with smaller drug–placebo differences. In a more recent multiple treatments meta-analysis of antipsychotic drug trials for acute treatment of schizophrenia exact same SMD of –0.33 (95% credible interval [CrI] = –0.43 to –0.22) for the placebo-associated improvements was computed (Leucht, Cipriani, et al., 2013). Similar to the findings with antipsychotic drug trials in schizophrenia, substantial placebo-associated mean improvements were documented also for the trials of bipolar mania. Two recent reviews, one involving a total of 20 single-agent and add-on studies (Sysko & Walsh, 2007), and the other with 38 single-agent studies (56 drug-placebo contrasts) indicated a placebo-associated response rate of 31% in trials of bipolar mania (Yildiz, Vieta, Tohen, & Baldessarini, 2011). Both reviews reported a secular trend for rising placebo effects for industry-supported studies (Sysko & Walsh, 2007; Yildiz, Vieta, Tohen, et al., 2011).

POTENTIAL EFFECT MODIFIERS IN RANDOMIZED CONTROLLED TRIALS AND STRATEGIES TO DIMINISH THEIR UNFAVORABLE IMPACTS

In this section each of the below factors are evaluated as potential effect modifiers in the context of RCTs of acute mania.

- The number of study sites
- Sample size
- Gender
- Age
- Psychotic and mixed features
- Trial completion rates
- Baseline disease severity
- Quality of ratings
- Study and illness duration
- Financial incentives affecting investigators and candidate patients

A recent meta-regression analysis investigating the phenomenon of placebo response in bipolar mania established that higher number of collaborating study sites was strongly associated with greater placebo-induced improvements (mean difference [MD]: 38 trials; $\beta = -0.11$, 95% CI: -0.15 to -0.06, $z = -4.67, p < .0001$) and diminished drug–placebo contrasts (SMD as Hedges' g: 48 trials; $\beta = 0.007$, 95% CI: 0.003 to 0.01, $z = 3.79, p = .00015$; Yildiz, Vieta, Tohen, et al., 2011). A finding missed in previous reviews owing to consideration of placebo and drug arms conjointly in the same regression model (Tarr et al., 2011). The finding indicating the number of study sites as an effect mediator has recently found support in antipsychotic treatment trials of schizophrenia spectrum disorders (Agid et al., 2013). In this comprehensive meta-analysis, the authors detected a significant increase in placebo response over the past few decades and explained this temporal effect by an increase of the number of sites per trial accompanied by a decrease in the number of academic sites (Agid et al., 2013; Leucht, Heres, et al., 2013). In light of these findings, we can propose the number of study sites as a critical factor contributing to the substantial noise encountered in the context of placebo-controlled RCTs.

Large studies do not only involve higher number of study sites but also large patient samples. For bipolar mania the meta-analysis described previously indicated that also a large sample size was associated with greater placebo-associated improvements (MD: 38 trials; $\beta = +0.06$, 95% CI: 0.04 to 0.08, $z = 6.47, p < .0001$) and smaller drug–placebo contrasts (SMD as Hedges' g: 48 trials; $\beta = -0.001$, CI: -0.003 to -0.0004, $z = -2.63$, $p = .008$; Yildiz, Vieta, Tohen, et al., 2011). In a database of 27 acute schizophrenia studies conducted between 1997 and 2008 it was reported that for each 1-point increase in the placebo mean change, the drug–placebo contrast decreased 0.4 points (Mallinckrodt et al., 2010). The authors also reported that as the percentage of patients randomized to placebo increased, mean placebo-induced improvements decreased (Mallinckrodt et al., 2010). In another meta-analysis of antipsychotic trials of schizophrenia, Agid and colleagues (2013) reported that greater placebo response was associated with the lower percentage of patients assigned to placebo when only studies published since 1998 were considered. However, the association was lost when the entire set of trials were considered (Agid et al., 2013). These opposing effect directions documented for the RCTs of bipolar mania versus schizophrenia may result from differences in trial, patient, and/or disease characteristics. For instance, for schizophrenia trials the percentage of patients randomized to placebo was reported in the range of 20% to 33% (Mallinckrodt et al., 2010), while it was about 47% for the RCTs of bipolar mania (Yildiz, Vieta, Tohen, et al., 2011). As mentioned earlier, current trends in the RCTs settings by compelling speedy completion and positive outcomes are likely to result in larger and larger trials yielding smaller contrasts through increased variance and noise.

Trial participants' age was also reported as an effect mediator in the context of placebo-controlled RCTs of bipolar acute mania (Yildiz, Vieta, Tohen, et al., 2011). This meta-regression analysis has documented that younger mean age of trial population was associated with lesser placebo effects (MD: 36 trials; $\beta = +0.92$, 95% CI: 0.33 to 1.15, $z = 3.07, p = .002$) and greater drug–placebo contrasts (SMD as Hedges' g: 46 trials; $\beta = -0.09$, CI: -0.13 to -0.04, $z = -4.03$, $p = .00006$; Yildiz, Vieta, Tohen, et al., 2011). Again, direction of effect was opposite to the antipsychotic trials of schizophrenia, for which younger age was associated with higher placebo responses (Agid et al., 2013).

Similarly, male gender was found to be associated with fewer placebo responses (MD: 35 trials; $\beta = -0.18$, 95% CI: -0.29 to -0.06, $z = -3.04$, $p = .002$) and greater drug–placebo contrasts (SMD as Hedges' g: 46 trials; $\beta = +0.02$, 95% CI: 0.007 to 0.03, $z = 3.49, p = .0005$) in the context of bipolar mania trials (Yildiz, Vieta, Tohen, et al., 2011). Gender effect in schizophrenia trials is questionable, as the most comprehensive recent review did not detect any sign of gender influence on the placebo-associated responses (Agid et al., 2013), while an earlier review had documented a 3-point increase in the mean placebo-associated improvements for each 10% increase in the female trial populations (Mallinckrodt et al., 2010). While disease-based specificity of the effect is questionable, given trial-level protection by randomization one would expect equal gender distribution in the treatment arms. Yet, as documented, nonsignificant differences in the distribution of male and female genders in the corresponding study arms yield a significant mediator effect when considered all together in the context of placebo-controlled RCTs. If such an effect can be verified in future regression models, trial designs for acute mania may call for more male participants but with a balanced study arm-based allocations.

Another proposed factor operating in the proposed vicious cycle is disease severity. Rising ethical standards and concerns on randomizing severe patients to placebo might have caused enrolment of progressively milder patients into clinical trials over time. The largest standard pairwise meta-analysis on antimanic treatment trials indicated that not placebo- but drug-associated improvements were predicted by increased disease severity (46 trials; $\beta = +0.26$, 95% CI: 0.13 to 0.40, $z = 3.80$, $p = .0002$; Yildiz, Vieta, Leucht, et al., 2011). The finding, being specific to active drugs, supported by the previous meta-analytic models, cannot solely be explained by a regression to the mean, but rather suggest a pharmacological response component in patients with more severe forms of bipolar mania (Tarr et al., 2011; Yildiz, Vieta, Leucht, et al., 2011). In that sense, it supports the assumption that patient populations experiencing more severe forms of mania would be enriched for drug responders. Another factor related to severity of manic episode is the presence of psychotic features. Impact of psychotic features was also specific to active drugs (MD: 40 trials; $\beta = +0.10$, 95% CI: 0.06 to 0.15, $z = 4.22$, $p = .00002$), with the effect being more influential, as it was also reflected on the enhanced drug–placebo contrasts (SMD as Hedges' g: 40 trials; $\beta = +0.85$, 95% CI: 0.43 to 1.28, $z = 3.91$, $p = .00009$; Yildiz, Vieta, Tohen, et al., 2011). In contrast with the effect of psychosis, another disease-specific modulator: mixed features decreased both drug-response and drug–placebo contrasts (MD: 45 trials; $\beta = -0.07$, 95% CI: -0.12 to -0.03, $z = -3.26$, $p = .001$; SMD as Hedges' g: 45 trials; $\beta = -0.59$, 95% CI: -0.99 to -0.19, $z = -2.92$, $p = .004$, respectively; Yildiz, Vieta, Tohen, et al., 2011). Neither presence of psychotic- nor mixed-features

had any impact on responses to placebo treatment. The sensitivity and specificity of the observed effects, as well as clinically distinct features of pure mania versus mania with mixed features, may validate consideration of patients with prominently mixed features, exclusively in independent trials. However, given recent modifactions in description of mixed features this finding needs to be replicated in future antimanic treatment trials. Given arm-based specificity of the effect, it is not surprising that a previous meta-regression model considering all study arms conjointly could only detect a trend toward a poorer outcome associated with mixed states (Tarr et al., 2011). Based on above summarized evidence, we may suggest inclusion of patients with moderate to severe forms of mania with or without psychotic features but with no prominent depressive components. Special care should be given to avoid patients who might have already entered the natural waning stage for the current episode as well as treatment-refractory patients.

Another factor associated with lower drug–placebo contrasts in bipolar mania trials was the higher dropout rates (Yildiz et al., 2011). If the drug-associated benefit and the resulting treatment effect is being modulated by disease severity either in the form of high baseline scores or presence of psychotic features, manic patients need to be exposed to the active drug long enough for accomplishment of the brain's adaptive response to drug-induced pharmacological alterations. The meta-analysis over 56 comparisons found that higher trial completion rates in drug arms were associated with both greater drug-associated benefit and drug–placebo contrasts (MD: 46 trials; $\beta = 0.08$, 95% CI: 0.04 to 0.13, $z = 3.99$, $p = .00007$; SMD as Hedges' g: 46 trials; $\beta = 0.006$, 95% CI: 0.002 to 0.009, $z = 2.86$, $p = .004$, respectively; Yildiz, Vieta, Tohen, et al., 2011). Considering that RCTs of acute mania involve already short study durations (three or four weeks), high rates of early dropouts are likely to mask actual magnitude of the true drug effects.

Evidence indicates that younger bipolar patients with short illness durations would be more likely to respond to pharmacologic treatment and less likely to respond to placebo (Yildiz, Vieta, Tohen, et al., 2011). Since diagnosis of bipolar disorder can technically be made only after the establishment of the first manic episode and an accurate documentation of age onset for the first mood episode is often barely obtainable, we did not attempt to extract data for illness duration. Nevertheless, present findings on the age effect as well as the clinical impression for obtaining better treatment responses in patients with more recent disease onset support the notion that younger patients with shorter illness durations may constitute better research samples with enhanced treatment contrasts. If this notion can find further support, a new illness duration related inclusion criterion may be considered.

Another potentially important factor mediating drug–placebo contrasts is the quality of ratings: both for baseline- and outcome-assessments. A recent methodologically sound study compared effect of site-based and centralized ratings on patient selection and placebo response in subjects with major depressive disorder (Kobak et al., 2010). That study established that 35% of the included subjects would not have been eligible to enter the study if the centralized rater's score was used to determine study entry. Further, the mean placebo change for the site-raters (~7.5) was significantly greater than the mean placebo change for centralized raters (~3.18, *p* < .001; Kobak et al., 2010). Although there is no published study investigating this issue in terms of manic symptom assessments, baseline score inflations, as well as expectancy effects (the tendency to see improvement over time), site-based ratings are likely to increase placebo-associated responses and diminish drug–placebo contrasts for the RCTs of bipolar mania as well. Given natural vulnerability of scale-based measurements, such inflations in baseline- and/or outcome-assessments can be easily mediated by the site investigators, site nurses, as well as study patients. For instance, the so-called *"professional"* patients seen in the catchment area of often-used trial sites might exaggerate their symptoms in order to be eligible for a study (Alphs et al., 2012). Similarly, site-investigators themselves may consciously or unconsciously inflate baseline scores in order to meet patient eligibility requirements, especially when sites are paid on a per-patient basis. For ensuring quality of ratings, interrater reliability should be checked at the beginning and also often during the study conduct. A centralized rater should synchronously watch the site investigators' ratings, and patient inclusion should be decided by their mutual agreement. Manic symptom improvements should be assessed by standardized use of a common metric such as the Young Mania Rating Scale (YMRS; Young, Biggs, Ziegler, & Meyer, 1978). Administration of different instruments with discrepancy in target symptoms, measurement items, and score ranges, may potentially increase variance and heterogeneity (Yildiz, Vieta, Correll, Nikodem, & Baldessarini, 2014).

Finally, regulations on investigator payments may have an impact on the study completion or dropout rates as such drug-effects and treatment contrasts. In industry-sponsored trials site investigators are often paid on a per-patient basis upon completion of one post-baseline evaluation. In such circumstances investigators may lose their motivation for dealing with extremely energy-demanding manic patients for the subsequent two or three weeks. Considering that the brain's adaptive response to pharmacotherapy necessitates longer exposure and previously documented negative influence of early dropouts on drug-associated responses, as well as drug-placebo contrasts, we propose a payment strategy facilitating constant investigator motivation throughout the study. Last but not least, employment of rescue medications in conduct of acute mania trials may call for special attention. The protocol-guided use of rescue medications is usually left to the yard staff since the site investigators are often occasionally on the yard. Given that manic patients would often cause sleepless and stressful shifts, the yard staff may tend to employ rescue medications at a maximum possibly allowed dose and rate. Given that exclusion of benzodiazepines as rescue medications from the trial protocols is not feasible, their employment by the site investigators, rather than the yard staff, on an exclusively as-needed basis may facilitate drug–placebo separation and reduce the risk of failure trials. Since manic patients often need constant extra care and timely handling during repeatedly encountered crisis, for enabling optimized and timely site evaluation and crisis management we suggest that the site investigators to stay on the yard through day and night shifts during the study conduct. Constant presence of the site investigators on the yard would not only optimize use of rescue medications but also award system systematically. Specific features of the manic syndrome such as inflated self-esteem, high energy, and increased tendency for pleasurable activities with diminished or no sleep make compatibility with a protocol-guided treatment in an inpatient unit very challenging both for the patients and staff. For minimizing early dropouts with limited use of pharmacological restraints while optimizing patients' comfort and compliance, employment of some recreational incentives with a negotiation-based award-promoting approach may help them to stay calm in the yard without harming themselves or others. Among such incentives may be special permissions for immediate family members' visits to the yard, occupation with safety-guarded energy-consuming games or activities, day and night television/video entertainment, Wi-Fi access, and special meals. One may argue against use of such recreational activities with concerns on enhanced placebo responses. However, our experience with the largest proof-of-concept academic trial in a manic patient sample with a mean syndromal severity of 63% of maximum possible score by the YMRS and psychotic features accompanying at a rate of 67% implied that employment of some recreational incentives increased study completion rates and enhanced drug–placebo contrasts (Yildiz et al., 2008).

In contrast, without such sensitive considerations, RCTs are left to patients with softer or already alleviated forms of manic syndrome or to the so called *"professional"* patients, yielding a group enriched for placebo responders. It is likely that a research population with more severe forms of manic syndrome would be enriched for real drug responders, but we need them to stay in the trial long enough to let the brain accomplish an adaptive response. The optimum and safe employment of such award mechanisms can be achieved only by the constant supervision of the site investigators. Quality and safety control by an independent monitor may also be considered. On condition that any indications of poor patient care and/or study conduct are identified, an action plan for further training or change of the investigators or research nurses or safety guards may be considered, and a central backup team may take position on the site in the meantime.

CONSIDERATION OF ALTERNATIVE DESIGNS

Placebo-controlled RCTs of mania constitute A-plus evidence, and they are actually the designs requested by the regulatory agencies. While we encourage the aforementioned approaches for improvement of quality and hopefully quantity of placebo-controlled RCTs of bipolar mania, in situations with limited sources alternative trial designs such as add-on or head to head trials may provide complementary clinical information if planned appropriately. As in the case of add-on trials, positive head to head trials designed for testing noninferiority may serve to provide rationale for a placebo-controlled monotherapy trial and accumulate data for future evidence synthesis. Head to head trials proving superiority over standard treatments might be another option although this approach, even more so, requires drugs that are truly more efficacious (Leucht, Heres, et al., 2013). The use of an early-response/nonresponse paradigm is another study design worth considering in order to enhance the selection of true drug responders, who can then participate in a double-blind, placebo-controlled discontinuation trial (Alphs et al., 2012; Correll, Malhotra, Kaushik, McMeniman, & Kane, 2003; Kinon et al., 2010). This strategy involves treating all patients with the experimental drug with or without an active control and then identifying those subjects who have at least a minimal prespecified level of improvement after two weeks of treatment. Because such patients represent a group enriched for drug responsiveness, they constitute an ideal subgroup to enter into a double-blind discontinuation study, where, following stabilization, patients are randomized to continued treatment or

placebo and time to destabilization is the endpoint (Alphs et al., 2012; Correll et al., 2003). The assumption underlying such a design would be that the early responders would include a greater proportion of patients who are truly "drug responsive," although it would also include some proportion of "placebo responders" (Alphs et al., 2012). Finally, investigator-initiated, large international trials to be funded by the National Institute of Mental Health, the FDA, the Department of Veterans Affairs, European Union Human Research Programs, and other medical research agencies by employing adaptive or sequential treatment strategies involving acute as well as maintenance phases would provide clinically very useful answers for the most critical research questions. Improvement of industry- or academia-initiated placebo-controlled RCTs together with employment of such alternative designs would likely change the face of placebo-associated responses, as well as the magnitude of the observed treatment contrasts in the trials of bipolar mania.

Finally, improvements in the individual RCTs would have extended impacts when combined via analytic evidence synthesis approaches. To enable the most informative and valid future evidence synthesis, each RCT effort should be registered before conduct and published upon completion by reporting quantifiable data on all outcome measures in a standardized manner. Further, by considering future evidence syntheses, each RCT report should report on the subgroups, such as those with or without psychotic or mixed features. In addition, outcome measures should involve important side effects encountered with use of antimanic drugs, again via a standardized approach: for example, data on patient's weight at baseline and end point, change in glucose or lipid levels, number of subjects who experience akathisia and those who need anti-Parkinsonian drugs, quantifiable data on extrapyramidal side-effect assessments, and suicidal thoughts or acts. Without accumulation of such data neither considerate evidence-based clinical decisions nor an evidence-based action plan for future research investments would be possible.

CLINICAL TRIALS OF BIPOLAR DEPRESSION

As reported in the previous chapters, available evidence on bipolar depression (BPD) is strikingly scarce. There are many possible reasons for this: The first is related to the fact that many clinicians and researchers have long assumed that major depressive episodes in bipolar or unipolar disorders share some common clinical characteristics and treatment response. This view also explains why antidepressants have long been the most common clinically employed treatment for BPD (Baldessarini et al., 2007). Moreover, this view explains the limited commercial interest in extending regulatory indications of antidepressants beyond "major depression" and the lack of specific trials aimed to establish antidepressant efficacy for BPD. The second reason may be related to safety issues. There are concerns that some drugs used to treat BPD (i.e., antidepressants), might induce mood switching, suicidality (i.e., suicidal thoughts or acts), or mood destabilization and rapid cycling (Bauer, Beaulieu, Dunner, Lafer, & Kupka, 2008; Undurraga et al., 2012). These concerns have led to routine exclusion of bipolar patients from most RCTs in major depression in the past 20 years (Undurraga & Baldessarini, 2012). Those allowing inclusion of patients with BPD did not usually select or stratify according to polarity (Geddes & Miklowitz, 2013). The third reason is related to clinical features of mood disorders (Baldessarini, 2013), which are typically characterized by clinical complexity, daily or weekly fluctuations in mood and behavior, and high risk of relapse or recurrence. Moreover, some of the available treatments can even worsen clinical course when prescribed or when discontinued, especially when discontinued abruptly (Baldessarini, Vieta, Calabrese, Tohen, & Bowden, 2010). This clinical complexity and lack of available RCT–based homogenous evidence on the treatment options for BPD address the importance of establishing standards for future RCTs with reliable and consistent diagnostic and clinical assessments, as well as outcome definitions. In addition, not only do the trial design factors have to meet high quality standards but also the trial conduct, as well as data reporting.

EVIDENCE ON EFFICACY AND SOURCES OF OUTCOME HETEROGENEITY

Meta-analytic reports on antidepressant use for BPD are often weak and inconsistent due to the paucity (involving only 4 to 12 trials) and substantial heterogeneity of the available RCTs (Gijsman, Geddes, Rendell, Nolen, & Goodwin, 2004; Sidor & MacQueen, 2012; Vázquez, Tondo, Undurraga, & Baldessarini, 2013). For this reason, their value in the context of BPD at present is highly questionable, as pointed out in the International Society for Bipolar Disorders (ISBD) task force report on the use of antidepressants in bipolar disorder, where the highest level of evidence was rated as B (Pacchiarotti et al., 2013). The situation is similar regarding other available treatments of bipolar depression, such as anticonvulsants, lithium, and antipsychotics (Cipriani et al., 2013; De Fruyt et al., 2012; Reinares et al., 2013; Vieta & Valentí, 2013). As reflected

on the attempts for evidence synthesis, available RCTs for BPD are for the most part weak, and the methodological quality of study designs and their reporting is highly heterogeneous. A recently published systematic review analyzed the methodology used in the individual RCTs of BPD in the past 20 years (Spanemberg et al., 2012). The authors included 30 RCTs in their analysis (all of them published in journals with an impact factor >3) and found striking results indicating the uneven and, in general, poor quality of available evidence. For example, almost half of considered RCTs were conducted with fewer than 50 patients; 70% of them failed to describe the method used in determining their sample sizes; 50% did not assess remission of depression as an outcome (they limited their analysis to response, usually defined as 50% reduction in a depressive symptoms scale); half had attrition rates over 20%; and last observation carried forward analysis was used in only two-thirds of the published reports (see Table 42.1 for further details).

The observed heterogeneity in BPD trials makes the comparison between outcomes (e.g., efficacy measures, tolerability) for different treatments and placebo difficult, as there is a lot of statistical noise. Moreover, high variability is associated with less statistical power (i.e., more false negative results; Ghaemi, 2009).

IS PLACEBO RESPONSE RISING IN ANTIDEPRESSIVE TREATMENT TRIALS?

There has been a steady increase in placebo-associated responses and an accompanying decrease in drug–placebo contrasts in antidepressant trials over the past three decades (Khan, Bhat, Kolts, Thase, & Brown, 2010; Undurraga & Baldessarini, 2012). Further, certain trial characteristics such as sample sizes or number of study sites were significantly associated with the higher placebo responses in the antidepressant trials (Undurraga & Baldessarini, 2012; Walsh, Seidman, Sysko, & Gould, 2002). This association has been observed particularly in the context of unipolar depression; however, unipolar and bipolar differentiation has been a matter of large debate in the past century, and most studies until mid-1980s did not differentiate between the two (Baldessarini et al., 2010; Benazzi, 2007; Khan et al., 2010).

POTENTIAL FACTORS CONTRIBUTING TO STATISTICAL HETEROGENEITY AND NOISE FOR BIPOLAR DEPRESSION TRIALS

Certain methodological characteristics of BPD trials and trial participants may contribute to heterogeneity, noise

Table 42.1. METHODOLOGICAL QUALITY OF PUBLISHED RANDOMIZED-CONTROLLED TRIALS IN BIPOLAR DEPRESSION

ITEM EVALUATED/DESCRIBED	NO. STUDIES (%)
Follow-up time (weeks)	
≤6	9 (30%)
6 to 8	13 (43.3%)
>8 weeks	8 (26.7%)
Placebo use	
Yes	20 (66.7%)
No	10 (33.3%)
Diagnostic assessment	
Structured diagnosis (SCID/MINI)	20 (66.6%)
Semistructured diagnosis	1 (3.3%)
Clinical diagnosis only	9 (30%)
Washout period	
Yes	11 (36.7%)
No	18 (60%)
Not described	1 (3.3%)
Inclusion criteria	
Cutoff score defined (HDRS, MADRS, etc.)	27 (90%)
Cutoff score is not defined	3 (10%)
Number of patients (Total)	
≤50	14 (46.7%)
50 to 100	5 (16.7%)
100 to 200	3 (10%)
>200 to 500	3 (10%)
≥500	5 (16.7%)
Sample size calculation	
Described	12 (40%)
Not described or not performed	18 (60%)
BD Subtypes	
BD Type I	6 (20%)
BD Type II	1 (3.3%)
Both	18 (60%)
Unclear	5 (16.7%)

ITEM EVALUATED/DESCRIBED	NO. STUDIES (%)
Type of statistical analysis	
Only LOCF	20 (66.7%)
LOCF + OC	2 (6.7%)
Other or unclear	8 (26.7%)
Assessed remission	
Yes	13 (43.3%)
No	17 (56.7%)
Manic switch	
Not assessed or not described	3 (10%)
Dropouts (follow-up)	
≤20%	13 (43.3%)
20% to 50%	14 (46,7%)
≥50%	2 (6.7%)
Unclear	1 (3.3%)
Type of sponsorship for the study	
Corporate sponsored	14 (46.7%)
Sponsored by institutions/foundations/government	10 (33.3%)
Not declared/unclear/unsponsored	6 (20%)

NOTE: Adapted from Spanemberg et al. (2012).

effect, and lower effect sizes (Henkel et al., 2012; Khan, Schwartz, Kolts, Ridgway, & Lineberry, 2007; Schalkwijk, Undurraga, Tondo, & Baldessarini, 2014; Undurraga & Baldessarini, 2012):

- Trial-durations
- Involved study arms: placebo versus active comparators
- Number of involved active treatment arms
- Sample sizes
- Degree of baseline disease severity
- Comparability in dosing strategies
- Involvement of ethnically distinct patient populations
- Number of study sites
- Frequency of assessments
- Employment or length of a wash-out phase via placebo or no treatment

STRATEGIES FOR DIMINISHING NOISE AND ENHANCING TREATMENT CONTRASTS IN BIPOLAR DEPRESSION TRIALS

Pragmatic trials in addition to placebo-controlled randomized controlled trials

The placebo-controlled, double-blind, parallel-group RCTs are the gold standard for establishment of efficacy for an experimental treatment, but they have an important limitation. That is, the patients are highly selected and homogeneous and therefore are unrepresentative of the typical bipolar patients who tend to have multiple comorbidities with heterogeneous presentations and are typically on multiple treatments (Post, 2009). The fact that rate of exclusions for potential subjects in a RCT is as high as 80% to 90% underscores how selective RCT patient populations can be (Post, 2010). In addition, for technical reasons most trials use monotherapy in their design, which is far from the usual clinical care. This situation makes outcome generalizability (i.e., external validity) of these types of studies a difficult and arguable exercise. On the other hand, they have good internal validity, and valid conclusions can be made regarding treatment efficacy.

To deal with the problem of generalizability, effectiveness trials (otherwise known as pragmatic or practical trials) have been proposed (March et al., 2005). This type of "clinically useful" oriented design compares clinically important interventions and allows the inclusion of more complex patients with comorbid psychiatric problems, as such being more akin to everyday clinical practice (though heterogeneity could reduce internal validity). This kind of design has been used in recent clinically useful studies such as STAR-D, STEP-BD, and CATIE (Post, 2010). A more comprehensive description of the problem with generalizability and judicious consideration of different trial designs are provided in Chapter 43 of this book.

Bipolar disorder subgroups

Bipolar type I and II have different clinical characteristics and treatment responses (Judd et al., 2003; Pacchiarotti et al., 2013). Consequently, clinical trials of bipolar depression may either be conducted for a specific bipolar type or may involve patients with both bipolar subtypes; however, in such circumstances a subgroup analysis of outcomes should be well documented.

Evaluation instruments

The most frequently used clinical scales to assess depressive symptom severity and treatment response are the Hamilton Rating Scale for Depression (HRSD), the Montgomery-Åsberg Depression Rating Scale (MADRS), and the Inventory for Depression Symptomatology (IDS), which were initially developed to evaluate unipolar major depressive disorder. Although the HRSD, with 23 items, considers atypical features, the HRSD–17 Items, MADRS, and IDS lack sensibility to correctly estimate "atypical" depressive symptoms such as anergy, hypersomnia, or hyperphagia, which are common in bipolar depression and partly encountered also in mixed manic-depressive states (Baldessarini et al., 2010). Moreover, most of them were developed in nonblind studies of hospitalized patients and are likely to be less sensitive to milder or subsyndromal forms (Tohen et al., 2009). Another scale recently developed for the dimensional measurement of bipolar depression is named as the Bipolar Depression Rating Scale (BDRS), which comprises items for assessment of atypical depressive and mixed symptoms (Berk et al., 2007).

Outcome definitions

Bipolar disorder is a complex illness, with variable course between and within life cycles of affected individuals. Clinical presentations such as mania, hypomania, depression, presence of psychotic and/or mixed manic-depressive features, subsyndromal depressive states, and rapid cycling course with variable interepisodic functionality and cognitive impairments, make clear-cut outcomes, which would cover all various forms of disease manifestation and course, difficult to define. The problem is even more significant if we consider that many of these clinical presentations can remit or change both in relation to treatment as well as spontaneously, as most are time limited.

In the light of this clinical complexity, the definition of clear-cut outcomes and treatment objectives (i.e., clinically meaningful outcomes) is mandatory. An expert consensus and standardization of outcome definitions and terminology is essential to make meaningful comparisons across studies, as well as combined analysis. Some commonly used outcomes in BPD trials based on available evidence and expert consensus are defined next (Martinez-Aran et al., 2008; Rush et al., 2006; Tohen et al., 2009):

RESPONSE

Response is typically defined as ≥50% reduction in the initial depression severity scores, as commonly measured via the HRSD, MADRS, IDS, or BDRS. It is a clinically useful definition, used to indicate whether to continue with the same drug, stop and change treatment, or adjust doses. The main problem of response is that it greatly depends on the baseline measure of symptom severity, and regression to the mean may contribute to an invalid impression of symptomatic improvement (Fava, Evins, Dorer, & Schoenfeld, 2003). Importantly, a time criterion in its definition should be employed to avoid misinterpretations by random mood fluctuations (two to four weeks has been recommended by a recent ISBD task force on the course and outcome nomenclature in bipolar disorders; Tohen et al., 2009). In addition, during assessment of response in the context of BPD trials, manic symptoms should also be evaluated using standardized scales to demonstrate that no switching or manic worsening has occurred, which would invalidate response as a clinically significant outcome.

REMISSION

Remission is typically based on the posttreatment depression severity scores. An upper limit for the depression score is defined under which the patient is defined as remitted (often if sustained for a period of time). Remission implies that the signs and symptoms of depression are absent or nearly absent. Differentiating between response and remission is important, as a patient could respond to a treatment without remitting (i.e., patients with residual depressive symptoms). These patients (responders but not remitters) experience more psychosocial impairment and have a higher likelihood of recurrence (Thase, 2003; Zimmerman et al., 2004). The definition of remission (i.e., cut-off scores and time intervals) is still a matter of debate. Unsurprisingly, lower cut-offs in depression severity rating scales scores have been associated with better functionality and fewer recurrences in depression (Zimmerman et al., 2004). Remission cut-offs with the most commonly used depression rating scales have been suggested by expert panels (Rush et al., 2006; Tohen et al., 2009). One of the main limitations of this concept is that it may not reflect the quantitative change in symptoms (i.e., patients who enter a study with low scores could have little change in their symptoms and still be counted or classified among the remitters; Tohen et al., 2009). Remission has implications for functional outcome, prognosis, and course (Zimmerman et al., 2004); as such, it should be employed as a primary outcome in BPD trials. Nevertheless, functionality should be measured as a separate outcome, as symptomatic remission in bipolar depression is not necessarily associated with a return to premorbid day-to-day functioning (Tohen et al., 2009).

RECOVERY

Recovery implies remission for an extended period of time, such that the possibility of relapse or roughening is no longer a concern and another affective episode is unlikely to occur in the near future. (*The Diagnostic and Statistical Manual of Mental Disorders* [fifth edition] defines it as two months, the same as the 2009 ISBD task force, which recommends 8 weeks as the sustained remission criteria).

RELAPSE AND RECURRENCE

Both concepts imply the clinical manifestation of the episode within the predefined time limits. The definition of relapse and recurrence depends on the natural course of the illness (in this case, the bipolar depressive episode). The ISBD has defined relapse as the early return of the syndrome (≤ 8 weeks), that is, before recovery, and recurrence as a late return of the syndrome (>8 weeks)—in other words, during or after recovery.

SWITCHING

The course of illness for a bipolar patient may involve immediate change or switching to the opposite pole (i.e., depression to mania or vice versa) or a return to a normal mood state (i.e., euthymia) prior to the next episode. Even though some drugs could induce switching, the attribution of treatment as the cause of this complication could be misleading as it could also correspond to the natural course of the illness. Tohen and colleagues (2009) have proposed the nomenclature "treatment-emergent affective switch" (TEAS) to avoid attributing causality and propose a definition of *definite* TEAS if occurring in less than eight weeks. In addition, they propose including the specific treatment if the switch emerges within less than two weeks from the beginning of treatment (e.g., antidepressant-associated TEAS).

SUBSYNDROMAL

The term *subsyndromal* is used to describe patients who fail to meet the full diagnostic criteria for a mood episode. Subsyndromal symptoms are associated with worse social and occupational functioning and may increase the risk of relapse (Judd et al., 2008; Marangell, 2004). Considering their prognostic relevance, subsyndromal symptoms should be measured. However, the symptom severity scales for depression have strong limitations regarding this point, as discussed later.

Table 42.2. RECOMMENDATIONS FROM THE INTERNATIONAL SOCIETY FOR BIPOLAR DISORDERS TASK FORCE REPORT ON THE NOMENCLATURE OF COURSE AND OUTCOME IN BIPOLAR DISORDERS

ITEM	MEASURE	CUANTIFICATION (SCORE, WEEKS, PERCENTAGE)
Symptomatic Response	HDRS, MADRS, IDS, BDRS	*% improvement* <25%, 25–49%, 50-74%, 75–100%
Symptomatic Remission	HDRS-17	≤5 or ≤7 points
	MADRS	≤5 or ≤7 points
	BDRS	≤8 points
Recovery	Time (weeks)	Remission ≥8 weeks
Relapse	Time (weeks)	New episode <8weeks from remission
Recurrence	Time (weeks)	New episode ≥8weeks from remission
Subsyndromal Depression	HDRS-17	8 to 14 points
	MADRS	8 to 14 points
	BDRS	9 to 16 points
Predominant polarity	Depressive episodes	2/3 total episodes being depressive
TEAS		
Definite & treatment specific	2 consecutive days (>50% time each day)	Full episode ≤ 2 weeks
Definite	2 consecutive days (>50% time each day)	Full episode ≤ 8 weeks
Likely	2 consecutive days (>50% time each day)	(>2 symptoms + YMRS >12) ≤ 12 weeks
Possible	2 consecutive days (>4 hrs each day)	(change mood or energy + YMRS >8) ≤ 12 weeks
Unlikely	Fleeting symptoms. Environmental or exogenous contribution	> 16 weeks

NOTE: Adapted from Tohen et al. (2009).

RAPID CYCLING

Rapid cycling was originally described by Dunner and Fieve (1974), who arbitrarily defined it as patients presenting four or more distinct episodes in one year. It has prognostic importance, as it has been associated with more severe depressive episodes, poorer response to treatment, worse functioning, higher substance abuse comorbidity, and greater suicidal risk (Cruz et al., 2008). Clinical trials aimed at evaluating a rapid cycling pattern should employ an adequate extension phase.

PREDOMINANT POLARITY

Predominant polarity is defined as patients having at least two-thirds of their lifetime episodes at one polarity or the other (Colom, Vieta, Daban, Pacchiarotti, & Sanchez-Moreno, 2006), that is, either predominantly depressed or predominantly manic. This course specifier has strong prognostic value, especially relevant to long-term therapeutic decisions and prediction of outcome. Predominant depression has been associated with depressive or mixed onset, occurrence of more mixed episodes, rapid cycling course, accompanying psychotic features, and higher suicidal risk (Baldessarini et al., 2012).

FUNCTIONAL OUTCOMES

Bipolar disorder can have important consequences in social, cognitive, and occupational functioning. These functional deficits have been traditionally associated with affective episodes but may also present during subsyndromal states and even during euthymia (Jaeger & Vieta, 2007). As previously stated, better functionality has been associated with symptomatic remission, but remission does not mean returning to a premorbid state of functioning, hence it should be measured as a separate outcome. There is a paucity of methods for measuring disability. Some of the most important ones are described next.

The recently developed Functioning Assessment Short Test measures six domains of functioning (autonomy, occupational and cognitive functioning, financial issues, interpersonal relationships, and leisure time) and may be a good instrument for clinical and research settings, since it is brief, has high reliability, and is intended specifically for bipolar patients (Rosa et al., 2007). In addition, the World Health Organization designed a tool aimed at identifying and classifying relevant domains of human experience affected by health conditions (Ayuso-Mateos et al., 2013). The International Classification of Functioning, Disability and Health has two core sets especially developed for bipolar disorder, which describe illness-associated functional problems (personal and environmental factors). Its main limitation is that it lacks validation in clinical settings. Another relevant tool is the World Health Organization Disability Assessment Schedule, which evaluates different domains of functioning and is a helpful research tool, although it may be too long to use in daily clinical practice (World Health Organization, 2013).

DATA ANALYSIS AND REPORTING

OUTCOME ANALYSIS AS INTENTION TO TREAT AND DROPOUT RATES

After defining the primary and secondary outcomes to be measured, the strategy for their analysis should be decided. Completer analyses have major limitations that include loss of power and loss of initial randomization as a consequence of dropouts (i.e., people who do not complete the study) not being aleatory (e.g., dropouts in one group as a consequence of adverse effects of medication or lack of efficacy). Therefore, samples of remaining subjects (i.e., completers) might be unrepresentative (Tierney & Stewart, 2005).

Intention to treat analysis includes analysis of data of all randomized participants, irrespective of how much of the treatment they received. In other words, it evaluates the treatment offer. This is intended to equalize the potential confounding factors for the entire sample but presents problems too. To account for incomplete data in this type of analysis, one of the most common strategies is to use the last observation carried forward (LOCF), where endpoint data is substituted with previous results. The LOCF imputation method has limitations as well, because it assumes that dropout is not related to treatment or to outcome and that a subject who discontinues treatment would have retained constant clinical status from the time of dropout to the planned endpoint (Schalkwijk et al., 2014; Siddique et al., 2008). Other analytical methods have been proposed to account for missing data, such as the mixed-effect modeling of repeated measures, or defined outcomes have been assessed even after subjects have dropped out of trials (Schalkwijk et al., 2014; Siddique et al., 2008).

Finally, dropout rates of over 20% pose serious threats to the validity of results obtained in trials (Schulz & Grimes, 2002). Regrettably, according to a recent systematic review, this seems to be the case in approximately half of the bipolar depression trials (Spanemberg et al., 2012).

LEVEL OF SIGNIFICANCE: P VALUE

As stated earlier, high variability observed in bipolar depression trials could lead to false-negative outcomes. On the other hand, making repeated analysis of data greatly augments the possibility of obtaining significant p values (typically $p < .05$), that is, false positives. For example, the chance of obtaining false positives (obtaining significance by chance) for a $p < .05$ will be 5% when making one comparison, 10% for two comparisons, 23% for five comparisons, and so on (Ghaemi, 2009). This could be corrected using different methods, such as the Bonferroni correction or the Holm-Bonferroni correction, but the importance of taking this into account is that, in order to avoid such kind of errors, researchers should choose one or a few primary outcome measures for which the study should be adequately powered.

On the other hand, in secondary analysis of infrequent events (such as subgroup analysis or analysis on adverse effects of a drug in a trial designed for efficacy outcomes), p values may show false negative results, owing to diminished statistical power by smaller groups (Ghaemi, 2009).

QUALITY OF REPORTING

A recently published systematic review on quality of reporting of RCTs on pharmacologic treatments of bipolar disorders stated that "a good part of the reporting quality…falls well below the required standards and also the practically feasible levels for many aspects, essential for adequate interpretation of methodological quality and clinical relevance" (Strech, Soltmann, Weikert, Bauer, & Pfennig, 2011. p. 1220). The lack of standardisation in RCTs reporting may influence their correct interpretation. Besides, vital information in guiding clinical decisions and for data pooling in the context of meta-analysis could be missing (Undurraga & Baldessarini, 2012). Furthermore, inadequate reporting and design have been associated with biased treatment effect estimates (Moher et al., 2010). As a result of this problem, the CONSORT statement was made in the 1990s and has been revised periodically ever since (Moher et al., 2010). It consists of a checklist of essential items that should be included in reports of RCTs and a diagram for documenting the flow of participants through a trial, intended to provide guidance to researchers on reporting of their RCTs. Importantly, many leading medical journals and major international editorial groups have supported this initiative.

Strech et al. (2011) systematically reviewed the literature to identify all RCTs involving pharmacologic treatment of bipolar disorder published between 2000 and 2008. They included 105 RCTs and assessed their quality of reporting based on the CONSORT statement (Moher et al., 2010): 25% of trials reported inadequately and 42% reported adequately. Reporting was especially poor for randomization procedures: only 16% of trials defined the generation of the random allocation sequence and 15% defined the method of allocation concealment. In addition, only 41% of trials reported on blinding measures for care providers and 46% for outcome assessors and only 2% reported how the success of blinding was evaluated. In addition, only 32% reported on description of sample size calculations. Furthermore, important variables such as education, duration of illness, and number of previous episodes were underreported (7%, 32%, and 42%, respectively). Finally, only 6% of trials reported number needed to treat (NNT) and 15% reported on the CI for the contrasts between groups.

When reporting outcomes, clinical applicability and ease of interpretation are important goals. Effect size estimations in general are easier to interpret and provide more information than hypothesis testing (p values), though they can be complementary. As reported previously, p value considered alone is not helpful to guide clinical decisions, as it can be clinically irrelevant and depend on design variables such as the sample size or on statistical analysis (e.g., repeated analysis leading to false positives). In addition, total scores assessed by the symptom severity scales are difficult to interpret if the clinician is not familiar with them, which is frequently the case. Alternative methods like simple effect size estimations such as Cohen's d have been proposed (Ghaemi, 2010; Martinez-Aran et al., 2008). Cohen's d is simply calculated as the difference between the study arms for change in scores divided by their pooled standard deviations. It is useful, as it corrects for the variation within the sample and gives values between zero and 1 or higher. It typically described as "small, 0.2," "medium, 0.5," or "large, 0.8" (Martinez-Aran et al., 2008). Other examples of effect size estimations are SMDs, risk ratio, odds ratio, absolute responder or remitter rates, NNT, and number needed to harm (NNH), each being described in a preceding chapter of this book. NNT and NNH are other clinically useful effect estimates that inform clinicians about how many patients one would need to treat with one intervention versus another to see a difference in an outcome (efficacy outcomes, such as response, remission, etc. or adverse outcomes such as tolerability, suicidal behaviors, etc.). In other words, they can quantify the clinical relevance of a statistically significant study result. Their main limitation is that they can only be calculated for binary variables. Continuous variables should use other effect size measures (or be converted to binary variables, e.g., yes/no response; Citrome, 2008). Effect sizes should routinely be accompanied by their corresponding CI or CrI, which is the estimate of precision. It is "the range of plausible values for the effect size" or the "likelihood that the real value for the variable would be captured in 95% of the trials" (Ghaemi, 2010). Of note, 95% CI is equivalent to p value of .05 (but gives more information).

In conclusion, evidence on the efficacy and safety of available treatments for bipolar depression is scarce and highly heterogeneous. Many factors contributing toward heterogeneity and statistical noise should be taken into account when interpreting existing trials and designing new clinical trials: longer trial durations, higher number of study arms, larger sample sizes, involvement of more study sites, lower baseline disease severity, possibility of doses adaptation, diversity of study populations and ethnic factors, high dropout rates, less placebo washout of previous drugs, and low frequency of symptomatic assessments. Moreover, bipolar disorder has complex clinical presentations that make establishing reliable and consistent diagnosis, clinical assessments, and (clinically relevant) outcome definitions extremely important. Notably, in light of current evidence, outcome assessments in bipolar depression should also consider functional status.

Regarding assessment methods, the most frequently used scales to assess depressive symptom severity and treatment response (i.e., HDRS, MADRS, IDS) were initially developed to evaluate unipolar major depressive disorder. Newer depression scales developed specifically for bipolar depression (e.g., BDRS) may be suitable for future trails of bipolar depression. Indeed, the only way to overcome the challenges posed by decreasing signal detection in depression RCTs may be the use of harder outcomes, such as specific biomarkers, which are yet to come (Vieta, 2014).

In addition, for statistical analysis of primary and secondary outcomes, a standard intention to treat approach should be adapted as it offers a better model than the completer analysis but nevertheless is far from being unbiased. It would be even better if new analytical methods such as mixed-effect modelling of repeated measures could be incorporated.

The last stage of research, reporting the results, is as important as methodological planning and statistical analysis. Regrettably, the reporting of results from bipolar depression trials is generally of poor quality and associated with biased estimates of treatment effects. Guidelines such as the CONSORT statement should be used as an aid when reporting. Clinical applicability and ease of interpretation, as well as possibility of future evidence synthesis, should be considered. In that sense, change in scores and their standard deviations for the entire sample, as well as subgroups, should constantly be reported and may better be accompanied by the standardized effect size estimations such as SMD or Cohen's *d* and responder and remitter rates, as these measures are easier to interpret and provide more information than hypothesis testing. NNT and NNH are also clinically oriented and easy-to-interpret outcome measures that should be incorporated into reporting whenever possible. Finally, as with bipolar mania trials, quantifiable data on the special subgroups such as bipolar I or II, psychotic versus nonpsychotic, with mixed features or rapid cycling course, as well as individual adverse effects, should be reported regularly with a standardized approach.

CLINICAL TRIALS OF BIPOLAR MAINTENANCE (OR PROPHYLAXIS) TREATMENT

Standardized designs have been established for studies of acute mania (and acute depression); however, no core design for maintenance therapy for BD has been agreed on by researchers in the field (Gitlin, Abulseoud, & Frye, 2010). Therefore, it is uncertain whether the results reported may be the product of differential efficacy between agents or between different designs, thus creating inconsistent results. Given the paucity of available maintenance trials and the diversity of their designs due to the patient populations examined and pursued outcome (i.e., antimanic or antidepressive prophylaxis as described by Grunze et al., 2013), more trials providing homogenous data on the measures of efficacy, as well as side effects, functionality, quality of life, and prevention of suicide are needed. Such studies will aid clinicians in providing more successful treatments for bipolar prophylaxis.

EARLY LITHIUM TRIALS

The early lithium trials have been heavily criticized due to the discrepancies between their strikingly positive results compared to those of subsequent comparative trials and naturalistic data. In 1995 Moncrieff published an article proposing that these discrepancies originate from the design of these early studies (i.e., discontinuation studies in which patients who had been receiving lithium were allocated to either continue receiving lithium or to placebo substitution; Moncrieff, 1995). Such studies fail to examine the efficacy of lithium prophylaxis in view of the substantial evidence that lithium withdrawal induces manic relapse (Dunner, 1998; Schou, 1993). Irrefutably, special care is imperative regarding the management of lithium withdrawal (Mander & Loudon, 1988).

PLACEBO-CONTROLLED MAINTENANCE TRIALS

In 1997 Bowden et al. reported data from the first placebo-controlled maintenance trial in bipolar I disorder, which has been conducted since 1973. Bipolar maintenance trial methodologies have evolved substantially during this time. Bowden et al. argued that this particular study, designed for submission to the regulatory agencies with considerations on the country-specific requirements, have had a strong influence on the study design. They also suggest that maintenance studies should be designed and executed to enroll patients with acute, severe forms of bipolar depression or bipolar mania, rather than recruiting patients with remission or milder forms of BD. They suggested that by paying greater attention to the frequency of manic and depressive episodes and the severity of an index episode, the statistical power of the study could be enhanced (Bowden et al., 1997).

Unlike the acute treatment trials, with over 50 trials for only acute bipolar mania being published, there is a surprising paucity of maintenance studies. In a recent review by Popovic, Reinares, Amann, Salamero, and Vieta (2011), which included all the RCTs assessing the effectiveness of drugs in the prophylactic treatment of BD compared to placebo, only 15 trials satisfied the inclusion criteria (Inclusion criteria were: a minimal duration of six months; patients over 18; while exclusion criteria were: small sample size (i.e., fewer than 17 subjects per arm); a study sample not exclusively composed of bipolar patients; those using rating scales not validated in patients with bipolar disorder. Since then, further two trials satisfying the same inclusion criteria have been published (Berwaerts, Melkote, Nuamah, & Lim, 2012; Marcus et al., 2011). It is noteworthy that some trials (e.g., McIntyre et al., 2010) were excluded because they did not have a long-term placebo group. Some of the RCTs used a three-arm design. Among the available 17 trials, there were 11 RCTs assessing drugs in monotherapy and 6 for combined treatment with mood stabilizers such as lithium and valproate. The studies were not homogeneous with respect to clinical characteristics of the sample (rapid-cycling course, manic/mixed states or depression, refractory patients or unbiased samples), sample size, and rates of study completion. In that regard, as discussed by Popovic et al. (2012), most studies enrolled enriched populations of patients who were currently or recently manic or mixed. Missing from most study designs was the recruitment of patients with index depressive episodes. Exclusion of depressed patients at enrollment may affect the polarity of mood episodes during the blinded relapse prevention phase since the study design was primarily configured to demonstrate efficacy in the delay or prevention of manic recurrence.

The absence of depressive index episodes in a compound whose primary spectrum of efficacy is in depression biases outcome against the drug, or vice versa. However, the main reason why some compounds have been studied only in the context of index mania is their failure to separate from placebo in acute bipolar depression trials; hence, the bias against index depression is actually caused by the high polarity index of the drug, indicating a stronger antidopaminergic action, which makes it more suitable for the treatment of mania and the prevention of subsequent manic episodes (Popovic et al., 2012).

The polarity index is a novel metric indicating the relative antimanic versus antidepressive preventive efficacy of drugs, and it was retrieved by calculating NNT for prevention of depression and NNT for prevention of mania ratio, emerging from the results of the RCTs. The metric aims to help clinicians to understand the prophylactic efficacy profile of drugs used for the treatment of bipolar disorder by translating results of clinical trials into real-world clinical practice (Popovic et al., 2014). According to Vieta (2014), in recent years we have started to measure the relative efficacy of drugs for bipolar disorder by means of the NNT (Popovic et al., 2011) and their profile according to the polarity index (Popovic et al., 2012), which is a useful measure that can be easily misunderstood (Alphs, Berwaerts, & Turkoz, 2013) since it actually provides advice on what not to use, rather than what to use, depending on the predominant polarity of manic and depressive episodes in a given patient (Baldessarini et al., 2012).

In fact, RCTs for maintenance treatment of bipolar disorder are not only scarce; they are completely lacking for various agents. Carbamazepine is a clear example; although it was the first agent after lithium to be advocated for long-term treatment of BD and two lithium-controlled studies indicate the drug's efficacy in relapse prevention, no maintenance trials exist. As for valproate and oxcarbazepine, the only existing maintenance trials are negative/failed, thus further studies are clearly needed. Future studies need to address the long-term effectiveness of agents such as carbamazepine, oxcarbazepine, and valproate, as well as some antipsychotics, which have not been assessed in long-term placebo-controlled studies. In fact, successful long-term management often requires combination treatment. Lack of evidence base for this strategy (e.g.,

lamotrigine as add-on treatment) should also be an object of future research.

DISCONTINUATION STUDIES

The methodological caveat of discontinuation studies is that findings may demonstrate "discontinuation effects" rather than preventing relapses. Additionally, because the rate of relapse is low in these studies they require a very large number of participants to reach adequate statistical power.

CONTINUATION STUDIES

Continuation trials involve patients who have responded to the relevant treatment in the acute phase and thus are enriched for the possibility of relapse in the subsequent continuation period. Since fewer participants are required, maintenance trials switched to continuation studies.

The lack of consistency in the designs of the placebo-controlled maintenance continuation studies listed in Table 42.3 has weakened the reliability and validity of these studies. Therefore the available evidence for the long-term treatment of bipolar disorder is lacking. More rigorous approaches should involve analyses of bipolar I and bipolar II subtypes or consideration of them in different trials as described in the studies outlined here. For example, quetiapine has recently been indicated by the FDA for monotherapy of bipolar I and bipolar II depression. Although no specific controlled trial addressed the efficacy and safety of quetiapine monotherapy in bipolar II, BOLDER (BipOLar DEpRession) studies I and II, and the EMBOLDEN continuation studies (described later) included sufficient bipolar II patients (Parker, 2012).

The two EMBOLDEN studies constitute a good example of the continuation of maintenance trials with an index episode of bipolar depression. These two RCTs are similar in design (i.e. multicenter, randomized, double-blind comparisons of the efficacy and safety of quetiapine monotherapy [300 mg or 600 mg daily] verses placebo in bipolar I or II disorder adults). The active comparator arm was lithium in EMBOLDEN I and paroxetine in EMBOLDEN II. The 26- to 52-week continuation phase consisted of patients who had achieved remission and were continued on the same dose of quetiapine or were switched to placebo. In their combined analysis, the authors demonstrated that both doses of quetiapine significantly increased the time to recurrence of any mood event. The subgroup analysis on bipolar II disorder was available, and the risk of recurrence of any mood event compared with placebo was significantly reduced in this subpopulation of patients with bipolar II

TRIAL (IN ORDER OF APPEARANCE IN TEXT)	PATIENT INCLUSION CRITERIA (MAINTENANCE PHASE)	DURATION (WEEKS)	NUMBER RANDOMIZED	DOSAGE (MG/DAY) OR PLASMA LEVELS/MEAN DOSAGE
Keck et al., 2007	Bipolar I ≥18 years YMRS≤10 MADRS≤13 No hospitalization in previous 3 months	100	ARI = 78 PLA = 83	ARI: 15–30mg/day Mean: 23.8 mg/day
Tohen et al., 20063	Bipolar I ≥18 years YMRS≤12 HDRS≤ 8 2 prior mixed or manic episodes in past 6 years	48	OLZ = 225 PLA = 136	OLZ: 5–20 mg/day
Tohen et al., 2004	Bipolar I 18-70 years YMRS≤12 HRSD-21≤ 8	72	LI/VPA + PLA = 48 LI/VPA + OLZ = 51	OLZ: 5–20 mg/day Mean: 12.5 mg/day LI: 0.66-0.86 mEq/l VPA: 60.1–73.8 μg/mL
Vieta et al., 2008a	Bipolar I ≥18 years YMRS≤12 HDRS≤ 12	104	QUE + LI/VPA = 336 PLA + LI/VPA = 367	QUE: 400 -800 mg/day Mean: 497 mg/day LI: 0.5–1.2 mEq/L VPA:50–125 μg/mL
Suppes et al., 2009	Bipolar I ≥18 years YMRS≤10 MADRS≤13	104	QUE + LI/VPA = 310 PLA + LI/VPA = 313	QUE: 400–800mg/day Mean: 519 mg/die LI: 0.5-1.2 mEq/L Mean: 0.71–0.74 mEq/L VPA: 50–125 μg/mL Mean: 68.91–71.38 μg/mL
Weisler et al.	Bipolar I YMRS ≤12 MADRS ≤12 Acute current or recent (past 26 weeks) manic, depressive, or mixed index episode treated with QUE	104	QUE = 404 LI = 364 PLA = 404	QUE: 300–800 mg/day Li: 0.6-1.2 mEq/L
Quiroz et al., 2010	Bipolar I 18–65 years Recent manic/mixed episode or stable patients with ≥1 mood episode in past 4 months	96	RLAI = 140 PLA = 136	RIS: 12.5–50 mg i.m. Mean:25mg
Macfadden et al., 2009	Bipolar I 18–70 years ≥4 episodes in the past year	52	RLAI + TAU = 65 PLA + TAU = 59	RLAT: 25–50mg/2 weeks
Bowden et al., 2010	Bipolar I ≥18 years Current or recent manic/mixed episode MRS≥14	24	ZIP + LI/VPA = 127 PLA + LI/VPA = 113	ZIP: 80–160 mg/day LI: 0.6–1.2 mEq/L Mean: 0.7–0.9 mEq/L VPA: 50–125 μg/mL Mean: 67.4–72.8
Bowden et al., 2003	Bipolar I ≥18 years Current or recent (hypo)mania ≥1 additional (hypo)manic and 1 depressive episode in the past 3 years	76	LAM: 59 LI: 46 PLA:70	LAM: 100–400mg/die LI: 0.8-1.1 mEq/L

(continued)

Table 42.3 CONTINUED

TRIAL (IN ORDER OF APPEARANCE IN TEXT)	PATIENT INCLUSION CRITERIA (MAINTENANCE PHASE)	DURATION (WEEKS)	NUMBER RANDOMIZED	DOSAGE (MG/DAY) OR PLASMA LEVELS/MEAN DOSAGE
Calabrese et al., 2003	Bipolar I ≥18 years Current or recent MDE ≥1 additional (hypo)manic and 1 depressive episode in the past 3 years	72	LAM: 221 LI: 121 PLA:121	LAM:50-400mg/die Mean:200mg/die LI: 0.8-1.1 mEq/L Mean: 0.8±0.3 mEq/L
Calabrese et al., 2000	Bipolar I and II Rapid cycling ≥18 years ≤14 HDRS ≤12 MRS <3 on item 3 HDRS stable for 4 weeks	26	LAM: 90 PLA: 87	LAM: 100–300 mg/day
Prien et al., 1973	Manic-depressive, manic type	24*	LI:101 PLA: 104	LI: 0.5-1.4 mEq/L
Bowden et al., 2000	Bipolar I 18-70 years Manic episode ≤3 months before randomization. MRS ≤11 DSS ≤13 GAS >60, No serious suicidal risk	52	VPA: 187 LI: 90 PLA:92	VPA: 71-125 µg/mL LI: 0.8-1.2 mmol/L
Vieta et al., 2008b	Bipolar I or II ≥18 years YMRS≤12 MADRS≤20 No acute phases in 6 months	52	OXC + LI=26 PLA + LI=29	OXC: 1200 mg/day LI:0.6 mEq/l
Marcus et al., 2011	Bipolar I YMRS ≥16 Current or recent manic/mixed episode Inadequate response to lithium or valproate YMRS ≥16 and ≤35% decrease from baseline at 2 weeks	52	ARI + LI/VPA=168 PLA + LI/VPA=169	ARI: 15-30mg/day
Berwaerts, 2012	Bipolar I 18 -65 years Current manic or mixed episodes At least 2 previous mood episodes (1 of which had to be a manic or mixed episode) within 3 years before screening YMRS ≥20 at baseline. No significant risk for suicidal or violent behavior; no borderline or antisocial personality disorder	Until the patients experienced recurrence	PALI=152 PLA=148 OLZ=83	PALI: 3- 12 mg/day OLZ: 5-20 mg/day

NOTE: Adapted from: Popovic et al. (2011).

ᵃ With a minimal duration of 6 months and in patients aged over 18.

with both doses of quetiapine (McElroy et al., 2010; Young et al., 2010). The strengths of these two EMBOLDEN studies are (a) the large patient population (*n* =1542 (565 bipolar II)) and (b) the continued treatment of responsive patients with quetiapine or placebo (using a randomized withdrawal design). Thus the authors were able to investigate the maintenance of effect associated with ongoing quetiapine treatment. Additionally, subgroup analyses for the bipolar subtypes were included and the study involved the largest bipolar II patient population studied to date in a continuation treatment study (McElroy et al., 2010).

OUTCOMES ASSESSMENTS AND RECOMMENDATIONS FOR FUTURE MAINTENANCE TRIALS [1]

The primary outcome measures in bipolar disorder maintenance trials vary greatly, making the comparison of efficacy of medication across studies difficult (Grunze et al., 2013). The majority of long-term studies use the results of Kaplan–Meier (KM) survival analyses based on time to intervention as the primary outcome. Other studies have used "any reason of failure" (i.e., new mood episodes, need for additional treatments, hospitalization, adverse events, withdrawal of consent, lost to follow-up) as primary outcomes. Some previous studies have used dropout for emerging new episodes (using *Diagnostic and Statistical Manual of Mental Disorders* [fourth edition] criteria/clinical rating scale thresholds). The problem with KM survival analytic techniques are that they measure the occurrence of a predefined event, for example, treatment emergent episode intervention, discontinuation, at baseline (absence of the event) and endpoint (occurrence of event) only (Grunze et al., 2013). Grunze et al. state that KM survival analytic techniques are not entirely appropriate considering that "completely healthy" between-episode states are unlikely given the subsyndromal fluctuations of mood, impaired functioning, and quality of life associated with bipolar disorder and also due to the failure to capture tolerability and impact on health data. Grunze et al. suggest that the reason for the popularity of the KM techniques is they are more sensitive to measuring differences than the more traditional counting of failures. Instead of KM analyses, some studies have used mean change over time of symptomatic rating scales such as the YMRS and MADRS (McIntyre, 2010; Tohen et al., 2003). The limitation of the change over time analyses is that only minor shifts of statistical means for all patients are captured using this method.

As indicated in Chapter 43 of this book, one option for assessing daily or weekly subsyndromal mood fluctuations versus full clinical relapse (in addition to repeated use of cross-sectional scales) is the National Institute of Mental Health Life Chart Method™ (NIMH-LCM™), which has both a clinician-rated and a self-rated version for assessing severity of mania and depression on a daily basis (Post & Yildiz, 2014). This scale can also track extremes of cycling, presence of dysphoric mania, and comorbid symptoms. In addition, it has a running tally of medications and a space for rating side effects with mild, moderate, or severe impact. Reliability is excellent, as severity of mania and depression is rated on the degree of functional impairment with which each phase is associated, making recall of severity relatively easy even at intervals of several weeks to a month between rating sessions. The scale has been validated against other measures and used productively in a number of studies, including long-term comparisons of lithium versus carbamazepine versus the combination for one year of prophylaxis for each phase; comparisons of lamotrigine, gabapentin, and placebo; and, most recently, detailed analyses of lamotrigine's long-term effects on mood stability (Post & Yildiz, 2014). Related longitudinal ratings that have been employed by the STEP-BD program are also endorsed, as such detailed description of the precise course of illness is particularly important in instances of extreme rapidity of cycling, which can even occur in bipolar outpatients in demanding professions.

One of the major assets of such detailed longitudinal ratings is the ability to simultaneously assess different thresholds for what one might consider as mild, moderate, or severe relapse, as well as employ modal measures such as that of area under the curve, signifying the magnitude and duration of mania and depression. Such a measure of area under the curve allows for precise intraindividual comparisons of the degree of symptomatology observed prior to and after a given experimental manipulation as a continuous variable, which should vastly increase the power to detect treatment difference compared with a single endpoint of percentage of relapse into a new episode.

Traditional designs in assessment of the efficacy of a prophylactic treatment have typically required patients to achieve substantial improvement or remission for a given period of time, then are randomized and followed up until the occurrence of a new episode or need for clinical intervention. While this has merits inpatient populations in whom this degree of wellness is readily achieved, it is far from ideal for those with highly treatment-resistant illness.

In order to enable future pooled analyses of bipolar maintenance trials' results, besides a standardized approach on the efficacy measures in terms of prophylaxis from emerging manic or depressive episodes, future RCTs should also quantify data on the important side effects such as weight gain or metabolic syndrome, undesirable neurological or cognitive effects, and TEAS, as well as quality of life, total life years gained, and functionality, in a standardized approach.

Given that BD is an especially heterogeneous condition, it might be wise to allow a limited degree of "preplanned diversity" into the maintenance trials, provided that equal allocation into study arms is maintained, objective outcome assessments are utilized, and, most important, similarity and transitivity of the trials are not jeopardized. More RCTs and more secondary outcomes in wisely planned designs may enable more effective clinical decision-making by utilizing advanced meta-analyses methods involving direct and indirect comparisons, sensitivity analysis, and meta-regressions. In order to achieve this we suggest (a) employment of the NIMH-LCM™ for detection of daily or weekly subsyndromal mood fluctuations in addition to weekly or biweekly assessments of mania and depression cross-sectionally via employment of standardized scales such as the YMRS and MADRS as appropriate; (b) employment of 52 weeks of study duration; (c) study designs that avoid withdrawal or discontinuation effects; (d) regular and standardized assessment and reporting of all important side effects such as weight gain or metabolic syndrome, undesirable neurological or cognitive effects, and TEAS, as well as quality of life, life years gained, and functionality; (e) regular reporting on the lifetime occurrence of depressive versus manic/mixed episodes and subgroup analysis on patients with predominantly depressive versus manic/mixed polarity; (f) regular reporting on the lifetime occurrence of psychotic features and subgroup analysis on patients with psychotic versus nonpsychotic features; and (g) regular reporting on the occurrence of rapid cycling features and subgroup analysis on patients with rapid cycling versus nonrapid cycling features.

Disclosure statement: Dr. Ayşegül Yildiz has received research grants from or served as a consultant to, or speaker for, Abdi Ibrahim, Actavis, AliRaif, AstraZeneca, Bristol-Myers Squibb, Janssen-Cilag, Lundbeck, Pfizer, Sanofi-Aventis, and Servier.

Dr. Eduard Vieta has received grants and served as consultant, advisor or CME speaker for the following entities: AstraZeneca, Bristol-Myers Squibb, Elan, Eli Lilly, Ferrer, Forest Research Institute, Gedeon Richter, Glaxo-Smith-Kline, Janssen-Cilag, Jazz, Johnson & Johnson, Lundbeck, Merck, Novartis, Otsuka, Pfizer, Roche, Rovi, Sanofi-Aventis, Servier, Shire, Solvay, Sunovion, Takeda, Teva, the Spanish Ministry of Science and Innovation (CIBERSAM), the Seventh European Framework Programme (ENBREC), and the Stanley Medical Research Institute.

Dr. Dina Popovic's work is supported by a Sara Borrell post-doctoral grant, provided by Carlos III Institute (CD13/00149), Spanish Ministry of Science and Innovation. Dr. Popovic has received research grants from, or served as a speaker for, Bristol-Myers Squibb, Merck Sharp & Dohme, and Janssen-Cilag.

Dr. Sarah Wooderson is employed by King's College London. This chapter presents independent research part-funded by the National Institute for Health Research (NIHR) Biomedical Research Centre at South London and Maudsley NHS Foundation Trust and King's College London. The views expressed are those of the author and not necessarily those of the NHS, the NIHR or the Department of Health. No external funding was used for this study.

Dr. Allan Young is employed by King's College London; Honorary Consultant SLaM. He has given paid lectures and been on advisory boards for all major pharmaceutical companies with drugs used in affective and related disorders. He has no share holdings in pharmaceutical companies. He was lead investigator for Embolden Study (AZ), BCI Neuroplasticity Study, and Aripiprazole Mania Study and has participated in investigator-initiated studies from AZ, Eli Lilly, Lundbeck, and Wyeth. Grant funding (past and present) includes: USA: National Institute of Mental Health, Brain and Behavior Research Foundation (NARSAD), Stanley Medical Research Institute; Canada: Canadian Institutes of Health Research, UBC-VGH Foundation, WEDC, CCS Depression Research Fund, MSFHR; UK: MRC; Wellcome Trust; Royal College of Physicians; BMA; NIHR.

This chapter presents independent research part-funded by the National Institute for Health Research (NIHR) Biomedical Research Centre at South London and Maudsley NHS Foundation Trust and King's College London. The views expressed are those of the author and not necessarily those of the NHS, the NIHR or the Department of Health.

Dr. Juan Undurraga has not disclosed any conflicts of interest.

REFERENCES

Agid, O., Siu, C. O., Potkin, S. G., Kapur, S., Watsky, E., Vanderburg, D., ... Remington, G. (2013). Meta-regression analysis of placebo response in antipsychotic trials, 1970-2010. *The American Journal of Psychiatry*, *170*(11), 1335–1344. doi:10.1176/appi. ajp.2013.12030315

Ahrens, B., Muller-Oerlinghausen, B., Schou, M., Wolf, T., Alda, M., Grof, E.,...et al. (1995). Excess cardiovascular and suicide mortality of affective disorders may be reduced by lithium prophylaxis. *Journal of Affective Disorders*, *33*(2), 67–75.

Alphs, L., Benedetti, F., Fleischhacker, W. W., & Kane, J. M. (2012). Placebo-related effects in clinical trials in schizophrenia: What is driving this phenomenon and what can be done to minimize it? *International Journal of Neuropsychopharmacology*, *15*(7), 1003–1014. doi:10.1017/S1461145711001738

Alphs, L., Berwaerts, J., & Turkoz, I. (2013). Limited utility of number needed to treat and the polarity index for bipolar disorder to characterize treatment response. *European Neuropsychopharmacology*, *23*(11), 1597–1599.

Ayuso-Mateos, J. L., Avila, C. C., Anaya, C., Cieza, A., Vieta, E., & Bipolar Disorders Core Sets Expert Group. (2013). Development of the international classification of functioning, disability and health core sets for bipolar disorders: Results of an international consensus process. *Disability and Rehabilitation*, *35*(25), 2138–2146. doi:10.3 109/09638288.2013.771708

Baldessarini, R. J. (2013). *Chemotherapy in psychiatry* (3rd ed.). New York: Springer Press.

Baldessarini, R. J., Leahy, L., Arcona, S., Gause, D., Zhang, W., & Hennen, J. (2007). Patterns of psychotropic drug prescription for U.S. patients with diagnoses of bipolar disorders. *Psychiatric Services*, *58*(1), 85–91. doi:10.1176/appi.ps.58.1.85-a

Baldessarini, R. J., Undurraga, J., Vázquez, G. H., Tondo, L., Salvatore, P., Ha, K.,...Vieta, E. (2012). Predominant recurrence polarity among 928 adult international bipolar I disorder patients. *Acta Psychiatrica Scandinavica*, *125*(4), 293–302. doi:10.1111/ j.1600-0447.2011.01818.x

Baldessarini, R. J., Vieta, E., Calabrese, J. R., Tohen, M., & Bowden, C. L. (2010). Bipolar depression: Overview and commentary. *Harvard Review of Psychiatry*, *18*(3), 143–157. doi:10.3109/10673221003747955

Bauer, M., Beaulieu, S., Dunner, D. L., Lafer, B., & Kupka, R. (2008). Rapid cycling bipolar disorder—Diagnostic concepts. *Bipolar Disorders*, *10*(1 Pt. 2), 153–162. doi:10.1111/ j.1399-5618.2007.00560.x

Benazzi, F. (2007). Is there a continuity between bipolar and depressive disorders? *Psychotherapy and Psychosomatics*, *76*(2), 70–76. doi:10.1159/000097965

Benedetti, F. (2009). *Understanding the mechanisms in health and disease.* New York: Oxford University Press.

Berk, M., Malhi, G. S., Cahill, C., Carman, A. C., Hadzi-Pavlovic, D., Hawkins, M. T.,...Mitchell, P. B. (2007). The Bipolar Depression Rating Scale (BDRS): Its development, validation and utility. *Bipolar Disorders*, *9*(6), 571–579. doi:10.1111/j.1399-5618.2007.00536.x

Berwaerts, J., Melkote, R., Nuamah, I., & Lim, P. (2012). A randomized, placebo- and active-controlled study of paliperidone extended-release as maintenance treatment in patients with bipolar I disorder after an acute manic or mixed episode. *Journal of Affective Disorders*, *138*(3), 247–258.

Bowden, C. L., Swann, A. C., Calabrese, J. R., McElroy, S. L., Morris, D., Petty, F.,...Gyulai, L. (1997). Maintenance clinical trials in bipolar disorder: Design implications of the divalproex-lithium-placebo study. *Psychopharmacology Bulletin*, *33*(4), 693–699.

Chang, C. K., Hayes, R. D., Perera, G., Broadbent, M. T., Fernandes, A. C., Lee, W. E.,...Stewart, R. (2011). Life expectancy at birth for people with serious mental illness and other major disorders from a secondary mental health care case register in London. *PLoS One*, *6*(5), e19590. doi:10.1371/journal.pone.0019590

Cipriani, A., Hawton, K., Stockton, S., & Geddes, J. R. (2013). Lithium in the prevention of suicide in mood disorders: Updated systematic review and meta-analysis. *BMJ*, *346*, f3646. doi:10.1136/bmj.f3646

Citrome, L. (2008). Compelling or irrelevant? Using number needed to treat can help decide. *Acta Psychiatrica Scandinavica*, *117*(6), 412–419. doi:10.1111/j.1600-0447.2008.01194.x

Colom, F., Vieta, E., Daban, C., Pacchiarotti, I., & Sanchez-Moreno, J. (2006). Clinical and therapeutic implications of predominant polarity in bipolar disorder. *Journal of Affective Disorders*, *93*(1–3), 13–17. doi:10.1016/j.jad.2006.01.032

Correll, C. U., Malhotra, A. K., Kaushik, S., McMeniman, M., & Kane, J. M. (2003). Early prediction of antipsychotic response in schizophrenia. *The American Journal of Psychiatry*, *160*(11), 2063–2065.

Cruz, N., Vieta, E., Comes, M., Haro, J. M., Reed, C., Bertsch, J., & Emblem Advisory Board. (2008). Rapid-cycling bipolar I disorder: Course and treatment outcome of a large sample across Europe. *Journal of Psychiatric Research*, *42*(13), 1068–1075. doi:10.1016/j. jpsychires.2007.12.004

De Fruyt, J., Deschepper, E., Audenaert, K., Constant, E., Floris, M., Pitchot, W.,...Claes, S. (2012). Second generation antipsychotics in the treatment of bipolar depression: A systematic review and meta-analysis. *Journal of Psychopharmacology*, *26*(5), 603–617. doi:10.1177/0269881111408461

Drexhage, R. C., Hoogenboezem, T. H., Versnel, M. A., Berghout, A., Nolen, W. A., & Drexhage, H. A. (2011). The activation of monocyte and T cell networks in patients with bipolar disorder. *Brain Behaviour and Immunity*, *25*(6), 1206–1213. doi:10.1016/j. bbi.2011.03.013

Dunner, D. L. (1998). Lithium carbonate: Maintenance studies and consequences of withdrawal. *Journal of Clinical Psychiatry*, *59*(6), 48–55; discussion 56.

Dunner, D. L., & Fieve, R. R. (1974). Clinical factors in lithium carbonate prophylaxis failure. *Archives of General Psychiatry*, *30*(2), 229–233.

Fava, M., Evins, A. E., Dorer, D. J., & Schoenfeld, D. A. (2003). The problem of the placebo response in clinical trials for psychiatric disorders: Culprits, possible remedies, and a novel study design approach. *Psychotherapy and Psychosomatics*, *72*(3), 115–127. doi:69738

Gitlin, M. J., Abulseoud, O., & Frye, M. A. (2010). Improving the design of maintenance studies for bipolar disorder. *Current Medical Research and Opinion*, *26*(8), 1835–1842.

Grunze, H., Vieta, E., Goodwin, G. M., Bowden, C., Licht, R. W., Möller, H. J.,...WFSBP Task Force on Treatment Guidelines for Bipolar Disorders. (2013). The World Federation of Societies of Biological Psychiatry (WFSBP) guidelines for the biological treatment of bipolar disorders: Update 2012 on the long-term treatment of bipolar disorder. *World Journal of Biological Psychiatry*, *14*(3), 154–219.

García-Rizo, C., Kirkpatrick, B., Fernandez-Egea, E., Oliveira, C., Meseguer, A., Grande, I.,...Bernardo, M. (2014). "Is bipolar disorder an endocrine condition?" Glucose abnormalities in bipolar disorder. *Acta Psychiatrica Scandinavica*, *129*(1), 73–74. doi:10.1111/ acps.12194

Geddes, J. R., & Miklowitz, D. J. (2013). Treatment of bipolar disorder. *Lancet*, *381*(9878), 1672–1682.

Ghaemi, S. N. (2009). *A clinician's guide to statistics and epidemiology in mental health: Measuring truth and uncertainty.* New York: Cambridge University Press.

Gijsman, H. J., Geddes, J. R., Rendell, J. M., Nolen, W. A., & Goodwin, G. M. (2004). Antidepressants for bipolar depression: A systematic review of randomized, controlled trials. *The American Journal of Psychiatry*, *161*(9), 1537–1547. doi:10.1176/appi.ajp.161.9.1537

Henkel, V., Casaulta, F., Seemuller, F., Krahenbuhl, S., Obermeier, M., Husler, J., & Moller, H. J. (2012). Study design features affecting outcome in antidepressant trials. *Journal of Affective Disorders*, *141*(2–3), 160–167. doi:10.1016/j.jad.2012.03.021

Hoertel, N., de Maricourt, P., & Gorwood, P. (2013). Novel routes to bipolar disorder drug discovery. *Expert Opinion on Drug Discovery*, *8*(8), 907–918. doi:10.1517/17460441.2013.804057

Hurko, O., & Ryan, J. L. (2005). Translational research in central nervous system drug discovery. *NeuroRx, 2*(4), 671–682. doi:10.1602/neurorx.2.4.671

Jaeger, J., & Vieta, E. (2007). Functional outcome and disability in bipolar disorders: Ongoing research and future directions. *Bipolar Disorders, 9*(1–2), 1–2. doi:10.1111/j.1399-5618.2007.00441.x

Judd, L. L., Schettler, P. J., Akiskal, H. S., Coryell, W., Leon, A. C., Maser, J. D., & Solomon, D. A. (2008). Residual symptom recovery from major affective episodes in bipolar disorders and rapid episode relapse/recurrence. *Archives of General Psychiatry, 65*(4), 386–394. doi:10.1001/archpsyc.65.4.386

Judd, L. L., Schettler, P. J., Akiskal, H. S., Maser, J., Coryell, W., Solomon, D., ...Keller, M. (2003). Long-term symptomatic status of bipolar I vs. bipolar II disorders. *International Journal of Neuropsychopharmacology, 6*(2), 127–137. doi:10.1017/S1461145703003341

Kemp, A. S., Schooler, N. R., Kalali, A. H., Alphs, L., Anand, R., Awad, G., ...Vermeulen, A. (2010). What is causing the reduced drug-placebo difference in recent schizophrenia clinical trials and what can be done about it? *Schizophrenia Bulletin, 36*(3), 504–509. doi:10.1093/schbul/sbn110

Khan, A., Bhat, A., Kolts, R., Thase, M. E., & Brown, W. (2010). Why has the antidepressant-placebo difference in antidepressant clinical trials diminished over the past three decades? *CNS Neuroscience and Therapeutics, 16*(4), 217–226. doi:10.1111/j.1755-5949.2010.00151.x

Khan, A., Schwartz, K., Kolts, R. L., Ridgway, D., & Lineberry, C. (2007). Relationship between depression severity entry criteria and antidepressant clinical trial outcomes. *Biological Psychiatry, 62*(1), 65–71. doi:10.1016/j.biopsych.2006.08.036

Kim, J. H., Jung, H. Y., Kang, U. G., Jeong, S. H., Ahn, Y. M., Byun, H. J., ...Kim, Y. S. (2002). Metric characteristics of the drug-induced extrapyramidal symptoms scale (DIEPSS): A practical combined rating scale for drug-induced movement disorders. *Movement Disorders, 17*(6), 1354–1359.

Kinon, B. J., Chen, L., Ascher-Svanum, H., Stauffer, V. L., Kollack-Walker, S., Zhou, W., ...Kane, J. M. (2010). Early response to antipsychotic drug therapy as a clinical marker of subsequent response in the treatment of schizophrenia. *Neuropsychopharmacology, 35*(2), 581–590. doi:10.1038/npp.2009.164

Kirsch, I. (2009). Antidepressants and the placebo response. *Epidemiologia e Psichiatria Sociale, 18*(4), 318–322.

Kobak, K. A., Leuchter, A., DeBrota, D., Engelhardt, N., Williams, J. B., Cook, I. A., ...Alpert, J. (2010). Site versus centralized raters in a clinical depression trial: Impact on patient selection and placebo response. *Journal of Clinical Psychopharmacology, 30*(2), 193–197. doi:10.1097/JCP.0b013e3181d20912

Laursen, T. M. (2011). Life expectancy among persons with schizophrenia or bipolar affective disorder. *Schizophrenia Research, 131*(1–3), 101–104. doi:10.1016/j.schres.2011.06.008

Leboyer, M., Soreca, I., Scott, J., Frye, M., Henry, C., Tamouza, R., & Kupfer, D. J. (2012). Can bipolar disorder be viewed as a multi-system inflammatory disease? *Journal of Affective Disorders, 141*(1), 1–10. doi:10.1016/j.jad.2011.12.049

Leucht, S., Arbter, D., Engel, R. R., Kissling, W., & Davis, J. M. (2009). How effective are second-generation antipsychotic drugs? A meta-analysis of placebo-controlled trials. *Molecular Psychiatry, 14*(4), 429–447. doi:10.1038/sj.mp.4002136

Leucht, S., Cipriani, A., Spineli, L., Mavridis, D., Orey, D., Richter, F., ...Davis, J. M. (2013). Comparative efficacy and tolerability of 15 antipsychotic drugs in schizophrenia: A multiple-treatments meta-analysis. *Lancet, 382*(9896), 951–962. doi:10.1016/S0140-6736(13)60733-3

Leucht, S., Heres, S., & Davis, J. M. (2013). Increasing placebo response in antipsychotic drug trials: Let's stop the vicious circle. *The American Journal of Psychiatry, 170*(11), 1232–1234. doi:10.1176/appi.ajp.2013.13081129

Leucht, S., Hierl, S., Kissling, W., Dold, M., Davis, J. M. (2012). Putting the efficacy of psychiatric and general medicine medication into perspective: Review of meta-analyses. *The British Journal of Psychiatry, 200*, 97–106.

Machado-Vieira, R., Salvadore, G., DiazGranados, N., Ibrahim, L., Latov, D., Wheeler-Castillo, C., ...Zarate, C. A. (2010). New therapeutic targets for mood disorders. *TheScientificWorldJournal, 10*, 713–726. doi:10.1100/Tsw.2010.65

Mallinckrodt, C. H., Zhang, L., Prucka, W. R., & Millen, B. A. (2010). Signal detection and placebo response in schizophrenia: Parallels with depression. *Psychopharmacology Bulletin, 43*(1), 53–72.

Mander, A. J., & Loudon, J. B. (1988). Rapid recurrence of mania following abrupt discontinuation of lithium. *Lancet, 2*(8601), 15–17.

Marangell, L. B. (2004). The importance of subsyndromal symptoms in bipolar disorder. *Journal of Clinical Psychiatry, 65*, 24–27.

March, J. S., Silva, S. G., Compton, S., Shapiro, M., Califf, R., & Krishnan, R. (2005). The case for practical clinical trials in psychiatry. *The American Journal of Psychiatry, 162*(5), 836–846. doi:10.1176/appi.ajp.162.5.836

Marcus, R., Khan, A., Rollin, L., Morris, B., Timko, K., Carson, W., & Sanchez, R. (2011). Efficacy of aripiprazole adjunctive to lithium or valproate in the long-term treatment of patients with bipolar I disorder with an inadequate response to lithium or valproate monotherapy: A multicenter, double-blind, randomized study. *Bipolar Disorders, 13*(2), 133–144.

Martinez-Aran, A., Vieta, E., Chengappa, K. N. R., Gershon, S., Mullen, J., & Paulsson, B. (2008). Reporting outcomes in clinical trials for bipolar disorder: A commentary and suggestions for change. *Bipolar Disorders, 10*(5), 566–579. doi:10.1111/j.1399-5618.2008.00611.x

Mathew, S. J., Manji, H. K., & Charney, D. S. (2008). Novel drugs and therapeutic targets for severe mood disorders. *Neuropsychopharmacology, 33*(9), 2080–2092. doi:10.1038/sj.npp.1301652

McElroy, S. L., Weisler, R. H., Chang, W., Olausson, B., Paulsson, B., Brecher, M., ...Investigators, E. I. (2010). A double-blind, placebo-controlled study of quetiapine and paroxetine as monotherapy in adults with bipolar depression (EMBOLDEN II). *Journal of Clinical Psychiatry, 71*(2), 163–174.

McIntyre, R. S. (2010). Aripiprazole for the maintenance treatment of bipolar I disorder: A review. *Clinical Therapeutics, 32*(1), S32–38.

McIntyre, R. S., Cohen, M., Zhao, J., Alphs, L., Macek, T. A., & Panagides, J. (2010). Asenapine in the treatment of acute mania in bipolar I disorder: A randomized, double-blind, placebo-controlled trial. *Journal of Affective Disorders, 122*(1–2), 27–38.

Moerman, D. (2002). *Meaning, medicine and the placebo effect.* New York: Cambridge University Press.

Moher, D., Hopewell, S., Schulz, K. F., Montori, V., Gotzsche, P. C., Devereaux, P. J., ...Altman, D. G. (2010). CONSORT 2010 explanation and elaboration: Updated guidelines for reporting parallel group randomised trials. *BMJ: British Medical Journal, 340.* doi:10.1136/bmj.c869

Moncrieff, J. (1995). Lithium revisited: A re-examination of the placebo-controlled trials of lithium prophylaxis in manic-depressive disorder. *The British Journal of Psychiatry, 167*(5), 569–573; discussion 573–564.

Pacchiarotti, I., Bond, D. J., Baldessarini, R. J., Nolen, W. A., Grunze, H., Licht, R. W., ...Vieta, E. (2013). The International Society for Bipolar Disorders (ISBD) task force report on antidepressant use in bipolar disorders. *The American Journal of Psychiatry, 170*(11), 1249–1262. doi:10.1176/appi.ajp.2013.13020185

Parker, G. (2012). *Bipolar II disorder: Modelling, measuring and managing* (2nd ed.). New York: Cambridge University Press.

Popovic, D., Reinares, M., Amann, B., Salamero, M., & Vieta, E. (2011). Number needed to treat analyses of drugs used for maintenance treatment of bipolar disorder. *Psychopharmacology (Berlin), 213*(4), 657–667.

Popovic, D., Reinares, M., Goikolea, J. M., Bonnin, C. M., Gonzalez-Pinto, A., & Vieta, E. (2012). Polarity index of pharmacological agents used for maintenance treatment of bipolar disorder. *European Neuropsychopharmacology, 22*(5), 339–346.

Popovic, D., Torrent, C., Goikolea, J. M., Cruz, N., Sánchez-Moreno, J., González-Pinto, A., & Vieta, E. (2014). Clinical implications of predominant polarity and the polarity index in bipolar disorder: A naturalistic study. *Acta Psychiatrica Scandinavica, 129*(5), 366–374.

Post, R. M. (2009). Myth of evidence-based medicine for bipolar disorder. *Expert Review of Neurotherapeutics, 9*(9), 1271–1273.

Post, R. M. (2010). Special issues of research methodology in bipolar disorder clinical treatment trials. In M. Hertzman & L. Adler (Eds.), *Clinical trials in psychopharmacology: A better brain* (2nd ed.). Hoboken, NJ: John Wiley.

Raz, A., Zigman, P., & de Jong, V. (2009). Placebo effects and responses: Filling the interstices with meaning. *PsycCRITIQUES, 54*, 33.

Reinares, M., Rosa, A. R., Franco, C., Goikolea, J. M., Fountoulakis, K., Siamouli, M.,…Vieta, E. (2013). A systematic review on the role of anticonvulsants in the treatment of acute bipolar depression. *International Journal of Neuropsychopharmacology, 16*(2), 485–496. doi:10.1017/S1461145712000491

Rosa, A. R., Sanchez-Moreno, J., Martinez-Aran, A., Salamero, M., Torrent, C., Reinares, M.,…Vieta, E. (2007). Validity and reliability of the Functioning Assessment Short Test (FAST) in bipolar disorder. *Clinical Practice and Epidemiology in Mental Health, 3*, 5. doi:10.1186/1745-0179-3-5

Rush, A. J., Kraemer, H. C., Sackeim, H. A., Fava, M., Trivedi, M. H., Frank, E.,…ACNP Task Force. (2006). Report by the ACNP Task Force on response and remission in major depressive disorder. *Neuropsychopharmacology, 31*(9), 1841–1853. doi:10.1038/sj.npp.1301131

Schalkwijk, S., Undurraga, J., Tondo, L., & Baldessarini, R. J. (2014). Declining efficacy in controlled trials of antidepressants: effects of placebo dropout. *The International Journal of Neuropsychopharmacology / Official Scientific Journal of the Collegium Internationale Neuropsychopharmacologicum (CINP), 17*(8), 1343–1352.

Schou, M. (1993). Is there a lithium withdrawal syndrome? An examination of the evidence. *The British Journal of Psychiatry, 163*, 514–518.

Schulz, K. F., & Grimes, D. A. (2002). Sample size slippages in randomised trials: Exclusions and the lost and wayward. *Lancet, 359*(9308), 781–785. doi:10.1016/S0140-6736(02)07882-0

Siddique, J., Brown, C. H., Hedeker, D., Duan, N., Gibbons, R. D., Miranda, J., & Lavori, P. W. (2008). Missing data in longitudinal trials—Part B, analytic issues. *Psychiatric Annals, 38*(12), 793–801.

Sidor, M. M., & Macqueen, G. M. (2011). Antidepressants for the acute treatment of bipolar depression: A systematic review and meta-analysis. *Journal of Clinical Psychiatry, 72*(2), 156–167. doi:10.4088/JCP.09r05385gre

Sidor, M. M., & MacQueen, G. M. (2012). An update on antidepressant use in bipolar depression. *Current Psychiatry Reports, 14*(6), 696–704. doi:10.1007/s11920-012-0323-6

Spanemberg, L., Massuda, R., Lovato, L., Paim, L., Vares, E. A., Sica da Rocha, N., & Cereser, K. M. (2012). Pharmacological treatment of bipolar depression: Qualitative systematic review of double-blind randomized clinical trials. *Psychiatric Quarterly, 83*(2), 161–175. doi:10.1007/s11126-011-9191-1

Strech, D., Soltmann, B., Weikert, B., Bauer, M., & Pfennig, A. (2011). Quality of reporting of randomized controlled trials of pharmacologic treatment of bipolar disorders: A systematic review. *Journal of Clinical Psychiatry, 72*(9), 1214–1221. doi:10.4088/JCP.10r06166yel

Sysko, R., & Walsh, B. T. (2007). A systematic review of placebo response in studies of bipolar mania. *Journal of Clinical Psychiatry, 68*(8), 1213–1217.

Tarr, G. P., Herbison, P., de la Barra, S. L., & Glue, P. (2011). Study design and patient characteristics and outcome in acute mania clinical trials. *Bipolar Disorders, 13*(2), 125–132. doi:10.1111/j.1399-5618.2011.00904.x

Thase, M. E. (2003). Evaluating antidepressant therapies: Remission as the optimal outcome. *Journal of Clinical Psychiatry, 64*(13), 18–25.

Tierney, J. F., & Stewart, L. A. (2005). Investigating patient exclusion bias in meta-analysis. *International Journal of Epidemiology, 34*(1), 79–87. doi:10.1093/ije/dyh300

Tohen, M., Frank, E., Bowden, C. L., Colom, F., Ghaemi, S. N., Yatham, L. N.,…Berk, M. (2009). The International Society for Bipolar Disorders (ISBD) Task Force report on the nomenclature of course and outcome in bipolar disorders. *Bipolar Disorders, 11*(5), 453–473. doi:10.1111/j.1399-5618.2009.00726.x

Tohen, M., Ketter, T. A., Zarate, C. A., Suppes, T., Frye, M., Altshuler, L.,…Baker, R. W. (2003). Olanzapine versus divalproex sodium for the treatment of acute mania and maintenance of remission: A 47-week study. *The American Journal of Psychiatry, 160*(7), 1263–1271.

Undurraga, J., & Baldessarini, R. J. (2012). Randomized, placebo-controlled trials of antidepressants for acute major depression: Thirty-year meta-analytic review. *Neuropsychopharmacology, 37*(4), 851–864. doi:10.1038/npp.2011.306

Undurraga, J., Baldessarini, R. J., Valentí, M., Pacchiarotti, I., Tondo, L., Vázquez, G., & Vieta, E. (2012). Bipolar depression: Clinical correlates of receiving antidepressants. *Journal of Affective Disorders, 139*(1), 89–93. doi:10.1016/j.jad.2012.01.027

Vázquez, G. H., Tondo, L., Undurraga, J., & Baldessarini, R. J. (2013). Overview of antidepressant treatment of bipolar depression. *International Journal of Neuropsychopharmacology, 16*(7), 1673–1685. doi:10.1017/S1461145713000023

Vieta, E. (2014). The bipolar maze: A roadmap through translational psychopathology. *Acta Psychiatrica Scandinavica, 129*(5), 323–327.

Vieta, E., & Cruz, N. (2012). Head to head comparisons as an alternative to placebo-controlled trials. *European Neuropsychopharmacology, 22*(11), 800–803.

Vieta, E., Grunze, H., Azorin, J. M., & Fagiolini, A. (2014). Phenomenology of manic episodes according to the presence or absence of depressive features as defined in DSM-5: Results from the IMPACT self-reported online survey. *Journal of Affective Disorders, 156*, 206–213.

Vieta, E., Pappadopulos, E., Mandel, F. S., Lombardo, I. (2011). Impact of geographical and cultural factors on clinical trials in acute mania: Lessons from a ziprasidone and haloperidol placebo-controlled study. *International Journal of Neuropsychopharmacology, 14*(8), 1017–1027.

Vieta, E., Thase, M. E., Naber, D., D'Souza, B., Rancans, E., Lepola, U.,…Eriksson, H. (2014). Efficacy and tolerability of flexibly-dosed adjunct TC-5214 (dexmecamylamine) in patients with major depressive disorder and inadequate response to prior antidepressant. *European Neuropsychopharmacology: The Journal of the European College of Neuropsychopharmacology, 24*(4), 564–574.

Vieta, E., & Valentí, M. (2013). Pharmacological management of bipolar depression: Acute treatment, maintenance, and prophylaxis. *CNS Drugs, 27*(7), 515–529. doi:10.1007/s40263-013-0073

Walsh, B. T., Seidman, S. N., Sysko, R., & Gould, M. (2002). Placebo response in studies of major depression: Variable, substantial, and growing. *JAMA, 287*(14), 1840–1847.

World Health Organization. (n.d.). WHO Disability Assessment Schedule 2.0: WHODAS 2.0. Retrieved from http://www.who.int/classifications/icf/whodasii/en/

Yildiz, A., Guleryuz, S., Ankerst, D. P., Ongur, D., & Renshaw, P. F. (2008). Protein kinase C inhibition in the treatment of mania: A double-blind, placebo-controlled trial of tamoxifen.

Archives of General Psychiatry, 65(3), 255–263. doi:10.1001/arch-genpsychiatry.2007.43

Yildiz, A., Vieta, E., Correll, C. U., Nikodem, M., & Baldessarini, R. J. (2014). Critical Issues on the Use of Network Meta-analysis in Psychiatry. *Harvard Review of Psychiatry, 22*(6), 367–372.

Yildiz, A., Vieta, E., Leucht, S., & Baldessarini, R. J. (2011). Efficacy of antimanic treatments: Meta-analysis of randomized, controlled trials. *Neuropsychopharmacology, 36*(2), 375–389. doi:10.1038/npp.2010.192

Yildiz, A., Vieta, E., Tohen, M., & Baldessarini, R. J. (2011). Factors modifying drug and placebo responses in randomized trials for bipolar mania. *International Journal of Neuropsychopharmacology, 14*(7), 863–875. doi:10.1017/S1461145710001641

Young, A. H., McElroy, S. L., Bauer, M., Philips, N., Chang, W., Olausson, B.,…Investigators, E. I. (2010). A double-blind, placebo-controlled study of quetiapine and lithium monotherapy in adults in the acute phase of bipolar depression (EMBOLDEN I). *Journal of Clinical Psychiatry, 71*(2), 150–162.

Young, R. C., Biggs, J. T., Ziegler, V. E., & Meyer, D. A. (1978). A rating scale for mania: Reliability, validity and sensitivity. *The British Journal of Psychiatry, 133*, 429–435.

Zimmerman, M., Posternak, M. A., & Chelminski, I. (2004). Implications of using different cut-offs on symptom severity scales to define remission from depression. *International Clinical Psychopharmacology, 19*(4), 215–220.

43.

CHALLENGES IN DESIGNING RELIABLE AND FEASIBLE TRIALS FOR TREATMENT OF BIPOLAR DISORDER

Robert M. Post and Ayşegül Yildiz

INTRODUCTION

A number of characteristics of bipolar disorder (BD) make it particularly difficult to study. BD is not only extremely pleomorphic but is complicated by more psychiatric comorbidities than virtually any other major psychiatric illness. This vast heterogeneity of illness presentation stands in absolute contradiction to the ideal requirements (for homogeneity) in the traditional randomized controlled clinical trials (RCTs; Leber, 2002; Post & Luckenbaugh, 2003). Moreover, episodes of BD are characterized by psychomotor behaviors of essentially opposite poles of manic hyperactivity and depressive slowness, lethargy, lack of motivation, and social withdrawal (Post, Keck, & Rush, 2002). Each type of episode can further vary in terms of severity and duration, yielding patterns ranging from isolated intermittent episodes to more rapid cycling, biphasic and triphasic mood alterations, and continuous cycling without a well interval.

In our recently collected outpatient series, 64.1% of patients had a pattern of rapid cycling (four or more episodes in a year prior to network entry), representing a substantial group with much faster patterns of recurrences (Nolen et al., 2004; Post, Chang, & Suppes, 2004). Further complicating the picture of the complexities of bipolar presentations are episodes that present as admixtures of mania and depression with several types of mixed states (Frye, 2008; Kupka et al., 2005; Suppes et al., 2005). It has been previously reported that 66% of women and 44% of men with BD type II experience some concurrent depressive symptoms during hypomania (Suppes et al., 2005).

Excluding hypomania, either phase of illness may have accompanying psychotic elements with hallucinations and delusions. Also, extremes of irritability, as well as anger attacks, are not uncommon during manic or depressive phases of illness. Superimposed on these diverse presentations is very high incidence of comorbidities; within the many US series, patients with BD have a comorbid anxiety disorder at a rate of 40% and an accompanying substance abuse disorder present at a similar rate (Kessler et al., 1994; McElroy et al., 2001). Substance abuse often begins early in bipolar adolescents, who are seven time more likely to adopt substance abuse compared with healthy age mates (Wilens et al., 2004).

EFFICACY–EFFECTIVENESS GAP

While the presence of each type of comorbidity—alcohol abuse, substance abuse, or a comorbid anxiety disorder—can yield a more difficult-to-treat bipolar subgroup with a less favorable prognosis, the complexity of illness presentations and the trial designs required to deal with them has led to a paucity of studies considering comorbidity in BD. Further, attempts to generate homogeneous patient populations for routine RCTs, which is critical for drug approval, have likely led to distinctive trial populations, at the expense of losing close comparison with the real-world clinical settings. While patients with specific comorbidities or rapid cycling patterns are explicitly excluded from regular RCTs, given the difficulties in dealing with severer forms of illness (such as suicidality in depressive or mixed phases or high energy, overactivity, reduced sleep, inflated mood, and poor insight in manic phases), patients experiencing erratic shifts in mood in such extreme levels are also often implicitly not considered as suitable candidates for the placebo-controlled RCTs. As a consequence, patient populations in the traditional RCTs are likely to be enriched for placebo rather than active drug responders. In support of this view, a recent report revealed a remarkably high percentage of exclusion in the process of potential subject selection during conduct of a regular RCT (Blanco et al., 2008).

The assessment of the degree of efficacy of a drug is therefore derived from highly selective subject populations and may not well reflect actual degree of effectiveness in the real-world treatment situations—the so-called efficacy–effectiveness gap. This has major implications for clinical decision-making. Many studies directed toward demonstrating efficacy for approval by the Food and Drug Administration (FDA) or some other regulatory body do not provide optimal assistance to patients and clinicians in choosing and sequencing alternatives in the face of inadequate response (Post et al., 2002; Post & Luckenbaugh, 2003). The accumulated RCTs evidence being grounded on such selected patient populations is limited in affording evidence-based treatment alternatives also for treatment-resistant cases. Recent estimates suggest that the majority of patients in the United States are treatment resistant, and a recent Scandinavian study suggested that only 5% of patients are excellent long-term responders to lithium monotherapy during 10-year follow-up (Kessing, Hellmund, & Andersen, 2012).

TRIALS FOR DRUG REGISTRATION VERSUS THOSE THAT ARE MOST CLINICALLY INFORMATIVE

If a patient does meet typical 50% improvement response criterion in a traditional RCT, additional information is often not provided about what treatment options may be required in order to achieve a more complete response or the ideal of a remission. For example, in our most recent meta-analytic data set of antimanic treatment trials, only half of the placebo-controlled studies reported on the remission rates, with the figure even less for the drug versus drug comparisons (Yildiz, Nikodem, Vieta, Correll, & Baldessarini, 2014). This is increasingly an important goal because considerable data indicate that residual manic or depressive symptomatology is a poor prognosis factor and augurs the likelihood of the emergence of a full-blown syndromal breakthrough episode at some point in the near future (Judd et al., 2002; Perlis et al., 2006).

Moreover, while there is wide recognition that multiple drugs used in combination are the norm for children and adult bipolar patients, the drugs are almost invariably initially studied for regulatory approval as monotherapy and only more recently as dual drug combinations. Clinical trial designs have not yet included those needed for elucidating the best sequences of drugs to be tried and the combinations most likely to be effective (Post & Luckenbaugh, 2003; Sachs, 2001).

NEED FOR DESIGNS THAT MORE OPTIMALLY INFORM CLINICAL PRACTICE

For these and a multitude of other reasons, many have strongly advocated for funding of more practical clinical trials, particularly for patients with BD. These studies are more typical of what has been considered services research and categorized more as effectiveness trials (March et al., 2005; Sachs, 2001; Slade & Priebe, 2001). Such trials involving patients with more complex and multiple comorbidities are particularly helpful in guiding routine clinical practice. In such trials, effectiveness and tolerability data can be rapidly acquired in a much less expensive open or assessor blind fashion with, for example, patients randomly exposed to one or another active treatment arm (Benson & Hartz, 2000; Concato, Shah, & Horwitz, 2000). A similar approach employed in the BALANCE study has successfully demonstrated the superiority of lithium and the combination of lithium and valproate over valproate alone for maintenance treatment of BD (Geddes et al., 2010).

Another approach to clinical utility would be to cross-over nonresponsive patients to the other agent in comparative studies. One could cross-over partial responders as well in order to achieve within-subjects comparability of the two treatments for both efficacy, effectiveness, and tolerability, particularly when both treatments are generally considered at equipoise.

The STEP-BD network has utilized a series of nested trials similar to those employed in the STAR-D trial, in which a given patient continues in the program and is exposed to additional options to either switch treatment or augment treatment in multiple sequences with the goal of bringing as many patients as possible into remission (Rush, 2007; Rush et al., 2000; Sachs, 2001).

Examining the effectiveness of complex combination treatments employed in observational naturalistic studies may provide a variety of preliminary and exploratory data and hypotheses about what might be the most optimal sequences to explore in more systematic sequential clinical trials. The most recent practical clinical trials have been disappointing in that adding lithium to treatment as usual (Nierenberg et al., 2013) or lamotrigine to the combination of lithium and valproate (Kemp et al., 2012) have shown little benefit.

Other methodological options include play the winner strategies, mirror images, and a variety of other approaches used in cardiology, oncology, and infectious diseases (Gelenberg, 1994; Gelenberg et al., 2008;

Lavori, Dawson, & Rush, 2000; Rush et al., 2000). In these other areas of medicine one often has data from RCTs examining the effectiveness of one combination of three or four drugs compared with another combination of agents. These kinds of studies have provided information about optimal combination treatments for congestive heart failure, lymphomas, and AIDs, to name just a few. Multiple drugs used in combination for treatment of BD are rarely systematically explored, even though complex combination therapy appears to be the norm in most academic and clinical practice settings. However, caution should be taken in designing such trials to facilitate homogenous data accumulation by employment of clinically most widely used combination treatments. Otherwise, heterogeneity in accumulated evidence may preclude use of advanced meta-analytic methods (Yildiz, Vieta, Correll, Nikodem, & Baldessarini, 2014). An example of a sequential treatments' design employing combination treatments of most clinical interest for treatment of bipolar depression is provided in a model in Figure 43.1a with, and 43.1b without, a placebo comparison.

"HIDDEN" HIGH DEGREES OF TREATMENT RESISTANCE

The overestimation of effectiveness of single agents in BD also has further unintended negative spin-offs. The degree of treatment resistance in the general population of patients with BD is underestimated (Gitlin, Swendsen, Heller, & Hammen, 1995; Goldberg, Harrow, & Leon, 1996; Kessing et al., 2012; Nolen et al., 2004; Post et al., 2004; Vestergaard, 1992). Lithium is still touted in many textbooks as being efficacious in some 50% to 80% of bipolar patients for acute treatment, while response rates (much or very much improved on the Clinical Global Impression Scale for use in Bipolar Illness [CGI-BP]; Spearing, Post, Leverich, Brandt, & Nolen, 1997) in long-term prophylaxis being close to 25% using "lithium monotherapy," but, in reality, such a designation often also allows antidepressants, benzodiazepines, and antipsychotics as necessary (Denicoff, Smith-Jackson, Bryan, Ali, & Post, 1997; Denicoff, Smith-Jackson, Disney, Ali, et al., 1997). Another example of this derives from the data of Calabrese and associates (2005) in rapid cycling bipolar patients, a not uncommon variant. In these instances, patients experienced only short-term mood stabilization to the combination of lithium and valproate in 25% of the observed cases and in only 17% of the intent-to-treat

population. Of those who were then randomized to either lithium or valproate monotherapy, approximately 50% relapsed on additional follow-up, suggesting that only some 10% to 12% of rapid-cycling patients may be responsive to either monotherapy.

The perception of the high degree of efficacy of lithium and related anticonvulsant mood stabilizers has been cited as one of the reasons that clinical trials of psychopharmacological agents in BD have been so consistently under funded in the past 40 years compared with other serious mental illnesses such as schizophrenia (Prien & Potter, 1990; Prien & Rush, 1996). Other reasons for the poor funding of clinical treatment research in BD are particularly pertinent to the topic of this chapter and include lack of agreed-upon study designs and outcome measures for long-term assessment of the illness.

CONTROVERSY ABOUT OPTIMAL DESIGNS AND RATING INSTRUMENTS

Review panels readily accept the appropriateness of the Hamilton Depression Rating Scale (HAMD) or Montgomery-Åsberg Depression Rating Scale (MADRS) for depression, the Yale–Brown Obsessive Compulsive Scale for obsessive-compulsive disorder, and the Positive and Negative Syndrome Scale or Brief Psychiatric Rating Scale for studies in schizophrenia, but there is less agreement on the most appropriate instruments for assessing the longitudinal course of BD. Repeated cross sectional measures with the Young Mania Rating Scale (YMRS) and HAMD are the norm and are widely used in acute clinical trials in mania and depression but often leave gaps in the more detailed assessment of the long-term course during prophylactic studies in rapidly fluctuating patients. Recent evidence synthesis methods enable multidimensional effectiveness assessments including the ones on cognition or memory or other measures of functionality as measures of disease severity or degree of clinical response. International health-care systems in their cost-effectiveness assessments have increasingly begun to employ such multidimensional comparative effectiveness analysis (Yildiz, Vieta, et al., 2014). This is important clinically because without employment of such multidimensional models, reimbursement strategies may approve the cheapest drugs if they are also effective. For example haloperidol, as the cheapest available antimanic treatment, may rank first in a model considering only efficacy and cost but much lower when the model includes additional data on functionality, quality of life,

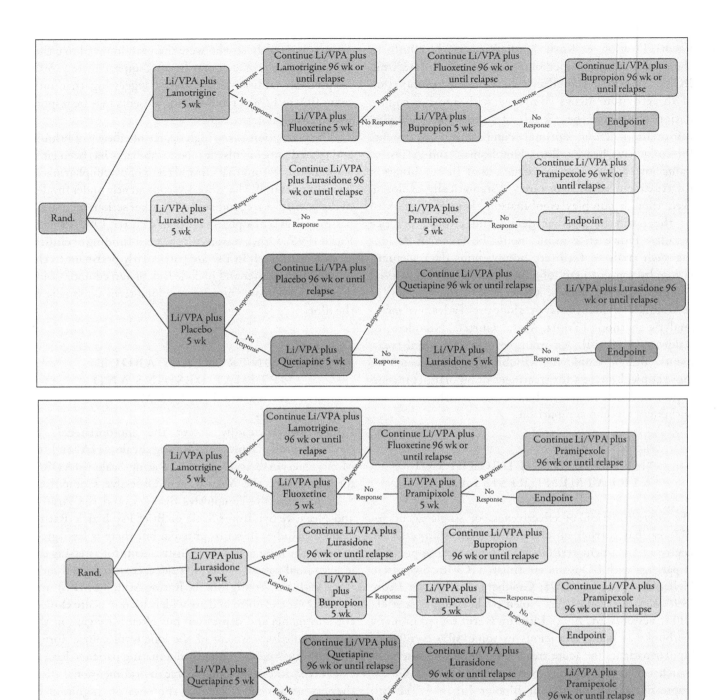

Figure 43.1 (a) Sequential treatments design involving a placebo comparison for bipolar depression. (b) Sequential treatments design for bipolar depression.

cognition, tardive dyskinesia, and total life years gained. Ideally, such a cost-effectiveness model for BD could include data on full clinical recovery or daily or weekly subsyndromal mood fluctuations, functionality, cognition, suicidality, metabolic, neurologic, and hormonal wellness, as well as treatment-emergent affective switches so long as the quantifiable data on these measures could be obtained.

One option for assessing daily or weekly subsyndromal mood fluctuations versus full clinical recovery (in addition to repeated use of cross-sectional scales) is the

National Institute of Mental Health Life Chart Method™ (NIMH-LCM™), which has both a clinician-rated and self-rated version for assessing severity of mania and depression on a daily basis (Leverich & Post, 1996, 1998). It can also track extremes of cycling, presence of dysphoric mania, and comorbid symptoms. In addition, it has a running tally of medications and a space for rating side effects with mild, moderate, or severe impact. Reliability is excellent, as severity of mania and depression is rated on the degree of functional impairment with which each phase is associated, making recall of severity relatively easy even at intervals of several weeks to a month between rating sessions (Denicoff et al., 2002; Denicoff, Smith-Jackson, Disney, Suddath, et al., 1997).

The scale has been validated against other measures and used productively in a number of studies including long-term comparisons of lithium versus carbamazepine versus the combination for one year of prophylaxis for each phase (Denicoff, Smith-Jackson, Disney, Ali, et al., 1997), comparisons of lamotrigine, gabapentin, and placebo (Frye et al., 2000; Obrocea et al., 2002), and, most recently, detailed analysis of lamotrigine's long-term effects on mood stability (Goldberg et al., 2008). Related longitudinal ratings that have been performed by the STEP-BD program are also endorsed (Sachs, 2001), as such detailed description of the precise course of illness is particularly important in instances of extreme rapidity of cycling, which can even occur in outpatients with bipolar disorder in demanding professions.

These recommendations for a frequent if not daily longitudinal measurement device in studies of long-term prophylaxis are also consistent with data from a variety of prospective follow-up studies, indicating that patients with BD are ill an average of some 50% of the time and spend three times more time depressed than manic (Judd & Akiskal, 2003; Kupka et al., 2007). Given the repeated observations that minor increases in symptomatology are often precursors to the occurrence of a more major episode, such fine-grained assessments are of great clinical importance, as well as necessary for capturing the nuances of mood fluctuations during clinical trials.

One of the major assets of such detailed longitudinal ratings is the ability to simultaneously assess different thresholds for what one might consider as mild, moderate, or severe relapse, as well as employ modal measures such as that of area under the curve, signifying the magnitude and duration of mania and depression. Such a measure of area under the curve allows for precise intraindividual comparisons of the degree of symptomatology observed prior to and after a given experimental manipulation as a continuous variable, which should vastly increase the power to detect treatment difference compared with a single endpoint of percentage of relapse into a new episode (Kraemer, 1991).

Traditional designs in assessment of the efficacy of a prophylactic treatment have typically required patients to achieve substantial improvement or remission for a given period of time, and then are randomized and followed up until the occurrence of a new episode or need for clinical intervention (Bowden et al., 2000; Calabrese, Shelton, Rapport, Kimmel, & Elhaj, 2002). While this has merits in patient populations in whom this degree of wellness is readily achieved, it is far from ideal for those with highly treatment-resistant illness.

In the epilepsies, for example, one does not require patients to be seizure-free in order to assess a single or adjunctive therapy but rather the reduction in seizure frequency with the addition of the new drug or placebo (Brodie, 1996). Similarly, assessing the reduction in area under the curve of manic and depressive symptomatology would appear to have considerable merit in those with high degrees of treatment resistance. This is typically the case when one is attempting to ascertain which treatments, adjuncts, or combinations are, in fact, most likely to stabilize the patient, rather than asking the question of how long a patient, once stabilized, can maintain this degree of improvement.

Using this strategy, one can begin to make statements about prevention of mania and depression based on relatively short time frames of observations (Post, Frye, Leverich, & Denicoff, 1998; Post & Leverich, 2008). In fact, it has been pointed out in the epilepsies that the higher the seizure frequency at baseline, the shorter the required trial duration for a clinical trial in order to demonstrate prophylactic efficacy of a given treatment agent. Similarly, given the considerable degree of treatment resistance in BD, attempts at developing new treatments for those difficult-to-treat patients should involve such rating and design strategies in patient populations with relatively high percentages of rapid and faster cycling patterns (making use of the most highly recurrent patients) rather than excluding them.

Highly sophisticated ways of analyzing such rapidly changing state data are discussed by Chassan et al. (1992). Since last observation carried forward analysis has many liabilities especially when there are missing data, the use of linear mixed (Hedeker, Mermelstein, & Demirtas, 2008) or related models (Salim, Mackinnon, & Griffiths, 2008) may be better to employ in analysis of such data.

CONSIDERATIONS ON MODEL RANDOMIZED CONTROLLED TRIAL DESIGNS

Klein et al. (2002), Kraemer and Pruyn (1990), and Brouwer and Mohr (1991) emphasized that one of the reasons that traditional placebo-controlled parallel group RCTs sometimes fail is that not enough preliminary work is done in advance of these large, extremely expensive trials (Kraemer & Pruyn, 1990; Kraemer et al., 1987; Lasagna et al 1994; Malakoff, 2008). They suggest that there should be adequate testing of likely effective doses and preliminary assessment of whether a given group is likely to be responsive. In these instances, initial pilot studies can be invaluable in avoiding potential negative outcomes in RCTs (Brouwers & Mohr, 1991; Klein et al., 2002; Lasagna, 1994; Laska, Klein, Lavori, Levine, & Robinson, 1994; Palmer & Rosenberger, 1999). Given the magnitude of investment in such RCTs, efforts in detecting and minimizing sources of noise, bias, false positive, or false negative results should be maximized. In Chapter 42 of this book, strategies for improving signal detection in classical placebo-controlled parallel group designs for the bipolar maintenance, depression, and mania trials are discussed. In designing RCTs with a minimum risk of false positive or false negative results, optimum sample size should be computed by use of actual effect estimates obtained through the pooled analysis of previously attained treatment effects aimed to achieve 80% to 90% power in obtaining significance. For pooled effect estimates a simple standard pairwise meta-analysis can be performed either manually or by employing commercial packages. These effect estimates and their standard deviations may then be placed in a formula to compute the required sample size per study arm, again either manually via use of appropriate statistical tests such as the Fischer's Exact Test or by employing the written programs. If a RCT has a less than 80% chance of detecting a true significance, then it is considered to result from the small sample size, named as type II error (a false negative result), also called a failed trial. Recently, as the number of RCTs with type II error are decreasing, the ones with potential type I error (detecting false significance for a true nonsignificance)—in other words, trials with larger-than-needed sample sizes—are getting more frequent. This may in part relate to the nature of funding by the manufacturers and the underlying rational of regulatory approval for their conduct. Given that with larger sample sizes obtaining significance for minor change in scores would be more likely, this trend in designing RCTs of larger samples is understandable. However, type I errors with false significance are as important as the type II errors with false negatives in delivering risk for clinically misleading information.

Another concern in terms of manifest or subtle (undetected) false negative (failure) and false positive trials is related to the potential sources of biases, such as randomization bias, allocation concealment or outcome assessment bias, or bias in dosing strategies or in patient or active comparator selection. Again, considering the huge amount of financial, physical, and intellectual investment, the goal for each RCT should be attaining of the most accurate and replicable results, and that goal can only be achieved through efforts in preventing any kind of biases.

Given the phasic nature of BD, RCTs are accumulated in three groups for bipolar depression, mania, and maintenance or prophylaxis. Consequently, accumulated evidence in each group is evaluated individually with their own candidate effect modifiers and source of bias, as well as noise. However, recently employed sequential treatment trials may include patients in acute phase of BD with longitudinal follow-up periods for prophylaxis yielding data for acute as well as maintenance phases. Such trial designs may or may not involve a placebo comparison and can be viewed as several RCTs following each other as illustrated in the Figure 43.1. Differences between adaptive and sequential treatment trial designs and their randomization and sample size estimation principles are provided in Chapter 44 of this book.

ALTERNATIVE DESIGNS FOR PILOT AND PROOF-OF-CONCEPT EFFICACY STUDIES

We suggest considering the usefulness of off-on-off-on designs and N of 1 trials to make preliminary assessments of potential drug efficacy more efficiently (Post & Luckenbaugh, 2003). These may be particularly useful in clinical research involving treatment refractory patients and examination of potential neurobiological mechanisms and predictors of clinical response to a given drug. In this case, all of the patients in the clinical trial are started on placebo (off) and then assigned to the active agent (on). Responders can be confirmed in a second off trial and then reconfirmed by re-responsiveness during the second on trial (i.e., the utilization of a B-A-B-A design). This type of design allows for the assessment of clinical responsivity in all of the patients studied rather than just half the population in the traditional placebo parallel group design without a crossover. It also deals well with illness heterogeneity, as each patient uses his or her own baseline as the control from which to assess responsivity. Moreover, in a traditional RCT there is no way to assess whether an individual patient has or has not responded to a drug (Chassan, 1992; Laska et al., 1994), particularly in instances where there are relatively high placebo response rates. The confirmation of responsivity during the second off and on phases mitigates this problem and, essentially, if the response and re-response is robust enough, "proves" that a given patient is actually a responder (Gaus & Hogel, 1995; McDermut et al., 1995; Post et al., 1998).

Once it has been established that a drug is effective in a series of N of 1 trials one could then move to comparative clinical trials in order to assess the wider percentage likelihood of response in different subgroups of patients and at the same time gain more robust tolerability data. We have done this using the double-blind B-A-B-A design with the dihydropyridine L-type calcium channel blocker nimodipine (McDermut et al., 1995; Pazzaglia et al., 1998; Pazzaglia, Post, Ketter, George, & Marangell, 1993; Post & Leverich, 2008), which has now been studied in a larger randomized, comparative trial involving some 200 subjects and showing that the nimodipine in combination with lithium was superior to combinations of it with valproate, carbamazepine, or lamotrigine (Chaudry et al., 2010).

The relative assets and liabilities of the traditional placebo parallel group RCT and that of the B-A-B-A designs are outlined in Table 43.1. One clear liability of the B-A-B-A design is that it is not traditionally FDA acceptable. However, the FDA has accepted the testing and approval of multiple adjunctive agents for those in the refractory epilepsies, and now more recently for adjunctive treatment in bipolar depression, so one would hope that other innovative designs would also increasingly be acceptable to the FDA.

In the face of a series of positive N of 1 studies, one may also be at a loss to decide the appropriate threshold for the number of such positive individual responders observed in order to consider a drug efficacious enough to promote the development of a large RCT or even, in some instances, directly win FDA approval. Busk and Serlin (1992) suggest that N of 1 trials can be aggregated to provide evidence of an overall drug effect even in special populations such as those with treatment resistance.

Statistical approaches to analyzing off-on-off-on data were made easier in patients with ultra-rapid fluctuations. Gentile, Roden, and Klein (1972) and others have made the argument that treating these within-subjects data on extreme mood fluctuations as emanating from the individual as "a random events generator" can lead to the appropriate application of analyses originally intended for completely independent events. Issues of autocorrelation can also be addressed in the beginning of the statistical analysis (Chassan, 1979).

Many of these approaches have been illustrated in some detail in McDermut et al. (1995) and overviewed in our papers on design issues in clinical trials for patients with BD (Post & Luckenbaugh, 2003; Post, 2010). These could involve chi squares for the percentage of days euthymic while on placebo versus on active drug; aggregating all of the data from each on-drug phase and each off-drug or placebo phase and then performing between group t tests on whatever rating scales are being used (Gentile et al., 1972); or, when there are substantial time trends in the data, considering Winer's Z approach, which calculates a mean symptomatology score for each separate phase and compares it sequentially to the next phase with a t value (Winer, 1971).

TRIAL DURATIONS IN THE TRADITIONAL RANDOMIZED CONTROLLED TRIALS IN MANIA AND DEPRESSION

Three weeks is considered the minimum if not ideal trial length for studies in acute mania. Six to eight weeks is consistently used in studies of acute bipolar depression. However, with the new studies of the rapidly acting antidepressants, such as IV ketamine or scopolamine, or even the older studies of sleep deprivation, more intensive ratings are required over short periods of time. Traditional durations of prophylactic studies have typically based on a long lead-in period in order to achieve mood stabilization and then durations of six months to 1.5 years for mood destabilization assessments in comparison to placebo. However, as noted previously, for the large group of patients with rapid or faster cycling patterns and a high degree of treatment resistance, trial durations can be markedly attenuated (Cochran, 1954).

CROSSOVER TRIALS FOR ENHANCING CLINICAL INFORMATICS AND STATISTICAL POWER

March et al. (2005) and many others have advocated for greater use of practical clinical trials in order to generate data more pertinent to clinical decision-making, as well as facilitate data acquisition with easier to perform and less expensive clinical trials. One of these approaches

TRADITIONAL PARALLEL GROUP RANDOMIZED CLINICAL TRIAL IN BIPOLAR ILLNESS		OFF-ON-OFF-ON (B-A-B-A) DESIGNS	
ASSETS	**LIABILITIES**	**ASSETS**	**LIABILITIES**
+ Meets FDA requirements	– Cumbersome, inflexible	+ Flexible, suitable for pilot studies	– Traditionally not FDA acceptable
+ Standard in literature	– Not appropriate for initial phases of drug discovery	+ Dose exploration possible	– Statistics not agreed upon
+ Minimizes time commitment for patients	– Requires large N; typically multiple centers	+ Smaller N possible to demonstrate efficacy	– Possible sequence or carryover effects
+ Standard statistics readily available	– Placebo exposure mandated for a portion of subjects	+ Placebo periods can be dropped in nonresponders	– Uncertain number of N-of-1 studies sufficient to demonstrate efficacy
+ Controls for group-oriented confounds	– Focus on overall group response	+ Less prone to type II errors	– Extended time commitment required of patients
+ Relatively easy interpretation of results	– Confounds individual and placebo response assessment	+ Less expensive	– "Off" trials risk illness exacerbation
+ Potential for demonstrating assay sensitivity	– Only half of patient population available for biological and predictor studies	+ Can be conducted at one site + Patient as own control	– Ethical issues with giving placebos
+ Less prone to type I errors	– Focused entry criteria and homogeneous samples	+ Wider entry criteria feasible	– Group-oriented effects more difficult to examine
+ Ability to stratify samples	– Dose schedule usually predetermined	+ Trial length can be individualized + Response can be confirmed in individuals	
	– Costly and difficult to manage	+ All patients available for biological predictor studies	
	– No guarantee of active medication exposure for all patients	+ Causality of side effects may be established and confirmed	
	– Ethical issues with giving placebos		
	– No comparative information for clinicians	+ Comparison of response to multiple medications possible + Potential for unplanned crossover effects + Suitable for high-risk populations with refractory illness	

NOTE: FDA = US Food and Drug Administration.

would be a randomization to two active agents for an initial examination of effectiveness and tolerability. Then, nonresponders to either treatment could be crossed over to the other treatment (Geller et al., 2012). In a potential third phase, nonresponders to either monotherapy could then be randomized to a combination of the two initially studied drugs compared with a third new intervention.

These kinds of practical clinical trial approaches not only more closely follow clinical decision-making but also would help to inform it and have been widely used in the STAR-D, STEP-BD, CATIE, and Stanley Foundation Bipolar Network attempts to study real patients more longitudinally and begin to ascertain what might be the most effective treatment approaches for eventually achieving sustained responses and remissions (Perlis et al., 2004; Greenhouse et al., 1991; Whitehead, 1991).

Another more formal alternative is to systematically crossover all patients to a given set of treatments. This kind of design has often been met with global statements that crossovers are discredited, partially based on the critique of Brown (1980). However, many statisticians have made the opposite argument and favor the more clinician- and patient-friendly characteristics of the crossover design compared with the traditional RCTs. Laska et al. (1994) make the point that the increased power of crossover designs and the ability to study all patients on an active agent for generating clinical and neurobiological markers and correlates of clinical response together outweigh any of the potential liabilities of crossover designs such as sequence or carryover effects.

An illustration of an even more complex example of such a study is that of Frye et al. (2000) and Obrocea et al. (2002). In these instances, all patients were exposed in a randomized, double-blind fashion to three different phases of treatment for an intended six weeks. This included exposure to a placebo, lamotrigine, and gabapentin. In this instance, there was a 53% (19/36) overall response for lamotrigine, 28% (10/36) for gabapentin, and 22% (8/36) for placebo, which were significantly different by Cochran's Q ($p = .014$). Post hoc analysis revealed that lamotrigine was superior to both gabapentin and placebo.

The crossover studies also demonstrate the increased statistical power derived from exposing all patients to each drug or phase, as opposed to the traditional RCTs. Figure 43.2 illustrates the differences in minimal sample size required for a given effect size. If one has a large effect size, for example, where d equals about 0.80, only 15 subjects would be required in a one sample crossover design study in order to achieve a two-tailed alpha = 0.05 and power = 0.80. However, in the traditional parallel group, two-sample design, 26 subjects/group (i.e., a total of 52, or more than three times that required in the crossover sample) would be required. With a medium effect size of 0.5, a one-sample design would require 34 subjects, but the two-sample design would require a total of 126 subjects, or 63 patients per group. The figure illustrates that the crossover trials need only about 25% of the number of patients that are needed in the parallel design trial (Schouten, 1999). This increased power of having all of the subjects exposed to each treatment in an intensive neurobiological research group in which one is examining a variety of measures that may be associated with prediction of clinical response or neuropathological effects of the illness interacting with drug effects is invaluable. Preliminary assessments of potential moderators or mediators of response (see later discussion) are also facilitated in designs allowing all patients enrolled in the study to be exposed to each treatment.

CARRYOVER EFFECTS

The multiple crossover trial discussed previously, as well as more simple single crossovers, bring about concerns about the effect of carryover on response rates and the greater potential for dropout with a longer study period,

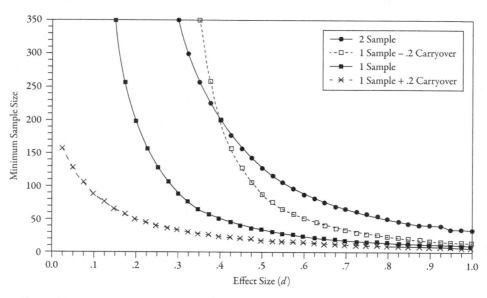

Figure 43.2 Minimal sample sizes; higher with small effect sizes and two sample studies.

as emphasized by Brown (1980). However, there are some additional advantages of the crossover design in which, in contrast to the parallel group trials, an investigator does not have to assume and demonstrate that the two randomized groups are similar on the basis of demographics, illness severity course, and pattern of presentation at baseline. In the repeated measures crossover trial, again, patients act as their own control throughout the study.

While carryover effects are clearly a potential problem in the crossover trial, it is also noteworthy that unintended carryover effects can still occur in parallel group studies in which treatment responsivity or nonresponsivity to previous drug exposures is rarely considered in the routine RCT designs (Gelenberg et al., 1989; Perlis et al., 2002).

In addition, statistical approaches can be used to take the carryover effects into account (Otto, 1992). Even if the possibility of a small to moderate carryover effect is taken into account for calculating the required sample size for a study, the crossover design still tends to require a smaller sample, as illustrated in Figure 43.2. When the carryover effect accounts for the equivalent of a small effect size, the crossover design still continues to require many fewer participants than the two-sample study until the total sample required reaches about 200. It is only when there is a substantial amount of carryover effect that the parallel group design begins to require a smaller sample size than the two-sample design.

LONG-TERM TREND FOR UNDERSTUDY OF BIPOLAR DISORDER COMPARED WITH OTHER MAJOR MENTAL DISORDERS

In 1989 and 1994 the NIMH-sponsored meetings in an attempt to elucidate the reasons for the relative deficit in the clinical trials portfolio in BD that had been long recognized and to develop potential solutions (Prien & Potter, 1990; Prien & Rush, 1996). However, there are still many measures indicating this funding deficit has persisted. One example may be the most recent network analysis by Leucht et al. (2013) constructed by 212 short-term studies of antipsychotics as monotherapy as identified in schizophrenia, while the most recent network analysis by Yildiz, Nikodem, et al. (2014), using comparable inclusion criteria, could identify only 57 studies as monotherapy for treatment of acute bipolar mania, a figure indicating a roughly 27% funding for BD relative to schizophrenia. Yet the lifetime prevalence of BD is 1.1% to 4.4% versus 0.4% to 0.8% for schizophrenia, so the real disparity is even much greater (Merikangas et al., 2007; Bhugra, 2005). The deficits in funding of studies in bipolar depression is even more striking; there are only 3 FDA-approved drugs for this indication.

In the 1994 meeting, John Rush summarized some of the recommendations from the two prior meetings which we and others have nicknamed "Rush's Rules" for easy recognition. Among the recommendations was the inclusion of bipolar-I, bipolar-II, and bipolar—not otherwise specified (NOS) subtypes in treatment studies of BD. Since bipolar-II has a lifetime prevalence double of bipolar-I (Merikangas et al., 2007) and a suicide rate equal to that of bipolar-I, its inclusion to RCTs of bipolar depression or maintenance studies was endorsed. Rush also recommended including patients with varying cycle frequencies, a theme we have previously mentioned in this chapter. He also advocated the development of a standardized outcome assessment package and a development of consensus on choices of acceptable longitudinal rating instruments. A critical recommendation was that the list of acceptable design strategies be broadened so that other approaches besides the traditional parallel group RCTs could be more widely used. These include crossover, mirror image, and equipoise stratified designs; head-to-head comparisons; and adaptive and the many other designs alluded to here and elsewhere that would provide more clinically useful information to treating physicians (Lavori et al., 2000, 2001). Also, as noted in the introduction, substance abuse as well as anxiety and other related comorbidities are common in BD, and the most cost-effective design strategies should be considered in these groups of patients in order to enhance clinical decision-making.

Many of these comments were reiterated by March et al. (2005), Post and Kowatch (2006), and many others, as well as most recently by Gelenberg et al. (2008) in recommending new design approaches in studies of unipolar depression. They recommended use of adaptive clinical trial designs in which clinical decisions and adjustments in clinical care are based on adaptive threshold-dependent algorithms that reflect individual patient's needs, as well as the mechanism of action of the drug being tested and the expected response times. In these instances, benchmarks are to be established in advance, such that time frames and symptomatic criteria for clinical decision-making, for example when to raise or lower a dose or augment or switch treatment strategies, are clearly delineated.

In spite of these consensus recommendations summarized here under the rubric of Rush's Rules, many of the most basic clinical comparisons have not yet been performed. Accumulated trial evidence for selecting the best initial or followup treatment options for acute bipolar depression does not even allow a reliable synthesis. The field is not only missing data on comparative efficacy assessments of individual treatment options for treatment of bipolar depression but also on drug class comparisons such as those with mood stabilizers versus atypical antipsychotics versus adjunctive antidepressants (Pacchiarotti et al., 2013). The undersized pharmacological-trials portfolio for BD has now carried over into the area of clinical treatment trials for childhood-onset BD (Geller et al., 2008; Post, 2012; Post, Chang, & Frye, 2013; Post & Kowatch, 2006).

One of the reasons that few of the recommendations of the prior NIMH and McArthur conferences on design strategies in BD have been carried out is that there is an apparent incompatibility between the use of designs and populations that are most clinically informative and the statistical and analytic requirements for a successful RCT. How one deals with the inclusion of BD-I, BD-II, and BD-NOS patients (and their comorbidities) in the same study feasibly and statistically is not readily apparent. While one approach might be to stratify for bipolar patients with and without a given comorbidity, this conflicts with the general recommendations to stratify for as few variables as possible in order to limit loss of power in a given study.

ASSESSING MODERATORS AND MEDIATORS

Kraemer, Stice, Kazdin, Offord, and Kupfer (2001), Kraemer, Wilson, Fairburn, and Agras (2002), Hinshaw (2007), and Gelenberg et al. (2008) discuss the importance of delineating moderators and mediators in efficacy studies. Problematically, however, is the concomitant need for extremely large Ns in order to accomplish this clinically critical task. Moreover, treating comorbidity as a potential moderator variable requires a second study to definitely demonstrate the effect (i.e., that patients with a given comorbidity would be less likely to respond to a given treatment than those without).

A moderator variable is thus something identified and measured prior to randomization as a pretreatment variable that might have an effect on the treatment outcome. This could include age, gender, psychiatric or medical comorbidity, and so on. In contrast, a mediator variable is one that would be observed over the course of the treatment trial that may influence the outcome. For example, the effectiveness of treatment of a mother's depression could influence the response of a child entered into a clinical trial of the efficacy of an agent for an externalizing disorder such

as attention deficit hyperactivity disorder or internalizing disorder such as anxiety or depression. While, for example, substance abuse comorbidity might be a presumed moderator variable in clinical treatment trials of those with BD, it is also possible that the degree of clinical improvement and mood stabilization observed during the trial could be a mediator variable for whether or not a primary substance abuse outcome is improved. In the case of comorbidities, separating moderator and mediator variables would appear to be of considerable importance and begin to allow better delineation of most appropriate treatments.

In many of these instances, including more representative patients in the clinical trial does appear to increase design complexity and potentially reduce statistical power for assessing the main efficacy outcome. This loss of homogeneity also makes evidence synthesis and meta-analyses more difficult. These design attributes and difficulties perhaps reflect the pharmaceutical industry's almost universal choice to deal with highly selective and more homogeneous patient populations in classical RCTs in their attempts to register a new drug. Leon (2008) and Kraemer and Kupfer (2006) also make the point that the increasing use of effect sizes and number needed to treat (NNT) or number needed to harm (NNH), as illustrated in Table 43.2, are highly dependent upon the population studied and that NNT and NNH may be virtually useless without appropriate weighing of these variables and the severity of the consequences of nontreatment. Hinshaw (2007) concluded that: "Treatment research in the future should explicitly consider the exploration of moderator and mediator variables, which can greatly aid the explanatory power of clinical trials and specify the critical next steps for intervention research." This is particularly important in BD clinical trials in which potential moderator and mediator variables are all too plentiful. In the face of establishing a moderator variable (which requires that there is a statistical interaction between the moderator variable and the predictor variable),

Table 43.2. SUMMARY OF EFFECT SIZE AND RELATED BENCH MARKS

	COHEN'S D	AVC	SRD	NNT
Small	0.20	0.56	0.11	8.89
Medium	0.50	0.64	0.28	3.62
Large	0.80	0.71	0.43	2.33

NOTE: Adapted from Leon (2008).
NNT = Number Needed to Treat
SRD = Success Rate Difference
Omit AVC

this also immediately raises the issue of how to better deal with that given moderator in the subsequent clinical trials. That is, if the presence of an anxiety disorder comorbidity is found to be an important moderator, for example, of less good response to lithium as the bulk of the evidence would now suggest, the next obvious pressing clinical question is to what sets of treatments such patients may, in fact, respond (Post et al., 1998).

Similarly, moderator variables have now been extended to include genotypes and single nucleotide polymorphism (SNP) profiles, which we all expect will soon help in the prediction of differential responsiveness of individuals to individual medication interventions. Here again we are faced with the need for rather large N clinical trials in order to begin to ascertain what is likely to be the first fruits of the molecular genetics revolution in the form of personalized medicine.

Both moderator and mediator tests are explanatory, exploratory, and comprise secondary analyses to generate hypotheses for the next set of potential series. Hinshaw quotes Kraemer et al. (2002) in indicating that all too often such analyses are viewed pejoratively as "fishing expeditions" and are looked at askance by both granting and manuscript review bodies. Instead, Hinshaw (2007) and Kraemer et al. (2002) emphasize the necessity of probing for subgroups for whom treatments optimally work (moderator variables) and examining the processes by which treatments exert effects (mediators). In this fashion, it is stressed that these kinds of examinations help bridge the large gap between theory and practice. Hinshaw (2007) states, "There is often a balance between the typical goal of an efficacy study—to generate internally valid conclusions regarding the precise effects of treatments on relative outcomes, which suggest narrow homogeneous samples—and the more ecologically valid objectives of effectiveness studies related to having diverse samples that yield (a) external validity and generalizability of findings and (b) tests of key moderator-defined subgroup."

CONCLUSION AND IMPLICATIONS

The classic placebo-controlled parallel group design of a RCT is the gold standard for demonstrating efficacy, acquiring FDA approval, and facilitating meta-analyses. Yet, as we have seen there is also the need for broadening the range of clinical trial designs in light of the vast heterogeneity of presentation of BD and fostering optimal clinical decision-making. We hope this discussion proves helpful for those seeking not only to construct optimal RCTs but other designs as well. We also hope that those designing future trials with both the standard, randomized controlled parallel group design and the many alternative designs noted will consider assimilating the suggestions listed here. These are aimed at facilitating evidence accumulation and enabling employment of standard and advanced meta-analytic evidence synthesis methods and, as well, creating a strong database for optimal clinical decision making.

Given diversities in clinical presentations of BD, rather than aiming trials on clinically rare types of patients, it may be wiser to allow a limited degree of preplanned diversity into the trial on condition that equal allocation into study arms is maintained and objective outcome assessments are utilized. If the considerations noted here are employed, alternative designs may not only include patient populations more similar to real-world clinical situations but may also eventually provide a strong basis for clinical decision-making by use of advanced meta-analytic computations involving direct and indirect comparisons, sensitivity analysis, and meta-regressions.

Consequently, we suggest (a) worldwide increases in nonprofit funding sources, especially given the roughly three to four times higher prevalence of BD as relative to schizophrenia and 18 times more frequent funding by profit versus nonprofit sources; (b) encouragement of technically competent investigator initiated RCTs conducted at selected academic study sites; (c) efforts to minimize unnecessary sources of heterogeneity or variations in terms of trial durations, end point or response definitions, and use of rescue medications; (d) constant study arm level outcome reporting via well-defined standard assessment tools; (e) unbiased outcome assessment strategies; (f) consistent reporting on study arm-based subgroup analyses (i.e., on bipolar patients with or without psychotic or mixed manic or depressive features, comorbid anxiety, or substance abuse disorders, or patients with different bipolar subtypes or cycling patterns); (g) adding objective quantifiable and standardized reporting of individual side effects, treatment emergent affective switches, as well as quality of life and functionality measures; and (h) considering patient populations with more severe and treatment refractory forms of illness on the condition that it is ethically justified with employment of utmost safety measures and optimized patient comfort.

Disclosure statement: Dr. Ayşegül Yildiz has received research grants from or served as a consultant to, or speaker for, Abdi Ibrahim, Actavis, AliRaif, AstraZeneca,

Bristol-Myers Squibb, Janssen-Cilag, Lundbeck, Pfizer, Sanofi-Aventis, and Servier.

Dr. Robert M. Post has not disclosed any conflicts of interest pertinent to this manuscript.

REFERENCES

Benson, K., & Hartz, A. J. (2000). A comparison of observational studies and randomized, controlled trials. *American Journal of Ophthalmology, 130*(5), 688.

Bhugra, D. (2005). The global prevalence of schizophrenia. *PLoS Medicine, 2*(5) e151–152.

Blanco, C., Olfson, M., Goodwin, R. D., Ogburn, E., Liebowitz, M. R., Nunes, E. V., & Hasin, D. S. (2008). Generalizability of clinical trial results for major depression to community samples: Results from the National Epidemiologic Survey on Alcohol and Related Conditions. *Journal of Clinical Psychiatry, 69*(8), 1276–1280.

Bowden, C. L., Lecrubier, Y., Bauer, M., Goodwin, G., Greil, W., Sachs, G., & von Knorring, L. (2000). Maintenance therapies for classic and other forms of bipolar disorder. *Journal of Affective Disorders, 59*(1), S57–S67.

Brodie, M. J. (1996). Antiepileptic drugs, clinical trials, and the marketplace. *Lancet, 347*(9004), 777–779.

Brouwers, P., & Mohr, E. (1991). Design of clinical trials. In E. Mohr & P. Brouwers (Eds.), *Handbook of clinical trials: The neurobehavioral approach* (pp. 187–212). Amsterdam: Swets & Zeitlinger.

Brown, B. W. Jr. (1980). The crossover experiment for clinical trials. *Biometrics, 36*(1), 69–79.

Busk, P. L., & Serlin, R. C. (1992). Meta-analysis for single case research design. In T. R. Kratochwill & J. R. Levin (Eds.), *Single case research design and analysis: New development for psychology and education* (pp. 187–212). Hillsdale, NJ: Lawrence Erlbaum Associates.

Calabrese, J. R., Shelton, M. D., Rapport, D. J., Kimmel, S. E., & Elhaj, O. (2002). Long-term treatment of bipolar disorder with lamotrigine. *Journal of Clinical Psychiatry, 63*(10), 18–22.

Calabrese, J. R., Shelton, M. D., Rapport, D. J., Youngstrom, E. A., Jackson, K., Bilali, S.,…Findling, R. L. (2005). A 20-month, double-blind, maintenance trial of lithium versus divalproex in rapid-cycling bipolar disorder. *The American Journal of Psychiatry, 162*(11), 2152–2161.

Chassan, J. B. (1979). Research design in clinical psychology and psychiatry. New York: John Wiley.

Chassan, J. B. (1992). Intensive design: Statistics and the single case. In M. Fava & J. F. Rosenbaum (Eds.), *Research designs and methods in psychiatry* (pp. 173–183). Amsterdam: Elsevier.

Chaudry, H. R., Khan, R. M., Shabbir, A., & Mufti, K. A. (2010). Nimodipine in the treatment of Bipolar Disorder. *Biological Psychiatry, 67*(95), p. 232S, Abstract #806.

Cochran, W. (1954). Some methods for strengthening the x^2 test. *Biometrics, 10*, 417–451.

Concato, J., Shah, N., & Horwitz, R. I. (2000). Randomized, controlled trials, observational studies, and the hierarchy of research designs. *New England Journal of Medicine, 342*(25), 1887–1892.

Denicoff, K. D., Ali, S. O., Sollinger, A. B., Smith-Jackson, E. E., Leverich, G. S., & Post, R. M. (2002). Utility of the daily prospective National Institute of Mental Health Life-Chart Method (NIMH-LCM-p) ratings in clinical trials of bipolar disorder. *Depression and Anxiety, 15*(1), 1–9.

Denicoff, K. D., Smith-Jackson, E. E., Bryan, A. L., Ali, S. O., & Post, R. M. (1997). Valproate prophylaxis in a prospective clinical trial of refractory bipolar disorder. *The American Journal of Psychiatry, 154*(10), 1456–1458.

Denicoff, K. D., Smith-Jackson, E. E., Disney, E. R., Ali, S. O., Leverich, G. S., & Post, R. M. (1997). Comparative prophylactic efficacy of lithium, carbamazepine, and the combination in bipolar disorder. *Journal of Clinical Psychiatry, 58*(11), 470–478.

Denicoff, K. D., Smith-Jackson, E. E., Disney, E. R., Suddath, R. L., Leverich, G. S., & Post, R. M. (1997). Preliminary evidence of the reliability and validity of the prospective life-chart methodology (LCM-p). *Journal of Psychiatric Research, 31*(5), 593–603.

Frye, M. A. (2008). Diagnostic dilemmas and clinical correlates of mixed states in bipolar disorder. *Journal of Clinical Psychiatry, 69*(5), e13.

Frye, M. A., Ketter, T. A., Kimbrell, T. A., Dunn, R. T., Speer, A. M., Osuch, E. A.,…Post, R. M. (2000). A placebo-controlled study of lamotrigine and gabapentin monotherapy in refractory mood disorders. *Journal of Clinical Psychopharmacology, 20*(6), 607–614.

Gaus, W., & Hogel, J. (1995). Studies on the efficacy of unconventional therapies: Problems and designs. *Arzneimittelforschung, 45*(1), 88–92.

Geddes, J. R., Goodwin, G. M., Rendell, J., Azorin, J. M., Cipriani, A., Ostacher, M. J.,…Juszczak, E. (2010). Lithium plus valproate combination therapy versus monotherapy for relapse prevention in bipolar I disorder (BALANCE): A randomised open-label trial. *Lancet, 375*(9712), 385–395. doi:10.1016/S0140-6736(09)61828-6

Gelenberg, A. J. (1994). Major complications of neuroleptic drug use. *Western Journal of Medicine, 160*(1), 55–56.

Gelenberg, A. J., Kane, J. M., Keller, M. B., Lavori, P., Rosenbaum, J. F., Cole, K., & Lavelle, J. (1989). Comparison of standard and low serum levels of lithium for maintenance treatment of bipolar disorder. *New England Journal of Medicine, 321*(22), 1489–1493.

Gelenberg, A. J., Thase, M. E., Meyer, R. E., Goodwin, F. K., Katz, M. M., Kraemer, H. C.,…Rosenbaum, J. F. (2008). The history and current state of antidepressant clinical trial design: A call to action for proof-of-concept studies. *Journal of Clinical Psychiatry.*

Geller, B., Luby, J. L., Joshi, P., Wagner, K. D., Emslie, G., Walkup, J. T.,…Lavori, P. (2012). A randomized controlled trial of risperidone, lithium, or divalproex sodium for initial treatment of bipolar I disorder, manic or mixed phase, in children and adolescents. *Archives of General Psychiatry, 69*(5), 515–528. doi:10.1001/archgenpsychiatry.2011.1508

Geller, B., Tillman, R., Bolhofner, K., & Zimerman, B. (2008). Child bipolar I disorder: Prospective continuity with adult bipolar I disorder; characteristics of second and third episodes; predictors of 8-year outcome. *Archives of General Psychiatry, 65*(10), 1125–1133. doi:10.1001/archpsyc.65.10.1125

Gentile, J. R., Roden, A. H., & Klein, R. D. (1972). An analysis-of-variance model for the intrasubject replication design. *Journal of Applied Behavior Analysis, 5*(2), 193–198.

Gitlin, M. J., Swendsen, J., Heller, T. L., & Hammen, C. (1995). Relapse and impairment in bipolar disorder. *The American Journal of Psychiatry, 152*(11), 1635–1640.

Goldberg, J. F., Bowden, C. L., Calabrese, J. R., Ketter, T. A., Dann, R. S., Frye, M. A.,…Post, R. M. (2008). Six-month prospective life charting of mood symptoms with lamotrigine monotherapy versus placebo in rapid cycling bipolar disorder. *Biological Psychiatry, 63*(1), 125–130.

Goldberg, J. F., Harrow, M., & Leon, A. C. (1996). Lithium treatment of bipolar affective disorders under naturalistic followup conditions. *Psychopharmacology Bulletin, 32*(1), 47–54.

Greenhouse, J. B., Stangl, D., Kupfer, D. J., & Prien, R. F. (1991). Methodologic issues in maintenance therapy clinical trials. *Archives of General Psychiatry, 48*(4), 313–318.

Hedeker, D., Mermelstein, R. J., & Demirtas, H. (2008). An application of a mixed-effects location scale model for analysis of Ecological Momentary Assessment (EMA) data. *Biometrics, 64*(2), 627–634.

Hinshaw, S. P. (2007). Moderators and mediators of treatment outcome for youth with ADHD: Understanding for whom and how interventions work. *Journal of Pediatric Psychology, 32*(6), 664–675.

Judd, L. L., & Akiskal, H. S. (2003). Depressive episodes and symptoms dominate the longitudinal course of bipolar disorder. *Current Psychiatry Reports, 5*(6), 417–418.

Judd, L. L., Akiskal, H. S., Schettler, P. J., Endicott, J., Maser, J., Solomon, D. A.,...Keller, M. B. (2002). The long-term natural history of the weekly symptomatic status of bipolar I disorder. *Archives of General Psychiatry, 59*(6), 530–537.

Kemp, D. E., Gao, K., Fein, E. B., Chan, P. K., Conroy, C., Obral, S.,...Calabrese, J. R. (2012). Lamotrigine as add-on treatment to lithium and divalproex: Lessons learned from a double-blind, placebo-controlled trial in rapid-cycling bipolar disorder. *Bipolar Disorders, 14*(7), 780–789. doi:10.1111/bdi.12013

Kessing, L. V., Hellmund, G., & Andersen, P. K. (2012). An observational nationwide register based cohort study on lamotrigine versus lithium in bipolar disorder. *Journal of Psychopharmacology, 26*(5), 644–652. doi:10.1177/0269881111414091

Kessler, R. C., McGonagle, K. A., Zhao, S., Nelson, C. B., Hughes, M., Eshleman, S.,...Kendler, K. S. (1994). Lifetime and 12-month prevalence of DSM-III-R psychiatric disorders in the United States: Results from the National Comorbidity Survey. *Archives of General Psychiatry, 51*(1), 8–19.

Klein, D. F., Thase, M. E., Endicott, J., Adler, L., Glick, I., Kalali, A.,...Bystritsky, A. (2002). Improving clinical trials: American Society of Clinical Psychopharmacology recommendations. *Archives of General Psychiatry, 59*(3), 272–278.

Kraemer, H. C. (1991). To increase power in randomized clinical trials without increasing sample size. *Psychopharmacology Bulletin, 27*(3), 217–224.

Kraemer, H. C., & Kupfer, D. J. (2006). Size of treatment effects and their importance to clinical research and practice. *Biological Psychiatry, 59*(11), 990–996.

Kraemer, H. C., & Pruyn, J. P. (1990). The evaluation of different approaches to randomized clinical trials: Report on the 1987 MacArthur Foundation Network I Methodology Workshop. *Archives of General Psychiatry, 47*(12), 1163–1169.

Kraemer, H. C., Pruyn, J. P., Gibbons, R. D., Greenhouse, J. B., Grochocinski, V. J., Waternaux, C., & Kupfer, D. J. (1987). Methodology in psychiatric research: Report on the 1986 MacArthur Foundation Network I Methodology Institute. *Archives of General Psychiatry, 44*(12), 1100–1106.

Kraemer, H. C., Stice, E., Kazdin, A., Offord, D., & Kupfer, D. (2001). How do risk factors work together? Mediators, moderators, and independent, overlapping, and proxy risk factors. *American Journal of Psychiatry, 158*(6), 848–856.

Kraemer, H. C., Wilson, G. T., Fairburn, C. G., & Agras, W. S. (2002). Mediators and moderators of treatment effects in randomized clinical trials. *Archives of General Psychiatry, 59*(10), 877–883.

Kupka, R. W., Altshuler, L. L., Nolen, W. A., Suppes, T., Luckenbaugh, D. A., Leverich, G. S.,...Post, R. M. (2007). Three times more days depressed than manic or hypomanic in both bipolar I and bipolar II disorder. *Bipolar Disorders, 9*(5), 531–535. doi:10.1111/j.1399-5618.2007.00467.x

Kupka, R. W., Luckenbaugh, D. A., Post, R. M., Suppes, T., Altshuler, L. L., Keck, P. E. Jr.,...Nolen, W. A. (2005). Comparison of rapid-cycling and non-rapid-cycling bipolar disorder based on prospective mood ratings in 539 outpatients. *The American Journal of Psychiatry, 162*(7), 1273–1280. doi:10.1176/appi.ajp.162.7.1273

Lasagna, L. L. (1994). Decision processes in establishing the efficacy and safety of psychotropic agents. In R. F. Prien & D. S. Robinson (Eds.), *Clinical evaluation of psychotropic drugs: Principles and guidelines* (pp. 13–28). New York: Raven Press.

Laska, E. M., Klein, E., Lavori, P. W., Levine, J., & Robinson, D. S. (1994). Design issue for the clinical evaluation of psychotropic drugs. In R. F. Prien & D. S. Robinson (Eds.), *Clinical evaluation of psychotropic drugs: Principles and guidelines* (pp. 29–67). New York: Raven Press.

Lavori, P. W., Dawson, R., & Rush, A. J. (2000). Flexible treatment strategies in chronic disease: Clinical and research implications. *Biological Psychiatry, 48*(6), 605–614.

Lavori, P. W., Rush, A. J., Wisniewski, S. R., Alpert, J., Fava, M., Kupfer, D. J.,...Trivedi, M. (2001). Strengthening clinical effectiveness trials: Equipoise-stratified randomization. *Biological Psychiatry, 50*(10), 792–801.

Leber, P. (2002). Not in our methods, but in our ignorance. *Archives of General Psychiatry, 59*(3), 279–280.

Leon, A. C. (2008). Implications of clinical trial design on sample size requirements. *Schizophrenia Bulletin, 34*(4), 664–669.

Leucht, S., Cipriani, A., Spineli, L., Mavridis, D., Orey, D., Richter, F.,...Davis, J. M. (2013). Comparative efficacy and tolerability of 15 antipsychotic drugs in schizophrenia: A multiple-treatments meta-analysis. *Lancet, 382*(9896), 951–962.

Leverich, G. S., & Post, R. M. (1996). Life charting the course of bipolar disorder. *Current Review of Mood and Anxiety Disorders, 1*, 48–61.

Leverich, G. S., & Post, R. M. (1998). Life charting of affective disorders. *CNS Spectrums, 3*, 21–37.

Malakoff, D. (2008). Clinical trials and tribulations: Allegations of waste: The "seeding" study. *Science, 322*(5899), 213.

March, J. S., Silva, S. G., Compton, S., Shapiro, M., Califf, R., & Krishnan, R. (2005). The case for practical clinical trials in psychiatry. *The American Journal of Psychiatry, 162*(5), 836–846.

McDermut, W., Pazzaglia, P. J., Huggins, T., Mikalauskas, K., Leverich, G. S., Ketter, T. A.,...Post, R. M. (1995). Use of single case analyses in off-on-off-on trials in affective illness: A demonstration of the efficacy of nimodipine. *Depression, 2*, 259–271.

McElroy, S. L., Altshuler, L. L., Suppes, T., Keck, P. E. Jr., Frye, M. A., Denicoff, K. D.,...Post, R. M. (2001). Axis I psychiatric comorbidity and its relationship to historical illness variables in 288 patients with bipolar disorder. *The American Journal of Psychiatry, 158*(3), 420–426.

Merikangas, K. R., Akiskal, H. S., Angst, J., Greenberg, P. E., Hirschfeld, R. M., Petukhova, M., & Kessler, R. C. (2007). Lifetime and 12-month prevalence of bipolar spectrum disorder in the National Comorbidity Survey replication. *Achieves of General Psychiatry, 64*(5), 543–552.

Nierenberg, A. A., Friedman, E. S., Bowden, C. L., Sylvia, L. G., Thase, M. E., Ketter, T.,...Calabrese, J. R. (2013). Lithium treatment moderate-dose use study (LiTMUS) for bipolar disorder: A randomized comparative effectiveness trial of optimized personalized treatment with and without lithium. *The American Journal of Psychiatry, 170*(1), 102–110. doi:10.1176/appi.ajp.2012.12060751

Nolen, W. A., Luckenbaugh, D. A., Altshuler, L. L., Suppes, T., McElroy, S. L., Frye, M. A.,...Post, R. M. (2004). Correlates of 1-year prospective outcome in bipolar disorder: Results from the Stanley Foundation Bipolar Network. *The American Journal of Psychiatry, 161*(8), 1447–1454.

Obrocea, G. V., Dunn, R. M., Frye, M. A., Ketter, T. A., Luckenbaugh, D. A., Leverich, G. S.,...Post, R. M. (2002). Clinical predictors of response to lamotrigine and gabapentin monotherapy in refractory affective disorders. *Biological Psychiatry, 51*(3), 253–260.

Otto, M. W. (1992). Statistical methods for clinical psychopharmacology trials. In M. Fava & J. F. Rosenbaum (Eds.), *Research designs and methods in psychiatry* (pp. 247–266.). Amsterdam: Elsevier.

Pacchiarotti, I., Bond, D. J., Baldessarini, R. J., Nolen, W. A., Grunze, H., Licht, R. W., Post, R. M. et al (2013). The International Society for Bipolar Disorders (ISBD) Task Force Report on Antidepressant Use in Bipolar Disorders. *The American Journal of Psychiatry, 170*(11), 1249–1262.

Palmer, C. R., & Rosenberger, W. F. (1999). Ethics and practice: Alternative designs for phase III randomized clinical trials. *Controlled Clinical Trials, 20*(2), 172–186.

Pazzaglia, P. J., Post, R. M., Ketter, T. A., Callahan, A. M., Marangell, L. B., Frye, M. A.,...Luckenbaugh, D. (1998). Nimodipine monotherapy and carbamazepine augmentation in patients with refractory recurrent affective illness. *Journal of Clinical Psychopharmacology, 18*(5), 404–413.

Pazzaglia, P. J., Post, R. M., Ketter, T. A., George, M. S., & Marangell, L. B. (1993). Preliminary controlled trial of nimodipine in ultra-rapid cycling affective dysregulation. *Psychiatry Research, 49*(3), 257–272.

Perlis, R. H., Miyahara, S., Marangell, L. B., Wisniewski, S. R., Ostacher, M., DelBello, M. P.,...Nierenberg, A. A. (2004). Long-term implications of early onset in bipolar disorder: Data from the first 1000 participants in the systematic treatment enhancement program for bipolar disorder (STEP-BD). *Biological Psychiatry, 55*(9), 875–881. doi:10.1016/j.biopsych.2004.01.022

Perlis, R. H., Ostacher, M. J., Patel, J. K., Marangell, L. B., Zhang, H., Wisniewski, S. R.,...Thase, M. E. (2006). Predictors of recurrence in bipolar disorder: Primary outcomes from the Systematic Treatment Enhancement Program for Bipolar Disorder (STEP-BD). *The American Journal of Psychiatry, 163*(2), 217–224.

Perlis, R. H., Sachs, G. S., Lafer, B., Otto, M. W., Faraone, S. V., Kane, J. M., & Rosenbaum, J. F. (2002). Effect of abrupt change from standard to low serum levels of lithium: A reanalysis of double-blind lithium maintenance data. *The American Journal of Psychiatry, 159*(7), 1155–1159.

Post, R. M. (2010). Special Issues of research methodology in bipolar disorders clinical treatment trials. In M. Hertzman & L. Alder (Eds.), *Clinical trials in psychopharmacology* (pp. 149–177). Hoboken, NJ: Wiley-Blackwell.

Post, R. M. (2012). The sorry state of treatment research in bipolar disorder: An ongoing but preventable catastrophe. *Journal of Nervous and Mental Disease, 200*(11), 924–927. doi:10.1097/NMD.0b013e31827189d4

Post, R. M., Chang, K., & Frye, M. A. (2013). Paradigm shift: Preliminary clinical categorization of ultrahigh risk for childhood bipolar disorder to facilitate studies on prevention. *Journal of Clinical Psychiatry, 74*(2), 167–169. doi:10.4088/JCP.12com08136

Post, R. M., Chang, K. D., & Suppes, T. (2004). Treatment of rapid-cycling bipolar disorder. *CNS Spectrums, 9*(2), 1–11.

Post, R. M., Frye, M. A., Leverich, G. S., & Denicoff, K. (1998). The role of complex combination therapy in the treatment of refractory bipolar illness. *CNS Spectrums, 3*, 66–86.

Post, R. M., Keck, P. Jr., & Rush, A. J. (2002). New designs for studies of the prophylaxis of bipolar disorder. *Journal of Clinical Psychopharmacology, 22*(1), 1–3.

Post, R. M., & Kowatch, R. A. (2006). The health care crisis of childhood-onset bipolar illness: Some recommendations for its amelioration. *Journal of Clinical Psychiatry, 67*(1), 115–125.

Post, R. M., & Leverich, G. S. (2008). *Treatment of bipolar illness: A casebook of clinicians and patients.* New York: W.W. Norton & Company.

Post, R. M., L'Herrou, T., Luckenbaugh, D. A., Frye, M. A., Leverich, G. S., & Mikalauskas, K. (1998). Statistical approaches to trial durations in episodic affective illness. *Psychiatry Research, 78*(1–2), 71–87.

Post, R. M., & Luckenbaugh, D. A. (2003). Unique design issues in clinical trials of patients with bipolar affective disorder. *Journal of Psychiatric Research, 37*(1), 61–73.

Prien, R. F., & Potter, W. Z. (1990). NIMH workshop report on treatment of bipolar disorder. *Psychopharmacology Bulletin, 26*(4), 409–427.

Prien, R. F., & Rush, A. J. (1996). National Institute of Mental Health Workshop Report on the Treatment of Bipolar Disorder. *Biological Psychiatry, 40*(3), 215–220.

Rush, A. J. (2007). STAR*D: What have we learned? *The American Journal of Psychiatry, 164*(2), 201–204.

Rush, A. J., Post, R. M., Nolen, W. A., Keck, P. E. Jr., Suppes, T., Altshuler, L., & McElroy, S. L. (2000). Methodological issues in developing new acute treatments for patients with bipolar illness. *Biological Psychiatry, 48*(6), 615–624.

Sachs, G. S. (2001). Design and promise of NIMH multicenter effectiveness trials: A STEP forward. *Bipolar Disorders, 3*(1), 16–17.

Salim, A., Mackinnon, A., & Griffiths, K. (2008). Sensitivity analysis of intention-to-treat estimates when withdrawals are related to unobserved compliance status. *Statistics in Medicine, 27*(8), 1164–1179.

Schouten, H. J. (1999). Planning group sizes in clinical trials with a continuous outcome and repeated measures. *Statistics in Medicine, 18*(3), 255–264.

Slade, M., & Priebe, S. (2001). Are randomised controlled trials the only gold that glitters? *The British Journal of Psychiatry, 179*, 286–287.

Spearing, M. K., Post, R. M., Leverich, G. S., Brandt, D., & Nolen, W. (1997). Modification of the Clinical Global Impressions (CGI) Scale for use in bipolar illness (BP): The CGI-BP. *Psychiatry Research, 73*(3), 159–171.

Suppes, T., Mintz, J., McElroy, S. L., Altshuler, L. L., Kupka, R. W., Frye, M. A.,...Post, R. M. (2005). Mixed hypomania in 908 patients with bipolar disorder evaluated prospectively in the Stanley Foundation Bipolar Treatment Network: A sex-specific phenomenon. *Archives of General Psychiatry, 62*(10), 1089–1096. doi:10.1001/archpsyc.62.10.1089

Vestergaard, P. (1992). Treatment and prevention of mania: A Scandinavian perspective. Neuropsychopharmacology, 7(4), 249–259.

Whitehead, J. (1991). *Sequential methods in clinical trials.* New York: Marcel Dekker.

Wilens, T. E., Biederman, J., Kwon, A., Ditterline, J., Forkner, P., Moore, H.,...Faraone, S. V. (2004). Risk of substance use disorders in adolescents with bipolar disorder. *Journal of the American Academy of Child & Adolescent Psychiatry, 43*(11), 1380–1386.

Winer, B. J. (1971). *Statistical principles in experimental design.* New York: McGraw Hill.

Yildiz, A., Nikodem, M., Vieta, E., Correll, C. U., & Baldessarini, R. J. (2014). A network meta-analysis on comparative efficacy and all-cause discontinuation of antimanic treatments in acute bipolar mania. *Psychological Medicine, in press.*

Yildiz, A., Vieta, E., Correll, C. U., Nikodem, M., & Baldessarini, R. J. (2014). Critical issues on use of network meta-analysis in psychiatry. *Harvard Review of Psychiatry, in press.*

44

SEQUENTIAL MULTIPLE ASSIGNMENT RANDOMIZED TRIALS

Fan Wu, Eric B. Laber, and Emanuel Severus[*]

INTRODUCTION

The management of bipolar disorder and other chronic conditions requires ongoing individualized treatment that is adaptive to the evolving heath status of each patient. The concept of individualized treatment is not new among clinical and intervention scientists; indeed, personalized medicine is discussed in one of the earliest texts on modern medicine (Osler, 1893). However, a more recent phenomenon is the construction of evidence-based (i.e., data-driven) adaptive treatment strategies known as dynamic treatment regimes (DTRs; Murphy, 2003; Robins, 2004). A DTR is a sequence of decision rules, one for each clinical decision point, that map up-to-date patient information to a recommended intervention. Because DTRs recommend treatment only if, when, and to whom it is needed, they have tremendous potential for improving patient outcomes while reducing cost and patient burden. These benefits are increasingly important due to increasing health-care costs and an aging population.

In this chapter we review Sequential Multiple Assignment Randomized Trials (SMARTs), a clinical trial design that produces high-quality data for estimating and evaluating DTRs. Our goal is to introduce the motivation and philosophical underpinnings for SMARTs and to discuss key scientific and practical considerations associated with designing a SMART. In a SMART patients are potentially randomized multiple times, with each randomization corresponding to a critical decision point in the treatment process. Figure 44.1 shows a schematic for a hypothetical SMART with two randomized stages; as depicted in this schematic, a SMART allows for randomizations and

treatment options to depend on intermediate patient outcomes (e.g., responder status). The use of multiple randomizations allows for efficient and statistically rigorous evaluation and comparison of DTRs (Lavori & Dawson, 2004; Murphy, 2005a). For example, in the context of bipolar depression, a simple DTR is (a) at baseline assign a mood stabilizer; (b) if after six weeks the subject exhibits at least a 50% improvement on the continuous symptom subscale for depression (SUM-D; Sachs, Guill, & McMurrich, 2002) over baseline and does not meet the *Diagnostic and Statistical Manual of Mental Disorders* (fourth edition; *DSM-IV*) criteria for (hypo)mania then continue current treatment; otherwise (c) augment the mood stabilizer with bupropion (BUP). An appropriately designed SMART (described later) facilitates estimation of the average cumulative clinical outcome under the foregoing DTR as well as comparison with alternative DTRs.

A large number of SMARTs have been completed or are currently in the field (e.g., The Methodology Center, 2014); recent funding calls for SMARTs from the National Institutes of Health suggest that this number will continue to increase (The Methodology Center, 2014). The Systematic Treatment Enhancement Program for Bipolar Disorder (STEP-BD) is a long-term, multisite pragmatic study of bipolar disorder (see Sachs et al., 2003, for details). A simplified version of Acute Depression Randomized Pathway (RAD) is a SMART embedded in STEP-BD. We use it as the basis for subsequent illustrative examples. Subjects enrolled in RAD, in addition to satisfying the enrollment criteria for STEP-BD, had to be at least 18 years of age and experiencing a major depressive episode. Figure 44.2 shows a schematic for RAD. In the first stage of RAD,

[*] Fan Wu is Graduate Student, Department of Statistics, North CarolinaStateUniversity, Raleigh, North Carolina27695, USA (E-mail fwu5@ncsu.edu).
Eric B. Laber is Assistant Professor, Department of Statistics, North CarolinaStateUniversity, Raleigh, North Carolina27695, USA (E-mail eblaber@ncsu.edu).
Emanuel Severus is consultant and Head of the Bipolar Disorders Outpatient Clinic, Department of Psychiatry and Psychotherapy, University Hospital Carl Gustav Carus, TU Dresden, Dresden, Germany (E-mail: Emanuel.Severus@uniklinikum-dresden.de).

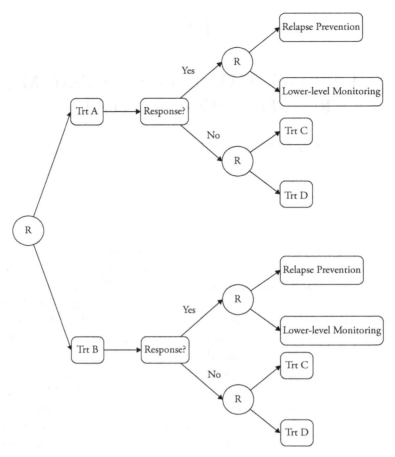

Figure 44.1 Schematic for a simple SMART with a step-down therapy for responders and treatment switch for nonresponders.

subjects are randomized to receive a mood stabilizer plus one of three treatments: (a) placebo, (b) BUP, or (c) paroxetine (PAR). The first-stage randomizations are not balanced: the probability of receiving placebo is 0.5 and 0.25 for BUP and PAR. After six weeks, subjects who experience at least a 50% improvement over the baseline SUM-D score and do not meet the criteria for (hypo)mania are deemed responders. Responders continue their first-stage treatment; nonresponders progress to the second stage wherein subjects receiving PAR or BUP in the first stage intensify their current treatment (dose increase) and subjects receiving a placebo are randomized with equal probability to BUP or PAR. As shown in Figure 44.2, it is possible for subjects to opt out of RAD and join another pathway of STEP-BD; however, for simplicity hereafter we assume all subjects remain in RAD.

In the remainder of this chapter we review the motivation and historical development of SMARTs, then discuss a template for designing a SMART. In the following section we discuss sample-size calculations for SMARTs and provide a brief annotated bibliography on estimation and inference. The chapter ends with concluding remarks.

MOTIVATION FOR SMARTs

Sequential randomized trials originated as a conceptual device to describe necessary conditions for making causal inference from observational longitudinal data (Robins, 1986, 1987). This line of thinking led to rich methodological developments for analyzing nonexperimental data (e.g., Murphy, 2001, 2003; Robins, 1989, 1993, 1997, 1998; Van Der Laan, 2006; Van Der Laan & Petersen, 2007). However, necessary conditions for causal inference are generally not testable using experimental data. Subsequently, a number of papers discussed SMART designs that ensure that these causal conditions hold (Lavori & Dawson, 2000, 2004; Murphy, 2005a).

As discussed previously, SMARTs sequentially randomize subjects over time. Sequential randomization allows for detection of delayed treatment effects. Such delayed effects will generally not be detected by concatenating multiple one-stage trials. Figure 44.3 illustrates this point with two hypothetical clinical trials for evaluating first- and second-line treatments for bipolar depression. The top two trials illustrate using two single-stage trials to

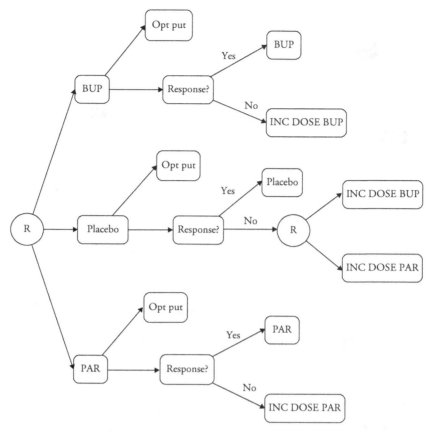

Figure 44.2 Schematic for the RAD arm of the STEP-BD study.

construct a two-stage treatment strategy. In the first trial, a mood stabilizer plus BUP is compared with a mood stabilizer + BUP + psychoeducation (PSY) using a simple two-arm randomized trial. In terms of mean SUM-D, BUP is marginally better than BUP + PSY; furthermore, because BUP is less expensive and burdensome than BUP + PSY, researchers recommend BUP as a first-line strategy. Then, in a follow-up study designed to find the optimal second-line treatment, researchers conduct a randomized trial wherein subjects are first given BUP, then nonresponders and responders are randomized to potential salvage and maintenance treatments (as depicted in the upper right of Figure 44.3). The results of this randomized trial suggest that the best second-line treatment is increased-dose BUP(INC DOSE BUP) for nonresponders and continuing first-stage treatment (BUP) or additional continuous mood monitoring (MM) + first-stage treatment (MM + BUP) for responders. For reasons of cost and patient burden, researchers conclude BUP should be given instead of MM + BUP to responders.

The bottom of Figure 44.3 shows a SMART for estimating the best first- and second-line treatments. Both the foregoing single-stage designs are embedded in the SMART design. However, the SMART does not abandon BUP + PSY after observing a marginal difference in interim SUM-D; this is because a SMART is designed to evaluate and compare entire sequences of treatments in terms of distal outcomes. Figure 44.3 shows that the optimal strategy from the SMART trial is quite different from that obtained by concatenating single-stage trials. Results of the SMART show that the best first-line treatment is BUP + PSY and the best second-line treatment is INC DOSE BUP + PSY for nonresponders and MM + BUP + PSY for responders. The final expected SUM-D score under this strategy is less for all subjects than the optimal strategy obtained by piecing together single-stage trials. The reason is that the SMART trial captures delayed effects of PSY: nonresponders benefited from continuing PSY in the second stage and responders learned to benefit from additional continuous MM because of PSY.

The delayed effect of PSY on additional continuous MM in the foregoing example demonstrates one way in which the second-stage treatment effect varies by first-stage treatment. In general, if the second-stage treatment effect varies by the first-stage treatment, SMARTs will be able to

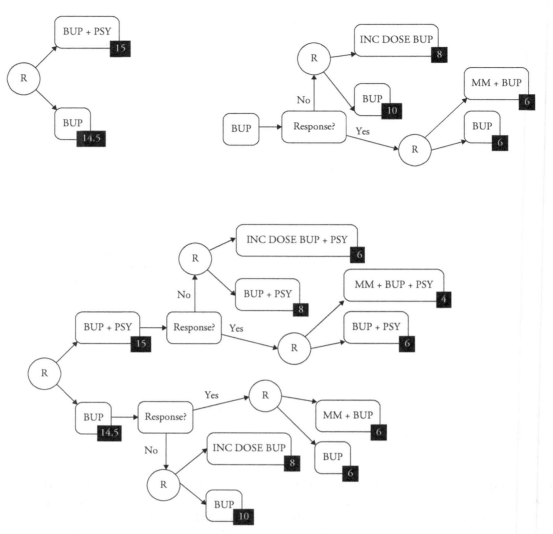

Figure 44.3 Schematic for piecing together a DTR using a sequence of one-stage trials and a corresponding SMART. The numbers at lower right corner show hypothetical mean SUM-D scores. Top left: Two-arm randomized trial comparing first line treatments: (i) mood stabilizer + bupropion + psychoeducation (BUP + PS Y); and (ii) mood stabilizer + bupropion (BUP). In the first stage comparison subjects receiving BUP had a lower mean SUM-D(14.5) than those receiving B UP + PS Y(15). Top right: Follow-up randomized trial comparing treatments among responders and nonresponders receiving BUP initially. Nonresponders are randomized to either mood stabilizer + increased-dosebupropion (INCDOSEBUP) or continuing BUP. Responders are randomized to either additional mood-monitoring + current treatment (MM+BUP) or just current treatment (BUP). Combining both trials the estimated optimal treatment strategy is to give BUP initially then INCDOSE BUP to nonresponders and either MM or MM + BUP to responders. Bottom: SMART for comparing first-and second-line treatments. Subjects receiving BUP + PSY initially have lowerlong-term SUM-D scores due to delayed effects of PSY. Patients receiving BUP + PSY initially utilize additional continuous mood-monitoring (MM) better than subjects receiving BUP. There commended treatment strategy based on the SMART is to recommend BUP + PSY initially and then MM + BUP + PSY to responders and INCDOSEBUP + PSY to nonresponders.

detect this dependence, whereas sequential one-stage trials will not. For a more technical treatment of these ideas, see Murphy (2005a).

DESIGNING A SMART

Designing a SMART requires prioritizing scientific questions to ensure sufficient statistical power. In this section we discuss three key steps in the design of a SMART: (a) identifying primary and secondary scientific questions, (b) identifying critical decision points, and (c) pruning the design. We have found these steps common to and useful in the design of several SMARTs. As a running example we consider the problem of designing a SMART in the context of bipolar depression. Because our focus is on design issues, our treatment of the underlying science is necessarily superficial.

STEP 1: IDENTIFYING PRIMARY AND SECONDARY SCIENTIFIC QUESTIONS

Though this is an obvious (and necessary) step, it is important not to postulate a design before identifying and focusing scientific questions. There is often a tradeoff between the complexity of the design and statistical efficiency; thus one should seek to construct a design producing data that can be used to address key scientific questions yet is as parsimonious as possible.

Suppose that our goal is to compare first- and second-line treatments for patients with bipolar depression. Our primary question of interest might be: Which is the best first line treatment for bipolar depression among (a) mood stabilizer alone (placebo); (b) mood stabilizer + BUP; and (c) mood stabilizer + (PAR)? Another primary question might be: What second-line treatment is best for nonresponders to first-line treatment? Initially we identify intensifying and switching treatment as viable second-stage treatment options among patients not responding to either BUP or PAR; under intensified treatment subjects would receive an increased dose of their first-line treatment whereas under a switch subjects receiving BUP as first line would switch to PAR and patients receiving PAR would switch to BUP. Patients receiving a placebo as a first-line treatment and not demonstrating an adequate response would be switched to either BUP or PAR.

After generating primary questions, it is important to identify secondary questions. Unlike primary questions, secondary questions are typically not considered in sample size or power calculations but are instead often viewed as exploratory or hypothesis generating. In the context of bipolar depression, a secondary question might be whether patients having experienced a (hypo)manic episode just prior to the major depressive episodes should receive an antidepressant in their first-line treatment in addition to a mood stabilizer. Randomization in the first stage to placebo, BUP, and PAR ensures that we can make this comparison through stratifying subjects by prior (hypo)mania status at enrollment and comparing first-line treatments across strata. A related but highly exploratory secondary question is whether there exists a subgroup of subjects experiencing substantial benefit (harm) from a first line antidepressant (BUP or PAR) relative to placebo. This secondary analysis falls under the heading of subgroup identification, which is currently an active area of research (Assmann, Pocock, Enos, & Kasten, 2000; Foster, Taylor, & Ruberg, 2011; Lipkovich, Dmitrienko, Denne, & Enas, 2011; Su, Tsai, Wang, Nickerson, & Li, 2009; Su, Zhou, Yan, Fan, & Yang, 2008).

A secondary analysis that is fundamental in the development of SMARTs is estimation of a DTR that optimizes a desirable clinical outcome. Formally, such a DTR is a sequence of functions, one for each decision point that maps up-to-date patient information to a recommended treatment. Estimation of a DTR should be contrasted with evaluating a small number of fixed (i.e., not data-driven) DTRs. There is a large literature on estimating DTRs primarily focused on regression-based approximate dynamic programming (Chakraborty, Murphy, & Strecher, 2010; Henderson, Ansell, & Alshibani, 2010; Laber, Lizotte, & Ferguson, 2014; Laber, Qian, Lizotte, Pelham, & Murphy, 2010; Murphy, 2005b; Nahum-Shani et al., 2012; Robins, 2004; Schulte, Tsiatis, Laber, & Davidian, 2014; Zhao, Zeng, Socinski, & Kosorok, 2011) or policy-search methods (Orellana, Rotnitzky, & Robins, 2010; Zhang, Tsiatis, Davidian, Zhang, & Laber, 2012; Zhang, Tsiatis, Laber, & Davidian, 2012, 2013; Zhao, Zeng, Rush, & Kosorok, 2012). Freely available software exists for many DTR estimation methods (e.g., see http://www4.stat.ncsu.edu/laber/software). Using Q-learning, a regression-based approximate dynamic programming algorithm (described later), we estimated the optimal DTR for patients with bipolar depression using data from RAD (for details see Wu, Laber, Lipkovich, & Severus, in press). The estimated optimal DTR is shown in Figure 44.4. It can be seen that patients with prior (hypo)mania immediately preceding the major depressive episode are not recommended to receive an antidepressant as a first-line treatment and that among patients not experiencing (hypo)mania before the major depressive episode, those over the age of 44.5 are recommended to PAR and those under 44.5 are recommended to BUP. Responders do not change from their first-line treatment. An important secondary question is whether an estimated optimal DTR is significantly better than standard of care or other fixed (non-data-driven) DTR. However, comparison of an estimated optimal DTR with a fixed (non-data-driven) DTR is a complicated statistical problem (Chakraborty, Laber, & Zhao, 2014; Laber et al. 2010).

STEP 2: IDENTIFYING CRITICAL DECISION POINTS

Randomization times in a SMART should correspond to critical decision points in the treatment process. Thus randomization times may not be fixed in calendar time but dictated by subject outcomes. In some settings the timing and/or criteria used to determine a treatment change are of primary interest, in which case these should be

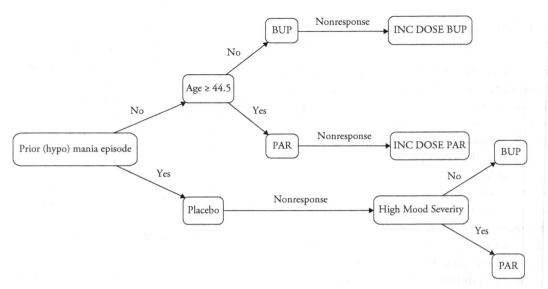

Figure 44.4 Estimated optimal DTR using data from RAD. Responders do not change from their first line treatment. High mood severity is defined as scale scores for mood elevation (SUM-M) exceeding 0.875.

considered as part of the treatment package. For example, there may be two competing definitions of response, for example strong (e.g., no more than two depressive or two manic symptoms present may be referred to as "remission") and weak (e.g., at least 50% improvement from baseline depression scale score without meeting *DSM-IV* criteria for hypomania or mania but not fulfilling the criteria for remission). In this case first-line randomizations might include all combinations of first-line treatments and responder definitions. Figure 44.5 shows the first stage of a SMART design comparing BUP and PAR with the strong and weakers ponder definitions. The number of arms in the first stage represents all combinations of first-line treatments and responder definitions. It is possible to compare the two responder definitions by pooling (marginalizing) over the first-line treatments and second-line treatments. Similarly, it is possible to compare the two first-line treatments by pooling (marginalizing) over the responder definitions and second-line treatments. The pooled comparisons are simple, two-group comparisons that, with equal randomization, will have half the total sample size in each group. However, other comparisons will require cutting the sample size significantly. For example, comparing all first-line treatment responder definition combinations pooling (marginalizing) over the second-stage treatments cuts the sample size to one-fourth the total sample size in each group, and so on. In some settings it may be prudent to consider a design that compares either responder definitions or first-line treatments but not both.

STEP 3: PRUNING THE DESIGN

In the beginning stages of designing a SMART it can be tempting to construct a very complex trial with many

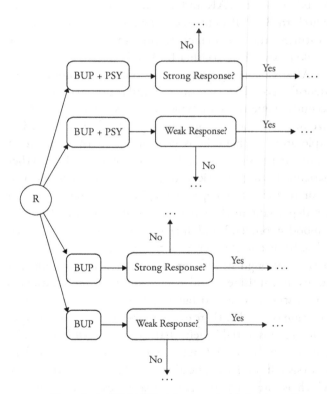

Figure 44.5 Hypothetical SMART with competing definitions of are sponder; "…" denotes subsequent randomizations. The number of first stage arms represents all combinations of first-line treatments and responder definitions.

possible treatment sequences in order to address a large number of primary and secondary questions. However, as the trial grows in complexity, statistical power diffuses. Thus it is often important to simplify an initial trial design to address a few key questions, even if this means leaving some questions to a follow-up study. A useful strategy is to experiment with cutting/combining treatment arms in an initial SMART design to see which questions can no longer be addressed after the cut/combination; cuts/combinations that eliminate questions of low importance should be considered so as to simplify the design.

SAMPLE SIZE, ESTIMATION, AND INFERENCE

For simplicity we restrict attention to a two-stage SMARTs with binary treatments at each stage. We assume that the data collected using the SMART will comprise n independent identically distributed trajectories of the form $\left(X_1, A_1, X_2, A_2, Y\right)$ where: $X_1 \in R^{p_1}$ denotes baseline (pre-randomization) subject covariates; $A_1 \in \{-1,1\}$ denotes the first-line treatment assignment; $X_2 \in R^{p_2}$ denotes interim subject information collected during the course of the first-line treatment but before the second-line treatment assignment; $A_2 \in \{-1,1\}$ denotes the second-line treatment; and $Y \in R$ denotes the outcome of interest coded so that higher values are better. The outcome Y need not correspond to a single measurement taken at the end of the study but could be a cumulative summary of the subject's health status over the entire study. The design of SMARTs require that the distribution of A_1 be completely determined by X_1 and the distribution of A_2 be completely determined by X_1, A_1 and X_2. For simplicity we assume that $P\left(A_1 = 1 | X_1\right) \equiv \frac{1}{2}$ and $P\left(A_2 = 1 | X_1, A_1, X_2\right) \equiv \frac{1}{2}$ with probability 1.

SAMPLE SIZE FORMULAE

A SMART should be sized to ensure proper power to answer a primary question of interest. For illustration we consider two primary questions of interest: (P1) comparison of first-line treatments and (P2) comparison of second-line treatments for responders. Sample size formulae for comparing fixed DTRs are given by Murphy (2005a; see also Oetting, Levy, Weiss, & Murphy, 2007). Define $\Delta = E\left(Y | A_1 = 1\right) - E(Y | A_1 = -1)$ to be the difference in the expected outcome under first-line treatments

1 and −1. To size a SMART for (P1), we want to find a sample size n so that we have sufficient power, say $1 - \beta$, to reject null hypothesis $H_0 : \Delta = 0$ in favor of the alternative $H_1 : \Delta \neq 0$ when Δ is sufficiently far from zero. Define the standardized effect size Cohen (1988),

$$\delta = \Delta / \sqrt{\frac{\left\{Var\left(Y | A_1 = 1\right) + Var\left(Y | A_1 = -1\right)\right\}}{2}}.$$ The required total sample size for a two-sided test of $H_0 : \Delta = 0$ at level α with power $(1-\beta)$ is $n = \frac{4\left(z_{\{1-\alpha/2\}} - z_{\{1-\beta\}}\right)^2}{\delta^2}$ where z_v is the $v \times 100$ percentile from a standard normal distribution. Application of this formula requires a postulated value of δ, which may be based on a combination of historical data and expert judgment.

Define $\Delta' = E(Y | Responder, A_2 = 1) - E(Y | Responder, A_2 = -1)$. To size a SMART for (P2) we find a sample size n' so that there is enough power, say $(1 - \beta')$, to reject $H_0 : \Delta' = 0$ in favor of $H_1 : \Delta' \neq 0$ when Δ' is sufficiently far from zero. Define the standardized effect size among responders as:

$$\delta' = \frac{\Delta'}{\sqrt{\frac{\left\{\begin{array}{c} Var\left(Y | Responder, A_2 = 1\right) \\ + Var\left(Y | Responder, A_2 = -1\right)\end{array}\right\}}{2}}},$$

and let ρ denote the marginalized probability of response $P\left(Responder\right)$. Then, the required sample size for power $(1 - \beta')$ of a two-sided test of $H_0 : \Delta = 0$ of level α' is $n' = \frac{4\left(z_{\{1-\alpha'/2\}} + z_{\{1-\beta\}}\right)^2}{\left\{(\delta')^2 \rho\right\}}$. Application of this sample size formula requires postulating both a standardized effect size and probability of response. Again, these can be based on a combination of historical data and expert judgment.

ESTIMATION

Define $H_1 = X_1$ and $H_2 = \left(X_1, A_1, X_2\right)$ so that H_t denotes the available information to the decision-maker at time $t = 1, 2$. A DTR is a pair of decision rules $\pi = \left(\pi_1, \pi_2\right)$, where $\pi_t :$ support $H_t = \{-1, 1\}$ so that a patient presenting with $H_t = h_t$ at time t is recommended treatment $\pi_t(h_t)$. This definition allows for decision rules with complex dependence on the evolving health status of each patient, as well as very simple decision rules like $\pi_1(h_1) = 1$ for all h_1. For any fixed (non-data-driven) decision rule π let $V(\pi)$ denote the expected outcome if all patients are assigned treatment according to π. A consistent and unbiased estimator of $V(\pi)$ is

$$\hat{V}(\pi) = \frac{\sum_{i=1}^{n} Y_i 1_{A_{1i}=\pi_1(H_{1i})} 1_{A_{2i}=\pi_2(H_{2i})}}{\sum_{i=1}^{n} 1_{A_{1i}=\pi_1(H_{1i})} 1_{A_{2i}=\pi_2(H_{2i})}} \qquad (1.3.1)$$

Where 1_u is one if u is true and zero otherwise. And $\{(H_{1i}, A_{1i}, H_{2i}, A_{2i}, Y_i)\}^n$ presents the data collected in the SMART. It can be seen that (1.3.1) is an average of the outcomes for patients that are observed to follow π (see Zhang et al., 2013, and references therein). An optimal DTR, say π^{opt}, satisfies $V(\pi^{opt}) \geq V(\pi)$ for all π. Thus an intuitive strategy for estimating π^{opt} is to search for the value $\hat{\pi}$ that maximizes (1.3.1). However, this is a non-smooth, non-convex optimization problem and may thus be computationally expensive (Zha et al., 2012; Zhang, Tsiatis, Davidian, et al., 2012; Zhang et al., 2013); furthermore, this approach does not easily allow exploratory analyses, which are often crucial in building high-quality models from observed data (Behrens, 1997; Velleman & Hoaglin, 1981). We next describe an alternative procedure, Q-learning, for estimating π^{opt} that builds on familiar regression models and allows exploratory model building and diagnostics.

Q-learning can be understood as a regression-based approximate dynamic programming algorithm. Define $Q_2(h_2, a_2) = E(Y | H_2 = h_2, A_2 = a_2)$ and $Q_1(h_1, a_1) = E(\max_{a_2} Q_2(H_2, a_2) | H_1 = h_1, A_1 = a_1)$ then it follows from dynamic programming Bellman (1957) $\pi^{opt}(h_t) = argmax_{a_t} Q_t(h_t, a_t)$ for $t = 1, 2$. The intuition for this is as follows: For a patient presenting with $H_2 = h_2$ then the best treatment in terms of the expected outcome is the value a_2 that maximizes $E(Y | H_2 = h_2, A_2 = a_2)$, thus $\pi_{opt}(h_2) = argmax_{a_2} Q_2(h_2, a_2)$.

Then it can be seen that $\max_{a_2} Q_2(H_2, a_2)$ is a random variable representing the outcome at stage 2 if patients are assigned second-line treatment using π^{opt}. Thus, $Q_1(h_1, a_1)$ is the expected final outcome for a patient presenting with $H_1 = h_1$, assigned first-line treatment $A_1 = a_1$, and second-line treatment according to π_2^{opt} and therefore $\pi_1^{opt}(h_1) = argmax_{a_1} Q_1(h_1, a_1)$.

Applying this dynamic programming solution requires the complete generative distribution, which is generally unknown in practice. Q-learning mimics dynamic programming by replacing the conditional expectations in the definitions of $Q_t(h_t, a_t)$, $t = 1, 2$ with regression models. The Q-learning algorithm is

(Q1)   Regress Y on H_2 and A_2 to obtain $\hat{Q}_2(h_2, a_2)$;

(Q2)   Define $\tilde{Y} = \max_{a_2} \hat{Q}_2(H_2, a_2)$;

(Q3)   Regress $\tilde{Y}$ on H_1 and A_1 to obtain $\hat{Q}_1(h_1, a_1)$.

The estimated optimal regime using Q-learning is $\hat{\pi}_t(h_t) = argmax_{a_t} \hat{Q}_t(h_t, a_t)$, $t = 1, 2$. Exploratory analyses and model diagnostics can be used to inform the regressions conducted in steps (Q1) and (Q3) (Chakraborty & Moodie, 2013 Laber, Linn, & Stefanski, 2014). Extensions of Q-learning exist to accommodate high-dimensional predictors (McKeague & Qian, 2014), censored data (Goldberg & Kosorok, 2012), and missing data (Shortreed, Laber, Stroup, Pineau, & Murphy, 2014), therefore making it an appealing choice in practice.

INFERENCE

Constructing confidence intervals or hypothesis tests for the optimal DTR is complicated by two factors: (a) the same data are used to both estimate and evaluate the DTR, and (b) the discreteness of treatment assignment is a non-smooth operation of the data. Consequently, standard methods for inference (e.g., the bootstrap or normal approximations) are not valid without modification (Chakraborty & Moodie, 2013; Chakraborty et al., 2010, 2014; Hirano & Porter, 2012; Laber et al., 2010; Moodie & Richardson, 2010; Robins, 2004). Fortunately, specialized inference procedures exist for many quantities of interest (Laber et al., 2010). Laber et al. derive local asymptotic confidence intervals for $Q_t(h_t, a_t)$, $t = 1, 2$. Chakraborty and Moodie (2013) use adaptive subsampling to produce valid confidence intervals for $Q_t(h_t, a_t)$, $t = 1, 2$ and later extended this methodology to produce prediction intervals for $V(\pi)$ (Chakraborty et al., 2014).

DISCUSSION

SMARTs are an efficient trial design for evaluating sequences of treatments and are thereby suited for developing DTRs for the treatment of chronic illnesses like bipolar disorder. Designing a SMART requires careful consideration of primary and secondary analyses, as well as statistical power. A large body of methodological work over the past two decades has created the necessary tools for analyzing data from SMARTs; more recently software implementing these methods has become widely available. We hope that clinical and intervention scientists will consider SMARTs as a mechanism for studying chronic illness and improving healthcare.

Disclosure statement: Dr. Emanuel Severus has no conflicts of interest to disclose. Dr. Fan Wu has no conflicts of interest to disclose.

Dr. Eric Laber has no conflicts of interest to disclose.

REFERENCES

Assmann, S. F., Pocock, S. J., Enos, L. E., & Kasten, L. E.(2000). Subgroup analysis and other (mis) uses of baseline data in clinical trials. *Lancet*, 355(9209), 1064–1069.

Behrens, J. T. (1997). Principles and procedures of exploratory data analysis.*Psychological Methods*, 2(2), 131.

Bellman, R. (1957). *Dynamic programming*. Princeton, NJ: Princeton University Press.

Chakraborty, B., & Moodie, E. E. (2013). *Statistical methods for dynamic treatment regimes*. New York: Springer.

Chakraborty, B., Laber, E. B., & Zhao, Y. (2014). Inference about the expected performance of a data-driven dynamic treatment regime.*Clinical Trials*, 11(4), 408–417.

Chakraborty, B., Murphy, S. A., & Strecher, V. (2010). Inference for non-regular parameters in optimal dynamic treatment regimes.*Statistical Methods in Medical Research*, 19(3), 317–343.

Cohen, J. (1988). *Statistical power analysis for the behavioral sciences*.New York: Psychology Press.

Foster, J. C., Taylor, J. M., & Ruberg, S. J. (2011). Subgroup identification from randomized clinical trial data.*Statistics in Medicine*, 30(24), 2867–2880.

Goldberg, Y., & Kosorok, M. R. (2012). Q-learning with censored data.*Annals of Statistics*, 40(1), 529.

Henderson, R., Ansell, P., & Alshibani, D. (2010). Regret-regression for optimal dynamic treatment regimes.*Biometrics*, 66(4), 1192–1201.

Hirano, K., & Porter, J. R. (2012). Impossibility results for nondifferentiable functionals. *Econometrica*, 80(4), 1769–1790.

Laber, E. B., Linn, K. A., & Stefanski, L. (2014). Interactive model building for Q-learning. *Biometrika* pp. 1–16.

Laber, E. B., Lizotte, D. J., & Ferguson, B. (2014). Set-valued dynamic treatment regimes for competing outcomes. *Biometrics*, 70(1), 53–61.

Laber, E. B., Qian, M., Lizotte, D. J., Pelham, W. E., & Murphy, S. A. (2010). Statistical inference in dynamic treatment regimes. Retrieved from http://arxiv.org/abs/1006.5831

Lavori, P. W., & Dawson, R.(2000). A design for testing clinical strategies: Biased adaptive within-subject randomization. *Journal of the Royal Statistical Society: Series A (Statistics in Society)*, 163(1), 29–38.

Lavori, P. W., & Dawson, R.(2004). Dynamic treatment regimes: practical design considerations.*Clinical Trials*, 1(1), 9–20.

Lipkovich, I., Dmitrienko, A., Denne, J., & Enas, G. (2011). Subgroup identification based on differential effect search—A recursive partitioning method for establishing response to treatment in patient subpopulations. *Statistics in Medicine*, 30(21), 2601–2621.

McKeague, I. W., & Qian, M. (2014). Estimation of treatment policies based on functional predictors. *Statistica Sinica* 24(3), 1461.

Moodie, E. E., & Richardson, T. S. (2010). Estimating optimal dynamic regimes: Correcting bias under the null. *Scandinavian Journal of Statistics*, 37(1), 126–146.

Murphy, S. A. (2003). Optimal dynamic treatment regimes.*Journal of the Royal Statistical Society: Series B*, 65(2), 331–355.

Murphy, S. A. (2005a). A generalization error for Q-learning.*Journal of Machine Learning Research*, 6, 1073.

Murphy, S. A. (2005b). An experimental design for the development of adaptive treatment strategies. *Statistics in Medicine*, 24(10), 1455–1481.

Murphy, S. A., Van Der Laan, M. J., & Robins, J. M. (2001). Marginal mean models for dynamic regimes.*Journal of the American Statistical Association*, 96(456), 1410–1423.

Nahum-Shani, I., Qian, M., Almirall, D., Pelham, W. E., Gnagy, B., Fabiano, G. A.,... Murphy, S. A. (2012). Q-learning: A data analysis method for constructing adaptive interventions. *American Psychological Association*, 17(4), 478.

Oetting, A. I., Levy, J. A., Weiss, R. D., & Murphy, S. A. (2007). Statistical methodology for a SMART design in the development of adaptive treatment strategies. *Causality and psychopathology: Finding the determinants of disorders and their cures*. Arlington, VA: American Psychiatric Publishing, Inc.

Orellana, L., Rotnitzky, A., & Robins, J. M. (2010). Dynamic regime marginal structural mean models for estimation of optimal dynamic treatment regimes, part I: Main content. *International Journal of Biostatistics*, 6(2).

Osler, W. (1893). *The principles and practice of medicine*. New York: D. Appleton and Company.

Robins, J. M. (1986). A new approach to causal inference in mortality studies with a sustained exposure period—Application to control of the healthy worker survivor effect. *Mathematical Modelling*, 7(9), 1393–1512.

Robins, J. M. (1987). Addendum to "A new approach to causal inference in mortality studies with a sustained exposure period application to control of the healthy worker survivor effect."*Computers & Mathematics with Applications*, 14(9), 923–945.

Robins, J. M. (1989). The analysis of randomized and non-randomized AIDS treatment trials using a new approach to causal inference in longitudinal studies. *Health Service Research Methodology: A Focus on AIDS*, 113, 159.

Robins, J. M. (1993). Information recovery and bias adjustment in proportional hazards regression analysis of randomized trials using surrogate markers. In *Proceedings of the Biopharmaceutical Section, American Statistical Association*. 24(3), 3.

Robins, J. M. (1997). Causal inference from complex longitudinal data. In *Latent variable modeling and applications to causality*(pp. 69–117). New York:Springer.

Robins, J. M. (1998).*Marginal structural models*. In *1997 Proceedings of the American Statistical Association, Section on Bayesian Statistical Science*(pp. 1–10). Robins, J. M. (1999). Testing and estimation of direct effects by reparameterizing directed acyclic graphs with structural nested models. In *Computation, causation, and discovery* (pp. 349–405) . Menlo Park, CA: AAAI Press.

Robins, J. M. (2004). Optimal structural nested models for optimal sequential decisions. In *Proceedings of the Second Seattle Symposium in Biostatistics*189–326.

Sachs, G. S., Guille, C., & McMurrich, S. L. (2002). A clinical monitoring form for mood disorders. *Bipolar Disorders*, 4(5), 323–327.

Sachs, G. S., Thase, M. E., Otto, M. W., Bauer, M., Miklowitz, D., Wisniewski, S. R., . . . Frank, E. (2003). Rationale, design, and methods of the systematic treatment enhancement program for bipolar disorder (STEP-BD). *Bipolar Psychiatry*, 53(11), 1028–1042.

Schulte, P. J., Tsiatis, A. A., Laber, E. B., & Davidian, M. (2014). Q-and a-learning methods for estimating optimal dynamic treatment regimes. *Statistical Science. in press.*

Shortreed, S., Laber, E., Stroup, S., Pineau, J., & Murphy, S. (2014). A multiple imputation strategy for sequential multiple assignment randomized trials. *Statistical in Medicine* 33(24), 4202–4214.

Su, X., Tsai, C.-L., Wang, H., Nickerson, D. M., & Li, B. (2009). Subgroup analysis via recursive partitioning. *Journal of Machine Learning Research, 10,* 141–158.

Su, X., Zhou, T., Yan, X., Fan, J., & Yang, S. (2008). Interaction trees with censored survival data. *International Journal of Biostatistics, 4*(1), 1–26.

The Methodology Center. (2014). Projects using SMARTs. State College: Pennsylvania State University. Retreived from http://methodology.psu.edu/ra/smart/projects

Van Der Laan, M. J. (2006). *Causal effect models for intention to treat and realistic individualized treatment rules.*

Van Der Laan, M. J., & Petersen, M. L. (2007). Causal effect models for realistic individualized treatment and intention to treat rules. *International Journal of Biostatistics, 3*(1), 3.

Velleman, P. F., & Hoaglin, D. C. (1981). *Applications, basics, and computing of exploratory data analysis.* Boston: Duxbury Press.

Wu, F., Laber, E. B., Lipkovich, I., & Severus. (in press). Estimating optimal treatment regimes in STEP-BD study using Q-learning. *Preprint,* pp. 1–26.

Zhang, B., Tsiatis, A. A., Davidian, M., Zhang, M., & Laber, E. (2012). Estimating optimal treatment regimes from a classification perspective. *Stat, 1*(1), 103–114.

Zhang, B., Tsiatis, A. A., Laber, E. B., & Davidian, M. (2012). A robust method for estimating optimal treatment regimes. *Biometrics, 68*(4), 1010–1018.

Zhang, B., Tsiatis, A. A., Laber, E. B., & Davidian, M. (2013). Robust estimation of optimal dynamic treatment regimes for sequential treatment decisions. *Biometrika, 100*(3), 681–694.

Zhao, Y., Zeng, D., Rush, A. J., & Kosorok, M. R. (2012). Estimating individualized treatment rules using outcome weighted learning. *Journal of the American Statistical Association, 107*(499), 1106–1118.

Zhao, Y., Zeng, D., Socinski, M. A., & Kosorok, M. R. (2011). Reinforcement learning strategies for clinical trials in nonsmall cell lung cancer. *Biometrics, 67*(4), 1422–1433.

45.

TRADITIONAL AND NOVEL RESEARCH SYNTHESIS APPROACHES TO SUPPORT EVIDENCE-BASED TREATMENT DECISIONS

Levente Kriston and Ayşegül Yildiz

INTRODUCTION

BACKGROUND

Choosing the best treatment option for bipolar disorder has become increasingly complex. Following the principles of *evidence-based medicine* (EBM), treatment decisions should be based on empirical research findings (Sackett, Rosenberg, Gray, Haynes, & Richardson, 1996). These findings may encompass a wide range of clinical study designs, including observational and experimental studies. However, to extract and use decision-relevant information from a continuously accumulating amount of clinical research data may easily become unmanageable for health-care providers and policymakers. In fact, as medical care providers trying to deliver best-treatment decisions we are, like in several other domains of modern society, "drowning in information but starved for knowledge" (Naisbitt, 1988).

For disentangling the challenge of information overload in EBM, evidence has to be synthesized. This *evidence or research synthesis* can be performed in several ways. A rather unstructured, subjective, and implicit approach to research synthesis is frequently described as *narrative review* (sometimes called literature review). Although they are frequently useful, the validity of narrative reviews can be difficult to assess. Based on the unsystematic approach and insufficient reporting, it is not always clear exactly which research question the authors of a narrative review address, how they search for and include evidence, and how they synthesize the findings and reach their conclusions. Thus narrative reviews usually do not fulfill the essential criterion of positivist science: reproducibility.

A research synthesis approach that uses an explicit and reproducible methodology is termed *systematic review*. A systematic review attempts to collect and summarize all the empirical evidence that fits prespecified criteria in order to answer a research question (Oxman & Guyatt, 1993). The fundamental characteristics of a systematic review include a clearly and specifically formulated research question; prespecified eligibility criteria for the inclusion of studies; a systematic, documented, and comprehensive search for studies that fulfill the eligibility criteria; a standardized approach for study inclusion; an assessment of the risk of bias in the included studies, individually as well as overall for the conducted review; data extraction; a systematic presentation of the characteristics of the studies; and a systematic, quantitative or qualitative, method of data synthesis (Egger, Smith, & Altman, 2001; Higgins & Green, 2011). Systematic reviews are performed with a view for minimizing bias and are likely to provide more reliable findings than narrative ones. Consequently, they increase trustworthiness of the conclusions and provide a solid basis for health-care decisions. Systematic reviews enable not only an objective appraisal of existing evidence that may resolve existing uncertainty regarding treatment effects but also may generate new research questions or demonstrate lack of evidence in specific health care domains (Egger et al., 2001; Higgins & Green, 2011). One of the major drivers of the systematic review methodology is the Cochrane Collaboration, an international network of researchers and clinicians for preparing, maintaining, and disseminating systematic reviews (Bero & Rennie, 1995; Friedrich, 2013). Systematic reviews of the Cochrane Collaboration follow a clearly defined and transparently documented standard (Higgins & Green, 2011) and are frequently referred to as *Cochrane Reviews*.

649

Systematic reviews that employ statistical methods to pool and summarize results of the included studies are called *meta-analyses* (Glass, 1976). By combining findings from all relevant studies, meta-analyses can reduce measurement error of single studies and provide more precise effect estimates for the considered treatment contrasts. They also facilitate exploration of possible differences across findings of the included studies (Higgins & Green, 2011). Actually, by strict meaning, meta-analysis describes the statistical data synthesis step within a systematic review (i.e., the quantitative combination of effect estimates from individual studies into a pooled summary estimate). Nonetheless, a systematic review that applies meta-analysis is often simply referred to as meta-analysis in the medical literature.

Conventionally, most systematic reviews and meta-analyses of treatments address the question of whether a treatment works in comparison to no treatment, an inactive treatment (e.g., placebo pill), or another active treatment (e.g., a widely accepted standard intervention). Thus they compare two treatment conditions with each other and are therefore frequently referred to as *pairwise meta-analysis*. But in everyday clinical practice, an answer to the question of whether a certain treatment works or not is only partially helpful. Clinical decision-making often involves multiple treatment alternatives and sometimes various combinations of them; as such, decision-makers are most interested in the relative benefits and harms of available treatment options. However, well-designed randomized controlled trials (RCTs) involving active treatment comparisons are rare in medical sciences overall and severe mental illnesses in particular, where available evidence is mostly based on placebo-controlled RCTs as requested by the regulatory agencies. At the policy level, this gap in available head-to-head evidence is often addressed by comparative effectiveness research programs (Sox & Greenfield, 2009). Statistically promising tools enabling simultaneous comparisons of multiple treatments, first introduced by Higgins and Whitehead (1996), have become just as popular. Evidence synthesis employing this kind of statistical analysis is termed *multiple treatment comparison meta-analysis, multiple-treatments meta-analysis, mixed treatment comparisons meta-analysis*, or *network meta-analysis* (Caldwell, Ades, & Higgins, 2005; Lumley, 2002; Mills, Thorlund, & Ioannidis, 2013; Salanti, 2012).

In this chapter we provide an overview of traditional and novel evidence synthesis methods. We focus primarily on meta-analysis but consider the whole systematic review process in its context. Since RCTs provide the strongest evidence for determination of benefits and harms

of interventions (Centre for Evidence Based Medicine, 2009), as regularly employed, we discuss meta-analyses that include RCTs. We describe both traditional (pairwise) and multiple treatments (network) meta-analysis by illuminating their underlying assumptions and providing a nontechnical introduction to their statistical procedures. We then deliver some guidance on the technical reporting, as well as the reading and interpretation of meta-analyses. Finally, we highlight future directions on the further development of evidence synthesis methods in general and meta-analysis in particular. In illustration of the described concepts, we employ a working example with real data on antimanic drug treatments for acute mania in bipolar disorder. Although the chapter may be helpful both for performing and reading meta-analysis, it can only offer an introduction. Interested readers are advised to consult the references provided at the end of the chapter for further details.

INTRODUCTION TO THE WORKING EXAMPLE

The treatment of acute mania is a major component in management of bipolar disorder. In this chapter we used an up-to-date (last search date: January 15, 2014) collection of RCTs that compared effectiveness of drug treatments with each other (head-to-head drug comparisons) as monotherapy in treating acute bipolar mania. Studies were included if they compared at least two drugs with each other. Placebo arms (if present) were ignored.

We included 32 trials in our exemplary dataset: 31 of them compared two drugs while 1 investigated three active treatments. Characteristics of the trials are displayed in Table 45.1.

The analyzed sample sizes ranged from 27 to 453 with a median of 178. The majority of the trials (22) had a duration of three weeks, with a range between one and eight weeks. In total, sexes were roughly evenly distributed among the included patients. The proportion of male patients ranged from 20.0% to 59.3% with a median of 48.4%. The median for the mean age of the study samples was 38.6 years with a rather limited range (29.4 to 44.4 years). The trials were fairly homogenous regarding mean baseline severity, expressed as Young Mania Rating Scale (YMRS) scores (median 30.8 points, range 23.8 to 42.4 points). In some of the studies, a substantial proportion of the included patients showed psychotic features (median 26.4%, range 0% to 57.4%). Most trials (25) reported adequate blinding, and the majority (24) were commercially funded.

Table 45.1 CHARACTERISTICS OF THE TRIALS INCLUDED IN THE WORKED EXAMPLE

STUDY	INVESTIGATED DRUGS	N	DURATION (WEEKS)	SEX (MALE %)	AGE (MEAN, YRS)	BASELINE SEVERITY[A]	PSYCHOTIC (%)[B]	BLINDING[C]	FUNDING
Berk, 1999	Lithium, olanzapine	30	4	56.7	30.7	35.8	n.r.	yes	Public
Bowden, 1994	Lithium, valproate	105	3	59.0	39.4	30.8	22.9	yes	Commercial
Bowden, 2000	Lithium, lamotrigine	152	6	50.0	37.7	33.0	50.0	yes	Commercial
Bowden, 2005	Lithium, quetiapine	205	3	57.6	38.4	33.0	24.9	yes	Commercial
Freeman, 1992	Lithium, valproate	27	3	22.2	n.r.	n.r.	n.r.	no	Public
Goldsmith, 2003	Lithium, lamotrigine	121	3	53.7	38.6	29.8	37.2	yes	Commercial
Ichim, 2000	Lithium, lamotrigine	30	4	53.3	32.7	37.4	0.0	yes	Public
Kakkar, 2009	Valproate, oxcarbazepine	60	3	55.0	29.4	34.2	n.r.	no	Public
Katagiri, 2012	Olanzapine, haloperidol	125	3	48.4	44.4	27.5	16.9	yes	Commercial
Keck, 2009	Lithium, aripiprazole	325	3	51.7	39.7	28.9	21.5	yes	Commercial
Kushner, 2006a	Lithium, topiramate	230	3	35.8	41.0	30.8	21.4	yes	Commercial
Kushner, 2006b	Lithium, topiramate	333	3	46.6	42.4	30.4	31.1	yes	Commercial
Li, 2008	Lithium, quetiapine	155	4	47.4	33.2	29.6	27.9	yes	Commercial
McElroy, 1996	Valproate, haloperidol	36	1	58.3	35.9	36.6	n.r.	no	Public
McIntyre, 2005	Quetiapine, haloperidol	201	3	36.7	42.3	33.2	40.7	yes	Commercial
McIntyre, 2009	Olanzapine, asenapine	385	3	59.2	39.4	28.4	29.7	yes	Commercial
McIntyre, 2010	Olanzapine, asenapine	390	3	53.6	38.4	29.6	36.3	yes	Commercial
Niufan, 2008	Lithium, olanzapine	140	4	47.1	32.6	33.2	13.6	yes	Commercial
Perlis, 2006	Olanzapine, risperidone	329	3	45.3	37.9	26.6	0.0	no	Commercial
Segal, 1998	Lithium, risperidone, haloperidol	45	4	22.2	33.3	27.3	n.r.	no	Commercial
Shafii, 2010	Lithium, olanzapine	40	3	n.r.	n.r.	36.8	n.r.	no	Public
Small, 1991	Lithium, carbamazepine	48	8	43.8	38.5	30.6	n.r.	yes	Public
Smulevich, 2005	Risperidone, haloperidol	298	3	54.0	39.7	31.7	34.6	yes	Commercial

Table 45.1 CONTINUED

STUDY	INVESTIGATED DRUGS	N	DURATION (WEEKS)	SEX (MALE %)	AGE (MEAN, YRS)	BASELINE SEVERITY[A]	PSYCHOTIC (%)[B]	BLINDING[C]	FUNDING
Tohen, 2002	Valproate, olanzapine	251	3	42.6	40.6	27.7	45.4	yes	Commercial
Tohen, 2003	Olanzapine, haloperidol	453	6	39.7	40.5	30.9	57.4	yes	Commercial
Tohen, 2008	Valproate, olanzapine	416	3	46.3	40.0	23.8	0.0	yes	Commercial
Vasudev, 2000	Valproate, carbamazepine	30	4	20.0	n.r.	42.4	n.r.	yes	Public
Vieta, 2005	Aripiprazole, haloperidol	347	3	38.3	41.8	31.3	0.0	no	Commercial
Vieta, 2010a	Quetiapine, paliperidone	388	3	58.9	39.0	27.4	21.5	yes	Commercial
Vieta, 2010b	Ziprasidone, haloperidol	350	3	59.3	37.8	34.1	32.1	yes	Commercial
Young, 2009	Aripiprazole, haloperidol	332	3	43.4	40.6	27.8	9.0	yes	Commercial
Zajecka, 2002	Valproate, olanzapine	120	3	51.7	38.5	35.7	34.8	yes	Commercial

NOTE. n.r. = not reported; *N* = number of randomized patients.

[A]Mean expressed as Young Mania Rating Scale score (if necessary transformed to range from 0 to 60). [B]Proportion of sample with psychotic features. [C]Blinding described and appropriate.

DATA REQUIREMENTS

The most widespread method of meta-analysis requires study-level data. Although approaches for using participant-level data from trials in so-called individual participant data meta-analyses are sometimes available (Riley, Lambert, & Abo-Zaid, 2010; Stewart et al., 2012), due to the limited access to complete data from clinical trials, such meta-analyses are not routinely performed. Study-level summary data is frequently obtainable from journal publications and other study reports, so their utilization is straightforward. Although not all of them are needed for the statistical data analysis, descriptive demographic (e.g., sex distribution and mean age of the sample) and clinical (e.g., mean disease severity, diagnostic subtype distribution) information about the investigated patient population is essential for interpreting the findings. Details on the examined treatment(s) (e.g., agents, treatment durations, dosage) are also needed for obtaining a thorough answer on the posed research question. In addition, often information on the internal validity (methodological rigor) of the included trials is obtained. Finally, summary outcome data should be available for all treatment arms separately (e.g., mean scores on disease severity scales, number of participants responding to each treatment) in order to be able to perform a meta-analysis. In several cases, the form of data presentation varies substantially across reports of the included trials so that calculation or imputation of missing data or transformation of reported data may be necessary (Egger et al., 2001; Higgins & Green, 2011).

In the conduct of meta-analysis, several different data types can be considered (Higgins & Green, 2011). Major data types include dichotomous or binary data (where each individual's outcome is one of two possible categories, e.g., response or nonresponse to treatment); continuous or interval-level data (where each individual's outcome is a measured quantity, e.g., a disease severity scale score); counts or rates (where each individual's outcome is the number of experienced events by the individual, e.g., number of adverse events); and time-to-event or survival data (where each individual's outcome is a time period until a prespecified event occurs but not all individuals experience the event during the observation, e.g., time to relapse). The availability and nature of the quantifiable data play a major role in determining which effect measure should be employed in the conduct of a meta-analysis.

EFFECT MEASURES

Although further alternatives are available, among of the most commonly employed effect measures for *binary data* are the risk ratio (RR, also called relative risk), odds ratio (OR), risk difference (RD), and number needed to treat (NNT). The calculation of these measures is displayed in Table 45.2.

Two of these measures are *relative* (risk ratio and odds ratio) and usually preferred for meta-analysis over the other options. While the risk ratio is easily interpretable as the factorial increase in the probability of experiencing an event in the experimental group compared to the control group, interpretation of the odds ratio may be challenging. If the event rate in the control group remains below 15%, odds ratios and risk ratios will yield largely similar values and odds ratios can be interpreted roughly as risk ratios. If the control group event rates are higher, odds ratios can be converted into risk ratios for interpretation, for example using the formulae in Table 45.2 (Grant, 2014). Both for odds ratio and risk ratio, values above 1 indicate an increased event rate in the experimental group, while values below 1 indicate more events in the control group. Thus whether a high or a low value points to superiority of the experimental intervention depends on the nature of the outcome. If the outcome is negative (e.g., death), values below 1 show benefits for the experimental intervention. If the outcome is positive (e.g., response to treatment), relative risks and odds ratios above 1 show superiority. For both outcome measures, statistical calculations are performed on the log scale and results are transformed back to the original scale for interpretation.

The risk difference and number needed to treat are *absolute* (but still comparative) measures and rather seldom used for meta-analysis, mainly due to their disadvantageous statistical characteristics. However, they are preferred by clinicians because of ease of interpretation. The risk difference corresponds to everyday language, while the number needed to treat can be interpreted as the expected number of individuals who need to receive the experimental rather than the control intervention for one additional person to either experience a beneficial or avoid an adverse outcome in a given time frame (Cook & Sackett, 1995). Frequently, after calculations were carried out on the relative measures (RR and OR), the overall results are often transformed into risk difference and number need to treat to enhance clinical interpretation of the findings.

In the case of *continuous outcomes,* effect measures (also called effect sizes) can be expressed as (standardized) mean differences. For this, both data collected at the

Table 45.2 CALCULATION OF COMMON EFFECT MEASURES FROM BINARY DATA

The Results of Trials Can be Expressed in A 2 × 2 Table:

	EVENT	NO EVENT	TOTAL
Control group	a1	b1	n1 (=a1 + b1)
Experimental group	a2	b2	n2 (=a2 + b2)

a1, b1, a2, b2 are number of individuals with the corresponding outcome (event or no event) in each treatment group (experimental or control intervention)

Risk of event in the control group *(rC)*	$rC = \dfrac{a1}{n1} = \dfrac{oC}{1+oC}$
Risk of event in the experimental group *(rE)*	$rE = \dfrac{a2}{n2} = \dfrac{oE}{1+oE}$
Odds of event in the control group *(oC)*	$oC = \dfrac{a1}{b1} = \dfrac{rC}{1-rC}$
Odds of event in the experimental group *(oE)*	$oE = \dfrac{a2}{b2} = \dfrac{rE}{1-rE}$
Risk ratio (relative risk) *(RR)*	$RR = \dfrac{rE}{rC} = \dfrac{a2/n2}{a1/n1} = \dfrac{OR}{1-rC \times (1-OR)}$
Odds ratio *(OR)*	$OR = \dfrac{oE}{oC} = \dfrac{a2/b2}{a1/b1} = \dfrac{a2 \times b1}{a1 \times b2} = \dfrac{RR \times (1-rC)}{1-RR \times rC} = \dfrac{RR-rE}{1-rE}$
Risk difference *(RD)*	$RD = rE - rC = \left(\dfrac{a2}{n2}\right) - \left(\dfrac{a1}{n1}\right)$
Number needed to treat *(NNT)*	$NNT = \dfrac{1}{RD} = \dfrac{1}{rE - rC}$

study endpoint and scores expressing change from baseline can be used. Data pooling on the attained treatment effects by employing the exact same outcome measure can be performed with the units of the original scale, resulting in a simple *mean difference* between the two groups. If different measures were employed to capture the same outcome (e.g., different symptom scales for measuring symptom severity), a uniform scale has to be employed that is named a *standardized mean difference* (SMD). The SMD is comparable across studies and expresses treatment effects relative to the observed variation in the trials, usually in units of standard deviation. Among various ways of standardization Cohen's *d* and Hedges' *g* are among those most commonly employed (Cohen, 1988;

Egger et al., 2001; Lipsey & Wilson, 2001). Although they are advantageous for calculation, their interpretation is not always straightforward due to their abstract nature. In spite of the fact that a general interpretation guideline ignores relevance by the clinical impact of distinct outcomes (e.g., death vs. symptom deterioration) and trial context, a rule of thumb describing SMD of 0.2, 0.5, and 0.8 as small, medium, and large effect sizes, respectively, is indiscreetly still widely applied (Cohen, 1988). It should be noted that for a meta-analysis using (standardized) mean difference as outcome, a measure of variability of the data in the trials is needed in addition to mean values, which is unfortunately not always reported in the original study reports.

DATA AGGREGATION

After the appropriate effect measure has been selected and the effect estimate for each trial has been calculated, the statistical data synthesis can be carried out. Several methods are available to perform a meta-analysis, but all use a *weighting* approach in data aggregation. Thus results from some trials may be more influential for the summary estimate than the others. Although one can think of a multitude of ways to determine the "importance" of each trial (e.g., by methodological rigor), in most cases the weights are derived from the precision of the estimates that a trial provides. The precision, on the other hand, is the inverse of the variance of the effect estimate in a trial, with the variance being the squared standard error of this estimate.

Traditionally, two basic effect models are available for meta-analysis. The *fixed effect model* assumes that a single true effect exists and each trial estimates this true effect with some measurement error. On the other side, the *random effects model* assumes that trial-specific treatment differences are from a common distribution around a global average. Consequently, while in a fixed effect model every source of variation is attributed to sampling error, random effects models allow for additional variation that is considered random due to lack of knowledge (Kriston, 2013). The choice between these models should be made a priori according to the characteristics of the considered trials rather than being based on the results. In general, while during the early years of meta-analysis fixed effects models were common, recently most analysts prefer random effects models, probably due to the more relaxed assumptions they require about the investigated treatment effects. Computations of the pooled effect estimates can be performed via several methods, which can be analytical (i.e., based on closed formulae) or iterative (e.g., restricted maximum likelihood). In random effects meta-analysis, while the analytic method by DerSimonian and Laird (1986) has been conventionally used for a long time, iterative approaches are continuously gaining a foothold, particularly for using complex models and data structures (Cornell et al., 2014).

Irrespective of the chosen model and the computational method, any analysis can be run by using *Bayesian statistics*. As opposed to the traditional, purely data-driven, so-called *frequentist* approach, the Bayesian approach aims for the formalized integration of prior beliefs (i.e., existing knowledge and expectations) and empirical data (Smith, Spiegelhalter, & Thomas, 1995; Sutton & Abrams, 2001). Additionally, in the Bayesian analysis probability statements on the research questions of clinical interest can be made directly, in a way, for example, to state the probability that patients receiving treatment A will have a better outcome than patients receiving treatment B. This leads to some important differences in the output by the two approaches; for example, in Bayesian statistics uncertainty around estimated parameters is quantified with credible intervals (CrI) instead of confidence intervals (CI). Still, although the two traditions have basically different backgrounds, the use of uninformative (also called vague or flat) priors in Bayesian statistics yields results that are often comparable to the frequentist output. With sufficient computing resources and advanced software becoming available, Bayesian meta-analysis is increasingly used, mainly due to its enormous conceptual and mathematical flexibility that enables investigating a wide range of models.

The results of a traditional, either frequentist or Bayesian, meta-analysis are usually displayed as *forest plots* that summarize essential qualitative and quantitative information graphically and numerically. Forest plots include effect estimates and confidence or credible intervals for both individual studies and for pooled summary estimates. In addition, information on weighting is provided in the form of differently sized blocks that draw the eye toward trials with larger weights, which dominate the calculation of the pooled estimate (Higgins & Green, 2011; Lewis & Clarke, 2001).

STATISTICAL HETEROGENEITY

In addition to estimating a summary effect, meta-analysis provides information about the variability of this effect across trials. On the one hand, 95% confidence intervals for the summary statistics are estimated in order to capture sampling variance. On the other hand, tests for *statistical heterogeneity* are performed to investigate whether variability in the results exceed the magnitude that would be expected due to chance (sampling error) alone. A commonly used test statistic is Cochran's Q that examines the null hypothesis that all studies estimate the same effect (Cochran, 1954). A frequently used descriptive measure of the percentage of statistical heterogeneity beyond the amount expected by or solely attributable to chance is the I^2 statistic (Higgins, Thompson, Deeks, & Altman, 2003). I^2 values above 50% to 60% indicate considerable heterogeneity. In random effects models, the τ^2 value is used to describe the variation of the trial-specific effects around the grand average. If the square root of the τ^2 (the between-trial standard deviation) approximates the magnitude of the summary effect, the observed results may not hold across all settings. For quantification of this uncertainty, a so-called *prediction interval* can be calculated that describes the range of effects that is likely to be expected in applications across individual settings (Kriston, 2013; Riley, Higgins, & Deeks, 2011). If the prediction interval contains the value of no effect (zero or 1 depending on effect measure), the observed average summary effect may not be generalizable to contexts beyond the included trials.

If a meta-analysis indicates low or no evidence of heterogeneity, confidence in the computed results would be high. On the contrary, statistical heterogeneity raises doubts concerning the findings, and attempts should be made to explain its sources. Often, statistical heterogeneity can be traced back to clinical and methodological heterogeneity. While *clinical heterogeneity or diversity* describes variation across the trials regarding characteristics of the investigated patient populations and interventions, *methodological heterogeneity or diversity* refers to variation across trials with regard to the applied methods. Attempts in exploration of the sources of heterogeneity involve considerations on those characteristics that can be associated with the observed treatment effects (i.e., whether the computed effect estimates varies across different categories or values). If it does, this characteristic is named a *treatment effect modifier or moderator*. Depending on preference and scaling of the possible moderators, subgroup and meta-regression analyses are frequently employed to explore heterogeneity (Higgins & Green, 2011; Higgins, Thompson, Deeks, & Altman, 2002; Kriston, 2013; Lau, Ioannidis, & Schmid, 1998; Thompson & Sharp, 1999; Thompson, 1994). *Subgroup analysis* is a division of the total set of trials into groups with a subsequent meta-analysis in each group and comparing summary effects between groups. In *meta-regression*, the effect size estimate in each trial is regressed on one or more possible effect moderators. To avoid data dredging, potential effect moderators should be defined a priori whenever possible (Higgins & Green, 2011). Although not aiming directly at exploration of statistical heterogeneity, a similar idea is followed in *sensitivity analyses,* in which the calculations are repeated using different (usually methodological) assumptions, in order to test whether the findings are robust and insensitive to the choices of the analyst.

THE SIMILARITY ASSUMPTION

It is generally accepted that research synthesis by meta-analysis makes sense only if all trials included for comparison are *sufficiently similar*. However, currently there is no consensus on the definition of "sufficiently similar". Indeed, meta-analyses are frequently criticized for "mixing apples with oranges". Eysenck (1978), in one of the first criticisms of meta-analysis stated that "the notion that one can distill scientific knowledge from a compilation of studies... dissimilar with respect to nearly all the vital parameters, dies hard" (p. 517). Smith, Glass, and Miller (1980), who belong to the pioneers of meta-analysis, responded by pointing out that "indeed the approach does mix apples and oranges, as one necessarily would do in studying fruits" (p. 47). Eysenck (1984), again, reacted with a comment stating that "adding apples and oranges may be a pastime for children learning to count, but unless we are willing to disregard the differences between these two kinds of fruit, the result will be meaningless" (p. 57). Later on, it became clear to at least some of the methodologists that "the definition of what study findings are conceptually comparable for purposes of meta-analysis is often fixed only in the eye of the beholder. Findings that appear categorically different to one analyst may seem similar to another" (Lipsey & Wilson, 2001, p. 3)—an insight that is still waiting to be widely accepted by the medical community.

The issue of similarity indeed is strongly related to the concept of clinical heterogeneity. Stating that trials are sufficiently similar equals the judgment that no substantial clinical heterogeneity among them is present that is associated with the treatment effect of interest. Technically, it means that either the distribution of treatment effect moderators across the trials are similar or their moderating effect is taken care of statistically as appropriate (e.g., via adjustment by meta-regression). It should be noted that clinical heterogeneity regarding variables that are not assumed to be associated with the outcome do not limit the validity of the meta-analytic findings but rather strengthen their generalizability. As exemplified earlier, empirical exploration of certain trial characteristics for their potential moderator effects is sometimes feasible by meta-regression and subgroup analyses, although these analyzes usually have insufficient power to detect even important differences (Thompson, 1994). Furthermore, given that undetected treatment effect moderators can always be present theoretically and the threshold for the maximum acceptable unexplained between-trial variation in the random effects model varies broadly, "whether or not to trust pooled effect estimates in a meta-analysis depends largely on the subjective relevance of clinical heterogeneity involved. No single analysis and interpretation strategy can be valid in every context or paradigm, thus, reflection of own beliefs on the role of heterogeneity is needed" (Kriston, 2013, p. 1). Accordingly, the question of whether the included trials are sufficiently similar to enable the drawing of valid conclusions is likely to remain a main focus of discussions about meta-analyses also in the future.

WORKED EXAMPLE ON TRADITIONAL META-ANALYSIS

Consider a meta-analysis aiming to investigate whether second-generation antipsychotics (SGAs) are more effective than mood stabilizers (MSs) for the treatment of acute mania in patients with bipolar disorder. Of the trials identified for our working example, 10 compared a MS with a SGA. These trials included a total of 1,712 patients with the sample size ranging from 30 to 416. The administered MSs were lithium (7 trials) and valproate (3 trials), while the investigated SGAs included olanzapine (6 trials), quetiapine (2 trials), aripiprazole (1 trial), and risperidone (1 trial). The outcome measure was the response to treatment defined as substantial improvement in mania symptoms (≥50% improvement as detected by the Young Mania Rating Scale) between the baseline and study endpoint. For three trials, data on the number of responders were not available and had to be estimated from the symptom change scores based on the assumption of normally distributed values. We chose odds ratio as the effect measure to compare the proportion of responders between MSs and SGAs and used random effects meta-analysis in a frequentist framework to pool findings of the original RCTs. Central results are displayed as a forest plot in Figure 45.1.

Trial weights indicate that the most precise trials contributed around 20% each to the pooled effect estimate. A statistically significant ($p = .023$) summary odds ratio of 1.33 (95%CI: 1.04 to 1.69) suggests a superiority of SGAs over MSs regarding response rates, even if only 2 of the 10 trials

yielded a significant result individually for themselves. Using an expected response rate of 0.47 (47%) for MSs (the median of MS response rates across the trials in the meta-analysis), the observed summary odds ratio of 1.33, and the formulae in Table 45.1 provides an estimated response rate of 0.54 (54%) for SGAs. This gives a risk difference of 7% and a number needed to treat of 14, suggesting a clinically moderate effect. Cochran's Q test for heterogeneity was not statistically significant ($p = .226$), and only limited between-trial heterogeneity was revealed ($\tau^2 = 0.034$ and $\tau = 0.184$ on the log-odds ratio scale, $I^2 = 23.6\%$). However, the 95% prediction interval (OR=0.79 to 2.21) suggests that superiority of SGAs over MSs is unlikely to be present across all individual settings; and even if the between-trial heterogeneity is limited, it still has a substantial impact on the conclusions of the meta-analysis. Although the average effect is statistically significant (the confidence interval of the summary odds ratio does not include one), individual effects vary too strongly (the prediction interval includes one), preventing a broad generalization of the results for the entire pool of settings considered. Briefly, SGAs are more effective than MSs at average but not in all settings.

We conducted some exemplary subgroup analyses according to the MS treatment (lithium vs. valproate), the SGA treatment (olanzapine vs. other), blinding (adequate vs. unclearly described), and funding (commercial vs. public). These analyses revealed no substantial effect moderation according to the administered treatments. Results were comparable for trials investigating lithium (7

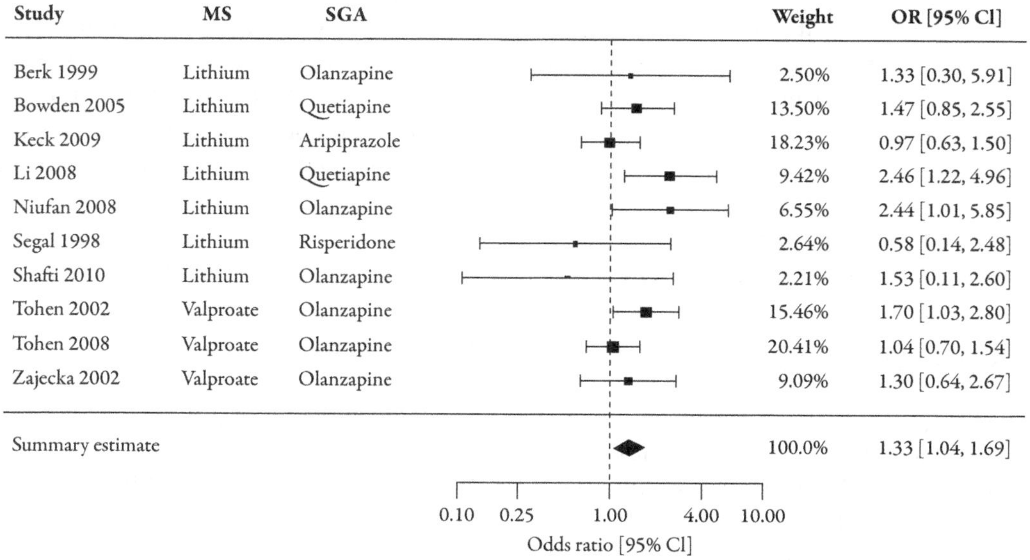

Study	MS	SGA		Weight	OR [95% CI]
Berk 1999	Lithium	Olanzapine		2.50%	1.33 [0.30, 5.91]
Bowden 2005	Lithium	Quetiapine		13.50%	1.47 [0.85, 2.55]
Keck 2009	Lithium	Aripiprazole		18.23%	0.97 [0.63, 1.50]
Li 2008	Lithium	Quetiapine		9.42%	2.46 [1.22, 4.96]
Niufan 2008	Lithium	Olanzapine		6.55%	2.44 [1.01, 5.85]
Segal 1998	Lithium	Risperidone		2.64%	0.58 [0.14, 2.48]
Shafti 2010	Lithium	Olanzapine		2.21%	1.53 [0.11, 2.60]
Tohen 2002	Valproate	Olanzapine		15.46%	1.70 [1.03, 2.80]
Tohen 2008	Valproate	Olanzapine		20.41%	1.04 [0.70, 1.54]
Zajecka 2002	Valproate	Olanzapine		9.09%	1.30 [0.64, 2.67]
Summary estimate				100.0%	1.33 [1.04, 1.69]

0.10 0.25   1.00   4.00 10.00

Odds ratio [95% CI]

Figure 45.1 Forest plot for traditional meta-analysis comparing response rates between mood stabilizers and second-generation antipsychotics in the worked example. MS=mood stabilizer; SGA = second-generation antipsychotic; OR = odds ratio (values above 1 indicate higher response rates in SGAs); CI = confidence interval

studies, OR = 1.37 [0.93; 2.02]) and valproate (3 studies, OR = 1.27 [0.93; 1.74]), as well as with olanzapine (6 studies, OR = 1.33 [0.99; 1.77]) and other SGAs (4 studies, OR = 1.32 [0.82; 2.13]). Confidence intervals were substantially overlapping for estimates in adequately blinded (8 studies, OR = 1.38 [1.08; 1.76]) and unclearly blinded (2 studies, OR = 0.56 [0.19; 1.63]) trials, as well as in commercially funded (8 studies, OR = 1.36 [1.05; 1.77]) and publicly funded (2 studies, OR = 0.87 [0.29; 2.57]) trials, although the fact that the general direction of the effect is opposite between these subgroups decreases the confidence in the findings to some degree. A meta-regression analysis investigating whether mean baseline mania severity is associated with the observed treatment effect (i.e., whether it is an effect moderator) led to a statistically not significant result ($p = .540$) suggesting that the observed summary estimate may hold across the whole severity spectrum of the included trials. A sensitivity analysis excluding trials in which responder data had to be estimated from symptom scores confirmed the results (7 studies, OR = 1.38 [1.02; 1.87]).

This independent analysis supports previous findings based on evidence from head-to-head RCTs (Tarr, Glue, & Herbison, 2011; Yildiz, Vieta, Leucht, & Baldessarini, 2011). However, some health-care professionals may claim that applicability of these findings is limited for several reasons. First, physicians usually prescribe drugs and not drug classes. Second, clinicians are mostly interested in the comparative effectiveness of all available treatment options. Third, ranking by efficacy among competing interventions may constitute a more practical and solid basis for treatment selection in routine practice. Meeting such clinical requests is possible in the domain of the so-called multiple treatments or network meta-analysis.

MULTIPLE TREATMENTS (NETWORK) META-ANALYSIS

INDIRECT EVIDENCE

Among k treatments, $(k \times (k-1))/2$ pairwise comparisons can be made. Consequently, comparing 10 health-care interventions with a traditional meta-analysis would require performing 45 meta-analyses of trials that directly compare the respective interventions. Although this may be tedious, it is possible and provides trustworthy *direct evidence* on the comparative performance of each pair treatments. However, challenges occur if some pairs of treatments had never been compared in a RCT. In this case, there is no data to analyze, and traditional pairwise meta-analysis is powerless.

To fill the gap caused by the paucity of direct head-to-head comparative evidence, using or, as in the original description, borrowing strength from *indirect evidence* has been proposed (Higgins & Whitehead, 1996). The basic assumption behind involvement of indirect evidence in the context of meta-analysis is transitivity, meaning that if both of two never directly compared treatments A and B have been compared to a third treatment C, the relation of A to C and the relation of B to C can be used to estimate the relation of A to B. Although it may sound convincing at first sight, everyday analogies advise some caution. For example, most people would agree that transitivity causes no problems in estimating height of persons (e.g., if Peter is 8 inches taller than Robert and Thomas is 14 inches taller than Robert, Thomas is likely to be around 6 inches taller than Peter). In contrast, transitivity is more challenging in some various other circumstances. As an extreme example, if the national basketball selection of Spain scores 8 points more than the German team in a game, and the French team scores 14 points more than Germany when they play against each other, most people would be cautious about being too confident that the French team will score 6 points more than Spain in their match. The question to decide is how to place RCT-based indirect comparisons between these two extreme positions of completely trustworthy and largely senseless transitivity.

A simple way to obtain indirect evidence on the relative performance of two treatments A and B using a common comparator C requires the effects of treatment A and B compared to C along with the standard error of these effects (Bucher, Guyatt, Griffith, & Walter, 1997; Song, Altman, Glenny, & Deeks, 2003). These can be based either on a single study or a meta-analysis of several trials. If d_{AC} and d_{BC} are treatment effects with standard errors $SE_{d(AC)}$ and $SE_{d(BC)}$, the relative effect of A versus B can be estimated as

$$d_{AB} = d_{AC} - d_{BC}$$

with standard error

$$SE_{d(AB)} = \sqrt{SE^2_{d(AC)} + SE^2_{d(BC)}}$$

and 95% confidence interval bounds

$$d_{AB} \pm 1.96 \times SE_{d(AB)}.$$

Calculations with relative effect measures using binary outcomes (risk ratio, odds ratio) should be performed on the log-scale. Using the equations (here shown for odds ratio),

$$\log(OR_{AB}) = \log(OR_{AC}) - \log(OR_{BC}) = \log\left(\frac{OR_{AC}}{OR_{BC}}\right)$$

and

$$\exp\left(\log\left(\frac{OR_{AC}}{OR_{BC}}\right)\right) = \frac{OR_{AC}}{OR_{BC}} = OR_{AB};$$

where *log* refers to the natural logarithm and *exp* to the exponential function, and transforming back and forth between the original and logarithmic scale may assist interpretation. For example, it can be seen that the indirectly estimated odds ratio for treatment A versus B is the ratio of the two odds ratios available from the direct comparisons with the common comparator C.

The principle of the "common comparator" can be extended to include more than three treatments. For example, if treatment A was compared to treatment B, B to C, and C to D, indirect evidence comparing A to D can be determined by calculating the indirect evidence for the A versus C comparison first and then repeating the method described previously using this A versus C (now indirect) and D versus C (still direct) information with C as a common comparator. As long as there is a "chain" of linked comparisons between two treatments, indirect evidence for the comparison of the two treatments building the starting point and the end of the chain can always be determined.

EVIDENCE NETWORKS

Mapping all comparative trials for a defined set of treatments provides an *evidence network*. For example, in an evidence network of treatments A, B, C, and D, all trials with A versus B, A versus C, A versus D, B versus C, B versus D, and C versus D comparisons are included (the inclusion of three- and four-arm trials is also possible), if such trials had been performed and identified for the research synthesis. An evidence network is usually presented graphically as a *network diagram* or *network plot*. A network diagram shows the investigated treatments as nodes, while RCTs comparing the respective treatments are displayed as lines (edges) connecting these nodes. Usually, both nodes and edges are used to convey further information. For example, the thickness of edges can be used to inform on the number of trials comparing the respective treatments, while the size of nodes can be defined according to the number of trials (or number of participants) in which the respective treatment was tested.

Depending on the availability of comparative trials, evidence networks can have several forms. A *connected network* is defined as a network in which direct or indirect comparison is possible for any pair of the treatments (i.e., it is possible to start from any node and follow the edges directly or through other nodes to reach any other node). For example, a set of three trials comparing treatments A versus B, B versus C, and C versus D, respectively, defines a connected network. A disconnected network contains "islands," so that neither direct nor indirect comparison is possible between treatments belonging to different islands. For example, a set of two trials with one comparing treatment A to B and another comparing C to D, respectively, defines a disconnected network. In any evidence network, *closed loops* are defined by available trials for a set of treatments in that it is possible to start at any treatment node, to follow the edges via intermediate nodes, and to reach to starting node again (without turning back). In a network of three treatments, a closed loop occurs when each treatment has been compared directly with both of the others (e.g., with three trials comparing A to B, B to C, and A to C, respectively). Closed loops play a particular role in evidence networks because they enable direct evidence on each comparison to be complemented by indirect evidence for the same comparison. A *star-shaped network* is seen when one treatment exists to which all other treatments have been compared in at least one RCT but no direct comparisons were performed for any pair of these remaining treatments. Thus a star-shaped network is a connected network without closed loops.

More often than not, evidence networks are unlike the aforementioned clear prototypes but are rather unstructured, containing more or less star-shaped subsets, closed loops of three or more treatments, and hardly connected or even fully disconnected treatment islands.

CONSISTENCY OF EVIDENCE

In a connected network of trials, for some treatment pairs direct comparisons will be available, and some treatments can be compared indirectly. For some treatment contrasts, both direct and indirect comparative evidence will be present. These treatment contrasts are informed by more than one source of evidence. Statistically, it means that more than one estimate will be available for the same effect. In these cases, it is possible to quantify the *consistency* of these estimates, that is, to measure to which degree they agree and to test whether any difference (disagreement) between them is attributable to chance or should be considered systematic. This investigation can be performed by determining the so called *inconsistency factor,* a quantitative measure of difference between two sources of evidence informing the same effect.

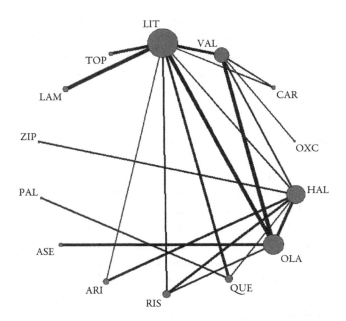

Figure 45.2 Evidence network in the worked example. The line width is proportional to the number of trials that compared each pair of treatments, and the size of each node is proportional to the number of comparisons (two-arm trials) in that each treatment was involved.

ARI = aripiprazole; ASE = asenapine; CAR = carbamazepine; HAL = haloperidol; LAM = lamotrigine; LIT = lithium; OLA = olanzapine; OXC = oxcarbazepine; PAL = paliperidone; QUE = quetiapine; RIS = risperidone; TOP = topiramate; VAL = valproate; ZIP = ziprasidone

In the frequentist framework, labeling evidence form direct comparisons of two treatments d_{dir} with standard error $SE_{d(dir)}$ and indirectly obtained evidence d_{ind} with standard error $SE_{d(ind)}$, the inconsistency factor can be calculated as

$$IF_{dir,ind} = d_{dir} - d_{ind}$$

with standard error

$$SE_{IF(dir,ind)} = \sqrt{SE_{d(dir)}^2 + SE_{d(ind)}^2}$$

and 95% confidence interval bounds

$$IF_{dir,ind} \pm 1.96 \times SE_{d(dir,ind)}.$$

As in the case of obtaining indirect evidence, calculations with relative effect measures using binary outcomes (risk ratio, odds ratio) should be performed on the log-scale. If the 95% confidence interval of the inconsistency factor does not include zero (1 on the original scale of risk ratio or odds ratio), the two investigated sources of evidence should be considered as statistically inconsistent.

While in a network of RCTs direct comparison of the two treatments A and B is possible only in a single way (by

comparing A to B), frequently more than one source of indirect evidence is available (e.g., using a common comparator C, using a common comparator D, using a comparison E vs. F when A vs. E and F vs. B comparisons have been performed, etc.). The concept of consistency can be easily generalized to compare two different sources of indirect evidence. Just like information from a direct and a specific indirect source may agree or not, agreement between estimates from two indirect comparisons can also be calculated. If the estimates from two indirect comparisons are d_{ind1} and d_{ind2}, the inconsistency factor can be determined as

$$IF_{ind1,ind2} = d_{ind1} - d_{ind2}$$

with standard error

$$SE_{IF(ind1,ind2)} = \sqrt{SE_{d(ind1)}^2 + SE_{d(ind2)}^2}.$$

Thus inconsistency can be quantified for any pair of estimates from direct or indirect comparisons. Still, it should be noted that, just like the tests used for exploring heterogeneity, the significance tests based on the inconsistency factors are also frequently underpowered to detect even substantial inconsistency.

WORKED EXAMPLE ON CALCULATIONS BY HAND IN AN EVIDENCE NETWORK

In the example dataset of head-to-head RCTs, 14 drugs were tested. The network of evidence is connected (see Figure 45.2).

Most comparisons have been made with the mood stabilizers lithium and valproate, the first-generation antipsychotic haloperidol, and the second-generation antipsychotic olanzapine. As evidence directly comparing these treatments is available, they build a few closed loops.

Comparative evidence for four other treatments (the mood stabilizer carbamazepine and the second-generation antipsychotics quetiapine, risperidone, and aripiprazole) is rather scarce, but each of them is still involved in at least one closed loop. Each of the five other treatments (the mood stabilizer oxcarbazepine; the second-generation antipsychotics asenapine, paliperidone, and ziprasidone; and the anticonvulsants lamotrigine and topiramate) has been compared to only one other drug.

For a moment, assume that we aim to get indirect evidence to estimate the relative effectiveness of lithium and olanzapine. Searching for a common comparator reveals that both were tested against valproate. A random effects meta-analysis of two trials on lithium versus valproate comparison provides an odds ratio of 1.89 [95% CI: 0.34; 10.43] (log OR = 0.6369, SE(log OR) = 0.8717). In a meta-analysis of three studies comparing olanzapine with valproate, we obtain an odds ratio of 1.27 [0.93; 1.74] (log OR = 0.2409, SE(log OR) = 0.1596). Using the formulae provided previously, we obtain the indirect estimate for the comparison of lithium and olanzapine as log OR = 0.6369–0.2409 = 0.3960. The standard error of this indirect estimate is SE(log OR) = $\sqrt{(0.8717^2+0.1596^2)}$ = 0.8862, leading to the 95% confidence bounds 0.3960±1.96 × 0.8862. Exponentiation of these values reveals an odds ratio of 1.49 [0.26; 8.44], indicating no statistically significant difference between lithium and olanzapine.

Both lithium and olanzapine were also tested against haloperidol. The only study comparing lithium to haloperidol shows an odds ratio of 1.71 [0.40; 7.29] (log OR = 0.5390, SE(log OR) = 0.7387). A meta-analysis of the two RCTs testing olanzapine versus haloperidol gives an odds ratio of 0.75 [0.53; 1.06] (log OR = –0.2893, SE(log OR) = 0.1784). The indirect estimate for the comparison of lithium with olanzapine is an odds ratio of 2.29 [0.52; 10.15] (log OR = 0.8283, SE(log OR) = 0.7599). The indirectly estimated odds ratio for the lithium versus olanzapine comparison using risperidone as common comparator is 1.57 [0.35; 7,15] (log OR = 0.4525, SE(log OR) = 0.7725). Note that it is possible to identify even more ways of quantifying indirect evidence for comparing lithium with olanzapine, for example through the path with aripiprazole and haloperidol as intermediate treatment nodes.

In our exemplary evidence network, three RCTs directly compared lithium with olanzapine. A traditional meta-analysis of these trials results in an odds ratio of 0.68 [0.29; 1.61] (log OR = –0.3843, SE(log OR) = 0.4383).

Even if neither of the direct nor any of the here displayed indirect comparisons indicates a statistically significant difference between lithium and olanzapine (all confidence intervals include 1), it is notable that while the direct comparison tends to support olanzapine, all performed indirect comparisons show some benefit for lithium. We can compute the inconsistency factors to check whether this apparent disagreement is statistically significant. The inconsistency of the evidence form direct comparisons and information from the indirect comparison using valproate as the common comparator can be determined as IF = –0.3843 – 0.3960 = –0.7803 with a standard error $\sqrt{(0.4383^2 + 0.8862^2)}$ = 0.9887, providing the 95% confidence interval for the inconsistency factor as –0.7803 ± 1.96 × 0.9887. Exponentiation of these values results in an inconsistency factor of 0.46 [0.07; 3.18], indicating that although the support for lithium from direct comparisons is at average only half as strong as from

the indirect comparison using valproate as the common comparator, the uncertainty of the inconsistency factor is very high (including the value of 1, i.e., no inconsistency) and thus limits any definite conclusion on inconsistency between direct and indirect evidence. Note that based on logarithmic identities, this inconsistency factor can also obtained as the ratio of the corresponding odds ratios (i.e., 0.68/1.49). Due to the fact that the standard errors of the other two indirect estimates (using haloperidol and risperidone as common comparators, respectively) are also rather large, uncertainty of the inconsistency factors in comparing them to the direct estimate (haloperidol, IF = 0.68/2.29 = 0.30; risperidone, IF = 0.68/1.57 = 0.43) is also very high and includes the value of no inconsistency (as such being statistically not significant). In summary, even if we could not obtain statistical evidence for inconsistency, the fact that all computed indirect evidence suggested benefit for lithium and the direct evidence favored olanzapine (with a doubled to tripled average benefit for olanzapine compared to lithium) may raise justified skepticism about the consistency of the whole body of evidence comparing these two treatments.

SIMULTANEOUS EVIDENCE SYNTHESIS VIA NETWORK META-ANALYSIS

If both direct and one or more indirect sources of evidence are available for a comparison in an evidence network, it is possible combine the estimates from these sources within traditional meta-analysis. Although it is imaginable to combine different sources of evidence for each comparison in an evidence network with distinct pairwise meta-analyses, it can be cumbersome if many treatments are compared and the network is complex with several possible sources of indirect evidence. It also raises some technical challenges, particularly for random effects models and in networks containing multiarm trials (that compare more than two treatments).

A simultaneous synthesis of the whole body of evidence in a network is possible with *network meta-analysis,* also called multiple treatment comparison meta-analysis, multiple-treatments meta-analysis, or mixed treatment comparisons meta-analysis (Caldwell et al., 2005; Lumley, 2002; Mills et al., 2013; Salanti, 2012). This method is based on the principles of meta-regression, requires the same input as traditional pairwise meta-analysis, and combines all direct and indirect evidence in a network of treatments. Network meta-analysis provides the output known from traditional meta-analysis for each comparison, including effect estimates, standard errors, and confidence or credible bounds, as well as an estimate of the between-trial variation in random effects models.

Network meta-analysis is commonly conducted by using the *Bayesian* approach because of its ability to deal with multi arm trials and to enable ranking of all considered treatments by efficacy or safety using probabilistic methods. Thus it makes it possible to determine the probability to which a certain treatment is the best, the second best, and so on. This information is usually displayed in so called *rankograms*. It also enables calculation of a single measure to summarize probabilistic ranking information, the *surface under the cumulative ranking curve* (SUCRA; Salanti, Ades, & Ioannidis, 2011). The SUCRA is a strongly aggregated statistic ranging from 0% (worst treatment) to 100% (best treatment). Such probability statements and SUCRA-based rankings are clinically attractive for global judgments. However, they are sometimes criticized for neglecting statistical uncertainty in their presentation (Ioannidis, 2009) and can be sensitive to small changes in the distribution of the effect estimates (Salanti et al., 2011). Further, high probabilities in low ranks do not necessarily indicate the most effective treatments, thus they should always be reported by accompanying effect-size measures.

Among the complexities of performing network meta-analysis in the context of the Bayesian approach is the necessity to define prior distributions for the modeled parameters and the simulation-based estimations with Markov Cain Monte Carlo algorithms. Thus expert statistical support for performing network meta-analyses is strongly recommended. Bayesian network meta-analysis applies a relatively complex statistical model (Dias, Sutton, Ades, & Welton, 2013), of which fit to the observed data can be measured using the deviance information criterion (Spiegelhalter, Best, Carlin, & Van Der Linde, 2002). The deviance information criterion is a fit measure that is adjusted for parsimony; that is, it prefers not only models that show little deviance form the data but also simple models with a low number of estimated parameters. In model comparisons, a lower value of the deviance information criterion indicates a better model. Roughly, a difference above 2 to 3 points is likely to be pragmatically relevant.

Network meta-analysis is being increasingly used for comparative effectiveness research in mental disorders. Notable examples include the investigation of second-generation antidepressants in major depression (Cipriani et al., 2009; Gartlehner et al., 2011); all antidepressants in primary care (Ramsberg, Asseburg, & Henriksson, 2012); psychological interventions for depression (Barth et al., 2013) and for posttraumatic stress disorder (Gerger et al., 2014); pharmacological and psychological interventions for persistent depressive disorder (Kriston, von Wolff, Westphal, Hölzel, & Härter, 2014) and for social anxiety disorder (Mayo-Wilson et al., 2014); commonly employed drugs for anxiety disorders in children and adolescents (Uthman & Abdulmalik, 2010) and for generalized anxiety disorder in adults (Baldwin, Woods, Lawson, & Taylor, 2011); treatments for smoking cessation (Mills et al., 2012); antimanic drugs for treatment of acute bipolar mania (Cipriani et al., 2011; Yildiz, Nikodem, Vieta, Correll, & Baldessarini, 2014); and antipsychotic drugs in schizophrenia (Hartling et al., 2012; Leucht et al., 2013).

ASSUMPTIONS IN NETWORK META-ANALYSIS

The assumptions behind network meta-analysis are very similar to the assumptions behind traditional pairwise meta-analysis but are required to hold across the entire set of trials (Caldwell et al., 2005). Although several different formulations of the assumptions are possible and they are not completely independent from each other, they can be broadly described with three terms: similarity, homogeneity, and consistency (Donegan, Williamson, D'Alessandro, & Tudor Smith, 2013; Jansen et al., 2011; Mills et al., 2013; Salanti, 2012).

The assumption of *similarity* (sometimes termed transitivity or comparability) can be simplified to the requirement that all trials should be clinically and methodologically sufficiently similar to each other to provide valid conclusions. In a set of similar trials, the true difference between treatment A and B in direct A versus B trials would be identical to (fixed effects model) or from the same common distribution as (random effects model) the A versus B difference estimated from indirect comparisons. This is equivalent to the assumption that there is either no imbalance in the distribution of effect moderators across the different treatment comparisons or that no moderators exist. As a way to comprehend this, one can imagine that all trials had examined all treatments of interest but that in each trial results for all but the actually reported two or three treatments had been randomly lost (Caldwell et al., 2005; Yildiz, Vieta, Correll, Nikodem, & Baldessarini, 2014). The specific assumption here is the similarity of the relative effects of treatments across the entire set of trials, irrespective of which treatments were actually evaluated (i.e., that the trials are "exchangeable" in their patient samples, design, conduct, and outcome measures). The similarity requirement cannot be fully validated by the data themselves, so well-informed clinical judgment is essential (Lu & Ades, 2004; Yildiz et al., 2014).

The assumption of *homogeneity* is analogous to the heterogeneity issues discussed in traditional meta-analysis earlier. It requires that no or only modest unexplained statistical heterogeneity is present among trials. It should be noted that this is not strictly a statistical assumption but rather a requirement for a convincing interpretation of the results in the context of network meta-analysis. Evaluation of homogeneity to a certain degree is possible by empirical means. As described for the context of traditional meta-analysis, tests for heterogeneity assessment can be performed also for network meta-analysis, and the estimate for the between-trial variability can be assessed for the computed treatment effects. In addition, fixed and random effects models can be compared globally using the deviance information criterion. If heterogeneity is identified, meta-regression known from traditional meta-analysis can be used for its exploration, although its application is considerably more complex in the context of network meta-analysis (Dias, Sutton, Welton, & Ades, 2013).

The assumption of *consistency* requires that estimates from different sources of evidence for a comparison agree. Broadly, consistency can be defined as homogeneity across comparisons. As noted previously, consistency of each comparison that is informed by at least two sources of evidence can be tested using inconsistency factors. In addition, global testing is also possible by comparing the deviance information criterion of models with and without the consistency restriction (Dias, Welton, et al., 2013). Several other methods have been described to investigate inconsistency (Dias, Welton, Caldwell, & Ades, 2010; Donegan, Williamson, D'Alessandro, & Tudor Smith, 2012; Krahn, Binder, & König, 2013; White, Barrett, Jackson, & Higgins, 2012), although their widespread application is somewhat limited by their complexity. Although the term *inconsistency* is commonly used to describe disagreement between direct and indirect sources of evidence, inconsistency among two or more sources of indirect evidence is also possible. It is relevant that testing of inconsistency requires that closed loops are present in an evidence network. Thus, for example, consistency checking for a star-shaped network is practically not possible. Tests for inconsistency checking yield substantial information only on the condition that the network involves a sufficient number of closed loops. Even then, the power of detecting inconsistency will strongly depend on the strategy to address the homogeneity assumption (Veroniki, Mavridis, Higgins, & Salanti, 2014). If some residual heterogeneity is tolerated by the analysts, it may weaken consistency tests and mask inconsistency.

Generally, all three assumptions require that there is either limited or no variability present in the evidence network regarding certain entities. For the similarity assumption, clinical and methodological variability across trials with regard to characteristics that are potential treatment effect modifiers should be minimal. For the homogeneity assumption, variability across estimates for the same treatment effects from different trials should be limited. For consistency, variability in treatment effects as estimated from different sources evidence (e.g., direct vs. indirect comparisons) should be low. Since the logic behind statistical testing allows rejection but not confirmation of the absence of variation, even if we do not identify significant dissimilarity, heterogeneity, or inconsistency, we still cannot claim that they are not there; in other words, "Absence of evidence is not evidence of absence" (Altman & Bland, 1995, p. 485). Moreover, statistical tests for testing the assumptions, if feasible at all, often have limited power.

WORKED EXAMPLE ON NETWORK META-ANALYSIS

We performed a Bayesian network meta-analysis in the example dataset including 14 drug treatments for acute mania (see trial characteristics and the evidence network described earlier). In 32 RCTs investigating these drugs, a total of 6,497 subjects were included.

In the basic model of random effects network meta-analysis consistency is assumed, so that from a set of effect estimates all other estimates can be calculated. Knowing the effects for a certain treatment compared to all other treatments, pairwise estimates for the other treatments can be determined. Figure 45.3 displays effect (odds ratio based on response) estimates for all treatments compared to lithium as reference.

No statistically significant difference was determined between lithium and all drugs but to-piramate. To-piramate was significantly less effective than lithium with an odds ratio of 0.47 [95% CrI: 0.25; 0.69], meaning that the odds of response in patients treated with topiramate is less than half of the odds of response in patients treated with lithium. Estimates from all pairwise comparisons (not shown in detail) revealed some further differences. Topiramate was also statistically significantly less effective than valproate (OR = 0.56, with 95% CrI [0.20; 0.86]), haloperidol (OR = 0.31 [0.16; 0.63]), olanzapine (OR = 0.33 [0.17; 0.65]), quetiapine (OR = 0.31 [0.15; 0.61]), risperidone (OR = 0.33 [0.15; 0.75]), aripiprazole (OR = 0.30 [0.14; 0.64]), and paliperidone (OR = 0.25 [0.09; 0.69]). Ziprasidone was outperformed by haloperidol (OR = 0.42 [0.21; 0.82]),

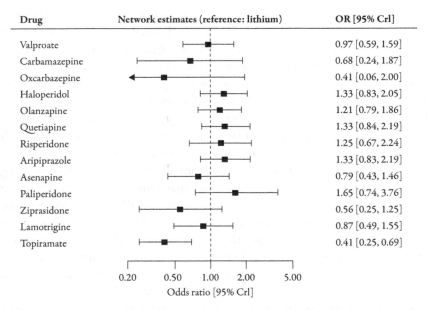

Drug	Network estimates (reference: lithium)	OR [95% CrI]
Valproate		0.97 [0.59, 1.59]
Carbamazepine		0.68 [0.24, 1.87]
Oxcarbazepine		0.41 [0.06, 2.00]
Haloperidol		1.33 [0.83, 2.05]
Olanzapine		1.21 [0.79, 1.86]
Quetiapine		1.33 [0.84, 2.19]
Risperidone		1.25 [0.67, 2.24]
Aripiprazole		1.33 [0.83, 2.19]
Asenapine		0.79 [0.43, 1.46]
Paliperidone		1.65 [0.74, 3.76]
Ziprasidone		0.56 [0.25, 1.25]
Lamotrigine		0.87 [0.49, 1.55]
Topiramate		0.41 [0.25, 0.69]

Odds ratio [95% CrI]

Figure 45.3 Effect (response odds ratio) estimates in random effects network meta-analysis for all treatments compared to lithium. OR = odds ratio (values above 1 indicate higher response rates in the drug named in the rows); CrI = credible interval

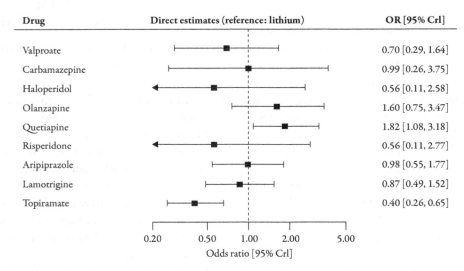

Drug	Direct estimates (reference: lithium)	OR [95% CrI]
Valproate		0.70 [0.29, 1.64]
Carbamazepine		0.99 [0.26, 3.75]
Haloperidol		0.56 [0.11, 2.58]
Olanzapine		1.60 [0.75, 3.47]
Quetiapine		1.82 [1.08, 3.18]
Risperidone		0.56 [0.11, 2.77]
Aripiprazole		0.98 [0.55, 1.77]
Lamotrigine		0.87 [0.49, 1.52]
Topiramate		0.40 [0.26, 0.65]

Odds ratio [95% CrI]

Figure 45.4 Effect (response odds ratio) estimates in random effects meta-analysis for all treatments that were directly compared to lithium. OR = odds ratio (values above 1 indicate higher response rates in the drug named in the rows); CrI = credible interval

aripiprazole (OR = 0.42 [0.18; 0.93]), and paliperidone (OR = 0.34 [0.11; 0.98]).

When direct comparisons on corresponding treatments were available, standard pairwise comparisons of drugs were possible. Figure 45.4 illustrates the treatment contrasts for drugs that were compared directly with lithium in at least one trial (estimated form a Bayesian analysis).

Direct comparisons involving lithium showed largely comparable effects to those shown in network meta-analysis, but quetiapine significantly outperformed lithium (OR = 1.82 [1.08; 3.18]). In other pairwise comparisons, results from direct comparisons were mostly either consistent with

the network estimates or not feasible due to lacking trials (not shown in detail). A notable exception is the statistically significant inferiority of asenapine to olanzapine (OR = 0.65 [0.43; 0.96]).

Rankograms are presented in Figure 45.5 (probability of each treatment to be the best, the second best, and so on) and Figure 45.6 (cumulative probability of each treatment to be the best, the second best, and so on).

Although none of the treatments can be convincingly classified as certainly the best or the worst, Figure 45.5 shows that while paliperidone had a rather high probability of taking the first or second rank, topiramate and

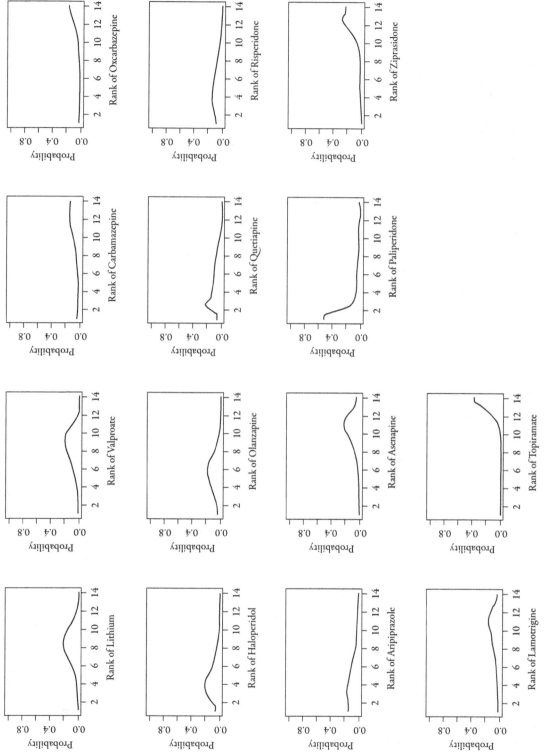

Figure 45.5 Rankogram for each treatment estimated from network meta-analysis.

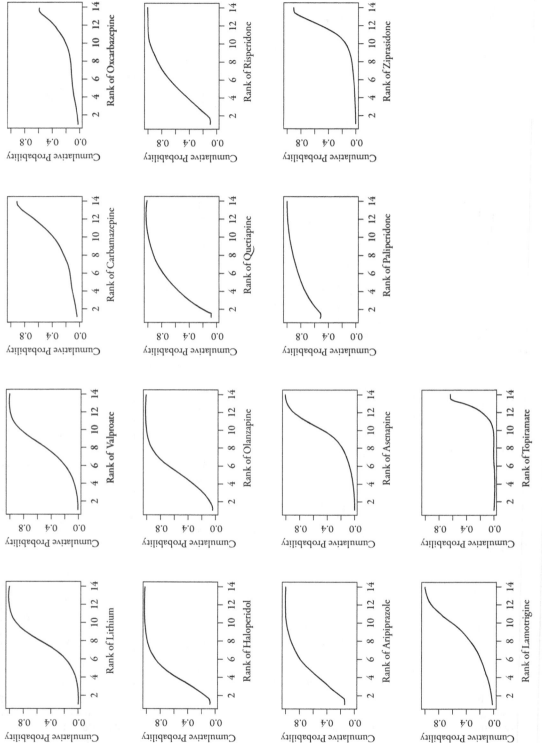

Figure 45.6 Cumulative rankogram for each treatment estimated from network meta-analysis.

ziprasidone were likely to take the last ranks. This impression is even strengthened by Figure 45.6, where a large area under the SUCRA indicates a better average rank. Numerically, we can use the SUCRA values (here expressed in percentages) for a global ranking of all investigated treatments from the best to the worst: paliperidone (85.0%), haloperidol (76.9%), aripiprazole (76.2%), quetiapine (74.7%), risperidone (69.9%), olanzapine (69.0%), lithium (49.2%), valproate (47.7%), lamotrigine (41.4%), asenapine (33.5%), carbamazepine (31.4%), ziprasidone (18.7%), oxcarbazepine (18.5%), and topiramate (7.9%). This reveals that a group of drugs consisting of the SGAs paliperidone, aripirazole, quetiapine, risperidone, and olanzapine, as well as the first-generation antipsychotic haloperidol are likely to be more effective than other treatments. While the anticonvulsants topiramate and oxcarbazepine and the SGA ziprasidone seem to be the least effective treatments, the remaining drugs, including lithium, ranked between the two groups. However, as indicated before, SUCRA-based rankings are sensitive to small changes in posterior distributions (e.g., in the breadth of the credible or confidence bounds) and thus should be evaluated together with point estimates (Salanti et al., 2011; Yildiz et al., 2014). Further caution should be taken in interpretation of the present findings, which is based on a network constructed by consideration of partial evidence of head-to-head comparisons by ignoring placebo arms (if exist) employed as a working example. The reported findings obtained in the worked example are somewhat different from the efficacy results obtained by employment of the entire evidence network (Yildiz et al., 2014).

In order to be able to decide whether the *similarity* assumption in our present network meta-analysis holds, we have to consult the trial characteristics (Table 45.1). The trials are fairly homogenous regarding demographic characteristics and baseline disease severity in the sample, whereas the proportion of patients with psychotic or mixed features shows some variability. However, no clear hypothesis exists concerning whether and/or how these factors may influence which head-to-head comparisons. In addition, none of the performed analyses suggested the presence of possible treatment effect modifiers over the network employed as a working example. A recent network meta-analysis considering the entire set of available RCTs (involving also drug–placebo comparisons) supported similarity of the included trials and network coherence via a number of meta-regression analyses, including presence of psychotic or mixed features (Yildiz et al., 2014).

Addressing the *homogeneity* assumption, the present network meta-analysis estimated the between-trial standard deviation to be 0.226 (log OR scale). This number is not easily interpretable but corresponds to a difference between an odds ratio of 1 and 1.26, suggesting rather reasonable heterogeneity. The deviance information criterion for this model was 118.8. As the deviance information criterion for the fixed effects model (119.5) was not substantially higher (meaning that a model without any between-trial variation did not offer a worse fit to the data), statistical heterogeneity was rather inconsiderable.

The *consistency* assumption can be tested in several ways. Here we can contrast effect estimates from the network meta-analysis with effects based on direct comparisons alone. Although there was a slight discrepancy between the two approaches regarding the statistical significance of some of the comparisons, credible intervals were substantially overlapping in all cases. Thus the fact that some comparisons popped up statistically significant in one but not in the other approach is likely to be traced back to power issues and to the rigid application of a constant threshold for significance rather than to the presence of considerable inconsistency. This judgment is supported also by examining a model without the consistency restriction. The deviance information criterion of this "inconsistency" model is 121.6, which is higher (i.e., not better) than the model making use of the consistency assumption. Further exploration of the consistency of the evidence network could be made by examining inconsistency factors in closed loops but were not performed here for each loop. Consistency of a few loops involving lithium and olanzapine were examined previously in frequentist analyses with the finding that direct comparisons between lithium and olanzapine showed stronger effects for olanzapine than the indirect evidence suggests. Still, this finding is accompanied by a very high degree of statistical uncertainty and without additional verification should be interpreted by caution.

In summary, we can conclude that the assumptions behind the network meta-analysis were sufficiently met in the working example. Although additional in-depth analyses may still increase or decrease our confidence, based on the performed calculations we see no reason to seriously doubt validity of the results for the considered data set of head-to-head RCTs. Based on the relative responder rate estimates (odds ratios) from the network meta-analysis and direct comparisons, as well as the probabilistic ranking information, we identified a group of antimanic drugs that are likely to be more effective than the remaining treatments within the considered evidence structure. However, as indicated earlier, the analyzed network is constructed a working example by employing only one-third of the available evidence (two-thirds of the entire data involves a placebo comparison) and considering only one effect size measure based on the binary data for responder rates. A complete data network constructed by involvement of drug-placebo comparisons and employing SMDs from symptom severity scales as the primary effect size measure while carefully examining similarity of the included RCTs offers a more sophisticated picture on the comparative efficacy and all-cause discontinuation rates of antimanic treatments (Yildiz et al., 2014).

REPORTING AND READING META-ANALYSES

For *reporting* both traditional and network meta-analysis, the Preferred Reporting Items for Systematic reviews and Meta-Analysis (PRISMA) statement should be considered (Moher, Liberati, Tetzlaff, Altman, & the PRISMA Group, 2009). A consolidated reporting guideline with a special focus on network meta-analysis has not been prepared yet, and current reporting practice has been found to be both heterogeneous and deficient (Bafeta, Trinquart, Seror, & Ravaud, 2014; Hutton et al., 2014). In fact, the

relatively high methodological complexity, the availability of several different statistical techniques, and the enormous amount of output leaves much space for a subjective and preference-based reporting of network meta-analyses. Usually reports are accompanied by extensive supplements (e.g., as web-only appendices) for additional numerical and graphical details. Currently, intensive research aims at developing comprehensive and standardized ways of communicating findings from network meta-analyses (Chaimani, Higgins, Mavridis, Spyridonos, & Salanti, 2013; Salanti et al., 2011; Tan et al., 2014).

Interpretation guidelines are available for the readers of both traditional meta-analyses (Greenhalgh, 1997; Leucht, Kissling, & Davis, 2009; Oxman, Cook, & Guyatt, 1994) and network meta-analyses (Jansen et al., 2011; Mills et al., 2012). A structured approach to the appraisal of empirical evidence from meta-analyses (and from other studies) is offered by the Grading of Recommendations Assessment, Development, and Evaluation (GRADE) system (GRADE Working Group, 2004; Guyatt et al., 2008), which has also been adapted to evidence from network-meta-analyses (Puhan et al., 2014; Salanti et al., 2014). A list of helpful questions to guide interpretation of findings from meta-analyses is provided in Box 45.1.

A particular challenge is posed by assessing the *applicability* of a meta-analytic finding to a specific decision-making situation (i.e., by transferring the research findings to the care of individual patients). Although some guidance is available (Atkins et al., 2011; Glasziou et al., 1998; Guyatt et al., 2011; Sackett, 1995), and methodological research attempts to tackle this issue exist (Kriston & Meister, 2014; Turner, Spiegelhalter, Smith, & Thompson, 2009), clinical judgment remains inevitable. Indeed, "identifying when it is appropriate to generalize from the abstract to the actual patient remains the central problem of any form of scientific clinical practice" (Smith & Egger, 1998, p. 289).

CONCLUSION AND FUTURE DIRECTIONS

In this chapter, we have reviewed and discussed pairwise and network meta-analysis for research synthesis. While providing an introduction, several important issues remained largely unaddressed, including the process of searching for evidence, the inclusion and exclusion of study reports, assessing risk of bias in the included studies, ways of dealing with missing and scarce data, available statistical software, and methods for addressing reporting bias in meta-analyses. Interested readers may consult the references at the end of the chapter or check one of the several text-books on evidence synthesis (Borenstein, Hedges, Higgins, & Rothstein, 2009; Center for Reviews and Dissemination, 2009; Cooper, 2009; Egger et al., 2001; Higgins & Green, 2011; Lipsey & Wilson, 2001).

Existing methods for research synthesis are being continuously refined, and new approaches arise at a high rate. As the amount of produced research findings increases, research synthesis will continue to play a central role in an evidence-based health care. Step by step, a couple of trends have become visible in recent years and are likely to take a more prominent role in the future.

First, methods have been developed and are becoming available for the synthesis of evidence obtained from *other study types than RCTs* and for research questions other than treatment effectiveness. These involve, among others, meta-analytic methods for epidemiological studies, prognostic trials, diagnostic accuracy studies, psychometric investigations, case studies, gene association studies, and health economic investigations. Although they all share the same idea of meta-analysis, methods developed for the synthesis of RCTs have to be somewhat modified and adapted to fulfill the needs of the various research fields.

Second, methods for *evidence linking* are being developed that are capable of incorporating considerably different sources of evidence, such as findings across several study types, expert knowledge, and theory. These models have frequently a rather high complexity, and it is likely to take some time until they become widely accepted and generally available. However, they can be a huge step toward the utilization of all available information in order to aid health-care decisions.

Third, current developments sometimes make use of statistical methods that *simulate data and different decision-making scenarios*. Particularly but not exclusively in health economics, the explicit modeling of the consequences of assumption-based decisions in research synthesis is being increasingly addressed to provide a robust base for decisions. In addition, these methods can aid decisions to identify research questions that are likely to add the most value to the existing body of evidence.

Fourth, *automated research synthesis* is winning place. Artificial intelligence systems are being developed to automatically identify and synthesize evidence to answer prespecified or user-defined research questions. If these systems are shown to yield trustworthy results, they can help us keep pace with the rapidly accumulating evidence and provide an always up-to-date summary of the available empirical findings.

Finally, *qualitative research synthesis* methods are being continuously refined. They separate from the rather subjective "narrative review" tradition in that they make use of the systematic review methodology but utilize qualitative research methods at the same time. They can be very helpful to address research questions beyond "Does this treatment work?" and investigate how, why, and under which conditions a specific treatment works. Particularly regarding complex interventions consisting of several interacting components and questions concerning translational and implementation science, qualitative research syntheses are likely to play a major role in future health policy decisions.

Of course this list does not intend to be comprehensive. Whichever way future methodological developments take, we should not forget that any research synthesis is only helpful if it reduces the amount of information we need to process for making good choices. Facing the rapidly increasing mass of produced systematic reviews and meta-analyses, in a rising number of cases preparing "overviews of reviews" and "meta-meta-analyses" have been found necessary. Although such enterprises can be undoubtedly helpful in some situations, we should be cautious not to amplify the information overload we were set out to tackle.

Disclosure statement: Dr. Kriston reports no conflicts to disclose.

Dr. Ayşegül Yildiz has received research grants from or served as a consultant to, or speaker for, Abdi Ibrahim, Actavis, AliRaif, AstraZeneca, Bristol-Myers Squibb, Janssen-Cilag, Lundbeck, Pfizer, Sanofi-Aventis, and Servier.

REFERENCES

Altman, D. G., & Bland, J. M. (1995). Absence of evidence is not evidence of absence. *BMJ, 311*(7003), 485.

Atkins, D., Chang, S. M., Gartlehner, G., Buckley, D. I., Whitlock, E. P., Berliner, E., & Matchar, D. (2011). Assessing applicability when comparing medical interventions: AHRQ and the Effective Health Care Program. *Journal of Clinical Epidemiology, 64*(11), 1198–1207. doi:10.1016/j.jclinepi.2010.11.021

Bafeta, A., Trinquart, L., Seror, R., & Ravaud, P. (2014). Reporting of results from network meta-analyses: Methodological systematic review. *BMJ, 348*, g1741.doi:10.1136/bmj.g1741

Baldwin, D., Woods, R., Lawson, R., & Taylor, D. (2011). Efficacy of drug treatments for generalised anxiety disorder: Systematic review and meta-analysis. *BMJ, 342*, d1199.

Barth, J., Munder, T., Gerger, H., Nüesch, E., Trelle, S., Znoj, H., ... Cuijpers, P. (2013). Comparative efficacy of seven psychotherapeutic interventions for patients with depression: A network meta-analysis. *PLoS Medicine, 10*(5), e1001454. doi:10.1371/journal.pmed.1001454

Bero, L., & Rennie, D. (1995). The Cochrane Collaboration: Preparing, maintaining, and disseminating systematic reviews of the effects of health care. *JAMA, 274*(24), 1935–1938. doi:10.1001/jama.1995.03530240045039

Borenstein, M., Hedges, L. V., Higgins, J. P. T., & Rothstein, H. R. (2009). *Introduction to meta-analysis* (1st ed.). Chichester, UK: John Wiley.

Bucher, H. C., Guyatt, G. H., Griffith, L. E., & Walter, S. D. (1997). The results of direct and indirect treatment comparisons in meta-analysis of randomized controlled trials. *Journal of Clinical Epidemiology, 50*(6), 683–691.

Caldwell, D. M., Ades, A. E., & Higgins, J. P. T. (2005). Simultaneous comparison of multiple treatments: Combining direct and indirect evidence. *BMJ, 331*(7521), 897–900. doi:10.1136/bmj.331.7521.897

Center for Reviews and Dissemination. (2009). *Systematic reviews: CRD's guidance for undertaking systematic reviews in health care.* York, UK: University of York. Retrieved from https://www.york.ac.uk/inst/crd/index_guidance.htm.

Centre for Evidence Based Medicine. (2009). *Oxford Centre for Evidence-based Medicine—Levels of evidence.* Oxford: University of Oxford. Retrieved from http://www.cebm.net/?o = 1025.

Chaimani, A., Higgins, J. P., Mavridis, D., Spyridonos, P., & Salanti, G. (2013). Graphical tools for network meta-analysis in STATA. *PloS One, 8*(10), e76654. doi:10.1371/journal.pone.0076654

Cipriani, A., Barbui, C., Salanti, G., Rendell, J., Brown, R., Stockton, S.,. . . Geddes, J. R. (2011). Comparative efficacy and acceptability of antimanic drugs in acute mania: A multiple-treatments meta-analysis. *Lancet, 378*(9799), 1306–1315. doi:10.1016/S0140-6736(11)60873-8

Cipriani, A., Furukawa, T. A., Salanti, G., Geddes, J. R., Higgins, J. P., Churchill, R.,. . . Barbui, C. (2009). Comparative efficacy and acceptability of 12 new-generation antidepressants: A multiple-treatments meta-analysis. *Lancet, 373*(9665), 746–758. doi:10.1016/S0140-6736(09)60046-5

Cochran, W. G. (1954). The combination of estimates from different experiments. *Biometrics, 10*(1), 101–129. doi:10.2307/3001666

Cohen, J. (1988). *Statistical power analysis for the behavioral sciences* (2nd ed.). Hillsdale, NJ: Lawrence Erlbaum Associates.

Cook, R. J., & Sackett, D. L. (1995). The number needed to treat: A clinically useful measure of treatment effect. *BMJ, 310*(6977), 452–454.

Cooper, H. M. (2009). *Research synthesis and meta-analysis: A step-by-step approach* (4th ed.). Los Angeles: SAGE.

Cornell, J. E., Mulrow, C. D., Localio, R., Stack, C. B., Meibohm, A. R., Guallar, E., & Goodman, S. N. (2014). Random-effects meta-analysis of inconsistent effects: A time for change. *Annals of Internal Medicine, 160*(4), 267–270. doi:10.7326/M13-2886

DerSimonian, R., & Laird, N. (1986). Meta-analysis in clinical trials. *Controlled Clinical Trials, 7*(3), 177–188.

Dias, S., Sutton, A. J., Ades, A. E., & Welton, N. J. (2013). Evidence synthesis for decision making 2: A generalized linear modeling framework for pairwise and network meta-analysis of randomized controlled trials. *Medical Decision Making, 33*(5), 607–617. doi:10.1177/0272989X12458724

Dias, S., Sutton, A. J., Welton, N. J., & Ades, A. E. (2013). Evidence synthesis for decision making 3: Heterogeneity—subgroups, meta-regression, bias, and bias-adjustment. *Medical Decision Making, 33*(5), 618–640. doi:10.1177/0272989X13485157

Dias, S., Welton, N. J., Caldwell, D. M., & Ades, A. E. (2010). Checking consistency in mixed treatment comparison meta-analysis. *Statistics in Medicine, 29*(7–8), 932–944. doi:10.1002/sim.3767

Dias, S., Welton, N. J., Sutton, A. J., Caldwell, D. M., Lu, G., & Ades, A. E. (2013). Evidence synthesis for decision making 4: Inconsistency in networks of evidence based on randomized controlled trials. *Medical Decision Making, 33*(5), 641–656. doi:10.1177/0272989X12455847

Donegan, S., Williamson, P., D'Alessandro, U., & Tudor Smith, C. (2012). Assessing the consistency assumption by exploring treatment by covariate interactions in mixed treatment comparison meta-analysis: Individual patient-level covariates versus aggregate trial-level covariates. *Statistics in Medicine.* doi:10.1002/sim.5470

Donegan, S., Williamson, P., D'Alessandro, U., & Tudor Smith, C. (2013). Assessing key assumptions of network meta-analysis: A review of methods. *Research Synthesis Methods, 4*(4), 291–323. doi:10.1002/jrsm.1085

Egger, M., Smith, G. D., & Altman, D. G. (Eds.). (2001). *Systematic reviews in health care: Meta-analysis in context.* London: BMJ.

Eysenck, H. J. (1978). An exercise in mega-silliness. *American Psychologist, 33*(5), 517. doi:10.1037/0003-066X.33.5.517.a

Eysenck, H. J. (1984). Meta-analysis: An abuse of research integration. *The Journal of Special Education, 18*(1), 41–59. doi:10.1177/002246698401800106

Friedrich, M. J. (2013). The Cochrane Collaboration turns 20: Assessing the evidence to inform clinical care. *JAMA, 309*(18), 1881–1882. doi:10.1001/jama.2013.1827

Gartlehner, G., Hansen, R. A., Morgan, L. C., Thaler, K., Lux, L., Van Noord, M.,. . . Lohr, K. N. (2011). Comparative benefits and harms of second-generation antidepressants for treating major depressive disorder: An updated meta-analysis. *Annals of Internal Medicine, 155*(11), 772–785. doi:10.7326/0003-4819-155-11-201112060-00009

Gerger, H., Munder, T., Gemperli, A., Nüesch, E., Trelle, S., Jüni, P., & Barth, J. (2014). Integrating fragmented evidence by network meta-analysis: Relative effectiveness of psychological interventions for adults with post-traumatic stress disorder. *Psychological Medicine, 44*(15), 3151–3164. doi:10.1017/S0033291714000853

Glass, G. V. (1976). Primary, secondary, and meta-analysis of research. *Educational Researcher, 5*(10), 3–8. doi:10.3102/0013189X005010003

Glasziou, P., Guyatt, G. H., Dans, A. L., Dans, L. F., Straus, S., & Sackett, D. L. (1998). Applying the results of trials and systematic reviews to individual patients. *ACP Journal Club, 129*(3), A15–A16.

GRADE Working Group (2004). Grading quality of evidence and strength of recommendations *BMJ, 328*(7454), 1490. doi:10.1136/bmj.328.7454.1490

Grant, R. L. (2014). Converting an odds ratio to a range of plausible relative risks for better communication of research findings. *BMJ, 348*, f7450. doi:10.1136/bmj.f7450

Greenhalgh, T. (1997). Papers that summarise other papers (systematic reviews and meta-analyses). *BMJ, 315*(7109), 672–675.

Guyatt, G. H., Oxman, A. D., Kunz, R., Woodcock, J., Brozek, J., Helfand, M.,. . . GRADE Working Group. (2011). GRADE guidelines: 8. Rating the quality of evidence—indirectness. *Journal of Clinical Epidemiology, 64*(12), 1303–1310. doi:10.1016/j.jclinepi.2011.04.014

Guyatt, G. H., Oxman, A. D., Vist, G. E., Regina, K., Falck-Ytter, Y., Alonso-Coello, P., Schünemann, H. J., & the GRADE Working Group (2008). GRADE: an emerging consensus on rating quality of evidence and strength of recommendations. *BMJ, 336*(7650), 924–926. doi:10.1136/bmj.39489.470347.AD

Hartling, L., Abou-Setta, A. M., Dursun, S., Mousavi, S. S., Pasichnyk, D., & Newton, A. S. (2012). Antipsychotics in adults with schizophrenia: Comparative effectiveness of first-generation versus second-generation medications: A systematic review and meta-analysis. *Annals of Internal Medicine, 157*(7), 498–511. doi:10.7326/0003-4819-157-7-201210020-00525

Higgins, J. P. T., & Green, S. (2011). *Cochrane handbook for systematic reviews of interventions, Version 5.1.0.* Oxford: Cochrane Collaboration. Retrieved from www.cochrane-handbook.org

Higgins, J. P. T., Thompson, S. G., Deeks, J. J., & Altman, D. G. (2003). Measuring inconsistency in meta-analyses. *BMJ, 327*(7414), 557–560. doi:10.1136/bmj.327.7414.557

Higgins, J. P., & Whitehead, A. (1996). Borrowing strength from external trials in a meta-analysis. *Statistics in Medicine, 15*(24), 2733–2749. doi:10.1002/(SICI)1097-0258(19961230)15:24<2733::AID-SIM562>3.0.CO;2-0

Higgins, J., Thompson, S., Deeks, J., & Altman, D. (2002). Statistical heterogeneity in systematic reviews of clinical trials: A critical appraisal of guidelines and practice. *Journal of Health Services Research & Policy, 7*(1), 51–61. doi:10.1258/1355819021927674

Hutton, B., Salanti, G., Chaimani, A., Caldwell, D. M., Schmid, C., Thorlund, K.,. . . Moher, D. (2014). The quality of reporting methods and results in network meta-analyses: An overview of reviews and suggestions for improvement. *PLoS One, 9*(3), e92508. doi:10.1371/journal.pone.0092508

Ioannidis, J. P. A. (2009). Ranking antidepressants. *Lancet, 373*(9677), 1759–1760; author reply, 1761–1762. doi:10.1016/S0140-6736(09)60974-0

Jansen, J. P., Fleurence, R., Devine, B., Itzler, R., Barrett, A., Hawkins, N.,. . . Cappelleri, J. C. (2011). Interpreting indirect treatment comparisons and network meta-analysis for health-care decision making: Report of the ISPOR Task Force on Indirect Treatment Comparisons Good Research Practices: Part 1. *Value in Health, 14*(4), 417–428. doi:10.1016/j.jval.2011.04.002

Krahn, U., Binder, H., & König, J. (2013). A graphical tool for locating inconsistency in network meta-analyses. *BMC Medical Research Methodology, 13*(1), 35. doi:10.1186/1471-2288-13-35

Kriston, L. (2013). Dealing with clinical heterogeneity in meta-analysis: Assumptions, methods, interpretation. *International Journal of Methods in Psychiatric Research, 22*(1), 1–15. doi:10.1002/mpr.1377

Kriston, L., & Meister, R. (2014). Incorporating uncertainty regarding applicability of evidence from meta-analyses into clinical decision making. *Journal of Clinical Epidemiology, 67*(3), 325–334. doi:10.1016/j.jclinepi.2013.09.010

Kriston, L., von Wolff, A., Westphal, A., Hölzel, L. P., & Härter, M. (2014). Efficacy and acceptability of acute treatments for persistent depressive disorder: A network meta-analysis. *Depression and Anxiety, 31*(8), 621–630. doi:10.1002/da.22236

Lau, J., Ioannidis, J. P., & Schmid, C. H. (1998). Summing up evidence: One answer is not always enough. *Lancet, 351*(9096), 123–127. doi:10.1016/S0140-6736(97)08468-7

Leucht, S., Cipriani, A., Spineli, L., Mavridis, D., Orey, D., Richter, F.,. . . Davis, J. M. (2013). Comparative efficacy and tolerability of 15 antipsychotic drugs in schizophrenia: A multiple-treatments meta-analysis. *Lancet, 382*(9896), 951–962. doi:10.1016/S0140-6736(13)60733-3

Leucht, S., Kissling, W., & Davis, J. M. (2009). How to read and understand and use systematic reviews and meta-analyses. *Acta Psychiatrica Scandinavica, 119*(6), 443–450. doi:10.1111/j.1600-0447.2009.01388.x

Lewis, S., & Clarke, M. (2001). Forest plots: Trying to see the wood and the trees. *BMJ, 322*(7300), 1479–1480.

Lipsey, M. W., & Wilson, D. (2001). *Practical meta-analysis* (1st ed.). Thousand Oaks, CA: SAGE.

Lu, G., & Ades, A. E. (2004). Combination of direct and indirect evidence in mixed treatment comparisons. *Statistics in Medicine, 23*(20), 3105–3124.

Lumley, T. (2002). Network meta-analysis for indirect treatment comparisons. *Statistics in Medicine, 21*(16), 2313–2324. doi:10.1002/sim.1201

Mayo-Wilson, E., Dias, S., Mavranezouli, I., Kew, K., Clark, D. M., Ades, A. E., Pilling, S. (2014). Psychological and pharmacological interventions for social anxiety disorder in adults: a systematic review and network meta-analysis. *Lancet Psychiatry, 1*(5), 368–376. doi:10.1016/S2215-0366(14)70329-3

Mills, E. J., Thorlund, K., & Ioannidis, J. P. A. (2013). Demystifying trial networks and network meta-analysis. *BMJ, 346*, f2914. doi:10.1136/bmj.f2914

Mills, E. J., Wu, P., Lockhart, I., Thorlund, K., Puhan, M., & Ebbert, J. O. (2012). Comparisons of high-dose and combination nicotine replacement therapy, varenicline, and bupropion for smoking cessation: A systematic review and multiple treatment

meta-analysis. *Annals of Medicine, 44*(6), 588–597. doi:10.3109/07853890.2012.705016

Mills, E. J., Ioannidis, J. P., Thorlund, K., Schünemann, H. J., Puhan, M. A., & Guyatt, G. H. (2012). How to use an article reporting a multiple treatment comparison meta-analysis. *JAMA, 308*(12), 1246–1253. doi:10.1001/2012.jama.11228

Moher, D., Liberati, A., Tetzlaff, J., Altman, D. G., & the PRISMA Group. (2009). Preferred reporting items for systematic reviews and meta-analyses: The PRISMA statement. *Annals of Internal Medicine, 151*(4), 264–269. doi:10.1059/0003-4819-151-4-200908180-00135

Naisbitt, J. (1988). *Megatrends: Ten new directions transforming our lives.* New York: Grand Central.

Oxman, A. D., Cook, D. J., & Guyatt, G. H. (1994). Users' guides to the medical literature. VI. How to use an overview. *JAMA, 272*(17), 1367–1371.

Oxman, A. D., & Guyatt, G. H. (1993). The science of reviewing research. *Annals of the New York Academy of Sciences, 703*, 125–133; discussion, 133–134.

Ramsberg, J., Asseburg, C., & Henriksson, M. (2012). Effectiveness and cost-effectiveness of antidepressants in primary care: A multiple treatment comparison meta-analysis and cost-effectiveness model. *PLoS ONE, 7*(8), e42003. doi:10.1371/journal.pone.0042003

Puhan, M. A., Schünemann, H. J., Murad, M. H., Li, T., Brignardello-Petersen, R., Singh, J. A., Kessels, A. G., Guyatt, G. H., & the GRADE Working Group. (2014). A GRADE Working Group approach for rating the quality of treatment effect estimates from network meta-analysis. *BMJ, 349*, g5630. doi:10.1136/bmj.g5630

Riley, R. D., Higgins, J. P. T., & Deeks, J. J. (2011). Interpretation of random effects meta-analyses. *BMJ, 342*, d549. doi:10.1136/bmj.d549

Riley, R. D., Lambert, P. C., & Abo-Zaid, G. (2010). Meta-analysis of individual participant data: Rationale, conduct, and reporting. *BMJ, 340*, c221. doi:10.1136/bmj.c221

Sackett, D. L. (1995). Applying overviews and meta-analyses at the bedside. *Journal of Clinical Epidemiology, 48*(1), 61–66; discussion 67–70.

Sackett, D. L., Rosenberg, W. M., Gray, J. A., Haynes, R. B., & Richardson, W. S. (1996). Evidence based medicine: What it is and what it isn't. *BMJ, 312*(7023), 71–72.

Salanti, G. (2012). Indirect and mixed-treatment comparison, network, or multiple-treatments meta-analysis: Many names, many benefits, many concerns for the next generation evidence synthesis tool. *Research Synthesis Methods, 3*(2), 80–97. doi:10.1002/jrsm.1037

Salanti, G., Ades, A. E., & Ioannidis, J. P. A. (2011). Graphical methods and numerical summaries for presenting results from multiple-treatment meta-analysis: An overview and tutorial. *Journal of Clinical Epidemiology, 64*(2), 163–171. doi:10.1016/j.jclinepi.2010.03.016

Salanti, G., Del Giovane, C., Chaimani, A., Caldwell, D. M., & Higgins, J. P. T. (2014). Evaluating the quality of evidence from a network meta-analysis. *PLoS One, 9*(7), e99682. doi:10.1371/journal.pone.0099682

Smith, G. D., & Egger, M. (1998). Incommunicable knowledge? Interpreting and applying the results of clinical trials and meta-analyses. *Journal of Clinical Epidemiology, 51*(4), 289–295.

Smith, M. L., Glass, G. V., & Miller, T. I. (1980). *The benefits of psychotherapy.* Baltimore, MD: John Hopkins University Press.

Smith, T. C., Spiegelhalter, D. J., & Thomas, A. (1995). Bayesian approaches to random-effects meta-analysis: A comparative study. *Statistics in Medicine, 14*(24), 2685–2699.

Song, F., Altman, D. G., Glenny, A.-M., & Deeks, J. J. (2003). Validity of indirect comparison for estimating efficacy of competing interventions: Empirical evidence from published meta-analyses. *BMJ, 326*(7387), 472. doi:10.1136/bmj.326.7387.472

Sox, H. C., & Greenfield, S. (2009). Comparative effectiveness research: A report from the Institute of Medicine. *Annals of Internal Medicine, 151*(3), 203–205. doi:10.7326/0003-4819-151-3-200908040-00125

Spiegelhalter, D. J., Best, N. G., Carlin, B. P., & Van Der Linde, A. (2002). Bayesian measures of model complexity and fit. *Journal of the Royal Statistical Society: Series B, 64*(4), 583–639. doi:10.1111/1467-9868.00353

Stewart, G. B., Altman, D. G., Askie, L. M., Duley, L., Simmonds, M. C., & Stewart, L. A. (2012). Statistical analysis of individual participant data meta-analyses: A comparison of methods and recommendations for practice. *PloS One, 7*(10), e46042. doi:10.1371/journal.pone.0046042

Sutton, A. J., & Abrams, K. R. (2001). Bayesian methods in meta-analysis and evidence synthesis. *Statistical Methods in Medical Research, 10*(4), 277–303.

Tan, S. H., Cooper, N. J., Bujkiewicz, S., Welton, N. J., Caldwell, D. M., & Sutton, A. J. (2014). Novel presentational approaches were developed for reporting network meta-analysis. *Journal of Clinical Epidemiology, 67*(6), 672–680. doi:10.1016/j.jclinepi.2013.11.006

Tarr, G. P., Glue, P., & Herbison, P. (2011). Comparative efficacy and acceptability of mood stabilizer and second generation antipsychotic monotherapy for acute mania—A systematic review and meta-analysis. *Journal of Affective Disorders, 134*(1–3), 14–19. doi:10.1016/j.jad.2010.11.009

Thompson, S. G. (1994). Why sources of heterogeneity in meta-analysis should be investigated. *BMJ, 309*(6965), 1351–1355.

Thompson, S. G., & Sharp, S. J. (1999). Explaining heterogeneity in meta-analysis: A comparison of methods. *Statistics in Medicine, 18*(20), 2693–2708.

Turner, R. M., Spiegelhalter, D. J., Smith, G. C. S., & Thompson, S. G. (2009). Bias modelling in evidence synthesis. *Journal of the Royal Statistical Society: Series A, 172*(1), 21–47. doi:10.1111/j.1467-985X.2008.00547.x

Uthman, O. A., & Abdulmalik, J. (2010). Comparative efficacy and acceptability of pharmacotherapeutic agents for anxiety disorders in children and adolescents: A mixed treatment comparison meta-analysis. *Current Medical Research and Opinion, 26*(1), 53–59. doi:10.1185/03007990903416853

Veroniki, A. A., Mavridis, D., Higgins, J. P. T., & Salanti, G. (2014). Characteristics of a loop of evidence that affect detection and estimation of inconsistency: a simulation study. *BMC Medical Research Methodology, 14*, 106. doi:10.1186/1471-2288-14-106

White, I. R., Barrett, J. K., Jackson, D., & Higgins, J. P. T. (2012). Consistency and inconsistency in network meta-analysis: Model estimation using multivariate meta-regression. *Research Synthesis Methods, 3*(2), 111–125. doi:10.1002/jrsm.1045

Yildiz, A., Nikodem, M., Vieta, E., Correll, C. U., & Baldessarini, R. J. (2014). A network meta-analysis on comparative efficacy and all-cause discontinuation of antimanic treatments in acute bipolar mania. *Psychological Medicine, advance online publication.*

Yildiz, A., Vieta, E., Correll, C. U., Nikodem, M., & Baldessarini, R. J. (2014). Critical issues on use of network meta-analysis in psychiatry. *Harvard Review of Psychiatry, 22*(6), 367–372. doi:10.1097/HRP.0000000000000025

Yildiz, A., Vieta, E., Leucht, S., & Baldessarini, R. J. (2011). Efficacy of antimanic treatments: Meta-analysis of randomized, controlled trials. *Neuropsychopharmacology, 36*(2), 375–389. doi:10.1038/npp.2010.192

INDEX

Page numbers followed by *f* and *t* indicate figures and tables, respectively. Numbers followed by *b* indicate boxes.

EMBOLDEN continuation studies, 614–617
emotion, expressed, 445
emotional instability, 474
emotionally unstable character disorder, 477
emotional processing, 211–212
emotion dysregulation, 450
emotion-regulation deficits, 173
EMPowerplus, 357
encephalopathy, 503
endocrine disorders, 499–500
endocrine system
    adverse effects associated with medications used to treat bipolar disorder, 394–400
    changes associated with bipolar disorder, 393–394
endogenous cannabinoid system, 420
endogenous opioid system, 419
endoplasmic reticulum stress, 107–108
energy metabolism, 152–153
English physicians, 7, 15t
environmental risk factors, 27–28
epidemiology, 21–23, 50
episodic aggressive behavior, 66
episodic mood lability, 64t
ERAT. see Early recovery adherence therapy
Esquirol, Jean-Étienne Dominique, 8, 15t
estimation, 645–646, 663–664, 664f
etanercept, 123
ethical considerations, 386
ethnic differences, 27
Europe, 6, 511t–512t, 513–514
European Medicines Agency, 599–600
European Network of Bipolar Research Expert Centre, 13
euthymia, 109
    cytokine abnormalities in, 117
    interepisode, 128
    maintenance of, 589, 590t
evaluation instruments, 608
everyday disability, 191–201
evidence
    consistency of, 659–660, 663, 667
    direct, 658
    indirect, 658–659
    methods for linking, 669
    simultaneous synthesis via network meta-analysis, 661–662
evidence-based assessment, 61–62, 62t, 63f, 69
evidence-based treatment decisions, 649–672
evidence networks, 659, 660–661, 660f
evidence or research synthesis, 649
excitotoxicity, 107–108
executive functioning, 194
exercise, 360, 396–397
experimental treatments, 465
expressed emotion, 445
extended phenotype, 173
extrapyramidal syndromes, drug-induced, 410–412

Falret, Jean-Pierre, 3, 8–9, 15t
family assessment, 177
Family Experience Study, 74
family-focused therapy, 439, 445–447
    with adolescents (FFT-A), 557
    in combination with pharmacotherapy, 446, 446t
    empirical support for, 446–447, 446t
    for youth, 447

family history, 28, 64t, 65–66
family interventions, 176–177
family studies, 28, 171–183, 182t
Fenton reaction, 83–84
Ferdinand VI, 7
Fieve, Ronald, 16t
fight or flight response, 137
FIND criteria, 67
Fischer's Exact Test, 628
fixed effects model, 655
FKBP5, 139
Flemming, Carl Friedrich, 10–11, 15t
[18F]-Fluorodeoxyglucose, 239
fluoxetine
    for bipolar depression, 290–291
    for bipolar II maintenance treatment, 314t
    olanzapine and fluoxetine combination (OFC), 307, 422
        for bipolar depression, 281–286, 283t, 284t, 289, 294–295
        for bipolar depression in children and adolescents, 553–554
        side effects of, 286, 287t
flupenthixol, 312, 313t, 427
flurazepam, 571t
folic acid supplements, 538–539
folie à double forme (insanity of double form), 8–9, 417
folie à formes alternes (insanity of alternative forms), 9
folie circulaire, 8–9, 417
Food and Drug Administration (FDA), 358, 493, 599–600
forest plots, 655, 657, 657f
fractional anisotropy, 206–207
France, 19th-century, 7–10
frequentist approach, 655
frontal cortex, 209–210
functional assessment, 194, 195t
functional capacity, 193
functional connectivity, 205, 207, 220
functional connectivity analysis, 207, 219, 219f
functional impairment
    in bipolar disorder, 191–193
    in elderly bipolar disorder, 575
functional magnetic resonance imaging (fMRI), 207, 219–220
    in at-risk populations, 334t–337t, 338
    in bipolar disorder, 211
    cognitive processing studies, 212–213
    emotional processing studies, 211–212
    of lithium effects, 215
    in offspring and unaffected twins of probands, 338–339
functional neurocircuitry, 243–244, 244f
functional outcome instruments, 192, 192t
functional rehabilitation, 199
Functioning Assessment Short Test, 610–611
funding for research, 625
future directions
    for cognitive behavioral therapy, 441
    for geriatric bipolar disorder, 579–580
    for psychoeducation, 441
for research, 585–671

GABA. see γ-Aminobutyric acid
gabaergic/glutamatergic system, 256, 418–419
gabapentin
    for anxiety disorders, 464
    for bipolar I disorder, 312, 312t, 313t

for bipolar II maintenance treatment, 314t
for elderly bipolar disorder, 573t, 577–578
evidence for efficacy of, 266, 312, 312t, 314t
for mania, 266
Gaddesden: John of, 6, 15t
galantamine, 423–424
Galen (Aelius Galenus of Pergamon), 4, 6, 15t
GAMIAN-Europe, 52
γ-Aminobutyric acid, 225, 227t, 229t, 230, 256, 418–419
Gao Lian (Kao Lien), 6, 15t
gastroenterological disorders, 503
gemischte Gemüthsstörungen (mixed mood disturbances), 10, 15t
gender differences
    co-occurrence of anxiety syndromes in mood disorders, 461, 462t
    and placebo response, 602–603
    in suicide attempts, 514
    in suicide rates, 515
gene expression studies, 118–119
generalized anxiety disorder, 25t, 460–461, 460t–461t, 462f, 463t
General Social Survey, 73
genetic risk factors, 28–29
genetics, 171–188
    and circadian abnormalities, 130
    inflammation-related genes, 119–120
    and MRI findings, 213
genetic studies, 28–29
    common variant association studies, 183–184
    family studies, 28, 171–183, 182t
    polygenic studies, 185
    rare variant association studies, 184–185
    twin studies, 28, 181–183
genome-wide association studies, 186
geriatric bipolar disorder. see Elderly
Germany, 19th-century, 10–12
gesture, suicide, 509–513
ghotrah (persecutory psychosis, paranoia), 6
glial cells, 254–255
global health, 509–513, 510t–513t
Global Program to Fight Stigma and Discrimination Because of Schizophrenia (Open-the-Doors), 77
glucocorticoid receptor, 138–139
glucocorticoid receptor gene GR, 139
glucocorticoids, 108
glutamate, 156, 225, 227t, 228, 229t, 230–232
glutamate/alpha-amino-3-hydroxy-5-methyl-4-isoxazolpropionate receptor gene GRIA2, 186
glutamate receptors, 156
glutamate-related agent–induced mania/hypomania, 421t
glutamatergic modulating agents, 294
glutamatergic neurotransmission, 255, 255f, 256
glutamatergic system, 156–157, 418–419
glutathione, 255
glutathione peroxidase, 83
glutathione S-transferase, 83
glycogen synthase kinase 3, 95–97, 99–100, 153–154, 403–404
glycogen synthase kinase 3 inhibitors, 153–154
glycogen synthase kinase 3α, 96

glycogen synthase kinase 3β, 96
Goodwin, Frederick K., 16t, 35
Grading of Recommendations Assessment, Development, and Evaluation (GRADE) system, 668
GRAPES mnemonic, 67
gray matter
    regional abnormalities, 209–211
    volumetric studies, 323, 339–340
Greece, ancient, 4–5, 10, 15t
Griesinger, Wilhelm, 9, 11, 16t
group therapy, 556–557
GSK. see Glycogen synthase kinase
Guislain, Joseph, 10
g value (Hedges' g), 654

Haber-Weiss reaction, 83–84
hallucinations, 5
haloperidol, 405
    depressogenic properties of, 427
    effects of, 660f, 661, 663–667, 664f, 665f, 666f
    for mania
        effect sizes, 268–276, 274t, 275t, 276
        evidence review, 265, 268, 269t, 272t–273t
        network meta-analysis of, 663–667, 664f, 665f, 666f
    neuroprotective effects of, 411
Hamilton Depression Rating Scale (Ham-D), 42, 625–626
Hamilton Rating Scale for Depression (HRSD), 608
harm avoidance, 438
harm reduction, 438
Hawthorne effect, 600
healthy lifestyle, 396–397, 397t, 438
Hecker, Ewald, 11, 16t
Hedges' g, 654
Heinroth, Johann Christian August Heinroth, 10, 15t
helper T cells (Th17), 99
hemoglobin A1C, 398
hepatitis C, 501–502
high-risk studies, 320–321
hippocampus, 210–211
Hippocratic tradition, 4–5, 15t
Hispanics, 27
histone deacetylase inhibitors, 163
historical overview
    of bipolar disorder diagnosis, 3–19, 15t–16t, 35
    of mood stabilizers, 404
    on therapeutic HPT axis hormones, 144
histrionic personality disorder, 475, 476b
HIV (human immunodeficiency virus), 500–501
Hoffmann, Friedrich, 6, 15t
homogeneity, 663, 667
homovanillic acid (HVA), 158
hormones
    in bipolar disorder, 159–160
    proof-of-concept studies of, 159–160
    risk factors for mania/hypomania, 421t
hospitalization, parent, 174–175
HPA axis. see Hypothalamic-pituitary-adrenal axis
HPT axis. see Hypothalamic-pituitary-thyroid axis
human immunodeficiency virus (HIV), 500–501
humoral theory, 4